BREAST CANCER MANAGEMENT

Application of Clinical and Translational Evidence to Patient Care

Second Edition

BREAST CANCER MANAGEMENT

Application of Clinical and Translational Evidence to Patient Care

Second Edition

Jean-Marc Nabholtz, M.D., M.Sc., Editor in Chief
*Professor of Medicine
Director
Cancer Therapy Development Program
Jonsson Comprehensive Cancer Center
University of California, Los Angeles
Chairman and Founder
Breast Cancer International Research Group
Los Angeles, California
U.S.A.*

Katia Tonkin, M.D., M.B.B.S., M.R.C.P., F.R.C.P.C.
*Senior Medical Oncologist
Cross Cancer Institute
Associate Professor
University of Alberta
Edmonton, Alberta
Canada*

David M. Reese, M.D.
*Director of Clinical Research
Breast Cancer International Research Group
Los Angeles, California
U.S.A*

Matti S. Aapro, M.D.
*Director
Multidisciplinary Institute of Oncology
Clinique de Genolier
Genolier, Switzerland
Consultant to the Scientific Director
European Institute of Oncology
Milan, Italy
Consultant
Division of Oncology
University Hospital
Geneva, Switzerland*

Aman U. Buzdar, M.D.
*Professor of Medicine
Deputy Chairman
Department of Breast Medical Oncology
University of Texas
M.D. Anderson Cancer Center
Houston, Texas
U.S.A.*

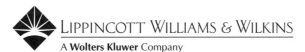

A **Wolters Kluwer** Company
Philadelphia · Baltimore · New York · London
Buenos Aires · Hong Kong · Sydney · Tokyo

Acquisitions Editor: Jonathan Pine
Managing Editor: Tanya Lazar
Developmental Editor: Brigitte P. Wilke
Supervising Editor: Allison Risko
Production Editor: Richard Rothschild, Print Matters, Inc.
Manufacturing Manager: Tim Reynolds
Cover Designer: David Levy
Compositor: Compset, Inc.
Printer: Edwards Brothers

© 2003 by Lippincott Williams & Wilkins, except for chapter 45, which is © by the authors
530 Walnut Street
Philadelphia, PA 19106 USA
LWW.com

All rights reserved. This book is protected by copyright. No part of this book may be reproduced in any form or by any means, including photocopying, or utilized by any information storage and retrieval system without written permission from the copyright owner, except for brief quotations embodied in critical articles and reviews. Materials appearing in this book prepared by individuals as part of their official duties as U.S. government employees are not covered by the above-mentioned copyright.

Printed in the USA

Library of Congress Cataloging-in-Publication Data

Breast cancer management : application of clinical and translational evidence to patient care / Jean-Marc Nabholtz, editor in chief . . . [et al.].—2nd ed.
  p. cm.
  Includes bibliographical references and index.
  ISBN 0-7817-4131-9
  1. Breast—Cancer—Treatment.   I. Nabholtz, Jean-Marc.

RC280.B8 B68396 2002
616.99'44906—dc21

2002030171

Care has been taken to confirm the accuracy of the information presented and to describe generally accepted practices. However, the authors, editors, and publisher are not responsible for errors or omissions or for any consequences from application of the information in this book and make no warranty, expressed or implied, with respect to the currency, completeness, or accuracy of the contents of the publication. application of this information in a particular situation remains the professional responsibility of the practitioner.

The authors, editors, and publisher have exerted every effort to ensure that drug selection and dosage set forth in this text are in accordance with current recommendations and practice at the time of publication. However, in view of ongoing research, changes in government regulations, and the constant flow of information relating to drug therapy and drug reactions, the reader is urged to check the package insert for each drug for any change in indications and dosage and for added warnings and precautions. This is particularly important when the recommended agent is a new or infrequently employed drug.

Some drugs and medical devices presented in this publication have Food and Drug Administration (FDA) clearance for limited use in restricted research settings. Is is the responsibility of health care providers to ascertain the FDA status of each drug or device planned for use in their clinical practice.

10 9 8 7 6 5 4 3 2 1

Acknowledgments

This book was only possible with the expert help of Wendy Schmidt, Editorial Assistant to Dr. Tonkin at the Cross Cancer Institute in Edmonton, Alberta, Canada. Without her careful attention to detail we would not have had such an excellent second edition.

We would like also to thank all the contributors and those individuals who helped them with their chapters.

Of course, without women with breast cancer, their families and supporters, none of the studies reported here could have been done. Their altruism and sacrifice has made the difference and will continue to improve survival outcome for all future generations of women diagnosed with breast cancer.

Contents

Part I Treatment Recommendations for Specific Stages of Breast Cancer

Section 1 Early Stage Disease: Radiation

1. Radiation Therapy for Breast Cancer: Radiotherapy Techniques to Decrease Treatment Morbidity 3
   Eugenio Vinés, Cécile Le Péchoux, and Rodrigo Arriagada

2. The Role of Radiation Therapy in Breast Cancer Management 25
   Bruce G. Haffty

3. Survival Impact of Locoregional Radiation in Stage I-II Breast Cancer: Evidence-Based Review 39
   Joseph Ragaz and John J. Spinelli

Section 2 Early Stage Disease—Surgery, Chemotherapy, and Hormones

4. Evolution in the Management of Ductal Carcinoma *in situ* through Randomized Clinical Trials 49
   Eleftherios Mamounas

5. Should Surgeons Abandon Routine Axillary Dissection for Sentinel Node Biopsy in Early Breast Cancer? 59
   Frederick L. Moffat, Jr. and David N. Krag

6. Surgical Considerations in Breast Cancer Patients Treated with Preoperative Chemotherapy 67
   Harry D. Bear

7. The Medical Oncology Perspective on Preoperative Chemotherapy for Early Operable Breast Cancer 85
   Charlotte N. Rees and Ian E. Smith

8. Adjuvant Treatment: Node-negative Breast Cancer 97
   Miguel Martin

9. Node-positive Breast Cancer 107
   Gul Atalay, Caroline Lohrisch, and Martine J. Piccart

Section 3 Metastatic Disease: Chemotherapy

10. The Taxanes: Paclitaxel and Docetaxel 147
    Jean-Marc Nabholtz, Alessandro Riva, Mary-Ann Lindsay, David M. Reese, and Katia Tonkin

11. Capecitabine 169
    Joyce A. O'Shaughnessy

12. Vinorelbine 179
    Laurent Zelek and Marc Spielmann

13. Liposomal Doxorubicin in the Treatment of Metastatic Breast Cancer 189
    Michael Smylie

14. High-Dose Chemotherapy and Autologous Stem Cell Transplantation for
    Metastatic Breast Cancer 195
    Edward A. Stadtmauer

Section 4 Metastatic Disease: Hormone Treatment

15. Aromatase Inhibitors in the Treatment of Breast Cancer 203
    Kellie L. Jones, Aman U. Buzdar, and Gabriel N. Hortobagyi

16. New Antiestrogens: Modulators of Estrogen Action 223
    Anthony Howell and S. J. Howell

Part II Translational Approaches: Current, Planned, and Most Promising

Section 1 Current

17. HER2/*neu* and Trastuzumab 245
    Mark D. Pegram and Dennis J. Slamon

18. Low-Dose Metronomic Antiangiogenic Chemotherapy: Preclinical and
    Clinical Applications in Breast Cancer 261
    Robert S. Kerbel and Giannoula Klement

19. Epidermal Growth Factor Receptor: Biology and New Therapeutics 273
    Sonia González and Jose Baselga

20. Dimming the Blood Tide: Angiogenesis, Anti-Angiogenic Therapy and
    Breast Cancer 287
    Kathy D. Miller and George W. Sledge, Jr.

21. Results from a Phase 1 Trial of *E1A* Gene Therapy in Breast and Ovarian
    Cancer: What's Next 311
    Naoto T. Ueno, Gabriel N. Hortobagyi, and Mien-Chie Hung

Section 2 Early Clinical and Preclinical

22. DNA Microarray Analysis of Breast Cancer: Toward Customized Anti-cancer
    Drug Therapy and Rational Drug Design 323
    John R. Mackey and Brent Zanke

23. Proteomics of Breast Cancer: Marker Discovery and Signal Pathway Profiling 331
    Hubert Hondermarck, Anne-Sophie Vercoutter-Edouart, Françoise Révillion,
    Jérôme Lemoine, Ikram El Yazidi-Belkoura, Victor Nurcombe, and
    Jean-Philippe Peyrat

24. Steroid and Growth Factor Receptors: Cross-Talk and Clinical Implications ... 345
    Richard J. Pietras

25. Cell Cycle Inhibitors in the Treatment of Breast Cancer 355
    Carolyn D. Britten

26. Predictive Molecular Markers: A New Window of Opportunity in the
    Adjuvant Therapy of Breast Cancer 367
    Angelo Di Leo, Fatima Cardoso, Sophie Scohy, and Martine J. Piccart

Part III   Anatomapathology and the Metastatic Process

27. Basic Biology of the Metastatic Process: Clinical Implications 383
    George N. Naumov, Ian C. MacDonald, Alan C. Groom, and Ann F. Chambers

28. Prognostic and Predictive Factors in Breast Cancer: An Evidence-Based
    Medicine Approach 391
    *Syed K. Mohsin, Valerie-Jean Bardou, Grazia Arpino, Gary C. Chamness,
    and D. Craig Allred*

29. Prognostic Factors in Invasive Breast Cancer Using Histology 411
    Sarah E. Pinder, Ian O. Ellis, Andrew H. S. Lee, and Christopher W. Elston

Part IV   Issues for the Practicing Oncologist

Section 1   Supportive Care and Quality of Life

30. Science and Alternative Therapy: The Past, Present, and Future 425
    Brent A. Bauer and Charles L. Loprinzi

31. Ethics and Hereditary Cancer: Issues for Women and Families with
    Hereditary Breast/Ovarian Cancer 437
    Lori d'Agincourt-Canning, Michael M. Burgess, and Barbara C. McGillivray

32. Hematopoietic Growth Factor Support in Breast Cancer 447
    Katia Tonkin, Douglas Stewart, and Stefan Gluck

33. Erythropoietin in the Management of Cancer Patients 457
    Alexander H.G. Paterson and Mary-Ann Lindsay

34. The Place of Bisphosphonates in the Management of Breast Cancer 463
    Alexander H.G. Paterson

35. Cutaneous Metastasis and Malignant Wounds 475
    Valerie Nocent Schulz

36. Chemotherapy-induced Nausea and Vomiting 489
    Sheryl Koski and Peter Venner

37. Quality of Life Data Interpretation: An Update on Key Issues in Advanced
    Breast Cancer 501
    Andrew Bottomley

38. The Internet, the Evidence, and the Health Consumer 511
    Lewis Rowett

Section 2   Prevention and Screening

39. Breast Screening 519
    Anthony B. Miller

40. Chemoprevention Studies in Italy and the United Kingdom 529
    Andrea Decensi, Jack Cuzik, and Umberto Veronesi

41. Breast Cancer Prevention: The U.S. Viewpoint 535
    D. Lawrence Wickerham and Joseph Costantino

Part V   Clinical Data Analysis: Current and Future Standards

42. Evidence Analysis: Historical and Contemporary Perspectives 551
    Jean-Marc Nabholtz, Linda Harris, David M. Reese, and Katia Tonkin

43. Clinical Practice Guidelines 557
    George P. Browman

44. RECIST: Response Evaluation Criteria in Solid Tumors 565
    Janet Dancey, Patrick Therasse, Susan G. Arbuck, and Elizabeth A. Eisenhauer

45. Need for Large-scale Randomized Evidence to Assess Moderate
    Benefits Reliably 575
    Richard Peto and Colin Baigent

46. Economic Evaluation Analysis in Breast Cancer Therapy: From Evidence
    to Practice 581
    Philip Jacobs, Katia Tonkin, and Barbara Conner-Spady

Part VI   High-Dose Chemotherapy

47. High-Dose Chemotherapy in the Adjuvant Therapy of Breast Cancer:
    The Argument for Further Investigation 589
    John Crown

Part VII   Summary Statement

48. The Future of Breast Cancer Medicine 601
    *Jean-Marc Nabholtz, Katia Tonkin, Matti S. Aapro, Aman U. Buzdar,
    and David M. Reese*

    Index 603

Contributors

Matti S. Aapro, M.D.
Director
Multidisciplinary Institute of Oncology
Clinique de Genolier
Genolier, Switzerland
Consultant to the Scientific Director
European Institute of Oncology
Milan, Italy
Consultant
Division of Oncology
University Hospital
Geneva, Switzerland

D. Craig Allred, M.D.
Professor of Pathology
Breast Center
Baylor College of Medicine
Houston, Texas
U.S.A.

Susan G. Arbuck, M.D.
Vice President Oncology
Bristol-Myers Squibb
Princeton, New Jersey
U.S.A.

Grazia Arpino, M.D.
Post-doctoral Fellow
Breast Center
Baylor College of Medicine
Houston, Texas
U.S.A.

Rodrigo Arriagada, M.D.
Institut Gustave Roussy
Villejuif, France
Instituto de Radiomedicina IRAM
Santiago, Chile

Colin Baigent, B.M.B.Ch., M.Sc.
Clinical Trial Service Unit and Epidemiological
   Studies Unit
University of Oxford
Department of Clinical Medicine
Radcliffe Infirmary
Oxford, United Kingdom

Valerie-Jean Bardou, M.D.
Visiting Post-doctoral Fellow
Breast Center
Baylor College of Medicine
Houston, Texas
U.S.A.

Jose Baselga, M.D.
Medical Oncology Service
Vall d'Hebron University Hospital
Barcelona, Spain

Brent A. Bauer, M.D., F.A.C.P.
Assistant Professor of Medicine
Mayo Medical School
Chair
Complementary and Integrative Medicine Program
Mayo Clinic
Rochester, Minnesota
U.S.A.

Harry D. Bear, M.D., Ph.D.
Chairman
Division of Surgical Oncology
Medical College of Virginia and Virginia
   Commonwealth University
Department of Surgery and the Massey Cancer Center
Richmond, Virginia
U.S.A.

Andrew Bottomley, Ph.D.
Coordinator
Quality of Life Unit
EORTC Data Center
Brussels, Belgium

Carolyn Britten, M.D., F.R.C.P.C.
Assistant Professor
Division of Hematology/Oncology
University of California, Los Angeles
Los Angeles, California
U.S.A.

George P. Browman, M.D.
Director
Program in Evidence-based Care
Cancer Care Ontario
Toronto, Ontario

CONTRIBUTORS

Professor
Department of Clinical Epidemiology and Biostatistics
Faculty of Health Sciences
McMaster University
Hamilton, Ontario
Chief Executive Officer
Hamilton Regional Cancer Centre
Cancer Care Ontario
Hamilton, Ontario
Canada

Michael M. Burgess, Ph.D.
Centre for Applied Ethics
University of British Columbia
Vancouver, British Columbia
Canada

Aman U. Buzdar, M.D.
Professor of Medicine
Deputy Chairman
Department of Breast Medical Oncology
University of Texas
MD Anderson Cancer Center
Houston, Texas
U.S.A.

Fatima Cardoso, M.D.
Translational Research Unit
Jules Bordet Institute
Brussels, Belgium

Ann F. Chambers, Ph.D.
Professor
Department of Oncology
University of Western Ontario
Senior Scientist
London Regional Cancer Centre
London, Ontario
Canada

Gary C. Chamness, Ph.D.
Professor
Breast Center
Baylor College of Medicine
Houston, Texas
U.S.A.

Barbara Conner-Spady, Ph.D.
Edmonton, Alberta
Canada

Joseph Costantino, Dr.P.H.
Associate Director
NSABP Biostatistical Center
Pittsburgh, Pennsylvania
U.S.A.

John Crown, M.D.
Consultant Medical Oncologist
St. Vincent's University Hospital
Dublin, Ireland

Lori d'Agincourt-Canning, M.A., M.Sc.
Centre for Applied Ethics
University of British Columbia
Vancouver, British Columbia
Canada

Janet Dancey, M.D., F.R.C.P.C.
Senior Investigator
Investigational Drug Branch
Cancer Therapy Evaluation Program
Division of Cancer Treatment and Diagnosis
National Cancer Institute
Rockville, Maryland
U.S.A.

Angelo Di Leo, M.D., Ph.D.
Associate Director
Chemotherapy Unit
Medical Director
Breast Office
Jules Bordet Institute
Brussels, Belgium

Elizabeth A. Eisenhauer, M.D., F.R.C.P.C.
Director
Investigational New Drug Program
National Cancer Institute of Canada Clinical Trials
  Group
Queen's University
Kingston, Ontario
Canada

Ian O. Ellis, M.D., F.R.C.Path.
Reader in Pathology
University of Nottingham
Nottingham City Hospital
Histopathology Department
Nottingham, United Kingdom

Christopher W. Elston, M.D., F.R.C.Path.
Consultant Histopathologist
Nottingham City Hospital
Histopathology Department
Nottingham, United Kingdom

Stefan Gluck, M.D., Ph.D.
Professor
Departments of Oncology, Medicine and
  Pharmacology and Therapeutics
Faculty of Medicine

University of Calgary
Senior Leader
Clinical Research Program
Tom Baker Cancer Centre
Calgary, Alberta
Canada

Sonia González, M.D.
Oncology Service
Vall d'Hebron University Hospital
Barcelona, Spain

Alan C. Groom, Ph.D.
Professor
Department of Medical Biophysics
University of Western Ontario
London, Ontario
Canada

Bruce G. Haffty, M.D.
Professor
Department of Therapeutic Radiology
Yale University School of Medicine
New Haven, Connecticut
U.S.A.

Linda Harris, M.L.S.
Librarian
Cross Cancer Institute
Edmonton, Alberta
Canada

Hubert Hondermarck, Ph.D.
Professeur de Biologie Cellulair
Universite des Sciences et Technologies de Lille
Lille, France

Gabriel N. Hortobágyi, M.D.
Department of Breast Medical Oncology
The University of Texas
M. D. Anderson Cancer Center
Houston, Texas
U.S.A.

Anthony Howell, M.D.
CRC Department of Medical Oncology
University of Manchester
Christie Hospital NHS Trust
Manchester, United Kingdom

S.J. Howell, M.B., B.S.
CRC Department of Medical Oncology
University of Manchester
Christie Hospital NHS Trust
Manchester, United Kingdom

Mien-Chie Hung, M.D.
Breast Cancer Research Program and
Departments of Molecular and Cellular Oncology
 and Surgical Oncology
The University of Texas
M. D. Anderson Cancer Center
Houston, Texas
U.S.A.

Philip Jacobs, D.Phil., C.M.A.
Professor
Department of Public Health Sciences
University of Alberta
Edmonton, Alberta
Canada

Kellie L. Jones, Pharm.D.
Department of Breast Medical Oncology
The University of Texas
M. D. Anderson Cancer Center
Houston, Texas
U.S.A.

Robert S. Kerbel, Ph.D.
Sunnybrook and Women's College Health Sciences
 Centre
Molecular and Cell Biology Research
Toronto, Ontario
Department of Medical Biophysics
University of Toronto
Toronto, Ontario
Canada

Giannoula Klement, M.D.
Sunnybrook and Women's College Health Sciences
 Centre
Molecular and Cell Biology Research
Toronto, Ontario
Canada

Sheryl Koski, M.D., F.R.C.P.C.
Department of Medicine
Cross Cancer Institute
Edmonton, Alberta
Canada

David N. Krag, M.D.
S.D. Ireland Professor of Surgical Oncology
Division of Surgical Oncology
Department of Surgery
University of Vermont College of Medicine
Burlington, Vermont
U.S.A.

Andrew H.S. Lee, M.D., M.R.C.Path.
Consultant Histopathologist
Nottingham City Hospital
Histopathology Department
Nottingham, United Kingdom

Jérôme Lemoine, Ph.D.
Laboratoire de Chimie Biologique
Université des Sciences et Technologies de Lille
Lille, France

Cécile Le Péchoux, M.D.
Radiation Oncologist
Department of Radiotherapy
Institut Gustave-Roussy
Villejuif, France

Mary-Ann Lindsay, Pharm.D.
Breast Cancer International Research Group
Edmonton, Alberta
Canada

Charles L. Loprinzi, M.D.
Professor of Medicine
Mayo Medical School
Vice Chair
Department of Oncology
Mayo Clinic
Rochester, Minnesota
U.S.A.

Ian C. MacDonald, Ph.D.
Associate Professor
Department of Medical Biophysics
University of Western Ontario
London, Ontario
Canada

John R. Mackey, M.D., F.R.C.P.C.
Chair
Northern Alberta Breast Cancer Program
Associate Professor
Medical and Experimental Oncology
University of Alberta
Canadian Leader
Breast Cancer International Research Group
Department of Medicine
Cross Cancer Institute
Edmonton, Alberta
Canada

Eleftherios Mamounas, M.D., M.P.H., F.A.C.S.
Integrated Medical Campus
Mt. Sinai Center for Breast Health
Mt. Sinai Cancer Center
Beachwood, Ohio
U.S.A.

Miguel Martin, M.D., Ph.D.
Head
Breast Cancer Section
Medical Oncology Department
Hospital Universitario San Carlos
Madrid, Spain

Barbara C. McGillivray, M.D.
Professor of Medical Genetics
University of British Columbia
Vancouver, British Columbia
Canada

Anthony B. Miller, M.B., F.R.C.P.
Head
Division of Clinical Epidemiology
Deutsches Krebsforschungszentrum
Heidelberg, Germany
Professor Emeritus
Department of Public Health Sciences
University of Toronto
Toronto, Ontario
Canada

Kathy D. Miller, MD.
Assistant Professor of Medicine
Division of Hematology and Oncology
Indiana University School of Medicine
Indianapolis, Indiana
U.S.A.

Frederick L. Moffat, Jr., M.D.
Associate Professor of Surgery
Division of Surgical Oncology
Daughtry Family Department of Surgery
University of Miami School of Medicine and
the Sylvester Comprehensive Cancer Center
Miami, Florida
U.S.A.

Syed K. Mohsin, M.D.
Assistant Professor
Breast Center
Baylor College of Medicine
Houston, Texas
U.S.A.

Jean-Marc Nabholtz, M.D., M.Sc.
Professor of Medicine
Director
Cancer Therapy Development Program
Jonsson Comprehensive Cancer Center
University of California, Los Angeles
Chairman and Founder
Breast Cancer International Research Group
Los Angeles, California
U.S.A.

CONTRIBUTORS

George N. Naumov, B.Sc. (Hons.)
Ph.D. Candidate
Department of Medical Biophysics
University of Western Ontario
London, Ontario, Canada
London Regional Cancer Centre
London, Ontario
Canada

Valerie Nocent Schulz M.D., M.P.H.
Palliative Medicine
University of Western Ontario
London Health Sciences Center
London Regional Cancer Center
St. Joseph's Health Center
London, Ontario
Canada

Victor Nurcombe, Ph.D.
Department of Anatomical Sciences
University of Queensland
Australia

Joyce A. O'Shaughnessy, M.D.
US Oncology Research
Dallas, Texas
U.S.A.

Alexander H.G. Paterson, M.D., F.R.C.P., F.A.C.P.
Tom Baker Cancer Centre
and University of Calgary
Calgary, Alberta
Canada

Mark Pegram, M.D.
Division of Hematology-Oncology
UCLA School of Medicine
Los Angeles, California
U.S.A.

Sir Richard Peto, F.R.S.
Professor of Medical Statistics and Epidemiology
Clinical Trial Service Unit and
Epidemiological Studies Unit
Department of Clinical Medicine
University of Oxford
Radcliffe Infirmary
Oxford, United Kingdom

Jean-Philippe Peyrat, Ph.D., Dr.S.
Centre de Lutte Contre le Cancer de Lille
Lille, France

Martine J. Piccart, M.D., Ph.D.
Translational Research Unit
Jules Bordet Institute
Brussels, Belgium

Sarah E. Pinder, M.D., F.R.C.Path.
Senior Lecturer
University of Nottingham
Nottingham City Hospital
Histopathology Department
Nottingham, United Kingdom

Joseph Ragaz, M.D.
British Columbia Cancer Agency
Vancouver, British Columbia
Canada

Charlotte N. Rees, M.D.
Royal Marsden Hospital
London, United Kingdom

David M. Reese, M.D.
Director of Clinical Research
Breast Cancer International Research Group
Los Angeles, California
U.S.A.

Françoise Révillion, Ph.D.
Centre de Lutte Contre le Cancer de Lille
Lille, France

Alessandro Riva, M.D.
Vice President
Clinical Research and Operations
Breast Cancer International Research Group
Paris, France

Lewis Rowett, Ph.D.
Executive Editor
Annals of Oncology
Viganello, Switzerland

Sophie Scohy, Ph.D.
Translational Research Unit
Jules Bordet Institute
Brussels, Belgium

Dennis J. Slamon, M.D., Ph.D.
Division of Hematology-Oncology
and Jonsson Comprehensive Cancer Center
University of California, Los Angeles
School of Medicine
Los Angeles, California
U.S.A.

Ian E. Smith, M.D., F.R.C.P.
Royal Marsden Hospital
London, United Kingdom

Michael Smylie, M.D.
Department of Medicine
Cross Cancer Institute
Edmonton, Alberta
Canada

John J. Spinelli, Ph.D.
British Columbia Cancer Agency
Vancouver, British Columbia
Canada

Edward A. Stadtmauer, M.D.
Associate Professor of Medicine
Director
Bone Marrow and Stem Cell Transplant Program
University of Pennsylvania Cancer Center
Philadelphia, Pennsylvania
U.S.A.

George W. Sledge, Jr., M.D.
Professor of Medicine, Pathology and Oncology
Division of Hematology and Oncology
Indiana University School of Medicine
Indianapolis, Indiana
U.S.A.

Marc Spielmann, M.D.
Head
Breast Cancer Unit
Institut Gustave-Roussy
Villejuif, France

Douglas Stewart, M.D.
Medical Oncologist and Associate Professor
Divisions of Medical Oncology and Hematology
University of Calgary and Tom Baker Cancer Centre
Calgary, Alberta
Canada

Patrick Therasse, M.D.
Director
European Organization for Research and Treatment of Cancer
Brussels, Belgium

Katia Tonkin, M.D., M.B.B.S., M.R.C.P., F.R.C.P.C.
Senior Medical Oncologist
Cross Cancer Institute
Associate Professor
University of Alberta
Edmonton, Alberta
Canada

Naoto T. Ueno, M.D.
Breast Cancer Research Program andDepartments
  Blood and Marrow Transplantation and
  Molecular and Cellular Oncology
The University of Texas
M. D. Anderson Cancer Center
Houston, Texas
U.S.A.

Peter Venner, M.D.
Department of Medicine
Cross Cancer Institute
Edmonton, Alberta
Canada

Anne-Sophie Vercoutter-Edouart, Ph.D.
Université des Sciences et Technologies de Lille
Lille, France

Eugenio Vinés, M.D.
Instituto de Radiomedicina IRAM
Santiago, Chile

D. Lawrence Wickerham, M.D.
Associate Chairman
NSABP Operations Center
Pittsburgh, Pennsylvania
U.S.A.

Ikram El Yazidi-Belkoura, Ph.D.
Université des Sciences et Technologies de Lille
Lille, France

Brent Zanke M.D., Ph.D., F.R.C.P.C.
Director
Cross Cancer Institute
Vice President
Alberta Cancer Board
Administration
Cross Cancer Institute
Edmonton, Alberta
Canada

Laurent Zelek, M.D.
Department of Medical Oncology
Hôpital Henri Mondor, Assistance Publique-Hôpitaux de Paris
Creteil, France

PART I

Treatment Recommendations for Specific Stages of Breast Cancer

SECTION 1

Early Stage Disease: Radiation

1

Radiation Therapy for Breast Cancer

Radiotherapy Techniques to Decrease Treatment Morbidity

Eugenio Vinés, Cécile Le Péchoux, and Rodrigo Arriagada

Almost since the discovery of X-rays and radium, and their early therapeutic use, some form of radiotherapy has been used against breast cancer. With the evolution of radiation oncology, breast radiotherapy has adopted multiple forms, from interstitial brachytherapy as the sole treatment for breast cancer (1) to an adjuvant to either radical or conservative surgery.

Although adjuvant irradiation to breast-conserving surgery is an almost unquestioned tool in the modern armamentarium, postmastectomy irradiation remains more controversial. On the one hand, the success of systemic treatments made irradiation seemingly superfluous as an addition to mastectomy; on the other, the increasing recognition of radiation late toxicity brought into question its therapeutic role (2–4).

Although not universally accepted (5,6), technological advances will probably take radiation therapy into a new era of improved treatment delivery and lesser side effects that will expand its role in years to come. In order to lend credibility to these newer treatment modalities, however, radiation oncologists must be willing to test not only generic treatments, but specific treatment schedules and techniques in a prospective, randomized fashion—still a difficult task to accomplish (7).

In the last ten years, much has been done to refine the role of irradiation both as an adjunctive to breast-conserving surgery and after mastectomy. Unresolved issues remain, such as patient selection, optimal treatment volumes, dose, fractionation, and technical aspects of irradiation. In this review, we will mainly focus on the evidence behind the technical aspects of breast cancer radiotherapy, and its potential influence on cancer-related outcomes and morbidity.

CONTRIBUTION OF RADIATION THERAPY TO LOCAL CONTROL

Locoregional Recurrence after Modified Radical Mastectomy

Local and regional recurrences after mastectomy pose an important clinical situation to the practicing clinician. Up to a 25% to 40% local recurrence rate has been reported in high-risk patients after radical mastectomy (8,9). These old data could be dismissed since the patterns of presentation have changed with the widespread use of screening mammograms—a shift to less advanced disease on presentation should reflect on lesser rates of locoregional recurrence. However, modern series continue to report similar

TABLE 1.1. Locoregional failure rates of modern series of patients treated with modified radical mastectomy and systemic therapy, with or without locoregional irradiation

Trial	Patient population	N	Systemic therapy	Follow-up	Isolated locoregional recurrence	Total locoregional recurrence
British Columbia (11)	Stages I-II Pre- and postmenopausal	154	CMF	150 months	33%	—
DBCCG 82b (10)	Stages II-III Premenopausal	856	CMF	114 months	32%	—
DBCCG 82c (13)	Stages II-III Postmenopausal	736	Tamoxifen	109 months	35%	—
ECOG (12)	Stages II-III Pre- and postmenopausal	2,098	CMF and CMF derivatives	10 years	12.6%	20.7%
MD Anderson (15)	Stages II-IIIa Pre- and postmenopausal	1,031	Doxorubicin-based	10 years	14%	19%
Duke (12)	Stages III-IV	21	High-dose chemotherapy/ BMT	4 years	53%	—
Stockholm (16)	Stages I-III	960	Without radiotherapy	15 years	26%	36%
			Pre or postoperative radiotherapy		6%	11%
FNCLCC (17)	Stages II	517	CMF Radiotherapy	14 years	—	35% 15%

rates of isolated and total locoregional recurrences after modified radical mastectomy alone (Table 1.1) (10–17).

Approximately 60% to 70% of locoregional recurrences occur in the chest wall, with 20% to 30% in the axilla, 10% to 40% in the supraclavicular lymph nodes, and 1% to 10% in internal mammary nodes (Table 1.2). Although it is somewhat less frequent than chest wall failure, prevention of recurrence in lymphatic draining basins is thought by many to significantly contribute to disease-free survival and overall survival by decreasing the risk of secondary dissemination (15,16,18). Of the regional sites, recurrence in internal mammary nodes is a matter of particular debate among radiation oncologists (19) because of its influence on treatment techniques and potential treatment-related morbidity. Recurrence in internal mammary nodes has been, however, elusive to demonstrate. Although surgical series report internal mammary node involvement in 20% more of women with positive axillary lymph nodes (20–22), internal mammary failure is uncommonly reported (Table 1.2). On the other hand, some studies suggest that women with central or medial tumors have increased rates of recurrence and death than lateral tumors (23,24), hypothesizing that this is due to higher rates of *untreated* metastasis to internal mammary nodes. Lacking direct evidence of potential harms or

TABLE 1.2. Patterns of locoregional failure after modified radical mastectomy and chemotherapy in modern series (failure rates are expressed as percentage of total locoregional failures)

Trial	N	Chest wall	Supra/infraclavicular	Axilla	Internal mammary
ECOG (14)	420	58%	37.6%	19.5%	0.9%
MD Anderson (15)	179	68%	47%	14%	8%
DBCCG 82c (13)	242	55.7%	15.2%	35.9%	—

benefits of internal mammary irradiation, this treatment is advocated by some authors (25) and discouraged by others (26).

Somewhat arbitrarily, a 10-year risk of locoregional recurrence above 10% is considered high enough to warrant adjuvant irradiation. This point is germane to the appropriate selection of patients for postmastectomy radiotherapy. In univariate analysis, factors such as tumor size, number of involved lymph nodes, and estrogen receptors are considered risk factors for locoregional recurrence after mastectomy (14,15). The question remains regarding which prognostic factors best help to define a "high-risk" population. While American retrospective studies point to metastasis in four or more axillary lymph nodes and tumors greater than 5 cm (14,15), modern randomized trials suggest significant locoregional recurrence rates even for patients with metastasis to one to three lymph nodes (10–17).

ROLE OF POSTMASTECTOMY IRRADIATION

It is now a well-established fact that postmastectomy irradiation at a total dose of 45 to 50 Gy in conventional fractionation decreases the risk of locoregional recurrence by a factor of approximately two-thirds (4). This increase in locoregional control is likely responsible for an increase in disease-free and overall survival (10–12), but it may be associated with an increased risk of cardiac toxicity in the long term (4). The subject of postmastectomy irradiation is dealt with in greater detail in Chapter 2.

Defining the Target for Postmastectomy Irradiation

A discussion on radiation target volumes is essential to understanding radiotherapy treatment techniques. In the following section we will summarize the rationales for treating specific areas in high-risk patients after a modified radical mastectomy. Target volume definitions derive from an accurate knowledge of the anatomy, patterns of spread of disease and patterns of failure after treatment. Whenever postmastectomy irradiation is indicated, there is ample evidence that the chest wall should be included in all cases (27), as it is the main site of locoregional failure.

Evidence supporting the treatment of lymph node areas is less compelling. One should consider treating a lymphatic drainage area if there is a significant risk of subclinical metastatic disease, or if there is a high risk of disease recurrence after a lymphatic dissection. Most of the lymphatic drainage of the breast is to the axillary lymph nodes. The importance of axillary lymph node involvement as a prognostic factor cannot be overstated, hence the use of routine axillary dissection in the management of these patients. Central and medial portions of the gland also drain directly to internal mammary lymph nodes (28). However, even in these centrally located tumors, the most important predictive factor is the axillary node involvement. Supraclavicular lymph nodes are the next echelon after axillary lymph nodes. Although they are not considered regional disease under the current staging system (29), supraclavicular failure is reported in at least 15% of patients with axillary metastasis (Table 1.2), and supraclavicular irradiation of subclinical disease is a common practice.

Currently available evidence supporting the treatment of lymph node areas stems from retrospective studies, as there are no published randomized trials of irradiation techniques (27).

ADJUVANT RADIATION AFTER BREAST-CONSERVING SURGERY

Essential to breast conservation, the routine use of breast irradiation is supported by multiple randomized studies and meta-analysis (4,30–37). Not all patients benefit from irradiation, as the local recurrence rate without radiotherapy is 30% to 40%. There have been efforts to refine the selection of patients for breast irradiation, with mixed results (38–42). Most trials were in favor of postoperative radiotherapy. In one trial (38), breast radiotherapy could be avoided in older patients when a quadrantectomy was performed. However, this kind of subgroup analysis needs confirmatory studies. To further complicate the issue, the presence of lymph node metastasis could in itself be an indication for adjuvant regional irradiation, if the theories for postmastectomy irradiation hold true.

The use of a boost to the primary tumor bed has been a practice among some radiation oncologists since the early 1970s. Only for the past 10 years or so has this practice been evaluated in a prospective, randomized fashion. Two trials report a benefit to adding a local tumor bed boost after breast irradiation (43,44), and the data are in keeping with previously published dose-response analysis (45,46).

In defining target volumes for breast-conserving radiotherapy, the main remaining controversy is the treatment of lymphatic areas. Rates of regional recurrence are probably similar to those observed after mastectomy (Table 1.2), and we would expect a similar situation regarding the indications for adjuvant irradiation.

THE PROBLEM OF LATE TOXICITY

Normal tissue tolerance is the major constraint to the success of therapeutic irradiation. Although we are accustomed to treat "normal tissues" as having homogeneous parameters of radiation tolerance, the answer is probably much more complex. Radiation tolerance doses are statistical abstractions that relate to the probability of causing clinically detectable damage at certain dose levels where there are significant interindividual variations (47). While total dose of irradiation is a major determinant of toxic late effects, fraction size is of paramount importance (48) with higher doses per fraction being associated with worse late toxicity. In general, fractional doses of 1.8 to 2 Gy are believed to be associated with acceptable late toxicity. In evaluating the adverse events possibly related to irradiation, one must consider the volume of irradiated normal tissues and dose employed. Radiation energy is less of an issue when it comes to late toxicity, as with lower radiation energies (less than 1 MV), higher surface doses, or "hot spots," are required to achieve adequate doses at the treatment depth, thereby resulting in high daily doses, which are ultimately responsible for toxic events.

Radiotherapy has not been universally accepted as an adjunct to mastectomy mostly because of data showing an increase in late noncancer mortality when irradiation has been used (2,4). Underlying mechanisms are unclear. While, classically, vascular changes are described in irradiated fields (49,50), perhaps suggesting tissue hypoxia as primarily responsible for radiation damage, studies do not reflect circulatory changes in the breast skin or the gland 2 to 5 years after 50 Gy of external beam irradiation (51). This does not rule out the possibility of vascular changes beyond this period, or the contributing influence of other types of injury, which may aggravate radiation-induced subclinical changes. Another possible mechanism is the loss of clonogenic units capable of repopulating injured tissue (52), ultimately leading to organ failure. Most of the reported toxicity and mortality observed with breast and chest wall irradiation is related to cardiovascular events, which has led some authors to point to internal mammary irradiation as the culprit (53). In Table 1.3 and Table 1.4 we describe the rates of radiation-related complications, attempting to correlate them with the treatment techniques that are most likely to be responsible for the toxicity.

CARDIAC TOXICITY

Irradiation to the mediastinum and heart is thought to be related to cardiac morbidity, heart failure, pericarditis, and coronary artery disease in patients irradiated for Hodgkin disease, seminoma, and breast cancer (2,4,54–56). In 1974, Stjernswärd analyzed the effects of irradiation as a complement to surgery in five controlled clinical trials (57). The results were remarkable: postoperative irradiation was associated with a 1% to 10% excess mortality in the different trials. It was hypothesized that the mortality was secondary to "the effects of irradiation on host immunity" (57). Later, a meta-analysis of randomized trials published by

TABLE 1.3. Cardiac complications in irradiated breast cancer patients (emphasis is placed on radiotherapy technical factors that can explain the presence or absence of cardiotoxicity)

Trial	Comparison reported	Relative risk of cardiac toxicity	Irradiation technique	Beam energy	Total dose/ dose per fraction	Other factors	Evidence level
Stockholm (61)	RT vs. no RT	3.2	"Deep tangential" fields covering IMN	^{60}Co	45 Gy / 1.8 Gy	Lung density corrections	III
Oslo II (60)	RT vs. no RT	11	Direct sternal field, 3 cm depth	^{60}Co	50 Gy / 2.5 Gy	NS	III
DBCCG (10,13,63)	RT vs. no RT	0.95 (95% CI: 0.17–1.5)	Direct IMN electron field. Treatment depth determined by US	6–17 MeV electrons	50 Gy / 2 Gy 48 Gy / 2.18 Gy	NS	II
PMH (64)	Left vs. Right side RT vs. age-matched population	1.14 Nonsignificant	Tangential fields. No IMN coverage	^{60}Co, 6 MV photons	40 Gy / 2.5 Gy	Cardiac risk factors accounted	III

DBCCG, Danish Breast Cancer Collaborative Group; IMN, internal mammary nodes; NS, not stated; PMH, Princess Margaret Hospital; RT, radiotherapy; US, ultrasound.

TABLE 1.4. Changes in pulmonary function after local/regional irradiation for breast cancer

Author	N	% complications	RT techniques	Energies	Dose/dose per fraction	Findings	Evidence level
Rothwell et al. (65)	184	3.8%*	Tangential CW fields Direct photon IMN field Anterior SC photon field Posterior axillary photon field	6 MV 60Co 6 MV 6 MV	40 Gy / 2.67 Gy	Greater risk of grade II-III pneumonitis with greater area of irradiated lung	III
Lingos et al. (66)	1,624	1%**	Tangential breast fields Anterior SC photon field Posterior axillary photon field	NS	45–50 Gy / 1.8–2 Gy	Higher risk of symptomatic pneumonitis with concomitant CT	III
Kimsey et al. (67)	34	5.8%†	Tangential breast fields Anterior SC photon field	60Co, 6MV, or mixed 60Co/8MV	45–50 Gy / 1.8–2 Gy 44–50 Gy / 2 Gy	Patients with clinical pneumonitis had >10% irradiated lung	III
Lind et al. (69)	105	3.8%*	Anterior CW/IMN electron field Anterior SC photon field Tangential breast fields Oblique IMN electron field	6–16 MeV 8 MV 4–8 MV 9–12 MeV	46 Gy / 2 Gy NS 50 Gy / 2 Gy NS	Risk increased with regional irradiation	III
Lind et al. (70)	613	2.4%*	Tangential breast fields "Partly wide" tangential fields to cover IMN, or Anterior mixed photon/electron IMN field Anterior SC photon field	6 or 15 MV‡ 6 or 15 MV‡	46 Gy / NS 46–50 Gy / NS	Risk increased with regional irradiation	III

CT, chemotherapy; CW, chest wall; IMN, internal mammary nodes; NS, not stated; RT, radiotherapy.
*Radiation pneumonitis requiring treatment.
**Clinical syndrome of radiation pneumonitis. Steroidal treatment given to 5 of 17 patients.
†Clinical radiation pneumonitis. No patient required treatment.
‡15 MV used for patients with large separation.

Cuzick et al. (3) confirmed the findings. At the time, it was suggested that the excess mortality in irradiated patients could be related to cardiovascular events. Furthermore, there is some data suggestive of an increased risk of cardiovascular events among women treated for cancer of the left breast (58,59), which has been ascribed, albeit without direct evidence, to the effect of irradiation.

In 1986, Høst and Loeb published long-term data on the Oslo trial of postoperative irradiation (60). In the second part of the trial, 1968 to 1972, patients treated with a radical mastectomy were randomized to lymphatic irradiation (sternal, supra and infraclavicular, and axillary regions) or no further treatment. Radiotherapy was carried out with direct (60) Cobalt (Co) fields, prescribed at a standard depth of 3 cm. There were no overall survival differences among groups, although irradiated stage I patients displayed a trend towards lower survival than unirradiated patients. When non-breast cancer death causes were analyzed, it was found that irradiated stage I patients had an exceedingly high rate of mortality from acute myocardial infarction than their unirradiated counterparts (10 of 170 vs. 1 of 186 patients, respectively).

In 1992, Rutqvist et al. (61) analyzed the cardiovascular morbidity findings in the Stockholm breast radiotherapy trial. Patients were randomized to preoperative irradiation, postoperative irradiation, or surgery alone. In all irradiated patients, the internal mammary nodes were treated, although specific techniques varied: some patients were treated using "wide tangential" fields covering both the preoperatively treated breast and both internal mammary chains. Later this technique was changed to "limited tangential fields" in which the tangential fields encompassed breast and ipsilateral internal mammary nodes only. An attempt was made to recreate radiation doses to the heart using computed tomography (CT) data from four patients. It was found that the highest cardiac dose was received by those patients treated with wide, left-sided cobalt fields, while electron fields and right-sided cobalt fields yielded intermediate and low cardiac doses, respectively. There was no difference in cardiac mortality in the overall population. When patients were analyzed by irradiated cardiac volume and compared with surgery alone, it was apparent that patients who received the highest cardiac doses had a significant excess of mortality from ischemic heart disease (Table 1.3).

In a retrospective comparison of patients treated with conservative surgery plus breast irradiation, and mastectomy alone, Rutqvist et al. (62) found no significant differences in rates of acute myocardial infarction at a median follow-up time of 9 years. Patients were mostly irradiated with tangential photon fields (^{60}Co, or 4–6 MV) to total doses of about 50 Gy using 2 Gy daily fractions. No attempt was made to cover internal mammary nodes in 88% of irradiated patients. Multivariate analysis of risk factors related to myocardial infarction only showed increasing patient's age to be significantly correlated with myocardial infarction.

Højris et al. (63) published an analysis of ischemic heart disease mortality in patients randomized to postmastectomy irradiation. Patients had been treated in two prospective randomized trials of adjuvant radiotherapy (10,13) and all patients received adjuvant CMF or tamoxifen. The radiotherapy technique included irradiation of chest wall and supraclavicular field by means of a direct photon field, specifically shielding the internal mammary chain. Internal mammary nodes were treated with a direct electron field, and the prescription depth was determined for each individual patient using ultrasound. Irradiation dose was 50 Gy in 25 daily fractions, or 48 Gy in 22 daily fractions. With a median follow up of 117 months, the analysis shows no differences in cumulative morbidity or mortality from ischemic heart disease by treatment allocated (RT versus no RT) or by laterality (Table 1.3).

In a retrospective review from the Princess Margaret Hospital, Vallis et al. analyzed 2,128 patients treated with conservative surgery and radiotherapy (64). The breast was irradiated using tangential photon fields (^{60}Co, or 6 MV photons) to a total dose of 40 Gy in 16 2.5-Gy fractions. Only 2.5% of patients received radiotherapy to internal mammary nodes. The analysis was carried out to assess a potential higher risk of cardiac disease in patients with left-sided cancers. Cardiac risk factors (smoking, hypertension, and prior cardiac history) were well balanced among patient groups. With a median follow-up of 10.2 years, no significant differences in the incidence of myocardial infarction were detected for left-sided versus right-sided breast cancers. The whole patient population was also compared to the age-matched general female population in Ontario for the study period: there was no increase in observed cardiac events among irradiated patients (Table 1.3).

From these data, it can be inferred that irradiation fields, namely internal mammary radiotherapy in itself, is not necessarily associated with increased cardiac toxicity. Nor is necessarily the use of doses per fraction of 2.5 Gy, as underscored by the Princess Margaret Hospital data (64). However, the data presented in Table 1.3 suggest an association between cardiac toxicity and the use of techniques that irradiate the heart to a high dose (i.e., a direct photon field for internal mammary nodes, or deep tangential fields).

Caution must be taken in interpreting cardiac toxicity in this setting. The latest Early Breast Cancer Trialists' overview on breast irradiation demonstrates a significant increase in non-breast cancer deaths among irradiated patients, probably due to excess cardiac mortality (4). Actually, the differences in non-breast cancer mortality are apparent largely beyond the 10th year of follow-up, approximately. As the studies that show no increase in cardiac events for irradiated patients have been reported with a median follow-up around 10 years, it is possible that with continuing observation, an excess cardiac mortality may be apparent in this population. On the other hand, it may well be that the increase in non-breast cancer mortality seen in the meta-analysis beyond 10 years of follow-up will decrease as modern trials continue to show no difference in cardiac mortality beyond that time limit. Certainly, continued follow-up and more prospective randomized trials are needed to settle the issue.

So far we have reviewed trials in which there was no adjuvant therapy, or which included CMF-based or tamoxifen systemic therapy. Nowadays, most patients will be offered doxorubicin-containing combinations, known to be potentially cardiotoxic. The interaction of anthracycline or taxane-containing chemotherapy regimens, or of biologic modifiers such as trastuzumab, and irradiation is yet to be evaluated.

PULMONARY MORBIDITY

Pulmonary toxicity is also a problem, apparently less related to mortality, but less extensively studied. Several articles relate lung radiation dosimetry to changes in pulmonary function tests (Table 1.4) (65–71). Although mortality from acute radiation pneumonitis is exceedingly rare, a contribution of late lung toxicity to late mortality is possible.

In a series of 184 patients from the United Kingdom, Rothwell et al. (65) correlated the incidence of radiation pneumonitis to irradiated lung volumes. Postoperative irradiation was delivered to the chest wall using tangential 6-MV photon fields. Whenever indicated, supraclavicular and axillary nodes were irradiated with anterior and posterior photon fields, respectively. Patients with medially located tumors, or with axillary nodal involvement also received direct anterior ^{60}Co irradiation to internal mammary nodes. There was a 3.8% incidence of severe radiation pneumonitis in the study population. No attempt was made to correlate symptoms with specific treatment techniques, but an association was found between the risk of pneumonitis and the "cross sectional area of irradiated lung" at the midplane of tangential fields. The use of a supraclavicular/axillary field in some patients was not addressed, as the authors only studied lung dose at the mid-tangential level. The authors stated that the use of a direct internal mammary field resulted in a greater area of irradiated lung than simple tangential fields.

In a retrospective analysis of 1,624 patients irradiated for stages I to II breast cancer, Lingos et al. (66) analyzed the incidence of radiation pneumonitis. Most patients were treated with tangential fields alone, or with the addition of a supraclavicular/axillary field. They found an incidence of clinical radiation pneumonitis of approximately 1%. In univariate analysis, the use of a supraclavicular/axillary field or the use of systemic chemotherapy was associated with the development of pneumonitis. Most notably, concurrent chemotherapy and radiotherapy resulted in 8.8% of cases of pneumonitis, compared to 1.3% when the two treatments were administered sequentially. Volumes of irradiated lung were analyzed in a case-control fashion using the "central lung distance" parameter as surrogate, but no correlation could be found to the risk of developing pneumonitis.

Kimsey et al. (67) prospectively studied 34 patients irradiated for stages I and II breast cancer. All patients were CT-planned to estimate the percentage of irradiated ipsilateral lung, and pulmonary function was measured before, during, and after irradiation. All patients were treated with tangential irradiation fields, and seven patients received also a supraclavicular field. Although most patients developed decreased pulmonary function tests by spirometry, these changes were transient. Only two patients developed clinical radiation pneumonitis, which resolved with no medical treatment. Remarkably, both patients with clinical radiation pneumonitis had an irradiated lung volume greater than 10%.

Hardman et al. (68) published a series of 110 patients irradiated for breast cancer and followed with serial pulmonary function tests. Nine patients developed distant metastasis within a year of irradiation, and were excluded from analysis. Of the remaining patients, 85 received locoregional irradiation (supraclavicular and axillary fields in addition to tangential breast/chest wall fields). Radiation doses were 45 Gy in 20 fractions using 4 to 6 MV photons. Of those, 24 patients developed respiratory symptoms after irradiation, but none was severe enough to warrant steroid treatment. Patients not receiving regional irradiation had fewer symptoms, but it was not statistically significant. In the analysis of serial pulmonary function tests, there was a significant decrease of 5% in forced expiratory volume in the first second (FEV_1), and significant decrease of approximately 8% in the CO_2 diffusion capacity at one year. Although a greater effect on pulmonary function is expected with regional irradiation, small patient numbers did not allow a meaningful comparison of the effect of irradiated volumes.

Lind et al. (69) studied pulmonary function and radiological changes in 105 stage II patients irradiated for breast cancer. Fifty-five patients had a modified radical mastectomy (MRM) and 50 patients underwent breast-conserving surgery (BCS). MRM patients were treated to chest wall and lymph nodes with a technique similar to that described by Højris et al. (63). Patients treated with BCS received tangential photon irradiation (4 to 6 MV) plus an oblique electron field to internal mammary nodes (36 patients) and supraclavicular/axillary irradiation (26 patients). Irradiation fields were treated at 2 Gy per fraction. Total dose was 46 Gy in MRM, and 50 Gy in BCS patients. CT scans were obtained at baseline and at 4 months after completion of treatment for measurement of lung density. Patients were also followed clinically, and pulmonary function tests (body plethysmography) were performed at baseline and at 5 months after treatment completion in 89 patients. Overall, using clinical assessment, four patients had severe pulmonary complications. Radiological changes (lung density of increasing severity) were correlated with regional irradiation, and also correlated with the risk of severe pulmonary complications ($p < 0.001$). The authors concluded that CT findings may be used as objective end points in assessing the severity of radiation-related lung complications.

A series of 613 patients receiving local or locoregional breast irradiation breast was reported by Lind et al. (70). Treatment of the intact breast or chest wall was carried out at 2 Gy per fraction to a total dose of 46 and 50 Gy, respectively. Patients who received internal mammary nodes (IMN) irradiation were treated either with deep tangential fields covering only the first three intercostal spaces, or with a separate anterior field consisting of a combination of photon and electron irradiation. All patients were CT-planned. The incidence of radiation pneumonitis was retrospectively evaluated from clinic visits. Radiation pneumonitis requiring steroids was seen in 2.4% of patients. In univariate analysis, regional irradiation was significantly associated with the development of pneumonitis, whereas the use of chemotherapy was of marginal significance. Multivariate analysis showed locoregional radiotherapy was significantly associated with the risk of pneumonitis. Interestingly, no patient treated with a separate anterior IMN field had radiation pneumonitis. Due to the small number of events (15 cases of radiation penumonitis), no conclusions could be drawn regarding specific radiotherapy techniques.

There is relatively little published on the time, course, and evolution of radiation-related pulmonary changes in breast cancer patients. In a small series of patients irradiated for lymphoma or breast cancer, Thews et al. (71) reported a relative 50% improvement of pulmonary function tests between 3 and 18 months after completion of irradiation, suggesting that studies with longer follow-up are needed to help ascertain the actual long-term effects of treatment.

SECOND MALIGNANCIES

Induction of second primary tumors is a well known, yet poorly understood, side effect of radiotherapy. In-field second primary malignancies are most frequently breast sarcoma, which seems to be related to integral dose (70,73), whereas an excess of contralateral breast cancers—presumed to be related to scattered radiation or increased risk due to the same factors that led to the initial malignancy—has been described in retrospective studies (74). Others have reported similar 15-year rates of second malignant tumors after mastectomy without irradiation or conservative surgery and breast irradiation (75). Lung cancers in formerly irradiated supraclavicular fields, and esophageal cancers in patients who received direct photon irradiation to internal mammary fields, have also been reported (75).

Lymphedema

Blocking of axillary lymphatic drainage by means of surgical removal of lymph nodes may result in arm or breast lymphedema. This disfiguring complication of axillary surgery may increase in frequency and severity with increasing extent of surgery and with the addition of supraclavicular and axillary irradiation (77). The assessment of lymphedema has been somewhat hampered by the varying definitions used in the literature and has been reported with an incidence of 0 to 56% depending on the types of treatment, length of follow up, and defining criteria (78).

Brachial Plexopathy

Brachial plexopathy is now a fairly uncommon complication of breast radiotherapy. Most reports relate this condition to the treatment of a supraclavicular/axillary field, especially when non-conventional fractionation regimens (i.e., fraction sizes more than 2 Gy) are used (79), or when overlap of fields is accepted (80).

COSMETIC RESULTS OF IRRADIATION

Not lethal, yet important, are the cosmetic results of breast-conserving treatments. As for surgery, there is some evidence that technical issues are in part responsible for poor cosmetic results after breast-conserving treatment (81–84). These relate to overlap of adjacent radiation fields that can lead to fibrotic areas, the use of higher doses per fraction, the use of a tumor bed boost (85), and the type of radiation technique used for the boost. Figure 1.1 is an example of a common cosmetic complication when a poor radiation technique is used.

Avoiding Toxicity Through Technique, Dose, and Fractionation

One elegant way to decrease radiation-related toxicity would be to identify patients that do not benefit from adjuvant irradiation who are routinely irradiated today on the presumption of subclinical disease. Evidence, so far, is lacking on predictive factors that would make this solution feasible.

The next best strategy is the identification of those patients who are especially sensitive to irradiation, since they probably make up the significant minority of cases that determine tolerance doses (47). Although cell lines derived from xeroderma pigmentosum or ataxia-telangetasia (ATM) cases are extremely sensitive to low doses of irradiation, the search for characteristic genetic constitutions associated with the "radiation sensitive" phenotype has

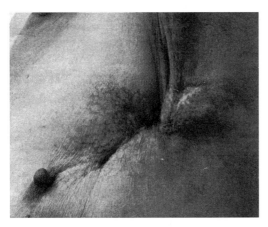

FIG. 1.1. Severe skin fibrosis and telangectasia 10 years after treatment for an early-stage breast cancer. Two main factors contributed to the poor cosmetic outcome in this patient: (a) Lumpectomy and axillary dissection were performed through the same incision; (b) A 14-Gy boost was given at a 3-cm depth with a direct ^{60}Co field, giving a high dose per fraction to the skin surface. See color plate.

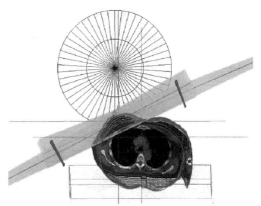

FIG. 1.2. Tangential irradiation fields for treatment of the intact breast. While two opposed fields would have a significant amount of divergence into the lung, it can be corrected with gantry rotation to minimize lung irradiation. The panel displays a tridimensional representation of the treatment fields.

not been successful. Notably, no ATM mutations have been demonstrated in patients displaying serious late effects to conventional irradiation in breast cancer (86,87).

So, the practicing radiation oncologist is faced with a two-headed dilemma in treating breast cancer. On one hand, many patients judged at risk of disease recurrence are overtreated. On the other hand, some of these patients will experience serious, even fatal, complications from the treatment. The compromise solution to which we still must conform is to minimize the risk of complications while keeping locoregional control rates high through judicious patient selection and treatment technique.

Irradiation of the Intact Breast

This is probably the most frequently encountered situation in clinical practice. The time-honored technique of choice is the use of tangential radiation fields to cover all of the breast tissue with a reasonable margin. Care must be taken to avoid divergence of the radiation beams towards the lung (Fig. 1.2) so as to limit the amount of irradiated pulmonary tissue. A gross estimate of the volume of irradiated lung can be made from simulation films by measuring the distance between the rib wall to the edge, at the midplane of the tangential fields (Fig. 1.3). A contemporaneous radiation oncology textbook accepts up to 3 cm of irradiated lung within standard tangential fields (88), which is likely to be associated with a relatively high risk of pulmonary complications. Although the evidence we have gathered regarding risk of pneumonitis is by no means conclusive, a safer approach would be to restrict central lung distances to less than 2 cm. Alternative treatment plans, such as the use of a third field to cover the medial portions of the breast using electrons or a mixture of photons and electrons may allow for appropriate coverage of the target volume while reducing lung doses (Fig. 1.4). For left-sided lesions, the anterior descending coronary artery has been shown to fall within standard tangential fields (89), so careful attention should be paid to the cardiac silhouette at the time of simulation.

When tissue inhomogeneities in electron density are incorporated in dosimetric calculations, it becomes apparent that the radiation dose received by the irradiated volume is more heterogeneous than that estimated by simple dosimetry (90–93). Not only the dose to the

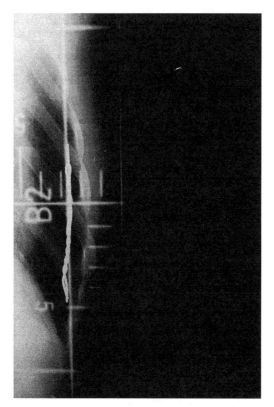

FIG. 1.3. Simulation film of a tangential breast irradiation field. The field is placed parallel to the chest wall. A graduated grid is placed in the center of the beam, so the central lung distance can easily be appreciated. Radiopaque surgical clips mark the tumor bed in the upper portion of the breast.

lung itself is significantly higher than estimated with simpler calculations, but also the dose to the chest wall. This can be quite significant with larger volumes of irradiated lung. Normally, wedge-compensating filters are used to make the dose distribution within the breast more homogeneous, which will also be modified by tissue density corrections.

Inhomogeneities due to contour variation also account for high-dose areas, especially in the extreme areas of the breast. Hot spots may result in higher acute toxicity, or in poor cosmetic results. These variations in dosimetry are only appreciated if the treatment is planned with multiple CT slices, which allows for some fine tuning of the treatment technique. Along these lines, three-dimensional CT-based calculations probably render a more accurate picture of the dose distribution through the breast, lung dosimetry, and other factors which could in turn be correlated to toxicity or treatment outcomes. Heterogeneities related to the different amount of tissue within the irradiated breast volume may be corrected by the use of compensator filters or by intensity modulation of radiation.

Recommended total dose to the breast is 45 to 50 Gy using conventional 1.8–2 Gy fractions. Although there is little direct evidence that fraction sizes are indeed associated with greater toxicity, some authors have identified fraction sizes

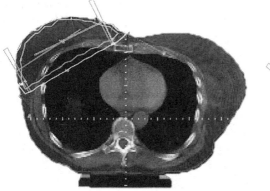
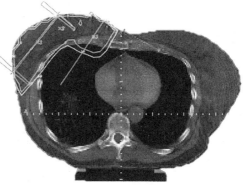

FIG. 1.4. Dosimetry of whole-breast irradiation in a patient with idiopathic lung fibrosis. The panel on the left **(A)** shows the amount of irradiated lung had a simple pair of tangential fields been used. On the right panel, **(B)** a three-field arrangement with two tangential fields, and a medial electron field has been used, thus significantly reducing the amount of irradiated lung.

TABLE 1.5. *Patterns of dose specification for tangential breast irradiation used in the literature*

Dose specification point	Reference	Comment
1.5–2 cm from medial field edge	"Several institutions"*	Using standard American techniques, it falls within lung tissue, when no heterogeneity corrections are used.
Lung-tissue interface	"Several institutions"*	Area of density heterogeneity not usually accounted in treatment planning.
Two thirds of the distance between the skin and the edge of the tangents at midplane	NSABP B-06 protocol	Free of dosimetric problems due to tissue heterogeneities. No evident advantage over ICRU point.
Isocenter	ICRU recommendation (96)	Allows for interinstitutional comparison of dose specification policies. There is usually a ± 5% inhomogeneity across the breast contour. Specification point must be modified if half-blocked fields are used.

ICRU, International Radiation Units and Measurement Commission.
*Common prescribing policy, not systematically analyzed in technical publications (95).

more than or equal to 2.67 Gy as significantly correlated with the incidence of radiation pneumonitis in combined modality therapy of lung cancer (93). Since little is to be gained in terms of disease control or morbidity with the use of large fraction sizes, we continue to recommend conventional fractionation regimens.

Another interesting issue is the need for standardization of a prescription point for breast radiotherapy. While typically the dose of irradiation is prescribed to "the isodose covering the target volume" (94), allowing for a broad range of variations in dose specification (Table 1.5) with the associated variations of hot spots and lung doses, a more accurate definition would allow better comparisons of reported data and results from different groups. The authors and others (95) favor the specification point put forward by the International Commission of Radiation Units and Measurements (ICRU) (96).

A boost dose to the primary tumor site has been shown to significantly reduce the incidence of local recurrence after breast-conserving treatment (43,44), with a possible detrimental effect on cosmetic outcome. Several techniques are available to deliver such radiotherapy boost and can be summarized as: a single electron beam field; multiple photon fields (so-called mini tangential fields, or a variation thereof); or a brachytherapy boost through an interstitial ^{192}Ir (Iridium) implant. These techniques seem to be equivalent in terms of local control (97–99), but the cosmetic results remain debatable. More recently, intraoperative radiotherapy has been proposed and is being evaluated as a boost dose or as exclusive postoperative radiotherapy in selected patients (100). Boost doses of 16 Gy in 2-Gy fractions, according to the ICRU definition, are favored, using appropriate electron energies whenever possible. Placement of surgical clips (Fig. 1.2) to determine the depth and extension of the tumor bed is especially useful in tailoring boost fields (101).

IRRADIATION OF THE CHEST WALL

The rationale for chest wall irradiation after a modified radical mastectomy has already been discussed. Technically, the considerations regarding pulmonary and cardiac morbidity are similar to those applying to whole-breast irradiation. For the sake of simplicity, the following discussion focuses on chest wall irradiation alone, dismissing the treatment of nodal areas. Standard tangential fields are often appropriate, but care must be exercised to cover the whole surgical scar, avoiding excessive lung irradiation. Beam energies more than or equal to 6 MV may require the use of bolus for a portion of the treatment in order to attain an adequate skin dose. An alternative technique involves the use of a direct electron field to cover the chest wall (63). Electron energy is chosen based on the depth of the chest wall, determined by ultrasound or CT scan. Both treatment techniques provide adequate coverage of the chest wall and surgical scar, while sparing the lung from unnecessary irradiation. Recommended total doses and doses per fraction are similar to whole-breast irradiation.

IRRADIATION OF LYMPHATIC DRAINAGE AREAS

Irradiation of the supraclavicular field is commonly done with an anterior photon field. The field is angled 12 to 15 degrees to avoid irradiating the spine and spinal cord. The lower border of the field is placed at the clavicle head, and the upper border is just above the clavicle (Fig. 1.5). When axillary lymph nodes are also a target, the supraclavicular field is widened to cover the medial portion of the humeral head. Alternatively, the field can be reduced, so the

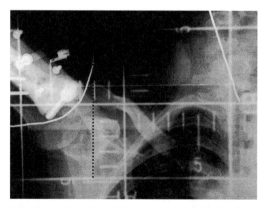

FIG. 1.5. Simulation film of an extended supraclavicular field covering both supraclavicular and axillary lymph nodes. The inferior border of the field is placed at the clavicular head, and the superior border is placed to cover the clavicle and palpable supraclavicular soft tissues. Care has been taken to place the medial border at the vertebral pedicles, to avoid unnecessary irradiation of the spinal cord. The lateral field border of an extended field is placed at the lateral border of the humeral head, to achieve adquate coverage of upper axillary nodes. In this situation, part of the humeral head and the acromioclavicular joint are blocked. The lateral edge of the field for treatment of supraclavicular nodes alone when no axillary treatment is intended is marked with a dotted line.

acromioclavicular joint can be blocked. Since supraclavicular/axillary irradiation may cause significant impairment of shoulder mobility (102), an effort must be made to block the acromioclavicular joint and the humeral head. An alternative technique is the use of a direct electron field to treat supraclavicular lymph nodes when no effort is made to irradiate axillary lymph nodes. The depth of supraclavicular nodes has been estimated in several studies of CT planning of breast irradiation (103,104). On average, supraclavicular nodes lie at a 3-cm to 4-cm depth from the anterior skin surface, hence the rationale to prescribe supraclavicular irradiation at a standard 3-cm depth. When patients are treated on a breast-angled board, the volume of irradiated upper lung increases proportionally to the steepness of the board angulation (Fig. 1.6).

Another important technical challenge—dealing with the addition of a supraclavicular field—that has to be met is the matching of this field to breast/chest wall tangential fields. A direct supraclavicular field, though matched on the skin, will diverge into the tangentials at depth. On the other hand, both tangential fields would diverge into the supraclavicular field, creating hot and cold spots at the junction. The classical solution to this problem is to attempt a geometric match plane at the junction of the three fields. A straight vertical edge is created for the lower border of the supraclavicular field by means of a beam splitter or with an asymmetric collimator. Coronal alignment of the tangential fields is obtained by alternatively rotating the treatment table. This still leaves us with some deep divergence of the tangential fields into the supraclavicular field that can be observed in the sagittal plane. Siddon et al. (105) proposed the use of a rotating block to accomplish the field match, and a number of techniques have been devised based on this principle (106–108). Alternatively, a monoisocentric technique can be used, which involves lesser technical complexity, but basically follows a similar principle of creating a vertical match plane at the junction of supraclavicular and tangential fields (109).

The need for a separate axillary field is rather controversial. Customarily, the midplane deliv-

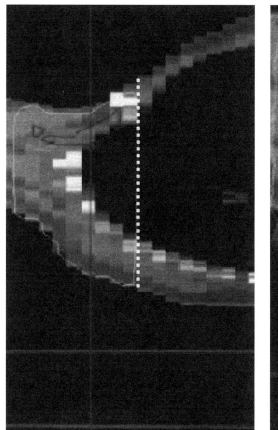 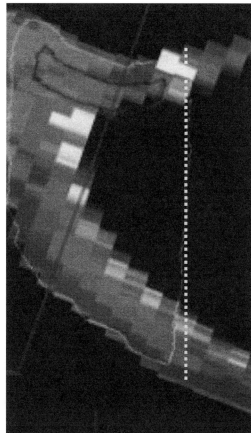

FIG. 1.6. A: Sagittal plane of a supraclavicular field with the patient lying flat on the treatment table or **B:** with an angled board showing the differences in irradiated lung with the two treatment setups.

ered to the upper level of the axilla from the supraclavicular field a posterior axillary field is calculated, and a posterior field is added to supplement the midplane dose up to 45 Gy to 50 Gy in 25 fractions. CT planning of supraclavicular/axillary fields suggests that the level III axillary lymph nodes (the stated target for a posterior axillary field) are at about the same depth as the supraclavicular lymph nodes, and so they may be adequately treated with a wide supraclavicular field alone (103,104). The most common indication for supplementary axillary irradiation in a dissected axilla is gross involvement of axillary fat, or "massive axillary involvement." However, some studies analyzing patterns of recurrence in this kind of patient treated without axillary irradiation fail to show an excess of isolated local recurrence (110–114), thus casting some doubt on the clinical indication, while others suggest higher axillary recurrence rates in patients with extranodal extension, or nodal metastasis at the axillary apex, when radiation is not used (115).

The internal mammary nodes are another controversial topic in breast radiotherapy (116,117). Retrospective studies suggest that irradiation of the internal mammary chain may confer a disease-specific survival advantage to high-risk patients (118,119). On the other hand, internal mammary irradiation, especially when old techniques with a direct photon field were used, may have been responsible for significant cardiac and pulmonary toxicity, to the point of offsetting the potential benefits of treatment. Current treatment

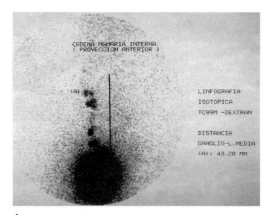

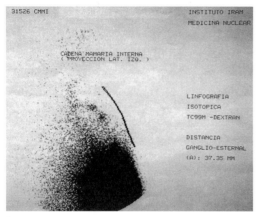

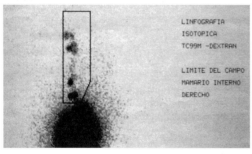

FIG. 1.7. Internal mammary lymphoscintigraphy. **A:** On the anterior projection, the midline (projected from sternal notch) has been marked, and the distance from midline to the uppermost internal mammary node (A) has been measured as 43.2 mm. **B:** Lateral projection. The anterior chest wall at midline is marked on the film, and the depth of lymph node (A) is measured as 37.3 mm. **C:** The standard internal mammary field and its relationship to the actual location of the lymph nodes.

techniques, especially the use of electron beam for most or all the internal mammary irradiation, is likely to be associated with the least amount of morbidity, as shown in two major randomized trials (63). If the internal mammary nodes are to be treated, it is advisable to localize them in a simple and predictable fashion. The internal mammary nodes are thought to be located mostly within the first three intercostal spaces, approximately 2.5 cm lateral to the midline, and at a depth of 2 cm (120); however, in individual patient measurements, these average distances show considerable variation (121). Techniques used to determine the position of internal mammary nodes commonly use as surrogate the chest wall/pleural interface as determined by ultrasound,[60] or the internal mammary vessels visualized with a contrast CT scan (122). A straightforward methodology used at the authors' institution involves the use of lymphoscintigraphy (Fig. 1.7), which allows visualization of internal mammary nodes in over 95% of patients (121). This may allow for better customization of radiation fields and optimal sparing of normal tissues.

DOSE AND FRACTIONATION ISSUES

There is little evidence from randomized trials regarding the optimal dosing schedule for breast cancer treatment. However, stated doses of 45 Gy to 50 Gy in 25 fractions to the whole breast followed by a 16-Gy boost to the tumor bed result in excellent local control rates, i.e., more than 90% at 10 years. Higher fractional doses have not been systematically tested in a prospective way. Kim et al. (123) retrospectively reviewed 418 patients irradiated after a radical mastectomy between 1958 and 1968. Patients were treated to 4,900 rad in 10 fractions, 4,410 rad in 9 fractions, 5,000 rad in 13 fractions, or 4,600 rad in 20 fractions. Local control rates with the three fractionation schedules were similar, but the incidence of clinically detected subcutaneous fibrosis ranged from 33% in patients treated with 490 rad per fraction to 17% in patients treated with lower fractionation schedules, supporting the notion that higher compli-

TABLE 1.6. *Indications for irradiation of breast, chest wall, and lymph nodes, with the evidence level supporting each recommendation*

Anatomical site	RT Indication	Level of evidence
Whole breast	Conservative surgery for infiltrating ductal carcinoma	I
	Conservative surgery for ductal carcinoma in situ	I
Chest wall (after MRM)	Metastasis in > 3 axillary lymph nodes	I
	Metastasis in 1–3 axillary lymph nodes	II
	Tumor > 5 cm	III
	T4	III
Internal mammary nodes	Medially located tumor and/or axillary lymph node metastasis	III
Supraclavicular nodes	Axillary lymph node metastasis	III
Axillary nodes	No axillary dissection	III
	Massive axillary involvement	III

cation rates are observed when high doses per fraction are used.

In summary, while breast or chest wall irradiation is supported by important amounts of evidence, the evidence for treating different nodal drainage areas is less compelling. Modern randomized trials that report a survival advantage to postmastectomy irradiation with little treatment-related morbidity have in common the application of techniques that spare vital organs such as the lung and heart and deliver comprehensive irradiation to lymphatics, thus lending indirect support to the claim of usefulness of nodal irradiation, and providing important information regarding the lack of deleterious side effects with long-term follow-up. Although the issue is not settled, the authors believe that irradiation of the breast and nodal areas can safely be done. Table 1.6 and Table 1.7 summarize the complex issues of treatment indications and techniques for the diverse clinical situations encountered in breast radiotherapy, and the evidence, or lack thereof, for each.

TECHNICAL INNOVATION

Intensity modulated radiation therapy (IMRT) may prove an answer to solve the complex problems of normal tissue overdose and selective avoidance of sensitive structures during irradiation (124). The technology is expensive, time-consuming, and not universally available. Due to its specifications, it may be associated with a higher integral radiation dose and, perhaps, second primary malignancies. Concerns have been raised that the radiotherapy community is adopting these technological advances—sometimes as a byproduct of pressures from industry—without

TABLE 1.7. *Recommended treatment techniques for each irradiated field, with the corresponding level of evidence supporting technical details*

Anatomical site	Treatment technique	Level of evidence
Whole breast	Tangential photon fields 45–50 Gy in 1.8–2 Gy fractions	III
Tumor bed after conservative surgery	Single electron field, or small tangential fields, or interstitial brachytherapy 16 Gy in 2 Gy fractions	I
Chest wall (after MRM)	Tangential photon fields, or single anterior electron field, or combination of both 45–50 Gy in 25 fractions	III
Internal mammary nodes	Mixed photon/electron beam Single anterior or oblique field	III
Supraclavicular nodes	Single anterior photon field	III
Axillary nodes	Single posterior photon field	III

proper testing or validation. One can only hope that randomized clinical trials comparing IMRT to conventional treatment techniques will be forthcoming.

CURRENT CLINICAL TRIALS

It is somewhat surprising that technique and dose-fractionation schedules, two of the most important determinants of radiation therapy, have not been extensively tested in randomized clinical trials. Systematic reviews of postmastectomy irradiation and postoperative non-small cell lung cancer irradiation have shown higher mortality rates in irradiated patients (2–4,125). They have been, however, dismissed because of "technical" factors (126). Yet, there are relatively few randomized trials evaluating treatment techniques in breast or other cancers.

A randomized trial including more than 1,000 of internal mammary node irradiation has been reported in abstract form by the Lyon group (127). So far, it shows no impact of internal mammary irradiation in terms of disease-free or overall survival. Data are not mature enough to draw conclusions at this point, and continued follow up is needed. The European Organization for Research and Treatment of Cancer (EORTC) is conducting a similar trial that will hopefully settle the question of internal mammary irradiation with a higher statistical power, as they are including 3,800 patients.

A similar trial (NCIC-CTG MA 20) is being conducted by the National Cancer Institute of Canada (NCIC) in which early-stage breast cancer patients are randomized to breast radiotherapy alone versus breast-plus-internal mammary/supraclavicular irradiation after conservative surgery. Approximately 300 patients have been randomized.

There is one trial evaluating fractionation that has completed accrual. It compared 39 Gy in 13 fractions to 42.9 Gy in 13 fractions to 50 Gy in 25 fractions for whole-breast irradiation after lumpectomy. The trial has only been reported in abstract form, and no toxicity data are available (128).

SUMMARY

Much has been learned over the past 50 years regarding the role of irradiation in breast cancer. However, as comparison of radiation techniques are not based on randomized studies, the level of evidence is not better than level III. With longer follow-up of treated patients and of clinical trials, it has become apparent that radiation therapy is a cause of significant morbidity, especially among long-term survivors probably cured from their disease. It is the role of radiation oncologists to prospectively design and test radiation treatment strategies to improve the quality of medical care.

REFERENCES

1. Keynes G. Conservative treatment of cancer of the breast. *Br Med J* 1937;2:643–649.
2. Cuzick J, Stewart H, Peto R, et al. Overview of randomized trials of postoperative adjuvant radiotherapy in breast cancer. *Cancer Treat Rep* 1987;71:15–29.
3. Cuzick J, Stewart H, Rutqvist L, et al. Cause-specific mortality in long-term survivors of breast cancer who participated in trials of radiotherapy. *J Clin Oncol* 1994;12:447–453.
4. Early Breast Cancer Trialists' Collaborative Group. Favourable and unfavourable effects on long-term survival of radiotherapy for early breast cancer: an overview of the randomised trials. *Lancet* 2000;355:1757–1770.
5. Glatstein EJ. Dr. Strange (high) Tech or how I learned to stop worrying and love my MLC/3D treatment planning, stereotactic LINAC. *Int J Radiat Oncol Biol Phys* 1999;45:1097–1101.
6. Halperin EC. Overpriced technology in radiation oncology. *Int J Radiat Oncol Biol Phys* 2000;48:917–918.
7. Arriagada R, Pignon J-P. Is meta-analysis a metaphysical or a scientific method? *Chest* 2000;118:832–834.
8. Spratt JS. Locally recurrent cancer after radical mastectomy. *Cancer* 1967;20:1051–1053.
9. Haagensen. The surgical treatment of mammary carcinoma. In: Haagensen CD (ed). *Diseases of the breast*. Philadelphia: WB Saunders, 1971.
10. Overgaard M, Hansen PS, Overgaard J, et al. Postoperative radiotherapy in high-risk premenopausal women with breast cancer who receive adjuvant chemotherapy. Danish Breast Cancer Cooperative Group 82b trial. *N Engl J Med* 1997;337:949–955.
11. Ragaz J, Jackson SM, Le N, et al. Adjuvant radiotherapy and chemotherapy in node-positive premenopausal women with breast cancer. *N Engl J Med* 1997;337:956–962.
12. Carter DL, Marks LM, Bean JM, et al. Impact of consolidation radiotherapy in patients with advanced breast cancer treated with high-dose chemotherapy and autologous bone marrow rescue. *J Clin Oncol* 1999;17:887–893.

13. Overgaard M, Jensen MB, Overgaard J, et al. Postoperative radiotherapy in high-risk postmenopausal breast-cancer patients given adjuvant tamoxifen: Danish Breast Cancer Cooperative Group DBCG 82c randomised trial. *Lancet* 1999;353:1641–1648.
14. Recht A, Gray R, Davidson NE, et al. Locoregional failure 10 years after mastectomy and adjuvant chemotherapy with or without tamoxifen without irradiation: Experience of the Eastern Cooperative Oncology Group. *J Clin Oncol* 1999;17:1689–1700.
15. Katz A, Strom EA, Buchholz TA, et al. Locoregional recurrence patterns after mastectomy and doxorubicin-based chemotherapy: implications for postoperative irradiation. *J Clin Oncol* 2000;18:2817–2827.
16. Arriagada R, Rutqvist LE, Mattson A, et al. Adequate locoregional treatment for early breast cancer may prevent secondary dissemination. *J Clin Oncol* 1995;13:2869–2878.
17. Laplanche A, Alzieu L, Delozier T, et al. Polyadenylic-polyuridylic acid plus locoregional radiotherapy versus chemotherapy with CMF in operable breast cancer: a 14 year follow-up analysis of a randomized trial of the Fédération Nationale des Centres de Lutte Contre le Cancer (FNCLCC). *Breast Cancer Res Treat* 2000;64:189–191.
18. Hellman S. Stopping metastasis at their source. *N Engl J Med* 1997;337:996–997.
19. Buchholz TA. Internal mammary lymph nodes: to treat or not to treat. *Int J Radiat Oncol Biol Phys* 2000;44:801–803.
20. Veronesi U, Cascinelli N, Bufalino R, et al. Risk of internal mammary lymph nodes metastasis and its relevance on prognosis of breast cancer patients. *Ann Surg* 1983;198:681–684.
21. Noguchi M, Otha N, Koyanski N, et al. Reappraisal of internal mammary nodes metastasis as a prognostic factor in patients with breast cancer. *Cancer* 1991;68:1918–1925.
22. Lacour J, Lê MG, Caceres E, et al. Radical mastectomy versus radical mastectomy plus internal mammary dissection. Ten years results of an international Cooperative Trial in breast cancer. *Cancer* 1983;51:1941–1943.
23. Lohrisch C, Jackson J, Jones A, et al. Relationship between tumor location and relapse in 6,781 women with early invasive breast cancer. *J Clin Oncol* 2000;18:2828–2835.
24. Zucali R, Mariani L, Marubini E, et al. Early breast cancer: Evaluation of the prognostic role of the site of the primary tumor. *J Clin Oncol* 1998;16:1363–1366.
25. Kuske RR. Adjuvant chest wall and nodal irradiation: maximize cure, minimize late cardiac toxicity. *J Clin Oncol* 1998;16:2579–2582.
26. Fowble B, Hanlon A, Freedman G, et al. Internal mammary node irradiation neither decreases distant metastasis nor improves survival in stage I and II breast cancer. *Int J Radiat Oncol Biol Phys* 2000;47:883–894.
27. Recht A, Edge SB, Solin LJ, et al. Postmastectomy radiotherapy: Guidelines of the American Society of Clinical Oncology. *J Clin Oncol* 2001;19:1539–1569.
28. Romrell LJ, Bland KI. Anatomy of the breast, axilla, chest wall, and related metastatic sites. In: Bland KI, Copeland EM III, eds. *The Breast. Comprehensive management of benign and malignant diseases,* 2nd ed. Philadelphia: WB Saunders, 1998.
29. Fleming ID, Cooper JS, Henson DE, et al., eds. *AJCC cancer staging manual,* 5th ed. Philadelphia: Lippincott-Raven, 1997.
30. Arriagada R, Lê MG, Rochard F, et al. Conservative treatment versus mastectomy in early breast cancer: patterns of failure with 15 years of follow-up data. Institut Gustave-Roussy Breast Cancer Group. *J Clin Oncol* 1996;14:1558–1564.
31. Veronesi U, Banfi A, Salvadori B, et al. Breast conservation is the treatment of choice in small breast cancer: long-term results of a randomized trial. *Eur J Cancer* 1990;26:668–670.
32. Fisher B, Anderson S, Redmond CK, et al. Reanalysis and results after 12 years of follow-up in a randomized clinical trial comparing total mastectomy with lumpectomy with or without irradiation in the treatment of breast cancer. *N Engl J Med* 1995;333:1456–1461.
33. Jacobson JA, Danforth DN, Cowan KH, et al. Ten-year results of a comparison of conservation with mastectomy in the treatment of stage I and II breast cancer. *N Engl J Med* 1995;332:907–911.
34. van Dongen, Voogd AC, Fentiman IS, et al. Long-term results of a randomized trial comparing breast-conserving therapy with mastectomy: European Organization for Research and Treatment of Cancer 10801 trial. *J Natl Cancer Inst* 2000;92:1143–1150.
35. Blichert-Toft M, Rose C, Andersen JA, et al. Danish randomized trial comparing breast conservation therapy with mastectomy: six years of life-table analysis: Danish Breast Cancer Cooperative Group. *J Natl Cancer Inst Monogr* 1992;11:19–25.
36. Early Breast Cancer Trialist's Collaborative Group. Effects of radiotherapy and surgery in early breast cancer - An overview of the randomized trials. *N Engl J Med* 1995;333:1444–1455.
37. Morris AD, Morris RD, Wilson JF, et al. Breast-conserving therapy vs. mastectomy in early-stage breast cancer: a meta-analysis of 10-year survival. *Cancer J Sci Am* 1997;3:6–12.
38. Veronesi U, Luini A, del Vecchio M, et al. Radiotherapy after breast-preserving surgery in women with localized cancer of the breast. *N Engl J Med* 1993;328:1587–1591.
39. Clark RM, Whelan T, Levine M, et al. Randomized clinical trial of breast irradiation following lumpectomy and axillary dissection for node-negative breast cancer: an update. Ontario Clinical Oncology Group. *J Natl Cancer Inst* 1996;88:1659–1664
40. Forrest AP, Stewart HJ, Everington D, et al. Randomised controlled trial of conservation therapy for breast cancer: 6-year analysis of the Scottish trial. Scottish Cancer Trials Breast Group. *Lancet* 1996;348:708–713.
41. Liljegren G, Holmberg L, Bergh J, et al. 10-year results after sector resection with or without postoperative radiotherapy for stage I breast cancer: a randomized trial. *J Clin Oncol* 1999;17:2326–2333.
42. Holli K, Saaristo R, Isola J, et al. Lumpectomy with or without postoperative radiotherapy for breast cancer with favourable prognostic features: results of a randomized study. *Br J Cancer* 2001;84:164–169.
43. Romestaing P, Lehingue Y, Carrie C, et al. Role of a 10-Gy boost in the conservative treatment of early breast cancer: results of a randomized clinical trial in Lyon, France. *J Clin Oncol* 1997;15:963–968.

44. Bartelink H, Horiot J-C, Poortmans P, et al. Recurrence rates after treatment of breast cancer with standard radiotherapy with or without additional radiation. *N Engl J Med* 2001;345:1378–1387.
45. Arriagada R, Mouriesse H, Sarrazin D, et al. Radiotherapy alone in breast cancer. I. Analysis of tumor parameters, tumor dose and local control: the experience of the Gustave-Roussy Institute and the Princess Margaret Hospital. *Int J Radiat Oncol Biol Phys* 1985; 11:1751–1757.
46. Van Limbergen E, Van der Schueren E, Van den Bogaert W, et al. Local control of operable breast cancer after radiotherapy alone. *Eur J Cancer* 1990; 26:674–679.
47. Peters LJ. Radiation therapy tolerance limits. For one or for all?—Janeway Lecture. *Cancer* 1996;77: 2379–2385.
48. Hall EJ. *Radiobiology for the radiologist,* 4th ed. Philadelphia: Lippincott, 1994.
49. Fajardo LF. *Pathology of radiation injury.* New York: Masson Publishing, 1982.
50. Turesson I, Nyman J, Holmberg E, Oden A. Prognostic factors for acute and late skin reactions in radiotherapy patients. *Int J Radiat Oncol Biol Phys* 1996; 36:1065–1075.
51. Perbeck LG, Celebioglu F, Danielsson R, et al. Circulation in the breast after radiotherapy and breast conservation. *Eur J Surg* 2001;167:497–500.
52. Rubin P, Constine LS, Williams JP. Late effects of cancer treatment: Radiation and drug toxicity. In: Perez CA, Brady LW, eds. *Principles and practice of radiation oncology,* 3rd ed. Philadelphia: Lippincott-Raven, 1997.
53. Harris JR, Hellman S: Put the "hockey stick" on ice. *Int J Radiat Oncol Biol Phys* 1988;15:497–499.
54. Annest LS, Anderson RP, Li W, Hafermann MD. Coronary artery disease following mediastinal radiation therapy. *J Thorac Cardiovasc Surg* 1983;85: 257–263.
55. Hanks GE, Peters T, Owen J. Seminoma of the testis: long-term beneficial and deleterious results of radiation. *Int J Radiat Oncol Biol Phys* 1992;24:913–919.
56. Kaufman J, Gunn W, Hartz AJ, et al. The pathophysiologic and roentgenologic effects of chest irradiation in breast carcinoma. *Int J Radiat Oncol Biol Phys* 1986; 12:887–893.
57. Stjernswärd J. Decreased survival related to irradiation postoperatively in early operable breast cancer. *Lancet* 1974;2:1285–1286.
58. Rutqvist LE, Johansson H. Mortality by laterality of the primary tumor among 55,000 breast cancer patients from the Swedish Cancer Registry. *Br J Cancer* 1990;61:866–868.
59. Paszat LF, MacKillop WJ, Groome PA, et al. Mortality from myocardial infarction after adjuvant radiotherapy for breast cancer in the Surveillance, Epidemiology, and End-Results Cancer Registries. *J Clin Oncol* 1998;16:2625–2631.
60. Høst H, Brennhovd IO, Loeb M. Postoperative radiotherapy in breast cancer—long-term results from the Oslo study. *Int J Radiat Oncol Biol Phys* 1986;12: 727–732.
61. Rutqvist LE, Lax I, Fornander T, Johansson H. Cardiovascular mortality in a randomized trial of adjuvant radiation therapy versus surgery alone in primary breast cancer. *Int J Radiat Oncol Biol Phys* 1992; 22:887–896.
62. Rutqvist LE, Liedberg A, Hammar N, et al. Myocardial infarction among women with early-stage breast cancer treated with conservative surgery and breast irradiation. *Int J Radiat Oncol Biol Phys* 1998;40: 359–363.
63. Højris I, Overgaard M, Christensen JJ, et al. Morbidity and mortality of ischaemic heart disease in high-risk breast-cancer patients after adjuvant postmastectomy systemic treatment with or without radiotherapy: analysis of DBCG 82b and 82c randomised trials. Radiotherapy Committee of the Danish Breast Cancer Cooperative Group. *Lancet* 1999;354:1425–1430.
64. Vallis KA, Pintilie M, Chong N, et al. Assessment of coronary heart disease morbidity and mortality after radiation therapy for early breast cancer. *J Clin Oncol* 2002;20:1036–1042.
65. Rothwell RI, Kelly SA, Joslin CAF. Radiation pneumonitis in patients treated for breast cancer. *Radiother Oncol* 1984;4:9–14.
66. Lingos TI, Recht A, Vicini F, et al. Radiation pneumonitis in breast cancer patients treated with conservative surgery and radiation therapy. *Int J Radiat Oncol Biol Phys* 1991;21:355–360.
67. Kimsey FC, Mendenhall NP, Ewald LM, et al. Is radiation treatment volume a predictor for acute or late effect on pulmonary function? A prospective study of patients treated with breast-conserving surgery and postoperative irradiation. *Cancer* 1994; 73(10):2549–2555.
68. Hardman PD, Tweeddale PM, Kerr GR, et al. The effect of pulmonary function of local and loco-regional irradiation for breast cancer. *Radiother Oncol* 1994; 30:33–42.
69. Lind PA, Svane G, Gagliardi G, Svensson C. Abnormalities by pulmonary regions studied with computer tomography following local or local-regional radiotherapy for breast cancer. *Int J Radiat Oncol Biol Phys* 1999;43:489–496.
70. Lind PA, Marks LB, Hardenbergh PH, et al. Technical factors associated with radiation pneumonitis after local +/- regional radiation therapy for breast cancer. *Int J Radiat Oncol Biol Phys* 2002;52:137–143.
71. Theuws JC, Seppenwoolde Y, Kwa SL, et al. Changes in local pulmonary injury up to 48 months after irradiation for lymphoma and breast cancer. *Int J Radiat Oncol Biol Phys* 2000;47:1201–1208.
72. Karlsson P, Holmberg E, Samuelsson A, et al. Soft tissue sarcoma after treatment for breast cancer—a Swedish population-based study. *Eur J Cancer* 1998; 34:2068–2075.
73. Taghian A, de Vathaire F, Terrier P, et al. Long-term risk of sarcoma following radiation treatment for breast cancer. *Int J Radiat Oncol Biol Phys* 1991; 21:361–367.
74. Boice JD Jr, Harvey EB, Blettner M, et al. Cancer of the contralateral breast after radiotherapy for breast cancer. *N Engl J Med* 1992;326:781–785.
75. Obedian E, Fischer DB, Haffty BG. Second malignancies after treatment of early-stage breast cancer: Lumpectomy and radiation therapy versus mastectomy. *J Clin Oncol* 2000;18:2406–2412.
76. Galper S, Gelman R, Recht A, et al. Second nonbreast malignancies after conservative surgery and radiation

therapy for early-stage breast cancer. *Int J Radiat Oncol Biol Phys* 2002;52:406–414.
77. Dewar JA, Sarrazin D, Benhamou E, et al. Management of the axilla in conservatively treated breast cancer: 592 patients treated at Institut Gustave-Roussy. *Int J Radiat Oncol Biol Phys* 1987;13:475–481.
78. Erickson VS, Pearson ML, Ganz PA, et al. Arm edema in breast cancer patients. *J Natl Cancer Inst* 2001;93:96–111.
79. Johansson S, Svensson H, Larsson LG, et al. Brachial plexopathy after postoperative radiotherapy of breast cancer patients—a long-term follow-up. *Acta Oncol* 2000;39:373–382.
80. Rawlings G, Arriagada R, Fontaine F, et al. Pléxite brachiale post-radiothérapique: expérience de l'Institut Gustave Roussy. *Bull Cancer* 1983;70:77–83.
81. de la Rochefordiere A, Abner AL, Silver B, et al. Are cosmetic results following conservative surgery and radiation therapy for early breast cancer dependent on technique? *Int J Radiat Oncol Biol Phys* 1992;23:925–931.
82. Dewar JA, Benhamou S, Benhamou E, et al. Cosmetic results following lumpectomy, axillary dissection and radiotherapy for small breast cancers. *Radiother Oncol* 1988;12:273–280.
83. Van Limbergen E, van der Schueren E, van Tongelen K. Cosmetic evaluation of breast conserving treatment for mammary cancer. 1. Proposal of a quantitative scoring system. *Radiother Oncol* 1989;16:159–167.
84. Van Limbergen E, Rijnders A, van der Schueren E, et al. Cosmetic evaluation of breast conserving treatment for mammary cancer. 2. A quantitative analysis of the influence of radiation dose, fractionation schedules and surgical treatment techniques on cosmetic results. *Radiother Oncol* 1989;4:253–267.
85. Vrieling C, Collette L, Fourquet A, et al. The influence of patient, tumor and treatment factors on the cosmetic results after breast-conserving therapy in the EORTC 'boost vs. no boost' trial. EORTC Radiotherapy and Breast Cancer Cooperative Groups. *Radiother Oncol* 2000;55:219–232.
86. Appleby JM, Barber JB, Levine E, et al. Absence of mutations in the ATM gene in breast cancer patients with severe responses to radiotherapy. *Br J Cancer* 1997;76:1546–1549.
87. Shayeghi M, Seal S, Regan J, et al. Heterozygosity for mutations in the ataxia telangiectasia gene is not a major cause of radiotherapy complications in breast cancer patients. *Br J Cancer* 1998;78:922–927.
88. Perez CA, Taylor ME. Breast: Stages Tis, T1, and T2 tumors. In Perez, CA, Brady LW, eds. *Principles and practice of radiation oncology,* 3rd ed. Philadelphia: Lippincott-Raven, 1998.
89. Storey MR, Munden R, Strom EA, et al. Coronary artery dosimetry in intact left breast irradiation. *Cancer J* 2001;7:492–497.
90. Fraass BA, Lichter AS, McShan DL, et al. The influence of lung density corrections on treatment planning for primary breast cancer. *Int J Radiat Oncol Biol Phys* 1988;14:179–190.
91. Solin LJ, Chu JC, Sontag MR, et al. Three-dimensional photon treatment planning of the intact breast. *Int J Radiat Oncol Biol Phys* 1991;21:193–203.
92. Mijnheer BJ, Heukelom S, Lanson JH, et al. Should inhomogeneity corrections be applied during treatment planning of tangential breast irradiation? *Radiother Oncol* 1991;22:239–244.
93. Roach M 3rd, Gandara DR, Yuo HS, et al. Radiation pneumonitis following combined modality therapy for lung cancer: analysis of prognostic factors. *J Clin Oncol* 1995;13:2606–2612.
94. Das IJ, Cheng CW, Fein DA, Fowble B. Patterns of dose variability in radiation prescription of breast cancer. *Radiother Oncol* 1997;44:83–89.
95. Kantorowitz DA. The impact of dose-specification policies upon nominal radiation dose received by breast tissue in the conservation treatment of breast cancer. *Int J Radiat Oncol Biol Phys* 2000;47:841–848.
96. ICRU (International Commission of Radiation Units and Measurements). Prescribing, recording, and reporting photon beam therapy. ICRU report 50: Washington DC, 1993.
97. Mansfield CM, Komarnicky LT, Schwartz GF, et al. Ten-year results in 1070 patients with stages I and II breast cancer treated by conservative surgery and radiation therapy. *Cancer* 1995;75:2328–2336.
98. Berberich W, Schnabel K, Berg D, Lamprecht E. Boost irradiation of breast carcinoma: teletherapy vs. brachytherapy. *Eur J Obstet Gynecol Reprod Biol* 2001;94:276–282.
99. Frazier RC, Kestin LL, Kini V, et al. Impact of boost technique on outcome in early-stage breast cancer patients treated with breast-conserving therapy. *Am J Clin Oncol* 2001;24:26–32.
100. Veronesi U, Orecchia R, Luini A, et al. A preliminary report of intreaoperative radiotherapy (IORT) in limited-stage breast cancers that are conservatively treated. *Eur J Cancer* 2001;37:2143–2146.
101. Rabinovitch R, Finlayson C, Pan Z, et al. Radiographic evaluation of surgical clips is better than ultrasound for defining the lumpectomy cavity in breast boost treatment planning: a prospective clinical study. *Int J Radiat Oncol Biol Phys* 2000;47:313–317.
102. Johansen J, Overgaard J, Blichert-Toft M, Overgaard M. Treatment of morbidity associated with the management of the axilla in breast-conserving therapy. *Acta Oncol* 2000;39:349–354.
103. Bentel GC, Marks LB, Hardenbergh PH, Prosnitz LR. Variability of the depth of supraclavicular and axillary lymph nodes in patients with breast cancer: is a posterior axillary boost field necessary? *Int J Radiat Oncol Biol Phys* 2000;47:755–758.
104. Goodman RL, Grann A, Saracco P, Needham MF. The relationship between radiation fields and regional lymph nodes in carcinoma of the breast. *Int J Radiat Oncol Biol Phys* 2001;50:99–105.
105. Siddon RL, Buck BA, Harris JR, Svensson GK. Three-field technique for breast irradiation using tangential field corner blocks. *Int J Radiat Oncol Biol Phys* 1983;9:583–588.
106. Lichter AS, Fraass BA, van de Geijn J, Padikal TN. A technique for field matching in primary breast irradiation. *Int J Radiat Oncol Biol Phys* 1983;9:263–270.
107. Chu JC, Solin LJ, Hwang CC, et al. A nondivergent three field matching technique for breast irradiation. *Int J Radiat Oncol Biol Phys* 1990;19:1037–1040.
108. Rosenow UF, Valentine ES, Davis LW. A technique for treating local breast cancer using a single set-up

point and asymmetric collimation. *Int J Radiat Oncol Biol Phys* 1990;19:183–188.
109. Klein EE, Taylor M, Michaletz-Lorenz M, et al. A mono isocentric technique for breast and regional nodal therapy using dual asymmetric jaws. *Int J Radiat Oncol Biol Phys* 1994;28:753–760.
110. Donegan WL, Stine SB, Samter TG. Implications of extracapsular nodal metastasis for treatment and prognosis of breast cancer. *Cancer* 1993;72:778–782.
111. Pierce LJ, Oberman HA, Strawderman MH, Lichter AS. Microscopic extracapsular extension in the axilla: is this an indication for axillary radiotherapy? *Int J Radiat Oncol Biol Phys* 1995;33:253–259.
112. Fisher BJ, Perera FE, Cooke AL, et al. Extracapsular axillary node extension in patients receiving adjuvant systemic therapy: an indication for radiotherapy? *Int J Radiat Oncol Biol Phys* 1997;38:551–559.
113. Mignano JE, Zahurak ML, Chakravarthy A, et al. Significance of axillary lymph node extranodal soft tissue extension and indications for postmastectomy irradiation. *Cancer* 1999;86:1258–1262.
114. Hetelekidis S, Schnitt SJ, Silver B, et al. The significance of extracapsular extension of axillary lymph node metastases in early-stage breast cancer. *Int J Radiat Oncol Biol Phys* 2000;46:31–34.
115. Voogd AC, de Boer R, van der Sangen MJ, et al. Determinants of axillary recurrence after axillary lymph node dissection for invasive breast cancer. *Eur J Surg Oncol* 2001;27:250–255.
116. Arriagada R, Lê MG. Adjuvant radiotherapy in breast cancer. The treatment of lymph node areas. *Acta Oncol* 2000;39:295.
117. Arriagada R, Guinebretière J-M, Lê MG. Do internal mammarynodes matter in the prognosis of axillary node-negative breast cancer? *Acta Oncol* 2000;39:307–308.
118. Fletcher GH, Montague ED. Does adequate irradiation of the internal mammary chain and supraclavicular nodes improve survival rates? *Int J Radiat Oncol Biol Phys* 1978;4:481–492.
119. Arriagada R, Le MG, Mouriesse H, et al. Long-term effect of internal mammary chain treatment. Results of a multivariate analysis of 1195 patients with operable breast cancer and positive axillary nodes. *Radiother Oncol* 1988;11:213–222.
120. Fletcher GH, Montague ED, Tapley N, Barker JL. Radiotherapy in the management of nondisseminated breast cancer. In: Fletcher GH, ed. *Textbook of radiotherapy,* 3rd ed. Philadelphia: Lea & Febiger, 1980.
121. Peñafiel P, Araya A, Hepp R, Solé C. Localización de la cadena mamaria interna para el tratamiento del cáncer mamario con radioterapia. *Alasbimn Journal* 1999;1:3.
122. Bentel G, Marks LB, Hardenbergh P, Prosnitz L. Variability of the location of internal mammary vessels and glandular breast tissue in breast cancer patients undergoing routine CT-based treatment planning. *Int J Radiat Oncol Biol Phys* 1999;44:1017–1025.
123. Kim JH, Chu FC, Hilaris B.The influence of dose fractionation on acute and late reactions in patients with postoperative radiotherapy for carcinoma of the breast. *Cancer* 1975;35:1583–1586.
124. Hurkmans CW, Cho BC, Damen E, et al. Reduction of cardiac and lung complication probabilities after breast irradiation using conformal radiotherapy with or without intensity modulation. *Radiother Oncol* 2002;62:163–171.
125. PORT Meta-analysis Trialists Group. Postoperative radiotherapy in non-small-cell lung cancer: systematic review and meta-analysis of individual patient data from nine randomised controlled trials. PORT Meta-analysis Trialists Group. *Lancet* 1998;352:257–263.
126. Machtay M, Kaiser LR, Glatstein E. Is meta-analysis really meta-physics? *Chest* 1999;116:539–542.
127. Romestaing P, Ecochard R, Hennequin C, et al. The role of internal mammary chain irradiation on survival after mastectomy for breast cancer—Results of a phase III SFRO trial (ESTRO proceedings). *Radiother Oncol* 2000;56 (suppl 1):306.
128. Yarnold JR, Bliss JM, Regan J, et al. Randomised comparison of a 13-fraction schedule with a conventional 25-fraction schedule of radiotherapy after local excision of early breast cancer: preliminary analysis. *Radiother Oncol* 1994;32 (suppl 1):101.

2
The Role of Radiation Therapy in Breast Cancer Management

Bruce G. Haffty

Radiation therapy plays a critical role in the management of breast cancer. Radiation therapy has clearly been established as an effective treatment modality in breast-conserving therapy, as adjuvant therapy in the postmastectomy setting, in the management of locoregional recurrence of disease, and as an effective tool in the palliation of patients with metastatic disease. Although radiation therapy is primarily a locoregional therapy, with its most significant impact on locoregional control of disease, there is substantial evidence that appropriate use of radiation therapy impacts on disease-free and overall survival in selected patients. In this chapter, the use of radiation therapy in the primary and adjuvant treatment of breast cancer, as well as in the management of locoregional relapse and in the palliation of breast cancer, will be presented.

THE ROLE OF SURGERY AND RADIATION

Surgery using either lumpectomy or other less-than-complete mastectomy procedures followed by radiation therapy (RT) to the intact breast is not only an acceptable, but the preferred, standard of care for the majority of women with early-stage invasive breast cancer (1–4). Numerous prospective randomized trials have clearly established breast-conserving surgery using lumpectomy followed by radiation to the intact breast as *the* alternative to mastectomy. Modern randomized trials have demonstrated that those patients treated conservatively, whether pathological node negative or node positive, have equivalent disease-free, distant metastasis-free, and overall survival rates to their counterparts treated by mastectomy. A meta-analysis of the randomized trials also confirms equivalent survival rates and disease-free survival rates for conservatively treated patients (5). Table 2.1 summarizes the results of several prospective randomized trials comparing conservative treatment to mastectomy. Relapses occurring in the conservatively treated breast can be effectively salvaged by mastectomy, without an overall compromise in survival rates (2,6–10).

The majority of patients with operable breast cancer are candidates for conservative surgery followed by radiotherapy (RT) to the intact breast; however, there are some relative contraindications and several factors may be predictive of adverse outcome following breast-conservation therapy. Factors which have been identified thus far as potential contraindications to breast conservation include, but are not limited to: pregnancy, history of prior irradiation, presence of collagen vascular disease, and technical and anatomical factors which may result in poor cosmetic outcome or increased complications (11–21).

Studies evaluating prognostic factors, which may result in an increased risk of local recurrence, have been widely reported. Gross multicentric or multifocal disease, detected clinically or mammographically, is generally considered to be a contraindication to breast conservation. Some individuals with two or more lesions can be considered for breast conservation, but patients with gross multicentric disease generally are treated better with mastectomy as they are at high risk of local recurrence. The increased incidence within breast recurrence is thought to be secondary to the presence of significant residual tumor burden following conservative surgery. In addition, the cosmetic result must be considered in evaluating patients with gross multicentric disease. This may be significantly compromised by the

TABLE 2.1. *Randomized trials of breast-conserving surgery (BCS) with radiation versus mastectomy*

Series	# Patient	Follow-up (Years)	Survival		Other Endpoints: DFS/Local Relapse	
			BCS	MAST	BCS	MAST
Milan I (4)	701	13	71%	69%	11[1]	7
NSABP-06 (2)	1529	12	63%	58%	50%[2]	49%
EORTC (9)	903	8	70%	70%	87%[3]	91%
NCI (5)	247	10	77%	75%	10%[4]	5%
DBCG (7)	905	6	79%	82%	70%[2]	66%
IGR (86)	179	10	80%	79%	5%[4]	10%

CS, conservative surgery with radiation; DBCG, Danish Breast Cancer Group; EORTC, European Organization for Research and Treatment of Cancer; MAST, mastectomy; 1, local relapse events; 2, disease-free survival; 3, local control; 4, locoregional relapse; NCI-US, National Cancer Institute - US; NSABP, National Surgical Adjuvant Breast and Bowel Project.

surgical removal of multiple lesions from the same breast. There have, however, been retrospective studies from institutions reporting selected patients with two synchronous ipsilateral breast masses and who underwent wide local excision of all gross disease and, subsequently, RT. Local recurrence rates were slightly higher in this group of patients. Thus only carefully selected patients with synchronous ipsilateral breast tumors should be offered breast-sparing procedures, provided the potential for increased risk of local recurrence is understood (20, 22).

The term "extensive intraductal component" is a pathologic entity that is defined as "invasive ductal carcinoma with an intraductal component comprising 25% or more of the primary invasive tumor with intraductal carcinoma in the surrounding normal breast tissue." Lesions composed of predominantly ductal carcinoma in situ with only focal areas of invasion can also be categorized as extensive intraductal component-positive tumors. Initial reports indicated that extensive intraductal component (EIC) was found to be a powerful predictor of local failure. It is important to note, however, that patients in these studies were treated at a time when microscopic assessment of the margins of resection was not routinely performed. In a more recent review, the relationship between microscopic margins of resection, the presence of extensive intraductal component, and ipsilateral breast tumor recurrence (IBTR) after breast-conserving therapy was evaluated. In that analysis, the 5-year rate of IBTR for all patients with negative margins was 2%, and for all patients with focally positive margins it was 9%. The data presented suggested that breast-conservation therapy can be considered in patients either with negative or focally involved margins whether or not EIC is present (23). In the subgroup of patients with greater than focally involved margins, their reported IBTR rate was high. It is apparent that patients with extensive intraductal component with diffusely involved margins, which can not be cleared on re-excision, are not optimal candidates for breast-conserving therapy. Whether or not EIC is present, the currently available literature suggests that achievement of a negative surgical margin is likely to result in a lower and more acceptable local relapse rate (17,23–25).

There are additional clinical and pathological factors that have been reportedly associated with higher local recurrence rates. Generally, there have been conflicting reports regarding both the clinical and/or pathological factors which may or may not be predictive of future

IBTR. Those factors typically predictive of a high rate of systemic metastasis, such as number of axillary lymph nodes involved, primary tumor size, lymph-vascular invasion, DNA ploidy, and high S-phase fraction, have not, however, been consistently shown to be predictive of IBTR.

There has been a relatively consistent association between young age at diagnosis, in itself a poor prognostic factor, and rate of local recurrence reported in several studies (21,26–28). Despite the highly significant correlation of young age and local recurrence in published series, there is no convincing evidence that young patients treated by breast-conserving surgery have a compromised survival, and we continue to offer young patients lumpectomy, followed by radiation therapy, as an acceptable standard of care. Similarly, there is no evidence that patients with strong family history and/or hereditary forms of breast cancer have a higher-than-normal rate of local recurrence, although data regarding the risk of local recurrence in patients with BRCA1 or BRCA2 positivity are limited (29–33).

In summary, it is apparent that in the vast majority of patients with operable breast cancer, provided adequate excision of the tumor can be obtained with an acceptable cosmetic result, breast-conservation surgery is an acceptable option.

Radiation therapy following breast-conservation surgery should be employed using careful treatment planning techniques that minimize treatment of the underlying heart and lung. In order to achieve the optimal cosmetic result, an effort should be made to obtain homogeneous dose distribution throughout the breast. Doses of 180 to 200 cGy per day to the intact breast for a total dose of 4,500 to 5,000 cGy are considered standard. Administration of a boost using an electron beam or interstitial implant to bring the tumor bed to a total dose of 6,000 to 6600 cGy is frequently employed. Although the necessity of a boost is controversial and has been the subject of debate, the majority of the radiation oncologists in the United States continue to use a boost. In a recently published randomized clinical trial, delivery of a boost of 10 Gy to the tumor bed after 50 Gy to the whole breast resulted in a statistically significant reduction in local recurrence, although the local recurrence rate in patients treated with or without the boost was quite acceptable (34). A larger, recently published randomized trial also confirmed a significant reduction in local relapse by the use of a boost. This reduction in local relapse was most significant in the subgroup of patients under age 50 (35).

The role of regional nodal irradiation is controversial in patients who have had breast-conserving therapy and axillary lymph node dissection. Patients with pathologically negative axillary nodes are generally treated to the breast only, eliminating radiation therapy to the internal mammary or supraclavicular fossa. In patients with node-positive disease, RT to the supraclavicular fossa and/or internal mammary chain may be considered, although the benefits are uncertain. Extrapolation from the results of recent randomized trials, indicating a survival benefit to regional nodal irradiation in the postmastectomy setting, indicates that regional nodal irradiation in node-positive conservatively treated patients may be beneficial (6,36–38). There is, however, continued controversy regarding the role of regional nodal irradiation. Two ongoing randomized trials, one from the European Organization for Research and Treatment of Cancer (EORTC) and the other from National Cancer Institute (NCI) Canada, are randomizing patients to radiation to the tangential fields alone versus radiation to the breast-chest wall and regional lymphatics. These trials will hopefully address the issue of the role of regional lymphatic irradiation in the era of anthracycline-based adjuvant chemotherapy.

Potential Groups of Patients in Whom Radiation Therapy Could be Avoided

For patients with invasive breast cancer, RT following lumpectomy remains the standard of care. Several prospective randomized trials have addressed the issue of lumpectomy alone versus lumpectomy with radiation, and have consistently shown RT to significantly reduce the risk of IBTR (2,39–42). These trials are summarized

TABLE 2.2. *Randomized trials of lumpectomy versus lumpectomy and radiation in early-stage invasive breast cancer*

Trial	# Patients	Follow-up	Local Relapse No Radiation	Local Relapse Radiation	Notes
NSABP (2)	1,400	12 years	35%	10%	Almost significant decrease in DFS/distant mets without RT
Milan III (42)	567	10 years	23.5%	5.8%	Used quadrantectomy
Uppsala (39)	381	5 years	18.4%	2.3%	Regional-distant metastasis —27 events vs. 19 events—not significantly different
Ontario (40)	837	8 years	35%	11%	Significant increase in distant metastasis observed in no-radiation arm.

in Table 2.2. Although there has been no clearly established survival benefit from RT to the intact breast following lumpectomy, local recurrence rates in patients treated with lumpectomy alone have been shown to be as high as 40% to 50%, despite the use of adjuvant systemic therapy. Furthermore, long-term data from trials randomizing conservatively treated patients to lumpectomy alone versus lumpectomy with irradiation are beginning to show a slight compromise in systemic recurrence and disease-free survival. A recently reported prospective single-arm trial attempted to employ lumpectomy alone in a highly selected group of patients with small tumors, negative margins and negative lymph nodes. Even in this select group of patients, the local recurrence rate approached 25%, even with relatively limited follow-up (43). There is an ongoing U.S. inter-group trial evaluating lumpectomy alone versus lumpectomy and RT in a select group of patients over 70 years of age with tumors less than 2 cm, positive estrogen receptors and negative pathologic margins. For patients with invasive carcinoma, the use of lumpectomy alone should only be recommended in the context of prospective trials.

Chemotherapy-Radiation Sequencing

The majority of patients undergoing lumpectomy followed by RT to the intact breast for invasive breast carcinoma will receive some form of systemic therapy, either cytotoxic chemotherapy and/or adjuvant hormonal treatment. In individuals prescribed cytotoxic chemotherapy, the optimal sequencing of radiation with chemotherapy remains an active area of investigation and an ongoing debate (44). There have been conflicting reports in the literature regarding the issue of delays in RT and local control rates. Although initial reports indicated a higher local recurrence rate for patients in whom definitive RT was delayed more than 16 weeks, a number of later series failed to confirm these findings (44–49). In addition, a randomized clinical trial addressing the issue of the sequencing of chemotherapy and RT from the Joint Center for Radiation Therapy (JCRT) indicated that although delaying RT resulted in a slightly higher local recurrence rate, more importantly, a delay in chemotherapy compromised distant metastasis (50). A recent update of this trial, however, failed to show any difference in the rate of systemic metastasis between the two arms. The vast majority of patients in this trial, however, were node positive. In the majority of node-positive patients where systemic cytotoxic chemotherapy is being considered, initiation of chemotherapy prior to radiation currently appears preferable. Concurrent chemo/radiotherapy, however, has also been employed, and although some studies reported an increased risk of acute reactions and complications with this approach, others have not. Clearly, concomitant chemo/radiotherapy may be considered in selected patients provided radiation is not administered with concomitant adriamycin-based chemotherapy.

For patients with node-negative disease, the issue of the timing of chemotherapy with RT is more controversial. Available data from randomized trials which were not specifically designed to answer this question, but were designed to address systemic chemotherapy issues, however, do not suggest a compromise in local control or systemic control by delaying either modality. Decisions regarding the timing of chemotherapy with RT are individualized, depending on risk factors for systemic and/or local disease, along with the patients' own preferences and application of available guidelines.

Alternatives to Whole-Breast Irradiation

As demonstrated in Table 2.2, for patients with invasive breast cancer, omission of irradiation results in high local relapse rates. A potential alternative to whole-breast irradiation is focused radiation to the tumor bed employing brachytherapy. Use of conformal radiation techniques, which can be directed at the lumpectomy site, has also been proposed. Early results from phase 1 and 2 trials evaluating radiation therapy to the tumor bed as an alternative to whole-breast irradiation show promise in selected patients (51–53). Typically, focused radiation is delivered over a relatively short period of time (4 to 5 treatment days), using temporary radioactive seeds in a two-plane implant, and encompassing the lumpectomy site and adjacent breast tissue. The Radiation Therapy Oncology Group (RTOG) has recently completed a phase 2 trial demonstrating acceptable short-term cosmesis and good local control for selected patients. Future trials employing this technique are in the planning stages, including the possibility of a three-arm randomized trial, comparing whole-breast irradiation to both brachytherapy and conformal radiation to the tumor bed.

Summary of Evidence-based Data Regarding the Conservative Management of Invasive Breast Cancer

- There is level I evidence that the conservative management of breast cancer by lumpectomy with irradiation results in equivalent survival and disease-free survival as mastectomy. Grade of evidence: A.
- There is level I evidence that radiation following lumpectomy significantly lowers the local relapse rate in the conservatively managed breast. Grade of evidence: A.
- There is level II evidence that a boost to the lumpectomy site following whole-breast irradiation significantly lowers the local relapse rate following whole breast irradiation. Grade of evidence: B.
- There is level I and level II evidence that the sequencing of chemotherapy with radiation has no significant impact on local control or survival. Grade of evidence: C.
- There is level III evidence that brachytherapy to the tumor bed may be a suitable alternative to whole-breast irradiation in selected cases. Grade of evidence: C.

MANAGEMENT OF DUCTAL CARCINOMA *IN SITU*

The role of lumpectomy alone versus lumpectomy with RT continues to be an active area of investigation and debate for patients with ductal carcinoma *in situ* (DCIS) (54–56). The National Surgical Adjuvant Breast and Bowel Project B-17 (NSABP-17) trial, which randomized patients with DCIS to lumpectomy versus lumpectomy and RT, clearly showed a benefit to RT in reducing the risk of local recurrence. The benefit of RT was noted in all subsets of patients, including those with low-grade–noncomedo-type DCIS. A randomized trial in Europe has recently reported similar results. As in the NSABP trial, all subgroups of patients benefited from RT with respect to reduction in the local relapse rate (Table 2.3). The radiation technique for DCIS is similar to that described above for invasive cancer, with 4,500 to 5,000 cGy to the whole breast, generally followed by a boost to the tumor bed.

There have been a number of retrospective series, with limited follow-up, reporting acceptable local recurrence rates in selected patients with DCIS treated by lumpectomy alone, without radiation. A recently published study employed careful treatment techniques with detailed attention to surgical margins. Based on their experience, the authors (57,58)

TABLE 2.3. *Studies in DCIS comparing lumpectomy to lumpectomy with radiation*

Study	# Patients	Follow-Up	Local Relapse Without RT	Local Relapse With RT
NSABP-17 (56)	818	43 Months	16.4% (50% of the events were invasive)	7% (25% invasive events)
EORTC (54)	1,010	4.25 Years	16% (48% of the events were invasive)	9% (45% of the events were invasive)

do not advocate radiation therapy in patients with DCIS that was excised with margins of 10 mm or more. Currently, we continue to offer RT to the majority of patients with DCIS, although results of ongoing trials and longer follow-up of patients treated with lumpectomy alone with careful attention to surgical margins is likely to identify a subset of patients with DCIS who may be treated with excision alone.

Radiation Therapy in Lobular Carcinoma *In Situ*

A proportion of patients with invasive breast cancer with ductal carcinoma *in situ* will have an associated histologic component of lobular carcinoma *in situ* (LCIS). Although data addressing this controversial area are limited, the available retrospective literature (11,58) indicates that there is no adverse impact with respect to local or systemic relapse of a component of LCIS. In general, if the underlying DCIS or invasive breast cancer is treated appropriately, the LCIS component does not impact on the management decision or outcome.

For patients with pure LCIS, there is no role for radiation following biopsy or lumpectomy. These patients may be managed surgically or observed. Although these patients have a high probability of subsequently developing a frankly invasive malignancy or DCIS and may benefit from chemoprophylaxis, there is no established role for radiation therapy for the patient with the histologic diagnosis of pure LCIS.

Summary of Evidence-based Data Regarding Radiation Therapy for *In Situ* Cancer

- There is level I evidence that radiation therapy to the breast, following lumpectomy, significantly improves the local control rate in patients with DCIS. Grade of evidence: A.
- There is level III evidence that lumpectomy alone (without irradiation) may be suitable in selected cases. Grade of evidence: B.
- There is level IV evidence that LCIS, as a component of DCIS or invasive disease, should not alter management of the underlying DCIS or invasive carcinoma. Grade of evidence: B.
- There is level IV and V evidence that there is no role for radiation therapy in the management of pure LCIS. Grade of evidence: B.

POSTMASTECTOMY RADIATION

A number of prospective and retrospective series in patients treated with mastectomy have demonstrated that patients with primary tumors greater than 5 cm in size and/or involvement of four or more lymph nodes have a high risk of locoregional failure following mastectomy (1,36–38,59–67). Even in patients who have undergone high-dose chemotherapy with or without stem cell rescue, locoregional failure is a significant problem without the use of postmastectomy radiation (68). Most current ongoing clinical trials evaluating dose-intensive chemotherapy, with or without bone marrow stem cell transplantation, routinely include postmastectomy RT to the chest wall and/or regional lymph nodes to minimize locoregional recurrence in patients who often have, relative to the average presentation, locally advanced cancer and multiple positive nodes.

The use of postmastectomy RT in patients with earlier stages of disease is more controversial. Three recently reported randomized clinical trials (36–38), however, demonstrated a disease-free survival and overall survival advantage with postmastectomy radiation in node-positive patients. In two of these trials, premenopausal patients were treated with mastectomy and CMF-based (cyclophosphamide, methotrexate and 5-FU) chemotherapy and were randomized to receive or not receive postmastectomy radiation to the chest wall and regional lymph nodes. In the third trial, postmenopausal women were treated with tamoxifen and randomized to postmastectomy radiation or observation. Long-term follow-up of these trials has shown an improvement in distant metastasis and overall survival, not only in patients with four or more positive nodes, but also in patients with one to three nodes. Thus, these trials have resurrected the issue of postmastectomy RT in patients with earlier stages of disease and limited nodal involvement. Although there are a number of controversies regarding the extent of axillary lymph node dissection, subset analysis, as well as RT techniques employed in these patients, these trials have highlighted the issue of considering postmastectomy radiation in patients with earlier stages of disease. Currently, there are plans for a randomized intergroup U.S. trial, addressing the issue of postmastectomy radiation in patients with one to three positive nodes. Hopefully, this trial will address the question of which subsets of patients with one to three nodes derive the greatest benefit from postmastectomy radiation using modern, currently accepted, radiation techniques and chemotherapy programs. The issue of postmastectomy radiation is covered more fully in this text in Chapter 3.

In those patients in whom postmastectomy RT is employed, careful treatment techniques and field arrangements that minimize overlap between adjacent fields and minimize the dose to underlying cardiac and pulmonary structures is required. Whether to include the internal mammary chain (IMC), supraclavicular fossa and/or axilla remains controversial and an unsettled issue. Although the randomized trials reported above employed techniques treating the internal mammary and axillary nodes, the risk-benefit of the extent of nodal irradiation is unclear. A current ongoing trial in Europe randomizing patients to tangential fields alone compared to tangential fields with IMC and supraclavicular radiation is ongoing, although the results of that trial will not be available for several years.

Summary of Evidence-based Data Regarding Postmastectomy Irradiation

- There is level I evidence that postmastectomy radiation improves the local-regional control rate for patients with node-positive and/or locally advanced breast cancer. Grade of evidence: A.
- There is level I evidence that postmastectomy radiation improves disease-free and overall survival for patients with four or more positive nodes. Grade of evidence: A.
- There is level II evidence that postmastectomy radiation improves disease-free and overall survival for patients with one to three positive nodes. Grade of evidence: B.
- There is level III and IV evidence suggesting that at least the chest wall should be included in the radiation field. However, there is no consistent evidence regarding the precise role of regional lymphatic irradiation. Ongoing trials may help to resolve these issues. Grade of evidence: C.

LOCOREGIONAL RECURRENCE OF DISEASE

Locoregional recurrence of disease remains a major clinical problem for patients with invasive breast cancer, and, to a lesser extent, DCIS. Depending on the patient's initial risk factors for and subsequent management of locoregional recurrence, rates as high as 50% have been reported in the literature. Appropriate surgery, systemic therapy, and radiation should be employed, as outlined in previous sections, in an effort to minimize the chance of locoregional recurrence. However, despite adequate and appropriate locoregional and systemic therapy, between 5% and 20% of patients can still experience locoregional recurrence of disease. With more than 150,000 new cases of breast cancer per year in the United States, locoregional recurrence remains a major problem facing the clinical oncologist. Locoregional recurrences can be classified into the following categories:

tumors in the ipsilateral breast following conservative surgery, postmastectomy chest wall recurrences, and regional nodal recurrences following conservative surgery or mastectomy.

Local Relapse Following Lumpectomy With or Without Radiation

The group of patients who develop a local failure after breast-conserving surgery for invasive breast cancer or DCIS usually develop their IBTR in the same quadrant as the initial primary tumor. Despite a more favorable prognosis for IBTR than other locoregional relapses, early IBTRs following lumpectomy and RT have been associated with a relatively high rate of systemic metastasis (9,69–72). For those patients who have undergone lumpectomy alone without radiation, re-excision at the time of local recurrence followed by RT may be an option, although there are limited data on this approach.

For patients experiencing an IBTR following lumpectomy with RT, mastectomy is the most commonly employed standard treatment modality. Although some studies have reported acceptable results with repeat wide local excision, or repeat wide local excision with additional radiation, selection criteria for this approach are unclear and long-term follow-up data are lacking. Studies from the University of Pennsylvania evaluating salvage mastectomy specimens of patients who sustained an IBTR failed to identify a subgroup of patients in whom local excision of the tumor bed provided adequate local control (73). There is a subgroup of patients, however, who are unwilling to consider salvage mastectomy. Based on available data, these patients may be managed by wide local excision with or without the addition of limited field re-irradiation, provided these patients are willing to accept a degree of uncertainty regarding this treatment approach (74,75).

Following definitive surgical treatment with salvage mastectomy for patients experiencing an IBTR, reconstruction with autologous tissue using a transverse rectus abdominus myocutaneous (TRAM) flap or other reconstructive technique may be considered. Acceptable long-term results in previously irradiated patients have been reported using these surgical techniques. Reconstruction with saline or silicon implants following radiation have traditionally been associated with a high rate of complications and should generally be avoided unless local expertise is established (76).

There are limited data regarding the role of systemic therapy following salvage mastectomy for IBTR. Although patients with early IBTRs have a relatively high rate of subsequent systemic metastasis, the benefit of adjuvant systemic therapy in this setting is unclear. Given the high rate of metastasis in more aggressive IBTRs, however, some patients and/or their oncologists may consider the use of adjuvant systemic therapy in those patients with aggressive early local recurrences. In those patients not previously on hormonal therapy with estrogen receptor positive recurrences, adjuvant tamoxifen may also be considered (77). For patients with late local recurrences—which may, in fact, represent new primary tumors and may be removed distant to the original tumor bed—evaluation of the tumor for prognostic factors such as tumor size, ER status, DNA ploidy, S phase fraction and other prognostic factors may aid the clinician in making a decision regarding the use of adjuvant systemic therapy. Owing to a lack of available data on adjuvant systemic therapy in the setting of an IBTR, the approach to these patients is, by necessity, highly individualized.

Postmastectomy Chest Wall Recurrences

Patients who develop a postmastectomy chest wall recurrence have a relatively high rate of subsequent systemic metastasis. Many of these patients will experience at least a long disease-free interval, and for those patients with isolated chest wall recurrences, long term 5- to 10-year disease-free survivals of more than 50% have been reported (46,77–81). It is therefore important to attempt to obtain adequate locoregional control in these patients who may experience a relatively long survival following chest wall recurrence. In patients suspected of having an isolated chest wall recurrence, a diagnostic biopsy is, at the very least, indicated. When feasible, excision of the mass should be attempted followed by comprehensive RT to involve the chest wall and/or regional lymph nodes. Radiation treatment techniques are generally similar to those employed with standard postmastectomy radiation therapy and consist of a photon and/or electron beam directed at the chest wall and adjacent lymph nodes. Treatment planning should strive for homogeneous dose distributions throughout the target area while minimizing the dose to the underlying cardiac and pulmonary structures. Conventional fractionation of 180 to 200 cGy a day to the area of locoregional recurrence and immediately adjacent areas at risk, to a total dose of 4,500 to 5,000 cGy, with a boost to the area of recurrence or gross residual disease to a dose of 6,000 to 6,500 cGy, usually results in acceptable long-term locoregional control.

For individuals experiencing a chest wall recurrence with previous breast and/or nodal RT, additional limited field RT may be considered. Re-irradiation to the chest wall with limited fields has been associated with acceptable long-term complications. Several reports regarding the use of hyperthermia with concomitant RT in this setting have also shown acceptable local control and complication rates (82,83).

Unfortunately, patients with chest wall recurrences following mastectomy have a relatively high rate of systemic metastasis. There remains, however, limited clinical trial data regarding the use of adjuvant systemic therapy in this setting. One randomized trial (81) has demonstrated disease-free survival benefit with the use of adjuvant tamoxifen following RT at the time of postmastectomy chest wall recurrence in patients with ER-positive tumors. Patients with ER-negative tumors and aggressive locoregional recurrences may be considered for cytotoxic chemotherapy given their relatively poor prognosis and high rate of distant metastasis, although the prospective, randomized trials addressing the use of adjuvant systemic therapy in this setting are nonexistent.

Treatment of Regional Nodal Recurrences

Regional nodal relapses following mastectomy or conservative surgery with RT have a relatively poor prognosis. Patients initially treated with a modified radical mastectomy experiencing an axillary recurrence have a favorable prognosis, whereas the majority of patients sustaining recurrences in the IMC region, supraclavicular fossa, and axilla following dissection and/or RT have a high rate of systemic metastasis. Nonetheless, adequate locoregional control in these patients at the time of regional relapse is an important goal. Following biopsy and/or surgical resection, when feasible, RT can provide adequate long-term locoregional control. Depending on the location of the regional relapse, RT to the nodal relapse and adjacent areas at risk can be accomplished using treatment techniques as previously described. Conventional doses of 180 to 200 cGy fractionation to total doses of 4,500 to 5,000 cGy with cone down to the area of residual disease to doses of between 5,000 to 6,000 cGy should result in adequate long-term locoregional control. These patients have an extremely high risk of systemic metastasis, but as with postmastectomy chest wall recurrences and IBTRs, there are limited data regarding the role of adjuvant systemic therapy in this setting. Again, owing to the lack of available data, adjuvant systemic therapy can be employed on an individualized basis. Receptor-positive patients who have not previously been on hormonal therapy are candidates for tamoxifen in addition to or instead of other systemic therapy.

The role of systemic therapy at the time of locoregional relapse has not yet been well defined. Given the significant numbers of patients who experience locoregional relapse, along with the relatively high rate of subsequent systemic disease in these patients, consideration of systemic therapy is reasonable. This area is clearly in need of well-designed multi-institutional trials to address the issue of adjuvant systemic therapy at the time of local relapse.

Summary of Evidence-based Data Regarding Management of Locoregional Relapses

- There is level III and IV evidence suggesting that mastectomy should be considered for patients experiencing an ipsilateral breast tumor

relapse in the previously irradiated breast. Grade of evidence: B.
- There is level IV and V evidence that re-excision, with or without additional radiation, may be acceptable in selected patients. Grade of evidence: C.
- There is level III evidence that radiation to the chest wall and/or regional lymphatic nodes should be considered for patients with postmastectomy chest wall or regional nodal relapse. Grade of evidence: B.
- There is level II evidence that hormonal therapy in addition to radiation is appropriate for patients with favorable receptor-positive chest wall relapses postmastectomy. Grade of evidence: B.

RADIATION THERAPY FOR PALLIATION OF METASTATIC DISEASE

Despite recent advances in early detection, diagnosis, and management of breast cancer, a significant percentage of patients will develop metastatic disease. Effective systemic therapy, in the form of cytotoxic chemotherapy and hormonal therapy, has given many patients with metastatic disease a prolongation in disease control, disease-free survival (DFS), and overall survival (OS). For patients developing symptomatic metastatic disease, radiation therapy to the involved symptomatic site remains a powerful and effective treatment modality which can substantially improve patient quality of life.

While palliation of symptomatic metastasis remains highly individualized, the goals of palliative radiation are clear: to provide effective relief of symptoms with acceptable toxicity. The total dose of radiation and the treatment schedule will be dependent on the extent and location of metastatic involvement, the patient's overall condition and prognosis, and logistical issues regarding travel to and from treatment. In general, courses of radiation ranging from 1 to 3 weeks are desirable to optimize quality of life, minimize the amount of time spent in therapy, and return as quickly as possible to routine activities and/or alternative systemic therapy.

Bone metastases are clearly the most common site of disease requiring palliative radiation in breast cancer patients. For the majority of these patients, the author favors a schedule of 30 Gy in 10 treatments or 20 Gy in 5 treatments, depending on the location and size of the radiation field. The author reserves single-fraction treatments for patients in whom transportation would create significant logistical problems. Randomized studies of all of these fractionation schemes, however, have demonstrated similar results with effective palliation (84,85). The most important emergent complication of spinal metastases is, of course, spinal cord or nerve compromise. Use of systemic steroids with radiation and occasionally surgical intervention remains a crucial "oncological emergency" to be recognized and treated appropriately.

Another site of metastatic disease, which is common in breast cancer and requires special consideration, is brain metastasis. For patients with multiple brain metastases, a course of radiation of 30 Gy in 10 treatments provides effective palliation. Patients with isolated metastasis may be considered for surgery, followed by whole-brain irradiation, or whole-brain irradiation in combination with a stereotactic radiosurgical boost. Radiosurgery as an adjunct to whole-brain irradiation is being used where available with increasing frequency in patients with isolated metastasis or in patients with a small number of lesions. It is particularly appealing in patients with a long disease-free interval and in whom other systemic disease is stable.

A relatively rare, but critical, problem in patients with metastatic breast cancer is the development of choroidal metastasis. Patients with metastatic breast cancer and visual problems should be completely evaluated with a thorough neurological and ophthalmologic exam, as well as brain imaging by CT scan and/or MRI. For patients with involvement of the choroid by metastatic breast cancer, radiation treatment to the involved eye provides effective palliation. Treatment with a lateral, en face or wedged pair field to the involved eye fractionated over 2 to 4 weeks will result in stabilization or improvement in vision in a majority of patients.

Summary of Evidence-based Data Regarding Radiation Therapy for the Palliative Treatment of Metastatic Disease

- There is level III, IV and V evidence that radiation therapy provides adequate palliation to patients with symptomatic metastatic breast carcinoma. Grade of evidence: A.
- There is level I, II and III evidence that a number of fractionation schemes, ranging from a single fraction of 7 to 8 Gy, to 20 Gy in 5 fractions, 30 Gy in 10 fractions or more protracted schedules, provide equivalent palliative benefit. Grade of evidence: B.

REFERENCES

1. National Institutes of Health Consensus Development Conference Statement: Adjuvant Therapy for Breast Cancer, November 1–3, 2000. *J Natl Cancer Inst Monogr* 2001;5–15.
2. Fisher B, Anderson S, Redmond CK, et al. Reanalysis and results after 12 years of follow-up in a randomized clinical trial comparing total mastectomy with lumpectomy with or without irradiation in the treatment of breast cancer. *N Engl J Med* 1995;333:1456–1461.
3. Haffty BG, Ward BA. Is breast-conserving surgery with radiation superior to mastectomy in selected patients? *Cancer J Sci Am* 1997;3:2–3.
4. Veronesi U, Banfi A, Salvadori B, et al. Breast conservation is the treatment of choice in small breast cancer: long-term results of a randomized trial. *Eur J Cancer* 1990;26:668–670.
5. Morris AD, Morris RD, Wilson JF, et al. Breast-conserving therapy vs mastectomy in early-stage breast cancer: a meta-analysis of 10-year survival. *Cancer J Sci Am* 1997;3:6–12.
6. Arriagada R, Le MG. Adjuvant radiotherapy in breast cancer—the treatment of lymph node areas. *Acta Oncol* 2000;39:295–305.
7. Blichert-Toft M, Rose C, Andersen JA, et al. Danish randomized trial comparing breast conservation therapy with mastectomy: six years of life-table analysis. Danish Breast Cancer Cooperative Group. *J Natl Cancer Inst Monogr* 1992;11:19–25.
8. Rutqvist LE. Radiation therapy as an adjunct to primary surgery in early stage breast cancer: biological and clinical rationale. *Semin Radiat Oncol* 1999;9:217–222.
9. van Dongen JA, Voogd AC, Fentiman IS, et al. Long-term results of a randomized trial comparing breast-conserving therapy with mastectomy: European Organization for Research and Treatment of Cancer 10801 trial. *J Natl Cancer Inst* 2000;92:1143–1150.
10. Veronesi U, Banfi A, Del Vecchio M, et al. Comparison of Halsted mastectomy with quadrantectomy, axillary dissection, and radiotherapy in early breast cancer: long-term results. *Eur J Cancer Clin Oncol* 1986;22:1085–1089.
11. Abner AL, Connolly JL, Recht A, et al. The relation between the presence and extent of lobular carcinoma in situ and the risk of local recurrence for patients with infiltrating carcinoma of the breast treated with conservative surgery and radiation therapy. *Cancer* 2000;88:1072–1077.
12. Chen AM, Obedian E, Haffty BG. Breast-conserving therapy in the setting of collagen vascular disease. *Cancer J* 2001;7:480–491.
13. Clark RM, Chua T. Breast cancer and pregnancy: the ultimate challenge. *Clin Oncol* (R Coll Radiol) 1989;1:11–8.
14. de la Rochefordiere A, Abner AL, Silver B, et al. Are cosmetic results following conservative surgery and radiation therapy for early breast cancer dependent on technique? *Int J Radiat Oncol Biol Phys* 1992;23:925–931.
15. Fowble B. Radiotherapeutic considerations in the treatment of primary breast cancer. *J Natl Cancer Inst Monogr* 1992;11:49–58.
16. Haffty BG, Fischer D, Rose M, et al. Prognostic factors for local recurrence in the conservatively treated breast cancer patient: a cautious interpretation of the data. *J Clin Oncol* 1991;9:997–1003.
17. Park CC, Mitsumori M, Nixon A, et al. Outcome at 8 years after breast-conserving surgery and radiation therapy for invasive breast cancer: influence of margin status and systemic therapy on local recurrence. *J Clin Oncol* 2000;18:1668–1675.
18. Recht A. Selection of patients with early stage invasive breast cancer for treatment with conservative surgery and radiation therapy. *Semin Oncol* 1996;23:19–30.
19. Schnitt SJ, Abner A, Gelman R, et al. The relationship between microscopic margins of resection and the risk of local recurrence in patients with breast cancer treated with breast-conserving surgery and radiation therapy. *Cancer* 1994;74:1746–1751.
20. Wilson LD, Beinfield M, McKhann CF, Haffty BG. Conservative surgery and radiation in the treatment of synchronous ipsilateral breast cancers. *Cancer* 1993;72:137–142.
21. Fourquet A, Campana F, Zafrani B, et al. Prognostic factors of breast recurrence in the conservative management of early breast cancer: a 25-year follow-up. *Int J Radiat Oncol Biol Phys* 1989;17:719–725.
22. Kurtz JM, Jacquemier J, Amalric R, et al. Breast-conserving therapy for macroscopically multiple cancers. *Ann Surg* 1990;212:38–44.
23. Gage I, Schnitt SJ, Nixon AJ, et al. Pathologic margin involvement and the risk of recurrence in patients treated with breast-conserving therapy. *Cancer* 1996;78:1921–1928.
24. Obedian E, Haffty BG. Negative margin status improves local control in conservatively managed breast cancer patients. *Cancer J Sci Am* 2000;6:28–33.
25. Smitt MC, Nowels KW, Zdeblick MJ, et al. The importance of the lumpectomy surgical margin status in long-term results of breast conservation. *Cancer* 1995;76:259–267.
26. de la Rochefordiere A, Asselain B, Campana F, et al. Age as prognostic factor in premenopausal breast carcinoma. *Lancet* 1993;341:1039–1043.

27. Harrold EV, Turner BC, Matloff ET, et al. Local recurrence in the conservatively treated breast cancer patient: a correlation with age and family history. *Cancer J Sci Am* 1998;4:302–307.
28. Vicini FA, Kestin LL, Goldstein NS, et al. Impact of young age on outcome in patients with ductal carcinoma-in-situ treated with breast-conserving therapy. *J Clin Oncol* 2000;18:296–306.
29. Gaffney DK, Brohet RM, Lewis CM, et al. Response to radiation therapy and prognosis in breast cancer patients with BRCA1 and BRCA2 mutations. *Radiother Oncol* 1998;47:129–136.
30. Pierce LJ, Strawderman M, Narod SA, et al. Effect of radiotherapy after breast-conserving treatment in women with breast cancer and germline BRCA1/2 mutations. *J Clin Oncol* 2000;18:3360–3369.
31. Turner BC, Harrold E, Matloff E, et al. BRCA1/BRCA2 germline mutations in locally recurrent breast cancer patients after lumpectomy and radiation therapy: implications for breast-conserving management in patients with BRCA1/BRCA2 mutations. *J Clin Oncol* 1999;17:3017–3024.
32. Verhoog LC, Berns EM, Brekelmans CT, et al. Prognostic significance of germline BRCA2 mutations in hereditary breast cancer patients. *J Clin Oncol* 2000;18:119S–124S.
33. Robson ME, Boyd J, Borgen PI, Cody HS, 3rd. Hereditary breast cancer. *Curr Probl Surg* 2001;38:387–480.
34. Romestaing P, Lehingue Y, Carrie C, et al. Role of a 10-Gy boost in the conservative treatment of early breast cancer: results of a randomized clinical trial in Lyon, France. *J Clin Oncol* 1997;15:963–968.
35. Bartelink H, Horiot JC, Poortmans P, et al. Recurrence rates after treatment of breast cancer with standard radiotherapy with or without additional radiation. *N Engl J Med* 2001;345:1378–1387.
36. Overgaard M, Jensen MB, Overgaard J, et al. Postoperative radiotherapy in high-risk postmenopausal breast-cancer patients given adjuvant tamoxifen: Danish Breast Cancer Cooperative Group DBCG 82c randomised trial. *Lancet* 1999;353:1641–1648.
37. Overgaard M, Hansen PS, Overgaard J, et al. Postoperative radiotherapy in high-risk premenopausal women with breast cancer who receive adjuvant chemotherapy. Danish Breast Cancer Cooperative Group 82b Trial. *N Engl J Med* 1997;337:949–955.
38. Ragaz J, Jackson SM, Le N, et al. Adjuvant radiotherapy and chemotherapy in node-positive premenopausal women with breast cancer. *N Engl J Med* 1997;337:956–962.
39. Sector resection with or without postoperative radiotherapy for stage I breast cancer: a randomized trial. Uppsala-Orebro Breast Cancer Study Group. *J Natl Cancer Inst* 1990;82:277–282.
40. Clark RM, Whelan T, Levine M, et al. Randomized clinical trial of breast irradiation following lumpectomy and axillary dissection for node-negative breast cancer: an update. Ontario Clinical Oncology Group. *J Natl Cancer Inst* 1996;88:1659–1664.
41. Liljegren G, Holmberg L, Adami HO, et al. Sector resection with or without postoperative radiotherapy for stage I breast cancer: five-year results of a randomized trial. Uppsala-Orebro Breast Cancer Study Group. *J Natl Cancer Inst* 1994;86:717–722.
42. Veronesi U, Marubini E, Mariani L, et al. Radiotherapy after breast-conserving surgery in small breast carcinoma: long-term results of a randomized trial. *Ann Oncol* 2001;12:997–1003.
43. Schnitt SJ, Hayman J, Gelman R, et al. A prospective study of conservative surgery alone in the treatment of selected patients with stage I breast cancer. *Cancer* 1996;77:1094–1100.
44. Haffty BG. Who's on first? Sequencing chemotherapy and radiation therapy in conservatively managed node-negative breast cancer. *Cancer J Sci Am* 1999;5:147–149.
45. Buchholz TA, Hunt KK, Amosson CM, et al. Sequencing of chemotherapy and radiation in lymph node-negative breast cancer. *Cancer J Sci Am* 1999;5:159–164.
46. McCormick B, Mendenhall NP, Shank BM, et al. Local regional recurrence and salvage surgery. American College of Radiology. ACR Appropriateness Criteria. *Radiology* 2000;215 (suppl):1181–1192.
47. Recht A. Radiotherapy-chemotherapy integration in breast-conservation therapy. *Front Radiat Ther Oncol* 1993;27:89–102.
48. Recht A, Harris JR, Come SE. Sequencing of irradiation and chemotherapy for early-stage breast cancer. *Oncology* (Huntingt) 1994;8:19–28; discussion 28, 31–32, 37.
49. Wallgren A, Bernier J, Gelber RD, et al. Timing of radiotherapy and chemotherapy following breast-conserving surgery for patients with node-positive breast cancer. International Breast Cancer Study Group. *Int J Radiat Oncol Biol Phys* 1996;35:649–659.
50. Recht A, Come SE, Henderson IC, et al. The sequencing of chemotherapy and radiation therapy after conservative surgery for early-stage breast cancer. *N Engl J Med* 1996;334:1356–1361.
51. Kuske RR, Jr. Breast brachytherapy. *Hematol Oncol Clin North Am* 1999;13:543–558, vi–vii.
52. Nag S, Kuske RR, Vicini FA, et al. Brachytherapy in the treatment of breast cancer. *Oncology* (Huntingt) 2001;15:195–202, 205; discussion 205–207.
53. Vicini FA, Chen PY, Fraile M, et al. Low-dose-rate brachytherapy as the sole radiation modality in the management of patients with early-stage breast cancer treated with breast-conserving therapy: preliminary results of a pilot trial. *Int J Radiat Oncol Biol Phys* 1997;38:301–310.
54. Julien JP, Bijker N, Fentiman IS, et al. Radiotherapy in breast-conserving treatment for ductal carcinoma in situ: first results of the EORTC randomised phase III trial 10853. EORTC Breast Cancer Cooperative Group and EORTC Radiotherapy Group. *Lancet* 2000;355:528–533.
55. Fentiman IS. Trials of treatment for non-invasive breast cancer. *Recent Results Cancer Res* 1998;152:135–142.
56. Fisher B, Dignam J, Wolmark N, et al. Lumpectomy and radiation therapy for the treatment of intraductal breast cancer: findings from National Surgical Adjuvant Breast and Bowel Project B-17. *J Clin Oncol* 1998;16:441–452.
57. Silverstein MJ, Lagios MD, Groshen S, et al. The influence of margin width on local control of ductal carcinoma in situ of the breast. *N Engl J Med* 1999;340:1455–1461.
58. Moran M, Haffty BG. Lobular carcinoma in situ as a component of breast cancer: the long-term outcome in patients treated with breast-conservation therapy. *Int J Radiat Oncol Biol Phys* 1998;40:353–358.
59. Arriagada R, Rutqvist LE, Le MG. Postmastectomy radiotherapy: randomized trials. *Semin Radiat Oncol* 1999;9:275–286.

60. Bartelink H. Post-mastectomy radiotherapy: recommended standards. *Ann Oncol* 2000;11 (suppl 3):7–11.
61. Cuzick J, Stewart H, Rutqvist L, et al. Cause-specific mortality in long-term survivors of breast cancer who participated in trials of radiotherapy. *J Clin Oncol* 1994;12:447–453.
62. Fowble B, Gray R, Gilchrist K, et al. Identification of a subgroup of patients with breast cancer and histologically positive axillary nodes receiving adjuvant chemotherapy who may benefit from postoperative radiotherapy. *J Clin Oncol* 1988;6:1107–1117.
63. Overgaard M. Overview of randomized trials in high risk breast cancer patients treated with adjuvant systemic therapy with or without postmastectomy irradiation. *Semin Radiat Oncol* 1999;9:292–299.
64. Overgaard M. Evaluation of radiotherapy in high-risk breast cancer patients given adjuvant systemic therapy. *Rays* 2000;25:325–330.
65. Overgaard M, Christensen JJ, Johansen H, et al. Evaluation of radiotherapy in high-risk breast cancer patients: report from the Danish Breast Cancer Cooperative Group (DBCG 82) Trial. *Int J Radiat Oncol Biol Phys* 1990;19:1121–1124.
66. Recht A, Bartelink H, Fourquet A, et al. Postmastectomy radiotherapy: questions for the twenty-first century. *J Clin Oncol* 1998;16:2886–2889.
67. Rutqvist LE, Cedermark B, Glas U, et al. Randomized trial of adjuvant tamoxifen combined with postoperative radiation therapy or adjuvant chemotherapy in postmenopausal breast cancer. *Cancer* 1990;66:89–96.
68. Marks LB, Rosner GL, Prosnitz LR, et al. The impact of conventional plus high dose chemotherapy with autologous bone marrow transplantation on hematologic toxicity during subsequent local-regional radiotherapy for breast cancer. *Cancer* 1994;74:2964–2971.
69. Fisher B, Anderson S, Fisher ER, et al. Significance of ipsilateral breast tumour recurrence after lumpectomy. *Lancet* 1991;338:327–331.
70. Fowble B. Ipsilateral breast tumor recurrence following breast-conserving surgery for early-stage invasive cancer. *Acta Oncol* 1999;38 (suppl 13):9–17.
71. Haffty BG, Reiss M, Beinfield M, et al. Ipsilateral breast tumor recurrence as a predictor of distant disease: implications for systemic therapy at the time of local relapse. *J Clin Oncol* 1996;14:52–57.
72. Veronesi U, Cascinelli N, Greco M, et al. Prognosis of breast cancer patients after mastectomy and dissection of internal mammary nodes. *Ann Surg* 1985;202:702–707.
73. Fowble B, Solin LJ, Schultz DJ, Weiss MC. Breast recurrence and survival related to primary tumor location in patients undergoing conservative surgery and radiation for early-stage breast cancer. *Int J Radiat Oncol Biol Phys* 1992;23:933–939.
74. Kurtz JM, Amalric R, Brandone H, et al. Results of wide excision for mammary recurrence after breast-conserving therapy. *Cancer* 1988;61:1969–1972.
75. Kurtz JM, Jacquemier J, Amalric R, et al. Is breast conservation after local recurrence feasible? *Eur J Cancer* 1991;27:240–244.
76. Forman DL, Chiu J, Restifo RJ, et al. Breast reconstruction in previously irradiated patients using tissue expanders and implants: a potentially unfavorable result. *Ann Plast Surg* 1998;40:360–363; discussion 363–364.
77. Rauschecker H, Clarke M, Gatzemeier W, et al. Systemic therapy for treating locoregional recurrence in women with breast cancer (Cochrane Review). *Cochrane Database Syst Rev* 2001;4:CD002195.
78. Mendenhall NP, Devine JW, Mendenhall WM, et al. Isolated local-regional recurrence following mastectomy for adenocarcinoma of the breast treated with radiation therapy alone or combined with surgery and/or chemotherapy. *Radiother Oncol* 1988;12:177–185.
79. Veronesi U, Marubini E, Del Vecchio M, et al. Local recurrences and distant metastases after conservative breast cancer treatments: partly independent events. *J Natl Cancer Inst* 1995;87:19–27.
80. Halverson KJ, Perez CA, Kuske RR, et al. Locoregional recurrence of breast cancer: a retrospective comparison of irradiation alone versus irradiation and systemic therapy. *Am J Clin Oncol* 1992;15:93–101.
81. Borner M, Bacchi M, Goldhirsch A, et al. First isolated locoregional recurrence following mastectomy for breast cancer: results of a phase III multicenter study comparing systemic treatment with observation after excision and radiation. Swiss Group for Clinical Cancer Research. *J Clin Oncol* 1994;12:2071–2077.
82. Lee HK, Antell AG, Perez CA, et al. Superficial hyperthermia and irradiation for recurrent breast carcinoma of the chest wall: prognostic factors in 196 tumors. *Int J Radiat Oncol Biol Phys* 1998;40:365–375.
83. van der Zee J, van der Holt B, Rietveld PJ, et al. Reirradiation combined with hyperthermia in recurrent breast cancer results in a worthwhile local palliation. *Br J Cancer* 1999;79:483–490.
84. Kirkbride P, Mackillop WJ, Priestman TJ, et al. The role of palliative radiotherapy for bone metastases. *Can J Oncol* 1996;6 (suppl 1):33–38.
85. Ratanatharathorn V, Powers WE, Moss WT, Perez CA. Bone metastasis: review and critical analysis of random allocation trials of local field treatment. *Int J Radiat Oncol Biol Phys* 1999;44:1–18.
86. Sarrazin D, Le MG, Arriagada R, et al. Ten-year results of a randomized trial comparing a conservative treatment to mastectomy in early breast cancer. *Radiother Oncol* 1989;14:177–184.

3

Survival Impact of Locoregional Radiation in Stage I–II Breast Cancer: Evidence-Based Review

Joseph Ragaz and John J. Spinelli

The 2002 review of the evidence-based survival impact of locoregional radiation (RT) in early cancer is the follow-up to our 2000 chapter, and includes critical data analysis of the Early Breast Cancer Trialists' Collaborative Group (EBCTCG) meta-analysis (1,2). Also added is a new meta-analysis restricted to patients with trials with adjuvant chemotherapy (3). Discussion also extends to include several individual trials permitting analysis of relative versus absolute gains of RT (4–8).

Very few issues in the modern era of breast cancer management have been as controversial as the role of locoregional radiation in the adjuvant setting. On the one hand, there are individual, newer trials showing a significant reduction of systemic recurrences and mortality by RT. On the other hand, we are facing the evidence-based reality of the Oxford-based meta-analysis showing no survival impact from RT as published in the past and updated in September 2000 (1,2). To increase the complexity of the issue, systemic therapy is undergoing evolutionary changes with the introduction of anthracylines, taxanes and Herceptin either in routine therapy or within the framework of randomized trials (9–14). These may increase the cure rates but also contribute towards RT-associated toxicity and thus add further complexity towards the overall impact of RT.

The orderly process of meta-analysis cannot be ignored as its very essence represents the epitome of the evidence-based approach assessing the outcome of any tested interventions. Yet, in regards to the EBCTCG radiation meta-analysis, attention has to be paid to modern-era RT trials, which are devoid of biases resulting from old techniques, poor planning, and inclusion of low-risk subsets. These may all substantially dilute the RT impact on mortality due to unnecessary toxicity and increase of non-breast cancer mortality. As before in these reviews (of this and the 2000 chapter), the outcome is defined as recurrences, both locoregional and systemic, with survival, including breast-cancer specific mortality as well as overall survival. Locoregional radiation is defined as adjuvant postmastectomy radiation treatment encompassing five fields, including the chest wall and nodal regions. Evidence will be categorized, whenever possible, into three categories (level I, level II, and level III), according to the strength of data supporting the given conclusions (Table 3.1) (15).

This review will discuss:

- EBCTCG analysis with critical comments regarding analysis of trials before and after 1975, separating trials of node-positive versus node-negative disease;
- Meta-analysis restricted to trials with adjuvant chemotherapy;
- Comments on interaction of outcome in positive RT trials versus (a) dose intensity of the chemotherapy and (b) cohorts at various risks for recurrence.

BACKGROUND

Radiotherapy has been considered a treatment modality primarily aimed at reducing local events. The Oxford overview of all radiation trials confirmed level I evidence for a substantial and significant reduction of locoregional events in virtually all randomized trials. However, the meta-analysis provided data showing that, despite a substantial reduction

TABLE 3.1. *Levels of scientific evidence about therapeutic interventions (adapted from Sacket et al., 15)*

LEVEL I EVIDENCE
i. Meta-analyses of homogeneous randomized trials
ii. Randomized controlled trials that are big enough to be either:
- positive with small risks of false-positive conclusions, or
- negative, with small risks of false-negative conclusions

LEVEL II EVIDENCE
Randomized controlled trials that are too small so that they show either:
- positive trends that are not statistically significant, with high chance for false-positive conclusions; or
- no impressive trends but high chance for false-negative conclusions

LEVEL III EVIDENCE
Formal comparison with historic controls

LEVEL IV EVIDENCE
Informal comparison with historic controls

LEVEL V EVIDENCE
Case series

of locoregional recurrences, overall survival was not improved. Of importance were observations of a reduction of systemic recurrences by RT, with a significant breast cancer mortality reduction, counterbalanced, however, in the overall survival analysis by increased cardiac deaths in irradiated patients (2). Increased cardiac mortality was due partially to the fact that the older kilovoltage RT machines were more cardiotoxic, but partially also due to cardiotoxicity not being recognized as a serious RT complication. Thus, compared to the RT techniques used at the present time, less cardiac shielding had been implemented in the early RT trials.

OXFORD OVERVIEW: A CRITICAL ANALYSIS

The above developments could help in understanding why the randomized RT trials initiated after 1975 and reported in the 1990s emerged with positive RT effects involving not only a reduction of locoregional recurrences, but also of systemic events and of overall mortality. The large heterogeneity of studies reviewed by the Oxford meta-analysis may preclude meaningful conclusions when compared to the more uniform use of RT equipment and planning techniques of newer trials. Also, a substantial proportion of trials in the EBCTCG meta-analysis included node-negative patients, many of whom had low-risk disease. These cohorts, due to lower number of events, derive preferentially more toxicity and less benefit, an observation common to outcomes of adjuvant chemotherapy in breast cancer or other malignancies.

It may be, therefore, important to establish the RT impact within the meta-analysis and focus on more homogeneous trials, such as those started before and after 1975, and evaluate the RT impact separately for trials with positive- versus negative-nodal status. This will enhance homogeneity of this meta-analysis, one of the prerequisites of accepting conclusions of any meta-analysis as level I evidence.

With this as the main objective, we recalculated the mortality impact of RT from the EBCTCG 2000 analysis by analyzing trials started before 1975 and after 1975, and according to the nodal status (16).

For the analysis (Table 3.2), the observed (O) and expected (E) numbers of all deaths expressing overall mortality and their variances were taken from the EBCTCG 2000 Lancet analysis (2) as the sum of breast cancer and non-breast cancer deaths, separate for each of the four cohorts. The "p" values were derived from the ratio of O to E to the standard deviation of O to E (estimated from the square root of the sum of the separate variances). The results were expressed as breast cancer and non-breast cancer deaths percentage (D%) from RT versus controls (CONTR) and applied in absolute numbers per 1,000 patients treated (net/1,000).

Results show that for trials started before 1975, RT showed a non-significant mortality increase, where $p = 0.34$ (10 more deaths per 1,000 treated cases); However, for patients enrolled in trials after 1975, there was a significant reduction of overall mortality due to RT, where $p = 0.001$ (avoidance of 32.8 deaths for each 1,000 treated) (Table 3.2A).

Table 3.2B shows results according to the nodal status. For node-negative cohorts, RT

TABLE 3.2. Re-analysis of the EBCTCG radiation (RT) meta-analysis 2000: Impact of locoregional radiation according to trials before and after 1975; and for node-negative and for node-positive trials (16)

TABLE 3.2A. Analysis of trials before and after 1975

	Breast Ca Deaths (%)		Non Breast Ca Deaths (%)		Overall Deaths /1,000		
	RT	CONTR	RT	CONTR	Net/1,000	O-E	p
RT<1975 (9,489 pts.)	43.5	46.8	18.3	14.0	+10.0	+15.6	0.34
RT>1975 (10,686 pts)	33.8	37.9	5.6	4.8	−32.8	−104.5	0.001

TABLE 3.2B. Analysis of impact of locoregional radiation according to the nodal status

	Breast Ca Deaths (%)		Non Breast Ca Deaths (%)				
	RT	CONTR	RT	CONTR	Net/1,000	O-E	p
N+ve (10,307 pts.)	47.1	51.6	8.6	7.0	−29.2	−121.6	0.00006
N−ve (9,868 pts.)	29.2	32.2	14.7	11.4	+3.3	+23.5	0.55

Breast cancer and non-breast cancer deaths % (D%) between RT versus controls (CONTR) are expressed in absolute numbers/1,000 patients treated (net/1,000). Avoided deaths = minus sign "−"; excess deaths = "+" sign.

resulted in a non-significant increase of deaths, where $p = 0.55$, or 3.3 excess deaths per 1,000 treated. For node-positive cases, however, there is a significant mortality reduction due to RT, where $p = 0.000006$, with 29.2 avoided deaths per 1,000 treated patients.

EBCTCG META-ANALYSIS: CONCLUSIONS

The Oxford-based EBCTCG meta-analysis shows a significant reduction of locoregional and systemic recurrences and a significant reduction of breast cancer mortality. Overall survival is not improved for all cases. However, patients in trials after 1975 and those with node-positive disease have a significant overall mortality reduction. (Evidence is level I for outcome results and survival categories, as discussed.)

ADJUVANT RT TRIALS: NEW TRIALS

More recently, several large randomized trials of postoperative wide-field RT have shown not only a significant reduction of locoregional recurrences due to RT, but also a substantial reduction of systemic events and of breast cancer mortality (5–8). Importantly, these trials introduced megavoltage equipment and improved RT planning in the late 1970s and 1980s, resulting in improved breast cancer cell kill and lower cardiotoxicity compared to the techniques used in the 1950s and 1960s. Also, adjuvant chemotherapy (CT) was used increasingly since the late 1970s, and several mechanisms have been offered to explain a positive CT/RT interaction (17,18). One of the important factors involves therapy of pre-existing systemic micrometastases which would otherwise contribute towards breast cancer death, regardless of local control by RT. Secondarily, chemotherapy can act as an effective radiosensitizer, improving the cell kill of RT in clones exposed to CT—a very important additional aspect favoring the combined chemo/radiation approaches in the therapy of solid tumors, in general. However, chemotherapy is considered less effective for bulky locoregional disease such as disease in the lymph nodes or chest wall (19), and may need RT to realize the curative potential of the adjuvant treatment.

Review of the New RT Trials

(For detailed description of each trial, see the appendix to this chapter).

Trial I. The Swedish Trial: Impact of Radiation in the Absence of Chemotherapy

One of the first modern era radiation trials using five-field radiation after mastectomy which showed RT benefit at long follow-up is the Swedish Stockholm trial as updated by Arriagada et al. (4).

Taking all patients (i.e., node-negative and node-positive, pre- and postmenopausal), locoregional recurrences were seen in 26% of controls versus 6% in RT arm (RR = 0.2, $p < 0.0001$); combined locoregional and distant metastases in 68% versus 55% (RR = 0.69, $p < 0.0001$); and deaths from any cause in 49% versus 44% (RR = 0.85, $p = 0.1$). Of importance is the analysis of distant metastases according to the nodal status. While not altered significantly in the node-negative patients, the rate of distant metastases was significantly reduced by RT in the node-positive cohorts (72% versus 54%, RR = 0.66, $p = 0.01$). Although overall survival was only minimally affected by RT in node-negative patients (RR = 0.92), the 20% mortality reduction reflecting the avoidance of systemic events by RT in the node-positive group was quite substantial and in line with the mortality reduction shown in the next generation trials from British Columbia and Denmark using adjuvant CT in conjunction with RT. Thus, the large Swedish Stockholm trial is one of the first radiation studies using megavoltage technique, just before the era of adjuvant chemotherapy, which showed a significant RT benefit in improving systemic recurrences and breast cancer mortality in node-positive cases.

Conclusion

This trial provides: level I evidence for reduction of locoregional recurrences in node-negative as well as node-positive patients; level I evidence for a reduction of systemic metastases in node-positive patients; and level II evidence for reduction of breast cancer mortality in node-positive cases.

Trial II. British Columbia Trial: Impact of Radiation in Association with Chemotherapy Schedules of Medium Dose Intensity

Results of the British Columbia trial (6) at 15 years follow-up (20) showed a significant reduction of locoregional and systemic recurrences by RT (RR = 0.44, $p = 0.003$; and RR = 0.66, $p = 0.006$, respectively), with a substantial and significant 29% improvement in breast cancer mortality (RR = 0.71, $p = 0.05$). The recent update of this trial showed not only a persistence of this benefit, but also more significance in improving overall survival, with a 30% reduction of overall mortality in patients randomized to RT (RR = 0.7, $p = 0.02$).(21) Subsets with one to three positive axillary nodes (N 1–3) benefited by a similar magnitude as the four or more nodes cases (RR of 0.65 versus 0.74, respectively).

Conclusion

This trial confirms, in patients eligible for the trial, a significant reduction of locoregional and systemic recurrences, with a resulting reduction of breast cancer and overall mortality. The benefits of RT were of similar magnitude among cases with one to three as for N4-positive nodes. The trial provides level I evidence for all outcomes.

Trial III. The Danish Premenopausal Study: RT Impact in Chemotherapy Schedules of Medium High Dose Intensity

Results of the Danish premenopausal trial (5) at 10 years showed a significant reduction of locoregional recurrences in patients from the RT arm and a significant improvement of overall survival. Table 3.2, Table 3.3, Table 3.4 and Table 3.5 show that the locoregional positive systemic recurrences, as well as overall survival rates, were all improved in the radiation arm. The RR reductions seen were of similar magnitude in all patients, as in various subsets including node-negative, 1 to 3 nodes and more than 4 nodes cohorts, as well as cases with 0 to 3, 3 to 9 or more than 10 lymph nodes removed (Tables 3.3, 3.4). These

TABLE 3.3. *Impact of RT: analysis of recurrences (locoregional and systemic) according to the nodal subsets*

Study	F/UP (years)	No RT	Recurrences (%) RT	Abs%
Arriagada et al., 1996 (4)	15			
All pts.		49	35	14
N-ve		34	26	12
N+ve		71	53	15
Overgaard et al., 1997 (5) pre	10			
All pts.		58	43	15
N-ve		34	22	12
N1–3		53	37	15
N4+		76	60	16
Ragaz et al., 1997 (6)	15			
All pts.		63	48	17
N1–3*		48	36	12
N4+*		83	62	21
Overgaard et al., 1999 (7) post	10			
All pts.		60	47	13
N-ve		53	34	19
N1–3		52	40	12
N4+		78	63	13

observations provide evidence for the survival improvement of RT for node-positive cohorts, and also that the relative odds reduction of events due to RT is constant across most subsets treated.

Conclusion

The Danish trial involving a very large number of cases showed, as in the British Columbia study, a significant reduction of recurrences (locoregional as well as systemic) and a reduction of overall mortality. Improvement was seen in subsets with high-risk node-negative disease, as well as in subsets with one to three and more than four positive nodes cases. The trial provides level I evidence for RT improvements of all outcomes in premenopausal breast cancer subsets as randomized.

Trial IV. The Danish Postmenopausal Study: RT Impact in the Presence of Tamoxifen

At 10-year follow-up, irradiated patients participating in the Danish postmenopausal trial (all ER-positive patients also randomized to tamoxifen; see the appendix to this chapter) had significantly less recurrences with 47% compared to 60% in cases without RT (7). Overall survival was also improved significantly (45% versus

TABLE 3.4. *Analysis of recurrences (locoregional and systemic) from the two Danish trials in subsets according to the number of nodes removed*

Study	F/UP (years)	No RT	Recurrences (%) RT	Abs%
Overgaard et al., 1997 (5) pre	10			
All pts.		58	43	15
Nodes removed				
N0–3		57	44	13
N3–9		58	41	17
N9+		57	44	13
Overgaard et al., 1999 (7) post	10			
All pts.		60	47	13
Nodes removed				
< 8		59	45	14
> 8		61	49	12

TABLE 3.5. Impact of RT: frequency of deaths for all patients

Study	F/UP (years)	Deaths (%) No RT	RT	Abs%
Arriagada et al., 1996 (4)	15	49	44	5
Overgaard et al.,* 1997 (5) pre	10	55	46	9
Ragaz et al.,* 1997(6)	15	54	46	8
Overgaard et al.,* 1999 (7) post	10	64	55	9

*Estimates from OS%

36%, $p = 0.03$). While all subsets had a substantial reduction of recurrences and improvement in overall survival (Tables 3.3, 3.4, 3.5), when compared to the premenopausal patients, in whom the survival benefit was seen already after the second year, the beneficial survival impact emerged substantially later in time, after 5 years, probably reflecting the slower rate of developing breast cancer events in the older patients.

Conclusion

This trial shows in postmenopausal patients treated with one year of tamoxifen a significant reduction of locoregional and distant recurrences and improvement of overall survival by RT. This trial provides level I evidence for cases eligible for the study.

Trial V. RT Impact in Chemotherapy Schedules of High Dose Intensity: The Pilot Study of the CALGB Trial with or Without Radiation

The summary results of the CALGB Duke high-dose chemotherapy requiring bone marrow transplant trial (8) indicate that, despite the high-dose chemotherapy, locoregional recurrences were seen in 27% versus 3% in unirradiated versus irradiated cases, and systemic recurrences were seen in 27% versus 9%, respectively (8). Thus, despite the intensive CT schedule used, locoregional micrometastases were not eliminated, local and systemic recurrences was not avoided, and RT was confirmed as a required adjuvant treatment modality.

Conclusion

In this study, there was a significant reduction of locoregional and distant recurrences by RT, despite the high-dose chemotherapy using anthracyclines and high-dose alkylators requiring stem cell transplant. This study provides level III evidence regarding RT impact on recurrences and no data on survival.

Meta-analysis of Randomized RT Trials Using Adjuvant Chemotherapy

Whelan et al. (3) recently published a meta-analysis of randomized trials using RT in addition to adjuvant systemic chemotherapy. Eighteen trials of both premenopausal and postmenopausal patients have been reviewed, with most patients having had modified radical mastectomy. RT was shown to reduce all types of recurrences with a 75% reduction of odds of locoregional recurrence (RR = 0.25, 95%; CI = 0.19, 0.34) and a 31% reduction of odds of any recurrence for systemic or locoregional, whichever was first (RR = 0.69, 95%; CI = 0.58 to 0.83). Overall mortality was also significantly reduced (with RR = 0.83, 95% CI = 0.74, 0.94).

Conclusion

This meta-analysis confirms beneficial impact of RT in trials with systemic therapy. As the technique involved overview of published literature and not of direct patient data, conclusions of this meta-analysis would constitute evidence at level II for beneficial RT effect on reducing recurrences and improving overall survival in breast cancer patients undergoing chemotherapy.

RADIATION IMPACT ON SYSTEMIC RECURRENCES/ BREAST CANCER MORTALITY

As seen in the appendix to this chapter, the reviewed trials show a substantial improvement of either systemic recurrences (including the Swedish, British Columbia, Danish and the CALGB trials) or of breast cancer mortality/ overall survival (the British Columbia and the Danish trials).

The unresolved issue is the more detailed interaction of local and systemic events, especially the impact of avoiding locoregional recurrences by RT and potential systemic dissemination as a result. The British Columbia trial provides evidence that most cases with locoregional events will eventually develop, in long-term follow-up of 15 years, a systemic recurrence (i.e., more than 80%), and will suffer a breast cancer death (23). Therefore, salvage RT or CT at the time of locoregional recurrence after mastectomy does not have the same curative potential as the same treatments delivered in the adjuvant setting. What was less clear until recently is a definitive answer to the question, "do systemic events originate from the locoregional recurrences or from the locoregional microscopical source (i.e. lymph nodes or chest wall) disseminating before the diagnosis of locoregional recurrence." In the latter case, both the locoregional, as well as systemic, recurrences would have a common source (i.e., the microscopical locoregional micrometastases) and both would be a secondary marker rather than a source of dissemination. Avoiding systemic recurrences by RT in the absence of locoregional failures has been reported in the British Columbia trial and other studies. Specifically, in the British Columbia trial, 23% of patients without RT had a locoregional recurrence at any point before or after systemic recurrence and only 17% as a first event, while as many as 61% had systemic disease if not irradiated (6). These data provide level I evidence for systemic recurrences occurring without locoregional recurrences and for RT preventing a significant proportion of those (34% event reduction, $p = 0.006$). Hence, counting only locoregional metastatic events and their avoidance may substantially underestimate the effect of RT on systemic disease and reducing mortality.

Accordingly, both locoregional and systemic recurrences originate from the same source, which, although microscopic, may be sufficiently extensive that it may be resistant to CT and demands RT. Thus, the locoregional recurrences are a marker rather than the source of systemic events.

CONCLUDING REMARKS

The main RT trials and adjuvant chemotherapy were initiated in the late 1970s, in the era of medium-intensity dose chemotherapy. A key current question is whether RT benefits would be seen with present-day CT schedules using increasingly higher dose intensity regimens, including anthracyclines and/or taxanes. While the definitive answer will come only from a new generation of randomized trials testing RT impact with contemporary CT (21,22), there are already data indicating that even with the highest dose intensity CT regimens currently available, relapses in high-risk cases treated without RT are substantial, and benefits of RT in those situations have been identified. Table 3.3 and Table 3.4 show that when reviewing the main recent trials, the relative risk of locoregional or systemic recurrences was reduced by RT of a similar magnitude (RR = 0.65 to 0.76) in all trials using chemotherapy regimens of different dose intensity, including the regimens utilizing no CT (4), medium DI as in the British Columbia or the Danish trials (5,6), full DI of the CMF trials (23), or high-dose CT requiring stem cell transplant (8).

These results indicate that, while the absolute relapse rates differ widely according to the underlying risk (i.e., nodal status, tumor size, etc.) across all chemotherapy DI utilized, the relative risk reductions due to RT among different trials remain constant. Thus, the RT gains, while similar in relative risk, will remain, in absolute terms, very substantial in patients with high recurrence risks, regardless of the CT schedules utilized, and will remain very low in cohorts at low risk for recurrence. These data, therefore, compel formation of policies where all chemotherapy-treated patients at high risk would be candidates for routine locoregional RT, with low-risk cohorts being candidates for either no routine RT or for trials assessing its impact on overall outcome.

While the new-generation radiation trials, which include the current CT regimens, are appropriate to determine the therapeutic ratio of RT interacting with anthracyclines, taxanes or Herceptines, the stratification in those trials for risk features and implementation of early stopping rules may demonstrate survival gains from locoregional RT in high-risk cohorts in a more timely fashion.

Outside the context of a randomized trial, it would also be appropriate to conclude that selected high-risk subsets should be offered RT, as RT in those situations may result in a substantial avoidance of breast cancer deaths. This evidence-based review, therefore, permits the conclusion that in high-risk stage I and II breast cancer subsets, it would be appropriate to use: RT routinely; no RT in low risk cases; and for intermediate risk patients, encouraged participation in randomized trials.

APPENDIX
OUTLINE OF INDIVIDUAL TRIALS

Trial I: The Swedish trial, Arriagada et al. (4) was launched in 1971 using megavoltage radiation technique, with 960 breast cancer patients treated with modified radical mastectomy. Patients were randomized to three groups: group I, preoperative RT; group II, postoperative RT; group III, surgical controls. Approximately 45% of all patients were premenopausal, and 60% of all cases were node negative. The radiotherapy schedule in both radiation arms included a total of 45 Gy over 5 weeks, using a five-field technique, which encompassed the chest wall, the axilla, supraclavicular area, and internal mammary nodes. As the interim analysis showed no difference between the pre- and the postoperative radiation arms, the two RT groups were merged, with the final analysis restricted to group I, radiation (RT), versus group II, controls. Analysis was reported at 15-year follow-up (5).

Trial II: The British Columbia study was a two-arm randomized trial, conducted between 1979 and 1986 (20). Eligibility included premenopausal node-positive breast cancer patients treated with mastectomy and adjuvant chemotherapy (CT) who were randomized to CT alone versus CT plus RT. RT was applied between the third and the fourth CT cycles (the sandwiched technique). All cases had a modified radical mastectomy with level I/level II axillary dissection and a median of 11 lymph nodes removed; all patients received megavoltage radiation with a cobalt source, with a planned dose of 3,750 cGy in 16 fractions over $3\frac{1}{2}$ weeks, encompassing all regional nodal areas including internal mammary fields. CT included: cyclophosphamide, 600 mg/m^2; methotrexate, 40 mg/m^2; and 5-FU, 600 mg/m^2, given every 3 weeks eight times. Long-term follow-up, over 15 years, was needed before the significance in favor of radiotherapy emerged (17).

Trial III: The Danish Breast Cancer Cooperative Group radiation trials took place between 1982 and 1989. Included were pre- and postmenopausal patients, with premenopausal patients receiving CMF chemotherapy reported separately [the Danish Breast Cancer Cooperative Group 82b trial (95)], and postmenopausal cases treated with tamoxifen reported separately [the DBCG 82c trial (7)]. The premenopausal study randomized 1,708 breast cancer patients, who had undergone mastectomy and adjuvant chemotherapy, into CT and RT versus CT alone. CT was a modified Bonadonna regimen, with cyclophosphamide, 600 mg/m^2; methotrexate, 40 mg/m^2; and 5-FU, 600 mg/m^2, given every 4 weeks. Of all patients, 135 had node-negative disease but a high-risk primary tumor (a tumor size greater than 5 cm or invasion of skin/pectoral fascia); remaining cases were node positive, with 1,061 having one to three positive axillary nodes, and 409 having more than four nodes involved. At mastectomy, a median of seven lymph nodes was removed, with 255, 1,042 and 409 patients having had zero to three, four to nine and more than nine nodes removed, respectively.

Trial IV: The Danish *postmenopausal* trial, as in the *premenopausal* study, started in 1982 (7). Until 1990, over 1,370 postmenopausal women with stage I and II breast cancer were randomized into groups with or without locoregional RT. All patients took 30 mg of tamoxifen per day for one year, as part of their systemic adjuvant therapy. Similar to the premenopausal cases, node-positive as well as node-negative cases were eligible; node positive cases were grouped into those with less than eight axillary nodes removed versus those with more than eight axillary nodes removed (8).

Trial V: The CALGB study of high dose intensity chemotherapy with bone marrow support provides some data regarding the RT effect in patients treated with high dose CT (8). This pilot study lead to the first large-scale, randomized, adjuvant high-dose chemotherapy trial requiring bone marrow/stem cell transplant in the adjuvant setting. Initiated by Peters et al. (24) from the CALGB group in the late 1980s for high-risk patients with stage II disease and more than ten 10 positive axillary nodes involved, it later became an Intergroup trial with several U.S. collaborative groups, including the Canadian Clinical Trials Group (NCIC-CTG), involved. Marks et al. (8) reported on the first 43 patients from this trial assessing the role of RT.

All patients were treated as a pilot study of the CALGB high-dose CT program using the Duke University phase I and II high-dose chemotherapy plus bone marrow transplant schedule. All cases had, after a modified radical mastectomy, induction chemotherapy with four cycles of cyclophosphamide 600, adriamycin 60, 5-fluorouracil 600 mg/m^2 (the CAF regimen). This was followed in cases randomized to the high-dose chemotherapy arm by cyclophosphamide 5,625 mg/m^2, cisplatin 165 mg/m^2, carmustine 600 mg/m^2 (the high-dose CDB regimen), with cytokines and stem cell transplant. Patients in the second arm were treated with the same CT but at lower doses (the lower dose CDB regimen), not requiring bone marrow/stem cell transplant, only cytokines. The first nine patients in the higher dose arm did not receive radiotherapy. Of those, three (33%) developed locoregional recurrence within the first 12 months, and three developed distant metastases. As a result, all subsequent 34 cases in the study had five-field radiation added at the end of the chemotherapy. At three years follow-up, these cases were updated and reported. Patients were well-balanced for prognostic factors, with a median of 13 positive nodes in both groups.

REFERENCES

1. Anonymous. Effects of radiotherapy and surgery in early breast cancer. An overview of the randomized trials. Early Breast Cancer Trialists' Collaborative Group. *N Engl J Med* 1995;333(22):1444–1455.
2. Anonymous. Favourable and unfavourable effects on long-term survival of radiotherapy for early breast cancer: an overview of the randomised trials. Early Breast Cancer Trialists' Collaborative Group. *Lancet* 2000;355(9217):1757–1770.
3. Whelan TJ, et al. Does locoregional radiation therapy improve survival in breast cancer? A meta-analysis. *J Clin Oncol* 2000;18(6):1220–1229.
4. Arriagada R, et al. Adequate locoregional treatment for early breast cancer may prevent secondary dissemination. *J Clin Oncol* 1995;13(12):2869–2878.
5. Overgaard M, et al. Postoperative radiotherapy in high-risk premenopausal women with breast cancer who receive adjuvant chemotherapy. Danish Breast Cancer Cooperative Group 82b Trial [see comments]. *N Engl J Med* 1997;337(14):949–955.
6. Ragaz J, et al. Adjuvant radiotherapy and chemotherapy in node-positive premenopausal women with breast cancer [see comments]. *N Engl J Med* 1997;337(14):956–962.
7. Overgaard M, et al. Postoperative radiotherapy in high-risk postmenopausal breast-cancer patients given adjuvant tamoxifen: Danish Breast Cancer Cooperative Group DBCG 82c randomised trial. *Lancet* 1999;353(9165):1641–1648.
8. Marks LB, et al. Post-mastectomy radiotherapy following adjuvant chemotherapy and autologous bone marrow transplantation for breast cancer patients with greater than or equal to 10 positive axillary lymph nodes. Cancer and Leukemia Group B. *Int J Radiat Oncol Biol Phys* 1992;23(5):1021–1026.
9. Levine MN, et al. Randomized trial of intensive cyclophosphamide, epirubicin, and fluorouracil chemotherapy compared with cyclophosphamide, methotrexate, and fluorouracil in premenopausal women with node-positive breast cancer. National Cancer Institute of Canada Clinical Trials Group [see comments]. *J Clin Oncol* 1998;16(8):2651–2658.
10. Gianni L, Capri G. Experience at the Istituto Nazionale Tumori with paclitaxel in combination with doxorubicin in women with untreated breast cancer. *Semin Oncol* 1997;24(1 suppl 3):1–3.

11. Henderson IC, et al. Improved disease free and overall survival from addition of sequential paclitaxel but not from the escalation of doxorubicin dose level in the adjuvant chemotherapy of patients with node-positive primary breast cancer. *Proc Am Soc Clin Oncol* 1999; 17:101a.
12. Slamon D, Leyland-Jones B, Shak S. Addition of Herceptin to first line chemotherapy for HER2 overexpressing metastatic breast cancer markedly increases anticancer activity: a randomized multinational controlled phase III trial. *Proc Am Soc Clin Oncol* 1998; 17:98a.
13. Slamon D, Pegram M. Rationale for trastuzumab (Herceptin) in adjuvant breast cancer trials. *Semin Oncol* 2001;28(1 suppl 3):13–19.
14. Cobleigh M, Vogel C, Tripathy D. Efficay and safety of Herceptin (humanized anti-HER2 antibody) as a single agent in 222 women with HER2 overexpression who relapsed following chemotherapy for metastatic breats cancer. *Proc Am Soc Clin Oncol* 1998;17:97a.
15. Sackett D. Rules of evidence and clinical recommendations on the use of antithrombotic agents. *Chest* 1989; 95(2 suppl):2–4.
16. Ragaz J, Spinelli JJ, Coldman AJ. Breast cancer survival advantage with radiotherapy. *Lancet* 2000;356 (9237):1270; discussion 1271.
17. Ragaz J, Spinelli JJ. Wide-field radiation as adjunct to adjuvant chemotherapy in high-risk cases with early breast cancer: do it or not? *Int J Cancer* 2000;87(3): 423–426.
18. Hellman S. Stopping metastases at their source. *N Engl J Med* 1997;337(14):996–997.
19. Schabel FM. Concepts for systemic treatment of micrometastases. *Cancer* 1975;35:15–24.
20. Chia S, Ragaz J, Jackson SEA. Locoregional recurrence in breast cancer: Marker or a source of systemic disease? Recurrence pattern analysis of the British Columbia randomized trial. *Proc Amer Soc Clin Oncol* 1998;17:168.
21. Pierce L. Randomized Trial of Locoregional Radiation in postmastectomy breast cancer patients with 1–3 positive axilalry lymph nodes. US and Candian Intergroup Trial. Personal communications, 2001.
22. Whelan T. Randomized Trial of Regional Radiation in patients with positive axillary nodes after partial mastectomy. Trial of the Canadian National Cancer Institute (the Ma-20). Personal communications, 2001.
23. Velez-Garcia E, Carpenter JT Jr, Moore M. Postsurgical adjuvant chemotherapy with or without radiotherapy in women with breast cancer and positive axillary nodes: a South-Eastern Cancer Study Group trial. *Eur J Cancer* 1992;28A(11):1833–1837.
24. Peters WP, Ross M, Vredenburgh JJ, et al. High-dose chemotherapy and autologous bone marrow support as consolidation after standard-dose adjuvant therapy for high-risk primary breast cancer. *J Clin Oncol* 1993; 11(6):1132–1143.

SECTION 2

Early Stage Disease—Surgery, Chemotherapy, and Hormones

4

Evolution in the Management of Ductal Carcinoma *in situ* through Randomized Clinical Trials

Eleftherios Mamounas

The clinical presentation, biological understanding, and management of non-invasive breast cancer have undergone significant changes during the past decade. As a result of the widespread use of high-quality mammography, the incidence of non-palpable, mammographically detected, localized ductal carcinoma *in situ* (DCIS) has been steadily increasing. This entity possesses an altogether different natural history than the previously encountered palpable DCIS, which is often associated with microinvasion and, occasionally, with axillary nodal involvement. The demonstration of favorable natural history for patients with mammographically detected DCIS challenged the need for radical surgical management, particularly as the efficacy of breast-conserving surgery was established for patients with invasive breast cancer (1). Randomized clinical trials both from the United States and Europe aimed to explore the role of breast-conserving surgery—with or without postoperative breast radiotherapy—and to define the role of tamoxifen in patients with DCIS.

ROLE OF LUMPECTOMY AND BREAST RADIOTHERAPY

The NSABP B-17 trial

The NSABP B-17 trial, the first randomized trial in patients with DCIS, was designed to evaluate the worth of breast irradiation following lumpectomy. Between 1985 and 1990, 818 patients with localized DCIS, detected by either physical examination or mammography, were randomized to receive either lumpectomy alone or lumpectomy followed by breast radiotherapy (Fig. 4.1). Lumpectomy for this study, as in previous NSABP studies, was considered the removal of the tumor and a sufficient amount of normal breast tissue so that the specimen margins were histologically tumor-free. Although axillary dissection was mandatory at the beginning of the study, it became optional subsequently, based on evidence indicating that it was not necessary in the treatment of DCIS. Results, originally reported after 5 years of follow-up and subsequently with 8 years of follow-up

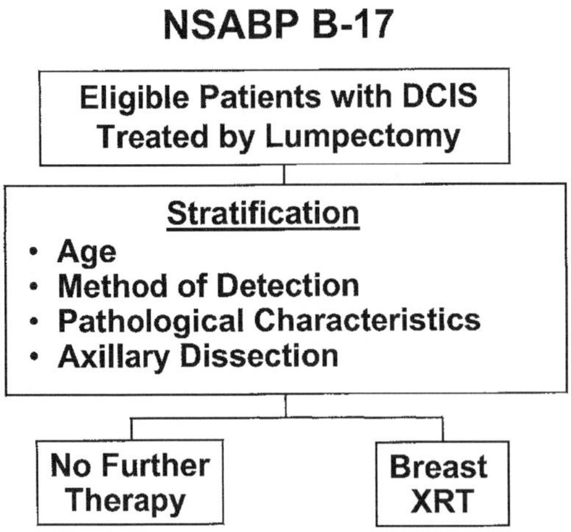

NSABP B-17

Eligible Patients with DCIS Treated by Lumpectomy

Stratification
- Age
- Method of Detection
- Pathological Characteristics
- Axillary Dissection

→ No Further Therapy
→ Breast XRT

FIG. 4.1. Schema of NSABP B-17 trial comparing lumpectomy alone to lumpectomy plus breast radiation in DCIS patients.

(2,3), were recently updated through 12 years of follow-up and continue to demonstrate that the addition of breast radiotherapy following lumpectomy significantly improves the event-free survival of these patients by decreasing the rate of all ipsilateral breast tumor recurrences (IBTR) by 58% (4). The event-free survival was 64% for women receiving post-lumpectomy radiotherapy, compared to 50% for women receiving lumpectomy alone (relative risk of failure: 0.63, $p = 0.00004$). After 12 years, the cumulative incidence of IBTR was 32% in women treated with lumpectomy alone, compared to 16% in women who received post-lumpectomy radiotherapy ($p < 0.000005$). The cumulative incidence of a non-invasive IBTR was 15% in women treated with lumpectomy alone and 8% in women treated with lumpectomy plus radiotherapy ($p = 0.001$) (Fig. 4.2). More importantly, the cumulative incidence of an invasive IBTR was 17% in the former group and 8% in the latter group, respectively ($p = 0.00001$) (Fig. 4.2). As was observed at 8 years, the cumulative incidence of first events other than IBTR was not significantly different in the two treatment groups: 18% in the group treated with lumpectomy alone and 21% in the group treated with lumpectomy and radiotherapy ($p = 0.99$). When the two treatment groups were combined, the cumulative incidence of contralateral breast

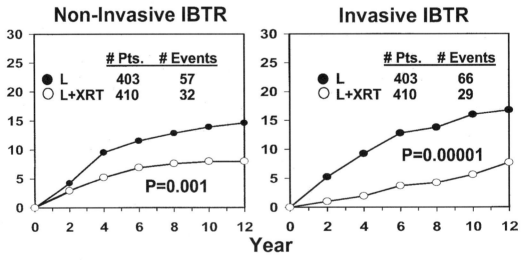

FIG. 4.2. Twelve-year cumulative incidence of invasive IBTR and non-invasive IBTR in the NSABP B-17 trial in patients treated with lumpectomy (*L*) or with lumpectomy and breast radiation (*L+XRT*). (Adapted with permission from Fisher B, Land S, Mamounas E, et al. Prevention of invasive breast cancer in women with ductal carcinoma in situ: an update of the National Surgical Adjuvant Breast and Bowel Project experience. *Semin Oncol* 2001;28:400–418.)

cancer was 7% (5% invasive and 2% non-invasive). Through 12 years of follow-up, the overall survival was 86% for women treated with lumpectomy alone and 87% for women who received radiotherapy after lumpectomy ($p = 0.80$). Fifty-eight percent of the deaths in each treatment group occurred before any breast cancer event. Locoregional or distant recurrences were uncommon, with only 17 (2.5%) occurring as first events in the 813 randomized patients with follow-up, 7 (2.2%) in the lumpectomy-alone group, and 10 (2.8%) in the lumpectomy-plus-radiotherapy group.

The EORTC Trial 10853

The EORTC randomized phase III trial was the second trial of local therapy in patients with DCIS to produce results (5). Between 1986 and 1996, 1,010 patients with clinically or mammographically detected DCIS measuring less than or equal to 5 cm were treated by complete local excision of the lesion and then randomly assigned to either no further treatment (n = 503) or to radiotherapy (n = 507). The radiotherapy regimen consisted of 50 Gy in 5 weeks to the whole breast. The median follow-up was $4\frac{1}{4}$ years. The 4-year local relapse-free survival rate was 84% in the group treated with local excision alone, compared to 91% in the group treated by local excision plus radiotherapy (hazard ratio 0.62, $p = 0.005$). The addition of radiotherapy resulted in similar reductions in the risk of invasive IBTR (40%, $p = 0.04$) and non-invasive IBTR (35%, $p = 0.06$). Contralateral breast cancer developed in 29 patients (21 [4%] in the radiotherapy group and 8 [2%] in the no-further-treatment group). The 4-year contralateral recurrence-free rate was 99% in the no-further-treatment group versus 97% in the radiotherapy group ($p = 0.01$). There were 24 patients who developed distant metastases. The 4-year metastasis-free rate was similar in the two groups: 98% in the no-further-treatment group and 99% in the radiotherapy group. There were 24 deaths, 11 of which occurred after an IBTR (7 deaths in the no further treatment group and 4 in the radiotherapy group).

The 4-year overall survival was 99% for both groups. These results are similar to those from the NSABP B-17 trial and provide further evidence supporting the role of radiotherapy for the treatment of localized DCIS.

PROGNOSTIC MARKERS FOR IBTR

Following the original and subsequent disclosure of the B-17 trial results, one commonly asked question was whether all patients with localized DCIS need breast radiotherapy following lumpectomy or whether there are subgroups with such a good prognosis that they could be treated with lumpectomy alone. To the opposite end, are there patients with more extensive or aggressive disease for whom breast conservation is not the best option and who may benefit from total mastectomy?

Attempts to answer these questions have been made by evaluating the effect of breast irradiation following lumpectomy on ipsilateral breast tumor recurrence in subsets of DCIS patients according to prognostic clinical and pathologic characteristics. Such evaluations have been attempted using data from randomized trials [NSABP B-17, EORTC 10853 (6–8)] and from non-randomized cohorts [Van Nuys experience (9,10)] with somewhat discordant results. In the B-17 trial (6), pathologic features were assessed centrally in a representative subgroup of 573 patients from the total cohort of randomized patients. Tumor characteristics, patient characteristics, and outcome were almost identical for the subset undergoing central pathology review and the total B-17 cohort. After five years of follow-up, presence of moderate/marked comedo-necrosis and uncertain/involved lumpectomy margins were the only statistically significant independent predictors—by multivariate analysis—of risk for ipsilateral breast tumor recurrence in patients treated with lumpectomy, with or without breast irradiation. When hazard rates of ipsilateral breast tumor recurrence were evaluated by categories of margin status and comedo necrosis combined, breast irradiation was found to be effective in all patient subgroups, although the absolute benefit was larger in the subgroups at higher risk for recurrence. Updated results of central pathology review from the B-17 trial were recently reported with 8 years of follow-up in an expanded cohort of 623 out of the 814 evaluable patients (7). With additional follow-up, the presence of marked/moderate comedo necrosis remained the only statistically significant independent predictor of risk for ipsilateral breast tumor recurrence in both treatment groups. Benefit from radiotherapy continued to be evident both in patients with moderate/marked comedo necrosis and in those with absent/mild comedo necrosis. At 8 years, breast radiation effected a 7% absolute reduction in the rate of breast tumor recurrence in the low-risk group.

In the EORTC 10853 trial, clinical and pathologic characteristics from patients with DCIS were related to the risk of recurrence. Pathologic features were derived from a central review of 863 of the 1,010 randomized cases (85%). The median follow-up was 5.4 years. Factors associated with a statistically significant increase in risk of local recurrence in the multivariate analysis were young age (less than or equal to 40 years), symptomatic detection of DCIS, growth pattern (solid and cribriform), involved margins, and treatment by local excision alone. The risk of invasive recurrence was not related to the histologic type of DCIS, but the risk of distant metastasis was significantly higher in poorly differentiated DCIS, compared with well-differentiated DCIS. Radiotherapy reduced the risk of recurrence in all subgroups. Although the numbers of events were too small for testing the effect of treatment on the different variables, the risk of recurrence with radiotherapy was particularly low in low-grade lesions (4%) or in lesions without necrosis (4%). On the other hand, even with radiotherapy, high recurrence rates were observed in the worst subgroups (i.e., 18% in cases with high nuclear grade, 16% in cases with necrosis, 17% in clinically detected cases). The study did not allow for identification of a safe margin width for treatment without radiotherapy, since the trial eligibility criteria did not require reporting of the margin width. Recurrence rates of 24% were observed in cases with close/involved margins and were even higher when margin status was not mentioned (up to 28%). Radiotherapy did not compensate for involved margins, as even with the application of radiotherapy, the recurrence rate was 20% in this group. However, even in the group of DCIS for which margins could be considered optimal (i.e., those patients who underwent a surgical re-excision in which no residual DCIS was found), a local recurrence rate of 18% was observed when these patients were treated with surgery alone.

The Van Nuys Prognostic Index (VNPI) as reported by Silverstein et al. (10), was devised by combining three statistically significant independent predictors of local tumor recurrence in a cohort of DCIS patients treated in two institutions. Initially, 254 patients treated with breast-conservation therapy at the Breast Center in Van Nuys between 1979 and 1995 were studied. Subsequently, 79 patients treated at the Children's Hospital in San Francisco between 1972 and 1987 were used to validate the initial results. Since comparable patients from both centers revealed nearly identical local recurrence-free survival rates in all subsets, the two groups were combined, yielding a final study group of 333 patients with a median follow-up of 79 months. Tissue was processed in a similar manner at both facilities. The margins were inked or dyed and specimens were serially sectioned at 2 mm to 3 mm intervals. The decision to proceed with mastectomy or breast-conserving surgery and the decision to add further treatment following breast-conserving surgery (i.e., breast irradiation) was not randomly assigned or dictated by a set protocol but was left at the discretion of the treating physician. By multivariate analysis, three statistically significant predictors of local recurrence were identified: tumor size, margin width, and histologic type, and each was given a score of one (best) to three (worst). Score one was given for tumors 15 mm or less in diameter, score two for tumors 16 mm to 40 mm in diameter and score three for tumors more than 40 mm in diameter. Similarly, score one was given for a margin width of 10 mm or greater, score two for a margin of 1 mm to 9 mm and score three for a margin of less than 1 mm. Finally, score one was given for non–high-grade tumors without comedo necrosis, score two for non–high-grade tumors with comedo necrosis and score three for high-grade tumors, irrespective of the presence or absence of comedo necrosis. The VNPI score was determined by adding the individual score from each category. Patients with VNPI score of three or four had similar outcomes (low-risk) and so did patients with scores five, six, or seven (intermediate-risk) and those with scores eight or nine (high-risk). However, each of these three groups (low-, intermediate- and high-risk) had statistically different local recurrence rates from one another. In addition, the authors concluded that patients with VNPI scores of three or four did not show a local disease-free survival benefit from breast irradiation following lumpectomy, but patients with VNPI five, six, or seven did. Patients with VNPI eight or nine also benefited from breast irradiation but their local recurrence rate was high with or without irradiation, making mastectomy possibly a better choice than breast conservation in this group of patients.

A number of methodological issues regarding the study of Silverstein have been raised (11), including: the retrospective nature of the study, the inclusion of patients treated at two institutions over a relatively long time period (1972–1995); and the potential variation over time in patient selection criteria, mammographic evaluation, extent of surgery, use of radiation, and specimen processing. Other investigators have shown that the rates of re-excision, specimen radiography, and postoperative mammography increase over time, with a resulting decrease in rates of local recurrence after lumpectomy and breast irradiation (12). Additional issues of concern center around the validity of the VNPI because of its retrospective development in a cohort of patients without unified or set local treatment criteria and its lacking of independent and prospective confirmation by other groups. Lastly, but perhaps more importantly, the appropriateness of examining and reporting treatment effects in relatively small subgroups of patients where therapy was not dictated by a set protocol has been challenged. A number of biases, some obvious and some more obscure, are introduced by such an approach, making the significance of the results questionable.

Despite the apparent differences between the prospective studies (NSABP B-17, EORTC 10853) and the retrospective Van Nuys experience in terms of identifying prognostic factors of recurrence, there are also significant similarities. Both include an assessment of margin status/width (a measure of the distance from the edge of the tumor to the edge of the lumpectomy specimen) and an assessment of grade/comedo necrosis (although grade was not an independent predictor in the NSABP/EORTC studies because of its close association with comedo necrosis). Pathologically evaluated tumor size was not an independent predictor in the NSABP and EORTC studies as it was in the VNPI, but mammographic tumor size was found to be an independent predictor in the 8-year update of the B-17 results (3). However, significant differences exist between the NSABP and EORTC studies and the Van Nuys experience in their respective treatment recommendations as outlined above. In that respect, treatment recommendations resulting from several well-designed and conducted randomized trials (level I evidence) bear considerably more weight than those reached by retrospective analysis of an arbitrarily defined cohort of patients with treatment selection at the discretion of the treating physician. Furthermore, although there are likely to be quantitative differences regarding the benefit from radiotherapy in different subsets of DCIS patients according to their risk for recurrence, no subgroups of patients were identified in the prospective randomized trials where the benefit from radiotherapy was absent.

ROLE OF TAMOXIFEN: THE NSABP B-24 TRIAL

Over the past three decades, a large body of scientific evidence has accumulated demonstrating benefit from tamoxifen administration in patients with resected operable invasive breast cancer (13). In these patients, tamoxifen not only reduces the risk for systemic recurrence and improves survival but also has a significant impact in reducing the rate of ipsilateral breast tumor recurrence following lumpectomy and breast irradiation (14,15). More importantly, tamoxifen has been found to reduce the incidence of second primary breast cancers in the contralateral breast by about 40% (13–19). The latter observation, along with preclinical evidence that tamoxifen inhibits both initiation and promotion of tumors in experimental animals (20,21), makes tamoxifen an attractive agent for patients with DCIS treated with lumpectomy and breast radiotherapy for possibly reducing the rate of development of subsequent ipsilateral or contralateral invasive breast cancers. Several trials were designed to test this hypothesis. The first to produce results was the NSABP B-24 trial (22). This trial evaluated the role of tamoxifen following lumpectomy and postoperative radiotherapy in patients with localized as well as more extensive DCIS. Between 1991 and 1994, 1,804 women with DCIS treated with lumpectomy and postoperative radiotherapy were randomized to receive either 20 mg of tamoxifen daily for five years or placebo (Fig. 4.3). Contrary to the B-17 trial, where lumpectomy margins were required to be free of DCIS for eligibility, in the B-24 trial patients were eligible whether the lumpectomy margins were free, involved, or of unknown status. As a result, in the B-24 trial, about 75% of the patients had free lumpectomy margins, about 16% had involved margins and in 9% the margins were unknown. Otherwise, the distribution of patient and tumor characteristics was similar between the two trials. More than 80% of the tumors were detected by mammography alone. At 5 years of follow-up, the addition of tamoxifen significantly reduced the incidence of all invasive and non-invasive breast cancers at any site by 37% (13.4% in the placebo group versus 8.2% in the tamoxifen group, $p < 0.001$). When the rate of all invasive breast cancer events was evaluated, tamoxifen resulted in a 43% reduction (7.2% in the placebo group versus 4.1% in the tamoxifen group, $p = 0.004$). The addition of tamoxifen also resulted in a non-significant reduction in the rate of non-invasive breast cancers (6.2% versus 4.2% respectively, $p = 0.08$). Tamoxifen's effect in reducing breast cancer events was evident both in the ipsilateral and in the contralateral breast. The cumulative incidence of contralateral breast cancers as first events was reduced by 52% in patients receiving tamoxifen, compared to those receiving placebo (3.4% versus 2.0% respectively, $p = 0.01$). Several patient and tumor characteristics were found to increase the rate of ipsilateral breast tumor recurrence, such as young age (under 50), involved/unknown lumpectomy margins, presence of comedo necrosis, and DCIS presentation with clinical findings. The effect of tamoxifen in reducing ipsilateral breast cancer was evident irrespective of age, margin status, or presence/absence of comedo necrosis. However, for women with clinically apparent DCIS at study entry, ipsilateral breast tumor recurrence rates were similar between the tamoxifen and placebo groups, although the number of patients in that category was small. Adverse effects from tamoxifen were similar to those observed in other tamoxifen clinical trials. The rate of endometrial cancer was 1.53 per 1,000 patients per year in the tamoxifen group, compared to 0.45 per 1,000 patients per year in the placebo group.

The B-24 results were recently updated through 7 years of follow-up (4) and continue to indicate a significant improvement in event-

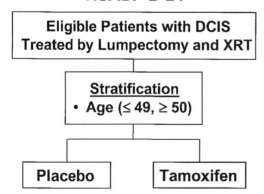

FIG. 4.3. Schema of NSABP B-24 trial comparing tamoxifen to placebo in DCIS patients treated with lumpectomy and breast irradiation.

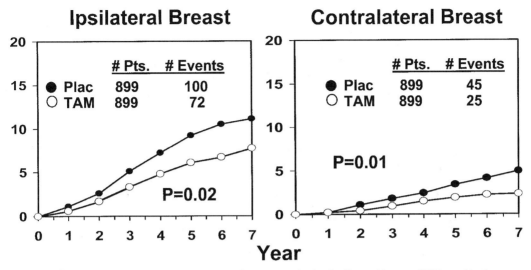

FIG. 4.4. Seven-year cumulative incidence of all events in the ipsilateral breast (IBT) and in the contralateral breast (CBT) in the NSABP B-24 trial (*Plac,* placebo; *TAM,* tamoxifen). (Adapted with permission from Fisher B, Land S, Mamounas E, et al. Prevention of invasive breast cancer in women with ductal carcinoma in situ: an update of the National Surgical Adjuvant Breast and Bowel Project experience. *Semin Oncol* 2001;28:400–418.)

free survival with the addition of tamoxifen (83% versus 77%, RR = 0.72, $p = 0.002$). This improvement is mainly the result of reductions in the rates of ipsilateral breast tumor (IBT) and contralateral breast tumor (CBT) development. At 7 years of follow-up, the cumulative incidence of any IBT in women treated with lumpectomy, radiotherapy, and placebo was 11.1%, compared to 7.7% in women treated with lumpectomy, radiotherapy, and tamoxifen ($p = 0.02$) (Fig. 4.4). This reduction in IBT was mainly the result of reduction in invasive IBT (5.3% and 2.6%, respectively). The cumulative incidence of non-invasive IBT was unaffected by tamoxifen administration (5.8% and 5%, respectively). The cumulative incidence of all CBT was also significantly reduced by tamoxifen (4.9% in the placebo group and 2.3% in the tamoxifen group, 53% reduction, $p = 0.01$) (Fig. 4.4). The reduction in invasive CBT from 3.2% to 1.8% was not significant ($p = 0.16$). There was, however, a significant reduction in noninvasive CBT (1.7% versus 0.5%, respectively, $p = 0.03$). As it was shown through 5 years of follow-up, the same patient and tumor characteristics continued to be associated with increased risk for IBT development through 7 years of follow-up. These included: age under 50, positive margins, presence of comedo necrosis, and presence of clinical findings at the time of detection. Through 7 years of follow-up, there were no differences in the overall survival between the two groups (95% for each group, $p = 0.78$). Seventy-five percent of the deaths in the placebo group and 76% of the deaths in the placebo group occurred before any breast cancer event.

The results from the B-24 trial continue to indicate a significant benefit from tamoxifen in patients with DCIS and provide level I evidence for this effect. When these results are viewed together with those demonstrating benefit from tamoxifen in women with prior invasive breast cancer (13–15) and in women with atypical hyperplasia and lobular carcinoma *in situ* (23), they support the use of tamoxifen in the majority of the spectrum of breast neoplasia.

The next logical question following disclosure of the B-24 results is whether the benefit from tamoxifen is limited to subsets of DCIS patients. Given the strong association between estrogen receptor expression and tamoxifen benefit in patients with invasive breast cancer, presence of a similar association needs to be investigated also in patients with DCIS. However, given that the effect of tamoxifen in patients with DCIS is evident both in the ipsilateral and the contralateral breast, tamoxifen may prove of benefit even in patients with estrogen-receptor negative DCIS.

RECENTLY COMPLETED, CURRENT AND FUTURE TRIALS

Several other randomized trials with similar designs to the NSABP B-17 trial, the NSABP B-24 trial and the EORTC 10853 trial have not yet produced results (24,25). The Swedish national trial compares sector resection alone to sector resection followed by breast radiotherapy, and the United Kingdom randomized trial investigates the role of breast radiotherapy and the role of tamoxifen following lumpectomy in a 2 times 2 factorial design (24).

In the United States, the Eastern Cooperative Oncology Group (ECOG) has initiated a registry of observation alone following lumpectomy in patients with low-risk DCIS. Eligible patients must have low/intermediate nuclear grade, non-comedo DCIS, of 2.5 cm or less in greatest diameter, or high nuclear grade, non-comedo DCIS, of 1.0 cm or less in greatest diameter. The tumor-free margin width after lumpectomy must be at least 3 mm. In addition, a recently initiated Intergroup study led by the Radiation Therapy Oncology Group (RTOG), evaluates the worth of adding breast irradiation to either tamoxifen or observation in a 2 times 2 factorial design for patients with unicentric, mammographically-detected, low/intermediate grade DCIS, of 2.5 cm or less in greatest diameter, with a 3 mm or more tumor-free margin width after lumpectomy. Both these trials will be useful in answering whether there are subsets of DCIS patients where breast irradiation can be omitted without increasing the rate of local recurrence in the ipsilateral breast.

SUMMARY

Randomized clinical trials have contributed significantly towards establishing the value of lumpectomy, breast irradiation, and tamoxifen in patients with DCIS. This paradigm shift has naturally resulted in several new questions. The most important ones center on the identification of patients who do or do not benefit from a certain intervention. Research efforts have so far focused on identifying patients who do not benefit from breast irradiation or who may need a mastectomy. The relationship between estrogen receptor expression and tamoxifen benefit is currently being investigated in the B-24 trial. Future research efforts will concentrate on the molecular characterization of these tumors so that therapy can be tailored appropriately. New biomarkers such as oncogene expression and tumor suppressor gene inactivation, as well as the presence of other genomic alterations, will play a significant role, not only as prognostic factors of recurrence and predictive factors of treatment effect, but also as potential targets for novel therapeutic interventions.

REFERENCES

1. Fisher B, Redmond C, Poisson R, et al. Eight-year results of a randomized clinical trial comparing total mastectomy and lumpectomy with or without irradiation in the treatment of breast cancer. *N Engl J Med* 1989;320:822–828.
2. Fisher B, Constantino J, Redmond C, et al. Initial results from a randomized trial evaluating lumpectomy and radiation therapy for the treatment of intraductal breast cancer. *N Engl J Med* 1993;328:1581–1586.
3. Fisher B, Dignam J, Wolmark N, et al. Lumpectomy and radiation therapy for the treatment of intraductal breast cancer: findings from National Surgical Adjuvant Breast and Bowel Project B-17. *J Clin Oncol* 1998;16:441–452.
4. Fisher B, Land S, Mamounas E, et al. Prevention of invasive breast cancer in young women with ductal carcinoma in situ: an update of the National Surgical Adjuvant Breast and Bowel Project Experience. *Semin Oncol* 2001;28:400–418.
5. Julien J-P, Bijker N, Fentiman IS, et al. Radiotherapy in breast-conserving treatment for ductal carcinoma in situ: first results of the EORTC randomised phase III trial 10853. *Lancet* 2000;355:528–533.
6. Fisher ER, Constantino J, Fisher B, et al. Pathologic findings from the NSABP Protocol B-17: Intraductal carcinoma (duct carcinoma in situ-DCIS). *Cancer* 1995;75:1310–1319.
7. Fisher ER, Dignam J, Tan-Chiu E, et al. Pathologic findings from the National Surgical Adjuvant Breast Project (NSABP) eight-year update of Protocol B-17: intraductal carcinoma. *Cancer* 1999;86:429–438.
8. Bijker N, Peterse JL, Duchateau L, et al. Risk factors for recurrence and metastasis after breast conserving

therapy for ductal carcinoma-in-situ: analysis of European Organization for Research and Treatment of Cancer Trial 10853.
9. Silverstein MJ, Lagios MD, Craig PH, et al. A prognostic index for ductal carcinoma in situ of the breast. *Cancer* 1996;77:2267–2274.
10. Silverstein MJ, Lagios MD. Use of predictors of recurrence to plan therapy for DCIS of the breast. *Oncology* 1997;11:393–410.
11. Schnitt SJ, Harris JR, Smith BL. Developing a prognostic index for ductal carcinoma in situ of the breast. Are we there yet? *Cancer* 1996;77:2189–2192.
12. Hiramatsu H, Bornstein BA, Recht A, et al. Local recurrence after conservative surgery and radiation therapy for ductal carcinoma in situ. Possible importance of family history. *Cancer J Sci Am* 1995;1:55–61.
13. Early Breast Cancer Trialists' Collaborative Group. Tamoxifen for early breast cancer: an overview of the randomized trials. *Lancet* 1998;351:1451–1467.
14. Fisher B, Constantino J, Redmond C, et al. A randomized clinical trial evaluating tamoxifen in the treatment of patients with node-negative breast cancer who have estrogen-receptor-positive tumors. *N Engl J Med* 1989; 320:479–484.
15. Fisher B, Dignam J, Bryant J, et al. Five versus more than 5 years of tamoxifen therapy for breast cancer patients with negative lymph nodes and estrogen receptor positive tumors. *J Natl Cancer Inst* 1996;88:1529–1542.
16. Baum M, Brinkley DM, Dossett JA, et al. Controlled trial of tamoxifen as a single adjuvant agent in the management of early breast cancer. Analysis at eight years by Nolvadex Adjuvant Trial Organisation. *Br J Cancer* 1988;57:608–611.
17. Breast Cancer Trials Committee, Scottish Cancer Trials Office. Adjuvant tamoxifen in the management of operable breast cancer: The Scottish trial. *Lancet* 1987; 2:171–175.
18. Rutqvist LE, Cedermark B, Glas U, et al. Contralateral primary tumors in breast cancer patients in a randomized trial of adjuvant tamoxifen therapy. *J Natl Cancer Inst* 1991;83:1299–1306.
19. CRC Adjuvant Breast Trial Working Party. Cyclophosphamide and tamoxifen as adjuvant therapies in the management of breast cancer. *Br J Cancer* 1988;57: 604–607.
20. Jordan VC. Effect of tamoxifen (ICI 46,474) on initiation and growth of DMBA-induced rat mammary carcinomata. *Eur J Cancer* 1976;12:419–424.
21. Jordan VC, Allen KE. Evaluation of the antitumor activity of the nonsteroidal antioestrogen monohydroxytamoxifen in the DMBA-induced rat mammary carcinoma model. *Eur J Cancer* 1980;16:239–251.
22. Fisher B, Dignam J, Wolmark N, et al. Tamoxifen in treatment of intraductal breast cancer: National Surgical Adjuvant Breast and Bowel Project B-24 randomised controlled trial. *Lancet* 1999;353:1993–2000.
23. Fisher B, Constantino JP, Wickerham DL, et al. Tamoxifen for prevention of breast cancer: report of the National Surgical Adjuvant Breast and Bowel Project P-1 Study. *J Natl Cancer Inst* 1998;90:1371–1388.
24. Recht A, Van Dongen JA, Fentiman IS, et al. Third Meeting of the DCIS Working Party of the EORTC (Fondazione Cini, Isola S. Giorgio, Venezia, 38 February 1994)-Conference Report. *Eur J Cancer* 1994; 30A:1895–1901.
25. Recht A, Rutgers EJTh, Fentiman IS, et al. The Fourth EORTC DCIS Consensus Meeting (Chateau Marquette, Heemskerk, The Netherlands, 23–24 January 1998)—Conference Report. *Eur J Cancer* 1998;34:1664–1669.

5

Should Surgeons Abandon Routine Axillary Dissection for Sentinel Node Biopsy in Early Breast Cancer?

Frederick L. Moffat, Jr. and David N. Krag

Regional lymph node status is the most significant pathological determinant of prognosis in breast cancer. Patients with nodal metastases are at much higher risk of breast cancer dissemination and mortality than pathological node-negative (pN-) patients, especially those with small primary tumors (1). Postoperative adjuvant systemic therapy significantly reduces the risk of development of systemic disease and death in pathological node-positive (pN+) patients. While pN- patients also benefit from adjuvant systemic therapy, the regimens used often differ from those employed for pN+ disease. The number of positive nodes is often a consideration in decisions regarding systemic adjuvant therapy. Detailed information on regional nodal status is therefore very important and is usually required for entry of patients into National Cancer Institute (NCI-US), other co-operative group-sponsored, and pharmaceutical industry clinical trials.

There is a great deal of enthusiasm among general and oncological surgeons for sentinel lymph node biopsy (SLNB), a term encompassing several technical variations on a new minimally invasive nodal staging operation. SLNB was brought to the attention of the entire surgical community by Morton et al. (2), who demonstrated that the first node(s) to receive lymph flow (and therefore metastasizing malignant cells) from a primary melanoma can be identified by peritumoral intradermal injection of vital blue dye.

Since that landmark paper, a wealth of published data has affirmed the validity of the sentinel lymph node (SLN) hypothesis in melanoma patients. There is now a consensus that, in the hands of experienced surgeons, SLNB in patients with clinical node-negative (cN-) melanoma is superior to either of the conventional options, these being observation alone or elective lymphadenectomy of at-risk nodal basins. This is valid only for melanoma, a disease in which, unlike breast cancer, occult nodal metastases are not only highly prejudicial to survival but almost invariably progress if left undisturbed.

Alex et al. (3) and Krag et al. (4) described a method of SLNB in which a radiocolloid, technetium Tc 99m sulfur colloid (^{99m}TcSC), was used as the SLN marking agent, and SLNB was performed using a gamma detection probe (GDP) to guide dissection directly to the SLN(s) by the shortest route from the overlying skin. A cutaneous hot spot denoting an underlying SLN was identified using the GDP, and SLNB was performed through an incision made at that point.

The use of blue dye alone, without radiocolloid, for labeling and identification of SLNs has been championed by Giuliano et al. (5–7). There is a modest but significant incidence of wound complications with this method due to the development of skin flaps while searching for blue-stained lymphatics (2). The surgical learning curve is significantly longer with blue dye alone as compared to radiocolloid with or without blue dye, and in the case of axillary SLNB, the extent of dissection required to find the SLN(s) can occasionally approach that of a standard lymphadenectomy. There is a very small incidence of permanent discoloration of skin and soft tissues with blue dye, and anaphylactic allergic reactions are seen in about 1% of cases in which isosulfan blue dye is used.

TABLE 5.1. Multicenter registry studies of SLNB in breast cancer

	No. Centers	No. Surgeons	No. Pts	SLN Localized	FN Rate
Wong 2001a (9)	N/A	148	1436	N/A	8.3%
Wong 2001b (10)	N/A	148	1415	90%	N/A
Dupont 2001 (11)	41	N/A	516	85%	N/A
Tafra 2001 (12)	N/A	48	529	87%	13%

N/A, not available.

EVIDENCE OF ACCURACY OF SLNB IN BREAST CANCER

Krag et al. (8) reported a prospective validation trial of SLNB in breast cancer. In this study, 11 surgeons in academic and community practice used a standardized SLNB technique in which radiocolloid was the sole SLN labeling agent. Numerous registry and single institution studies of SLNB in breast cancer patients using a variety of SLNB methodologies have since been published (Tables 5.1 and 5.2). There are also many reports on methodological variables such as type of radiocolloid, volume of radiocolloid injected, route of radiocolloid or blue dye injection (peritumoral/intraparenchymal, subdermal, intradermal), and time dependence of the various methods (36).

There has been a rapidly expanding literature on SLNB in breast cancer in which the results

TABLE 5.2. Single institution experience with SLNB in breast cancer

	No. Pts	No. pN+	SLN Localized	NPV	FN Rate
Blue Dye Only					
Giuliano 1994 (5)	174	62	66%	94%	11.9%
Giuliano 1996 (6)	114	25	64%	96%	8.0%
Giuliano 1997 (7)	107	42	93%	100%	0%
Guenther 1997 (13)	145	31	71%	96%	9.7%
Flett 1998 (14)	68	21	82%	94%	14.3%
Bobin 1999 (15)	100	42	83%	95%	5.0%
Morgan 1999 (16)	44	12	73%	91%	16.7%
Cserni 2000 (17)	70	39	83%	92%	7.7%
Haigh 2000 (18)	284	93	81%	98%	3.2%
Nos 2001 (19)	253	67	84%	96%	9.0%
Radiocolloid/GDP Only					
Alex 1996 (48)	70	21	71%	100%	0%
Veronesi 1997* (20)	163	85	98%	95%	4.7%
Roumen 1997 (21)	68	23	69%	97%	4.3%
Borgstein 1998 (22)	104	45	94%	98%	2.2%
Crossin 1998 (23)	50	8	84%	97%	12.5%
Minor 1998 (24)	42	7	98%	97%	14.3%
Snider 1998 (25)	80	14	88%	93%	7.0%
Rubio 1998 (26)	55	17	96%	95%	11.8%
Moffat 1999 (27)	70	20	89%	96%	10.0%
Offodile 1998 (28)	41	18	98%	100%	0%
Veronesi 1999* (29)	376	168	99%	94%	6.7%
Both Methods					
Albertini 1996 (30)	62	18	92%	100%	0%
Reintgen 1997 (31)	174	38	92%	99%	2.6%
Barnwell 1998 (32)	42	15	90%	100%	0%
Nwariaku 1998 (33)	119	27	81%	99%	3.7%
O'Hea 1998 (34)	60	20	93%	93%	15.0%
Hill 1999 (35)	104	47	92%	92%	10.6%

*Subdermal injection of radiocolloid (all other series were intraparenchymal/peritumoral).

and conclusions are significantly more variable than those in melanoma. Not surprisingly, therefore, there are significant differences of opinion between surgeons as to the routine use of SLNB and whether it can be substituted for routine axillary node dissection (AND) in clinical practice.

THE UNIVERSITY OF VERMONT MULTICENTER VALIDATION STUDY

The University of Vermont Multicenter Validation Study (8) was an NCI-sponsored prospective multi-center trial of SLNB in cN-, unifocal, invasive breast cancer utilizing a single method of SLN retrieval by 11 surgeons in both academic and community practice. Patients underwent SLNB using 1 mCi unfiltered ^{99m}TcSC in 4 mL normal saline injected peritumorally, and confirmatory AND was performed in all patients. Preoperative lymphoscintigraphy (LS) was not mandatory and blue dye was not used.

Of the 443 patients accrued, at least one cutaneous hot spot was localized in 413 patients (93.2%), and 114 patients proved to be pN+. SLNs were found outside the axilla (primarily in the internal mammary chain) in 8% of cases, and in 3% of all patients from whom one or more SLNs were removed, the positive SLNs were exclusively nonaxillary in location. The accuracy of the histological status of SLNs as compared to the axillary nodes was 97%, and the negative predictive value of SLNB was similarly favorable at 96%. However, among the 114 pN+ patients, the SLNs were negative for tumor in 13, a false-negative (FN) rate of 11.4%. All 13 patients with FN SLNBs had laterally situated cancers ($p = 0.004$). These FNs occurred most likely because of proximity of the axilla to the radioactive diffusion zone in the breast resulting from the intraparenchymal peritumoral injection of ^{99m}TcSC.

The radiocolloid diffusion zone in the breast significantly interferes with GDP localization of all SLNs (37,38), and is almost certainly an important factor for intersurgeon variation in FN rates. This diffusion zone, the size of which can vary markedly between patients, is an important factor in the surgical learning curve and FN rates. Nonetheless, SLN localization rates in this study and in single institution series in which radiocolloid/GDP methods are used generally exceed 90%.

The NCI, through collaboration between the National Surgical Adjuvant Breast and Bowel Project (NSABP) and the University of Vermont, is sponsoring the B-32 trial, a randomized phase 3 clinical trial comparing sentinel node resection to sentinel node resection plus conventional axillary dissection. Isosulfan blue dye is used in addition to radiocolloid, the blue dye being injected around the primary tumor intraoperatively, as SLN labeling with this marker is very time-dependent, unlike unfiltered ^{99m}TcSC. Suspicious nodes found during SLNB, which are deemed positive by palpation, are also removed and scored as SLNs.

MULTICENTER SLNB REGISTRY SERIES

There are now reports from multi-institutional SLNB registries in which participating academic and community surgeons underwent prior didactic and hands-on instruction in large animal models and, in some cases, initial direct supervision by training surgeons (Table 5.1). Most or all patients in these reports underwent concomitant AND.

The localization rates in these reports range from 85% to 90%, and FN rates from 8.3% to 13%, respectively. Once again, FN rates with SLNB were considerably in excess of the reported surgical understaging error rates of 2% to 3% for partial (levels I and II) axillary dissection, and 0% for total axillary lymphadenectomy (38).

SINGLE INSTITUTION SERIES IN WHICH CONFIRMATORY AND WAS PERFORMED

The surgical learning curve appears to be much longer when vital blue dye is used alone as compared to radiocolloid methods used with or without blue dye. Moreover, the dissection required to find blue-labeled nodes can be much more extensive without the aid of a GDP, as the dissection must trace blue-stained lymph vessels back towards the injection zone, as well as to SLNs, to ensure that any SLNs situated between the SLNB incision and the primary tumor are identified. The extent of dissection may occasionally approach that of AND.

In addition, localization rates tend to be lower when vital blue dye is used alone, ranging from 64% to 93%. By comparison, the localization rates for radiocolloid/GDP methods range from 71% to 99%, and for both methods used in combination, 81% to 100% (Table 5.2).

SLNB FN rates vary considerably, irrespective of the method used, and no method has a significant advantage over any other with respect to this very important statistic. For radiocolloid/GDP methods used alone, blue dye alone, and both nodal markers used in combination, FN rates ranged from 0% to 14.3%, 0% to 14.3% and 0% to 15%, respectively (Table 5.1). In general, the lowest reported rates are from single institution series, while higher rates predominate among multicenter studies.

SINGLE INSTITUTION STUDIES IN WHICH AND WAS NOT ROUTINELY PERFORMED

There are a few recent series reporting SLNB in breast cancer without confirmatory AND in most of the patients reported (31,35,39,40). These are from large academic institutions, which have invested considerable time and resources into developing SLNB for use in breast cancer. For the most part, these series consist of large numbers of patients operated upon consecutively by several surgeons in the institution. At varying times in the course of accruing patients, a number of variables such as type of radiocolloid, route of radiocolloid administration, type of GDP, etc., have been changed.

A number of guidelines and principles have been gleaned from these experiences, which may be of value to surgeons as they begin to learn how to do SLNB and acquire experience with this procedure.

The very low FN rates reported in some of these series, although calculated from only a subset of the patients studied, are a credit to the participating surgeons and institutions. However, it is by no means clear that these results can be replicated by the majority of surgeons in multiple institutions. Moreover, despite the authors' enthusiasm for SLNB without confirmatory AND, these reports do not include meaningful outcome data on long-term survival and regional disease control. These series offer no convincing evidence that SLNB should now replace AND in the management of breast cancer and should be considered evidence level 3, category C.

ONGOING METHODOLOGICAL DEVELOPMENTS IN SLNB FOR BREAST CANCER

SLNB is technically more challenging in breast cancer than melanoma, as noted above. The amount of dissection required when blue dye is used alone can be excessive, and the radioactive diffusion zone which results from intraparenchymal peritumoral injection of radiocolloid interferes significantly with GDP localization of some or all SLNs in individual patients.

A rapidly increasing number of communications in the peer-reviewed literature is focused on technical issues and modifications of existing methods (36). Krag et al. (37) and Linehan et al. (41) demonstrated superior SLN localization rates with unfiltered as compared to filtered ^{99m}TcSC. Krag et al. (37,42) have shown that the size of the radioactive diffusion zone does not vary significantly for volumes of radiocolloid injections above 4 mL, but larger volumes do improve SLN localization rates.

Alternative routes of radiocolloid administration are being investigated. Borgstein et al. (43) tested the hypothesis that the skin and parenchyma of the breast drain by the same lymphatic pathways to one or more common SLNs. In 30 consecutive patients, intradermally injected blue dye and peritumorally injected technetium Tc 99m colloidal albumin labeled the same lymph node(s). Confirmatory studies (44–46) have yielded similar results and excellent SLN localization rates. Intradermal, subdermal, and periareolar routes of injection avoid the problem of inadvertent injection of radiocolloid into the underlying pectoralis muscle or into breast biopsy cavities. With their expertise in radiocolloid injection and lymphoscintigraphy in melanoma, nuclear medicine physicians are more comfortable with these routes of administration. Moreover, the size of the diffusion zone at the injection site is much smaller and SLN radioactivity significantly greater than with peritumoral injection, which may facilitate superior SLN localization and reduced FN rates. The NSABP B-32 protocol has recently been modified to include an additional 0.2 mCi of unfiltered ^{99m}TcSC in 0.05 mL saline to be injected intradermally over the tumor.

Intradermal or subareolar injection of SLN labeling agents may contribute significantly to the simplification and standardization of the procedure and shortening of the surgical learning curve, expediting the evolution of a broad evidence-based consensus that SLNB should indeed replace AND as the standard nodal staging operation in breast cancer.

PROSPECTIVE RANDOMIZED COOPERATIVE GROUP TRIALS IN PROGRESS

Two prospective randomized cooperative group trials are open for accrual in the United States. The NSABP B-32 protocol randomly assigns patients with unifocal cN- breast cancer to SLNB plus AND or SLNB alone. The SLNs from patients, randomized to SLNB alone, are examined by a touch preparation technique intraoperatively. If the SLNs are found to be involved by tumor on touch preps or on subsequent paraffin section histology, AND is performed. The primary clinical endpoints are overall and disease-free survival, regional control, and morbidity. An ancillary pathology study conducted at all sites will determine the impact of occult metastases on survival. SLNs negative for metastases by routine H&E histopathology will be evaluated in a blinded fashion by immunohistochemistry using an anticytokeratin antibody cocktail. In addition, a detailed quality of life evaluation is being conducted at participating CCOP institutions. About 40% of the 5,400 patients required by the protocol have been accrued as of October, 2001. B-32 is now one of the fastest accruing breast cancer treatment trials under the aegis of NSABP.

Surgeons wishing to participate in NSABP B-32 are carefully trained and monitored through their early experience in a manner essentially identical to that employed in the University of Vermont trial. Experienced surgeon-trainers (core trainers) are sent out to train surgeons in their own institutions. The core trainer conducting the site visit meets with institutional operating room nursing staff, Nuclear Medicine, Radiology, and Pathology to discuss aspects of the protocol relevant to these personnel and departments. An exhaustive review of the protocol is undertaken on site with the surgeon(s) to be trained (maximum two surgeon trainees per site visit). The core trainer scrubs into at least one case with each surgical trainee to go over the SLNB technique prescribed by the protocol and to demonstrate the surgical steps to be taken in the event of initial failure of lymphatic mapping. The trainee is then required to complete 5 training cases of SLNB with immediate axillary dissection. These cases are reviewed in detail in a telephone interview with the core trainer. If it is ascertained that the surgeon trainee has the SLNB technique and B-32 protocol particulars well in hand, he or she is approved to accrue patients for randomization. Telephone reviews are then conducted after completion of the 10th, 20th, and 30th randomized cases for quality assurance.

The American College of Surgeons Oncology Group has chosen a different experimental design. A total of 7,600 patients with unifocal invasive clinical node-negative breast cancer are to be registered to undergo SLNB (protocol Z0010) in order to identify 1,900 pN+ patients for randomization (protocol Z0011). The two arms into which these 1,900 Z0011 patients are randomized are no further regional nodal surgery and AND. The primary clinical endpoints for Z0011 are essentially the same as those for NSABP B-32, the difference being that the

Z0011 study population is entirely pN+. The remaining 5,700 patients in protocol Z0010 (H&E-negative SLNs) undergo no further surgery, but their SLNs are analyzed in a blinded fashion by serial sections and immunohistochemistry. Patients in Z0010 will then be followed for survival.

Institutions wishing to participate in the ACoSOG are required to submit 20 cases in which SLNB and confirmatory AND have been performed. Approval for participation is given if the SLN localization rate is at least 90% and the FN rate no higher than 10%. There are no formal site visits for training surgeons, and the SLNB technique to be used is at the discretion of each participating surgeon.

Other prospective cooperative trials of SLNB in breast cancer are planned or underway elsewhere, such as the Medical Research Council ALMANAC trial in Great Britain.

CONCLUSION

There are several decades of data and experience with AND in cooperative trials groups. These demonstrate that the results obtained by breast surgeons in different practice settings in the United States and Europe are excellent and highly reproducible. Most importantly, the long-term survival and regional disease control outcomes with axillary dissection are well established. The same cannot be said of SLNB. Only a modest proportion of surgeons who currently manage breast cancer have had any experience with SLNB. Not only are the long-term results of SLNB alone not known, there is not even a consensus on how SLNB is best performed. This is a serious issue since the results to date with this new procedure remain highly variable. The variability in FN rates is especially troubling given that this is the most significant (albeit hard to measure) parameter of clinical accuracy.

In a survey of 1,000 randomly selected Fellows of the American College of Surgeons, Lucci et al. (47) reported that among the 410 respondents, 77% (316) performed SLNB in breast cancer patients. Of these, 90% used both blue dye and radiocolloid. It is encouraging to note that 55% performed SLNB as part of a clinical trial. Instruction in SLNB was obtained through courses by 35%, surgical oncology fellowships by 26%, and observation of colleagues by 31%. Over one-fourth of respondents (26%) were self-taught. Twenty-eight percent performed 10 or fewer SLNBs with concomitant AND before performing SLNB alone, and only 28% removed nonaxillary sentinel nodes identified by preoperative lymphoscintigraphy or intraoperative mapping of hot spots. These sobering data suggest a marked heterogeneity in expertise among surgeons who perform SLNB in breast cancer, and both highlight and heighten concerns about quality control and FN rates.

Clearly much remains to be done before SLNB can be considered a comparable or superior alternative for staging of the regional lymphatics in breast cancer. Most importantly, it remains to be established that SLNB results in the same cure rate and long-term control of regional nodal disease as AND does. Surgeons who have not yet begun to learn this technique now have the opportunity to participate in one of the cooperative group clinical trials now open for accrual. Participants in NSABP B-32 receive hands-on training in their own operating rooms and their experience is carefully monitored by their surgeon-mentors so that deficiencies or protocol violations are quickly identified and rectified. The randomized trials (B-32 and Z0011) offer the best opportunity to establish that performing SLNB alone in breast cancer patients will result in long-term treatment outcomes equivalent to those of AND while minimizing short- and long-term surgical morbidity.

REFERENCES

1. Dees EC, Shulman LN, Souba WW, et al. Does information from axillary dissection change treatment in clinically node-negative patients with breast cancer? An algorithm for assessment of impact of axillary dissection. *Ann Surg* 1997;226:279–287.
2. Morton DL, Wen D-R, Wong JH, et al. Technical details of intraoperative lymphatic mapping for early stage melanoma. *Arch Surg* 1992;27:392–399.

3. Alex JC, Weaver DL, Fairbank JT, et al. Gamma probe guided lymph node localization in malignant melanoma. *Surg Oncol* 1993;2:303–308.
4. Krag DN, Weaver DL, Alex JC, Fairbank JT. Surgical resection and radiolocalization of the sentinel node in breast cancer using a gamma probe. *Surg Oncol* 1993b;2:335–340.
5. Giuliano AE, Kirgan DM, Guenther JM, et al. Lymphatic mapping and sentinel lymphadenectomy for breast cancer. *Ann Surg* 1994;220:391–401.
6. Giuliano AE, Barth AM, Spivack B, et al. Incidence and predictors of axillary metastasis in T1 carcinoma of the breast. *J Amer Coll Surg* 1996;193:185–189.
7. Giuliano AE, Jones RC, Brennan M, et al. Sentinel lymphadenectomy in breast cancer. *J Clin Oncol* 1997;15:2345–2350.
8. Krag DN, Weaver DL, Ashkaga T, et al. The sentinel node in breast cancer. A multicenter validation study. *New Engl J Med* 1998a;339:941–946.
9. Wong SL, Edwards MJ, Chao C, et al. Sentinel lymph node biopsy for breast cancer: impact of the number of sentinel nodes removed on the false-negative rate. *J Amer Coll Surg* 2001a;192:684–691.
10. Wong SL, Edwards MJ, Chao C, et al. Predicting the status of the nonsentinel axillary nodes. A multicenter study. *Arch Surg* 2001b;136:563–568.
11. Dupont EL, Kamath VJ, Ramnath EM, et al. The role of lymphoscintigraphy in the management of the patient with breast cancer. *Ann Surg Oncol* 2001;8:354–360.
12. Tafra L, Lannin DR, Swanson MS, et al. Multicenter trial of sentinel node biopsy for breast cancer using both technetium sulfur colloid and isosulfan blue dye. *Ann Surg* 2001;233:51–59.
13. Guenther JM, Krishnamoorthy M, Tan LR. Sentinel lymphadenectomy for breast cancer in a community managed care setting. *Cancer J Sci Am* 1997;3:336–340.
14. Flett MM, Going JJ, Stanton PD, et al. Sentinel node localization in patients with breast cancer. *Br J Surg* 1998;85:991–993.
15. Bobin J-Y, Zinzindohoue C, Isaac S, et al. Tagging sentinel lymph nodes: a study of 100 patients with breast cancer. *Eur J Cancer* 1999;35:569–573.
16. Morgan A, Howisey RL, Aldape HC, et al. Initial experience in a community hospital with sentinel lymph node mapping and biopsy for evaluation of axillary lymph node status in palpable invasive breast cancer. *J Surg Oncol* 1999;72:24–31.
17. Cserni T, Boross G, Baltas BN, et al. Value of axillary sentinel nodal status in breast cancer. *World J Surg* 2000;24:341–344.
18. Haigh PI, Hansen NM, Qi K, Giuliano AE. Biopsy method and excision volume do not affect success rate of subsequent sentinel lymph node dissection in breast cancer. *Ann Surg Oncol* 2000;7:21–27.
19. Nos C, Freneaux P, Guilbert S, et al. Sentinel lymph node detection for breast cancer: which patients are best suited for the patent blue dye only method of identification. *Ann Surg Oncol* 2001;8:438–443.
20. Veronesi U, Paganelli G, Galimberti V, et al. Sentinel node biopsy to avoid axillary dissection in breast cancer with clinically negative nodes. *Lancet* 1997;349:1864–1867.
21. Roumen RMH, Valkenburg JGM, Geuskens LM. Lymphoscintigraphy and feasibility of sentinel node biopsy in 83 patients with primary breast cancer. *Eur J Surg Oncol* 1997;23:495–502.
22. Borgstein PJ, Pijpers R, Comans EF, et al. Sentinel lymph node biopsy in breast cancer: guidelines and pitfalls of lymphoscintigraphy and gamma probe detection. *J Amer Coll Surg* 1998;186:275–283.
23. Crossin JA, Johnson AC, Stewart PB, et al. Gamma probe guided resection of the sentinel lymph node in breast cancer. *Amer Surg* 1998;64:666–668.
24. Miner TJ, Shriver CD, Jaques DP, et al. Ultrasonographically guided injection improves localization of the radiolabeled sentinel lymph node in breast cancer. *Ann Surg Oncol* 1998;5:315–321.
25. Snider HS, Dowlatshahi K, Fan M, et al. Sentinel node biopsy in the staging of breast cancer. *Amer J Surg* 1998;176:305–310.
26. Rubio IT, Korourian S, Cowan C, et al. Sentinel lymph node biopsy for staging breast cancer. *Amer J Surg* 1998;176:305–310.
27. Moffat FL, Gulec SA, Sittler SY, et al. Unfiltered sulphur colloid and sentinel node biopsy for breast cancer: technical and kinetic considerations. *Ann Surg Oncol* 1999;6:746–755.
28. Offodile R, Hoh C, Barsky SH, et al. Minimally invasive breast carcinoma staging using lymphatic mapping with radiolabeled dextran. *Cancer* 1998;82:1704–1708.
29. Veronesi U, Paganelli G, Viale G, et al. Sentinel lymph node biopsy and axillary dissection in breast cancer: results in a large series. *J Natl Cancer Inst* 1999;91:368–373.
30. Albertini JJ, Lyman GH, Cox C, et al. Lymphatic mapping and sentinel node biopsy in patients with breast cancer. *JAMA* 1996;276:1818–1822.
31. Reintgen DS, Joseph E, Lyman GH, et al. The role of selective lymphadenectomy in breast cancer. *Cancer Control (MCC)* 1997;4:211–219.
32. Barnwell JM, Arredondo MA, Kollmorgen D, et al. Sentinel node biopsy in breast cancer. *Ann Surg Oncol* 1998;5:126–130.
33. Nwariaku FE, Euhus DM, Beitsch PD, et al. Sentinel lymph node biopsy, an alternative to elective axillary dissection for breast cancer. *Amer J Surg* 1998;176:529–531.
34. O'Hea BJ, Hill ADK, El-Shirbiny AM, et al. Sentinel lymph node biopsy in breast cancer: initial experience at Memorial Sloan-Kettering Cancer Center. *J Amer Coll Surg* 1998;186:423–427.
35. Hill ADK, Tran KN, Akhurst T, et al. Lessons learned from 500 cases of lymphatic mapping for breast cancer. *Ann Surg* 1999;229:528–531.
36. Keshtegar MRS, Ell PJ. Sentinel lymph node detection and imaging. *Eur J Nucl Med* 1999;26:57–67.
37. Krag DN, Ashkaga T, Harlow SP, et al. Development of sentinel node targeting technique in breast cancer patients. *Breast J* 1998b;4:67–74.
38. Moffat FL, Senofsky GM, Clark KC, et al. Axillary node dissection for early breast cancer: some is good but all is better. *J Surg Oncol* 1992;51:8–13.
39. Cox CE, Pendas S, Cox JM, et al. Guidelines for sentinel node biopsy and lymphatic mapping in patients with breast cancer. *Ann Surg* 1998;227:645–653.

40. Cox CE, Haddad F, Bass S, et al. Lymphatic mapping in the treatment of breast cancer. *Oncology* 1998;12:1283–1298.
41. Linehan DC, Hill ADK, Tran KN, et al. Sentinel lymph node biopsy in breast cancer: unfiltered isotope is superior to filtered. *J Am Coll Surg* 1999a;188:377–381.
42. Krag DN. Minimal access surgery for staging regional lymph nodes: the sentinel node concept. *Curr Probl Surg* 1998c;35:951–1018.
43. Borgstein PJ, Meijer S, Pijpers R. Intradermal blue dye to identify sentinel lymph node in breast cancer. *Lancet* 1997;349:1668–1669.
44. Borgstein PJ, Meijer S, Pijpers RJ, van Dienst PJ. Functional lymphatic anatomy for sentinel node biopsy in breast cancer. *Ann Surg* 2000;232:81–89.
45. Klimberg VS, Rubio IT, Henry R, et al. Subareolar versus peritumoral injection for location of the sentinel lymph node. *Ann Surg* 1999;229:860–865.
46. Linehan DC, Hill ADK, Akhurst T, et al. Intradermal radiocolloid and intraparenchymal blue dye injection optimize sentinel node identification in breast cancer patients. *Ann Surg Oncol* 1999b;6:450–454.
47. Lucci A Jr., Kelemen PR, Miller C III, et al. National practice patterns of sentinel lymph node dissection for breast carcinoma. *J Amer Coll Surg* 2001;192:453–458.
48. Alex JC, Krag DN. The gamma probe-guided resection of radiolabeled primary lymph nodes. *Surg Oncol Clin North Am* 1996;5:33–41.

6
Surgical Considerations in Breast Cancer Patients Treated with Preoperative Chemotherapy

Harry D. Bear

Since Haagensen (1) outlined criteria of inoperability for breast cancer, primary surgery, even radical mastectomy, has been considered inappropriate for certain patients, particularly those now staged as IIIB. For these women with locally advanced breast cancers (LABC), surgery failed to alter the clinical outcome because nearly all cases succumbed to systemic metastases. When effective chemotherapy became available in the 1970s, this became the primary or first treatment modality offered to these patients. The addition of chemotherapy for LABC has arguably increased survival for these patients, although it has not been shown convincingly that it is really the sequence of treatments, rather than the addition of effective systemic treatment at any time, that is responsible for this improvement.

As primary chemotherapy (also called neoadjuvant, induction or preoperative chemotherapy) improved, the responses of primary tumors became more impressive, and the survival of patients with LABC increased. Surgical attitudes about local treatment then evolved towards a more aggressive approach for patients who now had a reasonable chance at long-term survival. Recently, as a result of the dramatic shrinkage in local and regional disease induced by anthracycline-based chemotherapy, use of breast conservation in some of these patients has become feasible. Even more recently, the use of primary chemotherapy has been proposed for less advanced cancers, based partly on theoretical considerations related to the possibility of improved survival and to make breast conservation treatment (BCT) feasible in women with large primary tumors. For both locally advanced and early stage breast cancer, elimination of any surgical treatment of the primary tumor and/or lymph nodes after primary chemotherapy has also been described. The biologic and clinical rationale favoring primary or neoadjuvant chemotherapy is summarized in Table 6.1.

The surgical issues that will be addressed here relate to several key questions about patients with breast cancer who, for whatever reason, are treated with primary chemotherapy. These questions include: (a) Should women with LABC, either inflammatory or non-inflammatory, undergo mastectomy even if they respond well to chemotherapy, or can breast conservation be attempted? (b) In women with operable breast cancer, is it appropriate to use primary chemotherapy for the purpose of making breast conservation feasible? (c) If a complete clinical response (i.e., disappearance of palpable tumor) occurs with chemotherapy, is any surgical excision or lumpectomy necessary? (d) If lumpectomy is to be done, how does one ensure that the site of the original tumor is actually resected after a clinical complete response (CR)? (e) Is surgical/pathologic staging of the axillary nodes useful after chemotherapy? (f) Can the new technique of sentinel lymph node mapping be used instead of full axillary node dissection in the post-chemotherapy setting?

Prospective trials have been designed to evaluate the choice of local therapy after chemotherapy. However, in many series, the choice of local therapy was dependent on the response to systemic treatment and not a result of random allocation. Thus, it can be difficult to derive reliable conclusions about some aspects of surgical management. When the evidence is inconclusive, appropriate op-

TABLE 6.1. *Rationale for preoperative chemotherapy*

Biologic Rationale	
Removal of primary tumor may accelerate growth of micrometastases	
Serum growth factors	(Gunduz et al., 1979; Fisher et al., 1983) (78, 79)
Removal of source of angiostatins	(O'Reilly et al., 1994; O'Reilly et al., 1996) (80, 81)
Increased likelihood of chemoresistant clones with increased tumor burden	(Goldie and Coldman, 1979) (82)
Test of Skipper hypothesis, that primary and metastatic clones may respond differently to chemotherapy	(Skipper, 1971) (83)
Clinical Rationale	
Make unresectable tumors operable	(Hortobagyi et al., 1983; Hortobagyi, 1994; Gardin et al., 1995; Perez et al., 1997)(84–87)
Make breast conservation feasible for large tumors	(Mauriac et al., 1991; Schwartz et al., 1994; Scholl et al., 1994; Hortobagyi et al., 1995; Fisher et al., 1998; Bonadonna et al., 1998) (12, 31, 33, 38, 45, 88)
Allows objective assessment of response	(Fisher et al., 1998) (38)
More rapid assessment of new drugs and regimens	
Correlation of pathologic and molecular markers with response to treatment	

tions will be offered, based on what evidence does exist.

THE ROLE OF MASTECTOMY AFTER PRIMARY CHEMOTHERAPY FOR LABC

In a review of the history of primary chemotherapy for LABC, it is important to remember that the starting assumption during the 1950s through the 1970s was that surgery was contraindicated for most of these patients. Until effective systemic agents became available, the primary modality used in this setting was radiotherapy (2,3). This was moderately effective at controlling local disease, but since most of these patients succumbed fairly rapidly to systemic disease, long-term locoregional control was not a major issue.

When effective systemic therapy began to be used for patients with LABC, the most common approach to local therapy remained radiotherapy. With more prolonged survival, however, the inability of standard doses of radiation to control local disease became evident (4–6). This led to the use of higher doses of radiation and the reintroduction of surgery, including mastectomy. While higher doses of radiation can be more effective than standard doses, the morbidity also tends to be higher, with an increase in poor cosmetic outcome (5,7). A number of series have evaluated the choice of local treatment options in the context of LABC treated with neoadjuvant chemotherapy. We will consider inflammatory and non-inflammatory LABC separately, although some series include both types together.

NON-INFLAMMATORY LOCALLY ADVANCED BREAST CANCER

Once it had been shown that chemotherapy might improve survival in patients with LABC and could convert previously inoperable patients into surgical candidates, the possibility of breast conservation with good long-term local control began to be considered. Interpreting the literature in this area is hampered by the fact that some series mix widely varying groups of patients together, including some that are not really inoperable. The breast-conserving approach for LABC grew out of a historical convergence of the hopelessness of primary mastectomy for LABC, the rise of breast-conserving treatment (BCT) for early-stage breast cancer, and the dramatic tumor regressions seen with primary chemotherapy. In 1986, Héry et al. (5) reported on 25 patients with LABC treated with primary chemotherapy followed by breast and nodal irradiation. Unfortunately, almost one-fourth (24%) of these women later required mastectomy for local recurrences. A number of randomized trials have examined the issue of local treatment options for LABC after primary chemotherapy, but these have mostly been comparisons of mastectomy alone versus radiation alone (without even gross tumor excision). At the National Cancer Institute of Milan, mastectomy was compared to radiotherapy after three cycles of doxorubicin hydrochloride and vincristine, with more chemotherapy after local treatment (4). Although survival and other endpoints were not different between the treatment groups, all patients experienced a locoregional recurrence rate of approximately 30%. A United States trial conducted by the CALGB also evaluated mastectomy alone versus radiation alone after primary chemotherapy (8). Local treatment did not significantly affect survival or distant metastases, but only a selected subset of patients (91 out of 113) who became operable after chemotherapy was considered evaluable. And, although local control rates were similar in the two groups, local relapses rates were 19% and 27% for surgery and radiotherapy, respectively. Although not compared directly to breast-conserving treatment or to mastectomy alone, the highest local control rates have generally been obtained with the combination of mastectomy and radiation after chemotherapy (6,7,9). In 1992, however, the MD Anderson group reported on a retrospective analysis of mastectomy specimens from women who had undergone induction chemotherapy for locally advanced breast cancer, and concluded that 23% of the patients able to be evaluated could theoretically have undergone breast-conserving treatment (10). More recently, they have reported a high success rate for treatment of noninflammatory LABC with breast conservation following induction chemotherapy, as long as strict selection criteria were used (11). Schwartz et al. (12) have also reported on the selective use of BCT after chemotherapy for women presenting with LABC, with only one patient out of 55 experiencing local recurrence.

Pierce et al. (7) at the U.S. National Cancer Institute (NCI) reported a prospective series of patients with LABC treated with primary chemotherapy and then selected for BCT if they had a clinical CR and if multiple needle biopsies showed no tumor. These highly selected 31 patients (out of an initial group of 107) were then treated with radiation with 16% developing locoregional failure. This was higher than the local failure rate (4%) following mastectomy plus radiotherapy (RT) and led the authors to conclude that mastectomy was preferred treatment for these patients, regardless of local response to chemotherapy. The 16% recurrence rate is still lower than rates seen when radiation alone has been used less selectively. Moreover, the accuracy of needle biopsies in this report may be questioned, particularly in light of pathologic CR rates with chemotherapy in most recent series in the range of 10% or less. Thus, they probably underestimated the frequency and extent of residual disease in the breast. A more recent report of the NCI experience indicated that patients with noninflammatory LABC and negative biopsies after chemotherapy, and treated with RT alone had only a 4.5% rate of breast recurrence (13). In part, the forces that drive decisions about local therapy and understanding results in patients treated with primary chemotherapy relate to the prognostic relevance of response to chemotherapy (discussed in detail below). Because a poor response to chemotherapy indicates higher likelihood of distant failure and death, local control is less likely to be relevant in these patients. For this reason, if mastectomy is used only for patients who respond poorly to chemotherapy, one might get the impression that mastectomy is associated with a poor outcome. Conversely, if patients who respond poorly to chemotherapy are treated with radiation only, then one might erroneously conclude that mastectomy actually improves outcome.

For LABC patients with an incomplete response to primary chemotherapy, the choice of local treatment depends on technical operability. If a patient's tumor is inoperable after chemotherapy, then radiotherapy should be used, and mastectomy added later if the tumor becomes

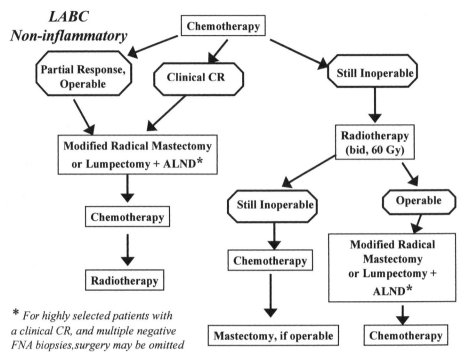

FIG. 6.1. Algorithm illustrating strategy for management of non-inflammatory locally advanced, inoperable breast cancer.
ALND, axillary lymph node dissection; LABC, locally advanced breast cancer.

operable after radiation. An alternative that can now be considered, after a trial of doxorubicin hydrochloride-based chemotherapy, would be taxane-based therapy, and then reassessment for operability (14–21). For patients who become operable after chemotherapy but who fail to meet the criteria for BCT (i.e., tumor size too large relative to breast size, presence of "grave signs," or evidence of multicentric disease), mastectomy should be performed, usually followed by radiation to the chest wall, particularly for positive nodes or a tumor more than 4 to 7 cm in diameter. For those who do meet standard BCT criteria, segmental mastectomy can be performed, and if negative margins can be achieved, the breast should then be irradiated. The grade of evidence for using BCT after chemotherapy for patients with LABC should be categorized as B. Until we have a good way to determine that a patient has had a complete pathologic CR, the use of radiation alone should probably not be considered standard treatment for most patients who present with a large mass. However, we have used this approach very selectively in a few patients, with aggressive twice-a-day radiotherapy to the breast, if there is no clinical evidence of residual tumor *and* multiple needle biopsies are negative. Our current treatment algorithm for noninflammatory LABC is shown in Figure 6.1. Although administration of additional chemotherapy after surgery is indicated as our standard, especially after an incomplete response, the data for this is soft. However, this question is beyond the scope of issues being addressed in this chapter.

INFLAMMATORY BREAST CANCER

Historically, this group of patients had the worst prognosis of all women with non-metastatic breast cancer, with 5-year survival rates of 10% or less. With aggressive systemic therapy, the expected 5-year survival for these women now approaches 50% (22). Local control was, relatively speaking, a less important problem when most of these women succumbed early to distant disease, but control of disease in the breast has now become a significant issue. It is generally agreed that these women should be treated with aggressive systemic chemotherapy and regional radiotherapy, but the role of mastectomy in these women is more controversial than for other patients with LABC. Many consider mastectomy-plus-radiation to be standard local therapy for inflammatory breast cancer. A 1996 report from M.D. Anderson (22) indicated that the results for patients with inflammatory breast cancer were similar with mastectomy plus RT compared to RT alone with an overall locoregional control rate of 82%. A more recent report from the same institution, however, suggested that local control and survival may actually be improved by the addition of mastectomy (23). The choice of local therapy in these 172 patients with inflammatory breast cancer was made according to criteria that evolved during the course of the experience reported. All patients were treated with primary doxorubicin hydrochloride-based chemotherapy. Patients who underwent mastectomy-plus-RT had a lower incidence of local recurrence (16.3%) than those treated with radiation alone (35.7%), but this advantage was confined to the patients with a partial response to chemotherapy. These authors also indicated an improvement in disease-free survival with mastectomy for patients who had either CR or PR to induction chemotherapy. Although they claim no systematic bias in favor of mastectomy, patients were not randomly allocated to locoregional treatment. Similar conclusions have been reached by other groups, and it has also been suggested that negative surgical margins may be particularly important in inflammatory breast cancer (24,25). The impact of negative margins was taken as evidence that an aggressive surgical approach is justified, but this correlation more likely reflects the response to chemotherapy rather than the adequacy of surgery. In some series, the decision to proceed to mastectomy was based on the response to systemic treatment, with patients achieving the best responses to chemotherapy chosen for mastectomy, while non-responders were relegated to radiation alone. Obviously, this would bias the results in favor of those treated with mastectomy (25–29). In contrast, in a group of patients with inflammatory breast cancer treated at the NCI who received radiation alone after pathologic CR to chemotherapy, the local recurrence rate was 38.9%, which was much worse than for noninflammatory LABC patients treated with breast conservation (13).

We have prospectively evaluated the use of accelerated super-fractionated radiation alone after chemotherapy in women with inflammatory breast cancer and found that most patients who had a CR to chemotherapy plus aggressive RT avoided mastectomy in the long-term (30). The overall breast preservation rate was 74%. Among 15 patients with a CR after induction chemotherapy, 87% remained locally controlled without mastectomy. It should be noted, however, that breast conservation was carefully chosen for those patients with no evidence of disease after chemotherapy plus RT, as determined by physical exam, mammography, and multiple fine needle aspiration biopsies. The latter technique, because of its ability to sample multiple areas of the breast tissue, might actually be more accurate than surgical or core needle biopsy.

Our own data suggest that breast conservation is feasible and safe in some of these patients, particularly if they have good response to induction chemotherapy, although this is the same group that apparently benefited most from mastectomy in the M.D. Anderson series. In the absence of definitive evidence on either side, the decision to perform or omit mastectomy for patients with inflammatory breast cancer must be individualized and based partly on philosophy. To some physicians and patients, the importance of breast conservation seems less relevant when overall survival is poor. On the other hand, as survival has improved, breast conservation has become a reasonable secondary objective, as long as it does not compromise survival. A suggested algorithm for inflammatory breast cancer, which we use as a guide to treatment decisions, is shown in Figure 6.2. Note that for women with a large mass and inflammatory changes, the local treatment follows the guidelines for other LABC patients, as shown in Figure 6.1. If a large mass, in addition to the inflammatory component, is present at diagnosis, we suggest lumpectomy or mastectomy as dictated by the residual mass after chemotherapy. Clearly, the role of BCT for inflammatory

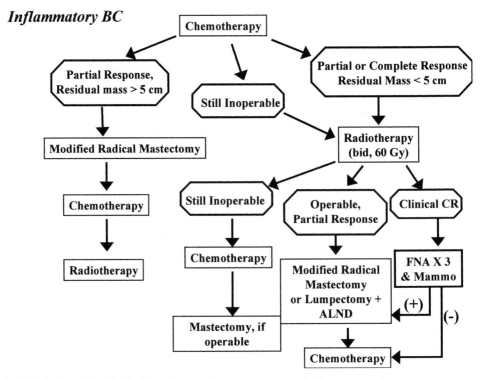

FIG. 6.2. Algorithm illustrating strategy for management of inflammatory breast cancer.

breast cancer remains unsettled. The existing evidence on this point is level III or IV, and the overall grade for recommending BCT for inflammatory breast cancer is category C.

USING PRIMARY CHEMOTHERAPY TO MAKE OPERABLE PATIENTS WITH LARGE BREAST CANCERS CANDIDATES FOR BREAST CONSERVATION

A number of non-randomized series have described use of preoperative chemotherapy in patients with operable breast cancers. As with LABC, many of these publications include patients ranging from stage II to stage IIIB and different endpoints are reported. The National Cancer Institute of Milan reported a series of 536 patients with tumors more than 2.5 cm in diameter. Using a variety of different chemotherapy regimens, 85% of these patients could be treated with breast conservation (lumpectomy plus radiation) (31). Although the rate of breast conservation in this report was high, many of these patients would likely have been considered suitable for BCT without prior chemotherapy in the United States. Despite a high rate of overall objective responses (76%), only 16% of the Milan patients had clinical CRs and only 3% had pathologic CR. Calais et al. (32) reported a prospective series of 158 patients with tumors more than 3 cm who were treated with primary chemotherapy. Subsequent therapy was determined according to response: patients with a clinical CR underwent radiation followed by more of the same chemotherapy as given initially; those with a partial response and tumor less than 3 cm after chemotherapy underwent lumpectomy plus radiation and more cycles of the same chemotherapy; non-responders underwent mastectomy plus radiation and then chemotherapy with different agents. Approximately 60% of the patients had objective responses and 20% had clinical CRs. BCT was possible in 49% of the patients, with only 7.8% experiencing local recurrences. Median follow-up at the time of this report was only 38 months. Not surprisingly, the 5-year survival rate was higher for responders (89.7%) than for non-responders who had mastectomies (57.3%). While this study could have been interpreted as showing that mastectomy was associated with decreased survival, the selection criteria for local treatment, rather than the local treatment itself, accounts for this difference.

A number of randomized trials have been carried out comparing primary chemotherapy to the more standard approach of adjuvant chemotherapy administered after local treatment. While these studies were not designed to address local therapy issues per se, they do offer important insights into the biology of local control after primary chemotherapy. Mauriac et al. (33) randomized 272 women with breast cancers more than 3 cm to modified radical mastectomy followed by chemotherapy versus chemotherapy followed by local treatment. In the latter group, 62.6% had BCT, and 44 patients had radiation only as local treatment (see below). In the early report of the trial, the preoperative chemotherapy group appeared to have an improved survival rate. It is important to note that chemotherapy was only given to patients in the primary mastectomy group if they were node-positive or ER-negative. Therefore, while *all* of the patients randomized to primary chemotherapy actually received chemotherapy, only 104 of the 138 primary mastectomy patients received drug treatment. This difference, rather than the sequence of treatments, probably accounts for the early survival difference. The more recent update with median follow-up of 124 months reveals that the survival advantage for the neoadjuvant group had disappeared (34). Local recurrence was higher in the primary chemotherapy group (23% isolated local recurrences as first site of relapse, versus 8.7% in the primary surgery group). This is not unexpected, but it doesn't necessarily mean that breast conservation is inappropriate for this group of patients. As discussed below, this high local recurrence rate was partly the result of inadequate local treatment, Scholl et al. (35) randomized 414 patients (T2 or T3, N0 or N1) to cyclophosphamide, Adriamycin, and 5-fluorouracil (CAF) in four cycles followed by radiation versus radiation followed by CAF in four cycles. Surgery was only used in patients who had a persistent mass after completing radiation, regardless of sequence. Breast conservation was possible in 82% of the primary chemotherapy group and in 77% of the primary radiation group. Survival at 5 years was also not significantly better in the primary chemotherapy group (86% versus 78%), despite the fact that the neoadjuvant chemotherapy patients received higher-intensity dose treatment, and 13% of the patients in the adjuvant group did not receive chemotherapy at all. In terms of local treatment, this series again shows that BCT is feasible in women with larger tumors, but can be achieved with either primary radiation or chemotherapy. The overall local recurrence rate for the primary chemotherapy group was 24%, and 37 out of 164 women initially treated with BCT eventually had mastectomies for ipsilateral breast tumor recurrences (IBTR); the 5-year actuarial breast preservation rate was 61%. In the United Kingdom, Powles et al. (36) carried out a randomized trial comparing neoadjuvant chemotherapy plus postoperative chemotherapy to standard chemotherapy given for the same number of cycles after surgery. The preoperative chemotherapy approach decreased the need for mastectomy (28% to 13%), but with only 200 patients in the trial, it is underpowered to reach any firm conclusions about outcomes.

The largest reported randomized trial comparing primary chemotherapy to standard postoperative chemotherapy was National Surgical Adjuvant Breast and Bowel Project (NSABP) Protocol B-18, in which 1,523 patients were randomized to preoperative or postoperative chemotherapy with four cycles of cyclophosphamide (AC) (37,38). Among 683 preoperative chemotherapy patients evaluatable for tumor response, the overall response rate to primary chemotherapy was 79%. Although 36% of patients had clinical CRs, only 13% had pathologic CRs, including 4% who had residual *in situ* disease only. Preoperative chemotherapy with four cycles of AC was associated with a statistically significant increase in the rate of BCT compared to primary surgical treatment (68% versus 60%), but survival at 5 years was virtually identical in the two treatment groups. This trial provides level I evidence for the conclusion that primary or preoperative chemotherapy is just as effective as standard postoperative adjuvant chemotherapy in terms of survival. Thus, it is considered safe to use neoadjuvant chemotherapy to shrink tumors and, where appropriate, to offer BCT to women with large operable tumors, without compromising survival. The IBTR rate was similar in both arms of this trial (7.9% for pre-op and 5.8% for post-op chemotherapy), but the IBTR rate was higher (15%) in the subset of patients who were converted to lumpectomy candidates by administering preoperative chemotherapy, even though negative margins were required in all patients (38). This might have been improved upon by the use of a radiation boost to the tumor bed (not allowed by the protocol) or by administration of tamoxifen citrate to pre-menopausal ER-positive women, whose risk for local recurrence was higher than for older women. The NSABP result raises questions about the biology of a tumor that shrinks during chemotherapy and the meaning of margins in this setting. We really don't know whether a particular patient's tumor actually shrinks, contracting toward the center, while other tumors really just become more indistinct, with residual tumor being left at the original tumor's perimeter (see Fig. 6.3).

The NSABP embarked on a second neoadjuvant chemotherapy trial, designed to determine whether sequential addition of docetaxel (given either preoperatively or postoperatively) after four cycles of AC would increase tumor response rates and overall survival (Fig. 6.4). Although survival endpoints have not been reached, preliminary results of clinical and pathologic response rates were recently presented at the 2001 San Antonio Breast Cancer Symposium. Briefly, the addition of docetaxel prior to surgery (group II) significantly increased clinical CR rates (64.8% versus 40.4%) and pathologic CR rates (25.6% versus 13.7%) compared to AC alone used in groups I and III. This, however, did not result in a significant increase in BCT.

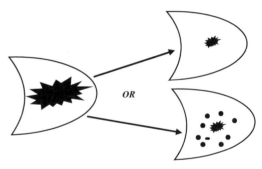

FIG. 6.3. Schematic showing alternative hypotheses about what happens during primary chemotherapy for a large breast cancer. In some cases, the tumor mass contracts inwards, leaving the surrounding tissue tumor-free. In other patients, the tumor may seem to disappear, but significant residual "rests" of tumor are left at the periphery of the original tumor mass.

An issue that has seldom been addressed in the literature is whether the cosmetic result of BCT is improved by using preoperative chemotherapy to shrink the tumor and reduce the amount of tissue to be removed at lumpectomy. While this seems plausible, the possibility that higher-than-usual doses of radiation may be needed to reduce the IBTR rate to acceptable levels after removal of a tumor that has been reduced in size by chemotherapy could negate much of this advantage. Future trials of preoperative chemotherapy should include careful assessment of the cos-

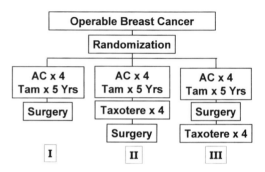

FIG. 6.4. Study schema for NSABP Protocol B-27. A, doxorubicin (Adriamycin); Taxotere, docetaxel; C, cyclophosphamide; Tam, tamoxifen.

metic outcome, as well as the local and systemic recurrence rates. The evidence available (levels I and II) provides category A support for using preoperative chemotherapy to make BCT feasible.

THE ROLE OF LUMPECTOMY IN PATIENTS WHO ARE CANDIDATES FOR BREAST CONSERVATION AFTER PRIMARY CHEMOTHERAPY

Based on NSABP Trial B-06 results, we know segmental mastectomy or lumpectomy, even with negative margins, leaves microscopic foci of cancer in the breast in at least 40% of patients (39,40). Addition of radiation therapy can reduce the incidence of IBTR from this theoretical 40% level to 10% or less. With positive margins, the IBTR rate has been shown to be higher than with negative margins (41). Thus, the purpose of lumpectomy can be viewed as reducing the tumor burden in the breast to a level that can be controlled with radiation. Can chemotherapy accomplish the same goal, particularly in patients with an apparent complete response to primary chemotherapy?

Some information relevant to this question can be extrapolated from the pathologic data in trials of preoperative chemotherapy. In virtually all of the trials reporting on the use of neoadjuvant chemotherapy followed by surgical excision of the primary lesion, only a small minority of patients (3% to 13%) were left without any residual invasive cancer in the breast (31,36–38). The theoretical issue that this raises is whether the residual cancer remaining in at least two-thirds of patients with a clinical CR after chemotherapy is analogous to the microscopic disease present after a lumpectomy with negative margins, or if the residual cancer is more like that remaining after an inadequate lumpectomy with positive margins. If the latter is true, then we would expect the rate of local recurrence to be higher, as in fact it was in women converted to BCT in NSABP B-18.

A number of trials, particularly from European centers, have documented experience with the use of radiation alone, without surgery, for local treatment of operable breast cancer treated initially with chemotherapy. However, while some of these trials were randomized, in prospective studies of neoadjuvant chemotherapy, few if any specifically address local treatment of operable breast cancer after chemotherapy. In the Calais trial cited earlier, 32 out of 158 patients had clinical CRs and were treated with radiotherapy alone, using 45 Gy to the whole breast and a 35-Gy brachytherapy boost to the tumor area (32). Only two of these 32 patients had a local recurrence, but median follow-up was only 38 months. Using a selective approach to local therapy, another French group used radiotherapy alone in 41 patients who had a clinical CR or near CR (42). With a median follow-up of only 30 months, they reported that three of these 41 had experienced a local recurrence. Interestingly, among the 64 patients who had residual tumor amenable to lumpectomy, there had been no local recurrences. Although this difference is small, it is actually the reverse of what one would expect, given the prognostic significance of response to chemotherapy. One of the most striking series supporting the omission of surgery for breast cancer also comes from France. Jacquillat et al. (43) reported on a prospective protocol in which 250 women with stage I to IIIB breast cancer were treated with neoadjuvant chemotherapy, followed by radiation alone to the breast, regardless of the response to chemotherapy (43). Two different radiation regimens were used, both biologically equivalent to 45 Gy to the whole breast, and an interstitial boost of 20 to 30 Gy was added, with the boost dose based on initial tumor size and residual disease. All patients achieved a clinical CR at the end of treatment, and no patient underwent initial mastectomy. With a median follow-up of over 5 years, the total IBTR rate was 9.2%, and the actuarial rate of breast preservation was 94%. The authors also indicate that, despite the aggressive radiotherapy regimen used, 88% of the patients had an excellent or good cosmetic result. Good cosmesis, however, has not been uniformly observed or even evaluated with the high doses of radiation often used in patients who do not undergo lumpectomy. The question as to whether either lumpectomy with moderate doses of radiation or omitting surgery and using more aggressive radiation produces better cosmetic outcomes remains open.

In a recent review (44), there was a tendency to observe increased local recurrence after neoadjuvant chemotherapy in those series' which included significant numbers of patients in whom radiotherapy was used as the only local treatment. In the CALGB trial cited earlier, 27% of patients who had radiotherapy as the sole treatment to the breast had local recurrences, even among those who had a good response to chemotherapy (8). In the prospective randomized trial described by Scholl et al. (35), the breast conservation rate was the same in both groups, and approximately half of the patients in each group were treated with radiotherapy as the only local treatment. While concluding that combined chemotherapy plus radiation can increase breast preservation in patients with T2 or larger tumors, the actuarial overall breast preservation rates in this trial were just over 60% at 5 years, even though approximately 80% of patients were treated initially with breast preservation. Despite using a radiation boost bringing the total dose up to 75 to 80 Gy in patients with CR and no surgery, the authors later noted that these patients, in particular, had high local recurrence rates (30% at 5 years), leading them to conclude that routine surgical excision should be considered, regardless of the response to primary chemotherapy (45). Baillet et al. (46) in Paris, having found that the cosmetic results of high-dose radiotherapy (45 Gy external beam plus 30 to 35 Gy interstitial boost) led to unsatisfactory cosmetic results, decided to decrease the boost selectively in patients with a good response to primary chemotherapy. In 135 patients with tumors more than 5 cm, 26 had failure in the breast, and the cosmetic results were considered excellent in only 66% of those alive at 5 years. In the Bourdeaux randomized trial of neoadjuvant versus adjuvant chemotherapy described previously, 44 patients who had a clinical CR after primary chemotherapy were selectively treated with radiation only, without breast surgery (33). At 124 months median follow-up, the total local recurrence in this subset was 34%, compared to 22.5% after lumpectomy plus radiation or mastectomy (34).

Even if lumpectomy after chemotherapy does not provide better cosmesis and/or improved local control, the resulting pathologic data provides important prognostic information relative to patient survival. Bonadonna (31), for example, found that the small subset of patients with a histologic complete response (no invasive or *in situ* cancer) had a better 8-year relapse-free survival (86%) than those with a good partial response but with residual microscopic disease (56%). Likewise, the M.D. Anderson series (11) found that patients with a histologic CR to induction chemotherapy had a higher likelihood of negative nodes, and those with no tumor in the breast or lymph nodes had a significantly higher overall survival at 5 years (89%) compared to those with a lesser response (64%). In NSABP B-18, clinical complete response was a significant predictor of disease-free, relapse-free, and distant disease-free survival (DFS, RFS, and DDFS), but not overall survival (38). Pathologic complete response was the most potent response parameter and the only one that came close to significance in predicting overall survival ($p = 0.06$). Patients who had a pathologic CR (no invasive cancer) had an overall 5-year survival of 87%, versus 77% to 78% for all other subsets in this arm of the study. The differences in DFS, RFS, and DDFS remained significant after adjusting for clinical tumor size, clinical nodal status, and age. However, in a Cox regression model, breast tumor response was a less powerful prognostic factor than tumor size or pathologic nodal status. As observed in the M.D. Anderson series, pathologic breast tumor response, and pathologic nodal status after chemotherapy were strongly related. Until recently, the importance of prognostication based on response to chemotherapy was largely theoretical since there was little that could be added to doxorubicin-based chemotherapy that would be likely to alter the outcome. With the demonstration of the efficacy of the taxanes against anthracycline-resistant breast cancer, there is now the potential for adding a systemic treatment that may improve outcomes in these poor prognosis patients (14–21). This question is currently being addressed in NSABP Protocol B-27, which may determine whether the addition of a taxane after doxorubicin plus cyclophosphamide will improve survival in those patients who have less than a complete response to the initial chemotherapy. The addition of a taxane did increase the pathologic CR rate by 87%, but no survival data are available. If survival is also improved by the sequential addition of docetaxel, this will be the first large trial to show that a change in therapy that increases the rate of pathologic CRs also results in improved survival. Despite the fact that local breast tumor response to chemotherapy is a powerful predictor of overall survival, it has not yet been demonstrated that improving the former will increase the latter. It also addresses the role of the taxane-docetaxel given pre- or postoperatively. If postoperative docetaxel improves survival, then it may be possible to determine whether a particular subset of patients (e.g., based on pathologic response to AC) benefits most from the additional chemotherapy.

Even in the selected subset of patients with a clinical CR, outcomes have not been uniformly favorable with the omission of surgery. This, along with the knowledge that very few patients receiving primary chemotherapy will be pathologically tumor-free and the importance of that pathologic information for predicting prognosis, makes it seem most prudent, at present, to proceed with at least lumpectomy, regardless of the clinical response to chemotherapy. However, this is an issue that could be specifically addressed in future trials. If we could identify patients likely to have a pathologic CR, then it might be appropriate to omit surgery in those patients. Another question that would then need to be addressed is the most reliable way to measure/predict response of the tumor to chemotherapy. Biologic and molecular markers that may predict response are currently being examined in ancillary trials to B-27. Candidates for measuring the response in a way that correlates with pathologic response include mammography, sonography, magnetic resonance imaging, and PET scanning of the breast, which are being actively investigated (47–50). A successor trial to B-27 will hopefully provide some data on whether such post-chemotherapy studies and/or needle biopsies are reliable predictors of breast tumor response. The evidence in favor of surgery, even after an apparent CR to chemotherapy, qualifies as category B.

WHERE LUMPECTOMY IS INDICATED AFTER CHEMOTHERAPY, DETERMINATION OF THE LOCATION AND EXTENT OF RESIDUAL TUMOR

Having made a case for either breast conservation or lumpectomy after primary chemotherapy when response to chemotherapy allows, it is important that the site of the primary tumor be located accurately. After a clinical CR, however, this may be difficult. A number of methods have been used successfully to overcome this problem. In many patients, the tumor site can be marked with small skin tattoos, similar to those used by radiation oncologists to mark treatment fields (31). Either a single spot over the center of the tumor or four spots marking the peripheral corners of the lesion can be used. The latter also helps to ensure that any measurements taken during the course of treatment will be comparable from week to week. Similarly, the use of a diagram drawn on a transparent grid to locate and outline the tumor has been suggested (51). Another successful method has been the use of mammographically or ultrasound-guided placement of a small clip(s) in or around the tumor before beginning treatment or before it disappears (52). Then, wire localization targeted on this clip can be used to guide tumor excision. In some patients, especially those with microcalcifications at the tumor site initially, a residual mammographic abnormality may remain after chemotherapy, even if no palpable tumor is present. This can be used for targeting of a needle as a guide to excision, without the need for a clip. Whatever the method used, if excision of the primary tumor site is deemed to be desirable, it is important to be sure that the appropriate tissue is removed. The evidence for any particular method of accomplishing this must be categorized as grade D.

THE ROLE OF SURGICAL AXILLARY LYMPH NODE STAGING AFTER CHEMOTHERAPY

Axillary lymph node dissection has generally been performed as standard treatment, firstly because pathologic node status is a strong predictor of prognosis and need for systemic therapy; secondly, because clinical assessment of the axillary nodes is inaccurate; and thirdly, because ALND provides good regional control without high-dose radiation to the axilla. It has been argued by some that the need for axillary node dissection and its attendant morbidity has decreased markedly (53–57). In part, this has resulted from the increasing use of adjuvant chemotherapy in node-negative as well as node-positive patients. It has also been argued that the use of preoperative chemotherapy may obviate the need for axillary node staging since chemotherapy is being given as primary treatment based on clinical staging, and in many regimens, additional chemotherapy and/or radiation are given to all patients who present with locally advanced breast cancer. Several reports on preoperative chemotherapy have, however, demonstrated that axillary node pathology profoundly impacts prognosis in such patients (31,38,58,59). In the Bonadonna report, 8-year, relapse-free survival varied from 75% in node-negative patients to 35% in patients with more than three positive nodes. A similar effect was seen in NSABP B-18 (38). A close association of nodal status with pathologic tumor response in the breast was also noted in NSABP B-18; 87% of patients with a pathologic CR in the breast had negative nodes. In fact, the M.D. Anderson group has argued that this association may make it possible to omit ALND in certain patients, although only 63% of their patients with a pathologic CR in the breast had negative nodes (60). This group has also suggested that axillary assessment with physical examination and ultrasound may identify patients with zero to three nodes involved, who may not need ALND if the axilla is to be irradiated (61). They have also suggested that a good partial response in the breast (more than 50% reduction in tumor size) correlates with a low rate of axillary node involvement and few positive nodes (86% node negative for clinical N0 patients and 65% for clinical N1 patients) (62). However, the number of patients in this latter study was small, and for some reason, six patients who had a pathologic CR in the breast (and who might have been expected to have the lowest rate of nodal involvement after chemotherapy) were excluded. Danforth et al. (13) similarly noted that only 2.4% of patients with a pathologic CR in the breast and clinically negative regional nodes had an axillary recurrence with the use of axillary radiation. If the pathologic response in the breast is a predictor of axillary nodal status, or if the breast pathology is used by itself to predict prognosis and to decide on the need for further treatment after primary chemotherapy, then ALND will add little important information. Furthermore, it seems clear that microscopic lymph node disease can be controlled with radiation, which, when added to breast radiation, causes little increase in morbidity (63–66). However, few patients have pathologic CRs with current regimens, and up to one-third of patients without tumor in the breast may still have cancer in the lymph nodes. Depending entirely on breast pathology at the present time would seem inappropriate for most patients treated with primary chemotherapy (category C evidence). The presence of tumor in both the breast and the axillary nodes may predict a worse prognosis than either alone (11). Although it seems clear that axillary node status after chemotherapy has prognostic significance, it is not clear how to treat it. Possibilities range from more of the same chemotherapy used preoperatively to chemotherapy with non–cross-resistant drugs (e.g., taxanes) or even to high-dose chemotherapy with stem cell transplant. Hopefully, the results of the NSABP B-27 trial will help to answer this question.

THE RELEVANCE OF SENTINEL NODE MAPPING AND BIOPSY IN PLACE OF FULL AXILLARY NODE DISSECTION AFTER CHEMOTHERAPY

In recent years, procedures for mapping the sentinel lymph nodes (SLN) have been described, and the pathologic status of the sentinel node(s) has been shown to be a highly accurate predictor of axillary node status (67–72). The sentinel nodes, identified by radionuclide tracers and/or by colored dyes, are felt to be the first nodes in the pathway of lymphatic spread. False-negative rates vary from a few percent to 11%, depending on the series quoted. For patients in whom primary chemotherapy is indicated, the idea of using SLN mapping as an alternative to axillary node dissection has some appeal, especially if decisions about subsequent additional therapy are going to be made on the basis of residual nodal metastases. One strategy to avoid the morbidity of ALND in patients receiving neoadjuvant chemotherapy would be to perform SLN biopsy (SLNB) prior to chemotherapy. If the SLN is pathologically negative before chemotherapy, there would be no need for ALND after chemotherapy. For those patients with a positive SLN at presentation, if surgery is indicated, lumpectomy or mastectomy plus ALND should be performed after chemotherapy. Bedrosian et al. (73) have shown that SLN could be identified prior to induction chemotherapy in 99% of 103 patients with T2 tumors. The false-negative rate of SLN was only 3%, similar to the rate in other series. However, performing surgical axillary nodal staging before induction chemotherapy makes it necessary to operate on these patients on two separate occasions. The accuracy of SLN status as an indicator of nodal pathology *after* chemotherapy hinges on two fundamental assumptions: (a) that nodal spread occurs sequentially, starting with the sentinel node; and (b) that regression of nodal disease occurs in reverse order during systemic treatment. While data from multiple studies seem to support the first assumption, the second has not been definitively established. If the sentinel node metastases regress while other nodes remain positive, then the pathologic status of the sentinel node will not accurately reflect the true nodal status. Data to support the use of SLN mapping to stage regional lymph nodes after chemotherapy have been accumulating gradually. At first, anecdotal reports of small numbers of patients undergoing SLN mapping and axillary node dissection after primary chemotherapy appeared. At least one of these, albeit involving only 14 patients, indicated that SLN biopsy had a high (21%) false-negative rate after chemotherapy (74). At M.D. Anderson, using a variety of mapping techniques, 51 patients underwent SLN biopsy after primary chemotherapy for stage II and III breast cancer (75). The SLN was falsely negative in three patients, but only 38 patients underwent complete axillary node dissection; the false-negative rate was 12%. By far, the largest series of SLN biopsy procedures after primary chemotherapy has been reported in abstract form only and was extracted from a subset of patients in NSABP Protocol B-27 (76). At the time of that report, data were available for 238 patients who had undergone SLN biopsy and ALND after neoadjuvant chemotherapy. Again, using a variety of techniques, the SLN was successfully identified in 84% of these patients, and among these patients, the SLN accurately predicted the overall nodal status in 96% of cases. The false-negative rate (11%) was essentially the same as in the M.D. Anderson experience and the multi-center trial reported by Krag et al. in the primary surgical setting (70). Even though the data are not definitive and the false-negative rate is in the range of 10%, SLNB may be useful in a proportion of these patients. This is particularly true in patients with a pathologic CR in the breast, in whom only a small percentage of patients would be expected to have positive nodes. In this scenario, only a very small number of patients with positive nodes after chemotherapy would be missed if SLNB was used. The levels of evidence supporting SLNB after chemotherapy remain in category C, but soon may reach category B.

SUMMARY

Conclusions about each of the issues and questions discussed here and the level of evidence for each are listed in Table 6.2. For noninflammatory LABC, a number of large trials provide fairly convincing evidence (levels II, III and IV; grade B) that BCT can be used selectively after neoadjuvant chemotherapy. The question of whether mastectomy is necessary for patients with inflammatory cancer remains controversial, with data on both sides (levels III and IV; category C). There is good evidence (levels I and II; category A), provided by a number of prospective randomized trials (especially NSABP Protocol B-18), that it is safe and appropriate to use primary chemotherapy to reduce the size of breast tumors in order to make

TABLE 6.2. *Summary of surgical issues after primary chemotherapy for breast cancer*

Question	Recommendation	Levels of evidence	Category or overall grade of evidence	Comments
Mastectomy for LABC (non-inflammatory)?	BCT may be used selectively.	II, III, IV	B	
Mastectomy for inflammatory breast cancer?	BCT may be used selectively, if no residual disease.	III, IV	C	If large mass present, should be resected by lumpectomy or mastectomy, as needed.
Can primary chemotherapy be used to facilitate BCT for large tumors?	Yes.	I, II	A	Uncertainty about post-chemotherapy margins and extent of residual disease may lead to higher IBTR rates than "standard" BCT for small cancers.
Is lumpectomy necessary after chemotherapy, even after a clinical CR?	Yes. (Might selectively eliminate lumpectomy for apparent CR patients, especially if pathologic CR could be predicted accurately.)	II, III	B	Prognostic information may be useful. Pathologic CR uncommon. Need for high-dose radiation if no surgery.
How does one find residual tumor after CR?	Tattoo, grid, clip or needle localization (mammographic or ultrasound guided) of residual mass or calcifications.	IV	D	
Role of surgical regional lymph node staging after primary chemotherapy	Should be used in most patients, especially in patients who do not have a CR in the breast. Might be omitted for few patients with pathologic CR in the breast and/or with negative sentinel node (see below).	III	C	Provides good regional control. Unclear how information will affect subsequent treatment at present.
SLNB after chemotherapy	Perhaps. Recent data encouraging.	III, IV	C	Less likely to miss positive nodes if path CR in breast. Unclear how information will affect subsequent treatment at present.

BCT feasible. For both locally advanced and early-stage breast cancer, the available data (levels II and III; category B) suggest that the tumor site should be excised, even after an apparent clinical CR, rather than using RT alone. Some results do indicate that surgery might be omitted in highly selected patients, but cosmetic outcomes, IBTR rates, and the utility of pathologic information have not been analyzed in a prospective randomized fashion. If the primary tumor site is to be excised, a number of techniques can be used to localize it accurately, but no real systematic study on this issue has been published (grade D). Data are inconsistent (level III) on the role of surgical staging of regional lymph nodes after chemotherapy, but for now, this should be done for most patients receiving primary chemotherapy (grade C). The potential role of SLNB after chemotherapy has appeal. Although the data available (levels III and IV) which justify its use in this setting are just beginning to emerge, it would certainly be a reasonable option in patients who have had a good clinical response to chemotherapy and do not have clinically enlarged lymph nodes (category C). A final note on the timing of surgery after chemotherapy: As long as one waits until the patient's leukocyte count has recovered to normal following the last dose of chemotherapy, the risk of complications should not exceed the expected rate for patients undergoing primary surgery (13,77). This generally takes 4 to 6 weeks.

REFERENCES

1. Haagensen CD, Stout AP. Carcinoma of the breast. II. Criteria of operability. *Ann Surg* 1943;118:859–868.
2. Zucali R, Uslenghi C, Kenda R, Bonadonna G. Natural history and survival of inoperable breast cancer treated with radiotherapy and radiotherapy followed by radical mastectomy. *Cancer* 1976;37:1422–1431.
3. Rubens RD, Armitage P, Winter PJ, et al. Prognosis in inoperable Stage III carcinoma of the breast. *Europ J Cancer* 1977;13:805–811.
4. DeLena M, Varini M, Zucali R, Rovini D. Multimodal treatment for locally advanced breast cancer: results of chemotherapy-radiotherapy versus chemotherapy-surgery. *Cancer Clin Trials* 1981;4:229–236.
5. Héry M, Namer M, Moro M, et al. Conservative treatment (chemotherapy/radiotherapy) of locally advanced breast cancer. *Cancer* 1986;57:1744–1749.
6. Perez CA, Graham ML, Taylor ME, et al. Management of locally advanced carcinoma of the breast: I. Noninflammatory. *Cancer* 1994;74:453–465.
7. Pierce LJ, Lippman M, Ben-Baruch N, et al. The effect of systemic therapy on locoregional control in locally advanced breast cancer. *Int J Radiat Oncol Biol Phys* 1992;23:949–960.
8. Perloff M, Lesnick GJ, Korzun A, et al. Combination chemotherapy with mastectomy or radiotherapy for Stage III breast carcinoma: a cancer and leukemia Group B study. *J Clin Oncol* 1988;6:261–269.
9. Hortobagyi GN, Ames FC, Buzdar AU, et al. Management of stage III breast cancer with primary chemotherapy, surgery, and radiation therapy. *Cancer* 1988;62:2507–2516.
10. Singletary SE, McNeese MD, Hortobagyi GN. Feasibility of breast-conservation surgery after induction chemotherapy for locally advanced breast carcinoma. *Cancer* 1992;69:2849–2852.
11. Kuerer HM, Newman LA, Smith TL, et al. Clinical course of breast cancer patients with complete pathologic primary tumor and axillary lymph node response to doxorubicin-based neoadjuvant chemotherapy. *J Clin Oncol* 1999;17:460–469.
12. Schwartz GF, Birchansky CA, Komarnicky LT, et al. Induction chemotherapy followed by breast conservation for locally advanced carcinoma of the breast. *Cancer* 1994;73:362–369.
13. Danforth DN, Zujewski J, O'Shaughnessy J, et al. Selection of local therapy after neoadjuvant chemotherapy in patients with stage IIIA,B breast cancer. *Ann Surg Oncol* 1998;5:150–158.
14. Holmes FA, Walters RS, Theriault RL, et al. Phase II trial of taxol, an active drug in the treatment of metastatic breast cancer. *J Natl Cancer Inst* 1991;83:1797–1805.
15. Valero V, Holmes FA, Walters RS, et al. Phase II trial of docetaxel: A new, highly effective antineoplastic agent in the management of patients with anthracycline-resistant metastatic breast cancer. *J Clin Oncol* 1995;13:2886–2894.
16. Seidman AD, Reichman BS, Crown JPA, et al. Paclitaxel as second and subsequent therapy for metastatic breast cancer: Activity independent of prior anthracycline response. *J Clin Oncol* 1995;13:1152–1159.
17. Ravdin PM, Burris HA III, Cook G, et al. Phase II trial of docetaxel in advanced anthracycline-resistant or anthracenedione-resistant breast cancer. *J Clin Oncol* 1995;13:2879–2885.
18. Gianni L, Munzone E, Capri G, et al. Paclitaxel in metastatic breast cancer: A trial of two doses by a 3-hour infusion in patients with disease recurrence after prior therapy with anthracyclines. *J Natl Cancer Inst* 1995;87:1169–1175.
19. Fountzilas G, Athanassiades A, Giannakakis T, et al. A phase II study of paclitaxel in advanced breast cancer resistant to anthracyclines. *Eur J Cancer* [A] 1996;32A:47–51.
20. Gradishar WJ. Docetaxel as neoadjuvant chemotherapy in patients with Stage III breast cancer. Phase II study: Preliminary results. *Oncology* 1997;11(Suppl. 8):15–18.
21. Archer CD, Lowdell C, Sinnett HD, et al. Docetaxel: Response in patients who have received at least two prior chemotherapy regimes for metastatic breast cancer. *Eur J Cancer* [A] 1998;34:816–819.
22. Valero V, Buzdar AU, Hortobagyi GN. Inflammatory breast cancer: Clinical features and the role of multimodality therapy. *Breast J* 1996;2:345–352.
23. Fleming RYD, Asmar L, Buzdar AU, et al. Effectiveness of mastectomy by response to induction chemotherapy for control in inflammatory breast carcinoma. *Ann Surg Oncol* 1997;4:452–461.
24. Curcio LD, Rupp E, Williams WL, et al. Beyond palliative mastectomy in inflammatory breast cancer—A reassessment of margin status. *Ann Surg Oncol* 1999;6:249–254.
25. Sener SF, Imperato JP, Khandekar JD, et al. Achieving local control for inflammatory carcinoma of the breast. *Surg Gynecol Obstet* 1992;175:141–144.
26. Hagelberg RS, Joly PS, Anderson RP. Role of surgery in the treatment of inflammatory breast carcinoma. *Am J Surg* 1984;148:124–131.
27. Schafer P, Alberto P, Forni M, et al. Surgery as part of a combined modality approach for inflammatory breast carcinoma. *Cancer* 1987;59:1063–1067.
28. Brun B, Otmezguine Y, Feuilhade F, et al. Treatment of inflammatory breast cancer with combination chemotherapy and mastectomy versus breast conservation. *Cancer* 1988;61:1096–1103.
29. Singletary SE. Editorial. Current treatment options for inflammatory breast cancer. *Ann Surg Oncol* 1999;6:228–229.
30. Arthur DW, Schmidt-Ullrich RK, Friedman RB, et al. Accelerated superfractionated radiotherapy for inflammatory breast carcinoma: Complete response predicts

outcome and allows for breast conservation. *Int J Radiat Oncol Biol Phys* 1999;44:289–296.
31. Bonadonna G, Valagussa P, Brambilla C, et al. Primary chemotherapy in operable breast cancer: Eight-year experience at the Milan Cancer Institute. *J Clin Oncol* 1998;16:93–100.
32. Calais G, Berger C, Descamps P, et al. Conservative treatment feasibility with induction chemotherapy, surgery, and radiotherapy for patients with breast carcinoma larger than 3 cm. *Cancer* 1994;74:1283–1288.
33. Mauriac L, Durand M, Avril A, Dilhuydy JM. Effects of primary chemotherapy in conservative treatment of breast cancer patients with operable tumors larger than 3 cm. Results of a randomized trial in a single centre. *Ann Oncol* 1991;2:347–354.
34. Mauriac L, MacGrogan G, Avril A, et al. Neoadjuvant chemotherapy for operable breast carcinoma larger than 3 cm: a unicentre randomized trial with a 124-month median follow-up. Institut Bergonie Bordeaux Groupe Sein (IBBGS). *Ann Oncol* 1999;10:47–52.
35. Scholl SM, Fourquet A, Asselain B, et al. Neoadjuvant versus adjuvant chemotherapy in premenopausal patients with tumours considered too large for breast conserving surgery: preliminary results of a randomised trial: S6. *Europ J Cancer* 1994;30A:645–652.
36. Powles TJ, Hickish TF, Makris A, et al. Randomized trial of chemoendocrine therapy started before or after surgery for treatment of primary breast cancer. *J Clin Oncol* 1995;13:547–552.
37. Fisher B, Brown A, Mamounas E, et al. Effect of preoperative chemotherapy on locoregional disease in women with operable breast cancer: findings from National Surgical Adjuvant Breast and Bowel Project B-18. *J Clin Oncol* 1997;15:2483–2493.
38. Fisher B, Bryant J, Wolmark N, et al. Effect of preoperative chemotherapy on the outcome of women with operable breast cancer. *J Clin Oncol* 1998;16:2672–2685.
39. Fisher B, Redmond C, Poisson R, et al. Eight-year results of a randomized clinical trial comparing total mastectomy and lumpectomy with or without irradiation in the treatment of breast cancer. *N Engl J Med* 1989;320:822–828.
40. Fisher B, Anderson S, Redmond CK, et al. Reanalysis and results after 12 years of follow-up in a randomized clinical trial comparing total mastectomy with lumpectomy with or without irradiation in the treatment of breast cancer [see comments]. *N Engl J Med* 1995;333:1456–1461.
41. Gage I, Schnitt SJ, Nixon AJ, et al. Pathologic margin involvement and the risk of recurrence in patients treated with breast-conserving therapy. *Cancer* 1996;78:1921–1928.
42. Bélembaogo E, Feillel V, Chollet P, et al. Neoadjuvant chemotherapy in 126 operable breast cancers. *Eur J Cancer* [A] 1992;28A:896–900.
43. Jacquillat C, Weil M, Baillet F, et al. Results of neoadjuvant chemotherapy and radiation therapy in the breast-conserving treatment of 250 patients with all stages of infiltrative breast cancer. *Cancer* 1990;66:119–129.
44. Kuerer HM, Hunt KK, Newman LA, et al. Neoadjuvant chemotherapy in women with invasive breast carcinoma: Conceptual basis and fundamental surgical issues. *J Am Coll Surgeons* 2000;190:350–363.
45. Scholl SM, Pierga JY, Asselain B, et al. Breast tumour response to primary chemotherapy predicts local and distant control as well as survival. *Eur J Cancer* [A] 1995;31A:1969–1975.
46. Baillet F, Rozec C, Ucla L, et al. Treatment of locally advanced breast cancer without mastectomy: 5- and 10-year results of 135 tumors larger than 5 centimeters treated by external beam therapy, brachytherapy, and neoadjuvant chemotherapy. *Ann N Y Acad Sci* 1993;698:264–270.
47. Vinnicombe SJ, MacVicar AD, Guy RL, et al. Primary breast cancer: Mammographic changes after neoadjuvant chemotherapy, with pathologic correlation. *Radiology* 1996;198:333–340.
48. Bassa P, Kim EE, Inoue T, et al. Evaluation of preoperative chemotherapy using PET with fluorine- 18-fluorodeoxyglucose in breast cancer. *J Nucl Med* 1996;37:931–938.
49. Abraham DC, Jones RC, Jones SE, et al. Evaluation of neoadjuvant chemotherapeutic response of locally advanced breast cancer by magnetic resonance imaging. *Cancer* 1996;78:91–100.
50. Herrada J, Iyer RB, Atkinson EN, et al. Relative value of physical examination, mammography, and breast sonography in evaluating the size of the primary tumor and regional lymph node metastases in women receiving neoadjuvant chemotherapy for locally advanced breast carcinoma. *Clin Cancer Res* 1997;3:1565–1569.
51. Margolese RG. Surgical considerations in preoperative chemotherapy of breast cancer—Recent results. *Cancer Res* 1998;152:193–201.
52. Kuerer HM, Newman LA, Buzdar AU, et al. Residual metastatic axillary lymph nodes following neoadjuvant chemotherapy predict disease-free survival in patients with locally advanced breast cancer. *Am J Surg* 1998;176:502–509.
53. Silverstein MJ, Gierson ED, Waisman JR, et al. Axillary lymph node dissection for T1a breast carcinoma: Is it indicated? *Cancer* 1994;73:664–667.
54. Morrow M. Axillary dissection: when and how radical? *Semin Surg Oncol* 1996;12:321–327.
55. Dent DM. Axillary lymphadenectomy for breast cancer—Paradigm shifts and pragmatic surgeons. *Arch Surg* 1996;131:1125–1127.
56. Cady B, Stone MD, Schuler JG, et al. The new era in breast cancer—Invasion, size, and nodal involvement dramatically decreasing as a result of mammographic screening. *Arch Surg* 1996;131:301–307.
57. Cady B. Is axillary lymph node dissection necessary in routine management of breast cancer? No. *Breast J* 1997;3:246–260.
58. McCready DR, Hortobagyi GN, Kau SW, et al. The prognostic significance of lymph node metastases after preoperative chemotherapy for locally advanced breast cancer. *Arch Surg* 1989; 124:21–25.
59. Machiavelli MR, Romero AO, Pérez JE, et al. Prognostic significance of pathological response of primary tumor and metastatic axillary lymph nodes after neoadjuvant chemotherapy for locally advanced breast carcinoma. *Cancer J Sci Am* 1998;4:125–131.
60. Kuerer HM, Newman LA, Buzdar AU, et al. Pathologic tumor response in the breast following neoadjuvant chemotherapy predicts axillary lymph node status. *Cancer J Sci Am* 1998b;4:230–236.

61. Kuerer HM, Newman LA, Fornage BD, et al. Role of axillary lymph node dissection after tumor downstaging with induction chemotherapy for locally advanced breast cancer. *Ann Surg Oncol* 1998a;5:673–680.
62. Lenert JT, Vlastos G, MIrza NQ, et al. Primary tumor response to induction chemotherapy as a predictor of histologic status of axillary nodes in operable breast cancer patients. *Ann Surg Oncol* 1999;6:762–767.
63. Fisher B, Redmond C, Fisher ER, et al. Ten-year results of a randomized clinical trial comparing radical mastectomy and total mastectomy with or without radiation. *N Engl J Med* 1985;312:674–681.
64. Delouche G, Bachelot F, Premont M, Kurtz JM. Conservation treatment of early breast cancer: long term results and complications. *Int J Radiat Oncol Biol Phys* 1987;13:29–34.
65. Baeza MR, Sole J, Leon A, et al. Conservative treatment of early breast cancer. *Int J Radiat Oncol Biol Phys* 1988;14:669–676.
66. Cabanes PA, Salmon RJ, Vilcoq JR, et al. Value of axillary dissection in addition to lumpectomy and radiotherapy in early breast cancer. *Lancet* 1992;339:1245–1248.
67. Veronesi U, Paganelli G, Galimberti V, et al. Sentinel-node biopsy to avoid axillary dissection in breast cancer with clinically negative lymph-nodes. *Lancet* 1997;349:1864–1867.
68. Turner RR, Ollila DW, Krasne DL, Giuliano AE. Histopathologic validation of the sentinel lymph node hypothesis for breast carcinoma. *Ann Surg* 1997;226:271–278.
69. Giuliano AE, Jones RC, Brennan M, Statman R. Sentinel lymphadenectomy in breast cancer. *J Clin Oncol* 1997;15:2345–2350.
70. Krag D, Weaver D, Ashikaga T, et al. The sentinel node in breast cancer—A multicenter validation study. *N Engl J Med* 1998;339:941–946.
71. Gulec SA, Moffat FL, Carroll RG, et al. Sentinel lymph node localization in early breast cancer. *J Nucl Med* 1998;39:1388–1393.
72. Veronesi U, Paganelli G, Viale G, et al. Sentinel lymph node biopsy and axillary dissection in breast cancer: Results in a large series. *J Natl Cancer Inst* 1999;91:368–373.
73. Bedrosian I, Reynolds C, Mick R, et al. Accuracy of sentinel lymph node biopsy in patients with large primary breast tumors. *Cancer* 2000;88:2540–2545.
74. Anderson BO, Jewell K, Eary JF, et al. Neoadjuvant chemotherapy contraindicates sentinel node mapping in breast cancer. *Proc ASCO* 1999;18:71a.
75. Breslin TM, Cohen L, Sahin A, et al. Sentinel lymph node biopsy is accurate after neoadjuvant chemotherapy for breast cancer. *J Clin Oncol* 2000;18:3480–3486.
76. Mamounas E, Brown A, Smith R, et al. Sentinel node biopsy (SNB) following neoadjuvant chemotherapy in breast cancer (BC): Results from NSABP B-27. Abstracts from the Society of Surgical Oncology 54th Annual Cancer Symposium, 2001:21–21.
77. Broadwater JR, Edwards MJ, Kuglen C, et al. Mastectomy following preoperative chemotherapy: Strict operative criteria control operative morbidity. *Ann Surg* 1991;213:126–129.
78. Gunduz N, Fisher B, Saffer EA. Effect of surgical removal on growth and kinetics of residual tumor. *Cancer Res* 1979;39:3861–3865.
79. Fisher B, Gunduz N, Saffer EA. Influence of the interval between primary tumor removal and chemotherapy on kinetics and growth of metastases. *Cancer Res* 1983;43:1488–1492.
80. O'Reilly MS, Holmgren L, Shing Y, et al. Angiostatin: A circulating endothelial cell inhibitor that suppresses angiogenesis and tumor growth. *Cold Spring Harbor Symp. Quant Biol* 1994;59:471–482.
81. O'Reilly MS, Holmgren L, Chen C, Folkman J. Angiostatin induces and sustains dormancy of human primary tumors in mice. *Nature Med* 1996;2:689–692.
82. Goldie JH, Coldman AJ. A mathematical model for relating the drug sensitivity of tumors to their spontaneous mutation rate. *Cancer Treat Rep* 1979;63:1727–1733.
83. Skipper HE. Kinetics of mammary tumor cell growth and implications for therapy. *Cancer* 1971;28:1479–1499.
84. Hortobagyi GN, Blumenschein GR, Spanos W, et al. Multimodal treatment of locoregionally advanced breast cancer. *Cancer* 1983;51:763–768.
85. Hortobagyi GN. Multidisciplinary management of advanced primary and metastatic breast cancer. *Cancer* 1994;74:416–423.
86. Gardin G, Rosso R, Campora E, et al. Locally advanced non-metastatic breast cancer: Analysis of prognostic factors in 125 patients homogeneously treated with a combined modality approach. *Eur J Cancer* [A] 1995;31A:1428–1433.
87. Perez EA, Foo ML, Fulmer JT. Management of locally advanced breast cancer. *Oncology* 1997;11(Suppl.9):9–17.
88. Hortobagyi GN, Buzdar AU, Strom EA, Ames FC, Singletary SE. Primary chemotherapy for early and advanced breast cancer. *Cancer Lett* 1995;90:103–109.

7

The Medical Oncology Perspective on Preoperative Chemotherapy for Early Operable Breast Cancer

Charlotte N. Rees and Ian E. Smith

Postoperative adjuvant chemotherapy is the conventional approach to the systemic management of early breast cancer. Definitive evidence shows that this approach significantly improves disease-free survival (DFS) and overall survival (OS) (1–3). During the last decade, there has been considerable interest in reversing treatments for patients with larger operable breast cancers, such that preoperative (neoadjuvant, primary, or induction) chemotherapy is given as first-line treatment prior to surgery to achieve down-staging and to increase the chance of conservative surgery (4). The origin of preoperative chemotherapy stems from its use in the treatment of locally advanced inoperable breast cancers where it leads to improvement in local control and survival (5,6). This approach was then extended to include large operable breast cancers where mastectomy was the recommended surgical option and patients were likely to be treated, in most instances, with postoperative adjuvant chemotherapy (7).

It has been found in animal models that the removal of the primary tumor may increase the growth of micrometastases; this was presumed to be due to the production of a growth factor, and the effect could be prevented by systemic chemotherapy given before tumor resection (10–12). More recently, an alternative explanation has been proposed: that tumors may release angiostatic factors which limit the growth of metastases by inhibiting new blood vessel formation and that removal of the primary may, therefore, promote angiogenesis and the growth of the metastases (13). Micrometastases have been identified using immunocytochemical techniques in the bone marrow of patients with primary breast cancer at presentation and are associated with a shorter DFS and OS (14).

Goldie and Coldman (15) proposed that as the number of tumor cells increases, the possibility of the development of chemo-resistant clones increases. This would favor the early administration of chemotherapy and may account for the failure of adjuvant chemotherapy in some instances.

SCIENTIFIC AND CLINICAL RATIONALE

The initial aim of preoperative chemotherapy was to use the primary as an *in vivo* measure of tumor response (8), ideally to down-stage the tumor and to potentially reduce the number of patients requiring mastectomy (9). The more fundamental aim, however, was to develop tumor response as a short-term surrogate marker for long-term outcome. The hope was that treatments could then be tailored to individual patients and that new therapies could be assessed more quickly than in the adjuvant setting.

THE EFFECT OF PREOPERATIVE CHEMOTHERAPY ON SURVIVAL

Randomized Studies

The earliest randomized studies looking at the effect of preoperative chemotherapy on survival suggested a small benefit, but this was not confirmed with long-term follow-up. The trials are summarized in Table 7.1.

In the first trial, 270 evaluable (N = 272 total entered) patients with operable breast carcinomas larger than 3 cm were randomized and treated by either initial mastectomy and adjuvant chemotherapy (group A) or preoperative

TABLE 7.1. *The effect of preoperative chemotherapy on survival, randomized controlled trials*

Study	Tumor stage (TMN)	Median follow-up years	Evaluable patients (n)	Preop Survival %	Postop survival %	Significance p value
Mauriac (16)	T2 (> 3cm),3, N0,1,M0	10	270	68	64	NS
Broet (19) Scholl (18)	T2,3,N0,1,M0	9	390	65	60	NS
Semiglazov (20)	T1,2,3,N0,1,2,M0	10	271	81	72	OS NS DFS p=0.04
Fisher (21,22)	T1,2,3,N0,1,M0	5	1,495	80	80	NS
Makris (24) Powles (23)	T1,2,3,4,N0,1,M0	4	286	80	82	NS

NS, not statistically significant.

chemotherapy followed by locoregional treatment adjusted by response (group B) (16). At the first analysis, with a median follow-up of 34 months, there was increased isolated local recurrences in group B, but group B had a significantly improved OS ($p = 0.04$). However, re-analysis at 124 months demonstrated no difference in DFS or OS between the two arms (17). Of note, 24% of the control arm (group A) did not receive adjuvant chemotherapy because at that time they were not considered to have any adverse prognostic features.

In a second French trial, S6, 390 evaluable (N = 414 total) patients received either radiation with or without surgery and adjuvant chemotherapy or preoperative chemotherapy followed by radiation with or without surgery (18). A statistically significant survival benefit (86% versus 78%, $p = 0.04$) in favor of the preoperative chemotherapy arm was seen at 5 years. There was no difference in DFS. A more recent analysis at 105 months confirmed a short-term survival benefit at 5 years (84% versus 77%, $p = 0.02$) in favor of the preoperative chemotherapy arm, but, at approximately 10 years, this was no longer significant (65% versus 60%, $p = 0.24$) (19).

A Russian trial of 271 patients with large breast cancers randomized to receive either preoperative chemotherapy followed by radiotherapy and chemotherapy or radiotherapy followed by postoperative chemotherapy demonstrated a 5-year DFS difference (81% versus 72%, $p = 0.04$) in favor of the preoperative chemotherapy arm, but OS was not statistically significant (20). They used an unusual regimen of thiotepa, methotrexate sodium, and 5-fluorouracil (TMF) for preoperative and postoperative chemotherapy.

The NSABP B-18 trial is the largest randomized trial comparing the effect of preoperative and postoperative chemotherapy on the outcome of women with operable breast cancer. In the trial, 1,523 patients (N = 1,495 evaluable) were randomly assigned to receive preoperative versus postoperative Adriamycin and cyclophosphamide (AC) chemotherapy (21,22). No difference in OS (80% both arms), DFS (67% both arms), or distant DFS (73% both arms) was seen at 5 years.

A further, smaller study examined the effect of preoperative chemo-endocrine therapy (methotrexate, mitoxantrone and tamoxifen citrate) on 309 women (N = 286 evaluable) with operable breast cancer (23). After a median follow-up of 48 months, there was no difference in OS or DFS (24).

The current weight of evidence suggests there is no survival benefit or disadvantage from the use of preoperative chemotherapy (level 1 evidence). There are now an increasing number of chemotherapy drugs that have, however, not been examined in this setting. It may be that the identification of short-term markers of response in the preoperative setting may predict for long-term outcome, and that individually tailored chemotherapy may have the potential to improve survival.

THE EFFECT OF PREOPERATIVE CHEMOTHERAPY ON THE REQUIREMENT FOR MASTECTOMY AND THE RISK OF LOCAL RECURRENCE

Non-Randomized Studies

Conservative surgery is the treatment of choice whenever possible in the management of early breast cancers, but for large, primary tumors, mastectomy remains the only surgical option. One of the initial aims of preoperative chemotherapy was to achieve tumor shrinkage and possibly negate the need for mastectomy. Results from non-randomized studies suggested that this could be achieved without increasing the local recurrence rate (25–27).

In a trial using infusional chemotherapy, 5-fluorouracil, epirubicin hydrochloride, and cisplatin (ECisF), eligible patients had to require mastectomy. Following preoperative chemotherapy, only 6% subsequently needed a mastectomy (28). Similarly, in an Italian series, only 15% of 536 patients required mastectomy following preoperative Adriamycin/CMF chemotherapy, although all were considered to require a mastectomy at the time of entry into the study (29).

However, there is also some evidence that patients with large operable breast cancers treated by preoperative chemotherapy followed by radiotherapy without subsequent surgery may be at a slightly increased risk of local relapse despite achieving clinical remission (21% versus 7% who had surgery, $p = 0.02$) (30).

Randomized Studies

The randomized trials are summarized in Table 7.2.

In the French Institut Bergonie trial (16) of 272 patients with breast cancers more than 3 cm, only 37% of patients in the preoperative arm required mastectomy, compared to 100% in the control arm. Of the patients who received preoperative chemotherapy, 23% developed locoregional relapse, compared to 9% in the postoperative arm, but 33% of the patients in the preoperative group received radiotherapy without surgical resection. The mastectomy rate in the preoperative arm rose to 55% at a median follow-up of 124 months due to local recurrence. Local recurrence was more likely to occur in those patients who received preoperative chemotherapy and radiotherapy alone.

TABLE 7.2. *The effect of preoperative chemotherapy on the requirement for mastectomy and the risk of local recurrence, randomized controlled trials*

Study	Median follow-up (years)	Evaluable patients (n)	Chemo regime pre & post	Mastectomy rate (%)	Local recurrence rate (%)
Mauriac (16,17)	10	270	EVcMMiTVd	[a]Preop 37 (1991) 55 (1999) [b]Postop 100	Preop 23 Postop 9
Scholl (18)	9	390	FAC	[c]Preop 18 Postop 23	Preop 27 Postop 19
Fisher (21,22)	5	1,495	AC	Preop 33 Postop 40 $p = 0.002$	Preop 7.9 Postop 5.8
Makris (24)	4	286	MMiMzTam	Preop 11 Postop 22 $p = 0.004$	Preop 2.7 Postop 3.5

E, epirubicin; Vc, vincristine; M, methotrexate; Mi, mitomycin C; T, thiotepa; Vd, vindesine; F, 5-fluorouracil; A, Adriamycin; C, cyclophosphamide; Mz, mitozantrone; Tam, tamoxifen.
[a]33% of patients received radiotherapy only following preoperative chemotherapy.
[b]24% of patients received no adjuvant chemotherapy.
[c]51% of preop patients received radiotherapy only and no surgery, 47% of postop arm received primary radiotherapy and no surgery.

In the S6 trial, there was a non-significant reduction in the mastectomy rate in favor of the preoperative chemotherapy arm, 18% versus 23% (18). Surgery was limited to those patients who had a persisting mass after radiotherapy in both arms. The postoperative chemotherapy arm received radiotherapy as their primary treatment. Fifty-one percent of patients in the preoperative chemotherapy arm and 46% in the postoperative chemotherapy arm had radiotherapy only. There was a non-significant difference in the 5-year local control rates (73% preoperative arm versus 81% postoperative arm, $p = 0.21$). The 5-year mastectomy rates were similar (39% preoperative versus 37% postoperative, $p = 0.95$).

In the NSABP B-18 trial, the frequency of lumpectomy was greater in the preoperative chemotherapy group (60% versus 67%, $p = 0.002$) (21). This was more pronounced in patients with tumors 5.1 cm or greater, with a frequency of 8% in the postoperative group, compared to 22% in the preoperative group (22). There was a non-significant difference in the risk of local recurrence between the two arms after 5 years (7.9% preoperative arm versus 5.8% in the postoperative arm, $p = 0.23$). Age was found to have a significant effect on the rate of recurrence in both arms (p less than 0.0001) and may be partly attributed to the fact that no patients less than 50, regardless of ER status, received tamoxifen. Patients who were down-staged with chemotherapy and underwent lumpectomy rather than mastectomy were statistically more likely to develop ipsilateral breast cancer recurrence than those who were initially planned to have a lumpectomy (14.5% versus 6.9%, $p = 0.04$).

In a further study of 293 patients with primary operable breast cancer, 11% of the preoperative group underwent mastectomy compared to 22% of the postoperative group ($p = 0.004$) (24). The local recurrence rate at a median follow-up of 48 months was not statistically significantly different between the two arms (2.7% for the preoperative arm and 3.5% for the postoperative arm).

In summary, there is considerable heterogeneity in the design of the studies. Two of the randomized studies have shown a significant reduction in the mastectomy rate following preoperative chemotherapy, and there may be a small increase in the risk of local recurrence, although it hasn't impacted survival to date. The need for mastectomy can be reduced, but not eliminated, with the use of preoperative chemotherapy. There is also some evidence that patients with large operable breast cancers treated by preoperative chemotherapy followed by radiotherapy without subsequent surgery may be at slightly increased risk of local relapse, despite achieving clinical remission. Surgical intervention is, therefore, advisable, despite apparent complete clinical response (cCR) (level of evidence: 2).

THE EFFECT OF PREOPERATIVE CHEMOTHERAPY ON TUMOR RESPONSE

It is now well established that preoperative chemotherapy is active in primary operable breast cancer with overall objective response rates generally higher than for patients with metastatic disease. The overall response rates range from 61% to 97% and cCR rates of 16% to 51% (Table 7.3) (17,18,20,22,24,25,27–29,31–34).

Non-Randomized Studies

The Milan group reported one of the largest prospective non-randomized studies with an overall response rate of 76% and a cCR rate of 16% (29). They also reported progression in only 3% of patients while on preoperative chemotherapy. In the final multivariate analysis at 8 years, the degree of tumor response and the achievement of complete remission, as confirmed by microscopic examination, were important prognostic markers.

The Marsden study using infusional epirubicin, cisplatin, and 5-FU (EcisF) reported an overall response rate of 98% and a cCR rate of 66% in an initial phase 2 study; the median time to achieve a response was 3 weeks, and the median number of courses needed to achieve complete remission was four (28). When this schedule was subsequently assessed in a larger

TABLE 7.3. *The effect of preoperative chemotherapy on tumor response*

Study	Chemotherapy regime	Evaluable patients (n)	Overall response (%)	Complete clinical response (cCR) (%)
Non-randomized				
Bonadonna (29)	A/E then CMF	536	76	16
Jacquillat (25)	VbTMF±A	250	71	30
Hortobagyi (32)	FAC	174	97	29
Calais (27)	MzVdCF/EVdCF	158	61	20
Belembaogo (31)	AVcCF±M	126	86	36
Smith (28)	ECisInfF	123	96	36
Cameron (33)	CAVcP	94	70	27
Amat (36)	D	54	72	18
Chollet (34)	AVrCF	50	88	51
Moliterni (35)	APx	41	91	N/A
Randomized				
Fisher (21,22)	AC	743	80	36
Scholl (18)	FAC	200	80	30
Makris (24)	MMiMzTam	144	84	22
Mauriac (16)	EVcMMiTVd	134	81	33
Semiglazov (20)	TMF	134	57	28

A, adriamycin; C, cyclophosphamide; Cis, cisplatin; D, docetaxel; E, epirubicin; F, 5-fluorouracil; InfF, infusional F; M, methotrexate; Mi, mitomycin C; Mz, mitozantrone; N/A, not available; P, prednisolone; Px, paclitaxel; T, thiotepa; Tam, tamoxifen; Vb, vinblastine; Vc, vincristine; Vd, vindesine; Vr, vinorelbine.

randomized phase 3 trial, response rates were lower, as discussed below.

Most recent chemotherapy schedules have included an anthracycline, and there have been a number of non-randomized studies using taxanes. In a non-randomized comparison between two consecutive studies, the response rate was 74% for single-agent anthracycline and 91% for an anthracycline/paclitaxel combination (35). A phase 2 study of single-agent docetaxel reported a response rate of 72% (36). The non-randomized studies are summarized in Table 7.3.

Randomized Studies

Data on tumor response from randomized trials comparing preoperative and postoperative chemotherapy are available. The largest trial, NSABP B-18, used AC in the preoperative chemotherapy arm and achieved an overall response rate of 80% and a cCR rate of 36% in 743 patients (21). Progression occurred in less than 3% of patients during chemotherapy. Other randomized studies (Table 7.3) have similar response rates (57% to 84%) and CCR rates (22% to 33%) to the NSABP B-18 trial.

Randomized Studies of Different Chemotherapy Regimens

In the last few years, randomized studies comparing different chemotherapy regimens have been designed in an attempt to improve tumor response rates with the hope that this may translate into a survival advantage. These studies are summarized in Table 7.4.

Four cycles of single-agent paclitaxel have been compared to four cycles of 5-fluorouracil, Adriamycin, and cyclophosphamide (FAC) with 87 patients in each arm. The overall response rate was 80% in both arms. The pathological complete remission (pCR) was 17% in the FAC arm and 8% in the paclitaxel arm.(37)

In the United Kingdom multi-center TOPIC 1 study, continuous infusional ECisF has been compared with AC bolus chemotherapy in 426 patients with operable cancers 3 cm or greater. Overall response rates were 77% and 75%, respectively, with cCR rates of 34% and 31% (38).

TABLE 7.4. *The effect of preoperative chemotherapy on tumor response. Randomized trials of different chemotherapy regimens*

Study	Chemo regimen	Evaluable patients (n)	Overall response (%)	Complete clinical response (cCR) (%)
Budzar (37)	Px x 4	87	80	27
	FACx 4	87	79	24
Smith (38)	ECisInfF x 6	213	77	34
	AC x 6	213	75	31
Hutcheon (39)	CVcAP x 8			
	CVcAP x 4	52	68	N/A
	then D x 4	52	94	N/A
			$p = 0.001$	
Luporsi (40)	FEC x 6	45	72	N/A
	ED X 6	45	84	N/A

A, Adriamycin; C, cyclophosphamide; Cis, cisplatin; D, docetaxel; E, epirubicin; F, 5-fluorouracil; InfF, infusional F; N/A, not available; P, prednisolone; Px, paclitaxel; Vc, vincristine.

In a smaller Scottish trial, 104 patients responding to cyclophosphamide, vincristine, Adriamycin, and prednisolone (CVAP), out of an original 158 (66%), were subsequently randomized to four further cycles of CVAP or docetaxel (39). The overall response rate was 68% in the CVAP arm and 94% in the docetaxel arm ($p = 0.001$).

In a further ongoing trial, six cycles of 5-fluorouracil, epirubicin (100 mg/m^2) and cyclophosphamide (FEC 100) were compared to six cycles of epirubicin/docetaxel in 90 patients, with overall response rates of 72% and 84%, respectively, and a pCR of 24% in both arms (40).

The largest trial, which has accrued 2,000 patients, is the NSABP B-27 study. This is a three-arm trial: (i) preoperative AC by 4, then surgery/radiotherapy; (ii) preoperative AC by 4, then docetaxel by 4, then surgery/radiotherapy; (iii) preoperative AC by 4, then surgery followed by docetaxel by 4, then radiotherapy (41).

Ongoing/Unreported Trials

In addition to those reported above, there are a number of ongoing or unreported trials. The United Kingdom TOPIC trial group is comparing AC with Navelbine/epirubicin for six cycles followed by surgery, adjuvant radiotherapy, and endocrine therapy as appropriate in the TOPIC 2 study (42). The accrual target is 400.

A Scottish Cancer Therapy Network trial (expected N = 700) is comparing AC with Adriamycin/docetaxel for six cycles followed by surgery and, if node-positive, further chemotherapy.

A three-arm Italian study is currently underway comparing two adjuvant chemotherapy protocols (Adriamycin, then cyclophosphamide, methotrexate, 5-fluorouracil [CMF] versus Adriamycin/paclitaxel then CMF) and a preoperative arm using Adriamycin/paclitaxel, then CMF.

In summary, preoperative chemotherapy is active in early breast cancer, and tumor progression on treatment is nearly always less than 5% (level of evidence: 1). Further progress of preoperative chemotherapy is dependent upon the design of more large, well-constructed, randomized controlled trials to establish whether any new treatments, when compared with current standard schedules, can improve response rates and survival.

POTENTIAL PREDICTIVE FACTORS FOR PREOPERATIVE CHEMOTHERAPY

Preoperative chemotherapy allows the primary tumor to be used as an *in vivo* model of tumor response. Its use may also identify surrogate clinical markers—e.g., tumor response or biologic markers—which may be shown to predict for long-term outcome. Adjuvant chemotherapy studies with DFS and OS as primary endpoints take many years to obtain useful information and delay the development of a new treatment. These predictive factors must be validated in well-designed prospective randomized trials. There is now evidence for possible clinical, pathological, and biological factors which could be used as surrogate predictive markers, and these will be discussed below.

Clinical Predictive Factors

Clinical tumor response is an important predictor of outcome following preoperative chemotherapy in breast cancer, although it doesn't always reach statistical significance (21,29,30,32,33,43,44). A high rate of complete clinical remission has been the key to success in a number of malignancies, including acute leukaemia, lymphoma, and germ cell tumors, and this has translated into improved survival. The important trials are summarized below and in Table 7.5.

The Milan study reported a significant correlation between RFS at 8 years and cCR using univariate analysis ($p = 0.0001$) and multivariate analysis ($p = 0.034$). At the Royal Marsden, clinical responders had improved DFS ($p = 0.009$) and OS ($p = 0.08$) compared to non-responders (30). In the NSABP B-18 study, DFS at 5 years was significantly increased in those patients who had a cCR ($p = 0.0014$) but OS was not ($p = 0.19$) (21). In the Institut Curie study, OS was correlated with overall clinical response ($p = 0.01$) (44).

Pathological Predictive Factors

Complete pathological response (pCR) of the primary tumor following preoperative chemotherapy is emerging as a clear-cut predictor of survival, with RFS and OS rates of over 80% (21,29,43). However, in practice, pCR rates are low, with most studies reporting response rates of 4% to 20% (21,29,35,36,43,44). The information is also only available following surgery and does not allow for alterations in the preoperative chemotherapy regimens. The most important trials are summarized below and in Table 7.5.

In the Milan study, it was shown by multivariate analysis that the nodal status was the most important factor ($p < 0.001$), followed by the degree of pathologic remission ($p = 0.034$) in influencing the RFS (29).

In the NSABP B-18 study, women who had a cCR and pCR to preoperative chemotherapy had a better DFS ($p = 0.0001$), RFS ($p < 0.0001$) and OS ($p = 0.06$) after 5 years (21). Following adjustment for tumor size, nodal status, and age, DFS and RFS remained significant, but OS was no longer significant ($p = 0.23$). There was a strong association between response to preoperative chemotherapy

TABLE 7.5. *The effect of complete clinical response and pathological response on survival.*

Study	Median Follow-up (years)	Pathological CR (pCR) (%)	Clinical CR (cCR) (%)	Clinical PR (cPR) (%)	No Response (%)	p value for pCR	p value for cCR
Hortobagyi (32)	5 OS IIIA	—	93	78	NR	—	0.6
	5 OS IIIB	—	88	44	24		0.01
Cameron (33)	7.5 OS	88	63[a]		33		0.005
Bonadonna (29)	8 RFS	86	56[a]		37	0.034[b]	—
Ellis (30)	5 OS	76	76	76	63	0.4	0.08
Fisher (21)	5 DFS	84	76	64	60	0.0001	0.0014
	5 OS	87	82	78	77	0.23[c]	0.19
Kuerer (48)	5 OS	89	64[d]			<0.01	—
Pierga (44)	10 OS	—	63[a]		47	—	0.01

NR, not reached.
[a]Overall clinical response, including patients with a cCR.
[b]Adjusted for tumor size and nodal status.
[c]Adjusted for tumor size, nodal status and age.
[d]Included all patients who did not achieve a pCR.

and pathologic nodal status ($p < 0.0001$) subsequent to therapy. Women with a pCR most frequently had microscopically negative nodes. It could be argued that the prognostic significance of the number of nodes still containing tumor after preoperative chemotherapy might simply reflect the number of nodes involved at presentation. However, in this study, there were more pathologically negative nodes in the preoperative arm than in the postoperative arm (59% versus 43%). Estimated relative risks indicated that breast tumor response was less important prognostically than pathologic nodal status ($p <$ than 0.0001) and clinical tumor size ($p < 0.0005$).

In a prospective study of neoadjuvant chemotherapy, 16% of patients achieved a pCR in the primary tumor and 12% of patients had no evidence of invasive carcinoma in the breast or axillary nodes (43). A pCR in the primary tumor was predictive of a complete axillary response ($p < 0.01$). Five-year OS and DFS rates were higher in the group that achieved pCR compared to patients who had less than a pCR ($p < 0.01$).

In the Royal Marsden study, there was no association between cCR and a pCR and survival. Pre-treatment palpable axillary nodes were a significant predictor of worsened DFS ($p = 0.0001$) and OS ($p = 0.0001$). Patients remaining node-positive post-chemotherapy had an inferior outcome compared with those becoming node-negative, DFS ($p = 0.03$), and OS ($p = 0.03$), but pathological axillary nodal status was not shown to predict for survival (30). Using data collected prospectively from 280 patients treated with preoperative chemotherapy, pCR was more likely in T1 or T2 tumors ($p = 0.0004$), in younger patients ($p = 0.008$), and in responders to chemotherapy ($p = 0.03$), particularly if a partial response was reached following two chemotherapy cycles ($p < 0.001$) (45).

Persistent pathological nodes following preoperative chemotherapy have also been shown to be a poor predictor of outcome (29,33,44,46).

In an M.D. Anderson series, 10-year survival figures following doxorubicin-based chemotherapy for women with stage III breast cancer were 65% for no nodes, 44% for one to three nodes, 32% for four to ten nodes and only 9% with more than ten nodes involved, but survival based on nodal groupings was not significantly statistically different (46).

In a Scottish study, 94 patients between 1984 and 1987 were treated with hormone therapy and cyclophosphamide, Adriamycin, vincristine, and prednisone (CHOP) preoperative chemotherapy given to those who failed to respond by 3 months. After 1987, patients were given CHOP only if they were ER negative and if they progressed on hormone therapy. The two key factors that predicted for poor survival were the number of involved axillary nodes following preoperative systemic therapy ($p < 0.00001$) and lack of response to preoperative therapy ($p < 0.05$), although the study did not have complete data regarding prechemotherapy nodal status (33).

In the Milan series, the 8-year relapse-free survival rate was 75% for node-negative patients, 51% with one to three nodes and 35% with less than three nodes involved. Cox regression analysis showed that nodal status at histology was the most important factor affecting RFS ($p < 0.001$) (29).

In a retrospective analysis of 488 patients who underwent surgery following preoperative chemotherapy, the tumor pathological response rate was 5% and was significantly correlated with clinical response ($p = 0.047$) (44). However, no correlation was made between histological response and survival, probably because of the low percentage of patients achieving pCR. The pathological nodal status also correlated with clinical response ($p = 0.04$). There was, in addition, a significant correlation between the number of axillary lymph nodes involved following preoperative chemotherapy and OS and DFS at 10 years ($p < 0.0001$).

Biological Predictive Factors

Breast cancer is an ideal model anatomically to study the biological effects of preoperative chemotherapy; the breast is accessible not only to clinical and radiological examination but also to serial sampling by fine-needle aspirate or

Tru-Cut biopsy. There is the potential to identify predictive biological markers of response and long-term outcome very early after the first course of treatment, thus enabling both individual tailoring of treatment and the more rapid evaluation of new therapies in the clinic.

The apoptotic index (AI), proliferation (Ki67 nuclear antigen), and Bcl-2 protein expression have been compared before and again 24 hours after ECisF or AC chemotherapy in 19 patients with operable breast cancer (47). Sequential Tru-Cut biopsies were taken 7 days prior to commencing chemotherapy and 24 hours after commencing treatment. Ten patients (59%) showed more than a 50% increase in AI 24 hours following chemotherapy. Overall there was a significant increase in apoptosis in the 24-hour biopsy ($p = 0.009$) but no significant difference in Ki67 or Bcl-2 expression. Of 13 clinical responders, nine (69%) showed a greater than 50% increase in AI, whereas three of four nonresponders (75%) showed no significant change in AI ($p = 0.22$).

A further study in which 57 patients were randomized to receive either two cycles of preoperative CMF chemotherapy or placebo followed by surgery and adjuvant chemotherapy confirmed that preoperative chemotherapy induces apoptosis. Samples were taken on entry into the study and at the time of surgery (48). The mean AI was 4.3% (range 1.1% to 7%) in the preoperative chemotherapy group, compared to 2.2% (range 1% to 4.1%) in the placebo group ($p < 0.05$). In the preoperative group, high AI levels were significantly associated with improved DFS and OS after a median follow-up of 44 months ($p < 0.05$).

A decrease in the proliferating fraction (PF) of less than 25% as measured by the proportion of tumor cells staining positive for Ki67 after one cycle of preoperative CEF (oral cyclophosphamide, epirubicin and 5-fluorouracil) chemotherapy has been shown to predict for a lower risk of disease recurrence (49). The recurrence rate was 21% for women with a decrease of more than 25% in PF, compared with 65% for women with a lower decrease in PF ($p = 0.033$).

Other studies have shown that tumors negative for cerbB-2 have higher response rates to preoperative chemotherapy ($p = 0.007$) and significantly better DFS ($p < 0.05$) (50,51). Higher response rates have been observed for tumors that are estrogen receptor (ER), progesterone receptor, (PgR) and Bcl-2 positive but did not reach statistical significance (50). ER and p53 expression have been shown to significantly predict for survival ($p < 0.05$) (52).

Two ancillary studies to the NSABP B-27 protocol have been implemented to evaluate serum and tumor biomarkers in relation to response and outcome (41). The first study evaluates the role of serum erbB-2 extracellular domain and serum erbB-2 antibodies. The second study will evaluate the following biomarkers: ER, PgR, proliferation markers, p53 oncogene mutations, erbB-2 overexpression, P-glycoprotein, and markers of apoptosis, e.g., Bcl-2. These studies should provide an excellent opportunity to gain insight into the biological effects of preoperative chemotherapy, particularly as the studies also evaluate the role of docetaxel in the adjuvant setting.

The design of future randomized controlled trials should ideally include the evaluation of potential biological predictive factors. Developments in molecular biology and micro-array technology will hopefully enable the identification of factors that can predict for response and outcome to preoperative chemotherapy and allow not only individualization of treatment but rapid evaluation of new treatments.

SUMMARY

Preoperative chemotherapy for primary operable breast cancer:

- Does not offer a survival benefit compared to adjuvant chemotherapy but is equivalent (level of evidence: 1)
- Reduces the requirement for mastectomy (level of evidence: 1)
- Does not significantly increase the risk of local recurrence (level of evidence: 2)
- Provides an *in vivo* model of response
- Has shown that clinical response is an important predictor for outcome (level of evidence: 1)

- Has shown that pathological complete response of the primary tumor and axillary nodes is an important predictor for outcome (level of evidence: 1)
- Offers the opportunity to identify predictive factors for response
- Offers the opportunity to evaluate new treatment modalities rapidly
- Offers the potential to individualize treatment according to response

CONCLUSION

Preoperative chemotherapy can be considered for patients with primary operable breast cancer amenable to breast-conserving surgery. Well-designed prospective randomized trials are required to evaluate new treatment modalities as they become available. These studies should incorporate the potential identification of predictive factors that may predict for outcome and allow the individualization of patient treatment in the future.

REFERENCES

1. Anonymous. Systemic treatment of early breast cancer by hormonal, cytotoxic, or immune therapy. 133 randomized trials involving 31,000 recurrences and 24,000 deaths among 75,000 women. Early Breast Cancer Trialists' Collaborative Group. *Lancet* 1992; 339:71–85.
2. Anonymous. Systemic treatment of early breast cancer by hormonal, cytotoxic, or immune therapy. 133 randomized trials involving 31,000 recurrences and 24,000 deaths among 75,000 women. Early Breast Cancer Trialists' Collaborative Group. *Lancet* 1992; 339:1–15.
3. Anonymous. Polychemotherapy for early breast cancer: an overview of the randomized trials. Early Breast Cancer Trialists' Collaborative Group. *Lancet* 1998; 352:930–942.
4. Fisher B, Anderson S, Redmond CK, et al. Reanalysis and results after 12 years of follow-up in a randomized clinical trial comparing total mastectomy with lumpectomy with or without irradiation in the treatment of breast cancer. *N Engl J Med* 1995;333:1456–1461.
5. De Lena M, Zucali R, Viganotti G, et al. Combined chemotherapy-radiotherapy approach in locally advanced (T3b-T4) breast cancer. *Cancer Chemother Pharmacol* 1978;1:53–59.
6. Hortobagyi GN, Blumenschein GR, Spanos W, et al. Multimodal treatment of locoregionally advanced breast cancer. *Cancer* 1983;51:763–768.
7. Goldhirsch A, Glick JH, Gelber RD, et al. International Consensus Panel on the treatment of primary breast cancer. V: Update 1998. Recent.Results. *Cancer Res* 1998;152:481–497.
8. Forrest AP, Levack PA, Chetty U, et al. A human tumour model. *Lancet* 1986;2:840–842.
9. Mansi JL, Smith IE, Walsh G, et al. Primary medical therapy for operable breast cancer. *Eur J Cancer Clin Oncol* 1989;25:(11)1623–1627.
10. Gunduz N, Fisher B, Saffer EA. Effect of surgical removal on the growth and kinetics of residual tumor. *Cancer Res* 1979;39:3861–3865.
11. Fisher B, Gunduz N, Coyle J, et al. Presence of a growth-stimulating factor in serum following primary tumor removal in mice. *Cancer Res* 1989;49:1996–2001.
12. Fisher B, Saffer E, Rudock C, et al. Effect of local or systemic treatment prior to primary tumor removal on the production and response to a serum growth-stimulating factor in mice. *Cancer Res* 1989;49:2002–2004.
13. O'Reilly MS, Holmgren L, Chen C, Folkman J. Angiostatin induces and sustains dormancy of human primary tumors in mice. *Nat Med* 1996;2:689–692.
14. Mansi JL, Gogas H, Bliss JM, et al. Outcome of primary-breast-cancer patients with micrometastases: a long-term follow-up study. *Lancet* 1999;354:197–202.
15. Goldie JH, Coldman AJ. A mathematic model for relating the drug sensitivity of tumors to their spontaneous mutation rate. *Cancer Treat Rep* 1979;63:1727–1733.
16. Mauriac L, Durand M, Avril A, Dilhuydy JM. Effects of primary chemotherapy in conservative treatment of breast cancer patients with operable tumors larger than 3 cm. Results of a randomized trial in a single centre. *Ann Oncol* 1991;2:347–354.
17. Mauriac L, MacGrogan G, Avril A, et al. Neoadjuvant chemotherapy for operable breast carcinoma larger than 3 cm: a unicentre randomized trial with a 124-month median follow-up. Institut Bergonie Bordeaux Groupe Sein (IBBGS). *Ann Oncol* 1999;10:47–52.
18. Scholl SM, Fourquet A, Asselain B, et al. Neoadjuvant versus adjuvant chemotherapy in premenopausal patients with tumors considered too large for breast conserving surgery: preliminary results of a randomized trial: S6. *Eur J Cancer* 1994;30A:645–652.
19. Broet P, Scholl SM, de la Rochefordiere A, et al. Short and long-term effects on survival in breast cancer patients treated by primary chemotherapy: an updated analysis of a randomized trial. *Breast Cancer Res Treat* 1999;58:151–156.
20. Semiglazov VF, Topuzov EE, Bavli JL, et al. Primary (neoadjuvant) chemotherapy and radiotherapy compared with primary radiotherapy alone in stage IIb-IIIa breast cancer. *Ann Oncol* 1994;5:591–595.
21. Fisher B, Bryant J, Wolmark N, et al. Effect of preoperative chemotherapy on the outcome of women with operable breast cancer. *J Clin Oncol* 1998;16:2672–2685.
22. Fisher B, Brown A, Mamounas E, et al. Effect of preoperative chemotherapy on local-regional disease in women with operable breast cancer: findings from National Surgical Adjuvant Breast and Bowel Project B-18. *J Clin Oncol* 1997;15:2483–2493.
23. Powles TJ, Hickish TF, Makris A, et al. Randomized trial of chemoendocrine therapy started before or after

surgery for treatment of primary breast cancer. *J Clin Oncol* 1995;13:547–552.
24. Makris A, Powles TJ, Ashley SE, et al. A reduction in the requirements for mastectomy in a randomized trial of neoadjuvant chemoendocrine therapy in primary breast cancer. *Ann Oncol* 1998;9:1179–1184.
25. Jacquillat C, Weil M, Baillet F, et al. Results of neoadjuvant chemotherapy and radiation therapy in the breast-conserving treatment of 250 patients with all stages of infiltrative breast cancer. *Cancer* 1990;66: 119–129.
26. Smith IE, Jones AL, O'Brien ME, et al. Primary medical (neo-adjuvant) chemotherapy for operable breast cancer. *Eur J Cancer* 1993; 29A:1796–1799.
27. Calais G, Berger C, Descamps P, et al. Conservative treatment feasibility with induction chemotherapy, surgery, and radiotherapy for patients with breast carcinoma larger than 3 cm. *Cancer* 1994;74:1283–1288.
28. Smith IE, Walsh G, Jones A, et al. High complete remission rates with primary neoadjuvant infusional chemotherapy for large early breast cancer. *J Clin Oncol* 1995;13:424–429.
29. Bonadonna G, Valagussa P, Brambilla C, et al. Primary chemotherapy in operable breast cancer: eight-year experience at the Milan Cancer Institute. *J Clin Oncol* 1998; 16:93–100.
30. Ellis P, Smith I, Ashley S, et al. Clinical prognostic and predictive factors for primary chemotherapy in operable breast cancer. *J Clin Oncol* 1998;16:107–114.
31. Belembaogo E, Feillel V, Chollet P, et al. Neoadjuvant chemotherapy in 126 operable breast cancers. *Eur J Cancer* 1992;28A:896–900.
32. Hortobagyi GN, Ames FC, Buzdar AU, et al. Management of stage III primary breast cancer with primary chemotherapy, surgery, and radiation therapy. *Cancer* 1988;62:2507–2516.
33. Cameron DA, Anderson ED, Levack P, et al. Primary systemic therapy for operable breast cancer—10-year survival data after chemotherapy and hormone therapy. *Br J Cancer* 1997;76:1099–1105.
34. Chollet P, Charrier S, Brain E, et al. Clinical and pathological response to primary chemotherapy in operable breast cancer. *Eur J Cancer* 1997;33:862–866.
35. Moliterni A, Tagliabue P, Tarenzi E, et al. Non-randomized comparison between primary chemotherapy (PC) with single agent anthracycline (A) or doxorubicin + paclitaxel (AT). *Proc Am Soc Clin Oncol* 2000;Abstract.
36. Amat S, Bougnoux P, Penault-Llorca F. Primary chemotherapy for operable breast cancer: High pathological response rate induced by docetaxel. *Proc Am Soc Clin Oncol* 2000;19:Abstract.
37. Buzdar AU, Singletary SE, Theriault RL, et al. Prospective evaluation of paclitaxel versus combination chemotherapy with fluorouracil, doxorubicin, and cyclophosphamide as neoadjuvant therapy in patients with operable breast cancer. *J Clin Oncol* 1999;17:3412–3417.
38. Smith I, A'Hern R, Howell A, et al. Preoperative continuous infusional ECisF (epirubicin, cisplatin and infusional 5 FU) v. Conventional AC chemotherapy for early breast cancer: A Phase III Multicentre Randomized Trial by the Topic Trial Group. *Proc Am Soc Clin Oncol* 2000;Abstract.
39. Hutcheon AW, Ogston KN, Heys SD, et al. Primary chemotherapy in the treatment of breast cancer: significantly enhanced clinical and pathological response with docetaxel. Proc *Am Soc Clin Oncol* 2000;Abstract.
40. Luporsi E, Vanlemmens L, Coudert B, et al. 6 Cycles of FEC vs 6 cycles of epirubicin-docetaxel (ED) as neoadjuvant chemotherapy in operable breast cancer patients; preliminary results of a randomized trial of Girec S01. *Proc Am Soc Clin Oncol* 2000; Abstract.
41. Mamounas EP. Overview of National Surgical Adjuvant Breast Project neoadjuvant chemotherapy studies. *Semin Oncol* 1998;25:31–35.
42. Gregory RK, Smith IE, A'Hern R. Results of a phase II randomized trial of preoperative navelbine-epirubicin (NE) v Navelbine-Mitooxantrone (NM) v adriamycin-cyclophosphamide (AC) chemotherapy for > 3cm early breast cancer. *Proc Am Soc Clin Oncol* 2001;20:21b Abstract.
43. Kuerer HM, Newman LA, Smith TL, et al. Clinical course of breast cancer patients with complete pathologic primary tumor and axillary lymph node response to doxorubicin-based neoadjuvant chemotherapy. *J Clin Oncol* 1999;17:460–469.
44. Pierga JY, Mouret E, Dieras V, et al. Prognostic value of persistent node involvement after neoadjuvant chemotherapy in patients with breast cancer. *Br J Cancer* 2000;83:1480–1487.
45. Verrill M, Ashley S, Walsh G, et al. Pathological complete response (pCR) in patients treated with neoadjuvant chemotherapy for operable breast cancer. *Breast Cancer Res Treat* 1998;50:328 Abstract.
46. Frye D, Buzdar AU, Hortobagyi GN. Prognostic significance of axillary nodal involvement after preoperative chemotherapy in stage III breast cancer. *Proc Am Soc Clin Oncol* 1995;14:95 Abstract.
47. Ellis PA, Smith IE, McCarthy K, et al. Preoperative chemotherapy induces apoptosis in early breast cancer. *Lancet* 1997;349:849
48. Shao ZM, Li J, Wu J, et al. Neo-adjuvant chemotherapy for operable breast cancer induces apoptosis. *Breast Cancer Res Treat* 1999;53:263–269.
49. Billgren AM, Rutqvist LE, Tani E, et al. Proliferating fraction during neoadjuvant chemotherapy of primary breast cancer in relation to objective local response and relapse-free survival. *Acta Oncol* 1999; 38:597–601.
50. Makris A, Powles TJ, Dowsett M, et al. Prediction of response to neoadjuvant chemoendocrine therapy in primary breast carcinomas. *Clin Cancer Res* 1997;3: 593–600.
51. Gregory RK, Powles TJ, Salter J, et al. Prognostic relevance of cerbB2 expression following neoadjuvant chemotherapy in patients in a randomised trial of neoadjuvant versus adjuvant chemoendocrine therapy. *Breast Cancer Res Treat* 2000;59:171–175.
52. Chang J, Powles TJ, Allred DC, et al. Predictive molecular markers for clinical outcome following primary chemotherapy for operable breast cancer. *Proc Am Soc Clin Oncol* 1998;Abstract.

8
Adjuvant Treatment: Node-negative Breast Cancer

Miguel Martin

The relative percentage of node-negative breast cancer (NNBC) to node-positive disease is progressively increasing in incidence in developed countries. This has, at least in part, resulted from mammography screening campaigns in at-risk populations and increased health education programs for whole populations of women in Western countries. At present, it is estimated that, in Spain, more than 50% of women with breast cancer are diagnosed before node involvement occurs, and it is expected that this proportion will increase in the next decade. In the United States, 61% of women currently present with NNBC, 30% present with a node-positive diagnosis, and the remainder present with metastatic disease (1). It is not unreasonable, therefore, to believe that NNBC will be the predominant form of presentation of the disease in all Western countries in the relatively near future. However, we still lack knowledge of prognostic and predictive factors, and therapeutic guidelines in patients with NNBC are more variable than in those with node-positive breast cancer. Thus, it remains increasingly important that further clinical studies be conducted in this relatively good prognosis group of patients to assess prognostic and predictive factors, as well as to determine optimum therapies using cytotoxic drugs, hormones, and, more recently, biological response modifiers such as trastuzumab (Herceptin) that, with fewer side effects, may offer an important risk-benefit ratio in NNBC.

Traditionally, NNBC, as opposed to node-positive breast cancer, has been considered to have a good prognosis and to be curable, in the majority of cases, with only locoregional therapy. As recently as 1985, the NIH Consensus Conference on Adjuvant Therapy of Breast Cancer concluded that the routine administration of systemic adjuvant therapy in node-negative patients could not be recommended. However, even by May 1988, the National Cancer Institute published a *Clinical Alert* describing the preliminary results from three major node-negative studies and concluded, "adjuvant hormonal or cytotoxic chemotherapy can have a meaningful impact on the natural history of node-negative breast cancer patients" (2).

There are certain crucial points that need to be taken into account at the time of deciding the most appropriate treatment for an individual patient with NNBC:

1. With local treatment alone, 60% to 70% of all NNBC patients will remain disease-free at 10 years.
2. About two-thirds of patients with NNBC, therefore, would not benefit from systemic adjuvant therapy after surgery (and radiation where indicated).
3. Those patients at high risk of recurrence require an adjuvant therapy that needs to be as effective as therapy recommended for patients with node-positive cancer, because patients with NNBC that have a relapse will die exactly as those with node-positive cancer.
4. The relative benefit of adjuvant therapy is the same in women with NNBC as in those with node-positive disease. However, the absolute benefit is less in the former group because of the lower risk of recurrence. This needs to be taken into account at the time of risk-benefit assessment and, as a result, the type of systemic treatment recommendation may differ from that for node-positive patients.

Designing a clinical trial of post-surgical adjuvant therapy for NNBC poses specific problems. The definition of the patient selection criteria, especially the criteria for high risk, is of crucial importance, since it facilitates interstudy comparisons and meta-analyses. Another relevant issue that has logistic and economic implications is the necessity for protracted follow-up before any differences in disease-free survival (DFS) and, especially, overall survival (OS) between study treatments become evident. Alternatively, validated surrogate endpoints for DFS and OS must be found and applied.

This chapter reviews, first, the prognostic and predictive factors of NNBC and, then, the outcome of NNBC patients with different adjuvant therapies. Evidence will be categorized, whenever possible, into three levels (I, II or III), according to the strength of data supporting the conclusions.

PROGNOSTIC/PREDICTIVE FACTORS AND DETERMINATION OF RISK OF RECURRENCE

Given that only one in three patients with NNBC presents with recurrence after local treatment, (3,4) it is fundamental to know the prognostic factors capable of predicting the recurrence of the disease (5–8).

Tumor size is, without doubt, one of the most studied prognostic factors and constitutes a variable that is independent of the rest of the other prognostic factors in NNBC patients (9). Risk of recurrence increases progressively with the size of the tumor. A classic study (4) indicated that the rate of recurrence over 20 years in patients with NNBC of less than 1 cm is 14%, rising to 31% in patients with tumors of 1 to 2 cm and to 39% in patients with tumors of 3 to 5 cm. A tumor size of 2 cm, or, more recently, 1 cm, is commonly used as a cut-off point in considering a patient with NNBC as having a high risk of recurrence based on this factor alone.

Pathological criteria such as histological and/or nuclear grade constitute other independent prognostic factors in NNBC. For some authors, the nuclear grade is a more potent prognostic factor that the histological grade, but both appear to possess independent prognostic capacities. The limitation of grade as an efficient prognostic factor rests in its subjectivity. There are definite issues of concordance of criteria with both intra- and interindividual variations for pathologists dealing with intermediate grade tumors, with fewer discrepancies arising in patients with well-differentiated or clearly undifferentiated tumors. Other studies (10) have also suggested that blood vessel invasion, in addition to size, was prognostic for long-term survival.

Hormone receptors remain prognostic, in addition to being the original and most widely used predictive factors that have been extensively investigated in women with NNBC (and, of course, node-positive disease). The presence of hormonal receptors is usually correlated to good histological differentiation and less aggressive clinical behavior. In most published large series from randomized trials, NNBC patients with positive receptors have been shown to have an OS and DFS significantly larger than those who do not express receptors (with an absolute difference of 5% to 10%). However, the value of studies of estrogen/progesterone receptors (ER/PgR) to discriminate outcome of groups of patients appears to decrease over time and almost disappears by 10 years of follow-up. Of additional benefit with respect to therapy, hormone receptors constitute a predictive factor in the response to adjuvant treatment with tamoxifen.

Histological subtype has also been investigated as a prognostic factor (11). Tubular and papillary carcinomas appear to have a less aggressive course than invasive ductal and lobular carcinomas. Colloid and medullar carcinomas have an intermediate prognosis. Some investigators exclude carcinomas of good prognosis (tubular and papillary) from adjuvant studies in NNBC unless the size exceeds 3 cm, but this criterion is not supported yet by conclusive data. This is, in part, due to the small numbers of patients in each subgroup and, therefore, a lack of prospective data based on histological subclassification. Similarly, observer variability makes determination of sub-groups liable to error in classification.

Patient age has been recognized, more recently, as an important prognostic factor. Women aged less than 35 years at diagnosis are considered, by many groups, at high risk for relapse (12). Whether age is truly an independent prognostic factor remains to be determined by further prospective studies.

Amongst the various biological factors, aneuploidy and a high fraction of cells in S-phase have been suggested as factors related to poor prognosis, although these have not always appeared as independent variables in multivariate studies. A similar situation exists with respect to p53 status (13,14), cathepsin-D levels (15), and c-erbB-2 status. Overexpression of c-erbB-2 is found in 20% of NNBC patients and appears in some studies to be associated with a poorer outcome (16–18).

Recently, markers of tumor angiogenesis and proteolysis have been reported as having independent prognostic value with respect to survival in NNBC (19,20); however, these preliminary results need to be confirmed in further studies.

Based on the most comprehensive evaluation of the literature, the St. Gallen Consensus Conference of 2001 (21) defined two groups with respect to risk of recurrence in women with NNBC (Table 8.1), instead of the three groups defined previously at the 1998 conference.

According to the St. Gallen criteria, more than half of all the patients with NNBC can be included in the average/high-risk group. Adjuvant therapy is justified in this group since the accumulated rate of recurrence at 10 years is around 40%.

On the other hand, it appears from the published literature that women with NNBC of less than 1 cm in diameter regardless of histologic grade, or 1 to 2 cm in diameter and histologic grade 1 have the same survival likelihood as age-matched women without breast cancer (22). Adjuvant therapy is not strongly recommended in the minimal/low-risk group, although the use of tamoxifen is acceptable.

The St. Gallen panel felt that nodal status and number of nodes remain the most important factor with respect to estimation of risk. Within NNBC, tumor size, histological plus nuclear grade, receptor status, lymphatic and/or vascular invasion, and age are factors that define groups with differential prognosis and can be used for treatment selection. Two new strategies were discussed by the panel at St. Gallen as having great potential for altering risk estimation, but both of these require further study. The first is sentinel node biopsy and the second is

TABLE 8.1. *Definition of risk categories for patients with node-negative breast cancer. St. Gallen Consensus Conference, 2001*

Risk category	Endocrine-Responsive[a]	Endocrine-Nonresponsive[a]
Minimal/low risk[b]	ER and/or PgR positive, and all of the following features: pT[c] ≤ 2 cm, and Grade 1[d], and age[e] ≥ 35 years	Not applicable
Average/high risk	ER and/or PgR positive, and at least one of the following features: pT[c] > 2 cm, or Grade 2–3[d], or age[e] < 35 years	ER and PgR negative

ER, estrogen receptor; PgR, progesterone receptor.

[a]Responsiveness to endocrine therapies is related to expression of ER and PgR in the tumor cells. The exact threshold of ER and/or PgR staining (with currently available immunohistochemical methods), which should be used to distinguish between endocrine-responsive and endocrine-nonresponsive tumor, is unknown. Even a low number of cells stained positive (as low as 1% of tumor cells) identify a cohort of tumors having some responsiveness to endocrine therapies. Probably, as is typical for biologic systems, a precise threshold does not exist. However, chosen empirically, approximately 10% positive staining of cells for either receptor might be considered as a reasonable threshold, accepted by most. Furthermore, it is clear that the lack of staining for both receptors confers endocrine non-responsiveness status.

[b]Some panel members recognize lymphatic and/or vascular invasion as a factor indicating greater risk than minimal or low. On the other hand, mucinous histologic type is associated with low risk of relapse.

[c]Pathologic tumor size (i.e., size of the invasive component).

[d]Histologic and/or nuclear grade.

[e]Patients with breast cancer at young age have been shown to be at high risk of relapse.

Reproduced with permission from Ciatto S, Cecchini S, Grazzini G, et al. Tumor size and prognosis of breast cancer with negative axillary nodes. *Neoplasma* 1990;37:179–184.

the use of preoperative systemic therapy, which leads to assessment of pathological features often using only FNA or core biopsy. Preoperative systemic therapy is likely to modify the characteristics of the primary tumor plus axillary nodes. However, use of preoperative treatment gives the clinician the unique opportunity to determine the clinical and pathological response to therapy, which also influences risk assessment.

There continues to be difficulty in assigning node-negative status (23). This is true using established surgical dissection of level I and II nodes and is made more complex by the use of sentinel node evaluation. The latter usually requires a learning curve to achieve a level of expertise by the surgeon, and it requires the pathologist to examine the sentinel node with special care, checking multiple levels and utilizing techniques such as immunohistochemical staining to rule out node positivity. These techniques are not considered routine when axillary dissection is performed. Thus, the assignment of NNBC and sub-classification into average/high-risk and minimal/low-risk categories continues to change with the evolution of new technologies. Our interventional strategies need to keep pace with these new developments (24).

SYSTEMIC ADJUVANT THERAPY IN NNBC

As commented earlier, NNBC had been considered, historically, as having a good prognosis with locoregional treatment alone. However, review of the published literature indicates a recurrence rate in the region of 30% at 10 years, which has prompted the conduct of controlled clinical trials with chemotherapy and tamoxifen. What follows are brief highlights of what appear to be the most important available published studies of adjuvant therapy in NNBC (25).

Adjuvant Hormone Therapy

The North American National Surgical Adjuvant Breast and Bowel Project (NSABP) B-14 study constitutes the most important trial of adjuvant hormone therapy (hormonotherapy) in NNBC because of its clear and appropriate methodology and sample size (26). The study included 2,664 patients with NNBC and positive estrogen receptors (ER) who were randomized to receive 20 mg of tamoxifen per day or placebo over a period of 5 years. The patients treated with tamoxifen had a 4-year DFS that was statistically greater to those treated with placebo (83% versus 77%), although the difference in OS was not statistically significant at the time of the first communication of the results. Published in 1989, the authors concluded, at that time, that the benefit due to tamoxifen, despite its small impact on DFS, constituted a notable advance in the treatment of such patients and, as such, warranted further studies. In a subsequent extension of the study, the patients that were disease-free following 5 years of treatment with tamoxifen were re-randomized to continue with tamoxifen or with placebo for a further 5 years. No additional benefit was observed with extending the treatment with tamoxifen to 10 years (27). The survival analysis at 10 years of follow-up demonstrated the maintenance of benefit in DFS in favor of tamoxifen compared to placebo (69% versus 57%) and at the same time showed a statistically significant benefit in OS in favor of hormone treatment (80% versus 76%).

The meta-analysis of the Early Breast Cancer Trialists' Collaborative Group (EBCTCG) reported in 1998 demonstrated that adjuvant tamoxifen increased OS at 10 years by 5.6% (standard deviation 1.3) with respect to the no-treatment group of women with NNBC (28). The benefit was clear in women with positive or unknown ER but not in those with negative receptors. According to the data of this meta-analysis, the improvement in DFS observed with tamoxifen was produced, essentially, in the first 5 years while the improvement in OS occurred over a period of 10 years. This is exactly the same result that the NSABP B-14 generated.

The panel of the 2001 St. Gallen Conference established that the combination of ovarian ablation (GnRH analogs) plus or minus tamoxifen is an alternative to chemotherapy-plus-tamoxifen in premenopausal, endocrine-responsive NNBC patients of average/high risk (22). This recommendation, however, is based on randomized trials carried out mainly in node-positive patients and in which the chemotherapy arm did not include anthracyclines.

Adjuvant Chemotherapy

In patients with NNBC considered at high risk for relapse, various studies assessed different protocols of adjuvant chemotherapy compared to observation only. More recently, CMF-like regimens were compared to doxorubicin-containing combinations and chemo/hormonal therapy was tested against tamoxifen alone. The taxanes and trastuzumab are currently being investigated as adjuvant therapy for NNBC patients in ongoing or ready-to-start randomized trials.

Chemotherapy Versus No Treatment

The great majority of the studies that have compared adjuvant chemotherapy to no treatment demonstrated a benefit in DFS and OS with chemotherapy. This does not include protocols that, by today's standards, would be considered suboptimal with respect to dose intensity. For example, a negative result was reported by the West Midlands Oncology Association in which 574 patients with NNBC were randomized to receive oral chlorambucil, methotrexate sodium and 5-fluorouracil (LMF), a regimen no longer used, versus observation alone. There were no differences in DFS or OS (29).

However, the Ludwig Breast Cancer Study Group (30) randomized 1,275 patients with NNBC to receive either a single cycle of CMF immediately postoperatively or no treatment. This minimal chemotherapy regimen produced a small, albeit statistically significant, benefit in DFS at 4 years (77% versus 73%) (30). This reveals the benefit of studies with large sample sizes, which allows for the observation of small, but statistically significant, differences in outcome.

The NSABP B-13 protocol randomized 679 patients with NNBC and negative ER to receive either chemotherapy treatment with methotrexate, 5-fluorouracil and folinic acid (MFL) or no treatment. At 4 years of follow-up, the DFS was significantly better in the group of patients that received chemotherapy (80% versus 71%) (31).

Similarly, the North American Intergroup (Eastern Cooperative Oncology Group [ECOG], Southwest Oncology Group [SWOG],and Cancer and Leukemia Group B [CALGB]) conducted a study in 536 women with NNBC. They used criteria of high-risk for recurrence (ER negative or ER positive plus tumor size more than 3 cm) and randomized patients to receive either six cycles of cyclophosphamide, methotrexate, 5-fluorouracil, and prednisone (CMFP) or no treatment. The DFS and OS rates at 10 years were 73% and 81%, respectively, among patients who received chemotherapy, compared with 58% and 71%, respectively, in the observation group (32,33).

The Istituto Nazionale Tumori of Milan initiated a study in women with NNBC and negative ER in 1980 (34). Ninety patients were included in the study and randomized to receive either 12 cycles of intravenous CMF or no treatment. The DFS at 12 years was significantly greater in the group that received chemotherapy (71% versus 43%) as was the OS rate (80% versus 50%). This often-quoted-but-small study has been criticized by some for achieving significance only as a result of the lower-than-expected outcome in the no-treatment group.

Two recently published Italian studies compared chemotherapy with observation in individuals with rapidly proliferating NNBC. Amadori et al. (35) randomized 281 node-negative patients with rapidly proliferating tumors, according to the thymidine labeling index, to receive six cycles of CMF or no further treatment after surgery plus or minus radiation. The 5-year DFS was 83% for patients treated with CMF, compared with 72% in the control group ($p = 0.0028$). CMF reduced both locoregional and distant metastases. Paradiso et al. (36) compared adjuvant $FE_{50}C$ (fluorouracil 500 mg/m² on day 1 and 8, epirubicin 50 mg/m² on day 1, and cyclophosphamide 500 mg/m² on day 1) to observation in 248 NNBC patients with fast-proliferating disease as determined on thymidine incorporation assay using an autoradiographic technique. Five-year disease-free survival (DFS) was 81% in the $FE_{50}C$ group and 69% in the control group ($p < 0.02$).

A further study (37) used an urokinase-type plasminogen activator (uPA) and a plasminogen activator/inhibitor type 1 (PAI-1) to divide patients into high-risk and low-risk groups. Their study used these factors prospectively and have shown that the high-risk group (high uPA and/or PAI-1) benefit from CMF chemotherapy with a 43.8% lower estimated probability of recurrence. These results were updated and confirmed at the San Antonio 2001 meeting (38).

The results of poly-chemotherapy studies were analyzed in a meta-analysis by the EBCTCG in 1998 (39). In women with NNBC, adjuvant chemotherapy significantly improved DFS and OS compared to no treatment in all age subgroups. The magnitude of benefit was clinically relevant (for example, the OS at 10 years increased from 71% to 78%). The benefit in DFS was observed within the first 5 years, while the difference in OS appeared after longer follow-up at the time of the 10-year analysis.

Anthracyclines Versus Non-anthracycline-based Chemotherapy

The role of the anthracyclines as adjuvant therapy in patients with NNBC has been explored by the North American Intergroup (Protocol INT 0102) (40). A total of 2,691 node-negative high-risk patients (ER and PR negative, tumors of 2 cm or more, or a high phase-S fraction) were randomized to receive oral CAF (cyclophosphamide, Adriamycin, and fluorouracil) or oral CMF (cyclophosphamide, methotrexate, 5-fluorouracil) with or without 5 years of tamoxifen. Both DFS and OS were statistically improved with CAF, although the benefit was small (absolute increase of 2% in OS and DFS at 5 years). The inclusion of tamoxifen showed an additional positive effect on DFS and OS, as one would predict, only in receptor-positive patients.

The Spanish Group for Breast Cancer Research (GEICAM) in 1987 initiated a randomized trial comparing CMF (cyclophosphamide 600 mg/m^2 i.v., methotrexate 60 mg/m^2 i.v., 5-fluorouracil 600 mg/m^2 i.v., on day 1 every 3 weeks for six cycles) with FAC (5-fluorouracil 500 mg/m^2 i.v., doxorubicin 50 mg/m^2 i.v., cyclophosphamide 500 mg/m^2 i.v., day 1 every 3 weeks for six cycles) in 998 women with operable breast cancer. Both regimens were found to be equi-myelotoxic. The patients were prospectively stratified with respect to nodal status (node-negative versus node-positive). In the subgroup of 415 patients with NNBC at a median follow-up of 73 months, FAC was statistically superior to CMF in terms of DFS and OS (73% versus 62%, and 85% versus 76%, respectively, at 7.5 years) (41).

The meta-analysis by the EBCTCG confirmed that combinations which included anthracyclines were moderately better than those without anthracyclines (absolute increment of 3% at 10 years) (39).

Taxanes Versus Non–taxane-containing Chemotherapy

Various currently ongoing studies in both the United States and Europe are assessing the role of taxanes as adjuvant therapy for high-risk NNBC patients. The American Intergroup is comparing four courses of standard AC (doxorubicin plus cyclophosphamide) to four courses of AT (doxorubicin 60 mg/m^2 plus Taxotere 60 mg/m^2) in operable breast cancer patients with or without involved lymph nodes. The GEICAM group began the Taxotere Adjuvant Rhône-Poulenc-GEICAM Trial in N0 breast cancer patients, or TARGET 0 study, in July 1999 to compare their standard therapy, FAC in six cycles, with TAC (Taxotere 75 mg/m^2, doxorubicin 50 mg/m^2, cyclophosphamide 500 mg/m^2) in six cycles as postoperative adjuvant therapy in women with NNBC using high-risk criteria as defined by the 1998 St. Gallen Consensus Conference.

Adjuvant Chemo/hormonal Therapy

The NSABP B-20 protocol (42) investigated the effect of combination chemotherapy (methotrexate plus fluorouracil, or CMF) with tamoxifen versus tamoxifen alone in 2,036 patients with NNBC and positive ER. The two chemo/hormonal combinations were better than tamoxifen alone (DFS at 5 years of 89% to 90% versus 85%), an improvement that was apparent in all age groups. The same cooperative group randomized 2,008 NNBC patients with ER-negative tumors to receive CMF plus placebo, CMF plus tamoxifen, AC plus placebo, or AC plus tamoxifen (43). No significant difference in DFS or OS was observed among the four groups in the first 5 years. A comparison between all CMF-treated and all AC-treated patients demonstrated no significant differences in DFS (87% at 5 years in both groups). Other publications have reviewed the use of chemo/hormonotherapy and have concluded that the magnitude of benefit depends on tumor size, age, and (self-evidently) hormone status (44).

The North American Intergroup INT 0102 trial discussed previously also demonstrated that the addition of tamoxifen to chemotherapy increased both DFS and OS, although only in the subset of patients with ER-positive tumors (40).

Summary

NNBC will constitute, without doubt, one of the epidemics of the next century. Adjuvant treatment for women with NNBC poses specific problems that are different from those that apply to women with node-positive breast cancer. For example, although the relative benefits of adjuvant treatments are similar in node-positive and NNBC patients, the absolute benefits are quantitatively less in individuals with NNBC. It is therefore necessary to calculate the risk/benefit ratio for each subgroup that is offered therapy (45). It follows, in addition, that in NNBC in particular, we need to precisely define the predictive factors for each at-risk subgroup. This would allow the more toxic therapy to be limited to those most likely to benefit and, more importantly, define appropriately the most effective treatment for each patient group requiring systemic adjuvant therapy. For the moment, we know that adjuvant chemotherapy benefits the average high-risk NNBC patient, both in terms of DFS and OS. In addition, it is established that tamoxifen, administered over 5 years, benefits NNBC patients with positive ER. The appropriate adjuvant treatment of minimum/low-risk NNBC patients remains more difficult to establish. Either tamoxifen or no adjuvant treatment are appropriate options for these hormone responsive individuals.

Available data in node-positive patients reveal that chemotherapy protocols should be used at optimum doses. There is, in addition, solid evidence from the EBCTCG overview that regimens that include anthracyclines have a small, additional benefit when compared to non-anthracycline regimens. Despite this, no general consensus guidelines exist with respect to standard adjuvant chemotherapy in women with NNBC. In the author's opinion, the option of an anthracycline-containing regimen should be offered to high-risk (however it is defined) patients who do not present with contraindications to their use. It has been demonstrated that the majority of women are likely to accept a higher risk of toxicity if, in exchange, they can obtain a therapeutic benefit, particularly survival improvement, however small. The risk/benefit ratio of chemotherapy and hormone therapy needs to be discussed with each individual patient with the knowledge of their risk factors such as age, co-morbidities, and concurrent medications and in the light of the individual's preferences (46,47).

Despite the best current chemotherapy or chemo/hormonal therapy, at least 15% to 20% of women with average/high-risk NNBC will continue to present with recurrent disease (Table 8.2). This highlights the continuing need to investigate potentially more active regimens. Undoubtedly, the taxanes are the next generation of pharmacological agents whose efficacy needs to be intensively explored. Trastuzumab (Herceptin), an anti-c-erbB-2 monoclonal antibody, provides further targeted therapy, such as hormones, whose efficacy as adjuvant therapy for

TABLE 8.2. Disease-free survival and overall survival after adjuvant tamoxifen, chemotherapy, or chemohormonal therapy in selected randomized NNBC trials

Reference (number of patients)	Prognostic Characteristics	Adjuvant Therapy	DFS (%)	OS (%)
NSABP B-14 (11,12) (n = 2843)	ER positive	Tamoxifen vs. no treatment	75 at 10 years vs. 69([a])	80 vs. 76([a])
Ludvig V (15) (n = 1275)	All	CMF x 1 vs. no treatment	77 at 4 years vs. 73([a])	NA
NSABP B-13 (16) (n = 679)	ER negative	MFL vs. no treatment	80 at 4 years vs. 71([a])	NA
Intergroup (17,18) (n = 536)	ER/PR negative or ER/PR positive plus T>3cm	CMFP vs. no treatment	73 at 10 years vs. 58([a])	81 vs. 71([a])
Istituto Nazionale Tumori (19) (n = 90)	ER-	CMF i.v. vs. no treatment	71 at 12 years vs. 43%([a])	80 vs. 50([a])
Amadori et al (20) (n = 281)	High TLI	CMF vs. no treatment	83 at 5 years vs. 72([a])	NA
National Oncology Institut of Bari (21) (n = 248)	High TLI	FEC vs. no treatment	81% at 5 years vs. 69%([a])	NA
Intergroup INT 0102 (23) (n = 2691)	ER/PR negative or ER/PR positive plus T>2cm/high SPF	CAF + tamoxifen vs. CMF + tamoxifen	87 at 5 years vs. 85([a])	93 at 5 years vs. 91([a])
GEICAM 8701 (24) (n = 415)	All	FAC vs. CMF	73 at 7.5 years vs. 62([a])	85 vs. 76([a])
NSABP B-20 (25) (n = 2036)	ER positive	MF or CMF + tamoxifen vs. tamoxifen	89–90 at 5 years vs. 85([a])	NA
NSABP B-23 (26) (n = 2,008)	ER negative	CMF or AC + tamoxifen vs. CMF or AC + placebo	87 at 5 years vs. 87	NA

SPF, S-phase fraction; T, tumor size; TLI, thymidine labeling index.
[a]Statistically significant difference.
For details of chemotherapy regimens, see text.

NNBC patients with c-erbB-2 overexpression warrants investigation. Trastuzumab, where appropriate, is particularly interesting in these patients because of its low side effect profile, which would make the risk/benefit ratio especially attractive to women with NNBC.

FINAL CONCLUSIONS WITH LEVEL OF EVIDENCE RECOMMENDATIONS

1. Adjuvant Hormone Therapy

   Tamoxifen clearly improves DFS and OS in ER-positive NNBC patients (level 1 evidence for both outcomes). Tamoxifen has no impact on DFS or OS of NNBC patients with hormone non-responsive tumors (level 1 evidence). The recommendation of ovarian ablation (surgical or chemical) plus or minus tamoxifen as an alternative to chemotherapy plus tamoxifen in premenopausal NNBC women is based on prospective randomized trials carried out largely in node-positive patients.

   Despite the survival benefits associated with tamoxifen therapy, a 10-year recurrence rate of more than 30% in NNBC patients remains unacceptable with today's standards in mind; it seems clear that NNBC, ER-positive patients, as a group, need additional adjuvant therapy to improve prognosis.

2. Adjuvant Chemotherapy

   Adjuvant chemotherapy improves long-term DFS and OS in high-risk NNBC with respect to no treatment (level 1 evidence).

   Doxorubicin-containing combinations are superior to CMF-type regimens in terms of both DFS and OS in high-risk NNBC patients (level I evidence).

There is still room for improvement, however, since the 5-year relapse rate in most studies is between 15% and 20%.

3. Adjuvant Chemo/hormonal Therapy

The evidence from the literature and the meta-analysis show that tamoxifen and chemotherapy are complementary, not competing, adjuvant treatments. The combination of chemotherapy and hormonotherapy increases DFS and OS when compared to either tamoxifen alone or chemotherapy alone, but as predicted, only in the subset of NNBC patients with hormone-receptor positive tumors (level 1 evidence).

REFERENCES

1. Ries LAG, Kosary CL, Hankey BF, et al., eds. *SEER Cancer Statistics Review 1973–95*. Bethesda, MD: National Cancer Institute, 1998.
2. Anonymous. Treatment Alert issued for node-negative breast cancer. *N Natl Cancer Inst* 1988;8:550–551.
3. Husbey RA, Ownby HE, Frederick J, et al. Node-negative breast cancer treated by modified radical mastectomy without adjuvant therapies: Variables associated with disease recurrence and survivorship. *J Clin Oncol* 1988;6:83–88.
4. Rosen PP, Groshen S, Kinne DW. Prognosis in T2N0M0 stage I breast carcinoma. A 20-year follow-up study. *J Clin Oncol* 1991;9:1650–1661.
5. Rosner D, Lane WW. Predicting recurrence in axillary-node negative breast cancer patients [see comments]. *Breast Cancer Res Treat* 1993;25:127–139.
6. Quiet CA, Ferguson DJ, Weichselbaum RR, Hellman S. Natural history of node-negative breast cancer: a study of 826 patients with long-term follow-up. *J Clin Oncol* 1995;13:1144–1151.
7. Gasparini G, Weidner N, Bevilacqua P, et al. Tumor microvessel density, p53 expression, tumor size, and peritumoral lymphatic vessel invasion are relevant prognostic markers in node-negative breast carcinoma [see comments]. *J Clin Oncol* 1994;12:454–466.
8. Costantino J, Fisher B, Gunduz N, et al. Tumor size, ploidy, s phase, and erb b-2 markers in patients with node-negative, er-positive tumors: findings from NSABP B-14 (meeting abstract). *Proc Asco* 1994;13:A59.
9. Ciatto S, Cecchini S, Grazzini G, et al. Tumor size and prognosis of breast cancer with negative axillary nodes. *Neoplasma* 1990;37:179–184.
10. Kato T, Kimura T, Miyakawa R, et al. Clinicopathologic features associated with long-term survival in node-negative breast cancer patients. *Surgery Today* 1996;26:105–114.
11. Voogd AC, Coebergh JW, Repelaer vDO, et al. The risk of nodal metastases in breast cancer patients with clinically negative lymph nodes: a population-based analysis [In Process Citation]. *Breast Cancer Res Treat* 2000;62:63–69.
12. Nixon NJ, Neuberg D, Hayes DF, et al. Relationship of patient age to pathologic features of the tumor and prognosis for patients with stage I or II breast cancer. *J Clin Oncol* 1994;12:888–894.
13. Silvestrini R, Benini E, Daidone MG, et al. p53 as an independent prognostic marker in lymph node-negative breast cancer patients. *J Natl Cancer Inst* 1993;85:965–970.
14. Rosen PP, Lesser ML, Arroyo CD, et al. p53 in node-negative breast carcinoma: an immunohistochemical study of epidemiologic risk factors, histologic features, and prognosis. *J Clin Oncol* 1995;13:821–830.
15. Ferrandina G, Scambia G, Bardelli F, et al. Relationship between cathepsin-D content and disease-free survival in node-negative breast cancer patients: a meta-analysis. *Br J Cancer* 1997;76:661–666.
16. Andrulis IL, Bull SB, Blackstein ME, et al. Neu/erbB-2 amplification identifies a poor-prognosis group of women with node-negative breast cancer. *J Clin Oncol* 1998;16:1340–1349.
17. Molland JG, Barraclough BH, Gebski V, et al. Prognostic significance of c-erbB-2 oncogene in axillary node-negative breast cancer. *Aust N Z J Surg* 1996;66:64–70.
18. Rosen PP, Lesser ML, Arroyo CD, et al. Immunohistochemical detection of HER2/neu in patients with axillary lymph node negative breast carcinoma. A study of epidemiologic risk factors, histologic features, and prognosis. *Cancer* 1995;75:1320–1326.
19. Linderholm B, Tavelin B, Grankvist K, Heriksson R. Vasculat endothelium growth factor is of high prognostic value in node-negative breast carcinoma. *J Clin Oncol* 1998;16:3121–3128.
20. Eppenberger U, Keung W, Schlaeppi JM, et al. Markers of tumor angiogenesis and proteolysis independently define high and low-risk subsets of node-negative breast cancer. *J Clin Oncol* 1998;16:3129–3136.
21. Goldhirsch A, Glick JH, Gelber RD, et al. Meeting Highlights: International Consensus Panel on the Treatment of Primary Breast Cancer. *J Clin Oncol* 2001;19:3817–3827.
22. Arnesson L-G, Smeds S, Fagerberg G. Recurrence-free survival in patients with small breast cancers. *Eur J Surg* 1994;160:271–276.
23. Mathiesen O, Carl J, Bonderup O, Panduro J. Axillary sampling and the risk of erroneous staging of breast cancer. An analysis of 960 consecutive patients. *Acta Oncol* 1990;29:721–725.
24. Parmigiani G, Berry DA, Winer EP, et al. Is axillary lymph node dissection indicated for early-stage breast cancer? A decision analysis. *J Clin Oncol* 1999;17:1465–1473.
25. Hebert-Croteau N, Brisson J, Latreille J, et al. Time trends in systemic adjuvant treatment for node-negative breast cancer. *J Clin Oncol* 1999;17:1458–1464.
26. Fisher B, Constantino J, Redmond C, et al. A randomized clinical trial evaluating tamoxifen in the treatment of patients with node-negative breast cancer who have estrogen-receptor-positive tumors. *N Engl J Med* 1989;320:479–484.
27. Fisher B, Digman J, Bryant J, et al. Five versus more than five years of tamoxifen therapy for breast cancer patients with negative lymph nodes and estrogen-receptor-positive tumors. *J Natl Cancer Inst* 1996;88(21):1529–1524.

28. Early Breast Cancer Trialists' Collaborative Group. Tamoxifen for early breast cancer: An overview of the randomised trials. *Lancet* 1998;351:1451–1467.
29. Morrison JM, Kelly KA, Howell A. West Midlands Oncology Association Trial on adjuvant chemotherapy in node-negative breast cancer. *Natl Cancer Inst Monogr* 1992;11:85–88.
30. The Ludwig Breast Cancer Study Group. Prolonged disease-free survival after one course of perioperative adjuvant chemotherapy for node-negative breast cancer. *N Engl J Med* 1989;320:491–496.
31. Fisher B, Redmond C, Dimitrov NV, et al. A randomized clinical trial evaluating sequential methotrexate and fluorouracil in the treatment of patients with node-negative breast cancer who have estrogen-receptor-negative tumors. *N Engl J Med* 1989;320:473–478.
32. Mansour EG, Gray R, Shatila AH, et al. Efficacy of adjuvant chemotherapy in high-risk node-negative breast cancer. *N Engl J Med* 1989;320:485–490.
33. Mansour EG, Gray R, Shatila AH, et al. Survival advantage of adjuvant chemotherapy in high-risk node-negative breast cancer: Ten-year analysis; An Intergroup study. *J Clin Oncol* 1998;16:3486–3492.
34. Zambetti M, Valagussa P, Bonadonna G. Adjuvant cyclophosphamide, methotrexate and fluorouracil in node-negative and estrogen receptor-negative breast cancer. *Ann Oncol* 1996;7:481–485.
35. Amadori D, Nanni O, Marangolo M, et al. Disease-free survival advantage of adjuvant cyclophosphamide, methotrexate, and fluorouracil in node-negative, rapidly proliferating breast cancer: a randomized multicenter Study. *J Clin Oncol* 2000;18:3125–3134.
36. Paradiso A, Schittulli F, Cellamare G, et al. A randomized clinical trial of adjuvant fluorouracil, epirubicin, and cyclophosphamide chemotherapy for patients with fast-proliferating, node-negative breast cancer. *J Clin Oncol* 2001;19:3929–3937.
37. Janicke F, Prechtl A, Thomssen C, et al. Randomized adjuvant chemotherapy trial in high-risk, lymph node-negative breast cancer patients identified by urokinase-type plasminogen activator and plasminogen activator inhibitor type 1. *J Natl Cancer Inst* 2001;93:913–920.
38. Harbeck N, Meisner C, Prechtl A, et al. Level-I evidence for prognostic and predictive impact of uPA and PAI-I in node-negative breast cancer provided by second scheduled analysis of multicenter Chemo-N_0 therapy trial. *Breast Cancer Res Treat* 2001;69(3):213 (A19).
39. Early Breast Cancer Trialists' Collaborative Group. Polychemotherapy for early breast cancer: An overview of the randomised trials. *Lancet* 1998;352:930–943.
40. Hutchins L, Green S, Ravdin P, et al. CMF versus CAF with and without tamoxifen in high-risk node-negative breast cancer patients and a natural history follow-up study in low-risk node-negative patients: First results of Intergroup trial INT 0102. *Proc ASCO* 1998;17:2.
41. Martín M, Villar A, Solé-Calvo A, et al. FAC versus CMF as adjuvant treatment for operable breast cancer: A GEICAM study. *Proc ASCO* 2001;20:32a.
42. Fisher B, Digman J, Wolmark N, et al. Tamoxifen and chemotherapy for lymph node-negative, estrogen receptor-positive breast cancer. *J Natl Cancer Institute* 1997;89:1673–1682.
43. Fisher B, Anderson S, Tan-Chiu E, et al. Tamoxifen and chemotherapy for axillary node-negative, estrogen receptor-negative breast cancer: findings from National Surgical Adjuvant Breast and Bowel Project B-23. *J Clin Oncol* 2001;19:931–942.
44. Styblo TM, Wood WC. Adjuvant chemotherapy in the node-negative breast cancer patient. *Surg Clin North Am* 1996;76:327–341.
45. Wood WC. Integration of risk factors to allow patient selection for adjuvant systemic therapy in lymph node-negative breast cancer patients. *World J Surg* 1994;18:39–44.
46. Hillner BE, Smith TJ. Efficacy and cost effectiveness of adjuvant chemotherapy in women with node-negative breast cancer. A decision-analysis model. *N Engl J Med* 1991;324:160–168.
47. Hillner BE, Smith TJ. A model of chemotherapy in node-negative breast cancer. *J Natl Cancer Inst Monogr* 1992;11:143–149.

9
Node Positive Breast Cancer

Gul Atalay, Caroline Lohrisch, and Martine J. Piccart

Throughout the history of adjuvant breast cancer treatment, patients have been subdivided into several risk categories, both for making recommendations with respect to choice of therapy and for enrollment into clinical trials. The choice of optimal adjuvant therapy requires a careful evaluation of prognostic and predictive factors, along with other factors such as the presence of co-morbid illness and patient preference. Nodal status and the number of nodes involved are the most important features for estimating risk of recurrence. The probability of recurrence is higher for women with node-positive (NP) disease and increases with each additional positive node. This chapter reviews adjuvant treatment modalities for NP breast cancer based on available evidence.

ENDOCRINE THERAPY

Following surgical removal of the primary tumor, the principle of adjuvant endocrine, or hormonal, therapy is to minimize exposure of any residual foci of breast cancer cells to estrogen, which may stimulate cellular proliferation. Almost two-thirds of breast cancers have nuclear receptors for estrogen (ER) and/or progesterone (PgR). Binding of estrogen and progesterone to their respective receptors results in molecular activation and secondary cell signaling. This complex multi-step pathway finally leads to upregulation of cell cycling through activation of nuclear transcription factors. The activation of this pathway can be inhibited in a variety of ways. These include removing circulating estrogens (ovarian ablation in premenopausal women, aromatase inhibitors in postmenopausal women) that compete with estrogen for receptor binding, but do not fully activate the secondary messenger cascade or treating patients with drugs such as tamoxifen or novel anti-estrogens. These therapeutic maneuvers are only effective in patients with ER-positive and/or PgR-positive disease.

TAMOXIFEN

The most comprehensive synthesis of data on tamoxifen (TAM) in early breast cancer trials comes from The Early Breast Cancer Trialists' Collaborative Group (EBCTCG) overview, last updated for trials initiated before 1990, comprising data finalized in 1995 to 1996 and published in 1998 (1). This systematic overview analyzed individual outcomes of 37,000 patients enrolled in 55 randomized clinical trials (RCTs) of adjuvant TAM compared with no adjuvant hormonal intervention, with an average follow-up of ten years. Trial data were unavailable for approximately 5,700 women in eight trials. Of those, 4,200 individuals were enrolled in three large trials of 5 years of TAM. ER status was positive in 18,000, negative in 8,000, and unknown in about 12,000 women. Analysis was divided according to whether TAM was given for 1 year, 2 years or about 5 years. Each trial compared tamoxifen to no hormonal therapy, with the primary outcomes of interest being recurrence and death from breast cancer. Using an intention to treat analysis, log-rank, observed-minus-expected, values were calculated for each study (TAM versus control) and combined for an estimate of overall effect.

Use of TAM was associated with a highly significant decrease in both recurrence and death with a significant trend of increased benefit with longer duration of therapy. Using 5 years of TAM, the 10-year proportional reductions in recurrence and mortality were 47% and 26%, respectively. These results were irrespective of age, menopausal status, daily dose (which in most cases was 20 mg per day), and additional chemotherapy (level I evidence). The proportional reductions in recurrence and mortality were 37% and 27%, respectively, for ER-unknown tumors, and 50% and 28%, respectively, for ER-positive tumors. For node-positive patients, relative risk reductions (RRR) of 43% for recurrence and 28% for mortality at 10 years were reported. The absolute survival improvement at 10 years was greater in the node-positive (NP) group when compared to the node-negative (NN) group (10.9% versus 5.6%).

The preliminary results, from 5 years use of TAM from the 2000 Oxford Overview with 15 years follow-up, confirm a significant decrease of similar magnitude in both death and recurrence among ER-positive cancers, again with a significant trend towards greater effect with longer treatment (2).

The magnitude of benefit from TAM after chemotherapy (CT) in premenopausal women is still being studied. Although the EBCTCG overview reports significant positive results in favor of TAM, the absolute number of premenopausal women studied to date is small. This issue is addressed in the chemo-endocrine section of this chapter.

Elderly Patients

The number of trials addressing the benefit of TAM in elderly women and the number of elderly patients enrolled in such trials are low. However, available evidence appears to support a reduction in recurrence and breast cancer mortality for this group. Twenty-year follow-up results of the EST 1178 trial (3) that compared TAM versus placebo for 2 years after mastectomy in 181 NP women older than 65 years of age with ER-positive or unknown tumors were recently reported. Significantly better disease-free survival (DFS; $p = 0.002$) and time to relapse (TTR; $p < 0.001$) were observed for TAM; however, due to death from other causes (40% of study population), there was no overall survival (OS) advantage for TAM, despite a substantial decrease in breast cancer-related mortality (60% versus 77%) (3).

Duration of Therapy

The optimal duration of TAM use has been addressed by EBCTCG meta-analysis and several large randomized trials, as summarized below.

It is clear from the last-published Oxford Overview that there is a highly significant trend towards greater effect with longer treatment (1 year versus 2 years versus 5 years). The proportional reductions in mortality were 12% for 1 year, 17% for 2 years and 26% for 5 years. The preliminary results from the 2000 Oxford Overview support this "greater effect with longer treatment" trend and show that the reduction in recurrence and mortality with 5 years of TAM use continues to increase during the 5- to 10-year follow-up period, despite discontinuation of the drug at 5 years (a carry-over effect).

A Danish trial evaluated (4) whether adjuvant TAM (30 mg per day) for 2 years is superior to TAM for 1 year in 1,779 postmenopausal, high-risk (NP or T more than 5 cm) breast cancer patients with either positive-ER or unknown-ER status. The difference between the two groups in terms of 5-year DFS and OS was not significant.

Two relatively large trials compared 5 years versus 2 years adjuvant TAM. A Cancer Research Campaign (CRC) trial included both NN and NP patients aged 50 years or older, irrespective of ER status, who initially received 2 years of adjuvant TAM. Of the 4,621 patients who were assigned to 2 years of TAM, only 2,937 disease-free patients were available for randomization, either to continue TAM for 3 more years or to stop treatment (5). Recently updated results at a median follow-up of 5.5 years reported a significantly reduced event-free-survival (EFS) rate for patients receiving 5 years of TAM (relative risk 0.75, 95%; confidence interval [CI] 0.65 to 0.86) without a significant OS benefit (6).

A Swedish trial randomized 3,545 NN and NP patients to adjuvant TAM for 2 years or 5 years. Two different doses of TAM were used (20 mg or 40 mg daily) by participating institutions. ER status was evaluated in 77% of patients, of whom 21% were ER-negative. This trial reported a greater OS and EFS benefit with longer treatment, restricted to women with ER-positive and erb-B2-negative tumors. The proportional benefit appeared to be similar in NN and NP subgroups (7,8).

Debate continues as to whether more than 5 years of adjuvant TAM provides additional protective benefit against breast cancer recurrence or death or is associated with lower survival due to cumulative serious adverse events. Thus far, no additional benefit has been observed for more than five years. However, the number of patients enrolled or reported in comparative trials, to date, is insufficient to draw definitive conclusions.

In the recent update of the National Surgical Adjuvant Breast and Bowel Project (NSABP) B-14 trial, which compared 5 years of TAM to placebo and then re-randomized patients who were disease free after 5 years of TAM to another 5 years of TAM or to placebo, there continues to be no additional benefit through 7 years of follow-up after re-randomization from TAM administered beyond 5 years in women with NN, ER-positive breast cancer (9).

Two Eastern Cooperative Oncology Group (ECOG) trials (E4181 [premenopausal] and E5181 [postmenopausal]) and the Scottish tamoxifen trial questioned the duration of TAM beyond 5 years (10,11). In the ECOG trials, 193 premenopausal and postmenopausal NP women who had already received 5 years of TAM were randomly assigned to continue or stop TAM. Five years after re-randomization, no statistically significant differences were found between the two groups in either DFS or OS. Patients with ER-positive tumors (73% in TAM and 67% in the observation arm) experienced a longer TTR with continued TAM treatment ($p = 0.014$); however, no significant survival advantage was present in this subgroup.

The Scottish trial, which began in 1978, initially compared adjuvant TAM for 5 years to TAM initiated at relapse and showed a highly significant benefit in terms of DFS ($p = 0.0002$) and OS ($p < 0.0001$) for the adjuvant TAM group, independent of nodal and menopausal status. The greatest benefit in DFS was observed in patients with ER levels at or greater than 100 fmol per mg protein (12). Three hundred and forty-two patients who were disease-free at 5 years in the adjuvant arm of the trial were entered into a TAM duration trial and re-randomized, either to continue TAM until relapse or death or to discontinue the drug. Six-year follow-up results demonstrated no added benefit in survival or freedom from recurrence in those continuing to take TAM beyond the initial 5-year period (hazard ratio [HR]: 1.27, favoring those randomized to stop TAM, indicating a non significant benefit in event-free survival) (13).

The initial 1978 trial and duration of TAM Scottish trials have both recently been updated at a median follow-up of 15 years. These updated results confirm the benefit of 5 years of adjuvant TAM over observation in terms of overall survival ($p = 0.006$), systemic relapse ($p = 0.07$) and death from breast cancer ($p = 0.02$), with the carry-over effect through 15 years of follow-up. No additional benefit was observed for those women randomly assigned to continue TAM beyond 5 years (14). The NSABP and the Scottish trials both demonstrated a trend toward a worse outcome with a longer duration of treatment and a higher incidence of endometrial cancer (but not endometrial cancer deaths) in continuing users.

A French trial randomized 3,733 NP and NN patients who were disease-free after 2 to 3 years of adjuvant TAM, to either stop or continue TAM for another 10 years. Approximately 65% of the patients in both arms had ER-positive tumors. The median treatment duration, at the time of analysis, was 30 months and 70 months in the short-term and long-term groups, respectively. Although no overall survival advantage was noted, patients benefited from longer treatment with improved DFS ($p = 0.0023$) when compared with the group that discontinued TAM. The significant improvement in DFS was observed in NP patients ($p = 0.001$) but not in the NN group. Longer treatment reduced the incidence of contralateral breast cancer and did not increase the number of endometrial cancers (15).

Given that, in NP disease, the majority of relapses occur within the first 5 years of diagnosis, it may be that little further reduction in recurrence rates occurs after 5 years of TAM. Any additional survival benefit due to reductions in systemic breast cancer relapse, new contralateral breast cancers, and cardiovascular deaths may be offset by the cumulative risks of endometrial cancer and thromboembolic events, which persist with continued use. Proponents of continuous TAM use, however, argue that the studies which have compared 5 years and more than 5 years of use are underpowered to detect small differences in outcome. The optimal duration of TAM treatment is likely to be definitively answered by two large British trials, ATLAS and aTTom. The ATLAS trial is randomizing approximately 20,000 women with ER-positive disease to continue for 5 more years or stop TAM after completion of 5 years. In the aTTom trial, women who receive TAM for varying lengths of time and remain disease free are randomly assigned either to discontinue TAM or receive it for an additional 5 years. The results of these trials will not be available for about 10 years. Based on currently available level I evidence, routine adjuvant TAM for longer than 5 years cannot be recommended.

Delayed Tamoxifen

With respect to the timing of tamoxifen treatment, a French trial attempted to answer the question, "Do women who remain free of recurrence still benefit from TAM if it is initiated a long time after surgery or radiotherapy?" In this study, 494 patients with a median interval of 5 years from their primary treatment were randomized to TAM for 5 years versus no treatment. Delayed TAM provided a significant overall DFS ($p = 0.01$) advantage over observation, but in the subgroup analysis, the survival benefit from delayed TAM was restricted to the NP ($p = 0.02$), and ER-positive/PgR-positive groups ($p = 0.001$ for ER positive, $p = 0.002$ for PgR positive group) (16).

Other Benefits

Contralateral Breast Cancer (CLBC)

The EBCTCG overview estimated that 5 years of TAM would lead to a 47% relative risk reduction in the incidence of contralateral breast cancer (CLBC). The preliminary data from the 2000 overview supports a carry-over effect for the reduction of CLBC (16% in years zero to 4 and 46% in years 5 to 10).

In the NSABP B-14 trial, there was a striking reduction in the CLBC incidence with 5 years of TAM use, and a persistent effect with longer treatment was anticipated; disappointingly, there was no difference in the incidence of CLBC between the two groups after the second randomization (to stop or continue TAM after 5 years).

Lipids and Cardiovascular Mortality

A reduction in serum low-density lipoprotein cholesterol (LOL), total serum cholesterol, and lipoprotein (a), and an increase in apolipoprotein-B levels have been demonstrated with TAM therapy (17,18). This surrogate marker effect probably contributes to the reduced incidence of coronary heart disease deaths reported in TAM-treated breast cancer patients compared with untreated controls (1,19,20). However, at present, there is no clear evidence that TAM decreases the incidence of coronary artery disease. This effect has not been demonstrated by the overview, but it must be remembered that not all studies systematically recorded this information.

Osteoporosis

By increasing bone mineral density, TAM is protective against osteoporosis in postmenopausal women (21–26). In premenopausal women treated with TAM, bone mineral density decreases. However, studies have concluded that the rate of loss is similar for breast cancer patients treated with TAM and placebo (22,27). The incidence of radiologic osteoporosis (using bone densitometry) in premenopausal breast cancer patients taking TAM compared with no TAM has only been examined in small prospective trials.

Negative Impact

An analysis of adjuvant TAM and survival impact was performed by MEDLINE and CAN-

CER literature searches for RCTs of TAM versus no TAM, which specifically recorded non-breast-cancer deaths. Over a 10-year period of follow-up, the relative risk of deaths from contralateral breast cancer (0.61) and cardiovascular events (0.75) favored TAM users, and the relative risk of death from endometrial cancer (7.5) and thromboembolic events (7.0) favored non-users (28).

The NSABP B-14 trial reported an annual hazard rate of endometrial cancer of 1.6 per 1,000 (23 cases) in TAM users compared with 0.2 per 1,000 (two cases) for placebo users (29). In the most recent update of this trial, the incidence of endometrial cancer, although small, was doubled in the group continuing TAM compared to the group that discontinued the drug (12 women [2.1%] versus six women [1.1%]) (9).

The EBCTCG overview estimated a fourfold excess incidence of endometrial cancer over 10 years and an excess of 1 to 2 per 1,000 endometrial cancer deaths with 5 years of TAM (1). Excluding deaths from endometrial and breast cancers, the relative risk of death was 0.99, suggesting that the risk of death from other causes is neither increased nor decreased by the use of TAM. The preliminary results from the 2000 Oxford Overview confirm that more cancers are prevented than caused by TAM. Overall, therefore, the benefits of 5 years of TAM in the majority of ER-positive breast cancer patients far outweigh any serious side effects associated with it.

AROMATASE INHIBITORS AND NOVEL-ANTIESTROGENS

Tamoxifen still remains the gold standard hormonal therapy for postmenopausal women with ER-positive breast cancer. However, numerous new hormonal agents have been developed and are in an advanced stage of adjuvant clinical trial evaluation, with early results already available for some agents. One important question being explored is the optimal sequence of hormonal agents. New avenues of investigation are exploring the value, if any, of switching to peripheral aromatase inhibitors (AIs) or selective estrogen receptor modifiers (SERMs) after adjuvant TAM, replacing TAM with these newer endocrine agents up-front, or combining TAM with new AIs (Table 9.1). The rationale is that the different mechanisms of action of these drugs and increased suppression of circulating estrogen, compared with TAM, may inhibit emergence of hormone-insensitive clones. Aromatase is an enzyme found in peripheral adipose tissue and breast cancer cells, which converts androstenedione to estrone and testosterone to estradiol, both active estrogens. Inhibition of aromatase effectively suppresses circulating and tumor estrogen levels in postmenopausal women, as this is the major source of estrogen production following menopause. Additionally, hormone-suppressing drugs with fewer side effects and lower risks of serious sequelae, such as venous thromboembolic disease and endometrial cancer, may be preferable to TAM even where only equivalence is established.

Aminoglutethimide

An RCT comparing TAM (20 mg per day for 5 years) to TAM and aminoglutethimide (AG; 250 mg twice a day for 2 years) in 2,021 postmenopausal women with ER-positive, NP (38%) or NN breast cancer found no difference in either relapse-free survival (RFS) (86%, 86%) or OS (94%, 95%) for the TAM or combination arms, respectively, with 49 months median follow-up (30). There was a higher rate of withdrawals in the TAM-plus-AG group due to more side effects (29% versus 21%). In an Italian RCT, 380 postmenopausal NP and NN patients who had received 3 years of adjuvant TAM were randomized to continue for another 2 years or switch to AG. Significantly longer overall survival was reported for the sequential hormonal treatment arm ($p = 0.005$) at a median follow-up of 61 months; however, this arm was associated with a higher incidence of drug-related side effects and treatment discontinuation ($p = 0.0001$) (31).

Given the need for concurrent hydrocortisone due to adrenal suppression and other significant toxicities associated with AG, coupled with the emergence of new peripheral AIs with

TABLE 9.1. *Ongoing and recently closed adjuvant RCTs of AIs and TAM in NP breast cancer*

Trial/Group	Accrual target/actual to date	Population	Comparison arms
ATAC	9,100 closed	Post local therapy Postmenopausal NN/NP	1. TAM 2. TAM + Anastrozole 3. Anastrozole
GABG-IV C ARNO	742 closed	RFS after 2 yr adjuvant TAM Postmenopausal and ≤70 years old NN or NP (0–9) ER (+)	1. TAM 30/day × 3 yr 2. Anastrozole 1/day × 3 yr
ABCSG 6A	1,700/812	RFS after 5 yr adjuvant TAM ± AG Postmenopausal NN and NP, ER (+)	1. No further therapy 2. Anastrozole 1/day × 3 yr
NCIC-CTG MA.17 and BIG 01–97	4,800/3,336	RFS after 5 yr adjuvant TAM	1. Letrozole 2.5/day × 5 yr 2. Placebo
ICCG and BIG 02–97	4,400/4,485 closed	RFS after 2–3 yr adjuvant TAM	1. TAM 20 mg/day × 2–3 yr 2. Exemestane 25 mg/day × 2–3 yr
IBCSG 18–98 and BIG 01–98	5,189/3,881	ER (+) Any nodal status	1. TAM × 5 yr 2. Letrozole × 5 yr 3. TAM × 2 yr → Letrozole × 3 yr 4. Letrozole × 2 yr → TAM × 3 yr
ABCSG 12	1,250/467	Premenopausal NN and NP ER (+)	1. OA (goserelin × 3 yr) + TAM × 3 yr 2. OA (goserelin × 3 yr) + Anastrazole × 3 yr
ABCSG 8	3,500/2,320	Postmenopausal ER (+) RFS after 2 yr of adjuvant TAM NN, NP	1. Anastrozole 1 mg/day/3 yr 2. TAM 20 mg/day/3 yr
NSABP B-33	3,000/44	Postmenopausal NN, NP DFS after 5 yr of adjuvant TAM	1. Exemestane 2 yr 2. Placebo 2 yr

ABCSG, Austrian Breast Cancer Study Group; ATAC, Adjuvant Tamoxifen Anastrozole Comparison; BIG, Breast International Group; GABG, German Adjuvant Breast Cancer Group; IBCSG, International Breast Cancer Study Group; ICCG, International Collaborative Cancer Group, NCIC-CTG, National Cancer Institute of Canada Clinical Trials Group; NSABP, National Surgical Adjuvant Breast and Bowel Project.

significantly improved side effect profiles, the further production and sale of this drug was recently discontinued.

New Aromatase Inhibitors

The new generation of steroidal and nonsteroidal AIs act peripherally, and thus do not suppress adrenal function like AG. The most frequently cited side effects are nausea and arthralgias. The risk of thromboembolic events is approximately half of that observed with TAM (32). By irreversibly (exemestane, formestane) or reversibly (anastrozole, letrozole) inhibiting peripheral and tumor aromatase, these drugs effectively reduce levels of circulating estrogens in postmenopausal women, thereby removing a growth stimulus for hormone-sensitive tumors. Several adjuvant efficacy trials comparing TAM, peripheral AIs, and the combination are ongoing, and a few are recently closed (Table 9.1). The ATAC (Arimidex, Tamoxifen, Alone, or in Combination) Trialists' Group trial, which randomized over 9,000 postmenopausal women with ER-positive or unknown disease to 5 years of adjuvant anastrozole or TAM or the combination of both, was recently reported (33). A significant improvement in recurrence-free survival was observed for anastrozole (HR 0.78; CI 0.65 to 0.93; $p = 0.0054$ for ER-positive patients). However, the absolute difference was only 2%, and there have been too few deaths to determine whether a survival advantage will emerge. Another encouraging finding was a significant reduction in the incidence of contralateral breast cancer with anastrozole compared to tamoxifen, which is known to reduce contralateral breast cancer by approximately 47%. Interestingly, the combination arm did no better than the tamoxifen arm; however, no definitive explanation has yet been put forward for this unexpected finding. A cautionary note when considering these results is that over half the enrolled patients have not yet received 5 years of adjuvant therapy, and thus these results are truly preliminary despite their promise.

Given their tolerability, previously established efficacy in hormone-sensitive metastatic breast cancer, and this new promising data in the adjuvant setting, the new AIs are likely to play an increasingly prominent role in adjuvant therapy. Until adjuvant trial results are mature, however, their routine use in the adjuvant setting cannot be recommended outside clinical trials.

Novel Anti-estrogens

Novel anti-estrogens have been developed with fewer or no estrogen agonist properties to eliminate the proliferative stimulus on the endometrium seen with TAM (34). These include agents such as raloxifene hydrocholoride and toremifene citrate.

There are no ongoing trials of adjuvant raloxifene. It is being compared to TAM in the NSABP P-02 (STAR) trial of primary prevention based on the observation—from the Multiple Outcome of Raloxifene Evaluation (MORE) trial of raloxifene versus placebo for the treatment of osteoporosis—of reduced breast cancer incidence with raloxifene (35).

In a Finnish study, the anti-estrogen toremifene (TOR) has been compared to TAM in postmenopausal NP breast cancer patients. The study is powered to demonstrate equivalence with endpoints of DFS, OS, and recurrence rate, and accrual of 1,480 patients was completed in July, 1999. After randomization of the first 900 patients with a balanced distribution of patient and tumor characteristics, no difference in recurrence (26.1% TAM versus 23.1% TOR, $p = 0.31$), or serious toxicity was observed at a mean follow-up of $3\frac{1}{3}$ years (36).

In two RCTs (target accruals 1,140 and 850), the International Breast Cancer Study Group (IBCSG) is comparing TOR (60 mg a day for 5 years) to TAM (20 mg a day for 5 years) in perimenopausal and postmenopausal NP patients who are also receiving either AC (Adriamycin, cyclophosphamide) chemotherapy or AC followed by CMF (cyclophosphamide, methotrexate, 5-fluorouracil) (37). Results of those trials should be available in the next 2 to 5 years.

There are no randomized trials of the pure antiestrogen faslodex reported as yet in the adjuvant node-positive breast cancer setting; however, early results in the metastatic hormone responsive disease are promising, as discussed in Chapter 16.

OVARIAN ABLATION

Ovarian ablation (OA) alone or in combination with other treatment modalities is discussed below in the section on higher dose intensity cyclophosphamide.

OTHER HORMONAL THERAPIES

Estrogen is the most well-studied hormonal stimulus for the growth of breast cancer microsatellites, which may give rise to future recurrences. However, as understanding of cell signaling, growth factors, growth factor receptors, and transcription regulation increases, modulation of some of these factors may provide additional protection against breast cancer recurrence. Examples under current clinical investigation include octreotide acetate and retinoids, with others likely to follow.

Octreotide, a somatostatin analogue, inhibits production of insulin-like growth factor, known to regulate cellular proliferation, and thus may provide additive or synergistic activity to TAM. The National Cancer Institute of Canada Clinical Trials Group (NCIC-CTG) is examining the value of combining TAM and octreotide in postmenopausal women with NN and NP breast cancer (NCIC-CTG MA-4). Target accrual is 850 patients with endpoints of RFS, OS, and quality of life.

Preclinical data have suggested synergy of fenretinide, a vitamin A analogue, with TAM (38). Retinoic acid is an endogenous compound that induces cellular differentiation, thus reducing the capacity of cells to proliferate. Various synthetic retinoids, including fenretinide, are being explored for their anti-cancer activity. An American Intergroup trial (INT 0151) is addressing the value of 5 years of fenretinide added to TAM (20 mg a day for 5 years) compared to TAM alone in NP, ER-positive postmenopausal breast cancer patients (39).

CHEMOTHERAPY

There are many cytotoxic drugs, either used singularly or in combination, that are active in breast cancer. The adjuvant regimens currently in common use are CMF and anthracycline-based combinations with or without taxanes. The oral Bonadonna schedule of CMF consists of: cyclophosphamide (C) 100 mg/m^2 by mouth on days 1 through 14; methotrexate (MTX) 40 mg/m^2 i.v. on days 1 and 8; and 5-fluorouracil (5-FU) 600 mg/m^2 i.v. on days 1 and 8 every 28 days. In many patients, C is given i.v. on days 1 and 8 (600 mg/m^2) to minimize nausea and improve compliance, although equivalence of the two regimens has never been established. Anthracycline-containing regimens in current use include AC (Adriamycin, 60 mg/m^2, and C, 600 mg/m^2 i.v. on day one every 21 days), FAC (5-FU 500 mg/m^2, Adriamycin 50 mg to 60 mg/m^2, C 500 mg to 600 mg/m^2 i.v. every 3 or 4 weeks), EC (epirubicin, 60 mg to 100 mg/m^2, and C 500 mg to 600 mg/m^2 i.v. day 1 every 21 days), and FEC (5-FU 500 mg to 600 mg/m^2, epirubicin 60 mg to 120 mg/m^2, C 500 mg to 600 mg/m^2 every 3 weeks or days 1 and 8 every 4 weeks). Many European centers give several cycles of Adriamycin (75 mg/m^2) followed by CMF, according to a schedule developed by Bonadonna.

The systematic overview of polychemotherapy by the EBCTCG provides a comprehensive review of adjuvant breast cancer therapy (40). It includes results from 18,000 women in 47 trials of prolonged polychemotherapy versus no CT, 6,000 women in 11 trials of anthracycline-containing regimens compared with CMF, and 6,000 women in 11 trials of shorter versus longer CT. The analysis of the entire group shows that polychemotherapy produces a highly significant proportional reduction in recurrence and mortality. While the reduction in recurrence is seen mainly during the first 5 years of follow-up, the reduction in mortality grows throughout the first 10 years.

Mortality and recurrence are significantly reduced for women both under 50 years of age (27% RRR, $2p < 0.00001$ and 35% RRR, $2p < 0.00001$, respectively) and over 50 years of age (11% RRR, $2p = 0.0001$ and 20% RRR, $2p < 0.00001$, respectively). These benefits are irrespective of ER status, menopausal status, and the added use of TAM (level I evidence). The absolute 10-year survival rate in women younger than 50 years is improved by 7% in NN and by 11% in NP patients, and the equivalent improvements for women aged 50 to 69 are 2% and 3%, respectively.

In women younger than 50 years of age, the benefits of CT appear to be similar in ER-positive and ER-negative subsets. In women aged 50 to 69 years, however, the reduction in recurrence is twice as large for ER-negative than ER-positive patients with a statistically significant difference between these effects.

In the relatively few trials that compared 6 months or less of polychemotherapy to longer durations of the same regimen, there was a non-significant improvement in recurrence (7%, $2p = 0.06$) and no improvement in survival with longer therapy (-1%, NS), regardless of the age group examined (less than 50 years, and all ages). Thus it has been concluded, given the absence of additional survival benefit, that longer than 3 to 6 months of chemotherapy is not required (level I evidence).

CMF

The classic CMF Bonadonna regimen was among the first polychemotherapy regimens to show DFS and OS benefits in the treatment of early breast cancer (41). An early study which explored the value of duration of classic CMF demonstrated similar overall survival for six cycles (76.9%) and 12 cycles (72.7%) among 466 node-positive breast cancer patients (42). Thus, six cycles of the Bonadonna schedule is considered by most clinicians as the standard reference regimen of CMF.

Direct comparison of the anthracycline-containing regimens with classical CMF in NP disease showed a significant DFS and 3% to 4% OS benefit favoring anthracyclines in the Oxford Overview and in several individual trials (those containing three-drug anthracycline-based regimens such as CAF and CEF) (43–45). The use of an anthracycline-based regimen is probably indicated in the high risk, NN setting as well. While CMF for high-risk women with breast cancer may be viewed as suboptimal, it remains the best-studied alternative to anthracycline-containing regimens in subsets of women with a low absolute risk of recurrence for whom CT is still recommended. It is also valid for high-risk women with contraindications to anthracycline use such as patients with a high risk of cardiotoxicity (i.e., elderly women with pre-existing cardiac dysfunction).

Interestingly, the absence of cross-resistance between CMF and anthracyclines has led to their sequential use in NP disease, particularly in Europe (46).

Anthracyclines Versus CMF

The last published EBCTCG overview analyzed 11 trials in which 6,000 women were randomized to anthracycline-containing regimens versus CMF. In these trials, the majority of women (70%) were less than 50 years old. Anthracycline-containing CT was superior in reducing recurrence (12% greater relative reduction, $2p = 0.006$) and death (11% greater relative reduction, $2p = 0.02$); however, the 99% confidence interval for this observation reached zero, and results from some large comparative trials were not available. Absolute improvements provided by anthracycline-based regimens over CMF were 3.2% ($2p = 0.006$) and 2.7% ($2p = 0.02$) in terms of recurrence and mortality, respectively, at 5 years.

Preliminary results of the updated EBCTCG overview with respect to randomized comparisons of anthracycline-containing and CMF regimens are now based on 14,000 women enrolled in 15 trials and continue to show a small but significant benefit with anthracyclines in terms of recurrence and death (2). For the NP subset in particular, the absolute benefit is in the range of 4% at 10 years.

The superior efficacy of anthracycline-based regimens over CMF is not only supported by the EBCTCG overview but also by several individual randomized trials (level 1 evidence). However the optimal anthracycline regimen has not been defined, since different anthracycline regimens with different dose intensities are included in the overview, and indeed there may be several equivalent anthracycline-containing regimens.

The trials that compared CMF and anthracycline regimens are summarized in Table 9.2 and several large trials are discussed below.

The largest direct comparison of CMF versus CAF (both at six cycles) was the US Intergroup Study 0102 which enrolled 4,406 NN, high-risk and low-risk patients. CAF was marginally superior to CMF in terms of both 5-year DFS (86% versus 84%, $p = 0.03$) and OS (92% versus 91%, $p = 0.03$) in 2,691 high-risk patients. However, CAF was also found to be more toxic (43).

The Danish-Swedish Breast Cancer Cooperative Group trial comparing nine cycles of CMF (600/40/600 mg/m^2 via i.v. on day 1 every 21 days) with nine cycles of CEF (600/60/600 mg/m^2 by i.v. on day 1 every 21 days) in a total 1,195 patients divided into three groups (group A, premenopausal, NN, grade II to III tumors; group B, premenopausal NP, ER-negative or unknown tumors; group C, postmenopausal NP, receptor-negative tumors). Six-year OS was superior for CEF in group A (CMF 83%, CEF 93%, $p < 0.01$) and in the combined premenopausal groups A and B (CMF 69%, CEF 76%, $p = 0.01$), but not for postmenopausal NP women (47). A criticism of this study is the use of an inferior comparative CMF regimen;

TABLE 9.2. *Randomized phase III adjuvant clinical trials of CMF versus anthracycline-based CT in NP breast cancer*

Trials	N	Population	Comparison arms[a]	Results
NSABP B-15	2,194	NP	4 × AC (60/600 q21d) 6 × CMF♦ 4 × AC → 3 CMF (750d1/40d1,8/600d1, 8 q28d)	No differences in DFS ($p = 0.5$) or OS ($p = 0.8$) between 3 arms
DBCG 89D/CSB II-3	1,195	NN/Prem/grade 2–3 NP/Prem/ER(-) or uk NP/Postm/ER neg	9 × CEF (600/60/600 q21d) 9 × CMF (600/40/600, q21d)	CEF superior to CMF only in NN/Prem (6-year OS: 83% vs. 93%, $p < 0.01$); no significant differences in node positive patients
GEICAM 8701	985	NP and NN	6 FAC (500/50/500 q21d) 6 CMF (600/60/600 q21d)	FAC better than CMF in terms of DFS (0.043) and marginally in OS ($p = 0.054$) in NN group only
NCIC MA.5	710	NP Prem	6 × CMF♦ 6 × Canadian CEF (500 d1, d8/60/75 d1–14, q28d)	CEF better than CMF in terms of 5-year DFS ($p = 0.009$) and 5-year OS ($p = 0.03$)
Belgian Study	777	NP ≤70 years	8 × HEC (100/830 q21d) 8 × EC (60/500 q21d) 6 × CMF♦	No statistically significant differences between HEC and CMF, in terms of DFS ($p = 0.80$) or OS ($p = 0.87$). HEC more effective than EC in terms of DFS ($p = 0.04$) and OS ($p = 0.05$)
ICCG	759	NP Prem	6 × FEC1 (600/50/600 q21d) or 6 × FEC2 (600 d1, d8/50/600 d1, d8 q28d) 6 × CMF1♦ or 6 × CMF2 (600/40/600 i.v., d1, d8, q28d)	CMF1 and FEC1 were similar in terms of DFS ($p = 0.61$) and OS ($p = 0.13$) FEC2 was superior to CMF2 in terms of DFS ($p = 0.03$) and OS ($p = 0.02$)
ONCO FRANCE	249	NP	12 × AVCF (30/1/300/400) 12 × CMF♦	Median OS at 16-years: 56% vs. 41% ($p = 0.01$) Median DFS at 16-years: 53% vs. 36% ($p = 0.006$)
SECSG 2	528	NP	6 × FAC (500/50/500 q21d) 6 × CMF (600/60/600 q21d)	Median OS at 5-years: 74% (67%–81%) vs. 68% (55%–81%)
GUN-3 Naples	220	NP, Stage II–III Pre & Postm; ER neg	6 × alternating CMF/EV (75/1,4 i.v., d1, d8, q21d) 6 × CMF♦	No differences in DFS ($p = 0.66$) and OS ($p = 0.58$)
BCSG 3 Austria[b]	245	NA	6 × CMFVA 6 × CMF	Nonsignificant differences
GABG 3 Germany[b]	288	NA	6 FEC 6 × CMF	Nonsignificant differences
Italian trial	207	Prem > 3LN T 1–3	6 × CMF♦ 4×EC(120/600 d1 q 21d)	No difference in DFS OS was superior to CMF in terms of OS (RR:1.45, $p = 0.0238$)
NSABC Israel Br 0283	202	NP Stage II	6 × CMF (500/40/600 i.v. d1, d8, q28d) → 4 × VA (50/5 q28d) 6 × CMF (500/40/600 i.v. d1, d8)	Postm 1–3NP: CMF better in terms of 4-years DFS (78% vs. 48%, $p < 0.05$) Prem ≥4NP: CMF-VA better in terms of DFS at 30 mo (76% vs. 28%, $p < 0.01$)
Czech	106	NN and NP	4 × AC (60/600, q21d) 4 × CMF (500 d1, d8/40 d1, d8/ 600 d1, d8, q28d)	No significant differences in terms of 3-year DFS (60% vs. 64%) or 3-year OS (82% vs. 80%)
SE Sweden BCGA	43	NP Prem	6 × AC (40 i.v. d1/200 oral d3–d6, q21d) 6 × CMF♦	Non significant differences (no p values provided)

[a]Doses are in mg/m^2.
[b]Reported results not available.

AVCF, doxorubicin + vincristine + cyclophosphamide + fluorouracil; CMF♦, CMF classical; ER, estrogen receptor; HEC, high-dose EC; NA, not available; NN, node negative; NP, node positive; Postm, postmenopausal; Prem, premenopausal; uk, unknown.

however, one could equally argue that the dose of epirubicin for each cycle was suboptimal, although nine cycles were used. The total dose of epirubicin was 540 mg/m^2 compared to 600 mg to 720 mg/m^2 planned dose for other epirubicin regimens (see later).

An NCIC-CTG trial comparing an intensive CEF regimen (oral C 75 mg/m^2 per day on days 1 through 14; E 60 mg/m^2 on days 1 and 8; 5-FU 500 mg/m^2 on days 1 and 8 for six cycles) to Bonadonna CMF reported a significant OS (77% and 70% for CEF and CMF, respectively; $p = 0.03$), and DFS (53% and 63% for CEF and CMF respectively; $p = 0.009$) benefit for CEF in 710 NP premenopausal and perimenopausal patients at a median follow-up of 59 months (44). This trial is discussed in the dose-intense CT section in more detail.

A recently published Belgian trial compared eight cycles of a full-dose EC regimen (epirubicin 100 mg/m^2 and cyclophosphamide 830 mg/m^2 on day 1 every 3 weeks) with six cycles of Bonadonna CMF and with eight cycles of a moderate-dose EC regimen (epirubicin 60 mg/m^2 and cyclophosphamide 830 mg/m^2 on day 1 every 3 weeks) in 777 NP breast cancer patients. The 4-year results suggested that the full-dose epirubicin-based regimen is as effective as CMF and more active than a moderate-dose epirubicin regimen with respect to EFS ($p = 0.04$) and OS ($p = 0.05$) (48).

A Spanish trial, Grupo Español de Investigación en Cáncer de Mama (GEICAM), which randomized 985 NP and NN women to either six cycles of FAC (500/50/500 mg/m^2) or six cycles of i.v. CMF (600/60/600 mg/m^2), was recently reported at a median follow-up of 7 years. The NN subgroup had a significant OS ($p = 0.043$) and a marginal DFS ($p = 0.054$) benefit in the FAC arm while the NP subset did not (49).

The NSABP B-15 adjuvant trial randomized 2,194 NP women with tumors non-responsive to TAM to four cycles of AC or six cycles of classical CMF or four cycles of AC followed 6 months later by three cycles of i.v. CMF. No DFS and OS difference was found between the three groups or for the comparison of four cycles AC and six cycles CMF (50). The NSABP B-23 trial showed no difference in EFS (83% versus 82%) or OS (90% versus 89%) at 5 years between four cycles of AC and six cycles of classical CMF in 2,008 NN patients with ER-negative tumors (51). In both of these trials, four cycles of AC were associated with less toxicity.

The Italian Cooperative Group Gruppo Oncologico Centro-Sud-Isole (GOCSI) randomized 466 premenopausal NP patients by using a 2 × 2 factorial design in order to evaluate the sequential regimen of Adriamycin followed by CMF versus CMF alone. Hazard ratios favored the sequential treatment arm in terms of relapse (HR 0.86, $p = 0.42$) and survival (HR 0.79, $p = 0.31$) but these results were not significant at a median follow-up of 5 years (52).

Among the several trials which have attempted to show improved outcomes by combining CMF and anthracyclines, one Italian study randomized 490 premenopausal and postmenopausal NP women to receive either 12 cycles of CMF or eight cycles of CMF followed by four cycles of doxorubicin. No differences were noted in RFS and OS, suggesting that the most active agent needs to be given up front (53). Another Italian study of similar size randomized NP premenopausal and postmenopausal women to receive either four cycles of doxorubicin followed by eight cycles of CMF (sequential regimen) or a total of 12 cycles of alternating doxorubicin (1 cycle) and CMF (2 cycles). Women who received the sequential treatment had a better RFS (42% versus 28%, $p = 0.002$) and OS (58% versus 44%, $p = 0.002$) at 10 years follow-up (46).

In summary, so far, two large trials comparing two-drug, relatively low-dose, anthracycline-based regimens versus classical CMF (NSABP B-15 in NP subset and NSABP B-23 in NN subset) have demonstrated equivalence in terms of DFS and OS. Both trials also suggested that AC was better tolerated than CMF when global toxicity was considered. Two other large trials (SWOG INT 0102 in NN subset and NCIC-CTG trial in NP subset) have demonstrated the superiority of the three-drug, relatively high-dose, anthracycline-based regimen over classical CMF at the expense of increased toxicity in the anthracycline-based CT arm. Several trials comparing CMF and anthracycline regimens are still ongoing and some were

TABLE 9.3. *Recently completed RCTs of CMF versus anthracycline-containing regimens in adjuvant breast cancer therapy*

Group/Trial	Accrual target/ actual to date	Population	Comparison arms[a]
GOIRC SANG 2B	631 closed	NP (1–3) NN, T2, 3 or T1c high risk	6 CMFEV alternating (Epi 40 days 1 and 8; Vincristine 1.4 day 1) 6 CMF (IV days 1 and 8 q28d)
NEAT	2,027 closed	NP and NN Any ER	4E → 4CMF (classical) 6 CMF (classical)

[a]All doses are in mg/m^2.
ER, estrogen receptor; NN, node negative; NP, node positive.
GOIRC, Italian Oncology Group for Clinical Research; NEAT, National Adjuvant Epirubicin Trial.

recently closed (Table 9.3). However, because they are relatively small, they may not individually show a significant difference between the two regimens if that difference is small, as suggested by the overview.

In light of the fact that only CEF or CAF have been able to surpass CMF in efficacy, the importance of 5-FU as part of the combination merits further examination. Another issue which may account for the superiority of CEF and CAF but an equivalence of AC to CMF is the duration or total dose of the anthracycline regimen. Whether four cycles of AC (4AC) is the optimal anthracycline regimen remains debatable.

Based on available evidence, therefore, longer/higher-dose anthracycline-containing regimens that include 5-FU are probably preferable in women with high-risk breast cancer until the equivalence of 4AC with them can be demonstrated in randomized trials. This is particularly the case for premenopausal women with NP disease. The added survival benefit of anthracyclines in postmenopausal women has not been established clearly, and they are best offered in the setting of a high-relapse risk to balance the cardiac toxicity, which tends to increase with age.

Taxanes

Taxanes have established activity in breast cancer and different side effects than anthracyclines with no intrinsic cardiomyopathy risk, but potentially significant neurotoxicity. The addition of taxanes may also increase the risk of severe neutropenia, febrile neutropenia, and serious infections; however, this remains to be proven. Large adjuvant RCTs are now underway or complete that compare taxane-based to anthracycline-based regimens, and to the combination of both either concurrently or sequentially.

Adjuvant taxane trials with reported results are summarized in Table 9.4.

The interim results from the collaborative trial (CALGB 9344) of the Cancer and Leuke-

TABLE 9.4. *Adjuvant taxane trials with reported results*

Taxane strategy	CALGB 9344 ODAC 1999 Paclitaxel sequential	CALGB 9344 NIH 2000 Paclitaxel sequential	NSABP B NIH 2000 Paclitaxel sequential	BCIRG 001 Asco 2002 Docetaxel combination
Median follow-up	30	52	34	33
Relapse risk reduction	22%	13%	7%	32%
Hazard ratio (relapse)	0.78	0.88	0.93	0.68
p value	0.002	0.03	0.38	0.001
Hazard ratio (death)	0.74	0.86	1.00	0.76
p value	0.006	0.56	0.98	0.11

mia Group B (CALGB), Eastern Cooperative Oncology Group (ECOG), Southwest Oncology Group (SWOG) and National Cancer Institute of Canada Clinical Trials Group (NCIC-CTG) suggested improved DFS (90%, 86%; $p = 0.008$) and OS (97%, 95%; $p = 0.04$) for patients randomized to 4AC followed by four cycles of paclitaxel (175 mg/m^2 every 21 days) compared to 4AC alone at median follow-up times of 22 months and 30 months (54). According to a subset analysis at 30 months of follow-up, the survival advantage appeared to be confined to the ER-negative subgroup, and at 52 months of follow-up, the improvement in OS previously observed for the trial population as a whole was no longer significant ($p = 0.07$). The relative decrease in recurrence, while still statistically significant, had dropped from 22% to 13% ($p < 0.05$) (55). This decrease in benefit over time could, arguably, relate at least in part to the low dose and duration of the 4AC regimen.

The results from the third interim analysis of NSABP B-28, which randomized 3,060 patients, were presented at the 2000 NIH Consensus Conference with 551 events and 269 deaths. They did not show a benefit from the addition of four cycles of paclitaxel to the standard 4AC regimen at a median follow-up of 34 months. A trend towards some benefit was observed with the addition of paclitaxel in women who were treated without additional TAM (56).

Interpretation of the impact of paclitaxel in both of these trials is confounded by the increased duration of treatment in the paclitaxel arm by 12 weeks, compared with the AC-alone arm. In addition, the adequacy of 4AC as the standard treatment in high-risk (NP) disease is questioned by many investigators (57).

The MD Anderson trial was better designed in that both the anthracycline-only and anthracycline-plus-taxane arms were of equal duration, and the anthracycline total dose was deemed adequate; however, it was limited in power, having randomized only 524 patients. At a median follow-up of 36 months, a 24% non-significant (NS) reduction in RFS was observed, favoring four paclitaxel cycles followed by four FAC cycles over eight cycles of FAC (58). A large ongoing NCIC-CTG trial, in which all three treatment arms have the same duration, is now exploring the value of four-cycle paclitaxel after 4AC, compared with six-cycle CEF and six high-dose EC cycles with growth factor support (G-CSF) followed by four cycles of paclitaxel and erythropoietin (NCIC MA-21).

The recently reported results of the BCIRG 001 trial, which compares TAC (docetaxel, Adriamycin, and cyclophosphamide) to FAC, has shown a significant improvement both in DFS and OS for patients with one to three nodes in the TAC arm at a median follow-up of 33 months (59). Of note, febrile neutropenia and amenorrhea were more frequent in the TAC arm. The results of this trial with longer follow-up are awaited with interest, since they will help in further clarification of the impact of adjuvant taxane-based regimens.

In summary, we have insufficient data to make meaningful conclusions about the benefit of the taxanes in early breast cancer (BC). The results of the BCIRG 001 trial are very encouraging, but the follow-up is still short, and the history of CALGB 9344 calls for caution with respect to early optimism.

Fortunately, a wealth of evidence about the efficacy of adjuvant taxanes should be available within the next 5 years as results mature in ongoing adjuvant and neoadjuvant paclitaxel and docetaxel RCTs (Table 9.5). Metastatic trials suggest better response with single-agent docetaxel than with single-agent doxorubicin, and with anthracycline-docetaxel combinations than with AC (60,61). If this proves to be the case in the adjuvant setting and has tolerable side effects, a substantial change in adjuvant CT practice is likely to follow.

Chemotherapy plus Trastuzumab

The addition of Herceptin (trastuzumab), an anti-human epidermal growth factor receptor-2 (HER-2) antibody, to chemotherapy has demonstrated improved survival compared to chemotherapy alone in patients with metastatic breast cancer overexpressing HER-2 (62–64). Based

TABLE 9.5. Ongoing or recently closed adjuvant RCTs with taxanes in NP breast cancer

Group/Trial	Accrual target/ actual to date	Population	Comparison arms[a]
BIG 02–98	2,730/2,890 closed	NP	4 A (75 q21d) → 3 CMF (Bonadonna) 4 AC (60/600) → 3 CMF (B) 3 A → 3 D (100 q21d) → 3 CMF (B) 4 AD (50/75 q21d) → 3 CMF (B)
FNCLCC + Belgium	2,000 closed	NP	6 FEC 100 (500/100/500 q21d) 3 FEC 100 → 3 D (100 q21d)
ECOG 1199	5,000/NA	NP or high-risk NN	4AC → 4D q 3 wks 4AC → 4P q 3 wks 4AC → 12D q wk 4AC → 12 P q wk
GONO MIG 5	1,000/735	NP	6 CEF (600/60/600 q21d) 4 EP (90/175 q21d)
ICCG C/14/96	800/370	NP Postmenopausal	6 E (50 d1,8 q28) 4 E → 3 D (100 q21d)
NCIC-CTG MA.21	1,200/215	NP, high-risk NN < 60 years old	6CEF (60 d1,8) 6EC(120 q2wk) + G-CSF → Ep+4P 4AC (60 d1 q21d) → 4P
Intergroup S9623	1,000/602 closed	4–9 NP	3 A → 3 P → 3 CY 4 AC → High dose with SCT
CALGB 9741	2,005 closed	NP	4 A → 4P → 4C (each q 3 wks) 4 A → 4P → 4C (each q 2 wks + G-CSF) 4 AC → 4P (each q 3 wks) 4 AC → 4P (each q 2 wks + G-CSF)
UK TACT	3,340/NA	Operable invasive early breast cancer	8FEC 4FEC → 4 D 4 E → 4 CMF
US community based	3,000/NA	NP	4EC → 4D or 4P q 3 wks 8ED or 8 EP q 3 wks
BCIRG TAX 316	1,000/1,491 closed	NP, <65 years	DAC × 6 FAC × 6
E 2197	2,778/2,958 closed	NP NN HR	ADX4 ACX4
NSABP B-30	4,000/2,387	NP	AC → D AC ACD
SBG 2001	1,100/not yet started	NP	Dose escalated FECX7 Std dose FE100CX7 Dose escalated FECX4+3P Std FE100CX4+3P
BCRIG 005	3,000/1,700 (June 2002)	NP	6DAC (75/50/500) 4AC (60/600) → 4D

[a]All drug doses are in mg/m^2.
D, docetaxel; E, epirubicin; ECOG, Eastern Cooperative Oncology Group; ECTO, European Cooperative Trial in Operable Breast Cancer; Ep, erythropoietin; FNCLCC, Fédération Nationale des Centres de Lutte contre le Cancer; GONO MIG, Gruppo Oncologico Nord Ovest - Mammella Intergruppo; NN, node negative; NP, node positive; P, paclitaxel; pRR, pathologic response rate.

on these findings, trastuzumab is now being incorporated into several adjuvant breast cancer trials (65). The NSABP B-31 trial, the NCCTG (North Central Clinical Treatment Group) N-9831 trial, the BCIRG 006 trial and the Breast International Group (BIG) 01 HERA are among those trials investigating the role of trastuzumab in the adjuvant setting. These carefully designed trials will determine also the risk/benefit ratio associated with the use of this innovative anticancer agent in early breast cancer. This topic is discussed in detail in Chapter 17.

Negative Impact

There were no excess non-breast cancer deaths for polychemotherapy versus no CT in the EBCTCG overview (death ratio 0.89; p = NS).

This was true for both vascular (hazard ratio 0.99) and other neoplastic (hazard ratio 0.75) deaths. For women younger than 50, the number of deaths from causes other than breast cancer was low and there was no significant difference in the incidence according to adjuvant CT versus none.

An approximate 1% incidence of toxic deaths as a result of adjuvant chemotherapy is generally accepted. This complication arises primarily in association with febrile neutropenia and sepsis, the incidence of which varies among the different chemotherapy regimens and comorbidity of the treated group. In addition, there are troublesome short-term side effects reported with cytotoxic drugs, including alopecia, nausea, vomiting, diarrhea, chemical cystitis and conjunctivitis, myalgias, arthralgias, neuropathy, fatigue, symptomatic anemia, and others, depending on the agents. Permanent menopause can also occur with some regimens, which may have beneficial impact on the risk of breast cancer recurrence but a negative impact in terms of quality of life and the subsequent risk of both osteoporosis and coronary artery disease.

Of greater concern are two possible long-term toxicities: cardiotoxicity and secondary leukaemia. Anthracyclines are associated with a dose-dependent risk of congestive cardiomyopathy. The risk is small (less than 5%) with cumulative doses up to 450 mg/m^2 of doxorubicin, but rise exponentially thereafter. The risk is somewhat lower with epirubicin at equieffective doses. Although small, there is a risk of secondary leukemia with both anthracyclines and alkylator-based CT, and this risk increases with dose escalation (66,67). The conditional probabilities of developing acute leukaemia following epirubicin-containing and non–epirubicin-containing regimens (CMF and AC) were recently reported as 1.5% and 0.3%, respectively, after a median follow-up of 5 years (68).

The EBCTCG meta-analysis reported a 20% reduction in annual odds of developing contralateral breast cancer (CLBC) with CT, which is marginally significant when translated into absolute benefit. It does, however, provide reassurance that CT does not increase the risk of CLBC.

In deciding whether or not to offer adjuvant chemotherapy, the absolute relapse risk, risk reduction, and risk of serious side effects must be considered individually. Although the benefit of CT in NP breast cancer is clearly evident for women younger than 50 (11% mortality reduction), it is more modest in women 50 to 69 years old (3% absolute mortality reduction). There is an upper age limit for most trials, so the magnitude of benefit and toxicity observed in these trials cannot be easily generalized to women older than 69.

Women aged 50 to 65 with a relatively high risk of relapse, and women with ER-negative tumor(s), who are unlikely to derive significant benefit from adjuvant TAM, can expect a higher relative benefit from CT. In these individuals, the potential adverse sequelae of CT are more justifiable. In contrast, for older women with endocrine-responsive disease, the added benefit of CT to TAM may be viewed by some as too low to justify the added toxicity. For women older than 70, competing causes of death become more significant, and tolerance to CT tends to decline. These factors should be strongly weighed against prognostic factors in the consideration to offer CT to elderly women. The recently reported results of the large American Intergroup trial 0100 exploring the benefit of CAF in a tamoxifen-treated NP postmenopausal population showed a 5% absolute survival gain with combined modality at a median follow-up of $7\frac{1}{3}$ years (69). The price to pay for this improvement in the combined treatment group included 23 (2.1%) cases of congestive heart failure (CHF), 9 (0.8%) cases of acute myelogenous leukemia and myelodysplastic syndrome (AML/MDS), and 24 (2.2%) cases of pulmonary emboli, deep venous thromboses and cerebrovascular accidents. This trial is discussed in detail under the topic Chemoendocrine Treatment below.

For premenopausal women, especially those who are in the younger age group, the decision to offer CMF or anthracycline-based CT should also take into account absolute relapse risk. Given the mounting evidence of a small but real benefit of anthracycline-containing CT over CMF, young patients with NP disease should be offered anthracycline-containing CT (in the absence of pre-existing cardiac disease or significant cardiac risk factors), given their high risk of relapse. Prospective evaluation of HER-2 (cerbB-2/human epidermal growth factor receptor-2) and other predictive factors may define a population for which anthracyclines are definitively superior, and thus enable individual tailoring of CT regimens.

DOSE-INTENSIVE/DOSE-DENSE CHEMOTHERAPY

Although adjuvant CT and hormonal therapy reduce recurrence of and death from NP breast cancer, relapses still occur with unacceptably high frequency. Whether escalating drug doses (increasing dose intensity) and/or reducing the interval between cycles (increasing dose density) are associated with improved outcome has been the subject of numerous RCTs (70). With the advent of colony-stimulating growth factors, which shorten the duration of neutropenia, delivery of higher drug doses with shorter intervals has become more feasible (71). Nevertheless, any additional benefit observed with dose-dense and dose-intense therapies must be viewed in light of increased short-term and long-term toxicity. True dose-dense and dose-intense RCTs have addressed the benefit of increased doses of anthracyclines or C or both (Table 9.6).

Anthracyclines

Suboptimal Anthracycline Dose Intensity

In many early trials, the high-dose arms contained what are currently considered conventional CT doses, while the low-dose arms had inferior or suboptimal doses (Table 9.5). These studies, summarized below, effectively demonstrated that there is a threshold dose and intensity below which DFS and OS are compromised (70,72–76).

The CALGB 8541 study compared three dose intensities of CAF in 1,550 NP breast cancer patients and found inferior DFS and OS in the low-dose arm (300/30/300 mg/m² every 4 weeks in four cycles) compared with the moderate-dose (400/40/400 mg/m² every 4 weeks in six cycles) and high-dose arms (600/60/600 mg/m² every 4 weeks in four cycles) at 9 years of follow-up ($p = 0.0001$) (72). The high-dose HD arm of the CALGB 8541 trial contained the same total dose of doxorubicin but increased dose intensity compared to the moderate-dose ID arm. There were no differences between the ID and HD arms in terms of DFS and OS. By today's standards, the low-dose arm had suboptimal doses of all three drugs, and the other two arms had doses within the conventional range. Thus, the results of this trial support the concept of a threshold level below which treatment is less effective and compromises survival. Grade IV leukopenia was substantially higher in the high-dose arm compared to the moderate-dose arm (66% and 17%, respectively), but the frequency of other toxicities was similar.

The French Adjuvant Study Group (FASG 01) enrolled 602 premenopausal/postmenopausal NP women and found that $6FEC_{50}$ (where the subscript denotes the dose of epirubicin in mg/m²) significantly improved DFS compared to $3FEC_{50}$ or $3FEC_{75}$ at a mature follow-up of 8 years. OS was marginally better for the $6FEC_{50}$ group compared to $3FEC_{50}$ group in pair-wise comparisons ($p = 0.006$) (73).

In another study from the same group (FASG 05), $6FEC_{50}$ was inferior to $6FEC_{100}$ in terms of DFS ($p = 0.03$) and OS ($p = 0.007$) in 565 premenopausal/postmenopausal NP breast cancer patients aged below 65 (75). The absolute improvements in DFS and OS were 11.5% (from 54.8% to 66.3%) and 12.1% (from 65.3% to 77.4%), respectively.

Taken together, these trials speak in favor of a dose-response curve at the low end of dose intensity for both doxorubicin and epirubicin in adjuvant breast cancer therapy.

An Intergroup RCT (ECOG, CALGB, and SWOG) compared CAF to a dose-dense, optimized 16-week schedule of weekly chemotherapy (77). In the 16-week regimen, total doses of doxorubicin and 5-FU were 13% and 60% higher, respectively, than in CAF, and two additional drugs (methotrexate and vincristine) were given. With 3.9 years follow-up, 4-year RFS and OS were similar for both groups. The 16-week schedule was not conventionally statistically superior to CAF in women with one to three positive nodes, (RFS, CAF 73.6%, 16

TABLE 9.6. *Reported adjuvant RCTs of conventional versus low-dose CT, and of dose-intense or dose-dense versus conventional dose CT for NP breast cancer*

				Low-dose versus conventional dose chemotherapy				
Trial/Group	Population	n	Drug intensified	Comparative doses	5y DFS	p value	OS	p value
CALGB 8541	NP	1,550	Adriamycin	30 mg/m² d1 q28d × 6 (1)	56%	1 vs. 2/3 <0.0001	72%	1 vs. 2/3 0.04
				60 mg/m² d1 q28d × 4 (2)	61%	2 vs. 3 0.85	77%	2 vs. 3 0.11
				40 mg/m² d1 q28d × 6 (3)	66%		78%	
FASG	NP Premenopausal	595	Epirubicin	50 mg/m² d1 q21d × 6 (1)	64.2%	1 vs. 2/3 0.03	82.6%	1 vs. 2/3 NS
				50 mg/m² d1 q21d × 3 (2)	55.6%	2 vs. 3 NS	74.9%	2 vs. 3 NS
				75 mg/m² d1 q21d × 3 (3)	55.2%		79.5%	
FASG	≥4 NP or 1–3 NP and ER - Premenopausal	565	Epirubicin	50 m/m² d1 q21d × 6	54.8%	0.03	65.3%	0.009
				100 mg/m² d1 q21d × 6	66.3%		77.4%	

				Dose-dense or dose-intense versus conventional dose chemotherapy				
Trial/Group	Population	n	Drug intensified	Comparative doses	5y DFS	p value	OS	p value
CALGB 8541	NP	1,023	Adriamycin	60 mg/m² d1 q28 × 4	61%	0.85	77%	0.11
				40 mg/m² d1 q28d × 6	66%		78%	
Intergroup	NP and ER (-)	646	Adriamycin 5-FU	Adria 15mg/m²/wk	62.7%	2p = 0.19	71.4%[a]	2p = 0.10
				5-FU 250 mg/m²/wk	67.5%	1p = 0.09	[a]	1p = 0.05
				Adria 20 mg/m²/wk			78.1%	
				5-FU 600 mg/m²/wk			[a]	
Intergroup 9344	NP	3,170	Adriamycin	60 mg/m² d1 q21d × 4	—	NS	—	NS
				75 mg/m² d1 q21d × 4	—		—	
				90 mg/m² q2d × 4 (45 mg/m2 d1,2)	—			
NSABP B22	NP	2,305	Cyclophosphamide	600 mg/m² × 4	62%	0.3	78%	0.95
				1,200 mg/m² × 2	60%		77%	
				1,200 mg/m² × 4	64%		77%	
NSABP B25	NP	2,548	Cyclophosphamide	1,200 mg/m² × 4	62%	NS	81%	NS
				2,400 mg/m² × 2	66%		80%	
				2,400 mg/m² × 470%			82%	
NCIC MAS	NP/high risk NN Premenopausal	716	Epirubicin	CMF (Bonadonna) × 6	53%	0.009	70%	0.03
				CEF (E 60 mg/m² d1,8 q28d) × 6	63%		77%	
Belgian trial	NP	777	Epirubicin and C	CMF (Bonadonna) (1)	78%[b]	1 vs. 2 vs. 3 NS	91%[c]	1 vs. 2 vs. 3 NS
				E 60 mg/m², C 500 mg/m² d1 q21d (2)	72%[b]		89%[c]	
				E 100 mg/m², C 830 mg/m² d1 q21d (3)	80%[b]	2 vs. 3 0.04	92%[c]	2 vs. 3 0.05

[a]Four-year recurrence-free survival.
[b]Three-year event-free survival.
[c]Three-year overall survival.
ER, estrogen receptor; NN, node negative; NP, node positive.

week 82.1%, 2p = 0.085; OS, CAF 77.7%, 16 week 86.8%, 2p = 0.052) and less so in women with more than 3 positive nodes. Treatment-related morbidities were different: Three toxic deaths were encountered in the CAF arm, and the 16-week schedule was substantially more complicated to deliver.

High Dose Intensity Anthracyclines

A collaborative RCT (CALGB 9344) compared three different doses of doxorubicin (60, 75, or 90 mg/m^2 i.v. day 1 every 21 days) in four cycles of AC, followed by a second randomization in each arm to four cycles of paclitaxel versus no further treatment (54). In an interim analysis based on 540 events, the doxorubicin dose had no impact on DFS or OS. The analysis of the actual dose received in each group after adjustment for toxicity has not been presented; however, in the 90 mg/m^2 doxorubicin group, the doxorubicin was delivered as 45 mg/m^2 for two days rather than as a single bolus. Whether this compromised any superior efficacy associated with the higher dose is unknown.

Cyclophosphamide

Suboptimal Doses of Cyclophosphamide

In a retrospective study, Bonadonna demonstrated that patients who received less than 85% of the intended dose intensity of CMF had inferior relapse-free survival compared to patients who received 85% or more (78). This concept has not been explored in a prospective trial in the adjuvant setting. In the metastatic setting, i.v. CMF given once every 3 weeks (dose-intensity of cyclophosphamide: 200 mg/m^2/week) resulted in poorer survival compared to the Bonadonna schedule of oral cyclophosphamide, which is given for 14 days every 4 weeks (dose intensity 350 mg/m^2/week) in a randomized trial (79).

Higher Dose Intensity/density Cyclophosphamide

The NSABP B-22 trial compared standard doses of C (4 × 600 mg/m^2) in AC to regimens that were dose-intense (2 × 1,200 mg/m^2) and dose-intense plus dose-dense (4 × 1,200 mg/m^2) (80). Patients were stratified by age (less than 50 versus 50 or more years), as well as by number of positive nodes, estrogen receptor level, and type of surgery. At 5 years follow-up, no OS or DFS differences were observed for the three groups or for subsets of patients with one to three NP (55% of study population), four to nine NP (30% of study population), or more than 10 NP (14% of study population) disease. Toxicity, in particular, severe infection, septic episodes, and vomiting were higher in the arm with both dose intensity and dose density, as might be expected. The frequency of AML and MDS following CT was similar in all arms (one, three, and two cases, respectively). A subsequent NSABP trial (B-25), reported no differences in DFS and OS at 5 years between three higher-than-conventional C doses (4 × 1,200 mg/m^2; 2 × 2,400 mg/m^2; 4 × 2,400 mg/m^2) with G-CSF support or also in combination with doxorubicin (AC every 3 weeks) (81). Twenty-two cases of AML and MDS have occurred in this trial (incidence 0.87%, similar frequency in each arm), with cytogenetics typical of post-alkylator and post-topoisomerase II-inhibitor leukemia occurring in six and three cases, respectively.

Thus far, several well-conducted randomized trials have failed to show an advantage for escalating the dose of cyclophosphamide beyond 600 mg/m^2 every 3 weeks in association with doxorubicin or of increasing the duration of CMF beyond six cycles when using the Bonadonna regimen. Higher doses are clearly associated with excess short-term and long-term toxicity, however.

Anthracyclines-Cyclophosphamide-Paclitaxel

Taxanes are being intensively studied in the adjuvant setting, following their established activity in metastatic breast cancer. However, at present, the results of most of these trials are unavailable. As described in the chemotherapy section of this chapter, results from three randomized trials in which paclitaxel was added to anthracycline-based regimens have all failed to demonstrate a survival advantage for adding paclitaxel to date. However, follow-up is short and mature results of these and other trials are awaited. Of note, none of these trials have explored dose intensification of taxanes, and the benefit of standard doses needs to be established before the value of increased doses can be explored.

One closed Intergroup study with a 2 by 2 design (CALGB 9741) is exploring the use of sequential CT using doxorubicin, paclitaxel, and cyclophosphamide or concurrent doxorubicin and cyclophosphamide followed by paclitaxel at 14-day or 21-day intervals in women with NP stage II or IIIA breast cancer. The results are awaited with interest.

Anthracyclines Versus CMF

A few trials have compared high-dose anthracyclines to CMF. The NSABP B-15 trial demonstrated equivalence of four cycles of AC with six cycles of CMF (6CMF); however, whether 4AC is the optimal anthracycline regimen remains debatable, since more dose-intense anthracycline regimens have proven superior to CMF in RCTs.

The question of whether higher doses of anthracyclines (than in 4AC) are superior to CMF has been addressed by several trials with apparently conflicting results. A Canadian NCIC-CTG study (NCIC-CTG MA5) compared six cycles of an intensive CEF regimen (epirubicin 60 mg/m^2 on days 1 and 8 every 4 weeks) to classical 6CMF and reported a 19% RRR in mortality (OS 77% versus 70%, $p = 0.03$) and 29% RRR in recurrence (DFS 53% versus 63%, $p = 0.009$) for CEF among 710 NP premenopausal patients at a median follow-up of 59 months (44). Whether the superiority of the CEF schedule is due to the increased dose-intensity of anthracyclines or the substitution of methotrexate by epirubicin remains unanswered. The delivered dose intensities of epirubicin and methotrexate were 77% and 88%, respectively.

In contrast, there was no difference in OS between six cycles of classical CMF and eight cycles of full-dose EC (HEC arm, 100/830 mg/m^2 on day 1 every 3 weeks) in the Belgian trial (85% and 86%, respectively) with 50 months median follow-up; however, the HEC arm was superior to the moderate-dose arm (EC, 60/500/m^2 on day 1 every 3 weeks for 8 cycles) in both EFS ($p = 0.04$) and OS ($p = 0.05$) (48). Possible explanations for the lack of superiority of HEC over CMF in the Belgian trial include the absence of 5-FU in the anthracycline arm, a less favorable patient population in terms of chemotherapy effectiveness (40% of patients were postmenopausal), and the administration of TAM to 40% of the patients (an effective adjuvant modality that makes additional benefits from chemotherapy more difficult to detect).

Not surprisingly, dose-intense/dose-dense CT schedules are associated with increased toxicity. For example, in the NCIC trial, an increased rate of hospitalization for febrile neutropenia (8.5% versus 1.1% in CEF and CMF arms, respectively) and increased rate of secondary leukemia were reported in the CEF group (44). Five cases of secondary leukemia among 359 patient (1.4 %) have occurred in the CEF arm, although classic post-topoisomerase II-inhibitor cytogenetics were only observed in one case. Three cases of AML were reported in the Belgian study, all in the HEC arm (1.2%) (48). The increased rate of AML and MDS noted in the Scandinavian Breast Group Study SBG 9401 with nine cycles of tailored FEC is also noteworthy (82). A recent report analyzing the risk of acute leukemia in 1,463 premenopausal NP patients enrolled in four NCIC-CTG adjuvant therapy trials demonstrated that the conditional probability of developing acute leukemia was 1.8% for CEF as opposed to 0.3% for non–epirubicin-containing regimens (AC or CMF) (68). The NSABP group has recently reviewed data from all its adjuvant trials in which regimens containing doxorubicin and cyclophosphamide were used, for a total of 8,533 patients. Thirty-nine cases of AML/MDS were reported. The incidence correlated particularly with cyclophosphamide dose intensity, with a cumulative incidence of AML/MDS at 5 years of 1.04% (95% CI 0.64% to 1.67%) for patients receiving more intense regimens, compared to 0.22% (95% CI 0.12% to 0.43%) for those treated with standard AC (83).

Until the efficacy of dose intense regimens has been confirmed, they should be used judiciously, preferably in a controlled trial setting,

TABLE 9.7. Ongoing and recently closed adjuvant RCTs of dose-dense or-intense CT in NP breast cancer

Trial/Group	Accrual target/ actual to date	Population	Comparative arms
ABCSG 10	400/111	Pre/postmenopausal NN and NP	4 EC (60/600 mg/m^2 d1 q21d) → 4 CMF (600/40/600 mg/m^2 d1 q21d) → TAM (5 yrs) 4 EC (60/600 mg/m^2 d1,2 q21d) → 4 CMF (600/40/600 mg/m^2 d1,22 q21d) → TAM (5 yrs)
GABG IVE	375 closed	Postmenopausal, <70 >10 NP	4 EC → 3 CMF 4 E (120 mg/m^2) + Hormonal therapy
OCSGL	380/51 trial interrupted	>10 NP 2–3 NP, high risk	6 FEC (E 50 mg/m^2 q21d) 6 FEC (E 60 mg/m^2 d1,8 q28d) 6 EC, G-CSF (E 120 mg/m^2 C 830 mg/m^2 q21d)
INT 0137	3,176 closed	Pre/postmenopausal 1–3NP NN high risk	6 AC (54 mg/m^2/1.2 g/m^2 q21d) + G-CSF 4 A (81 mg/m^2 q21d) + G-CSF → 3 C 2.4 g/m^2 q21d + G-CSF
NCIC-CTG MA-21	2,500/215	Pre/post menopausal, ≤60 NP, high risk NN	6CEF (75 mg/m^2 po d1–14 ; 60 mg/m^2 d1,8; 500 mg/m^2 d1,8) 6 EC (120 mg/m^2 d1; 830 mg/m^2 d1 14d with Epo and G-CSF) then 4 paclitaxel (175 mg/m^2 q 21d) 4AC (60 mg/m^2; 600/m^2 q21d) then 4 paclitaxel (175 mg/m^2 q21d)
GONO MIG 1	1,200/1,214 closed	NP NN high risk	6 FEC (600/60/600 mg/m^2 d1, 8 q21d) 6 FEC q14d + G-CSF

NN, node negative; NP, node positive; OCSGL, Oncological Center Study Group in Lodz.

given their increased toxicity. Several large ongoing and recently closed trials (Table 9.7) may establish superior efficacy of dose-intense and dose-dense over conventional-dose CT, but at present these strategies cannot be recommended as routine therapy, even in very high-risk disease. Other scientific approaches of interest with respect to dose-dense-intense CT administration include optimizing the duration of exposure to cytotoxic drugs, selecting the most promising drug combinations, and targeting the population most likely to benefit from dose intensification.

CHEMOENDOCRINE THERAPY

The essential question in considering combined therapy for NP breast cancer is whether, in women with strong indications for CT (premenopausal and postmenopausal women with ER-negative tumors or high-risk features), the addition of hormonal therapy further improves outcome, and whether CT adds further benefits in women for whom adjuvant hormonal therapy is indicated (postmenopausal women with ER-positive tumors and other low-risk features for relapse, and premenopausal women with ER-positive tumors who have chosen ovarian ablation). According to the Oxford Overview, the addition of TAM to CT significantly decreases the risk of recurrence and significantly improves survival in ER-positive women compared to CT alone. CT plus TAM decreased the annual odds of recurrence and death by 52%, plus or minus 8%, and 47%, plus or minus 9%, respectively, compared to CT alone in patients with ER-positive tumors (1). In women over 50 years of age, CT provided significant proportional reductions in recurrence and mortality with or without TAM. The number of patients under 50 years of age enrolled in the trials of CT plus TAM versus TAM was small and may be the reason why no significant reduction in recurrence and mortality has been demonstrated with the addition of TAM to CT in this subgroup by the overview (65).

Although not yet published, the 2000 Oxford Overview confirms these figures (2). Based on these findings, the anti-cancer activity of CT and tamoxifen appear to be complementary and additive. In the absence of contraindications, all patients with ER-positive tumors receiving adjuvant CT should also receive tamoxifen.

Postmenopausal Women

ER-positive and Low-risk Tumors

The decision to use tamoxifen alone or in combination with chemotherapy in postmenopausal women with NP disease must be made on an individual basis, taking into consideration factors such as absolute risk, age, patient comorbidity, and personal preference. Despite the significant benefit demonstrated by the Oxford Overview in terms of recurrence and mortality when both CT and TAM are given in hormone receptor positive disease, the administration of CT to all postmenopausal women remains controversial. Most individual RCTs comparing adjuvant CT or hormonal therapy to chemoendocrine therapy have suggested equivalence. Those that demonstrated a DFS and/or OS advantage for the combination were also associated with a higher toxicity profile for CT plus TAM versus TAM alone (Table 9.8).

Several trials of chemoendocrine treatment versus endocrine treatment in postmenopausal women are discussed below.

The IBCSG VII study used a 2 by 2 design which accrued 1,266 NP postmenopausal women between 1986 and 1993 (84). All patients received TAM (5 years), and randomization was to no CT (group A, n = 306), early CMF (group B, n = 302), delayed CMF (group C, n = 308), or early-plus-delayed CMF (group D, n = 296). CMF was given according to the

TABLE 9.8. *Adjuvant RCTs of TAM versus TAM plus CT in postmenopausal ER-positive and negative, NP breast cancer*

Trial/Group	N	ER status	Intervention A (TAM)	Intervention B (CT + TAM)	% 5 yr DFS A	% 5 yr DFS B	% 5 yr OS A	% 5 yr OS B
NCIC-CTG 1997 (89)	705	+	TAM 30 mg/d × 2 yr	6 CMF i.v. d1 q21d + TAM 30 mg/d × 2 yr	61	64 $p = 0.80$	80	82 $p = 0.94$
ICCG 1999 (85)	604	±	TAM 20 mg/d × 4 yr	6 Epi 50 mg/m² d1, 8 i.v. q4w + TAM 20 mg/d × 4 yr	62.1	73.7 $p = 0.02$	77	80.6 $p = 0.46$
INT0100 (69,86)	1,477	+	TAM 20 mg/d × 5 yr	CAF + T / CAF → T	67	76 $p = 0.0002$	79	84 $p = 0.006$
IBCSG 1997 (84)	1,266	±	A: TAM 20 mg/ d × 5 yr	B: TAM + CMF mo 1,2,3 / C: TAM + CMF mo 9, 12,15 / D: TAM + CMF mo 1,2, 3,9,12,15	A: 55 C: 59	B: 64 D: 63 $p = N/A$	A: 77 C: 74	B: 74 D:76 $p = 0.70$
Gelber meta-analysis 1996 (94)	503	±	TAM × 12 mo + prednisone	12 CMF + TAM × 12 mo + prednisone	33.5	44.8 $p = 0.02$	44.9	55.1 $p = NS$
	72	±	TAM × 24 mo	8 AC + TAM × 24 mo	35.1	45.7 $p = N/A$	51.3	54.3 $p = N/A$
	91	±	TAM × 36 mo	12 CMFVP + TAM × 36 mo	53.2	68.2 $p = 0.04$	59.6	75.0 $p = 0.11$
	59	+	TAM × 12 mo	6 CMF + TAM × 12 mo	62.0	46.6 $p = N/A$	65.5	60.0 $p = N/A$
	593	+	TAM × 12 mo	12 CMFVP + TAM × 12 mo	66.8	68.7 $p = NS$	77.0	74.1 $p = NS$
	113	±	TAM × 24 mo	24 CMF + TAM × 24 mo	38.8	50.0 $p = NS$	71.6	58.7 $p = 0.06$
	210	+	TAM × 60 mo	6 CMF, 4 Epi + TAM × 60 mo	76.0	80.0 $p = 0.10$	89.4	90.6 $p = 0.70$
	1,233	±	TAM × 12 mo	8 CMF + TAM × 12 mo	60.2	67.9 $p = N/A$	75.0	76.4 $p = N/A$
	1,226	<60y + / >60y ±	TAM × 60 mo	4 AC or 17 PF or 17 PAF all with TAM × 60 mo	79.7	88.0 $p = 0.0004$	91.4	94.2 $p = 0.04$

ICCG, International Collaborative Group; N/A, not available; NS, non significant; PAF, L-PAM, Adriamycin, and 5-FU; PF, L-phenylalanine (L-PAM) and 5-FU; TAM, tamoxifen.

Bonadonna regimen. Analysis of DFS and OS was carried out using the intention-to-treat principle (ITT) on 1,212 evaluable patients after 60 months median follow-up. There was no significant difference in 5-year OS ($p = 0.70$ for the comparison of all four groups) despite better DFS for the comparisons of any CMF (groups B, C, D) or early CMF (groups B and D) versus TAM alone (group A). For the entire study group, early CMF significantly improved 5-year DFS compared to group A (no CT) and group C (delayed CMF; 64% versus 57%, $p = 0.01$), while delayed CMF did not (compared to groups A and B). Patients with ER-negative tumors who received delayed CMF did not have a significant increased risk of relapse compared with TAM alone. Thus the benefit of adding CT is maximized when it is given early. For patients with ER-positive disease (77% of the study group), there was a relative risk reduction for recurrence of 33%) for early CT (hazard ratio 0.67; 95% CI 0.50 to 0.91), 21% for late CT (hazard ratio 0.78; 95% CI 0.58 to 1.04), and 36% for both early and delayed CT (hazard ratio 0.64; 95% CI 0.47 to 0.88), compared to tamoxifen alone (group A). The lack of OS improvement with the addition of CMF in this RCT suggests that the actual benefit is small and may not always warrant the attendant toxicity.

A separate efficacy and tolerability analysis of the IBCSG VII trial, including 608 patients in groups A and B only, was reported recently. The outcome of patients who were 65 or more years old (172 of 608) was compared to younger postmenopausal women in this report. For older patients, 5-year DFS for CMF plus TAM versus TAM alone were identical; however, for younger patients, early CMF plus TAM was significantly better than TAM (61% versus 53%, $p = 0.008$). More women in the older age group experienced grade 3 toxicity compared to younger patients, and as a result, older women received a suboptimal CMF dose intensity (85).

A study of similar magnitude, INT0100, compared 5 years of TAM (n = 361) to six cycles of CAF (C, 100 mg/m^2 days 1 through 14; A, 30 mg/m^2 days 1 and 8; 5-FU, 500 mg/m^2 days 1 and 8 every 28 days) plus TAM, with TAM beginning either with (CAFT, n = 546) or after (CAF plus T, n = 563) CT in NP, receptor-positive postmenopausal women. An interim analysis demonstrated a significantly better DFS for the combination (data for CAFT and CAF plus T combined) compared with TAM and was reported in 1997 (86). According to recently updated results with 7.3 years median follow-up, the significant DFS benefit of the combination persists (absolute improvement of 9% at 5 years). More importantly, a significant OS benefit was also demonstrated for the addition of CT, with an absolute improvement of 5% at 5 years. The survival curves diverge after the first 4 years of follow-up and remain separated beyond year 5. The benefits of combined modality treatment must be balanced against increased toxicity, which is summarized in Table 9.9 (69). The question with respect to optimal timing for TAM administration has been answered by a recent report of the 8-year outcome of the two arms of this study (sequential versus concurrent CAF and TAM). The results show a 18% DFS advantage when TAM is administrated sequentially after CAF (87).

The other positive trial is the NSABP B-16 trial, which randomized 1,245 NP, receptor-

TABLE 9.9. *Intergroup Trial 0100: Treatment Related Events (69)*

	Year 1			Year 2			
	Deaths	GI toxicity	Thromboembolic events	CHF	AML/MDS	Thromboembolic events	Uterine cancer
CAFT (n = 1,084)	n = 4	27%	3.3%	2.1%	0.8%	2.2%	1.1%
TAM (n = 354)	n = 0	0.5%	0%	0.31%	0%	2%	1.1%

AML/MDS, acute myelogenous leukemia/myelodysplastic syndrome; CAFT, cyclophosphamide, adriamycin, 5-FU, and tamoxifen; CHF, congestive heart failure; GI, gastrointestinal; TAM, tamoxifen.

positive women over 50 years of age to the comparison of TAM alone (20 mg per day for 5 years) or TAM given concurrently with CT, the latter consisting of either four cycles of AC (doxorubicin 60 mg/m^2 i.v. and cyclophosphamide 600 mg/m^2 i.v. every 21 days) or 17 cycles of PF (L-PAM 4 mg/m^2 by mouth and 5-FU 300 mg/m^2 i.v. on days 1 through 5 every 6 weeks). PAF (with doxorubicin 30 mg/m^2 i.v. on days 1 and 21 every 6 weeks) replaced PF after 1985. Three-year DFS and OS were significantly better in the AC-plus-TAM arm compared to the TAM alone arm (DFS was 84% versus 67%, $p = 0.0004$ and OS was 93% versus 85%, $p = 0.04$). The DFS of PAF-TAM or PF-TAM arms were also significantly better when compared to TAM alone, but without a significant survival advantage (88).

In general, studies which showed equivalence for chemoendocrine therapy versus endocrine therapy alone are limited by being either small, and therefore underpowered, or by the use of inferior chemotherapy regimens or suboptimal duration of TAM.

The NCIC-CTG compared CMF and TAM (30 mg a day for 2 years) to TAM in a RCT of 705 postmenopausal, ER-positive or PgR-positive patients stratified by local therapy received, number of positive nodes, level of hormone positivity, and time since menopause (89). Of the 353 CT-randomized patients, 84% completed the six cycles of CMF (i.v. on day 1 every 21 days). No differences in 5-year DFS (64% and 61%, $p = 0.8$), loco-regional RFS (56% and 49%, $p = 0.72$), or OS (82% and 80%, $p = 0.94$) were observed between the CT-plus-TAM and TAM arms, respectively. Two toxic deaths occurred in the combination arm. Although the CMF regimen used in this trial has been shown to be inferior to oral Bonadonna-CMF in metastatic disease, they have never been directly compared in the adjuvant setting (79). Nevertheless, proponents of chemoendocrine therapy might argue that the lack of superiority of the combination arm may be related to delivery of an inferior CT regimen.

A multicenter RCT, conducted by the International Collaborative Cancer group (ICCG), compared low-dose epirubicin (Epi) plus TAM (n = 301) to TAM alone (n = 303) in postmenopausal patients (90). Analysis of RFS and OS was performed using intention to treat (ITT), with a median follow-up of 4.8 years. Seventy-five percent of the patients had ER-positive (50%) or ER-unknown disease; 38% had four to nine positive axillary nodes, and 58% had more than nine positive nodes. Of the patients randomized to the combination, 79% completed all cycles with a 95% total dose intensity of Epi; 31 patients received no CT. Non-significant trends favoring the combination were observed in 5-year RFS (73.7% and 62.1%) and OS (80.6% and 77%). There was no subset analysis according to the number of involved nodes. Toxicity was higher in the combination arm: one sudden death; two CHF; eight of the nine with thromboembolic complications; and five hematologic malignancies (two AML, three other).

In a SWOG (7827) study, 892 receptor-positive and NP postmenopausal patients were randomized to TAM (20 mg a day for 1 year) or CMFVp (cyclophosphamide 60 mg/m^2 a day by mouth for 1 year; methotrexate 15 mg/m^2; 5-FU, 400 mg/m^2 i.v. weekly for 1 year; vincristine 0.625 mg/m^2 i.v. weekly for 10 weeks; and prednisone in decreasing doses from 30 mg/m^2 a day for 10 weeks) or CMFVp plus TAM. At a median follow-up of $6\frac{1}{2}$ years, no DFS and OS differences were observed between the three arms (91). Recently reported 15-year results continue to show no significant difference in both DFS and OS between the three arms (92).

The FASG 07 trial, randomizing 335 NP, receptor-positive postmenopausal women to either six cycles of FEC (500/50/500/m^2 i.v. every 21 days) plus TAM (30 mg a day for 3 years) or TAM alone showed a significant DFS advantage for the FEC arm ($p = 0.047$) at a median follow-up of 48 months (93).

In 1996, a systematic overview reviewed the available data from earlier RCTs of TAM alone versus CT plus TAM in women older than 50 who had axillary NP breast cancer (94). Nine trials, comprising 3,920 women with an average follow-up of 7 years, were analyzed using quality-adjusted time without symptoms or toxicity (Q-TWiST) for RFS and OS. Four trials were restricted to ER-positive tumors, and four included both ER-negative and ER-positive tumors. No difference in quality-adjusted survival time was found with the addition of CT to TAM compared to TAM alone. Patients treated with CT/TAM gained 5.4 months of RFS and 2 months of OS (pNS); however, this was at the expense of 2 to 24 months of CT. In five of these trials, TAM was given for only 1 or 2 years, which we know from the EBCTCG overview is inferior to longer therapy. On the one hand, this analysis strengthens the argument that CT might provide only marginal additional benefit in ER-positive, postmenopausal women who receive adequate TAM treatment (only four of nine trials); however, because many of the CT regimens were also substandard, one could also argue that the question has not been adequately tested so far.

A few trials in postmenopausal NP breast cancer have compared chemoendocrine therapy to CT alone, rather than hormonal therapy (95,96). These studies show either borderline superiority for the combination arm or no difference. In a subset of 259 women 50 years or older with high-risk breast cancer (one to three NP and ER-negative or four or more 4 NP) from an RCT of the German Gynecological Adjuvant Breast Group (GABG), superior DFS ($p = 0.01$) and a trend towards improved survival were observed in the AC/TAM arm compared with AC alone (95). However, for the entire study population (n = 471), no significant difference was observed in either endpoint.

Given that TAM is associated with a larger magnitude of benefit than CT in postmenopausal women, until evidence suggests otherwise, the treatment plan for postmenopausal women should always include a hormonal agent if the ER status is positive. Since the addition of CT to tamoxifen in postmenopausal, ER-NP women results in a small survival advantage, consideration to add CT should be made for each individual on the basis of absolute risk, keeping in mind the added toxicity and small magnitude of benefit. Because the benefits may be limited, it is important to allow a woman to make an informed decision about CT.

It should be noted that, in general, large comparative trials with an anthracycline-based regimen have consistently shown improved DFS and OS over tamoxifen alone, whereas CMF-containing trials of similar magnitude have not. Studies that enrolled patients with four or more positive nodes were not sufficiently powered to allow subset analyses in ER-positive, high–node-burden disease, a group which might derive the largest absolute benefit from combined modality therapy. Nevertheless, in this setting, the addition of anthracycline-based chemotherapy to TAM may be preferable. Several recently closed and ongoing chemoendocrine studies in NP patients are summarized in Table 9.10 and they will hopefully contribute sufficient patient numbers to reach a confident conclusion about the value of combined therapy over single modality treatment.

ER-negative Tumors

In the IBCSG VII trial (TAM versus TAM plus three different CMF schedules), DFS was shorter for patients with ER-negative tumors compared with ER-positive tumors in all groups (ER negative, 51%, 51%, 38%, 42%; ER positive, 57%, 69%, 64%; 70% for groups A, B, C, D, respectively) (84). This highlights the overall worse short-term prognosis of ER-negative tumors. TAM is not effective in ER-negative disease, and the incremental value of adding it to CT is likely to be negligible. Although some comparative studies addressing this question have included ER-negative patients, analysis of these subsets involves small numbers and unreliable statistical comparisons (84,90,96). In addition, the prevention study confirms that TAM does not prevent ER-negative cancers, and the expected reduction in contralateral breast cancer associated with adjuvant TAM has not yet shown an impact on overall survival of women with ER-negative breast tumors. Thus, CT is the adjuvant systemic therapy of choice for women with NP, ER-negative tumors, and there is no role for TAM.

Premenopausal Women

Tamoxifen and Chemotherapy

Within the premenopausal group there are still very limited data about women randomized to

TABLE 9.10. *Ongoing or recently closed adjuvant RCTs of chemoendocrine therapy in NP breast cancer*

Group/Trial	Accrual target/ actual to date	Population	Comparison arms[a]
ABCSG 09	660/281	ER (+) NN, NP; Grade 3	TAM 20 mg × 5 yr TAM + 4 EC (60/600 q21d)
EORTC 10901	1,816/1,863 closed	NN, NP Any ER status	CT + TAM 20 mg × 3 yr CT only 6 CMF/FAC/CAF/CEF or 4 AC/EC
GABG IVD	700/829 closed	ER (−); ≤ 70 yr NN, 1–3 NP ER (-); ≤ 70 yr 4–9 NP	3 CMF 3 CMF → TAM × 5 yr 4 EC → 3 CMF 4 EC → 3 CMF → TAM × 5 yr
IKA-IKMN[b]	500/110 closed, low accrual	NP	TAM 30 mg × 3 yr 4 EC → TAM × 3 yr
NCIC-CTG MA.12	672 closed	Pre and perimeno NP, high risk NN Any ER status	CT → TAM CT → placebo
UKCCCR-ABC	1,991 closed	NP and NN Any ER status	TAM TAM + CT
GFEA 08	326 closed	NP, >65 years, ER (+)	TAM 30 mg/d × 3 yr TAM + Epi 30 wkly × 2q3w × 8
GEICAM 9401	485 closed	NP Any ER status (Sequential vs concomitant)	4 EC → TAM (20 mg/d × 5 yr) 4 EC + TAM
ICCG C/4/87	697 closed	Postmenopausal NP Any ER status	TAM Epirubicin + TAM

[a]All doses are in mg/m^2 unless stated otherwise.
[b]Receptor status not available.
EORTC, European Organization for the Research and Treatment of Cancer; GEICAM, Grupo Espanol de Investigacian en Cancer de Mama; GFEA, Groupe Français d'Etude Adjuvante; IKA, Integraal KankerAmsterdam; UKCCCR, United Kingdom Co-ordinating Committee on Cancer Research.

receive CT alone or CT plus tamoxifen. Despite this, it is current practice to prescribe TAM following adjuvant CT for premenopausal women who have hormone-receptor-positive tumors, on the basis of the EBCTCG findings. However, the Oxford Overview examined the benefit of TAM (independent of CT) in younger women of all risks (NP and NN), and individual studies of CT versus CT/TAM in NP disease have failed to demonstrate an advantage for the combination. The volume of mature evidence is small, and several large studies addressing the value of TAM in premenopausal women following CT are still accruing patients and were not included in the overview. Thus, future results of trials such as the NCIC-CTG MA-12 (placebo or TAM after adjuvant CT in premenopausal and perimenopausal high-risk NN and NP breast cancer), the EORTC 10901 (CT followed by TAM or observation) and ICCG C/9/91 (FEC 50 or 75 followed by hormone or no hormone therapy) may provide more reliable estimates of the benefit of TAM in this subgroup.

Ovarian Ablation

It is logical to anticipate that the value of ovarian ablation (OA), if any, would be seen in a population whose hormonal milieu changes most significantly as a result of ablation and whose tumors are most likely to be stimulated by hormones. That is, premenopausal women with ER- or PgR-positive disease. Since the first example of OA for early breast cancer was reported in the *Lancet* in 1896, numerous randomized trials have addressed the role of OA in this disease (97).

Ovarian Ablation Versus No Adjuvant Therapy

In the absence of CT, ovarian ablation is associated with a significant protective effect against recurrence and breast cancer mortality in premenopausal women (98).

The EBCTCG meta-analysis comprehensively reviewed RCTs beginning before 1990 which compared OA with no hormonal maneuver, and for which at least 15 years of follow-up was available (8). Data were retrieved for 12 of 13 trials, all of which began before 1980 and all of which induced ablation surgically or by irradiation, corresponding to 96% of patients randomized in such studies. Menopausal status was not defined in these studies and age (less than 50 and 50 or older) was used as a surrogate for menopausal status. Of the 12 available trials, seven of them compared OA with no adjuvant therapy, four trials compared CT with or without ablation, and one study had a 2 by 2 factorial design for CT and OA. Log-rank, observed-minus-expected values were calculated for RFS and OS in each trial, and these were combined to determine an overall effect. Results from four studies of adjuvant ablation with luteinizing hormone-releasing hormone (LHRH) analogues were not available.

The EBCTCG found that, for women younger than 50 years (n = 2102), the proportional risks of death and recurrence are decreased by 18% and 18.5%, respectively, compared to control. The absolute risk reductions in recurrence and survival were 6% ($2p = 0.0007$) and 6.3% ($2p = 0.001$), respectively, and the corresponding numbers needed to treat (NNT) to avoid one recurrence and one death were about 17 and 16 women, respectively. In the NP group, RFS was 24% in the control group and 37.4% in the OA group ($2p = 0.0002$), a difference of 3.8 events per 100 women treated (NNT 7.5). OS at 15 years was 29.2% in the control and 41.7% in the ablation groups ($2p = 0.0007$), a difference of 3.9 deaths per 100 women (NNT 8).

No significant differences in RFS or OS were observed between the OA and control groups among the 1,354 randomized patients over the age of 50 (1,018 deaths and 48 additional recurrences without death) (98). This is not surprising, given that the estrogen levels in this predominantly perimenopausal and postmenopausal age group are likely to be similar to castrate levels before OA takes place.

A recently presented Vietnamese trial randomized 709 premenopausal patients to either adjuvant oophorectomy plus tamoxifen (combined endocrine therapy) or the same treatment at the time of relapse. A significantly longer DFS and OS were observed for women receiving adjuvant treatment at a median follow-up of 3 years (99). The benefit was confined to the women with ER-positive disease.

Ovarian Ablation With or Without TAM Versus Chemotherapy

The question of whether OA is an equivalent, inferior, or superior treatment to CT in premenopausal women has been the subject of several RCTs. Unfortunately, their interpretation is limited by the immaturity of results and some design limitations such as suboptimal CT regimens and inadequate use of TAM in women with ER-positive tumors in the CT arms.

Among the trials comparing OA to CMF (cyclophosphamide, methotrexate and 5-FU) chemotherapy, the Scottish trial randomized 332 premenopausal women with NP breast cancer to 6 months of CMF (oral C) or OA and showed no difference in EFS and OS after a maximum follow-up of 12 years. ER assays were done in 81% of primary tumors, but those results did not play a part in the randomization procedure. The analysis of patient outcome with respect to ER suggested that OA improved survival in patients having a high ER content, while CMF was more beneficial in patients whose tumors were ER poor (100).

A Scandinavian trial compared OA to nine cycles of CMF (intravenous C) in 732 hormone receptor positive breast cancer patients who were NP or had T3 tumors. Five-year DFS and OS rates were found to be similar. Of note, amenorrhea occurred in 68% patients treated with CMF (101).

The Zoladex Early Breast Cancer Research Association Trial (ZEBRA) compared six cycles of classical CMF with goserelin acetate, an LHRH (luteinizing hormone-releasing hormone) agonist/analogue, for 2 years in 1,640 premenopausal NP patients with any receptor type. According to the preliminary results, a similar DFS was observed in the two arms; however, in the ER-negative subset, comprising 25% of the patients, DFS was significantly better in the group treated with CMF. Survival data are not yet available. Eighty percent of patients in the CT arm remained amenorrheic at 3 years, while two-thirds of patients in the goserelin arm regained their menses by 1 year following completion of goserelin treatment (102). Quality of life data from the same trial suggest a better overall tolerance for goserelin versus CMF during the treatment period (103).

A German trial randomized 600 perimenopausal/premenopausal, NP, receptor-positive women to either leuprolide acetate for 2 years or six cycles of CMF. An interim analysis from 227 patients revealed no significant difference between the two arms in terms of DFS and OS. With only two years follow-up, these findings are clearly not mature (103).

A Danish-Swedish trial, Danish Breast Cancer Group (DBCG) 89-D, randomized 732 receptor-positive, premenopausal, high-risk patients (NP and/or tumor greater than 5 cm) to OA or nine cycles of CMF (C 600 mg/m^2, M 40 mg/m^2, F 600 mg/m^2 i.v. on day 1 every 3 weeks). DFS and OS differences between the two arms were not significant after a follow-up of 68 months, indicating that the ablation of functioning ovaries had a comparable effect to CMF type CT in terms of DFS and OS in premenopausal receptor positive patients (105).

Several trials have compared OA plus tamoxifen (combined endocrine treatment) to CT (Table 9.11). Early results of an Austrian Breast Cancer Study Group (ABCSG V) trial comparing i.v. CMF to the combination of OA (using goserelin for 3 years) and TAM (20 mg a day for 5 years) in ER-positive breast cancer patients (1,045 randomized, 157 recurrences, 56 deaths) showed no difference in OS with a median follow-up of 42 months, despite better RFS ($p < 0.02$) in the OA group (106). In this study, patients who became amenorrheic following CMF had a significantly longer DFS and OS than those who did not. A subset analysis of the NP population at the time of study maturity may provide some insight into the relative benefits of these therapies in NP disease. A recent report of this trial confirmed a significantly improved RFS in the goserelin plus TAM arm ($p < 0.02$) compared to the CMF arm at a median follow-up of 60 months, without a significant difference in terms of OS (107).

TABLE 9.11. *Results of RCTs of OA plus TAM versus CT in NP premenopausal women*

Trial	Population	N	Comparison arms	Results	Median follow-up (months)
ABCSG 5	NN/NP (54%) ER (+) Premenopausal	1,088	OA (goserelin) × 3 yr + TAM × 5 yr CMF d1, 8 q28d × 6 (intravenous C)	RFS better for endocrine therapy ($p < 0.02$) OS equivalent	60
GROCTA 02	NP, ER (+) Peri/premenopausal	240	OA (goserelin or surgery or radiation) × 2 yr + TAM × 5 yr (30 mg/day) 6 × CMF (classical oral C)	DFS and OS are equivalent	89
FASG 06	NP (1–3) ER (+) premenopausal	333	TAM + OA (triptorelin) (30 mg/day) × 3 yr FEC50X6	DFS and OS are equivalent (too few events so far)	54
French trial	NP ER (+)	162	OA (surgery or pelvic RT) + TAM FAC	DFS and OS are equivalent (but underpowered) closed due to poor accrual	94

ABCSG, Austrian Breast Cancer Study Group; FASG French Adjuvant Study Group; GROCTA, Italian Cooperative Group for Chemohormonal Therapy of Early Breast Cancer.

The Italian Breast Cancer Adjuvant Study Group [Italian Cooperative Group for Chemohormonal Therapy of Early Breast Cancer (GROCTA) 02 trial] trial compared six cycles of oral CMF with 2 years of OA (surgical, by radiation, or by LHRH analogue goserelin) and 5 years of 30 mg per day of TAM in 240 NP premenopausal/perimenopausal women with ER-positive tumors. No difference has been reported between the two arms in terms of 5-year DFS and OS at a median follow-up of 76 months. Again, the patients who became amenorrheic following CMF treatment had a significantly longer OS. The method of OA used did not impact on the probability of relapse or death (108). A recent update confirmed these results at a median follow-up of 89 months (109).

A French study, French Adjuvant Study Group (FASG) 06, compared an anthracycline-based regimen [six cycles of FEC-50 (5-FU, epirubicin 50 mg/m^2, cyclophosphamide)] to 3 years of 30 mg a day TAM and triptorelin in 333 receptor-positive, NP, premenopausal women. FEC induced amenorrhea in 42% of patients. With a median follow-up of 54 months, the number of events was too low to demonstrate a significant DFS and OS with any degree of power; however, it was suggested that complete hormonal blockade may be a valuable alternative to CT for selected premenopausal women with receptor-positive tumors and NP disease (110).

A French trial compared adjuvant OA (by surgery or radiotherapy) plus tamoxifen to FAC (5-FU, Adriamycin and cyclophosphamide) in 162 NP, receptor-positive, premenopausal patients. While no DFS and OS differences were observed between the two arms, a trend toward improved survival favoring total estrogen blockade was reported. This trial was closed due to low accrual (111).

So far, the findings from trials of OA versus CT suggest similar efficacy of the two modalities in women with NP, ER-positive breast cancer. The benefit from adjuvant CMF may be mediated, in part, by chemotherapy-induced amenorrhea. Because many of these trials are small, used for NP-disease CMF-based chemotherapy, and have short follow-up, more mature and pooled data are needed to identify any overall efficacy and toxicity differences for the two modalities. The impact of these regimens needs to be explored in conjunction with tamoxifen.

Ovarian Ablation in the Presence of Chemotherapy

Given that cytotoxic therapy frequently suppresses ovarian function, it is predicted that the magnitude of benefit of OA would be less in women who also received CT. In the Oxford Overview, the incremental survival benefit of OA in the presence of CT was found to be smaller than when OA was the sole adjuvant therapy given; however, these observations were based on small numbers (98). For women less than 50 years old (NP and NN), the benefit attributable to OA compared to control was 10% and 8% for DFS and OS, respectively, in patients who had both OA and CT, compared with 25% and 24%, respectively, for OA alone. Both treatment approaches were statistically better than their respective control arms ($2p < 0.001$). This suggests that some of the benefit of CT derives from induction of transient or permanent ovarian suppression. The Overview did not address the benefits of combined therapy in NP disease specifically, but several trials have examined this population. The most recent overview, which is not yet published, suggests that, in the presence of chemotherapy, there is no added survival benefit to OA. ER status was defined only in four trials (750 patients) of ablation plus CT versus the same CT alone, and there was a trend in terms of DFS and OS, favoring the addition of ovarian ablation in women with ER-positive tumors. These studies are underpowered by the inclusion of all premenopausal women, whether or not they become amenorrheic from CT. Most trials, summarized later, also did not include tamoxifen in the systemic treatment (CT) alone arm, which makes them difficult to interpret in the context of today's standard of care.

The potential benefit of OA added to CT and/or tamoxifen in the subset of women who maintain ovarian function after CT is unknown. A retrospective analysis of 3,700 premenopausal/perimenopausal women treated in four IBCSG trials of adjuvant CMF (various schedules) indicated that patients younger than 35 years with ER-positive tumors who did not become amenorrheic following CMF have a very high risk of relapse and death. Therefore, for this subgroup of patients, CT alone may be an inadequate modality of adjuvant treatment, and an additional form of hormonal maneuver such as OA or tamoxifen might be required (112).

SWOG compared adjuvant CMFVp (n = 140; C, 60 mg/m^2 a day for 1 year; MTX, 15 mg/m^2; 5-FU, 400 mg/m^2 i.v. weekly for 1 year; vincristine, 0.625 mg/m^2 i.v. weekly for 10 weeks; and prednisone, in decreasing doses, from 30 mg/m^2 a day for 10 weeks) to CMFVp with surgical OA (n = 148) in NP, premenopausal women with ER-positive tumors (113). Stratification was according to the number of involved nodes and type of primary surgery. With a median follow-up of 7.7 years, with power to detect only a 15% difference in relapse and death using intention to treat, OS was 71% and 73% ($p = 0.70$) for the CT and combination arms (43 and 38 deaths), respectively, with no significant difference in toxicity. Recently, 15-year results were reported, and they continue to show no difference in both DFS and OS (92).

The IBCSG Trial II randomized 327 premenopausal women with more than four positive nodes and any ER status to 12 cycles of CMFp versus surgical oophorectomy followed by 12 cycles of CMFp and found no OS and DFS difference between the two groups with 10 years of follow-up (114). For the subset of 107 ER-positive patients, there was a non-significant OS trend favoring the combination (combination 41%, CMFp 30%; $p = 0.12$).

The INT 0101 trial randomized 1,503 premenopausal, NP, receptor-positive women to six cycles of CAF (C, 100 mg/m^2 by mouth on days 1 through 14; A, 30 mg/m^2 i.v. on days 1 and 8; 5-FU, 500 mg/m^2 i.v. on days 1 and 8 every 28 days), 6CAF plus 5 years of goserelin (3.6 mg s.c. every 28 days) for 5 years (CAF+Z), and 6CAF plus goserelin plus 20 mg a day of TAM for 5 years (CAF+ZT). Seven-year DFS rates were 58%, 64%, and 73%, respectively. A significant DFS advantage has been shown for CAF+ZT when compared to CAF+Z. The addition of Z to the CAF arm did not show a DFS advantage over CAF alone ($p = 0.095$). OS at 7 years was similar for the three arms of the study. The addition of goserelin in patients less than 40 years of age, and the addition of tamoxifen in patients more than 40 years of age significantly improved 5-year DFS in exploratory subset analyses. An unforeseen weakness of this trial is the lack of a chemotherapy-plus-TAM treatment arm, as the value of TAM in premenopausal women was not established when the trial was designed (115).

An International Breast Cancer study Group trial (IBCSG 11–93) investigated the role of four cycles of adjuvant CT (Adriamycin cyclophosphamide [AC] or epirubicin cyclophosphamide [EC]) in addition to OA and 5 years of TAM for premenopausal NP women with ER-positive (+) tumors. The trial closed before target accrual was met due to low enrollment; a total of 174 patients were randomized to OA followed by adjuvant CT and 5 years of TAM versus OA followed by 5 years of TAM arms. No significant DFS and OS difference was observed at a median follow-up of 4.1 years (116).

Several RCTs investigating the role of chemoendocrine treatment included both premenopausal and postmenopausal women. The IBCSG trials I through IV enrolled premenopausal and postmenopausal NP women in four different trials comparing different combinations of CMF and hormonal therapy (TAM in postmenopausal women, OA in premenopausal women) (114). For the comparison of observation versus TAM plus prednisone (P) versus CMF plus TAM plus P, 10-year OS rates were 45%, 53%, and 61%, respectively ($p = 0.04$) for patients with one to three positive nodes (n = 86, 83, 89 for the three treatment arms, respectively), and 25%, 26%, and 35% ($p = 0.27$) for four or more positive nodes (n = 70, 70, 65). There was insufficient power to make separate statistical comparisons between the hormone and hormone/CT arms.

The German Breast Cancer Study Group (GBCSG) trial compared three and six cycles of CMF (500/40/600 mg/m^2 i.v. days 1 and 8 every 28 days), with (n = 184) and without (n = 189) TAM (30 mg per day for 2 years), in 473 premenopausal and postmenopausal NP women. The proportion of ER-negative tumors was 37% and 39%, respectively (96). A recent update, based on 10 years follow-up, demonstrates no significant difference in EFS and OS with respect to treatment duration, while treatment with tamoxifen resulted in an NS improvement in outcome (117).

A combined Cancer Research Campaign (CRC), Swedish, and Italian group reported results of a RCT of OA (goserelin monthly for 26 months), OA and TAM (20 mg per day for 2 years), TAM alone, or no hormonal intervention, using a 2 by 2 factorial design. This trial enrolled approximately 2,500 premenopausal NN and NP breast cancer patients. The use of elective unspecified adjuvant CT was permitted according to the standard at the participating institutions. From the available data, it is not clear whether CT, which was given to 43% of the patients, was equally distributed. A recent report of this trial showed that goserelin significantly prolonged both EFS (RR = 0.80, 95% CI 0.70 to 0.92, $p < 0.001$), and OS (RR = 0.82, 95% CI 0.67 to 0.99, $p = 0.04$) (118). Further follow-up may clarify the issue of efficacy of TAM in amenorrheic women.

All together, these trials suggest that the addition of OA to CT in premenopausal women does not improve survival, the same conclusion reached by the most recent Oxford Overview, as yet unpublished. The inclusion of premenopausal women who developed amenorrhea during CT, a group for which there is unlikely to be any added benefit of ovarian ablation, is a clear confounder in these trials. The ideal trial design, in which only women without CT-induced amenorrhea are randomized to ovarian ablation or not, is being planned by a large intergroup collaboration and will hopefully adequately address the issue of the value of adding OA to CT.

In summary, for premenopausal women who have ER-positive, NP breast cancer associated with a non-extreme recurrence risk (up to 10 involved nodes, low-grade, small size tumor, etc.), either OA or CT can be recommended, given that cumulative evidence from several large studies suggests equivalence. CT may be preferable in women with a higher nodal burden, given a higher absolute risk of recurrence, and the cytotoxic activity against micrometastases characteristic of CT. The results of several recently closed trials (Table 9.12) may provide more definitive consensus as to the value of combining CT and hormonal therapy (OA or TAM). Given that this is still an unsettled issue, whenever possible, women with high-risk disease should be considered for a therapeutic randomized trial.

Among several questions that remain to be answered by well-designed RCTs are the optimal role of OA with other forms of adjuvant therapy, the definition of particular subgroups most likely to benefit from OA alone or added to CT and/or TAM, the comparison of LHRH analogues with other endocrine therapies, the optimal duration of treatment with the LHRH analogues, and the long-term morbidity of OA.

Premenopausal women with ER-negative tumors should not be offered OA as an equivalent alternative to CT for the same reasons that ta-

TABLE 9.12. *Recently closed adjuvant RCTs of OA versus OA + CT in premenopausal NP breast cancer*

Group/trial	Target/actual accrual	Population	Comparison arms
UKCCCR-ABC	2,144 closed	Pre/perimenopausal NP and NN Any ER status	TAM TAM + OA
FNCLCC	1,000 closed	After adjuvant CT NP and NN	OA (RT/LHRH agonist/surgery) Control
GABG IVB	700/776 closed	NN and 1–3 NP Any ER status 4–9 NP	3CMF 3CMF → OA (Goserelin × 2 yr) 4EC → CMF 4EC → CMF → OA (Goserelin × 2 yr)
IBCSG 11–93	760/174 closed due to low accrual	NP ER (+)	OA → TAM × 5 yr OA → 4AC or 4 EC → TAM × 5 yr

moxifen is not adequate in postmenopausal women with ER-negative disease.

Negative Impact. No difference in the incidence of non-breast cancer deaths was noted between the control and OA groups in randomized trials of OA versus no adjuvant therapy in the Oxford Overview.

Ovarian ablation can be achieved through irradiation, surgical oophorectomy, or the use of an LHRH agonist. Apart from a small mortality risk associated with any surgical procedure, these procedures do not carry risks of life-threatening complications. Sequelae related to early menopause are the only significant long-term morbidities. In contrast, a 1% mortality risk is generally accepted with CT. Additionally, significant, although usually short-lived, morbidities are common with CT, including alopecia, nausea, vomiting, fatigue, infection, stomatitis, diarrhea, neuropathy, and various others, depending on the regimen. Serious and long-term sequelae include the risk of alkylator- and anthracycline-induced leukemias, anthracycline-induced cardiotoxicity, and premature menopause.

Estrogen is cardioprotective, and thus women with prematurely induced menopause have increased risk of cardiac disease compared with premenopausal age-matched controls. However, with 15 years of follow-up, the OS benefit, which takes into account death from all causes (including breast cancer and cardiovascular causes), continues to favor OA and CT over no adjuvant therapy (98). Longer follow-up may demonstrate a late convergence in the survival curves attributable to higher incidence of cardiovascular events in the treated groups.

Premature menopause is also associated with an increased risk of osteoporosis (OP). The incidence of OP in older trials is hard to interpret in light of currently available preventative measures, including supplemental calcium and bisphosphonates, which substantially reduce the risk of OP in postmenopausal women (119,120).

HIGH-DOSE TREATMENT AND STEM CELL TRANSPLANTATION

The risk of breast cancer relapse after adjuvant systemic therapy increases with increasing number of positive nodes at diagnosis (121). In an attempt to ameliorate this adverse risk, investigators have explored the role of high-dose CT with hematopoietic stem cell harvest and rescue reinfusion (SCT) in women with multiple positive nodes. There are a few RCTs comparing high-dose regimens with SCT to less myeloablative doses of CT drugs that are still accruing patients (Table 9.13). Several RCTs have been reported, and these are summarized below. The only positive transplant trial reported so far has been discredited in the light of trial misconduct (122). Given the yet-to-be-established benefit and the higher potential treatment-related mortality and long-term sequelae, high-dose CT with SCT cannot currently be recommended outside an RCT.

The CALGB 9082 trial compared high-dose alkylating agents with SCT to intermediate doses of the same drugs in 738 women with 10 or more positive nodes (123). The median number of involved nodes was 14, and 19% had more than 20 involved. After four cycles of CAF, patients were randomized to high-dose (HD) cyclophosphamide, cisplatin, and BCNU (CPB) with SCT or intermediate dose (ID) CPB with transplantation allowed at the time of relapse. With 37 months median follow-up, the actuarial 5-year event-free survivals (EFS) were 68% and 64% ($p = 0.7$), and OS rates were 78% and 80% ($p = 0.1$), for the HD and ID arms, respectively. The lower number of relapses in the HD arm was balanced by higher treatment-related mortality (29 in 394 deaths; 3% within 100 days of transplant). A recent update presented at the 2001 ASCO meeting, at a median follow-up of 5.1 years, continues to show no significant difference in EFS (61% versus 60%, $p = 0.49$) or OS (70% versus 72%, $p = 0.23$) between the HD and ID arms, respectively.

A Dutch trial randomized 885 stage II and III patients with 4 or more LNs involved to either conventional CT (five cycles of $FE_{90}C$) or four cycles of $FE_{90}C$ plus HD CT with CTC (cyclophosphamide 6 g/m^2, thiotepa 480 mg/m^2, carboplatin 1,600 mg/m^2) and peripheral blood progenitor cell (PBPC) transplantation (124). Of note, the patients on the standard dose CT arm were not allowed to cross over to the HD CT arm at progression. Disease-free survival

TABLE 9.13. *Recently closed and ongoing adjuvant RCTs of high dose CT with stem cell transplant (SCT) in NP breast cancer*

Trial/ group	Accrual target/ actual to date	Population	Comparison arms	Comments
Dutch (129)	97	> 10 NP	4 FEC + RT + TAM 4 FEC → STAMP V + SCT	Results negative for DFS and OS ($p = 0.8$)
MDA Trial	78 closed early, low accrual	> 10 NP	8 FAC 8 FAC → high dose CT × 2 with SCT	Results negative 62%, 48% DFS ($p = 0.35$) 77%, 58% OS ($p = 0.23$)
Intergrp (CALGB 9082) (123)	875	≥ 10 NP stage II, III	CAF (600/60/1,200) → C 1.9 g/m² × 3d, CDDP 55 × 3d, BCNU 600 + SCT + TAM + RT 1 CAF → C 300 × 3d, CDDP 30 × 3d, BCNU 90 + TAM + RT	Results negative 61 vs. 60% EFS $p = 0.49$ 70 vs. 72% OS $p = 0.23$
SBG 9401 (82,125)	525	> 70% relapse risk and NP	9 FEC individual dose (5-FU 600/E 38–120/C 450–1,800/m²) with G-CSF 3 FEC → C 1.5 g/m², thio 125, carbo 200 d1–4 + SCT + RT + TAM	Results negative 3 yr RFS 72% (tailored arm) vs. 63% (CTCb) $p = 0.013$ (log rank) 3 yr OS $p = NS$
South Africa (122)	154	≥ 10 NP ≥ 7 NP and T > 5cm high risk	C 4.4 g/m² + mitox 45 + VP16 1.5 g/m² + SCT CAF (600/50/600) or CEF (600/70/600)	Results positive for high dose arm
IBCSG 15–95	210/344 closed	≤ 65 yr and ≥ 10 NP or ≥ 5 NP & ER – or ≥ 5 NP and T3	EC (200 /4 g/m²) → SCT, TAM 4 AC (50/600) or EC (90/600) q3w → 3 CMF (Bonadonna) + TAM	No results
PEGASE 01 (126)	314 closed	≥ 8 NP	3 FEC$_{100}$ (500/100/600) 3 FEC$_{100}$ + SC harvest → Mitox 45 C 200 × 2d, mel 140 + SCT	3 yr DFS 55% (ID) vs. 70% (HD) $p < 0.03$ 3 yr OS $p = NS$
GABG-IV EH-93	320/307	≥ 9 NP	4 EC (90/900) → 3 CMF 4 EC (90/900) → C 6 g/m², thio 0.6 g/m², mitox 40 + SCT	No results
MCG (127)	398 closed 9/98	≥ 3 NP	3E (120) → 6 CMF C 7 g/m², harvest → Vcr; MTX 8 g/m² E 120 → Mel 140 + thio 0.6 g/m² + SCT	Preliminary results are negative
ICCG C/10/92	300/281 closed	NA	6 FEC (FEC d1 q 3wk) + (FEC d1,8 q 4wk) × 5 3 FEC (FEC d1 q 3wk) + (FEC d1,8 q 4wk) × 2 C 6 g/m²/thio 500 /carbo 800 4d IVCI + SCT	No results
ACCOG I	600/605 closed	>4 NP	4 A → 8 CMF 4 A → C 6/m²/thio 800 + SCT	No results
ACCOG II B	Not activated	After neoadj AC or AT NP	8 CMF C 6 g/m² + thio 800 + SCT	No results
ABCSG 11	240/108	NP, NN high risk	6 ET (90/200 q21d) + G-CSF → TAM 20 mg/5y 3 ET (90/200) + C 1,500 /thio125 /carbo 1,500 d-7 to –4 + uromitexan 1,500 d -7 to -3 + SCT + TAM	No results
GABG-IMA	300/87	≤ 50 yr and ≥ 10 NP and stage III	3 EC (45/500 d1, 2 q15) → C 2 g/m²/ carbo 500 → thio 200 /mitox 20 d1–3 + SCT 3 EC → 3 CMF (Bonadonna i.v.)	No results
GABG-IMA	320/121	≤ 60 yr and ≥ 10 NP and stage II	VIPE (VP16 500,os 4 g/m²; CDDP 50;Epi 50 d1) HD-VIC (VP16 500; Ifos 4g/m²; carbo 500 d1–3) 4 EC (90/600 q21d) → 3 CMF (500/40/ 600 d1,8 q28)	No results

continued

TABLE 9.13. Continued

Trial/ group	Accrual target/ actual to date	Population	Comparison arms	Comments
INT 0121	541 closed	NP stage II, III	CAF (100 po d1–14/30 d1,8/500 d1,8) CAF → C 6 g/Thio 800 i.v. 96 h + SCT	No results
INT S9623	1,000/602	4–9 NP	A 80 d1, 15,29 + T 200/24 h d43,57,71 + C 3 g/m² d85,99,113 + G-CSF AC (80/600) d1,22,43,64 → STAMP I or V + SCT	No results
NWSAT	885 closed	≥ 4 NP II, III	5 FEC 4 FEC → C 6 g/m², thio 0.48 g/m², carbo 1.6 g/m² SCT	3 yr DFS 72 (HD) % vs. 65% $p = 0.057$ 3 yr OS $p = 0.31$
BCIRG 002 TAX 321	476/NA closed early	≥ 4 NP	DAC(75/50/500) × 6 DAC (75/50/500) × 4 → MCV → HD + AuPSCT	No results

Doses are in mg/m² unless otherwise indicated.

A, Adriamycin; ACCOG, Anglo-Celtic Cooperative Oncology Group; AuPSCT, Autologous peripheral stem cell transplantation; carbo, carboplatin; CDDP, cisplatin; E, Epirubicin; ifos, ifosfamide; IMA, Interdisziplinäre Mammakarzinom-Arbeitsgruppe; INT, Intergroup; IVCI, Intravenous continuous infusion; MCG, Michelangelo Cooperative Group; MCV, mitoxantrone + cyclophosphamide + vinorelbine; MDA, M.D. Anderson; mel, melphalan; mitox, mitoxantrone; NA, Not Available; NWSAT, Netherlands Working Party for Autotransplantation in Solid Tumors; T, paclitaxel; thio, thiotepa; Vcr, vincristine.

and OS were significantly better in the transplant arm in a planned analysis of the first 284 patients. However, the analysis on the whole trial population (n = 885) at a median follow-up of 3 years showed a marginal benefit in RFS ($p = 0.057$) and no OS ($p = 0.31$) advantage for the HD arm. So far, no AML or MDS have been reported. Four patients died from causes other than breast cancer in the HD arm (n = 442) and one non-breast cancer related death occurred in the standard dose arm (n = 443).

The Scandinavian Breast Cancer Study Group (SBG) randomized 525 patients with high-risk NP breast cancer (more than a 70% risk of relapse within 5 years) to tailored and escalated FEC with G-CSF and prophylactic antibiotics (as standard dose CT) or to conventional FEC with stem cell mobilization, followed by high-dose CT (C 6 g/m², thiotepa 0.5 g/m², and carboplatin 0.8 g/m²) with SCT (82,125). All patients received locoregional radiotherapy and TAM for 5 years. At a follow-up of 38 months, 81 versus 113 relapses and 60 versus 82 deaths were observed in the tailored FEC and HD arms, respectively. The 3-year DFS favored the control arm (72% versus 63%, $p = 0.013$, log-rank) and OS was not different ($p = 0.12$, log-rank). In fact, the patients in the tailored FEC arm received greater cumulative doses of CT (3 times the dose of 5-FU, 5 times more epirubicin and 1.4 times more cyclophosphamide) compared to those in the HD arm. Of note, nine patients in the tailored FEC arm developed AML and MDS, compared to none in the transplant arm. In reality, this trial compares two intensive treatment regimens, with and without stem cell rescue, rather than HD and standard dose CT.

The French Pegase 01 trial randomized 314 patients less than age 60 with less than seven involved nodes to either HD CT and PBPC transplant or no further chemotherapy following four cycles of $FE_{100}C$. Preliminary results demonstrated an improved DFS ($p < 0.003$) at 3 years in favor of the HD arm without an OS advantage (126). One may question the adequacy of only four cycles of FEC as a control arm.

An Italian trial (MCG, Michelangelo Cooperative Group) of similar size compared standard sequential CT with HD CT plus SCT in breast cancer patients below age 60 with involvement of more than three LN and found no OS advantage for the HD CT arm at 5 years of follow-up (127).

Three additional smaller trials were reported to be negative, but they were clearly underpowered since they enrolled less than 100 patients each (128–130).

A recommendation for routine adjuvant high-dose CT with SCT cannot be made on the basis of one small flawed positive trial and four additional immature or small trials that suggest equivalence. Although enthusiasm for this treatment strategy has waned slightly in view of the negative results, mature results from a number of ongoing large pivotal trials will be available within a few years (Table 9.13). It is hoped that together these data will provide a definitive conclusion about the value or the lack of value of this kind of aggressive therapy for high-risk NP breast cancer.

SUMMARY OF EVIDENCE

Adjuvant therapy for node positive breast cancer

1. **Endocrine Therapy**
   - **Tamoxifen**

     There is level I, grade A evidence to support a survival advantage with the use of tamoxifen for 5 years in ER-positive, node-positive breast cancer in women 50 to 69 years of age. The amount of data available for women younger than 50 and older than 69 with ER-positive disease is too small to constitute level I evidence of benefit; however, it is standard practice to prescribe tamoxifen to all women with ER-positive disease, regardless of age, and confirmatory evidence from ongoing trials is expected.

     Current level I, grade A evidence does not support the use of more than 5 years of tamoxifen at present; however, large trials addressing this question are ongoing.
   - **Aromatase inhibitors**

     There is currently no mature evidence to support the routine use of aromatase inhibitors in the adjuvant setting. Adjuvant aromatase inhibitors should be currently reserved for the clinical trial setting for the time being.
   - **Ovarian ablation**

     Level I, grade A evidence supports a survival advantage for ovarian ablation versus no adjuvant therapy in ER-positive node positive breast cancer among women younger than 50.

     Level I, grade A evidence supports no added benefit of ovarian ablation in women with node-negative or node-positive breast cancer who are treated with chemotherapy. Whether there is benefit for women who do not become amenorrheic following chemotherapy is not known.

2. **Polychemotherapy**

   There is level I, grade A evidence to support a survival benefit with 3 to 6 months of polychemotherapy over no chemotherapy in node-positive breast cancer, regardless of ER status. Polychemotherapy in standard doses should be offered to premenopausal and postmenopausal NP patients with receptor-negative breast cancer and to NN patients with high risk factors.

   Level I, grade A evidence supports superiority of anthracycline regimens of adequate dose intensity that are longer than 3 months and include fluorouracil over CMF regimens in terms of survival.

   Level I, grade B evidence supports equivalence of 4AC and classical CMF (six cycles) in node-positive breast cancer.

   Level I, grade B evidence supports a dose intensity threshold for anthracyclines below which survival is compromised.

   The evidence regarding the role of adjuvant paclitaxel is immature; however, there are indications that taxanes might further improve survival compared to anthracyclines. Level III evidence supports a small advantage of AC followed by paclitaxel in ER-negative node-positive breast cancer. It is unclear whether this advantage derives from longer overall CT duration or the addition of a non-cross-resistant drug following AC.

   There is no evidence available yet to judge the benefit and toxicity associated with adjuvant docetaxel or adjuvant trastuzumab added to standard chemotherapy, plus or minus tamoxifen. Trials addressing these questions are ongoing,

3. **Chemoendocrine Therapy**

   Polychemotherapy should be combined with tamoxifen in all patients with receptor-

positive tumors. Despite the small absolute numbers of young women studied, level II evidence supports the use of tamoxifen in young women with ER-positive tumors who receive chemotherapy.

Level I to II, grade B evidence supports a modest survival advantage and increased toxicity with the addition of anthracycline-based regimens but not CMF to TAM in postmenopausal women. Many of the studies exploring the combination of CT and TAM are flawed by virtue of suboptimal CT regimens or use of less than 5 years of TAM; therefore, this question remains inadequately addressed.

4. **Dose-dense-intense Adjuvant Chemotherapy**

Evidence supports no survival or disease-free survival advantage to doseintense or dosedense doxorubicin (level II) or cyclophosphamide (level I, grade A) AC over standard AC.

5. **High-dose Therapy with Stem Cell Support**

Level I, grade A evidence supports no survival advantage with respect to the use of more dose-intensive myeloablative regimens including HDCT with SCS in high-risk, node-positive breast cancer.

REFERENCES

1. Early Breast Cancer Trialists' Collaborative Group. Tamoxifen for early breast cancer: an overview of the randomized trials. *Lancet* 1998;351:1451–1467.
2. Peto R. Fifth main meeting of the Early Breast Cancer Trialists' Collaborative Group. Oxford, UK—September 2000 (unpublished data).
3. Cummings FJ, Gray R, Tormey D. Adjuvant tamoxifen versus placebo in older women with node-positive breast cancer: Twenty-year follow up of EST 1178 *Proc Am Soc Clin Oncol* 2001;20, 32a:124.
4. Andersen J, Andersson M, Andersen KW, at al. A randomized phase III trial of adjuvant endocrine therapy with tamoxifen for one year (TAM1) vs tamoxifen for two years (TAM2) in postmenopausal high risk patients with estrogen receptor positive or estrogen receptor unknown breast cancer. A DBCG study. *Eur J Cancer* 1998;S41–42:168.
5. Trials Working Party of Cancer Research Campaign Breast Cancer Trials Group. Preliminary results from the Cancer Research Campaign Trial evaluating tamoxifen duration in women aged fifty years or older with breast cancer. *J Natl Cancer Inst* 1996;88:1834–1839.
6. Potyka I Houghton J, Baum J, et al. Duration of tamoxifen therapy in the management of early operable breast cancer for postmenopausal patients—results from the CRC trial after completion of trial therapy. *The Breast* 2001;10(suppl 1):P50.
7. Swedish Breast Cancer Cooperative Group. Randomized trial of two versus five years of adjuvant tamoxifen for postmenopausal early stage breast cancer. *J Natl Cancer Inst* 1996;88:1543–1549.
8. Nordenskjold B, Carstensen J, Rutqvist L, et al. Prolonged follow-up of the Swedish randomized trial of two versus five years of adjuvant tamoxifen for postmenopausal early stage breast cancer and relationships to hormone receptor and ERBB2 levels. *Proc Am Soc Clin Oncol* 2000;72a:276.
9. Fisher B, Dignam J, Bryant J, Wolmark N. Five versus more than five years of tamoxifen for lymph node-negative breast cancer: Updated findings from the National Surgical Adjuvant Breast and Bowel Project B-14 randomized trial. *J Natl Cancer Inst* 2001;93:684–690.
10. Stewart HJ, Forrest AP, Everington D, et al. Randomized comparison of 5 years of adjuvant tamoxifen with continuous therapy for operable breast cancer. *Br J Cancer* 1996;74:297–299.
11. Tormey DC, Gray R, Falkson HC. Postchemotherapy adjuvant tamoxifen therapy beyond five years in patients with lymph node-positive breast cancer. *J Natl Cancer Inst* 1996;88:1828–1833.
12. Breast Cancer Trials Committee, Scottish Cancer Trials Office (MRC), Edinburgh. Adjuvant tamoxifen in the management of operable breast cancer: the Scottish trial. *Lancet* 1987;2:171–175.
13. Stewart HJ, Forrest AP, Everington D, at al. Randomized comparison of 5 years adjuvant tamoxifen with continuous therapy for operable breast cancer. The Scottish Cancer Trials Breast group. *Br J Cancer* 1996; 74:297–299.
14. Stewart HJ, Prescott RJ, Forrest AP. Scottish Adjuvant Tamoxifen Trial: a randomized study updated to 15 years. *J Natl Cancer Inst* 2001;93;6:456–462.
15. Delozier T, Spielmann M, Mace-Lesec'h J, et al. Tamoxifen adjuvant treatment duration in early breast cancer: Initial results of a randomized study comparing short-term treatment with long-term treatment. *J Clin Oncol* 2000;18:3507–3512.
16. Delozier T, Switsers O, Genot JY. Delayed adjuvant tamoxifen; ten years results of a collaborative randomized controlled trial in early breast cancer (TAM-02 trial). *Ann Oncol* 2000;11:515–591.
17. Love RR, Wiebe DA, Feyzi JM, et al. Effects of tamoxifen on cardiovascular risk factors in postmenopausal women after 5 years of treatment. *J Natl Cancer Inst* 1994;86:1534–1539.
18. Gotto AM. Results of recent large cholesterol-lowering trials and implications for clinical management. *Am J Cardiol* 1997;79:1663–1666.
19. McDonald CC, Stewart HJ. Fatal myocardial infarction in the Scottish Adjuvant tamoxifen trial. The Scottish Breast Cancer Committee. *BMJ* 1991;303:435–437.
20. Rutqvist LE, Mattsson A. Cardiac and thromboembolic morbidity among postmenopausal women with early-stage breast cancer in a randomized trial of adjuvant tamoxifen. The Stockholm Breast Cancer Study Group. *J Natl Cancer Inst* 1993;85:1398–1406.
21. Powles TJ, Hickish T, Kanis J, et al. Effect of tamoxifen on bone mineral density measured by dual-energy x-ray absorptimometry in healthy premenopausal and postmenopausal women. *J Clin Oncol* 1996;14:78–84.

22. Love RR, Mazess RB, Tormey DC, et al. Bone mineral density in women with breast cancer treated with adjuvant tamoxifen for at least two years. *Breast Cancer Res Treat* 1988;12:297–301.
23. Love RR, Mazess RB, Barden HS, et al. Effects of tamoxifen on bone mineral density in postmenopausal women with breast cancer. *N Engl J Med* 1992;326: 852–856.
24. Fornander T, Rutquist LE, Sjoberg HE, et al. Long-term adjuvant tamoxifen in early breast cancer: effect on bone mineral density in postmenopausal women. *J Clin Oncol* 1990;8:1019–1024.
25. Turken S, Siris E, Seldin D. Effect of tamoxifen on spinal bone density in women with breast cancer. *J Natl Cancer Inst* 1989;81:1086–1088.
26. Ryan WG, Wolter J, Bagdade JD. Apparent beneficial effect of tamoxifen on bone mineral content in patients with breast cancer: A preliminary study. *Osteoporosis Int* 1992;2:39–41.
27. Gotfredsen A, Christiansen C, Palshof T, et al. The effect of tamoxifen on bone mineral content in premenopausal women with breast cancer. *Cancer* 1984; 53:853–857.
28. Ragaz J, Coleman A. Survival impact of adjuvant tamoxifen on competing causes of mortality in breast cancer survivors, with analysis of mortality from contralateral breast cancer, cardiovascular events, endometrial cancer, and thromboembolic episodes. *J Clin Oncol* 1998;16:2018–2024.
29. Fisher B, Costantino JP, Redmond CK, et al. Endometrial cancer in tamoxifen-treated breast cancer patients: findings from the National Surgical Adjuvant Breast and Bowel Project (NSABP B-14). *J Natl Cancer Inst* 1994;86:527–537.
30. Samonigg H, Jakesz R, Hausmaninger D, et al. Tamoxifen versus tamoxifen plus aminoglutethimide for stage I and II receptor-positive postmenopausal node-negative or node-positive breast cancer patients: four-year results of a randomized trial of the Austrian Breast Cancer Study Group (ABCSG). *Proc Am Soc Clin Oncol* 1999;18:68a (abstract 253).
31. Boccardo F, Rubagotti A, Amoroso D, et al. Sequential tamoxifen and aminoglutethimide versus tamoxifen alone in the adjuvant treatment of postmenopausal breast cancer patients: Results of an Italian Cooperative Study. *J Clin Oncol* 2001;19:4209–4215.
32. Nabholtz JM, Bonneterre J, Buzdar AU, et al. Preliminary results of two multi-center trials comparing the efficacy and tolerability of Arimidex (anastrazole) and tamoxifen in postmenopausal women with advanced breast cancer. *Breast Cancer Res Treat* 1999;57(1):31 (abstract 27).
33. Baum M, on behalf of the ATAC Trialists' Group. The ATAC (Arimidex, Tamoxifen, Alone, or in Combination) adjuvant breast cancer trial in postmenopausal (PM) women. *Breast Cancer Res Treat* 2001;69(3): 210 (abstract 8).
34. Gradishar WJ, Jordan VC. Clinical potential of new antiestrogens. *J Clin Oncol* 1997;15:840–852.
35. Cummings SR, Eckert S, Krueger KA, et al. The effect of raloxifene on risk of breast cancer in postmenopausal women: results from the MORE randomized trial Multiple Outcome of Raloxifene Evaluation. *JAMA* 1999;281(23):2189–2197.
36. Holli K, Valavaara R, Blanco G, et al. Safety and efficacy results of a randomized trial comparing adjuvant toremifene and tamoxifen in postmenopausal patients with node positive breast cancer *J Clin Oncol* 2000; 18:3487–3494.
37. Holli K. Adjuvant Trials of Toremifene vs tamoxifen: The European experience. *Oncology* 1998;5S:23–27.
38. Awada A, Piccart M. New agents in development for cancer therapy. Consultant series no 18. Gardiner-Caldwell Communications Limited, Cheshire, UK, 1997: pp 71.
39. Piccart MJ, Goldhirsch A, et al. An overview of recent and ongoing adjuvant clinical trials for breast cancer. Second edition. Breast International Group-aisbl. Moreau PCE s.a., Mollem, Belgium, March 2000.
40. Early Breast Cancer Trialists' Collaborative Group. Polychemotherapy for early breast cancer: an overview of the randomised trials. *Lancet* 1998;352:930–942.
41. Bonadonna G, Brusamolino E, Valagussa P, et al. Combination chemotherapy as an adjuvant treatment in operable breast cancer. *N Engl J Med* 1976;294: 405–410.
42. Tancini G, Bonadonna G, Valagussa P, et al. Adjuvant CMF in breast cancer. Comparative 5 year results of 12 versus 6 cycles. *J Clin Oncol* 1983;1:2–10.
43. Hutchins L, Green S, Ravdin P, et al. CMF versus CAF with and without tamoxifen in high-risk node-negative breast cancer patients and a natural history follow-up study in low-risk node-negative patients: first results of Intergroup trial INT 0102. *Proc Am Soc Clin Oncol* 1998;17:1a (abstract 2).
44. Levine MN, Bramwell VH, Pritchard KI, et al. Randomized trial of intensive cyclophosphamide, methotrexate, and fluorouracil in premenopausal women with node-positive breast cancer: National Cancer Institute of Canada Clinical Trials Group. *J Clin Oncol* 1998;16:2651–2658.
45. Carpenter JT, Velez-Garcia E, Aron BS, et al. Five-year results of a randomised comparison of cyclophosphamide, doxorubicin (adriamycin), methotrexate and fluorouracil (CAF) vs cyclophosphamide, methotrexate and fluorouracil (CMF) for node positive breast cancer: A Southeastern Cancer Study Group Study. *Proc Am Soc Clin Oncol* 1994;13:66 (abstract 68).
46. Bonadonna G, Zambetti M, Valagussa P, et al. Sequential or alternating doxorubicin and CMF regimens in breast cancer with more than three positive nodes. Ten year results. *JAMA* 1995;273(7):542–547.
47. Mouridsen HT, Andersen J, Anderson M, et al. Adjuvant anthracycline in breast cancer. Improved outcome in premenopausal patients following substitution of methotrexate in the CMF combination with epirubicin. *Proc Am Soc Clin Oncol* 1999;18:68a (abstract 254).
48. Piccart MJ, Di Leo A, Beauduin M, et al. Phase III trial comparing two dose levels of epirubicin combined with cyclophosphamide with cyclophosphamide, methotrexate, and fluorouracil in node-positive breast cancer. *J Clin Oncol* 2001;19(12):3103–3110.
49. Martin M, Villar A, Solé-Calvo A, et al. FAC versus Adjuvant treatment for Operable Breat cancer. *Proc Am Soc Clin Oncol* 2001;20:32a (abstract 126).
50. Fisher B, Brown AM, Dimitrov NV, et al. Two months of doxorubicin-cyclophosphamide with and without interval reinduction therapy compared with 6 months

of cyclophosphamide, methotrexate, and fluorouracil in positive-node breast cancer patients with tamoxifen-nonresponsive tumours: results from the National Surgical Adjuvant Breast and Bowel Project B-15. *J Clin Oncol* 1990;8:1483–1496.
51. Fisher B, Anderson S, Wolmark N, et al. Chemotherapy with or without tamoxifen for patients with ER- negative breast cancer and negative nodes: results from NSABP B23. *Proc Am Soc Clin Oncol* 2000; 19:72a (abstract 277).
52. Bianco AR, Costanzo R, Di Lorenzo G, et al. The Mam-1 GOCSI trial: a randomised trial with factorial design of chemo-endocrine adjuvant treatment in node-positive (N+) early breast cancer (EBC). *Proc Am Soc Clin Oncol* 2001;20:27a (abstract 104).
53. Moliterni A, Bonadonna G, Valagussa P, et al. Cyclophosphamide, methotrexate, and fluorouracil with and without doxorubicin in the adjuvant treatment of resectable breast cancer with one or three positive axillary nodes. *J Clin Oncol* 1991;9:1124–1130.
54. Henderson IC, Berry D, Demetri G, et al. Improved disease-free and overall survival from the addition of sequential paclitaxel but not from the escalation of doxorubicin dose level in the adjuvant chemotherapy of patients with node-positive primary breast cancer. *Proc Am Soc Clin Oncol* 1998;17:101a (abstract 390).
55. Henderson CI. Adjuvant chemotherapy: Taxanes—the "Pro" position. Program and abstracts of the NIH Consensus Development Conference; Adjuvant Therapy for Breast Cancer November 1–3, 2000, Bethesda, Maryland.
56. Mamounas EP. NSABP B-28. Initial results. Program and abstracts of the NIH Consensus Development Conference; Adjuvant Therapy for Breast Cancer; November 1–3, 2000, Bethesda, Maryland.
57. Piccart MJ. Taxanes in the adjuvant setting: Why not yet? NIH Consensus Development Conference on Adjuvant Therapy for Breast Cancer. November 1–3, 2000, Bethesda, Maryland.
58. Thomas E, Buzdar A, Theriault R, et al. Role of Paclitaxel in adjuvant therapy of operable breast cancer: preliminary results of prospective randomized clinical trial. *Proc Am Soc Clin Oncol* 2000;20:74a (abstract 285).
59. Naboltz JM, Pienkowski T, Mackey J, et al. Phase III trial comparing TAC (docetaxel, doxorubicin, cyclophosphamide) with FAC (5-fluororuracil, doxorubicin, cyclophosphamide) in the adjuvant treatment of node positive breast cancer patients: interim analysis of the BCIRG 001 study. *Proc Am Soc Clin Oncol* 2002;21:36a (abstract 141).
60. Nabholtz JM, Falkso C, Campos D, et al. Doxorubicin and Docetaxel (AT) is superior to standard doxorubicin and cyclophosphamide as 1st line CT for MBC: randomized phase III trial. *Breast Cancer Res Treat* 1999;57:84 (abstract 330).
61. Di Leo A, Piccart MJ. Paclitaxel activity, dose, and schedule: data from phase III trials in metastatic breast cancer. *Semin Oncol* 1999;26(Suppl 8):27–32.
62. Slamon D, Leyland-Jones B, Shak S, et al. Addition of Herceptin (Humanized anti-her2 antibody) to first line chemotherapy for her2 overexpressing metastatic breast cancer markedly increases anticancer activity: a randomized multinational controlled phase III trial. *Proc Am Soc Clin Oncol* 1998;17:98a (abstract 377).
63. Norton L, Slamon D, Leyland-Jones B, et al. Overall survival advantage to simultaneous chemotherapy plus the humanized anti-HER2 monoclonal antibody Herceptin in HER2-overexpressing metastatic breast cancer. *Proc Am Soc Clin Oncol* 1999;127a (abstract 483).
64. Cobleigh MA, Vogel CL, Tripathy D, et al. Efficacy and safety of herceptin (humanized anti-her2 antibody) as a single agent in 222 women with her2 overexpression who relapsed following chemotherapy for metastatic breast cancer. *Proc Am Soc Clin Oncol* 1998;17:97a (abstract 376).
65. Gebhart-Piccart MJ. Herceptin: the future in adjuvant breast cancer therapy. *Anticancer Drugs* 2001; 12(suppl 4).
66. Tucker MA, Meadows AT, Boice JD Jr, et al. Leukemia after therapy with alkylating agents for childhood cancer. *J Natl Cancer Inst* 1987;78:459–464.
67. Chambers SK, Chopyk RL, Chambers JT, et al. Development of leukemia after doxorubicin and cisplatin treatment for ovarian cancer. *Cancer* 1989;64: 2459–2461.
68. Crump M, Tu D, Shepherd L, et al. risk of acute leukemia following adjuvant epirubicin-based adjuvant chemotherapy for breast cancer. *Breast Can Res Treat* 2001;69(3):247 (abstract 243).
69. Albain K, Green S, Ravdin P, et al. Overall survival after cyclophosphamide, adriamycin, 5-FU, and tamoxifen (CAFT) is superior to T alone in postmenopausal receptor (+), node (+) breast cancer: New findings from phase III Southwest Oncology Group Intergroup Trial S8814 (INT-0100). *Proc of Am Soc Clin Oncol* 2001;20:24a (abstract 94).
70. Biganzoli L, Piccart MJ. The bigger the better? or what we know and what we still need to learn about anthracycline dose per course, dose density and cumulative dose in the treatment of breast cancer [editorial]. *Ann Oncol* 1997;8:1177–1182.
71. Del Mastro L, Garrone O, Sertoli MR, et al. A pilot study of accelerated cyclophosphamide, epirubicin and 5-fluorouracil plus granulocyte colony stimulating factor as adjuvant therapy in early breast cancer. *Eur J Cancer* 1994;30A:606–610.
72. Budman DR, Berry DA, Cirrincione CT, et al. Dose and dose intensity as determinants of outcome in the adjuvant treatment of breast cancer. *J Natl Cancer Inst* 1998;90:1205–1211.
73. Fumoleau P, Bremond A, Kerbrat P. Better outcome of premenopausal node-positive breast cancer patients treated with 6 cycles vs 3 cycles of adjuvant chemotherapy; Eight year follow up results of FASG 01. *Proc Am Soc Clin Oncol* 1999;18:67 (abstract 252).
74. Bonadonna G, Valagussa P. Dose-response effect of adjuvant chemotherapy in breast cancer. *N Engl J Med* 1981;304:10–15.
75. Hryniuk W, Levine MN. Analysis of dose intensity for adjuvant chemotherapy trials in stage II breast cancer. *J Clin Oncol* 1986;4:1162–1170.
76. French Adjuvant Study Group. Benefit of a high-dose epirubicin regimen in adjuvant chemotherapy for node-positive breast cancer patients with poor prognostic factors: 5-year follow-up Results of French adjuvant Study Group 05 Randomized Trial. *J Clin Oncol* 2001;19(3):602–611.
77. Fetting JH, Gray R, Fairclough DL, et al. Sixteen-week multidrug regimen versus cyclophosphamide,

doxorubicin, and fluorouracil as adjuvant therapy for node-positive, receptor-negative breast cancer: an Intergroup study. *J Clin Oncol* 1999;16:2382–2391.
78. Bonadonna G, Valagussa P. Dose-response effect of adjuvant chemotherapy in breast cancer. *N Engl J Med* 1981;304:10–15.
79. Engelsman E, Klijn JCM, Rubens RD, et al. "Classical" CMF versus a 3-weekly intravenous CMF schedule in postmenopausal patients with advanced breast cancer. *Eur J Cancer* 1991;27:966–970.
80. Fisher B, Anderson S, Wickerham DL, et al. Increased intensification and total dose of cyclophosphamide in a doxorubicin-cyclophosphamide regimen for the treatment of primary breast cancer: findings from National Surgical Adjuvant Breast and Bowel Project B-22. *J Clin Oncol* 1997;15:1858–1869.
81. Fisher B, Anderson S, De Cillis A, et al. Further evaluation of intensified and increased total dose of cyclophosphamide for the treatment of primary breast cancer: Findings from NSABP B-25. *J Clin Oncol* 1999;17:3374–3388.
82. Bergh J, Wiklund T, Erikstein B, et al. Tailored fluorouracil, epirubicin, and cyclophosphamide compared with marrow supported high-dose chemotherapy as adjuvant treatment for high-risk breast cancer: a randomised trial. *Lancet* 2000;356:1384–1391.
83. Smith RE, Bryant J, DeCellis A, et al. Acute myeloid leukemia and myelodysplastic syndrome following doxorubicin-cyclophosphamide adjuvant therapy for operable breast cancer: the NSABP experience. *Breast Can Res Treat* 2001;69(3):209 (abst 2).
84. International Breast Cancer Study Group. Effectiveness of adjuvant chemotherapy in combination with tamoxifen for node positive postmenopausal breast cancer patients. International Breast Cancer Study Group. *J Clin Oncol* 1997;15(4):1385–1394.
85. Crivellari D, Bonetti M, Castiglione-Gertsch M, et al. Burdens and benefits of adjuvant cyclophosphamide, methotrexate, and fluorouracil and tamoxifen for elderly patients with breast cancer: The International Breast Cancer Study Group Trial VII. *J Clin Oncol* 2000;18:1412–1422.
86. Albain K, Green S, Osborne K, et al. Tamoxifen (T) versus cyclophosphamide, adriamycin and 5-FU plus either concurrent or sequential T in postmenopausal, receptor (+), node (+) breast cancer: a Southwest Oncology Group phase III intergroup trial (SWOG-8814, INT-0100). *Proc Am Soc Clin Oncol* 1997;16:128a (abstract 450).
87. Albain KS, Green SJ, Ravdin PM, et al. Adjuvant chemohormonal therapy for primary breast cancer should be sequential instead of concurrent: initial results from intergroup trial 0100(SWOG-8814). *Proc Am Soc Clin Oncol* 2002;21:37a (abstract 143).
88. Fisher B, Redmond C, Legault-Poissons. Postoperative chemotherapy and tamoxifen compared with tamoxifen alone in the treatment of positive-node breast cancer patients aged 50 years and older with tumors responsive to tamoxifen: results from NSABP B-16. *J Clin Oncol* 1990;8:1005–1018.
89. Pritchard KI, Paterson AHG, Fine S, et al. Randomized trial of cyclophosphamide, methotrexate, and fluorouracil chemotherapy added to tamoxifen as adjuvant therapy in postmenopausal women with node-positive estrogen and/or progesterone receptor-positive breast cancer: A report of the National Cancer Institute of Canada Clinical Trials group. *J Clin Oncol* 1997;15:2302–2311.
90. Wils JA, Bliss JM, Marty M, et al. Epirubicin plus tamoxifen versus tamoxifen alone in node positive postmenopausal patients with breast cancer. A randomized trial of the International Collaborative Cancer Group. *J Clin Oncol* 1999;17:1988–1998.
91. Rivkin SE, Green S, Metch B, et al. Adjuvant CMFVP versus tamoxifen versus concurrent CMFVP and tamoxifen for postmenopausal, node positive, and estrogen receptor positive breast cancer patients: A Southwest Oncology Group Study. *J Clin Oncol* 1994; 10:2078–2085.
92. Rivkin SE, Green S, Altman SJ. Adjuvant chemo and endocrine therapy for node positive breast cancer. 15 year results of Southwest Oncology Group (SWOG) Study 7827. *Proc Am Soc Clin Oncol* 2001;20:26a (abstract 105).
93. Fargeot P, Roche H, Kerbrat B, et al. DFS advantage of CE therapy vs tamoxifen alone in node positive, positive hormone receptors operable postmenopausal breast cancer patients: results of FASG-07 Randomized Trial. On behalf of the French adjuvant study Group. *Proc Am Soc Clin Oncol* 2000;19:87a (abstract 332).
94. Gelber RD, Cole BF, Goldhirsch A, et al. Adjuvant chemotherapy plus tamoxifen compared with tamoxifen alone for postmenopausal breast cancer: meta-analysis of quality-adjusted survival. *Lancet* 1996; 347:1066–1071.
95. Kaufmann M, Jonat W, Abel U, et al. Adjuvant randomized trials of doxorubicin/cyclophosphamide versus doxorubicin/cyclophosphamide/tamoxifen and CMF chemotherapy versus tamoxifen in women with node-positive breast cancer. *J Clin Oncol* 1993;11: 454–460.
96. Schumacher M, Bastert G, Bojar H, et al. Randomized 2 × 2 trial evaluating hormonal treatment and the duration of chemotherapy in node-positive breast cancer patients. *J Clin Oncol* 1994;12:2086–2093.
97. Beatson GT. On the treatment of inoperable cases of carcinoma of the mamma: suggestions for a new method of treatment, with illustrative cases. *Lancet* 1896;ii:104–107.
98. Early Breast Cancer Trialists' Collaborative Group. Ovarian ablation in early breast cancer: overview of the randomized trials. *Lancet* 1996;348:1189–1196.
99. Love RR, Duc NB, Binh NG, et al. Oophorectomy and tamoxifen adjuvant therapy in premenopausal Vietnamese and Chinese women with operable breast cancer. *J Clin Oncol* 2001;20, 26a:99.
100. Scottish Cancer Trials Breast Group, Guy's Hospital. Adjuvant ovarian ablation versus CMF chemotherapy in premenopausal women with pathological stage II breast carcinoma: Scottish trial. *Lancet* 1993;341: 1293–1298.
101. Ejlertsen B, Dombernowsky P, Mouridsen HT, et al. Comparable effect of ovarian ablation and CMF chemotherapy in premenopausal hormone receptor positive breast cancer patients. *Proc Am Soc Clin Oncol* 1999;18:66a.

102. Kaufmann M. Zoladex (Goserelin) vs CMF as adjuvant therapy pre/ perimenopusal, node-positive, early breast cancer: preliminary efficacy results from the Zebra study. *The Breast* 2001;10(suppl 1): P53.
103. de Haes H, Olschewski M, Schumacher M, et al. Early benefits in quality of life observed in Zoladex treated versus CMF treated pre/perimenopausal patients with node-positive early breast cancer. *Proc Am Soc Clin Oncol* 2001;20:35a (abstract 138).
104. Wallwiener D, Possinger K, Bonadr G, et al. Leuprorelin acetate vs CMF in the adjuvant treatment of premenopausal women with ER/PR-positive breast cancer: interim results of the Table Study. *Proc Am Soc Clin Oncol* 2001;20:34a (abstract 132).
105. Ejlertsen B, Dombernowsky P, Mouridsen T, et al. Comparable effect of ovarian ablation and CMF chemotherapy in premenopausal hormone receptor positive breast cancer patients (PRP). *Proc Am Soc Clin Oncol* 1999;18:66a (abstract 248).
106. Jakesz R, Hausmaninger H, Samonigg H, et al. Comparison of adjuvant therapy with tamoxifen and goserelin versus CMF in premenopausal stage I and II hormone-responsive breast cancer patients: four-year results of Austrian Breast Cancer Study Group (ABCSG). *Proc Am Soc Clin Oncol* 1999;18:67a (abstract 250).
107. Jakesz R, Hausmaniger H, Samonigg E, et al. Complete endocrine blockade with tamoxifen and goserelin is superior to CMF in the adjuvant treatment of premenopausal, lymph node positive and negative patients with hormone responsive breast cancer. *The Breast* 2001;10(suppl 1):S26.
108. Boccardo F, Rubagotti A, Amaroso M, et al. Cyclophosphamide, methotrexate, and fluorouracil versus tamoxifen plus ovarian suppression as adjuvant treatment of estrogen receptor-positive pre-/perimenopausal breast cancer patients: results of the Italian Breast Cancer adjuvant Study Group 02 Randomized Trial. *J Clin Oncol* 2000;18:2718–2727.
109. Boccardo F, Rubagotti A, Amaroso M. CMF vs tamoxifen plus ovarian suppression as adjuvant treatment of ER positive (ER+) pre/perimenopausal breast cancer patients. *The Breast* 2001;10(suppl 1):S62.
110. Roche HH, Kerbrat P, Bonneterre J, et al. Complete hormonal blockade versus chemotherapy in premenopausal early stage breast cancer patients with positive hormone-receptor and 1–3 node positive tumor: results of the FASG 06 Trial. *Proc Am Soc Clin Oncol* 2000;19:72a, 279.
111. Roché H, Mihura J, de Lafontan B, et al. Castration and tamoxifen versus chemotherapy (FAC) for premenopausal, node and receptor positive breast cancer patients: A randomized trial with a 7 years median follow up. *Eur J Cancer* 1996;(suppl 2), PP-5–6:35.
112. Aebi S, Gelber S,Castiglione-Gertsch R, et al. Is chemotherapy alone adequate for young women with oestrogen receptor-positive breast cancer. *Lancet* 2000; 355:1869–1874.
113. Rivkin SE, Green S, O'Sullivan J, et al. Adjuvant CMFVP versus adjuvant CMFVP plus ovariectomy for premenopausal, node-positive, and estrogen receptor-positive breast cancer patients: A Southwest Oncology Group study. *J Clin Oncol* 1996;14(1): 46–51.
114. Castiglione-Gertsch M, Johnsen C, Goldhirsch A, et al. The International (Ludwig) Breast Cancer Study Group Trials I-IV: 15 years of follow-up. *Ann Oncol* 1994;5:717–724.
115. Davidson N, O'Neill A, Vukov A, et al. Effect of chemohormonal therapy in premenopausal node (+) receptor (+) breast cancer: An Eastern Cooperative Group phase III Intergroup trial. *Proc Am Soc Clin Oncol* 1999;18:67a.
116. Thurlimann B, Price K, Gelber RD, et al. Endocrine therapy alone with ovarian function suppression plus tamoxifen versus endocrine therapy plus chemotherapy: is chemotherapy useful for premenopausal women with node-positive, endocrine responsive breast cancer? First results of IBCSG trial 11–93. *The Breast* 2001;10(suppl 1):S10.
117. Sauerbrei W, Bastert G, Bojar H. Randomized 2 × 2 trial evaluating hormonal treatment and the duration of chemotherapy in node-positive breast cancer patients: an update based on 10 years' follow-up. *J Clin Oncol* 2000;18:94–101.
118. Baum M, Houghton J, Odling-Smee W, et al. Adjuvant Zoladex in premenopausal patients with early breast cancer: results from the ZIPP trial. *The Breast* 2001;10(supp 1):P64.
119. Filipponi P, Pedetti M, Fedeli L, et al. Cyclical IV clodronate in postmenopausal osteoporosis: results of a long-term clinical trial. *Bone* 1996;18:179–184.
120. Reid IR, Watti DJ, Evans MC, et al. Continuous therapy with pamidronate, a potent bisphosphonate, in postmenopausal osteoporosis. *J Clin Endocrinol Metab* 1994;79:1595–1599.
121. Fisher B, Bauer M, Wickerman DL, et al. Relation of number of positive axillary nodes to the prognosis of patients with primary breast cancer. An NSABP update. *Cancer* 1983;52:1551–1557.
122. Bezwoda WR. Randomized controlled trial of high dose chemotherapy versus standard dose chemotherapy for high risk, surgically treated, primary breast cancer. *Proc Am Soc Clin Oncol* 1999;18:2a.
123. Peters WP, Rosner G, Vredenburgh E, et al. Updated results of a prospective, randomized comparison of two doses of combination alkylating agents (AA) as consolidation after CAF in high-risk primary breast cancer involving ten or more axillary lymph nodes (LN). *Proc Am Soc Clin Oncol* 2001; 20:21a (abstract 81).
124. Rodenhuis S, Bontenbal M, Beex L, et al. Randomized phase II study of high-dose chemotherapy with cyclophosphamide, thiotepa and carboplatin in operable breast cancer with 4 or more axillary lymph nodes. *Proc Am Soc Clin Oncol* 2000;19:74a (abstract 286).
125. The Scandinavian Breast Cancer Study Group 9401. Results from a randomized adjuvant breast cancer study with high dose chemotherapy with CTCb supported by autologous bone marrow stem cells versus dose escalated and tailored FEC therapy. *Proc Am Soc Clin Oncol* 1999;18:2a.
126. Roché H, Pouillart P, Meyer N, et al. Adjuvant high dose chemotherapy improves early outcome for high risk (N>7) breast cancer patients: The Pegase 01 Trial. *Proc Am Soc Clin Oncol* 2001;20:26a (abstract 102).

127. Gianni A, Bonadonna G. Five years results of the randomized clinical trial comparing standard high-dose myeloablative chemotherapy in the adjuvant treatment of cancer with >3 positive nodes. *Proc Am Soc Clin Oncol* 2001;20:21a (abstract 80).
128. Hortobagyi GN, Buzdar AU, Theriault RL, et al. Randomized trial of high-dose chemotherapy and blood cell autografts for high-risk primary breast carcinoma. *J Natl Cancer Inst* 2000;92:3, 225–233.
129. Rodenhuis S, Richel DJ, van der Wall E, et al. Randomised trial of high-dose chemotherapy and haemopoietic progenitor- cell support in operable breast cancer with extensive axillary lymph node involvement. *The Lancet* 1998;352:515–521.
130. Tokuda Y, Tajima M, Igarashi T, et al. Randomized phase III study of high-dose chemotherapy (HDC) with autologous stem cell support as consolidation in high-risk postoperative breast cancer. Japan Clinical Oncology Group. (JGOG208) *Proc Am Soc Clin Oncol* 2001;20:38a (abstract 148).

SECTION 3

Metastatic Disease: Chemotherapy

10
The Taxanes: Paclitaxel and Docetaxel

Jean-Marc Nabholtz, Alessandro Riva, Mary-Ann Lindsay,
David M. Reese, and Katia Tonkin

Among the new chemotherapeutic agents developed for the treatment of breast cancer in the last decade, the taxanes have emerged as the most important. Both paclitaxel and docetaxel have significant activity as single agents and are now being investigated as part of combination or sequential regimens, both in the metastatic and adjuvant settings. The integration of the taxanes with other cytotoxic compounds and with novel targeted therapies will continue to be an area of intense investigation in the coming years.

Paclitaxel was the first taxane to be evaluated for the treatment of advanced breast cancer. The drug is a complex plant alkaloid that was initially extracted from the bark of the Pacific yew tree, *Taxus brevifolia,* in 1971, although its development was hindered for some time by scarce supply (1). Subsequently, paclitaxel was found to have a wide spectrum of antineoplastic activity against solid tumors (2). Paclitaxel is now produced by partial biosynthesis from precursor compounds (3).

To provide a renewable source of taxane, docetaxel was synthesized in 1986 using a precursor extracted from the needles of the European yew, *Taxus baccata* (4). A semisynthetic analogue of paclitaxel that differs from the parent compound by two chemical modifications, docetaxel also has substantial activity *in vitro* and *in vivo* against a variety of tumor cell lines (5). In general, docetaxel appears to be very potent in preclinical tumor models and to have a favorable pharmacokinetic profile compared to paclitaxel.

Mechanistically, the taxanes exert a cytotoxic effect by adversely affecting microtubule function. Both agents promote and stabilize tubulin assembly in microtubules, preventing microtubule depolymerization. This stabilization inhibits the reorganization of the microtubule complex that ordinarily occurs during the cell cycle, leading ultimately to apoptosis. For both drugs, longer durations of exposure increase cytotoxicity. Resistance to the taxanes is not well understood, but may occur via P-glycoprotein expression or tubulin mutations. There appears to be significant but incomplete clinical cross-resistance between paclitaxel and docetaxel (6).

While they are structurally closely related, the pharmacokinetics of the taxanes differ somewhat. Plasma clearance of paclitaxel displays nonlinear kinetics; thus, alterations in dose and schedule result in disproportionate changes in the area under the curve (AUC) of the drug. In contrast, docetaxel pharmacokinetics are linear, so the concentration of the drug changes predictably with changes in dose. Both drugs are metabolized in the liver by cytochrome P-450 enzymes (7).

The remainder of this chapter summarizes the clinical development and current use of the taxanes for the treatment of breast cancer and outlines future directions for clinical research utilizing these drugs.

TAXANES IN ADVANCED BREAST CANCER

The initial clinical development of paclitaxel began in the mid-1980s with a series of phase 1 studies in various malignancies. Subsequently, docetaxel was introduced, and clinical trials of this agent were initiated in 1992. Both drugs have followed the traditional pathway for development of new anti-neoplastic agents.

Paclitaxel Monotherapy

Phase 1 Trials

The original phase 1 trials evaluating paclitaxel were performed using a variety of doses and schedules. These regimens used short daily infusions over 5 days every 3 weeks, single infusions over 1 to 6 hours every 3 weeks, and prolonged infusions of 24 to 120 hours every 3 weeks (8–21). In general, each schedule has a different maximum tolerated dose and toxicity profile, which led to the evaluation of multiple different monotherapy programs in the phase 2 setting. The principal toxicities of paclitaxel when delivered every 3 weeks include: myelosuppression (in particular neutropenia), fatigue, myalgia and arthralgia, neuropathy, and alopecia. In addition, hypersensitivity reactions characterized by cutaneous flushing, bronchospasm, hypotension, bradycardia, and angioedema can occur; these reactions may be severe and life-threatening in 2% of patients. Premedication with corticosteroids and antihistamines (H_1 and H_2 blockers) is, therefore, mandatory prior to administration of paclitaxel. Less common severe side effects include nausea, vomiting, and mucositis.

More recently, paclitaxel has been given on a weekly schedule (22–25). A dose of 80 mg/m² appears to be optimal, producing a lower incidence of neutropenia and alopecia than every-3-weeks schedules.

Phase 2 Trials

A wide variety of infusion times have been evaluated using paclitaxel in a range of doses (135 mg to 250 mg/m²) (Table 10.1). In trials using short, 3-hour infusion times, objective response rates of 32% to 60% have been reported for patients without prior chemotherapy for metastatic disease (26–29), compared with 6% to 42% for those previously exposed to anthracyclines (27,30–34). Median time to progression in these studies was usually 3 to 4 months, and toxicity was mild at the lower doses.

Several trials have investigated longer infusion schedules (24 to 96 hours) (Table 10.2) (20,35–41). These studies generally reported higher response rates (32% to 62%) and time to progression (4 to 6 months) than those achieved with 3-hour infusion times, particularly in patients who had received prior anthracyclines.

TABLE 10.1. *Phase 2 trials of single-agent 3-hour paclitaxel in advanced breast cancer*

Author	Dose (mg/m²)	N	ORR (%)	TTP (months)	Median survival (months)
First-line therapy					
Seidman (26)	250	25	32	NR	NR
Mamounas (27)	250	82	43	NR	NR
Bonneterre (28)	225	101	44	NR	NR
Davidson (29)	225	30	60	7.0	12.8
After anthracyclines					
Vermorken (30)	250–300	33	6	NR	NR
Gianni (33)	175–225	50	38	5.0	11.0
Seidman (26)	175	41	21	NR	NR
Fountzilas (34)	175	33	42	5.6	9.4
Michael (32)	175	24	25	4.1	6.3
Vici (31)	135–175	41	22	5.0	9.0

NR, not reported; ORR, objective response rate; TTP, time to progression.

TABLE 10.2. *Phase 2 trials of single-agent paclitaxel using prolonged infusion times*

Author	Dose (mg/m^2)	N	ORR (%)	TTP (months)	Median survival (months)
First-line therapy					
24-hour infusion					
Reichman (37)	250	26	62	NR	NR
Holmes (36)	250	14	57	NR	NR
Rivera (38)	150–175	68	19	7.0	NR
Swain (35)	135	19	32	NR	NR
After anthracyclines					
24-hour infusion					
Seidman (40)	200–250	76	33	7.0	NR
Holmes (36)	250	6	33	NR	NR
Abrams (39)	135–175	172	23	NR	NR
96-hour infusion					
Wilson (20)	140	33	48	6.3	9.8
Constenla (41)	125	20	30	4.0	NR

NR, not reported; ORR, objective response rate; TTP, time to progression.

With these regimens, severe neutropenia is more common, although there is a lower incidence of neuropathy.

To definitively address the impact of dose and schedule on efficacy and toxicity, several randomized trials were subsequently performed (Table 10.3) (42–46). The registration trial of paclitaxel in metastatic breast cancer compared the 135 mg and 175 mg/m^2 doses, both given as a 3-hour infusion (42). There was no significant difference in response rates (22% versus 29%, respectively) or in time to progression in the group receiving the higher dose (4.2 versus 3 months). A second randomized trial evaluated the impact of infusion time, comparing 3-hour and 24-hour infusions at the 175 mg/m^2 dose level in 521 patients (43). Response rates and time-to-progression were nearly identical on both arms; the 3-hour regimen produced less febrile neutropenia and fewer severe infections, although neurotoxicity was more common in this group. Based on these data, 3-hour infusional paclitaxel was adopted as standard therapy.

Three additional randomized trials subsequently evaluated the effects of paclitaxel dose

TABLE 10.3. *Randomized trials evaluating different paclitaxel doses and schedules*

Author	Setting	Regimens	N	ORR (%)	TTP or TTF (months)	Median Survival (m)
Nabholtz (42)	Second-line MBC	135 mg/m^2 (3 h)	471	22	3.0	10.5
		175 mg/m^2 (3 h)		29	4.2	11.7
				$p = 0.11$	$p = 0.02$	$p = 0.32$
Peretz (43)	Second-line MBC	175 mg/m^2 (3 h)	521	29	No difference	NR
		175 mg/m^2 (24 h)		31		NR
				$p = $ NS		
Smith (45)	First-line LABC or MBC	250 mg/m^2 (3 h)	563	44	6.3	21.1
		250 mg/m^2 (24 h)		54	7.2	21.9
				$p = 0.02$	$p = 0.95$	$p = 0.96$
Winer (44)	First- or second-line MBC	175 mg/m^2 (3 h)	475	21	3.8	9.8
		210 mg/m^2 (3 h)		28	4.1	11.8
		250 mg/m^2 (3 h)		22	4.8	11.9
				$p = 0.64$	$p = 0.03$	$p = 0.48$
Holmes (46)	First- or second-line MBC	250 mg/m^2 (3 h)	179	23	4.5	11.0
		140 mg/m^2 (24 h)		29	7.5	10.0
				$p = $ NS	$p = $ NS	$p = $ NS

LABC, locally advanced breast cancer; MBC, metastatic breast cancer; NR, not reported; NS, not significant; ORR, objective response rate; TTF, time to treatment failure; TTP, time to progression.

and schedule on efficacy and toxicity. In one trial involving 475 patients, doses of 175 mg/m^2, 210 mg/m^2, and 250 mg/m^2 given over 3 hours were compared (44). Response rates (21% to 28%) were not significantly different among the treatment arms, although there was a modest prolongation in time to progression (4.8 versus 3.8 months) in the highest dose group compared with the lowest. Toxicity, however, also increased with increasing dose. The National Surgical Adjuvant Breast and Bowel Project (NSABP) B-26 trial compared 3-hour and 24-hour infusions using a dose of 250 mg/m^2 (45). The response rate was higher in the 24-hour arm (54% versus 44%), but time to progression and median overall survival did not differ. In addition, there was significantly greater neutropenia and fatigue in the 24-hour group. Another trial compared a 3-hour infusion at 250 mg/m^2 with a 96-hour infusion at 140 mg/m^2 (46). Response rates were identical, although toxicity was again increased in the 96-hour arm. Overall, these results suggest that, while response rates may be somewhat improved, there is no clinically significant advantage to prolonged paclitaxel infusions, especially in light of trade-offs in terms of toxicity and inconvenience.

The administration of paclitaxel on a weekly schedule has also been investigated. In the largest phase 2 study, involving 212 patients with heavily pretreated metastatic breast cancer, the response rate was 22%, with 42% of patients experiencing disease stabilization (47). The median survival was 12.8 months. Therapy was well tolerated, with only 15% of patients experiencing grade 3/4 hematologic toxicity and 9% of patients developing grade 3/4 neuropathy. These data suggest that weekly paclitaxel has reasonable activity and probably a more favorable toxicity profile than the standard regimen of 175 mg/m^2 over 3 hours. Randomized trials comparing weekly to 3-week schedules are currently in progress.

Phase 3 Trials Comparing Paclitaxel and Standard Chemotherapy

The utility of single-agent paclitaxel compared with standard first-line chemotherapy for the treatment of metastatic breast cancer has been evaluated in three randomized trials (Table 10.4). The European Organization for Research and Treatment of Cancer (EORTC) studied paclitaxel 200 mg/m^2 over 3 hours every 3 weeks versus doxorubicin 75 mg/m^2 every 3 weeks as first-line therapy for metastatic disease (48). Doxorubicin produced significantly greater response rates (41% versus 25%) and increased progression-free survival (7.5 versus 3.9 months), although there was no difference in overall median survival. However, by design, patients failing one drug crossed over to the other, which likely obscured any potential survival differences. Of note, approximately 15% of patients failing dox-

TABLE 10.4. *Phase 3 trials comparing single-agent paclitaxel with standard chemotherapy as first-line therapy in metastatic breast cancer*

Author	Regimens	N	ORR (%)	TTP (months)	Median survival (months)
Paridaens (48)	P 200 mg/m^2 (3 h)	331	25	3.9	15.6
	D 75 mg/m^2		41	7.5	18.3
			$p = 0.003$	$p < 0.001$	$p = NS$
Sledge (49)	P 175 mg/m^2 (24 h)	739	33	5.9	22.2
	D 60 mg/m^2		34	6.2	20.1
	P + D (150/50 mg/m^2)		46	8.0	22.4
			$p = NS$	$p < 0.05$	$p = NS$
Bishop (50)	P 175 mg/m^2 (3 h)	209	29	5.3	17.3
	CMFP		35	6.4	13.9
			$p = NS$	$p = NS$	$p = 0.07$

CMFP, cyclophosphamide, methotrexate, 5-fluorouracil, prednisone; D, doxorubicin; NR, not reported; NS, not significant; ORR, objective response rate; P, paclitaxel; TTP, time to progression.

orubicin subsequently responded to paclitaxel, suggesting there is not complete clinical cross-resistance between these agents. Doxorubicin was more toxic than paclitaxel in terms of hematologic, gastrointestinal, and cardiac side effects, while paclitaxel produced a greater incidence of neurotoxicity. Neutropenia, febrile neutropenia, documented infections, and hospital admission for serious adverse events were more frequently observed in the doxorubicin arm.

In contrast to these data, in a three-arm trial, the American Intergroup reported that treatment with single-agent paclitaxel or doxorubicin resulted in essentially identical response rates (33% versus 34%), time to progression (5.9 versus 6.2 months), and median survival (49). However, it should be noted that the dose of doxorubicin used in this study (60 mg/m^2) was lower than that used in the EORTC trial (75 mg/m^2). A crossover was also built into this study, with 20% of those failing doxorubicin experiencing an objective response to paclitaxel. Both paclitaxel-containing arms had a greater incidence of grade 4 toxicity, particularly neutropenia and its complications.

The third trial compared paclitaxel (175 mg/m^2 every 3 hours) with cyclophosphamide, methotrexate sodium, 5-fluorouracil, and prednisone (CMFP) (50). In this study, response rates (29% versus 35%) and progression-free survival (5.3 versus 6.4 months) were similar, although there was a trend towards improved overall survival (17.3 versus 13.9 months, $p = 0.068$) in the group receiving paclitaxel. One potential explanation for the fact that survival was increased without corresponding improvements in response rate or time to progression is that a greater percentage of patients in the paclitaxel group (33% versus 21%) responded to subsequent anthracycline. These patients had increased survival, suggesting that the sequence of paclitaxel followed by an anthracycline is superior to a CMF-based program followed by anthracycline. Paclitaxel produced significantly less severe leukopenia, febrile neutropenia, documented infections, thrombocytopenia, mucositis, and nausea or vomiting. Alopecia, peripheral neuropathy, and myalgia or arthralgia were more frequent in the paclitaxel group.

Conclusion

There is level I evidence in favor of doxorubicin over paclitaxel in terms of response rate and time to progression. Given the lack of a significant survival advantage, the clinical choice to use single-agent paclitaxel instead of an anthracycline for the first-line treatment of metastatic breast cancer is reasonable, in particular for patients already exposed to anthracyclines in the adjuvant setting or unable to tolerate anthracyclines due to cardiac disease. Paclitaxel is an acceptable alternative to CMF-based regimens in previously untreated patients and for those who have failed standard chemotherapy, including anthracyclines.

Docetaxel Monotherapy

Phase 1 Trials

The clinical development of docetaxel began in the early 1990s. Initially, various schedules and doses were investigated, including 1-hour infusions every 3 weeks (51,52), daily infusions for 5 days every 3 weeks (53), and prolonged infusions (2, 6, or 24 hours) (54,55). The consensus was that a dose of approximately 100 mg/m^2 as a 1-hour infusion every 3 weeks provided the most favorable ratio of efficacy to toxicity. Common toxicities using this dose and schedule include myelosuppression (neutropenia), mucositis, fatigue, skin rash and fluid retention. Taxane-specific side effects, such as neurotoxicity and nail changes, also occur, although they are not usually severe. Subsequently, hypersensitivity reactions were also described, which led to the use of steroid prophylaxis (56).

As with paclitaxel, weekly docetaxel has recently been investigated in the phase 1 setting (57,58). Initial studies suggested a toxicity threshold of 40 mg/m^2 per week, below which there is a limited incidence of neutropenia and alopecia (although fatigue and nail changes can be significant with long-term treatment). Beyond this dose, the standard toxicities of docetaxel become apparent, precluding further dose escalation (59).

TABLE 10.5. *Phase 2 trials of docetaxel monotherapy in advanced breast cancer*

Author	Dose (mg/m^2)	N	ORR (%)	TTP (months)	Median survival (months)
First-line therapy					
Coleman (66)	100	47	64	4.6	11.2
Fumoleau (65)	100	37	68	7.2	NR
Hudis (63)	100	37	54	6.1	NR
Chevallier (64)	100	31	68	8.6	16+
Ten Bokkel Huinink (60)	100	8	38	NR	NR
Trudeau (61)	75–100	48	55	NR	NR
Dieras (62)	75	31	52	5.6	NR
After prior chemotherapy					
Alexopoulos (73)	100	45	67	8.0	11.5
Vorobiof (68)	100	28	43	NR	NR
Ten Bokkel Huinink (60)	100	24	58	NR	NR
O'Brien (70)	75–100	331	46	NR	6.5
Salminen (75)	75–100	31	48	7.0	NR
Shapiro (71)	75–100	23	48	NR	8.0
Taguchi (67)	60	47	40	NR	NR
Ikeda (72)	60	22	27	6.0	12.1
Adachi (69)	60	72	44	NR	NR
Taguchi (74)	60	64	56	NR	NR
Anthracycline-resistant					
van Oosterom (77)	100	129	50	6.0	NR
Ferraresi (81)	100	56	53	NR	NR
Bonneterre (76)	100	51	29	NR	NR
Ravdin (79)	100	42	50	6.5	NR
Valero (78)	100	34	53	7.5	9.0
Bonneterre (80)	75–100	825	23	4.0	9.8

NR, not reported; ORR, objective response rate; TTP, time to progression.

Phase 2 Trials

Numerous phase 2 trials of docetaxel monotherapy, most using a dose of 100 mg/m^2, established the efficacy of this agent in advanced breast cancer (Table 10.5) (60–81). These trials reported response rates of 30% to 68%, and demonstrated that docetaxel has substantial activity both as first-line therapy and in patients previously treated with chemotherapy, including anthracyclines. The consistency of the results obtained in these trials is probably due to the uniform use of 1-hour infusions and a relatively narrow range of doses (60 mg to 100 mg/m^2). In these trials, the most common side effects included neutropenia, febrile neutropenia, alopecia, and fatigue; severe neurotoxicity was generally rare, as were allergic reactions. Fluid retention was usually manageable with 3-day steroid prophylaxis.

Weekly docetaxel has also been evaluated in the phase 2 setting. Three separate trials in patients with metastatic disease used doses of 35 mg to 40 mg/m^2, given weekly for 6 consecutive weeks followed by a 2-week rest period. Response rates in these trials ranged from 34% to 41%, with responses in both first-line and salvage treatment (82–84). Median survival ranged from 10 to 13 months. Acute toxicity, including myelosuppression, was mild; fatigue was the most common clinically significant side effect. These data suggest that weekly docetaxel is active and has a favorable toxicity profile. The treatment can be administered with minimal hematologic toxicity, and is particularly suitable for use in elderly patients or those who are poor candidates for combination chemotherapy. Data from randomized trials comparing weekly to standard therapy are not available.

Phase 3 Trials

Four phase 3 trials tested single-agent docetaxel against various standard therapies for metastatic breast cancer (Table 10.6) (85–88).

TABLE 10.6. *Phase 3 trials comparing single-agent docetaxel with standard chemotherapy in advanced breast cancer*

Author	Regimens[a]	N	ORR (%)	TTP (months)	Median survival (months)
CMF failure, first- or second-line					
Chan (85)	D 100	326	48	6.1	15.0
	A 75		33	4.9	14.0
			$p = 0.008$	$p = 0.45$	$p = 0.39$
Anthracycline failure					
Nabholtz (86)	D 100	392	30	4.5	11.4
	MMC 12 + VBL 6		12	2.6	8.7
			$p < 0.0001$	$p = 0.001$	$p = 0.01$
Sjöström (87)	D 100	283	42	6.3	10.4
	MTX 200 + 5-FU 600		21	3.0	11.1
			$p < 0.0001$	$p < 0.001$	$p = $ NS
Bonneterre (88)	D 100	172	43	NR	NS
	VIN 25 + CI 5-FU 750		39		
			$p = $ NS		

[a]Doses are in mg/m^2.
A, doxorubicin; CI, continuous infusion; D, docetaxel; 5-FU, 5-fluorouracil; MMC, mitomycin-C; MTX, methotrexate; NR, not reported; NS, not significant; ORR, overall response rate; TTP, time to progression; VBL, vinblastine; VIN, vinorelbine.

In a study of 326 patients who had failed prior CMF-based regimens, docetaxel was compared with doxorubicin as either first- or second-line therapy (85). Docetaxel produced higher response rates (48% versus 33%, $p = 0.0008$) and time to progression (6.1 versus 4.9 months), although the latter was not statistically significant. Overall survival was similar in both groups (15 versus 14 months). Approximately 25% of patients in each group crossed over to the other treatment after disease progression. Hematologic toxicity was greater in the doxorubicin arm, leading to more frequent dose reductions and treatment delays. In addition, congestive heart failure occurred only in those who received anthracycline. These data suggest that docetaxel has at least equivalent (and perhaps superior) efficacy when compared with doxorubicin, as well as an acceptable toxicity profile.

The other three randomized phase 3 trials evaluated docetaxel against various combination regimens in patients who had progressed after treatment with anthracyclines. These regimens included mitomycin-C plus vinblastine sulfate, methotrexate plus 5-fluorouracil, and vinorelbine tartrate plus continuous-infusion 5-fluorouracil (86–88). In the trials involving mitomycin-C–vinblastine and methotrexate-5-fluorouracil, docetaxel use resulted in statistically significant increases in overall response rates and time to progression. In addition, there was a statistically significant advantage in overall survival in the mitomycin-C–vinblastine study (11.4 versus 8.7 months, $p = 0.01$). It should be noted that in the methotrexate-5-fluorouracil study, a crossover design was employed, potentially obscuring any survival advantage that may have emerged with docetaxel. No difference in response rate was detected in the comparison with vinorelbine-continuous infusion 5-fluorouracil, although there was a trend towards improved time to progression and overall survival with docetaxel.

Conclusion

In the aggregate, these randomized studies establish docetaxel as perhaps the most active single agent for the treatment of advanced breast cancer. There is level I evidence for a survival benefit of docetaxel as second-line therapy (against mitomycin-C–vinblastine) after anthracycline failure. Docetaxel monotherapy also represents a reasonable first-line choice for the therapy of metastatic disease, and in this setting it may be considered a standard of care, particularly in patients already exposed to anthracycline. It is also a standard therapy for patients who have progressed on anthracyclines.

TAXANE MONOTHERAPY

There is compelling evidence to support the use of either of the taxanes as single agents, both as first-line and salvage therapy for advanced breast cancer. While data from direct comparisons of docetaxel with paclitaxel are not available, the evidence suggests that docetaxel may have a practical advantage over paclitaxel. Docetaxel has maximum efficacy when infused over 1 hour. In contrast, paclitaxel has maximum effect when given via longer infusions (24 hours). The toxicity profiles of the two drugs also differ and should be taken into account when choosing therapy. Finally, there is evidence from phase 2 trials that weekly administration of taxanes has good activity and probably an improved toxicity profile. Randomized trials comparing weekly with every-3-week administration are eagerly awaited to assess the relative efficacy and toxicity of weekly taxanes for the treatment of breast cancer.

Taxanes in Combination Regimens for Advanced Disease

In light of their activity as single agents, it was logical to combine the taxanes with other active compounds for the treatment of advanced breast cancer. Most studies have focused on the combination of taxanes with anthracyclines, since these agents have the greatest efficacy, a demonstrated lack of clinical cross-resistance, and, with the exception of myelosuppression, largely non-overlapping toxicity profiles. More recently, paclitaxel and docetaxel have been combined with other active drugs such as capecitabine, gemcitabine hydrochloride and vinorelbine.

Paclitaxel-Anthracycline Combinations

A series of phase 2 trials was performed to evaluate the efficacy and toxicity of paclitaxel in combination with either doxorubicin or epirubicin hydrochloride (Table 10.7) (89–102). The initial studies using paclitaxel and doxorubicin reported high response rates (42% to 94%), suggesting that this combination is highly active in patients with untreated advanced breast cancer. As anticipated, the principal acute toxicities of this regimen include neutropenia and mucositis. Unexpectedly, however, there was also a high incidence of congestive heart failure (more than 20%) in some of these trials (95,96). The risk of cardiac toxicity was especially high at cumulative doxorubicin doses above 360 mg/m^2.

Additional investigation uncovered a previously unknown pharmacokinetic interaction between paclitaxel and doxorubicin. Paclitaxel given by short infusion decreases the hepatic clearance of doxorubicinol, the metabolite of doxorubicin, resulting in an increase in the AUC of the anthracycline (103). The effect on doxorubicin pharmacokinetics appears to be sequence- and schedule-dependent; the AUC increases substantially if paclitaxel precedes doxorubicin, or if the interval between infusions is less than an hour. To circumvent this problem, strategies limiting the cumulative dose of doxorubicin to 360 mg/m^2, incorporating a significant time interval (16 to 24 hours) between infusions of the drugs, and using prolonged infusions of one or both drugs have been recommended (97,98). While these approaches lower the risk of cardiac toxicity, the regimens appear to be either less effective or impractical. Thus, the continued development of effective paclitaxel-doxorubicin combinations is problematic.

The combination of epirubicin and paclitaxel also appears quite active based on phase 2 trials (Table 10.7) (99–102). However, there appears to be a pharmacokinetic interaction whereby paclitaxel increases exposure (AUC) to epirubicin and its metabolites. In addition, epirubicin decreases the clearance of paclitaxel by approximately 30% (102). Thus, it is not clear whether the substitution of epirubicin for doxorubicin will substantially lower the risk of cardiac toxicity or prove to be a therapeutically rational alternative.

TABLE 10.7. Selected phase 2 trials of paclitaxel-anthracycline combinations

Author	Regimen[a]	N	ORR (%)	TTP (months)	Survival (months)
Schwartsmann (94)	D 60 P 250 (3 h)	25	80	NR	NR
Frassineti (93)	D 50 P 130–250 (3 h)	32	78	NR	NR
De Lena (92)	D 50 P 120–250 (1 h)	34	82	11.8	27.8
Conte (99)	E 90 P 135–225 (3 h)	49	84	NR	NR
Pazos (90)	D 60 P 200 (1 h)	76	76	13.4	21.0
Sparano (91)	D 60 P 200 (3 h)	48	52	7.3	21.6
White (100)	E 75 P 200 (3 h)	34	50	6.3	11.2
Fisherman (98)	D 60–75 (72 h) P 160–200 (72 h)	39	72	9.0	23.0
Gehl (95)	D 50–60 P 155–200 (3 h)	29	83	11.0	18.0
Gianni (96)	D 60 P 125–200	32	94	NR	NR
Lluch (89)	D 50 P 175 (3 h)	73	78	10.0	NR
Rischin (101)	E 75 P 175 (3 h)	43	54	6.9	17.9
Graselli (102)	E 90 P 175 (3 h)	27	76	10.0	29.0
Holmes (97)	D 48–60 (24 h) P 125–160 (24 h)	48	69	9.6	20.5

[a]Doses are in mg/m^2.
D, doxorubicin; E, epirubicin; ORR, objective response rate; P, paclitaxel; TTP, time to progression.

Five randomized phase 3 trials have compared paclitaxel-anthracycline combinations to standard chemotherapy for the treatment of advanced breast cancer (Table 10.8) (49,104–107). In the largest of these, the American Intergroup study, 739 patients were randomized to paclitaxel over 24 hours, doxorubicin, or both; patients assigned to monotherapy crossed over to the other agent at the time of progression (49). While overall response rates (46% versus 33% to 34%, $p = 0.007$) and time to progression (8.0 versus 5.9 to 6.2 months, $p = 0.009$) were improved in the combination arm compared to doxorubicin alone, median survival did not differ. These results were not deemed promising enough to incorporate this regimen in the adjuvant setting. A second study tested the incorporation of a significant time interval (24 hours) between infusions of the two drugs and compared paclitaxel-doxorubicin with standard FAC (5-fluorouracil, doxorubicin, cyclophosphamide) in 267 women with metastatic breast cancer (104). Overall response rates, time to progression, and median survival rates were superior in the taxane arm; this was the first trial to demonstrate a statistically significant survival advantage with taxane-anthracycline therapy. However, it should be noted that there was a low rate of cross-over to taxanes among patients treated with FAC, which may account for the survival difference. The incidence of significant cardiotoxicity was less than 1%, probably because paclitaxel was infused 24 hours after doxorubicin.

Two trials conducted by the EORTC and AGO Breast Cancer Group reported similar response rates, time to progression, and overall survival when comparing paclitaxel-anthracycline with anthracycline-cyclophosphamide (105,106). The EORTC trial compared AC with doxorubicin-paclitaxel (without a significant time interval between infusions) to attempt to capitalize on the

TABLE 10.8. Randomized trials of paclitaxel-anthracycline combinations as first-line therapy in metastatic breast cancer

Author	Regimens[a]	N	ORR (%)	TTP (months)	Survival (months)
Jassem (104)	AT: A50 + T220	267	68	8.3	23.3
	FAC: F500 + A50 + C500		55	6.2	18.3
			$p = 0.03$	$p = 0.03$	$p = 0.01$
Sledge (49)	T 175	739	33	5.9	22.0
	A 60		34	6.2	20.1
	AT: A50 + P150		46	8.0	22.4
			$p = NS$	$p < 0.05$	$p = NS$
Biganzoli (105)	AT: A60 + T175	275	58	NR	NR
	AC: A60 + C600		54		
			$p = NS$		
Carmichael (107)	ET: E75 + T200	705	67	6.5	13.8
	EC: E75 + C600		56	6.7	13.7
			$p = NR$	$p = 0.72$	$p = 0.92$
Luck (106)	ET: E60 + T175	560	46	NR	NR
	EC: E60 + C600		40		
			$p = NS$		

[a]Doses are in mg/m^2.
A, doxorubicin; C, cyclophosphamide; E, epirubicin; F, 5-fluorouracil; ORR, objective response rate; T, paclitaxel; TTP, time to progression.

pharmacokinetic interaction between the drugs for efficacy; the total dose of doxorubicin was limited to 360 mg/m^2 to lower the risk of cardiac toxicity. However, while the incidence of CHF was low in both arms, the relative dose intensity of doxorubicin was significantly decreased in patients on the taxane arm, owing to a high incidence of febrile neutropenia and asymptomatic declines in left ventricular ejection fraction. Since the dose of doxorubicin may affect outcome, this reduction could have obscured any potential efficacy benefit.

More recently, in the United Kingdom a randomized trial involving 705 patients compared epirubicin and cyclophosphamide (EC) and epirubicin and Taxol (ET) (107). While response rates were improved in the taxane arm (67% versus 56%), there was no difference in progression-free or overall survival.

Finally, the Hellenic Cooperative Oncology Group performed a study comparing sequential epirubicin and paclitaxel with up-front combination therapy using these drugs (108). Response rates were not statistically different (55% versus 42%, $p = 0.10$); likewise, time-to-progression and median overall survival were comparable. The significance of this trial is unclear, since neither arm of this trial used standard doses of epirubicin or paclitaxel.

Docetaxel-Anthracycline Combinations

Docetaxel has also been intensively investigated in conjunction with anthracyclines for the treatment of advanced breast cancer. The initial dose-finding study defined the recommended 3-weekly doses as docetaxel 75 mg/m^2 with doxorubicin 50 mg/m^2, or docetaxel and doxorubicin, both at 60 mg/m^2 (109). Three phase 2 trials subsequently explored the efficacy and toxicity of these doses, while a third study evaluated docetaxel (75 mg/m^2) and doxorubicin (50 mg/m^2) with cyclophosphamide (500 mg/m^2) (TAC) (110–113). This latter trial was performed to define a regimen that could be directly compared with standard FAC in both the metastatic and adjuvant settings.

Efficacy data from these trials were very promising (Table 10.9). Response rates ranged from 57% to 79%, with favorable times to progression and survival. The high response rates were maintained in patients with unfavorable prognostic features, such as multiple metastatic sites, visceral lesions, and prior exposure to ad-

TABLE 10.9. Selected phase 2 trials of docetaxel-anthracycline combinations

Author	Regimen[a]	N	ORR (%)	TTP (months)	Survival (months)
Baltali (112)	A 60 T 80	42	79	8.0	NR
Nabholtz (113)	T 75 A 50 C 500	47	77	9.8	>24
Dieras (111)	A 50 T 75	39	74	NR	NR
Sparano (110)	A 60 T 60	51	57	7.6	27.5
Milla-Santos (120)	E 130 T 100	32	88	16.3	20.1
Mavroudis (118)	E 70 T 90	54	66	11.5	NR
Viens (119)	E 60–110 T 75	62	69	9.1	22.7
Pagani (117)	E 90 T 75	68	66	4.5	NR

[a]Doses are in mg/m^2.
A, doxorubicin; C, cyclophosphamide; E, epirubicin; F, 5-fluorouracil; ORR, objective response rate; T, docetaxel; TTP, time to progression.

juvant chemotherapy. In general, toxicity was manageable. Myelosuppression (neutropenia) was the most common side effect, with 85% to 100% of patients developing grade 3/4 neutropenia and 30% to 40% experiencing febrile neutropenia at some point in the course of treatment. However, neutropenia with these regimens tends to be of brief duration, and severe infections were infrequent. Most importantly, there was no evidence of a pharmacokinetic interaction between docetaxel and doxorubicin; the incidence of congestive heart failure in these trials was 0% to 4%, a rate which would be anticipated with the use of doxorubicin alone. Indeed, additional studies have confirmed no direct pharmacokinetic interaction between docetaxel and doxorubicin (114–116).

Epirubicin has also been combined with docetaxel (Table 10.9) (117–120). In phase 2 trials, response rates and survival times comparable to those achieved with doxorubicin have been reported: The toxicity profile of the epirubicin-docetaxel combination was also comparable. However, further evaluation of this combination is required to determine if there are significant clinical differences between epirubicin and doxorubicin in conjunction with docetaxel.

The results obtained in phase 2 trials of docetaxel with anthracyclines prompted several randomized studies comparing these combinations with standard therapy (Table 10.10) (121–123). One randomized phase 3 trial compared standard AC with AT (doxorubicin and docetaxel) in 429 patients with untreated metastatic breast cancer (121). Response rates (59% versus 47%) and median time to progression (37 versus 32 weeks) were significantly improved in the group receiving AT, although median survival did not differ (22.5 versus 21.7 months). The advantage in terms of response was maintained in patients with poor prognosis features, including the presence of visceral metastases, liver or lung lesions, and the involvement of three or more sites. One potential explanation of the lack of survival advantage with AT is the fact that a significant percentage of patients receiving AC crossed over to a taxane (in particular, docetaxel) after disease progression. The only significant difference in toxicity between the two groups was the incidence of hematologic toxicity. Of patients receiving AT, 96% experienced grade 3/4 neutropenia, compared with 82% in the AC arm. In addition, the incidence of febrile neutropenia was higher in those receiving AT (33% versus

TABLE 10.10. *Randomized trials of docetaxel-anthracycline combinations as first-line therapy for metastatic breast cancer*

Author	Regimens[a]	N	ORR (%)	TTP (months)	Survival (months)
Nabholtz (121)	AT: A50 + T75	429	59	8.7	22.5
	AC: A60 + C600		47	7.4	21.7
			$p = 0.009$	$p = 0.05$	$p = 0.26$
Mackey (122)	TAC: T75 + A50 + C500	484	55	7.2	21.0
	FAC: F500 + A50 + C500		44	6.8	22.0
			$p = 0.02$	$p = 0.51$	$p = 0.93$
Bonneterre (123)	ET: E75 + T75	142	63	7.8	NR
	FEC: F500 + E75 + C500		34	5.9	
			$p < 0.05$	$p = 0.05$	

[a]Doses are in mg/m^2.
A, doxorubicin; C, cyclophosphamide; E, epirubicin; F, 5-fluorouracil; ORR, objective response rate; T, docetaxel; TTP, time to progression.

10%). However, severe infections occurred infrequently, probably reflective of the fact that neutropenia with the AT regimen is usually of short duration.

A second randomized phase 3 trial evaluated the TAC and FAC regimens as first-line treatment for metastatic disease (122). Results were generally consistent with those observed in the AT versus AC trial. TAC produced higher response rates (55% versus 44%), although median time to progression (31 versus 29 weeks) and overall survival (21 versus 22 months) did not differ. Again, the superiority in response rates was maintained in patients with poor-prognosis disease. The lack of improvement in TTP, compared with the AT versus AC trial, may, in part, have occurred from the inclusion of a patient population with more advanced disease and greater prior exposure to anthracyclines.

One randomized phase 2 trial has evaluated the ET regimen in comparison with standard FEC as first-line therapy in 142 patients with metastatic breast cancer (123). Preliminary data indicate that response rates (63% versus 34%) and time to progression (7.8 versus 5.9 months) are superior with ET; survival data are not yet mature. Febrile neutropenia and asthenia occurred more commonly in patients receiving ET.

Conclusion

There is level I evidence that docetaxel-anthracycline regimens yield higher response rates and time to progression when compared to standard chemotherapy programs. There is, as yet, no compelling evidence for an advantage in overall survival.

OTHER COMBINATION REGIMENS

In addition to the anthracyclines, paclitaxel and docetaxel have been evaluated in combination with other new agents for the treatment of advanced breast cancer. Based on potential mechanistic synergies, paclitaxel and vinorelbine have been tested in the phase 2 setting. A series of trials established response rates of 38% to 60%, both in treatment-naïve and pretreated patients (124–130). The primary toxicities of the paclitaxel-vinorelbine regimen include myelosuppression (neutropenia), peripheral neuropathy, and alopecia. No randomized trials comparing this combination with other regimens are available.

Docetaxel has also been combined with vinorelbine in the phase 2 setting (131). In one trial, 42 patients received the combination as first-line therapy and 15 as salvage treatment. The response rates were 64% and 53%, respectively; times to progression were 12 months and 9.8 months. As anticipated, grade 3/4 neutropenia was the most frequent serious toxicity, occurring in 32% of patients; 7% of patients developed sepsis.

More recently, the taxanes have been combined with gemcitabine (132–135). One trial utilized paclitaxel, while three trials studied the docetaxel-gemcitabine combination. Response rates in these relatively small trials ranged from 36% to 79%. The combinations were well tolerated, with myelosuppression (neutropenia and, less frequently, thrombocytopenia) being the major toxicity. Another regimen that has shown activity incorporates gemcitabine, epirubicin, and paclitaxel (GET) (136). In a phase 2 trial this program produced a 92% response rate (including 31% complete responses) in 36 untreated patients with metastatic breast cancer. Based on these data, a large-scale phase 3 trial comparing GET with ET has been initiated.

Of particular interest, the taxanes have been evaluated in combination with capecitabine, an orally administered 5-FU pro-drug that has single-agent activity in metastatic breast cancer (see Chapter 11). Final data are now available from a randomized phase 3 trial comparing capecitabine-docetaxel with docetaxel alone in 511 patients previously treated with an anthracycline (137). Approximately one-third of patients received study therapy as first-line treatment for metastatic disease, while two-thirds received it as second- or third-line treatment. Patients received 2,500 mg/m^2 capecitabine daily for 14 days with 75 mg/m^2 of docetaxel on day 1 in the combination arm, and 100 mg/m^2 docetaxel in the monotherapy group. In this study, combination therapy significantly improved response rates (42% versus 34%), time to progression (6.1 versus 4.2 months), and overall survival (14.5 versus 11.5 months). Patients receiving the combination did experience a higher incidence of gastrointestinal toxicity (diarrhea, nausea, vomiting) and hand-and-foot syndrome, necessitating dose reductions in 65% of patients; there was a greater incidence of myelosuppression and febrile neutropenia in the group receiving docetaxel alone. This trial is the first to report a survival advantage of a combination regimen over docetaxel monotherapy. Moreover, the improvement in survival in spite of the high incidence of capecitabine dose reductions suggests that a lower starting dose of capecitabine may maintain efficacy, while reducing the toxicity of the combination.

Conclusion

There is level I evidence that the capecitabine-docetaxel combination has enhanced efficacy compared to single-agent docetaxel, including an overall survival advantage. This combination is now a reasonable treatment option for patients who have disease progression on anthracyclines. The data also provide a rationale for the further exploration of capecitabine-taxane combinations in both the metastatic and adjuvant settings.

There is level II evidence that taxanes in conjunction with vinorelbine or gemcitabine give improved response rates compared to taxane alone, but there is to date no comparative evidence suggesting these regimens are superior to taxane monotherapy or taxane-anthracycline combinations.

TAXANES IN THE ADJUVANT SETTING

Given their activity in advanced disease, there has been tremendous interest in developing the taxanes for the adjuvant treatment of early stage breast cancer. Two generations of large-scale phase 3 trials have been performed. The first generation of studies—for example, the CALGB 9344 trial—involves regimens with and without taxanes, given either in combination or in sequence. More recent trials, in contrast, contain a taxane in all treatment arms (Table 10.11).

The trials first initiated, including CALGB 9344 and NSABP B-28, compare standard four-course AC with AC followed by four cycles of paclitaxel. Preliminary results from the CALGB study, after a 20-month median follow-up, suggested that the addition of paclitaxel to AC increased disease-free and overall survival (138). These results were confirmed after 30 months' median follow-up, although the benefits seemed to be restricted to patients with hormone receptor-negative disease, using a subset analysis. However, additional follow-up (median 52 months) indicated that the advantage was preserved only for disease-free survival and not overall survival (139). Results from the NSABP B-28 trial (median follow-up 34

TABLE 10.11. Selected adjuvant trials incorporating taxanes

Trial	Regimens[a]
Paclitaxel	
CALGB 9344	AC (60/600) × 4
	AC (60/600) × 4 → paclitaxel (175) × 4
NSABP B-28	AC (60/600) × 4
	AC (60/600) × 4 → paclitaxel (225) × 4
Italian Cooperative Group	CEF (600/60/600) × 6
	ET (90/175) × 6
CALGB 9741	Doxorubicin (60) × 4 → paclitaxel (175) × 4 → cyclophosphamide (600) × 4 (q3w)
	Doxorubicin (60) × 4 → paclitaxel (175) × 4 → cyclophosphamide (600) → 4 (q2w, with G-CSF)
	AC (60/600) × 4 → paclitaxel (175) × 4 (q3w)
	AC × 4 (60/600) → paclitaxel (175) × 4 (q2w, with G-CSF)
Docetaxel	
First Generation	
BCIRG 001	TAC (75/50/500) × 6
	FAC (500/50/500) × 6
ECOG 2197	AC (60/600) × 4
	AT (60/60) × 4
BIG 2–98	Doxorubicin (75) × 4 → CMF (oral) × 3
	Doxorubicin (75) × 3 → docetaxel (100) × 3 → CMF (oral) × 3
	AC (60/600) × 4 → CMF (oral) × 3
	AT (50/75) × 4 → CMF (oral) × 3
ICCG	Epirubicin (50; day 1, 8) × 6
	Epirubicin (50; day 1, 8) × 3 → docetaxel (100) × 3
Italian Adjuvant Group	Epirubicin (120) × 4 → CMF × 4
	Epirubicin (120) × 4 → docetaxel (100) × 4 → CMF × 4
French Cooperative Adjuvant	FEC (50/100/500) × 6
	FEC (50/100/500) × 3 → docetaxel (100) × 3
Second Generation	
BCIRG 005	TAC (50/75/500) × 6
	AC (60/600) × 4 → docetaxel (100) × 4
NSABP B-30	ATC (50/75/500) × 4
	AC (60/600) × 4 → docetaxel (100) × 4
	AT (50/75) × 4
Intergroup (ECOG 1199)	AC (60/600) × 4 → paclitaxel (175) × 4 (q 3w)
	AC (60/600) × 4 → paclitaxel (80) × 12 (weekly)
	AC (60/600) × 4 → docetaxel (100) × 4 (q 3w)
	AC (60/600) × 4 → docetaxel (35) × 12 (weekly)

[a]All doses are in mg/m^2.

AC, doxorubicin plus cyclophosphamide; AT, doxorubicin plus docetaxel; ATC, doxorubicin, docetaxel, cyclophosphamide; BCIRG, Breast Cancer International Research Group; BIG, Breast International Group; CALGB, Cancer and Leukemia Group B; CEF, cyclophosphamide plus epirubicin plus 5-fluorouracil; CMF, cyclophosphamide plus methotrexate plus 5-fluorouracil; ECOG, Eastern Cooperative Oncology Group; ET, epirubicin plus paclitaxel; FAC, 5-fluorouracil plus doxorubicin plus cyclophosphamide; FEC, 5-fluorouracil plus epirubicin plus cyclophosphamide; ICCG, International Collaborative Cancer Group; NSABP, National Surgical Adjuvant Breast and Bowel Project; TAC, docetaxel plus doxorubicin plus cyclophosphamide.

months) showed equivalent survival in both treatment groups. Clearly, mature results from these trials will be required to determine if there is potential value in using sequential therapy with AC followed by paclitaxel.

The first trial developed with docetaxel in early breast cancer was the NSABP B-27 study, initiated in 1995. This trial examines three different regimens in the neoadjuvant setting: AC for four cycles followed by surgery; AC for four cycles followed by docetaxel for four cycles prior to surgery; and AC for four cycles followed by surgery and then docetaxel for four courses (140). Preliminary results indicate a high clinical objective response rate (85%) in all three arms. However, the clinical complete response rate was substantially greater (65% versus 40%) in the group receiving docetaxel after AC (and prior to surgery) than in the group receiving AC alone. More importantly, the pathologic complete response rate in the former was also significantly greater (26% versus 14%). Since the presence of pathologic complete response has previously been a predictor of survival, these results are provocative, and final data regarding disease-free and overall survival are eagerly awaited.

Several adjuvant trials incorporating docetaxel are either completed or in progress (Table 10.11). These studies utilize docetaxel both sequentially and in combination with standard programs. The first adjuvant trial using docetaxel was reported at the 2002 meeting of the American Society of Clinical Oncology (141). This planned 33-month interim analysis from BCIRG 001, which compares TAC with FAC in 1,491 node-positive patients, indicates that TAC improves disease-free survival when compared with FAC (relative risk [RR] of relapse, 0.68; $p = 0.001$). This effect was seen in the overall population and in patients with one to three positive nodes (RR, 0.50; $p = 0.001$). Disease-free survival was improved in patients with both hormone receptor-positive disease (RR, 0.50; $p = 0.0002$) and hormone receptor-negative disease (RR, 0.68; $p = 0.02$) as well as in patients with either HER-2-positive tumors (RR, 0.59; $p = 0.02$). In addition, there was an overall survival advantage in the group with one to three positive nodes; the relative risk of death in this group was 0.46 for those receiving TAC ($p = 0.006$). No differences in disease-free or overall survival emerged between treatment arms in those patients with more than four positive axillary nodes.

While preliminary, these results are the first to suggest a survival advantage with the use of docetaxel in the adjuvant setting. The fact that the effect of docetaxel appears most pronounced in those with a lower tumor burden (one to three positive nodes) is intriguing and may imply that our current approach to adjuvant therapy—in which the highest risk patients receive the most aggressive therapy—should be revisited. Perhaps those patients with the lowest tumor burden have the greatest chance of cure and will benefit the most from aggressive therapy.

Conclusion

In summary, numerous trials are in progress using the taxanes in the adjuvant setting. The preliminary results currently available are encouraging, and suggest a role for the taxanes for the treatment of early stage breast cancer.

There is level II evidence for the use of paclitaxel following standard AC in terms of disease-free and overall survival. There is preliminary level I evidence for the superiority of TAC over FAC for disease-free and overall survival in patients with one to three involved nodes. However, additional data are required to fully understand the role of each taxane in the management of early breast cancer.

INTEGRATION OF TAXANES WITH BIOLOGIC THERAPIES

Trastuzumab, a humanized anti-HER-2 antibody, represents the first targeted biologic therapy for the treatment of breast cancer. Approximately 25% to 30% of primary breast tumors overexpress the HER-2 protein, a transmembrane receptor involved in normal and neoplastic cell growth; 20% exhibit HER-2 gene amplification (142). HER-2 protein overexpression and gene amplification are associated with aggressive breast tumor behavior, resulting in shortened disease-free and overall survival (143–145).

The antibody is active both as a single agent and in combination with chemotherapy, including taxanes (146,147). In the pivotal international randomized trial, trastuzumab in combination with paclitaxel was superior to paclitaxel alone for the treatment of HER-2-overexpressing metastatic breast cancer (147). Combination therapy produced greater response rates (38% versus 16%) and time to progression (6.9 versus 3.0 months). There was also an increase in median survival (22.1 versus 18.4 months), but this was not statistically significant. There were no significant differences in serious toxicity; in particular, the incidence of congestive heart failure was comparable (1% to 2%), although the incidence of asymptomatic declines of left ventricular ejection was greater in the group treated with antibody-plus-paclitaxel.

Several other pertinent observations emerged from this trial. First, trastuzumab has the greatest activity in patients with high-level HER-2 overexpression (three positive by immunohistochemistry) or gene amplification. In fact, patients whose tumors display gene amplification as detected by fluorescence *in situ* hybridization (FISH) analysis have the greatest likelihood of responding to trastuzumab (148). In addition, the combination of trastuzumab with anthracyclines results in an unacceptably high incidence of cardiac toxicity; 16% of patients in the pivotal trial treated with anthracycline-cyclophosphamide plus trastuzumab developed congestive heart failure (147).

There is now substantial interest in combining trastuzumab with docetaxel. This is based on several observations. As noted previously, docetaxel may be the single most active agent against advanced breast cancer. In addition, preclinical experiments suggest that the combination of docetaxel and trastuzumab is particularly active. *In vitro* and *in vivo* studies reveal a potent synergistic cytotoxic effect of trastuzumab in conjunction with the platinum salts, docetaxel, and vinorelbine (149–151). In comparison, in the same *in vitro* system, the effect with paclitaxel is additive.

Preliminary results from several phase 2 trials using docetaxel in combination with trastuzumab are now available. In a study involving 21 patients with metastatic breast cancer, 16 of whom had received chemotherapy for metastatic disease, the overall response rate was 45% (152). The treatment regimen in this trial consisted of 75 mg/m^2 of docetaxel every three weeks along with standard weekly trastuzumab (loading dose of 4 mg per kg and then 2 mg per kg weekly). Two additional trials used weekly docetaxel (35 mg/m^2) with standard trastuzumab and noted response rates of 50% to 63% (153,154). A final phase 2 trial of weekly docetaxel-trastuzumab as first- or second-line therapy in patients with HER-2-overexpressing metastatic breast cancer reported a response rate of 63% and median time to progression of 9 months (155). In all of these trials, the main toxicity was myelosuppression, as would be expected from single-agent treatment with docetaxel. Thus far, there have been no cases of significant cardiac dysfunction, although longer follow-up and evaluation of additional patients previously exposed to anthracyclines in the adjuvant setting is required.

Another approach attempting to capitalize on potential synergies uses triple therapy with docetaxel, platinum, and trastuzumab (TCH). This regimen has the advantage of avoiding cardiac toxicity associated with the use of trastuzumab in conjunction with anthracyclines. The BCIRG and members of the UCLA Community Oncology Research Network conducted two parallel phase 2 trials of TCH in patients with HER-2-overexpressing advanced breast cancer (156). In both studies, 75 mg/m^2 of docetaxel every three weeks and standard trastuzumab were administered; 75 mg/m^2 of cisplatin was used in the first study, whereas carboplatin to an AUC of six was given in the second. Prior chemotherapy was permitted in the carboplatin trial but not the cisplatin study. Sixty-two patients were enrolled in each trial. The response rates were 77% (TcisH) and 64% (TcarboH) among first-line patients with FISH-positive tumors. Of note, the times to progression were 12.7 and 17 months, respectively. Principal toxicities included febrile neutropenia, nausea and vomiting, and diarrhea; one patient in each trial developed symptomatic congestive heart failure.

A second study of TCH was performed in patients with HER-2-overexpressing locally advanced or inflammatory breast cancer (157). In this study, standard weekly trastuzumab, with 3 weekly dosages of 70 mg/m^2 docetaxel and 70 mg/m^2 of cisplatin was administered for four cycles prior to surgery. Preliminary results indicate a pathologic complete response rate of 22% in 27 evaluable patients. Approximately 60% of patients were pathologically node-negative, a much higher rate than would be expected in this population if definitive surgery had been performed without neoadjuvant therapy. There was minimal hematologic toxicity due to the use of prophylactic G-CSF and erythropoietin; one patient developed congestive heart failure.

TABLE 10.12. *Adjuvant trials incorporating trastuzumab in patients with HER2-positive early breast cancer*

Trial	Regimens
NSABP B-31	AC (60/600) × 4 → paclitaxel (175) × 4
	AC (60/600) × 4 → paclitaxel (175) × 4 + trastuzumab × 1 year
American Intergroup	AC (60/600) × 4 → paclitaxel (80) weekly × 12
	AC × 4 → paclitaxel (80) weekly × 12 → trastuzumab × 1 year
	AC × 4 → paclitaxel (80) weekly × 12 + trastuzumab × 1 year
BCIRG 006	AC (60/600) × 4 → docetaxel (100) × 4
	AC (60/600) × 4 → docetaxel (100) × 4 + trastuzumab × 1 year
	TCH (75/AUC 6) × 6 → trastuzumab × 1 year
HERA	Chemotherapy[a] → observation
	Chemotherapy[a] → trastuzumab × 1 year
	Chemotherapy[a] → trastuzumab × 2 years

[a]Acceptable chemotherapy in the HERA trial includes AC, EC, FAC, FEC, CMF, ET, or AT.
AC, doxorubicin plus cyclophosphamide; AUC, area under the curve; BCIRG, Breast Cancer International Research Group; HERA, HER2 Adjuvant Trial; NSABP, National Surgical Adjuvant Breast and Bowel Project; TCH, docetaxel plus platinum salt (cisplatin or carboplatin) plus trastuzumab.

Conclusion

There is level III evidence that docetaxel-trastuzumab–based combinations have significant activity in patients with HER-2-overexpressing metastatic breast cancer. These combinations also appear feasible and safe. However, additional evidence is required before these combinations could be adopted as standard therapy.

Taxanes and Trastuzumab in the Adjuvant Setting

Several studies of adjuvant therapy now incorporate taxanes with trastuzumab (Table 10.12). The NSABP and the American Intergroup are conducting studies using AC followed by paclitaxel, with or without the addition of trastuzumab. BCIRG 006, in contrast, compares AC followed by docetaxel, AC followed by docetaxel with concurrent trastuzumab, and docetaxel-carboplatin-trastuzumab (TCH), where six cycles of chemotherapy are administered with trastuzumab given both during chemotherapy and for a year following. The Breast International Group (BIG) is conducting a three-arm trial in which patients receive chemotherapy (standard regimens to be chosen by participating centers) followed by either observation, trastuzumab for one year, or trastuzumab for two years. Data from these trials, when available, will help clarify the role of trastuzumab in conjunction with taxane-containing chemotherapy in the adjuvant setting.

OVERALL CONCLUSIONS

There is no doubt that the taxanes are the most important cytotoxic agents introduced for the treatment of breast cancer in the last decade. There is level I evidence for the use of taxanes as standard treatment in metastatic breast cancer after disease progression on prior chemotherapy. In addition, there is level I evidence for the use of single-agent taxanes, or a taxane in combination with anthracyclines, as first-line therapy for metastatic disease. However, short-infusion paclitaxel in combination with anthracyclines should be used with caution because of the potential risk of cardiac toxicity.

There is an emerging role for the taxanes in the treatment of early breast cancer. However, more data are required to fully assess their role in the adjuvant and neoadjuvant settings. Within the next 2 to 5 years, an evaluation of the role of the taxanes in the adjuvant setting and in combination with biologic therapies such as trastuzumab will be available and will help us to understand to what extent the taxanes may affect the natural history of breast cancer.

REFERENCES

1. Wani MC, Taylor HL, Wall ME, et al. Plant antitumour agents. VI. The isolation and structure of Taxol, a novel antileukemic and antitumour agent from Taxus brevifolia. *J Am Chem Soc* 1971;93:2325–2327.
2. Greenlee RT, Hill-Harmon MB, Murray T, et al. Cancer Statistics, 2001. *CA Cancer J Clin* 2001;51:15–36.
3. Hezari M, Croteau R. Taxol biosynthesis: an update. *Planta Med* 1997;63:291–295.
4. Lavelle F, Gueritte-Voegelein F, Guenard D. Le Taxotere: des aiguilles d'if a la clinique. *Bull Cancer* 1993;80:326–338.
5. Bissery MC, Nohynek S, Sanderink GJ, et al. Docetaxel (Taxotere): a review of preclinical and clinical experience. Part 1: preclinical experience. *Anticancer Drugs* 1995;6:339–368.
6. Dorr RT. Pharmacology of the taxanes. *Pharmacotherapy* 1997;17(5 pt 2):96S–104S.
7. Vaishampayan U, Parchment RE, Jasti BR, et al. Taxanes: an overview of the pharmacokinetics and pharmacodynamics. *Urology* 1999;54(6A suppl):22–29.
8. Legha SS, Tenney DM, Krakoff IR. Phase I study of Taxol using a 5 day intermittent schedule. *J Clin Oncol* 1986;4:762–766.
9. Grem JL, Tutsch KD, Simon KJ, et al. Phase I study of Taxol administered as a short i.v. infusion daily for 5 days. *Cancer Treat Rep* 1986;71:1179–1184.
10. Donehower RC, Rowinsky E, Grochow LB, et al. Phase I trial of Taxol in patients with advanced cancer. *Cancer Treat Rep* 1987;71:1171–1177.
11. Wiernik PH, Schwartz EL, Strauman JJ, et al. Phase I clinical and pharmacokinetic study of Taxol. *Cancer Res* 1987;47:2486–2493.
12. Schiller HJ, Storer B, Tutsch K, et al. Phase I trial of 3-hour infusion of paclitaxel with or without granulocyte colony-stimulating factor in patients with advanced cancer. *J Clin Oncol* 1994;12:241–248.
13. Kris MG, O'Connell JP, Gralla RJ, et al. Phase I trial of Taxol given as a 3-hour infusion every 21 days. *Cancer Treat Rep* 1986;70:605–607.
14. Brown T, Halvin K, Weiss G, et al. A phase I trial of Taxol given by a 6-hour infusion. *J Clin Oncol* 1991;9:1261–1267.
15. Wiernik PH, Schwartz EL, Einzig A, et al. Phase I trial of Taxol given as a 24-hour infusion every 21 days: responses observed in metastatic melanoma. *J Clin Oncol* 1987;5:1232–1239.
16. Ohmura T, Zimet AS, Coffey VA, et al. Phase I study of Taxol in a 24-hour infusion schedule. *Proc Am Soc Clin Oncol* 1985;26:167.
17. Hurwitz CA, Relling MV, Weitman SD, et al. Phase I trial of paclitaxel in children with refractory solid tumors: a Pediatric Oncology Group study. *J Clin Oncol* 1993;11:2224–2229.
18. Rowinsky EK, Burke PJ, Karp JE, et al. Phase I and pharmacodynamic study of Taxol in refractory adult acute leukemias. *Cancer Res* 1989;49:4640–4647.
19. Sarosy G, Kohn E, Stone DA, et al. Phase I study of Taxol and granulocyte colony-stimulating factor in patients with refractory ovarian cancer. *J Clin Oncol* 1992;10:1165–1170.
20. Wilson WH, Berg S, Bryant G, et al. Paclitaxel in doxorubicin-refractory or mitomycin-refractory breast cancer: a phase I/II trial with 96-hour infusion. *J Clin Oncol* 1994;12:1621–1629.
21. Spriggs DR, Tondini C. Taxol administered as a 120 hour infusion. *Invest New Drugs* 1992;10:275–278.
22. Luftner D, Flath B, Printz B, et al. Weekly fractionated paclitaxel in metastatic breast cancer–dose optimizing study. *Eur J Cancer* 1997;33:S196 (abstract 694).
23. Breier A, Ledbedinsky C, Pelayes L, et al. Phase I/II weekly paclitaxel 80 mg/m^2 in pre-treated breast and ovarian cancer. *Proc Am Soc Clin Oncol* 1997;16:163a (abstract 568).
24. Change A, Boros L, Asbury Y, et al. Dose-escalation study of weekly 1-hour paclitaxel administration in patients with refractory cancer. *Semin Oncol* 1997;24(5 Suppl 17):S17-69–S17-71.
25. Seidman AD, Hudis CA, Albanel J, et al. Dose-dense therapy with weekly 1-hour paclitaxel infusions in the treatment of metastatic breast cancer. *J Clin Oncol* 1999;16:3353–3361.
26. Seidman AD, Hudis CA, Tiersten A, et al. Phase II trial of paclitaxel by 3-hour infusion as initial and salvage chemotherapy for metastatic breast cancer. *J Clin Oncol* 1995;13:2575–2581.
27. Mamounas E, Brown A, Fisher B, et al. 3-hour high-dose Taxol infusion in advanced breast cancer: a NSABP phase II study. *Proc Am Soc Clin Oncol* 1995;14:206.
28. Bonneterre J, Tubiana-Hulin M, Chollet PH, et al. Taxol (paclitaxel) 225 mg/m^2 by 3-hour infusion without G-CSF as first-line therapy in metastatic breast cancer (MBC). *Proc Am Soc Clin Oncol* 1996;15:179.
29. Davidson NG. Single agent paclitaxel as first-line treatment of metastatic breast cancer: the British experience. *Semin Oncol* 1996;23(suppl 11):6–10.
30. Vermorken D, Ten Bokkel Huinink WW, Mandjes IAM, et al. High dose paclitaxel with granulocyte colony-stimulating factor in patients with advanced breast cancer refractory to anthracycline therapy: a European Cancer Center trial. *Semin Oncol* 1995;22:16–22.
31. Vici P, Di Lauro S, Conte L, et al. Paclitaxel activity in anthracycline refractory breast cancer patients. *Tumori* 1997;83:661–664.
32. Michael M, Bishop JF, Levi JA, et al. Australian multicentre phase II trial of paclitaxel in women with metastatic breast cancer and prior chemotherapy. *Med J Aust* 1997;166:530–533.
33. Gianni L, Munzone E, Capri G, et al. Paclitaxel in metastatic breast cancer: a trial of two doses by a 3-hour infusion in patients with disease recurrence after prior therapy with anthracyclines. *J Natl Cancer Inst* 1995;87:1169–1175.
34. Fountzilas G, Athanassiades A, Giannakakis T, et al. A phase II study of paclitaxel in advanced breast cancer resistant to anthracyclines. *Eur J Cancer* 1996;32A:47–51.
35. Swain SM, Honig SF, Tefft MC, et al. A phase II trial of paclitaxel (Taxol) as first line treatment in advanced breast cancer. *Invest New Drugs* 1995;13:217–222.
36. Holmes FA, Walters RS, Theriault RL, et al. Phase II trial of Taxol: an active drug in the treatment of meta-

static breast cancer. *J Natl Cancer Inst* 1991;83: 1797–1805.
37. Reichman BS, Seidman AD, Crown JPA, et al. Paclitaxel and recombinant human granulocyte colony-stimulating factor as initial chemotherapy for metastatic breast cancer. *J Clin Oncol* 1993;11:1943–1951.
38. Rivera E, Holmes FA, Frye D, et al. Phase II study of paclitaxel in patients with metastatic breast carcinoma refractory to standard treatment. *Cancer* 2000;89: 2195–2201.
39. Abrams JS, Vena DA, Baltz J, et al. Paclitaxel activity in heavily pretreated breast cancer: a National Cancer Institute Treatment Referral Center trial. *J Clin Oncol* 1995;13:2056–2065.
40. Seidman AD, Reichman BS, Crown JP, et al. Paclitaxel as a second and subsequent therapy for metastatic breast cancer: activity independent of prior anthracycline response. *J Clin Oncol* 1995;15:1152–1159.
41. Constenla M, Lorenzo I, Garcia-Arroyo FR, et al. Phase II trial of paclitaxel 96-hour infusion with G-CSF in anthracycline-resistant metastatic breast cancer. *Proc Am Soc Clin Oncol* 1997;16:165a.
42. Nabholtz J-M, Gelmon K, Bontenbal M, et al. Multicenter, randomized comparative study of two doses of paclitaxel in patients with metastatic breast cancer. *J Clin Oncol* 1996;14:1858–1867.
43. Peretz T, Sulkes A, Chollet P, et al. A multicenter randomized study of two schedules of paclitaxel (PTX) in patients with advanced breast cancer (ABC). *Eur J Cancer* 1995;31(suppl 5):S75a.
44. Winer E, Berry D, Duggan D, et al. Failure of higher dose paclitaxel to improve outcome in patients with metastatic breast cancer—results from CALGB 9342. *Proc Am Soc Clin Oncol* 1998;17:101a (abstract 388).
45. Smith RE, Brown AM, Mamounas EP, et al. Randomized trial of 3-hour versus 24-hour infusion of high-dose paclitaxel in patients with metastatic or locally advanced breast cancer: National Surgical Adjuvant Breast and Bowel Project Protocol B-26. *J Clin Oncol* 1999;17:3403–3411.
46. Holmes FA, Valero V, Buzdar A, et al. Finals results: randomized phase III trial of paclitaxel by 3-hr versus 96-hr infusion in patient (pt) with metastatic breast cancer (MBC): the long and short of it. *Proc Am Soc Clin Oncol* 1998;17:110a (abstract 426).
47. Perez EA, Vogel CL, Irwin DH, et al. Multicenter phase II trial of weekly paclitaxel in women with metastatic breast cancer. *J Clin Oncol* 2001;19:4216–4223.
48. Paridaens R, Biganzoli L, Bruning P, et al. Paclitaxel versus doxorubicin as first-line single-agent chemotherapy for metastatic breast cancer: a European Organization for Research and Treatment of Cancer randomized study with cross-over. *J Clin Oncol* 2000;18:724–733.
49. Sledge GW, Neuberg D, Ingle J, et al. Phase III trial of doxorubicin (A) versus paclitaxel (T) versus doxorubicin + paclitaxel (A + T) as first-line therapy for metastatic breast cancer (MBC): an intergroup trial. *Proc Am Soc Clin Oncol* 1997;16:1a (abstract 2).
50. Bishop J, Dewar J, Toner G, et al. Initial paclitaxel improves outcome compared with CMFP combination chemotherapy as front-line therapy in untreated metastatic breast cancer. *J Clin Oncol* 1999;17:2355–2364.
51. Extra JM, Rousseau F, Bruno R, et al. Phase I and pharmacokinetic study of Taxotere (RP 56976; NSC 628503) given as a short intravenous infusion. *Cancer Res* 1993;53:1037–1042.
52. Taguchi T, Furue H, Niitani H, et al. Phase I clinical trial of RP 56976 (docetaxel), a new anticancer drug. *Gan To Kagaku Ryoho* 1994;21:1997–2005.
53. Pazdur R, Newman RA, Newman BM, et al. Phase I study of Taxotere: five-day schedule. *J Natl Cancer Inst* 1992;84:1781–1788.
54. Burris H, Irvin R, Kuhn J, et al. Phase I clinical trial of Taxotere administered as either a 2-hour or 6-hour intravenous infusion. *J Clin Oncol* 1993;11:950–958.
55. Bisset D, Setanoians A, Cassidy J, et al. Phase I and pharmacokinetic study of Taxotere (RP 56976) administered as a 24-hour infusion. *Cancer Res* 1993; 53:523–527.
56. Riva A, Fumoleau P, Roche H, et al. Efficacy and safety of different corticosteroid premedications in breast cancer patients treated with Taxotere. *Proc Am Soc Clin Oncol* 1997;16:188a (abstract 660).
57. Hainsworth JD, Burris HA, Erland JB, et al. Phase I trial of docetaxel administered by weekly infusion in patients with advanced refractory cancer. *J Clin Oncol* 1998;16:2164–2168.
58. Luck HJ, Donne S, Glaubitz M, et al. Phase I study of weekly docetaxel in heavily pretreated breast cancer patients. *Eur J Cancer* 1997;33:703a.
59. Loffler TM. Is there a place for 'dose-dense' weekly schedules of the taxoids? *Semin Oncol* 1998;25 (suppl 12):32–34.
60. Ten Bokkel Huinink WW, Prove AM, Piccart M, et al. A phase II trial with docetaxel (Taxotere) in second line treatment with chemotherapy for advanced breast cancer. A study of the EORTC-ECTG. *Ann Oncol* 1994;5:527–532.
61. Trudeau M, Eisenhauer EA, Higgins BP, et al. Docetaxel in patients with metastatic breast cancer: a phase II study of the National Cancer Institute of Canada Clinical Trials Group. *J Clin Oncol* 1996; 14:422–428.
62. Dieras V, Chevallier B, Kerbrat P, et al. A multicentre phase II study of docetaxel 75 mg/m^2 as first-line chemotherapy for patients with advanced breast cancer: a report of the Clinical Screening Group of the EORTC. *Br J Cancer* 1996;74:650–656.
63. Hudis CA, Seidman AD, Crown JP, et al. Phase II and pharmacologic study of docetaxel as initial chemotherapy for metastatic breast cancer. *J Clin Oncol* 1996;14:58–65.
64. Chevallier B, Fumoleau P, Kerbrat P, et al. Docetaxel is a major cytotoxic drug for the treatment of advanced breast cancer: a phase II trial of the Clinical Screening Co-operative Group of the EORTC. *J Clin Oncol* 1995;13:314–322.
65. Fumoleau P, Chevallier B, Kerbrat P, et al. A multicentre phase II study of the efficacy and safety of docetaxel as first-line treatment of advanced breast cancer: a report of the Clinical Screening Group of the EORTC. *Ann Oncol* 1996;17:2341–2354.
66. Coleman RE, Howell A, Eggleton SP, et al. Phase II study of docetaxel in patients with liver metastases from breast cancer. The UK study group. *Ann Oncol* 2000;11:541–546.
67. Taguchi T, Hirata K, Kuni Y, et al. An early phase II study of RP 56976 (docetaxel) in patients with advanced/recurrent breast cancer. *Gan To Jagaku Ryoho* 1994;21:2624–2632.

68. Vorobiof DA, Chasen MR, Moeken R, et al. Phase II trial of single agent docetaxel in previously treated patients with advanced breast cancer (ABC). *Proc Am Soc Clin Oncol* 1996;15:130 (abstract 185).
69. Adachi I, Wantabe T, Takashima S, et al. A late phase II study of RP 56976 (docetaxel) in patients with advanced or recurrent breast cancer. *Br J Cancer* 1996; 73:210–216.
70. O'Brien ME, Leonard RC, Barrett-Lee PJ, et al. Docetaxel in the community setting: an analysis of 377 breast cancer patients treated with docetaxel (Taxotere) in the UK. UK Study Group. *Ann Oncol* 1999; 10:205–210.
71. Shapiro JD, Millward MJ, Rischin D, et al. Activity and toxicity of docetaxel (Taxotere) in women with previously treated metastatic breast cancer. *Aus NZ J Med* 1997;27:40–44.
72. Ikeda H, Koshiba R. Efficacy of docetaxel for anthracycline-resistant metastatic breast cancer. *Gan To Kagaku Ryoho* 2001;28:637–641.
73. Alexopoulos CG, Rigatos G, Efremidis AP, et al. A phase II study of the effectiveness of docetaxel (Taxotere) in women with advanced breast cancer previously treated with polychemotherapy. Hellenic Cooperative Interhospital Group in Oncology. *Cancer Chemother Pharmacol* 1999;44:253–258.
74. Taguchi T, Mori S, Abe R, et al. Late phase II clinical study of RP 56976 (docetaxel) in patients with advanced/recurrent breast cancer. *Gan To Jagaku Ryoho* 1994;21:2624–2632.
75. Salminen E, Bergman M, Huhtala S, et al. Docetaxel: standard recommended dose of 100 mg/m² is effective but not feasible for some metastatic breast cancer patients heavily pretreated with chemotherapy. A phase II single-center study. *J Clin Oncol* 1999;17:1127–1131.
76. Bonneterre J, Guastalla JP, Fumoleau P, et al. A phase II trial of docetaxel in patients with anthracycline resistant metastatic breast cancer. *Breast Cancer Res Treat* 1995;37:89 (abstract 305).
77. van Oosterom AT. Docetaxel (Taxotere): an effective agent in the management of second-line breast cancer. *Semin Oncol* 1995;22(6 suppl 13):22–28.
78. Valero V, Holmes F, Walters RS, et al. Phase II trial of docetaxel: a new, highly effective anti-neoplastic agent in the management of patients with anthracycline-resistant metastatic breast cancer. *J Clin Oncol* 1995;13:2886–2894.
79. Ravdin PM, Burris HA, Cook G, et al. Phase II trial of docetaxel in patients with anthracycline-resistant or anthracenedione-resistant breast cancer. *J Clin Oncol* 1995;13:2879–2885.
80. Bonneterre J, Spielman M, Guastalla JP, et al. Efficacy and safety of docetaxel (Taxotere) in heavily pretreated advanced breast cancer patients: the French compassionate use programme experience. *Eur J Cancer* 1999; 35:1431–1439.
81. Ferraresi V, Milella M, Vaccaro A, et al. Toxicity and activity of docetaxel in anthracycline-pretreated breast cancer patients: a phase II study. *Am J Clin Oncol* 2000;23:132–139.
82. Burstein HJ, Manola J, Younger J, et al. Docetaxel administered on a weekly basis for metastatic breast cancer. *J Clin Oncol* 2000;18:1212–1219.
83. Stemmler HJ, Gutschow K, Sommer K, et al. Weekly docetaxel (Taxotere) in patients with metastatic breast cancer. *Ann Oncol* 2001;12:1393–1398.
84. Hainsworth JD, Burris HA, Yardley DA, et al. Weekly docetaxel in the treatment of elderly patients with advanced breast cancer: a Minnie Pearl Cancer Research Network phase II trial. *J Clin Oncol* 2001;19:3 500–3505.
85. Chan S, Friedrichs K, Noel D, et al. Prospective randomized trial of docetaxel versus doxorubicin in patients with metastatic breast cancer. The 303 Study Group. *J Clin Oncol* 2000;17:2341–2354.
86. Nabholtz J-M, Senn HJ, Bezwoda WR, et al. Prospective randomized trial of docetaxel versus mitomycin C plus vinblastine in patients with metastatic breast cancer progressing despite previous anthracycline-containing chemotherapy. *J Clin Oncol* 1999;17:1413–1424.
87. Sjöström J, Blomqvist C, Mouridsen H, et al. Docetaxel compared with sequential methotrexate and 5-fluorouracil in patients with advanced breast cancer after anthracycline failure: a randomized phase III study with crossover on progression by the Scandinavian Breast Group. *Eur J Cancer* 1999;35:1194–1201.
88. Bonneterre J, Monnier A, Roche H, et al. Taxotere versus 5-fluorouracil + Navelbine in patients with metastatic breast cancer as 2nd line chemotherapy. *Breast Cancer Res Treat* 1997;50:261 (abstract 564).
89. Lluch A, Ojeda B, Colomer R, et al. Doxorubicin and paclitaxel in advanced breast carcinoma: importance of prior adjuvant anthracycline therapy. *Cancer* 2000; 89:2169–2175.
90. Pazos C, Mickiewicz E, Di Notto MR, et al. Phase II trial of doxorubicin/taxol in metastatic breast cancer. Argentine Multicenter Taxol Group. *Breast Cancer Res Treat* 1999;55:91–96.
91. Sparano J, Hu P, Rao RM, et al. Phase II trial of doxorubicin and paclitaxel plus granulocyte colony-stimulating factor in metastatic breast cancer: an Eastern Cooperative Oncology Group Study. *J Clin Oncol* 1999;17:3828–3834.
92. De Lena M, Latorre A, Calabrese P, et al. High efficacy of paclitaxel and doxorubicin as first-line therapy in advanced breast cancer: a phase I-II study. *J Chemother* 2000;12:367–373.
93. Frassineti GL, Zoli W, Silvestro L, et al. Paclitaxel plus doxorubicin in breast cancer: an Italian experience. *Semin Oncol* 1997;24:S17-19–S17-25.
94. Schartsmann G, Mans DR, Menke CH, et al. A phase II study of doxorubicin/paclitaxel plus G-CSF for metastatic breast cancer. *Oncology* (Huntingt) 1997; 11(4 suppl 3):24–29.
95. Gehl J, Boesgaard M, Paaske T, et al. Combined doxorubicin and paclitaxel in advanced breast cancer: effective and cardiotoxic. *Ann Oncol* 1996;7:687–693.
96. Gianni L, Munzone E, Capri G, et al. Paclitaxel by 3-hour infusion in combination with bolus doxorubicin in women with untreated metastatic breast cancer: high antitumor efficacy and cardiac effects in a dose-finding and sequence-finding study. *J Clin Oncol* 1995;13:2688–2699.
97. Holmes FA, Valero V, Walters RS, et al. Paclitaxel by 24-hour infusion with doxorubicin by 48-hour infusion as initial therapy for metastatic breast cancer: phase I results. *Ann Oncol* 1999;10:403–411.
98. Fisherman JS, Cowan KH, Noone M, et al. Phase I/II study of 72 hours infusional paclitaxel and doxorubicin with granulocyte colony stimulating factor in patients with metastatic breast cancer. *J Clin Oncol* 1996;14:774–782.

99. Conte PF, Baldini E, Gennari A, et al. Dose-finding study and pharmacokinetics of epirubicin and paclitaxel over 3 hours: a regimen with high activity and low cardiotoxicity in advanced breast cancer. *J Clin Oncol* 1997;15:2510–2517.
100. White J, Howells A, Jones A, et al. A multicentre phase II pilot study of epirubicin and Taxol (paclitaxel) in patients with advanced breast cancer. *Clin Oncol* (R Coll Radiol) 2000;12:256–259.
101. Rischin D, Smith J, Millward M, et al. A phase II trial of paclitaxel and epirubicin in advanced breast cancer. *Br J Cancer* 2000;83:438–442.
102. Grasselli G, Vigano L, Capri G, et al. Clinical and pharmacologic study of the epirubicin and paclitaxel combination in women with metastatic breast cancer. *J Clin Oncol* 2001;19:2222–2231.
103. Gianni L, Vigano L, Locatelli A, et al. Human pharmacokinetic characterization and in vitro study of the interaction between doxorubicin and paclitaxel in patients with breast cancer. *J Clin Oncol* 1997;15:1906–1915.
104. Jassem J, Pienkowski T, Pluzanska A, et al. Doxorubicin and paclitaxel versus fluorouracil, doxorubicin and cyclophosphomide as first-line therapy for women with metastatic breast cancer: results of a randomized phase III multicenter trial. *J Clin Oncol* 2001;19:1707–1715.
105. Biganzoli L, Cufer T, Bruning P et al. Doxorubicin (A)/taxol (T) versus doxorubicin/cyclophosphamide (C) as first line chemotherapy in metastatic breast cancer (MBC): a phase III study. *Proc Am Soc Clin Oncol* 2000;19:73a (abstract 282).
106. Luck HJ, Thomssen C, Untch M, et al. Multicentric Phase III study in first line treatment of advanced metastatic breast cancer (ABC). Epirubicin/paclitaxel (ET) versus epirubicin/cyclophosphamide (EC). A study of the AGO Breast Cancer Group. *Proc Am Soc Clin Oncol* 2000;19:73a (abstract 280).
107. Carmichael J. UKCCR trial of epirubicin and cyclophosphamide (EC) versus. epirubicin and Taxol (ET) in the first line treatment of women with metastatic breast cancer (MBC). *Proc Am Soc Clin Oncol* 2001;20:22a (abstract 84).
108. Fountzilas G, Papadimitriou C, Dafni U, et al. Dose-dense sequential chemotherapy with epirubicin and paclitaxel versus the combination, as first-line chemotherapy, in advanced breast cancer: a randomized study conducted by the Hellenic Cooperative Oncology Group. *J Clin Oncol* 2001;19:2232–2239.
109. Misset JL, Diéras V, Gruia G, et al. Dose-finding study of docetaxel and doxorubicin in first-line treatment of patients with metastatic breast cancer. *Ann Oncol* 1999;10:553–560.
110. Sparano JA, O'Neill A, Schaefer PL, et al. Phase II trial of doxorubicin and docetaxel plus granulocyte-colony stimulating factor in metastatic breast cancer: Eastern Cooperative Oncology Group study E1196. *J Clin Oncol* 2000;18:2369–2377.
111. Diéras V, Barthier S, Beuzeboc P, et al. Phase II study of docetaxel in combination with doxorubicin as 1st line chemotherapy of metastatic breast cancer. *Breast Cancer Res Treat* 1998;50:262 (abstract 266).
112. Baltali E, Ozisik Y, Guler N, et al. Combination of docetaxel and doxorubicin as first-line chemotherapy in metastatic breast cancer. *Tumori* 2001;87:18–19.
113. Nabholtz J-M, Mackey JR, Smylie M, et al. Phase II study of docetaxel, doxorubicin, and cyclophosphamide as first-line chemotherapy for metastatic breast cancer. *J Clin Oncol* 2001;19:314–321.
114. Gianni L, Vigano L, Locatelli A, et al. Human pharmacokinetic characterization and in vitro study of the interaction between doxorubicin and paclitaxel in patients with breast cancer. *J Clin Oncol* 1997;15:1906–1915.
115. Schüller J, Czejka M, Kletzl H, et al. Doxorubicin (DOX) and Taxotere® (TXT): a pharmacokinetic (PK) study of the combination in advanced breast cancer. *Proc Am Soc Clin Oncol* 1998;17:205a (abstract 790).
116. Bellot R, Robert J, Dieras V, et al. Taxotere (T) does not change the pharmacokinetic (PK) profile of doxorubicine and doxorubicinol (Dx-ol). *Proc Am Soc Clin Oncol* 1998;17:221a (abstract 853).
117. Pagani O, Sessa C, Nole F, et al. Epidoxorubicin and docetaxel as first-line chemotherapy in patients with advanced breast cancer: a multicentric phase I-II study. *Ann Oncol* 2000;11:985–991.
118. Mavroudis D, Alexopoulos A, Ziras N, et al. Frontline treatment of advanced breast cancer with docetaxel and epirubicin: a multicenter phase II study. *Ann Oncol* 2000;11:1249–1254.
119. Viens P, Roche H, Kerbrat P, et al. Epirubicin-docetaxel combination in first-line chemotherapy for patients with metastatic breast cancer: final results of a dose-finding and efficacy study. *Am J Clin Oncol* 2001;24:328–335.
120. Milla-Santos A, Milla L, Rallo L, et al. High-dose epirubicin plus docetaxel at standard dose with lenograstim support as first-line therapy in advanced breast cancer. *Am J Clin Oncol* 2001;24:138–142.
121. Nabholtz JM, Falkson G, Campos D, et al. A phase III trial comparing doxorubicin (A) and docetaxel (T) (AT) to doxorubicin and cyclophosphamide (AC) as first line chemotherapy for MBC. *Proc Am Soc Clin Oncol* 1999;18:125a (abstract 485).
122. Mackey J, Paterson A, Dirix L, et al. Final results of the phase III randomized trial comparing docetaxel (T), doxorubicin (A) and cyclophosphamide (C) to FAC as first line chemotherapy for patients (pts) with metastatic breast cancer (MBC). *Proc Am Soc Clin Oncol* 2002;21:25a (abstract 137).
123. Bonneterre JM, Dieras V, Tubiana-Hulin M, et al. Epirubicin/docetaxel (ET) versus 5FU/epirubicin/cyclophosphamide (FEC) combinations as first line chemotherapy in patients with metastatic breast cancer [MBC]. *Breast Cancer Res Treat* 2001;69:215 (abstract 27).
124. Michelotti A, Gennari A, Salvadori B, et al. Paclitaxel and vinorelbine in anthracycline-pretreated breast cancer: a phase II study. *Ann Oncol* 1996;7:857–860.
125. Tortoriello A, Facchini G, Caponigro F, et al. Phase I/II study of paclitaxel and vinorelbine in metastatic breast cancer. *Breast Cancer Res Treat* 1998;47:91–97.
126. Ellis GK, Gralow JR, Pierce HI, et al. Infusional paclitaxel and weekly vinorelbine chemotherapy with concurrent filgrastim for metastatic breast cancer: high complete response rate in a phase I-II study for doxorubicin-treated patients. *J Clin Oncol* 1999;17:1407–1412.
127. Romero Acuna L, Langhi M, et al. Vinorelbine and paclitaxel as first-line chemotherapy in metastatic breast cancer. *J Clin Oncol* 1999;17:74–81.
128. Vici P, Amodio A, Di Lauro L, et al. First-line chemotherapy with vinorelbine and paclitaxel as simultaneous infusion in advanced breast cancer. *Oncology* 2000;58:3–7.

129. Martin M, Lluch A, Casado A, et al. Paclitaxel plus vinorelbine: an active regimen in metastatic breast cancer patients with prior anthracycline exposure. *Ann Oncol* 2000;11:85–89.
130. Cocconi G, Mambrini A, Quarta M, et al. Vinorelbine combined with paclitaxel infused over 96 hours (VI-TA-96) for patients with metastatic breast cancer. *Cancer* 2000;88:2731–2738.
131. Kornek GV, Ulrich-Pur H, Penz M, et al. Treatment of advanced breast cancer with vinorelbine and docetaxel with or without human granulocyte colony-stimulating factor. *J Clin Oncol* 2001;19:621–627.
132. Murad AM, Guimaras RC, Aragao BC, et al. Phase II trial of the use of paclitaxel and gemcitabine as a salvage treatment in metastatic breast cancer. *Am J Clin Oncol* 2001;24:264–268.
133. Fountzilas G, Nicolaides C, Bafaloukos D, et al. Docetaxel and gemcitabine in anthracycline-resistant advanced breast cancer: a Hellenic Cooperative Oncology Group phase II study. *Cancer Invest* 2000;18:503–509.
134. Mavroudis D, Malamos N, Alexopoulos A, et al. Salvage chemotherapy in anthracycline-pretreated metastatic breast cancer patients with docetaxel and gemcitabine: a multicenter phase II trial. Greek Breast Cancer Cooperative Group. *Ann Oncol* 1999;10:211–215.
135. Laufman LR, Spiridonidis CH, Pritchard J, et al. Monthly docetaxel and weekly gemcitabine in metastatic breast cancer: a phase II trial. *Ann Oncol* 2001;12:1259–1264.
136. Conte P, Salvadori B, Donati S, et al. Gemcitabine, epirubicin, and paclitaxel combinations in advanced breast cancer. *Semin Oncol* 2001;28(2 Suppl 7):15–17.
137. Vukelja S, Moiseyenko V, Leonard R, et al. Xeloda (capecitabine) plus docetaxel combination therapy in locally advanced/metastatic breast cancer: latest results. *Breast Cancer Res Treat* 2001;69:269 (abstract 352).
138. Henderson IC, Berry D, Demetri G, et al. Improved disease-free survival (DFS) and overall survival (OS) from the addition of sequential paclitaxel (T) but not from the escalation of doxorubicin (A) dose level in the adjuvant chemotherapy of patients (pts) with node positive primary breast cancer (BC). *Proc Am Soc Clin Oncol* 1998;17:101a (abstract 390).
139. NIH Development Conference Statement: Adjuvant Therapy for Breast Cancer. *J Natl Cancer Inst Monographs* 2001;30:5–15.
140. National Surgical Adjuvant Breast and Bowel Project investigators. The effect on primary tumor response of adding sequential Taxotere to Adriamycin and cyclophosphamide: preliminary results from NSABP B-27. *Breast Cancer Res Treat* 2001;69:210 (abstract 5).
141. Nabholtz J-M, Pienkowski T, Mackey J, et al. Phase III trial comparing TAC (docetaxel, doxorubicin, cyclophosphamide) with FAC (5-fluorouracil, doxorubicin, cyclophosphamide) in the adjuvant treatment of node positive breast cancer patients: interim analysis of BCIRG 001 Study. *Proc Am Soc Clin Oncol* 2002.
142. Pauletti G, Dandekar S, Rong H, et al. Assessment of methods for tissue-based detection of the HER-2/neu alteration in human breast cancer: a direct comparison of fluorescence in situ hybridization and immunohistochemistry. *J Clin Oncol* 2000;18:3651–3664.
143. Slamon DJ, Godolphin W, Jones LA, et al. Studies of the HER-2/neu proto-oncogene in human breast and ovarian cancer. *Science* 1989;244:707–712.
144. Toikkanen S, Helin H, Isola J, et al. Prognostic significance of HER-2 oncoprotein expression in breast cancer: a 30-year follow-up. *J Clin Oncol* 1992;10:1044–1048.
145. Andrulis IL, Bull SB, Blackstein ME, et al. Neu/erbB-2 amplification identifies a poor-prognosis group of women with node-negative breast cancer. *J Clin Oncol* 1998;16:1340–1349.
146. Vogel CL, Cobleigh MA, Tripathy D, et al. Efficacy and safety of trastuzuamb as a single agent in first-line treatment of HER2-overexpressing metastatic breast cancer. *J Clin Oncol* 2002;20:719–726.
147. Slamon D, Leyland-Jones B, Shak S, et al. Use of chemotherapy plus a monoclonal antibody against HER2 for metastatic breast cancer that overexpresses HER2. *New Engl J Med* 2001;344:783–792.
148. Mass R, Press M, Anderson S, et al. Improved survival benefit from Herceptin (trastuzumab) and chemotherapy in patients selected by fluorescence in situ hybridization. *Breast Cancer Treat Res* 2001;69:213 (abstract 18).
149. Pegram M, Hsu S, Lewis G, et al. Inhibitory effects of combinations of HER-2/neu antibody and chemotherapeutic agents used for the treatment of breast cancer. *Oncogene* 1999;18:2241–2251.
150. Pegram MD, Finn RS, Arzoo K, et al. The effect of HER-2/neu overexpression on chemotherapeutic drug sensitivity in human breast and ovarian cancer cells. *Oncogene* 1999;15:537–547.
151. Konecny G, Pegram MD, Beryt M, et al. Therapeutic advantage of chemotherapy drugs in combination with Herceptin against human breast cancer cells with HER-2/neu overexpression. *Breast Cancer Res Treat* 1999;57:114a (abstract 467).
152. Kuzur ME, Albain KA, Huntington M, et al. A phase II trial of docetaxel and trastuzumab in metastatic breast cancer patients overexpressing HER-2. *Proc Am Soc Clin Oncol* 2000;19:131a (abstract 512).
153. Uber KA, Nicholson BP, Thor AD, et al. A phase II trial of weekly docetaxel (D) and Herceptin (H) as first- or second-line treatment in HER2 over-expressing metastatic breast cancer. *Proc Am Soc Clin Oncol* 2001;19:50b (abstract 1949).
154. Meden H, Beneke A, Hesse T, et al. Weekly intravenous recombinant humanized anti-Her2 monoclonal antibody (trastuzumab) plus docetaxel in patients with metastatic breast cancer (MBC): a pilot study. *Proc Am Soc Clin Oncol* 2001;19:60b (abstract 1987).
155. Esteva FJ, Valero V, Booser D, et al. Phase II study of weekly docetaxel and trastuzumab for patients with HER2-overexpressing metastatic breast cancer. *J Clin Oncol* 2002;20:1800–1808.
156. Nabholtz JM, Pienlowski T, Northfelt D, et al. Results of two open label multicentre phase II pilot studies with Herceptin in combination with docetaxel and platinum salts (cis or carboplatin) as therapy for advanced breast cancer (ABC) in women with tumors over-expressing the HER2-neu proto-oncogene. *Eur J Cancer* 2001;37(suppl 6):190 (abstract 695).
157. Hurley JE, Doliny P, Velez P, et al. High rate of axillary node clearance with neoadjuvant Herceptin, Taxotere, and cisplatin in locally advanced and inflammatory breast cancer. *Breast Cancer Treat Res* 2001;69:300 (abstract 516).

11
Capecitabine

Joyce A. O'Shaughnessy

Since its synthesis in 1957, 5-fluorouracil (5-FU) has been an important agent in the treatment of metastatic and early stage breast cancer. 5-FU is generally given as an intravenous bolus as part of combination chemotherapy regimens, although continuous infusion schedules of single-agent 5-FU help circumvent the short half-life of the drug and have shown significant activity against both untreated and heavily pretreated metastatic breast cancer (1). However, administration of 5-FU by continuous intravenous infusion is inconvenient for patients and is associated with a significant incidence of central venous catheter complications (2).

Capecitabine is a rationally designed, oral, tumor-activated fluoropyrimidine carbamate which is converted to 5-FU preferentially at the tumor site following a series of three enzymatic reactions (Fig. 11.1). Capecitabine, unlike oral 5-FU, is highly orally bioavailable, and, following intestinal absorption, is hydrolyzed first in the liver by carboxylesterase to produce 5'-deoxy-5-fluorocytidine, which is then deaminated on the pyrimidine ring by cytidine deaminase to 5'-deoxy-5-fluorouridine (Fig. 11.1) (3). Finally, the prodrug is converted to 5-FU by thymidine phosphorylase (TP), which is generally expressed at higher levels in most human cancers, including breast cancer, compared with the corresponding normal tissues (4).

Thymidine phosphorylase (TP) is a potent angiogenic factor that correlates with aggressive tumor biology and higher grade cancers, raising the possibility that part of capecitabine's antitumor activity might be mediated by an antiproliferative effect on tumor-associated neovasculature (5). Capecitabine's primary mechanism of action, however, is the same as that of 5-FU, namely the inactivation of thymidylate synthase (TS) by 2'-deoxy-5'-fluorouridine-5'-monophosphate (FdUMP) and interference with RNA processing via incorporation of 5'fluorouridine-5'-triphosphate (FUTP) into RNA (6).

5-Fluorouracil is catabolized into inactive metabolites by dihydropyrimidine dehydrogenase (DPD), which is also overexpressed in some human cancers (7). Intriguing preclinical data suggest that the antitumor activity of capecitabine against a variety of human cancer xenografts in mice is positively associated with higher ratios of TP to DPD (8). In addition, a recent study in patients with early-stage node-positive and node-negative breast cancer showed a correlation between the level of TP expression in the primary tumor and the effectiveness of adjuvant 5'-doxifluridine (DFUR) administered postoperatively (9). Doxifluridine is the capecitabine metabolite that is converted to 5-FU by TP. Standardization of protein and RNA-based assays for TP, DPD and TS is underway and will likely lead to the rational selection of capecitabine therapy for patients with breast cancer who are most likely to benefit.

Pharmacokinetic studies with oral capecitabine have shown peak plasma concentrations of 5-FU within 1.5 to 2 hours after capecitabine administration which then decline with half-lives in the range of 0.7 to 1.2 hours (10). Fasting conditions increase both the rate and extent of absorption of capecitabine, causing a 13% increase in the 5-FU area under the curve (AUC) (10,11). In patients with mild to moderate hepatic dysfunction, the AUCs of capecitabine, 5'DFUR and 5-FU are increased by 48%, 20% and 15%, respectively (12). Caution is needed, therefore, when administering capecitabine to patients with impaired hepatic dysfunction.

A recent study has examined the safety of capecitabine in colon cancer patients in relation to their renal function. Patients with an estimated creatinine clearance of 30 mL to 50

Enzymatic Activation of Capecitabine

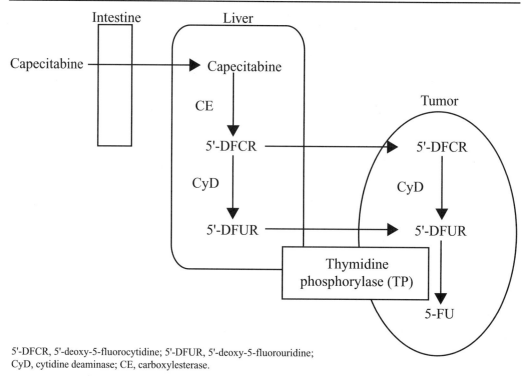

5'-DFCR, 5'-deoxy-5-fluorocytidine; 5'-DFUR, 5'-deoxy-5-fluorouridine;
CyD, cytidine deaminase; CE, carboxylesterase.

FIG. 11.1. Capecitabine has excellent oral bioavailability and is absorbed through intestines intact. It is then converted in the liver (middle box) to 5'DFCR and to 5'-DFUR, and then 5'-DFUR is converted to 5-FU preferentially at the tumor site. 5-FU, 5-fluorouracil.

mL per minute experienced a higher incidence of grade 3/4 toxicities than did patients with a creatinine clearance above 50 mL per minute, calculated according to the Cockroft and Gault formula (13,14). It is therefore recommended that in patients with moderate renal impairment (30 mL to 50 mL per min), the starting dose of capecitabine be reduced to 75% of the standard starting dose. Patients with severe renal impairment with a calculated creatinine clearance less than 30 mg per minute have even more pronounced toxicity with capecitabine (14). This has led to the recommendation by some investigators that capecitabine not be administered to patients with severe renal impairment (14).

PHASE 2 STUDIES OF SINGLE AGENT CAPECITABINE

The standard intermittent schedule of capecitabine of 1,250 mg/m^2 given twice a day for 14 days with a 7-day rest was chosen on the basis of phase 1 and 2 studies (15). Several phase 2 studies have subsequently defined the safety and efficacy of single-agent capecitabine in patients with metastatic breast cancer. Table 11.1 summarizes the phase 2

TABLE 11.1. Single-agent capecitabine phase 2 studies in metastatic breast cancer

Capecitabine dose/schedule	N	Prior therapy	ORR	Ref.
2,500 mg/m² daily on days 1–14	162	Anthracyclines and paclitaxel	20%	16
2,500 mg/m² daily on days 1–14	74	Anthracyclines and a taxane	24%	18
2,500 mg/m² daily on days 1–14	68	Anthracyclines and a taxane	25%	20
1,657 mg/m² daily on days 1–21 (every 28 days)	46	36% anthracycline 54% alkylator 64% 5-FU	28%	22
2,500 mg/m² daily on days 1–14 vs. i.v. CMF	61 32	46% adjuvant CT 80% adjuvant CT	30% 16%	23
2,500 mg/m² daily on days 1–14 vs. Paclitaxel 175 mg/m²	22 20	Anthracyclines Anthracyclines	36% 21%	24

CMF, cyclophosphamide/methotrexate/5-fluorouracil; 5-FU, 5-fluorouracil; ORR, objective response rate.

data for capecitabine when administered as a single agent.

The pivotal phase 2 trial that led to FDA approval of capecitabine was a multicenter study in patients with anthracycline- and paclitaxel-pretreated metastatic breast cancer. Standard-dose capecitabine was associated with an objective response rate of 20% (95% confidence interval [CI], 14% to 28%) in the 135 patients with measurable disease (16). In the 42 patients whose metastatic breast cancer had progressed while receiving anthracycline and paclitaxel, the objective response rate with capecitabine was 29%. An additional 40% of patients achieved stable disease for a median of 3.5 months. The median duration of response was 8.1 months and the median survival duration for the entire treated population (n = 162) was 12.6 months. Patients who had an objective response or stable disease with capecitabine had similar survival rates, indicating that stabilization of metastatic breast cancer confers clinical benefit. Of the 51 patients in this study who had considerable tumor-related pain at study entry, 47% experienced a durable 50% reduction in pain intensity as measured by the Memorial Visual Analog Scale (16).

Adverse events associated with capecitabine included grade 3 hand-and-foot syndrome (9.9%), grade 3/4 diarrhea (14%), grade 3/4 stomatitis (2.5%), and transient grade 3/4 hyperbilirubinemia (10%). Grade 4 adverse events were uncommon (3.4% of patients), as was neutropenia (grade 4 in 1.8% of patients), and alopecia did not occur. Close monitoring of coagulation parameters or phenytoin levels is required in patients taking coumadin or phenytoin because capecitabine may elevate the plasma concentrations of these two agents (17).

A second phase 2 study of capecitabine using the standard intermittent schedule was conducted in 74 patients with metastatic breast cancer previously treated with an anthracycline and either paclitaxel or docetaxel. The objective response rates were similar in the paclitaxel- and docetaxel-pretreated patients at 27% and 21%, respectively (18). The median durations of response and overall survival were nearly identical to those described in the initial pivotal phase 2 study. In addition, the adverse event profile was comparable in this study; 42% of patients in both trials required a 25% reduction in the capecitabine dose due to toxicity. Patients who underwent dose reductions were generally those who were benefiting from therapy and therefore received the agent over many cycles. No loss of clinical benefit was observed in patients requiring a 25% dose reduction (19). A single 25% dose reduction was generally sufficient to prevent a clinically significant recurrence of the adverse event.

These phase 2 studies established the significant antitumor activity of capecitabine in anthracycline- and taxane-pretreated metastatic breast cancer. A third phase 2 study of standard-dose capecitabine on the intermittent schedule in 68 anthracycline- and taxane-pretreated metastatic breast cancer patients also demonstrated an objective response rate of 25%, with an additional 47% of patients obtaining disease stabilization (20).

To evaluate the effect of dose on efficacy, a retrospective review from the M.D. Anderson Cancer Center of capecitabine dosing patterns was conducted in metastatic breast cancer patients who received starting doses between less than 2,100 mg/m^2 per day and 2,625 mg/m^2 per day. The mean starting dose was 2,230 mg/m^2 per day, and the mean tolerated starting dose was 2,035 mg/m^2 per day (21). No difference in antitumor activity or time-to-progression was noted within this range of capecitabine starting doses. The incidence of adverse events, including diarrhea, stomatitis and hand-and-foot syndrome, was lower with the lower starting doses. The investigators concluded that, due to an improved therapeutic index, this analysis supports a standard starting dose of 2,000 mg/m^2 per day.

A recent phase 2 study has explored lower-dose capecitabine (1,657 mg/m^2 daily for 3 weeks followed by a 1-week rest) in 50 patients with measurable metastatic breast cancer. Patients had been treated with no more than one prior chemotherapy regimen (anthracycline 36%, alkylating agent 54%, 5-FU 64%) (22). The objective response rate was 28% (95% CI: 16% to 43.5%) in 46 evaluable patients. An additional 24% of patients had stable disease for at least 6 months. Grade 3/4 hand-and-foot syndrome occurred in 18% of patients and an isolated and reversible elevation in serum bilirubin occurred in 10% of patients. Diarrhea and mucositis were rare. Thus, this dose and schedule of capecitabine has promising antitumor activity with a favorable safety profile and warrants further investigation.

RANDOMIZED PHASE 2 STUDIES OF CAPECITABINE VERSUS STANDARD CHEMOTHERAPY

Two randomized phase 2 studies have compared standard-dose, intermittent schedule capecitabine with single-agent paclitaxel or with intravenous CMF (cyclophosphamide, methotrexate and 5-FU).

In the first study, capecitabine was evaluated as first-line therapy for women greater than age 55 with measurable metastatic disease and was compared to a reference treatment of i.v. CMF (600/40/600 mg/m^2) given every 3 weeks (23). The 95 patients in this study had a median age of 69 and 70 years on the capecitabine and CMF arms, respectively; approximately one-fourth of the patients on each arm had been previously treated with adjuvant chemotherapy. The overall response rate in the capecitabine-treated group was 30% (95% CI: 19% to 43%), while in the CMF group the response rate was 16% (95% CI: 5% to 33%). There was no difference in median time to disease progression or overall survival. Alopecia and myelosuppression were less common with capecitabine than with CMF, while hand-and-foot syndrome and diarrhea were more common with capecitabine. Thirty-four percent of patients treated with capecitabine required treatment interruption and/or dose reduction, and 16% of patients discontinued treatment due to toxicity. A 25% dose reduction was generally effective in preventing the recurrence of treatment-related adverse events. Overall, capecitabine was found to have significant antitumor activity as first-line therapy for older women with metastatic breast cancer.

In the second study (24), 42 women with metastatic breast cancer previously treated with an anthracycline were randomized to standard-dose intermittent schedule capecitabine or to treatment with paclitaxel, 175 mg/m^2 over 3 hours given every 3 weeks. Accrual to this study was closed prematurely because of the difficulty encountered in randomizing women to an oral versus an intravenous therapy. In contrast to the first trial, the median age in this study was 52 years. The objective response rate observed with capecitabine treatment was 36% (95% CI: 17% to 59%) and with paclitaxel was 21% (95% CI: 6% to 46%). A higher percentage of patients treated with paclitaxel developed grade 3 or 4 toxicity (58% versus 22%). This discrepancy was mainly due to a higher incidence of neutropenia in the paclitaxel arm.

In summary, the objective response rate observed with capecitabine in anthracycline- and taxane-pretreated metastatic breast cancer has been demonstrated to be 20% to 25% in several phase 2 studies. The two randomized phase 2 studies above indicate that the response rate of capecitabine as first- or second-line therapy for metastatic breast cancer is approximately 30% to 36%. These data suggest that capecitabine is an acceptable treatment choice in patients with previously treated metastatic breast cancer, and its use may be considered a standard of care in this setting.

CAPECITABINE AND TAXANE COMBINATIONS

Studies of human breast cancer xenografts in nude mice have shown that both paclitaxel and docetaxel increase the tumor expression of TP by at least six-fold 4 to 6 days after taxane exposure (25). Further preclinical animal studies have shown synergistic antitumor activity against human breast cancer xenografts when capecitabine is combined with either paclitaxel or docetaxel. Interestingly, combining a taxane with either 5-FU or UFT (a fixed combination of Tegafur plus uracil) led to only additive antitumor activity. A recent in vivo study has also demonstrated that administering docetaxel on day 8 and capecitabine on days 1 to 14 to mice bearing human MX-1 breast cancer xenografts resulted in more potent and synergistic antitumor activity than did administering docetaxel on day 1 or day 15 in a 3-week regimen (26). In total, these preclinical data suggest a favorable biological interaction between the taxanes and capecitabine.

The synergistic effects of the taxanes and capecitabine may be due to upregulation of TP by the taxanes, leading to greater conversion of capecitabine to 5-FU at the tumor site. Data from the MX-1 human breast cancer xenograft model also suggest that the combination of day-8 docetaxel with capecitabine and its intermediate metabolite, 5′-deoxy-5-fluorouridine (5′d FUrd), has potent antitumor effects that may be separate from those mediated by enhanced TP expression (26).

Some clinical data confirm the clinical relevance of TP upregulation by capecitabine. Eight women with locally advanced breast cancer were treated with three cycles of docetaxel, (60 mg/m^2 given every 3 weeks), and tumor levels of TP were assessed on biopsies obtained prior to and after chemotherapy. Six of eight tumors demonstrated a significant increase in TP expression as determined by immunohistochemistry following docetaxel treatment (27). Thus, upregulation of TP appears to occur in a majority of human breast cancers in patients following docetaxel treatment.

To explore the feasibility and tolerability of combination therapy, a phase 1 study of docetaxel and capecitabine was conducted in 33 patients with advanced solid tumors. Two regimens were found to be tolerable: docetaxel 100 mg/m^2 on day 1 with capecitabine 825 mg/m^2 twice a day on days 1 to 14, and docetaxel 75 mg/m^2 on day 1 with capecitabine 1,250 mg/m^2 twice a day on days 1 to 14 (28). Each cycle was 3 weeks in length. No pharmacokinetic interactions between the two drugs were observed, and the associated toxicities were largely nonoverlapping. Dose-limiting toxicities were asthenia and neutropenia. Five patients with a variety of solid tumors had a complete or partial response.

Several phase 1 or 2 studies of paclitaxel in combination with capecitabine have also been conducted (Table 11.2). In one trial, 19 patients with metastatic breast cancer were treated with paclitaxel 175 mg/m^2 every three weeks and escalating doses of capecitabine in two divided daily doses for 14 days with a seven-day rest. The recommended combination doses were paclitaxel 175 mg/m^2 and capecitabine 1,650 mg/m^2 per day for 14 days (29). As anticipated, the dose-limiting toxicities of this combination were hand-and-foot syndrome and neutropenia. No major pharmacokinetic interactions between capecitabine and paclitaxel were observed. Nine of the 16 patients with measurable disease (56%) had an objective response.

Another phase 1 study combined paclitaxel (175 mg/m^2) with continuous administration of capecitabine in 17 patients with advanced solid tumors. The recommended dose of capecitabine was 1,331 mg/m^2 per day continuously (30). Major toxicities observed in this study included myelosuppression and diarrhea; significant hand-and-foot syndrome was not seen, probably

TABLE 11.2. Combination capecitabine and taxane studies

Regimen	N	Prior therapy	ORR	OS (mo)	Ref.
Capecitabine 2,500 mg/m^2 days 1–14 + Docetaxel 75 mg/m^2 day 1	511	Anthracyclines	42%	14.5	33
vs. Docetaxel 100 mg/m^2 day 1			30% $p = 0.006$	11.5 $p = 0.01$	
Capecitabine 1,650–2,000 mg/m^2 days 1–14 Paclitaxel 175 mg/m^2 day 1	16	Anthracyclines	56%	NR	29
Capecitabine 2,000 mg/m^2 days 1–14 Paclitaxel 175 mg/m^2 day 1	44	Anthracyclines	62%	NR	31
Capecitabine 1,650 mg/m^2 days 1–14 Paclitaxel 175 mg/m^2 day 1	37	None (n = 26) 2nd-line (n = 11)	49%	NR	32
Capecitabine 1,800 mg/m^2 days 1–14 Docetaxel 30 mg/m^2 weekly	12	Anthracyclines	50%	NR	34

NR, not reported; ORR, objective response rate; OS, overall survival.

owing to the relatively low dose of capecitabine. In addition, no pharmacokinetic interactions between the two drugs were observed.

A phase 2 study of paclitaxel (175 mg/m^2 every 3 weeks) with capecitabine (2,000 mg/m^2 per day for 14 days) was conducted in 73 patients with locally advanced or metastatic breast cancer that had progressed following anthracycline-based chemotherapy. In the 44 patients with measurable disease, the objective response rate was 62% (31). Ten percent of the patients developed grade 3 hand-and-foot syndrome and 11% had grade 3 or 4 neutropenia. Overall, this combination was generally well tolerated. A third phase 2 study of paclitaxel (175 mg/m^2) with capecitabine (1,650 mg/m^2 on days 1 to 14) showed an objective response rate of 49% in 37 patients (32). In this trial, 26 patients received the combination as first-line and 11 as second-line treatment for metastatic disease.

A large phase 2 study has recently led to FDA approval of capecitabine in combination with docetaxel for metastatic breast cancer patients who have been previously treated with an anthracycline. Five hundred eleven patients with advanced breast cancer were randomized to receive treatment with either single-agent docetaxel (100 mg/m^2 every 3 weeks) or with combined docetaxel (75 mg/m^2 every 3 weeks) plus capecitabine (1,250 mg/m^2 twice a day for 14 days) (33). The median age of the patients treated in this multination, global study was 52 years. In excess of 80% of patients in both groups had visceral metastatic disease, 60% had three or more sites of metastatic disease, and two-thirds of patients received study therapy as second- or third-line therapy for metastatic disease. The investigator-assessed objective response rates were 42% for combined docetaxel and capecitabine and 30% for docetaxel alone ($p = 0.006$). Median time to disease progression was significantly superior with the combination at 6.1 months versus 4.2 months for single-agent docetaxel ($p = 0.0001$). With a minimum of 15 months follow-up for all patients, overall survival significantly favored combination docetaxel and capecitabine; median overall survival with the combination was 14.5 months versus 11.5 months with docetaxel ($p = 0.0126$).

The one-year survival rates were 57% (95% CI: 51% to 63%) with the combination versus 47% (95% CI: 41% to 53%) with docetaxel alone. The survival curves separated markedly early in the course of therapy in this heavily tumor-burdened group of patients. In addition, the survival advantage of the combination was seen in the first-line, second-line, and third-line therapy patient subgroups. There were no imbalances in post-study cytotoxic, hormonal, or biologic therapies with two-thirds of patients receiving additional cytotoxic therapy. Fifteen percent of patients in the docetaxel treatment group received capecitabine at the time of disease progression. Neutropenia, neutropenic fever, arthralgias, and myalgias were more common with docetaxel alone, while diarrhea, stomatitis, and hand-and-foot syndrome were more common with the combination. No significant difference in quality of life was seen comparing the combination to single-agent docetaxel, although there was a trend towards improved quality of life after several months of therapy with the combination. Thus, the combination of docetaxel and capecitabine is the only cytotoxic therapy that has been demonstrated to provide a survival advantage over treatment with single-agent docetaxel or any other chemotherapy agent or combination in anthracycline-pretreated metastatic breast cancer patients.

An ongoing phase 1 and 2 study of weekly docetaxel (30 mg/m^2) plus capecitabine (1,800 mg/m^2 on days 1 to 14) on a 21-day cycle has shown a 50% response rate in the first 12 patients with anthracycline-pretreated metastatic breast cancer (34). Excessive lacrimation, asthenia, and nail loss have been observed. Further data are required to determine the potential role of this weekly regimen in clinical practice.

Summary

Single-agent Agent Capecitabine

- Level II evidence exists from several well-conducted phase 2 studies demonstrating that capecitabine has significant antitumor activity in anthracycline- and taxane-pretreated metastatic breast cancer patients. The objective response rates and clinical toxicities associated with capecitabine have been consistently documented in many phase 2 trials.
- Level III evidence exists from two retrospective studies as well as level II evidence from one prospective phase 2 study that lower doses of capecitabine—1,875 mg/m^2 to 2,100 mg/m^2 daily for 2 weeks or 1,657 mg/m^2 daily for 3 weeks—produce objective response and disease control rates similar to the FDA-approved dose of 2,500 mg/m^2.
- There is level III evidence available from a large retrospective analysis of renal function and the safety of capecitabine in colon cancer patients showing that patients with moderate renal impairment (calculated creatinine clearance 30 mL to 50 mL per minute) should be treated with a lower starting dose of capecitabine (1,900 mg/m^2 per day) and that capecitabine should be avoided in patients with a very low creatinine clearance (less than 30 mL per minute).

Capecitabine-Taxane Combination Therapy

- Level I evidence demonstrates that combined docetaxel and capecitabine produces greater overall response rates, time to disease progression, and overall survival in anthracycline-pretreated metastatic breast cancer patients than does docetaxel alone. The U.S. FDA has approved capecitabine in combination with docetaxel as treatment for anthracycline-pretreated metastatic breast cancer patients.
- Level II evidence demonstrates the significant antitumor activity and acceptable safety of combined paclitaxel given every 3 weeks and capecitabine.

FUTURE STUDIES

Adjuvant

Because of the significant overall survival advantage that has been demonstrated with combined capecitabine-docetaxel compared with full-dose docetaxel alone in anthracycline-pretreated metastatic breast cancer patients, this regimen will be evaluated in three adjuvant or neoadjuvant chemotherapy trials in patients with operable breast cancer.

The NSABP will compare doxorubicin and cyclophosphamide (AC) for four cycles followed by docetaxel for four cycles with AC followed by docetaxel-capecitabine as preoperative therapy in patients with operable breast cancer. US Oncology will conduct a study using the same regimens as adjuvant therapy in node-positive or high-risk node-negative breast cancer patients. Finally, CALGB is conducting an adjuvant phase 3 trial of single-agent capecitabine compared with the physician's choice of either four cycles of AC or six cycles of oral classical CMF in early stage breast cancer patients 65 years or older.

Metastatic Breast Cancer

Capecitabine is now an established part of the therapeutic armamentarium for patients with metastatic breast cancer. As noted above, the most pressing question is whether the overall survival advantage associated with capecitabine-docetaxel treatment in metastatic disease will improve the disease-free and overall survival of early-stage breast cancer patients who are treated with standard anthracycline-based chemotherapy. In regards to the further development of capecitabine in metastatic breast cancer, several phase 2 trials are underway which combine weekly docetaxel or paclitaxel with capecitabine on 21-day or 28-day cycles. These trials will help determine the efficacy and toxicity of these regimens and may lead to randomized studies.

Another area of substantial interest is combining capecitabine with biologic agents. For example, other ongoing phase 2 trials utilize capecitabine alone or in combination with docetaxel with trastuzumab, an anti-HER-2 antibody. A large, randomized phase 3 trial is being conducted comparing capecitabine alone to combined capecitabine and anti-vascular endothelial growth factor antibody, bevacizumab, (rhuMAb-VEGF) as therapy for anthracycline- and taxane-pretreated metastatic breast cancer patients. This latter study is one of the first to evaluate the effectiveness of an antiangiogenic therapy in the treatment of advanced breast cancer.

REFERENCES

1. Bunnell CA, Winer EP. Oral 5-FU analogues in the treatment of breast cancer. *Oncology* 1998;12:39–43 (suppl 7).
2. Hansen RM, Ryan L, Anderson T, et al. Phase III study of bolus versus infusion fluorouracil with or without cisplatin in advanced colorectal cancer. *J Natl Cancer Inst* 1996;88:668–674.
3. MacKean M, Planting A, Twelves C, et al. Phase I and pharmacologic study of intermittent twice-daily oral therapy with capecitabine in patients with advanced and/or metastatic cancer. *J Clin Oncol* 1998;16:2977–2985.
4. Fox SB, Westwood M, Moghaddam A, et al, The angiogenic factor platelet-derived endothelial growth factor/thymidine phosphorylase is up-regulated in breast cancer epithelium and endothelium. *Br J Cancer* 1996;73:275–280.
5. Takehayashi Y, Akiyama S, Akiba S, et al. Clinicopathologic and prognostic significance of an angiogenic factor, thymidine phosphorylase, in human colorectal carcinoma. *J Natl Cancer Inst* 1996;88:1110–1117.
6. Pinedo HM, Peters GF. Fluorouracil; Biochemistry and pharmacology. *J Clin Oncol* 1988;6:1653–1664.
7. Mori K, Hasegawa M, Nishida M, et al. Expression levels of thymidine phosphorylase and dihydropyrimidine dehydrogenase in various human tumor tissues. *Int J Oncol* 2000;17(1):33–38.
8. Ishikawa T, Sekiguchi F, Fukase Y, et al. Positive correlation between the efficacy of capecitabine and doxifluridine and the ratio of thymidine phosphorylase to dihydropyrimidine dehydrogenase activities in tumours in human cancer xenografts. *Cancer Res* 1998;58:685–690.
9. Takahashi H, Maeda Y, Watanabe K, et al. Correlation between elevated intratumoral thymidine phosphorylase and prognosis of positive breast carcinoma undergoing adjuvant doxifluridine treatment. *Int J Oncol* 2000;17:1205–1211.
10. Reigner B, Verweij J, Dirix L, et al. Effect of food on the pharmacokinetics of capecitabine and its metabolites following oral administration in cancer patients. *Clin Cancer Res* 1998;4:941–948.
11. Judson IR, Beale PJ, Trigo JM, et al. A human capecitabine excretion balance and pharmacokinetic study after administration of a single oral dose of 14C-labelled drug. *Invest New Drugs* 1999;17:49–56.
12. Reigner B, Glynne Jones R, Cassidy J, et al. Hepatic dysfunction due to liver metastases does not affect the bioactivation of Xeloda. *Proc Amer Soc Clin Oncol* 1998;17:224a (abstract 863).
13. Cockroft DW, Gault MH. Prediction of creatinine clearance from serum creatinine. *Nephron* 1976;16:31–41.
14. Cassidy J, Twelves C, Van Cutsem E, et al. First-line oral capecitabine therapy in metastatic colorectal cancer; a favorable safety profile compared with i.v. 5-fluorouracil (5-FU)/leucovorin. *Ann Oncol* 2002;4:566–575.
15. Findlay M, Cutsem E, Kocha W, et al. A randomized phase II study of Xeloda™ (capecitabine) in patients with advanced colorectal cancer. *Proc Am Soc Clin Oncol* 1997;16:227a.
16. Blum JL, Jones SE, Buzdar AM, et al. Multicenter phase II study of capecitabine in paclitaxel-refractory metastatic breast cancer. *J Clin Oncol* 1999;17:485–493.
17. Blum JL. The role of capecitabine, an oral enzymatically activated fluoropyrimidine, in the treatment of metastatic breast cancer. *The Oncologist* 2001;6:56–64.
18. Blum JL, Buzdar AM, Dieras V, et al. Phase II trial of Xeloda (capecitabine) in taxane-refractory metastatic breast cancer. *Proc Am Soc Clin Oncol* 1999;18:107a (abstract 403).
19. O'Shaughnessy J, Blum J. A retrospective evaluation of the impact of dose reduction in patients treated with

Xeloda (capecitabine) *Proc Amer Soc Clin Oncol* 2000; 19:104a (abstract 400).
20. Reichardt P, von Minckwitz G, Luck Hj, et al. Capecitabine: An active and well tolerated treatment option for patients with metastatic breast cancer recurring after taxane-containing chemotherapy. Results of a multicenter phase II trial. *Breast Ca Res Treat* 2000; 64:83 (abstract 331).
21. Michaud LB, Gauthier MA, Wojdylo JR, et al. Improved therapeutic index with lower dose capecitabine in metastatic breast cancer (MBC) patients (pts). *Proc Amer Soc Clin Oncol* 2000;19:104a (abstract 402).
22. Kusama M, Sano M, Ikeda T, et al. A phase II study of Xeloda™ (capecitabine) in patients with advanced metastatic breast carcinoma—The Cooperative Study Group of capecitabine for breast carcinoma. *Proc Am Soc Clin Oncol* 2001;20:446 (abstract 1924).
23. O'Shaughnessy JA, Blum J, Moiseyenko V, et al. Randomized, open-label, phase II trial of oral Capecitabine (Xeloda®) vs. a reference arm of intravenous CMF (cyclophosphamide, methotrexate and 5-fluorouracil) as first-line therapy for advanced/metastatic breast cancer. *Ann Oncol* 2001;12:1247–1254.
24. Moiseenko VM, O'Reilly, Dalbot DC, et al. A comparative randomized phase II study of Xeloda (capecitabine) and paclitaxel in breast cancer progressing after anthracycline antibiotics. *Vopr Onkol* 2000;46:285–289.
25. Sawada N, Ishikawa T, Fukase Y, et al. Induction of thymidine phosphorylase activity and enhancement of Capecitabine efficacy by Taxol/Taxotere in human cancer xenografts. *Clin Cancer Res* 1998;4:1013–1019.
26. Fujimoto-Ouchi K, Tanaka Y, Tominaga T. Schedule dependency of antitumor activity in combination therapy with capecitabine/5 fluorouridine and docetaxel in breast cancer models. *Clin Cancer Res* 2001;4:1079–1086.
27. Kurosumi M, Tabei T, Suemasu K, et al. Enhancement of immunohistochemical reactivity for thymidine phosphorylase in breast carcinoma cells after administration of docetaxel as a neoadjuvant chemotherapy in advanced breast cancer patients. *Oncol Rep* 2000; 5:945–948.
28. Pronk LC, Vasey P, Sparreboom A, et al. A phase I and pharmacokinetic study of the combination of capecitabine and docetaxel patients with advanced solid tumours. *Br J Cancer* 2000;83:22–29.
29. Villalona-Calero, MA, Blum JL, Jones SE, et al. A phase I and pharmacologic study of capecitabine and paclitaxel in breast cancer patients. *Ann Oncol* 2001; 12:605–614.
30. Villalona-Calero MA, Weiss GR, Burris HA, et al. Phase I and pharmacokinetic study of the oral fluoropyrimidine capecitabine in combination with paclitaxel in patients with advanced solid malignancies. *J Clin Oncol* 1999;17:1915–1925.
31. Perez-Manga G, Constenla M, Guillem V, et al. Efficacy and safety of capecitabine (Xeloda®) in combination with paclitaxel in patients with locally advanced or metastatic breast cancer preliminary results of a phase II study. *Breast Cancer Res Treat* 2000;64;124 (abstract 535).
32. Meza LA, Amin B, Horsey M, et al. A phase II study of capecitabine in combination with paclitaxel as first or second line therapy in patients with metastatic breast cancer (MBC). *Proc Amer Soc Clin Oncol* 2001;20: 70b (abstract 2029).
33. O'Shaughnessy J, Miles D, Vukelja S, et al. Superior survival with docetaxel/capecitabine combination therapy in anthracycline-pretreated patients with advanced breast cancer: phase III trial results. *J Clin Oncol* (submitted).
34. Tonkin K, Scarfe AG, Koske S, et al. Preliniary results of a phase I/II study of weekly docetaxel (Taxotere®) combined with intermittent capecitabine (Xeloda®) for patients with anthracycline pre-treated metastatic breast cancer. *Proc Am Soc Clin Oncol* 2001;20:67b (abstract 2016).

12
Vinorelbine

Laurent Zelek and Marc Spielmann

The laboratory data that showed vinca alkaloids produced an antileukemic effect in mice prompted intense research which has led to the clinical use of vincristine sulfate, vinblastine sulfate, vindesine and, later, vinorelbine tartrate (VNB, Pierre Fabre Médicament, Boulogne, France). VNB differs chemically from other vinca alkaloids through an original synthesis process that generates substitutions on the catharantine moiety. Its antitumor activity, demonstrated in experimental studies, led to clinical studies which have confirmed its value in a broad spectrum of malignancies, including breast cancer.

Like other vinca alkaloids which exhibit selective activity against mitotic microtubules, VNB binds to tubulin, thereby interfering with microtubule assembly. Differences between neurons and other cell types in their tubulin-associated protein content probably account for the decreased neurotoxicity (peripheral neuropathy) of VNB compared to that of other vinca alkaloids.

VNB concentration in plasma decays according to a three-compartment model with a long terminal phase elimination half-life: $T_{1/2}\alpha = 2–6$ minutes; $T_{1/2}\beta = 1.9 \pm 0.8$ hours; $T_{1/2}\gamma = 40 \pm 18$ hours. There is initial high protein binding (80%) that decreases to 50% after 96 hours. The pharmacokinetic profile of VNB is not strikingly different from that of other vinca alkaloids. Its metabolism and elimination have been studied in animals and humans following the administration of radiolabelled VNB. In summary: (a) intense hepatic extraction occurs and less than 60% of the infused dose is recovered in the vascular effluent within the first two hours; (b) biliary excretion is active with a concentration in bile that is 7,000-fold higher than in the effluent; (c) less than 12% of VNB is found in urine within 72 hours (1).

SINGLE-AGENT ACTIVITY

At least thirteen phase 2 studies (2–14) have investigated the activity of single-agent VNB against breast cancer and are summarized in Table 12.1. The commonest scheduling was weekly dosing (2–4) starting at a dose of 30 mg/m^2 per week. Alternative schedules such as 5-day continuous infusion have been proposed but were not demonstrated to be superior to weekly VNB (5,6); using a three consecutive day schedule is not recommended because of hematological toxicity (7).

Response rates ranging from 34% (4) to 50% (3) are consistently reported with a median time to treatment failure of about 6 months and a median survival exceeding 1 year (2–4), even when given as second-line therapy after failure with anthracyclines (4). No other vinca alkaloid has attained this level of activity in breast cancer; only anthracyclines and taxanes exhibit comparable potency as second-line treatment for metastatic breast malignancies.

These trials consistently reported excellent tolerance and low toxicity. The main side effect documented was grade 3/4 neutropenia which occurred in 75% of patients but fever was not invariable. Furthermore, quality of life analyses suggested that patients with advanced breast cancer receiving weekly VNB maintained a satisfactory score and that, in some respects, VNB could be considered comparable to or even better than other salvage agents (8).

Single-agent VNB has also been evaluated in patients known to be at risk of more severe chemotherapy-induced side effects, i.e., elderly patients with advanced breast cancer or those

TABLE 12.1. *Clinical trials with single-agent vinorelbine*

Author (ref.)	Main selection criterion	Regimen	Patients (n =)	Main grade 3–4 toxicities (%)	Response rate (complete responses)	Median time to progression
Phase trials						
Fumoleau (2)	First-line stage IV	VNB 30 mg/m^2/week	157	Neutropenia (72%)	41% (7%)	6 mos
Weber (4)	First- and second-line stage IV	VNB 30 mg/m^2/week	107	Neutropenia	34% (11%)	34 weeks
Toussaint (5)	Stage IV, up to third-line	VNB 8 mg/m^2 d1 (bolus) followed by: 5.5–10 mg/m^2/d, d1 to 4 (continuous infusion)	64	Neutropenia (52.2%)	36% (3%)	6 mos
Vogel (10)	> 60 years old stage IV	VNB 30 mg/m^2/week	56	Neutropenia 80%	38% (4%)	6 mos
Garcia-Conde (3)	First-line stage IV	VNB 30 mg/m^2/week	54	Neutropenia (71%)	50% (2%)	9 mos
Ibrahim (6)	Stage IV, salvage therapy	VNB 8 mg/m^2 d1 (bolus) followed by: 11 mg/m^2/d, d1 to 4 (continuous infusion)	47	Neutropenia Mucositis	16% (2/44)	4.3 mos
Livingstone (13)	Stage IV, taxane-refractory	VNB 30 mg/m^2/week + G-CSF	40	Neutropenia (58%)	25%	13 weeks
Zelek (15)	Stage IV after failure with taxanes	VNB 30 mg/m^2/week without G-CSF	40	Neutropenia (52.5%) Neuropathy (12.5%)	25% (0%)	6 mos
Trillet-Lenoir (17)	First-line; locally advanced or stage IV	VNB 60 to 80 mg/m^2/ week	36	Neutropenia (14%) Nausea, vomiting (14%)	30% (1/36)	NA
Sorio (9)	> 65 years old stage IV	VNB 30 mg/m^2 d1 & 8 (d1 = d21)	25	Neutropenia (37%)	30% (0)	5 mos
Fazeny (16)	Stage IV after failure with taxanes	VNB 30 mg/m^2 d1 & 15 (then q 21d after 4th cycle)	14	Neuropathy (4/14 pts)	0%	—
Udom (14)	Stage IV, two prior regimens	VNB 25 mg/m^2 q 14d	20	Neutropenia (grade 1–3: 35%) Neutropenic fever (1/20 pts)	35% (0%)	4 mos
Randomized trial						
Jones (12)	Stage IV after failure with anthracyclines	VNB 30 weekly versus MEL 25 d1 (q28d)	115 64	Neutropenia (75%) Neutropenia (69%) Thrombopenia (59%)	16% (5%) versus 9% (2%)[a]	35 weeks versus 31 weeks[a]

[a]Statistically significant difference.
MEL, melphalan; NA, data not available; TTP, time to progression; VNB, vinorelbine.

with liver metastases. In patients older than 60 years with advanced breast cancer, findings reported are similar to those found in younger patients, especially regarding tolerance; no pharmacokinetic rationale justifies reducing the dose of VNB in elderly patients (9,10). In patients with liver metastases, a VNB dose reduction is warranted in the event of severe liver failure but is not mandatory in patients with moderate hepatic insufficiency (11).

Of particular interest is the study by Jones et al. (12) which is the only one to have compared single-agent VNB to a more conventional salvage regimen after failure with first-line anthracycline-based therapy. A total of 150 patients were randomized to receive either weekly VNB at a starting dose of 30 g/m^2 per week or intravenous melphalan given every 28 days at a dose of 25 mg/m^2. Despite the moderate dose intensity delivered (19.3 mg/m^2 per week), essentially limited by delays in hematological recovery, VNB proved to be significantly more effective than melphalan, whatever the endpoints considered: (a) one-year survival was 35.7% versus 21.7% ($p = 0.034$); (b) median time to progression was 12 versus 8 weeks ($p < 0.001$); and (c) the objective response rate was 16% (complete responses: 5%) versus 9% (complete responses: 2%) ($p = 0.06$). Although all patients had previously received anthracycline-based chemotherapy (CT), tolerance remained acceptable. In particular, only 10% of patients had to be admitted for febrile neutropenia whereas 75% experienced grade 3/4 neutropenia. Moreover, it is noteworthy that quality of life was not impaired with VNB. This randomized study is among the very few that demonstrate a survival benefit with second-line CT in metastatic breast cancer; taxanes were in the investigational arm in all the others.

More recent studies (13–15) confirm that single-agent VNB should continue to be included in the most active regimens after failure with taxanes. Dose intensity appears to be a crucial issue, and the suboptimal schedule of the only negative trial (16) probably explains its results. With weekly schedules, however, objective responses have been reported at 25% with delivered dose intensities of 27.7 mg/m^2 per week plus G-CSF (13) and 22.5 mg/m^2 per week without G-CSF (15). In this population, the limiting toxicity is not only hematologic but also neurologic (peripheral neuropathy or ileus) (15,16). Given this critical adverse effect, caution should be exercised when using G-CSF to maximize dose intensity.

These latter studies demonstrate that VNB continues to be one of the most active salvage therapies after failure with gold-standard regimens including taxanes. The absence of cross-resistance with other agents and a favorable tolerance profile make VNB highly attractive for combination regimens.

MULTIAGENT REGIMENS INCLUDING VINORELBINE

The results of the first prospective randomized phase 3 trial comparing a two-drug combination with VNB (VNB 25 mg/m^2 days 1 and 8 plus doxorubicin 50 mg/m^2 day 1) versus a standard FAC regimen were published relatively recently (18). A total of 177 patients (of whom 170 were evaluable) were randomly assigned to one of the two treatment arms. As response rates (74% and 75%) and median survival (17.3 and 17.8 months) were similar in each arm, the authors concluded that the activity of VNB plus doxorubicin was equivalent to that of a standard three-drug schedule. The unbalanced demographic—that only 25% of the patients in the control arm had previously received adjuvant therapy versus 52% in the investigational arm—should be understood to disadvantage VNB since exposure to adjuvant therapy reduces the likelihood of achieving a response to a first-line metastatic regimen (19). Although the authors did not find that previous adjuvant therapy had an adverse effect on response, the study population is too small to really appreciate the impact of prior exposure to anthracyclines. Noteworthy are the improved response rates and survival obtained in patients treated with VNB plus doxorubicin in the subgroup with liver metastases.

Two other trials with a doxorubicin-based control arm have been published (20,21). The most recent from Namer et al. (21) compared VNB plus mitoxantrone (MV) versus FAC. The authors concluded that MV represents a chemotherapy combination with equivalent efficacy to standard FAC/FEC and improved results for patients who have previously received adjuvant chemotherapy (OR rate 33% versus 13%, $p = 0.025$; PFS 8 months versus 5 months, $p = 0.0007$). Toxicity must be balanced to allow for increased hematological suppression and risk of febrile neutropenia with MV compared with a higher risk of subjectively unpleasant side-effects such as nausea/vomiting and alopecia with FAC/FEC. The National Cancer Institute of Canada trial (20) comparing VNB plus doxorubicin versus doxorubicin alone found no significant difference in response rates, time to failure, or survival. Because of the weak statistical power of these trials, there is still no definitive answer to whether VNB plus anthracycline regimens are superior to standard regimens in selected subgroups as suggested by Namer et al. (21). The last randomized trial of interest (22) compared VNB (25 mg/m^2 days 1 and 5) plus fluorouracil (750 mg/m^2 per day day 1 to 5) versus Taxotere (100 mg/m^2 every 21 days). Taxane-based regimens can now be regarded as the gold standard in second-line

TABLE 12.2. Vinorelbine-containing regimens

Author (ref.)	Main selection criterion	Regimen[a]	Patients (n =)	Main grade 3–4 toxicities (% of patients)	Response rate (complete responses)	Median time to progression
(i) Vinorelbine + anthracycline						
Adenis (25)	Neo-adjuvant stage II & III	VNB 25 mg/m² d1 & 8 MXT 10 mg/m² d1	104	Neutropenia (83%)	64% of downstaging allowing conservative surgery	—
Spielmann (23)	First-line stage IV	VNB 50 d1 & 8 DOX 50 d1	89	Neutropenia (41%)	74% (21%)	12 mos
Llombart-Cussac (27)	First-line stage IV	VNB 25 mg/m² d1 & 8 MXT 10–12 mg/m² d1	66	Neutropenia (46%)	49% (6%)	7 mos
Nistico (29)	First-line stage IV	VNB 25 mg/m² weekly EPI 90 mg/m² weekly + G-CSF	52	Neutropenia (39%)	77% (19%)	10 mos
Baldini (28)	First-line stage IV	VNB 25 mg/m² d1 & 8 EPI 90 mg/m² d1	51	Neutropenia (70%)	61.7% (8.5%)	10 mos
Chollet (26)	Neo-adjuvant T<3cm with adverse prognostic factors	VNB 25 mg/m² d1 & 4 THP 20 mg/m² d1 to 3 CPM 300 mg/m² d1 to 4 5-FU 400 mg/m² d1 to 4	50	Neutropenia (81%) Anemia (25%) Thrombopenia (20%)	88% (51%) including pCR 30%	—
Blomqvist (24)	Stage IV dose-finding study	VNB 15 d1; 20 d1; 20 d1 & 8 (3 levels) EPI 60 d1	40	Neutropenia (75%)*	60% (20%)*	5.1 mos[a]
(ii) Vinorelbine + fluorouracile						
Dieras (30)	First-line stage IV	VNB 30 mg/m² d1 & 5 5-FU 750 mg/m² d1 to 5 (inf)	63	Neutropenia (90%) Mucositis (37%)	61.6% (12.6%)	8.4 mos
Kornek (34)	First- and second-line stage IV	VNB 40 mg/m² d1 & 14 5-FU 400 mg/m² d1 to 5 (iv) LLV 100 mg/m² d1 to 5 + G-CSF	53	Neutropenia (36%) Mucositis (6%)	1st-line: 59% (13%) 2nd-line: 19% (0%)	1st-line: 10.5 mos 2nd-line: 7 mos
Nole (32)	First-line stage IV Phase I-II with dose-escalation	VNB 25–30 mg/m² d1 & 3 5-FU 350 mg/m² d1 to 3 (iv) LV 100 mg/m² d1 to 3	45	Neutropenia (77%)	62% (18%)	10 mos
Zambetti (31)	Previously treated stage IV	VNB 20 mg/m² d1 & 6 5-FU 700 mg/m² d1 to 5 (inf)	28	Neutropenia (20%)	61% (14%)	8 mos
(iii) Vinorelbine + alkylating agents						
Campisi (36)	Anthracycline-resistant stage IV (phase I-II)	VNB 25 or 30 mg/m² d1, 25 mg/m² d1 & 8 IFM 1,500–2,000 mg/m² d1 to 3	42	Neutropenia (33%)	36.5% (4.8%)	7 mos
Fabi (35)	Second-line stage IV	VNB 30 mg/m² d1 & 8 TTP 12 mg/m² d1 & 8	33	Neutropenia (72%) Anemia (48%)	28% (6%)	9 mos
(iv) Vinorelbine + mitomycin						
Vici (36)		VNB 25 mg/m² d1 & 8 MMC 15 mg/m² d1	60	Neutropenia (17%)	40% (5%)	7 mos
Scheithauer (37)	Second-line stage IV	VNB 30 mg/m² d1 MMC 10 mg/m² d1	34	Neutropenia (12%) Thrombopenia (15%)	35% (6%)	6.3 mos

Study	Setting	Regimen	N	Toxicity	Response (CR)	Duration
(v) Vinorelbine + CDDP						
Ray-Coquard (39)	Previously treated stage IV	VNB 6 mg/m² d1 (i.v.), 6 mg/m² d1 to 5 (inf) CDDP 20 mg/m² d1 to 5	58	Neutropenia (78%) Thrombopenia (12%) Neuropathy (5%)	41% (3%)	9.2 mos
Shamseddine (40)	Previously treated stage IV	VNB 25 mg/m² d1 & 8 CDDP 30 mg/m² d1 to 3	23	Thrombopenia (27%) Neutropenia (9.2%)	61% (26%)	4 mos
(vi) Vinorelbine + taxanes						
Romero Acuna (44)	First-line stage IV	VNB 30 mg/m² d1 & 8 TXL 135 mg/m² d1	49	Neutropenia (46/49) Neuropathy (grade 1/2 : 67% ; no grade 3)	60% (7%)	7 mos
Michelotti (41)	Stage IV anthracycline-pretreated	VNB 25 mg/m² d1 & 8 or 3 TXL 135 mg/m² d1	37	Neutropenia (97%)	38%	6.5 mos
Tortoriello (43)	Pretreated stage IV Phase I/II study	VNB 30 mg/m² d1 TXL 90–210 mg/m² d1 +/- G-CSF	34	Neutropenia (2 pts at the 5th dose level) Neuropathy (3 pts at the 6th dose level)	38% (9%)	12 mos
Ellis (45)	Stage IV anthracycline-pretreated	VNB mg/m² d 8 & 15 TXL mg/m² d1 to 4 (inf) + G-CSF	32	Neutropenia Neuropathy (6%)	50% (22%)	6.1 mos
Budman (46)	Stage IV Phase I dose-finding study	VNB 7–13 mg/m² d1,2,3 TXL 135–200 mg/m² d3 +/- G-CSF	28	Neutropenia (G-CSF required after 1st dose level) myalgia, fatigue (with VNB 13 mg/m²/d + TXL 200 mg/m²)	12/25	NA
Fumoleau (42)	First-line stage IV Phase I dose-finding study	VNB 20–22.5 mg/m² d1 & 5 TXT 60–100 mg/m² d1	27	Neutropenic fever (3 pts at 3rd dose level)	66% (80% OR at the highest dose level)	NA
(vii) Vinorelbine + trastuzumab						
Burstein (52)	Stage IV	VNB 25 mg/m²/week + trastuzumab 4 mg/kg x1, 2 mg/kg/week thereafter	40	Neutropenia (43%) Neuropathy (grade 1–2: 48%) Heart failure (grade 2: 3/40 pts)	75% (3/40)	22 weeks -1st line: 34 weeks -2nd line: 16 weeks
(viii) Randomized trials – order of size						
Norris (20)	First- and second-line stage IV	VNB 25 mg/m² d1 & 8 DOX 50 mg/m² d1 versus DOX 70 mg/m² d1	151	Neutropenia (86)	35% (NA)	6.9 mos
Namer (21)	First-line stage IV	VNB 25 mg/m² d1 & 8 MXT 12 mg/m² d1 versus 5-FU 500 mg/m² d1 DOX or EPI 50 mg/m² d1 CPM 500 mg/m² d1	152 142	Neutropenia (87) Neutropenia (NA)	30% (NA) 35.5% (NA)	6.4 mos 8 mos
			139	Neutropenia (NA)	33.3% (NA)	5 mos[b]

Continued

TABLE 12.2. Continued

Author (ref.)	Main selection criterion	Regimen[a]	Patients (n)	Main grade 3–4 toxicities (% of patients)	Response rate (complete responses)	Median time to progression
(viii) Randomized trials – order of size (cont.)						
Blajman (18)	First-line stage IV	VNB 25 mg/m² d1 & 8 DOX 50 mg/m² d1 versus 5-FU 500 mg/m² d1 DOX 50 mg/m² d1 CPM 500 mg/m² d1	85 85	Neutropenia (7%) Neutropenia (7%)	75% (6) 74% (13)	17.8 mos 17.3 mos
Bonneterre (22)	Stage IV after failure with anthracyclines	NVB 25 mg/m² d1 & 5 5-FU 750 mg/m² d1 to 5 (inf) versus TXT 100 mg/m² d1	45 46	Neutropenia (65%) Neutropenia (78%)	44% 54%	6 mos 8 mos

[a]At highest dose level.
[b]In pretreated patients ($p = 0.0007$), in naive patients (no adjuvant chemotherapy), FAC/FEC is significantly better (9 vs 6 months).

CDDP, cisplatinum; CPM, cyclophosphamide; DOX, doxorubicin; EPI, epirubicin; 5-FU, fluorouracil; IFM, ifosfamide; inf, infusional; i.v., intravenous bolus; LLV, L-leucovorin; LV, leucovorin; MMC, mitomycin; MXT, mitoxantrone; THP, pirarubicin; TTP, Thiotepa; TXL, paclitaxel; TXT, docetaxel; VNB, vinorelbine.

therapy: the objective response rate and the duration of response were 44% and 6 months, and 54% and 8 months, respectively.

A variety of pilot studies have been published in which VNB was combined with various cytotoxics: anthracyclines, taxanes, fluorouracil, ifosfamide, and mitomycin (23–49). They are listed in Table 12.2. They all demonstrated excellent feasibility and encouraging response rates. Whatever the regimen considered, neutropenia was the most frequent limiting toxicity with grade 3/4 occurring in about 75% of the patients; it chiefly led to deferral of treatment and/or dose reductions rather than to febrile neutropenia, which was observed in no more than 10% of patients.

VNB-containing regimens are rarely used as neo-adjuvant treatment (25,26). The provocative pathologic response rate of 30% yielded in the series by Chollet et al. (26) is among the highest ever reported in the literature at the expense of severe, although not life-threatening, hematological toxicity. Further investigations are needed to corroborate these results.

Recent trials published (41–49) combined taxanes with VNB. A solid biological rationale supports such combinations since it has been suggested that resistance to taxanes could be mediated *in vitro* by excess depolymerized tubulin produced by vinca alkaloids, thereby increasing the likelihood of cell death (50). The absence of cross-resistance with taxanes and encouraging response rates after failure with taxanes observed in two studies (13,15) should be emphasized. All published trials have demonstrated the feasibility of taxane-VNB regimens despite severe but manageable hematologic toxicity; the incidence of neuropathy is below what could have been expected (Table 12.2). As weekly taxanes have proved capable of reversing resistance to conventional every-3-week schedules in some patient groups, it may be interesting to combine them with weekly VNB as a salvage regimen. Preliminary results with such schedules are, however, conflicting (48,49). Amid the wide variety of schedules combining taxanes and VNB, no particular one has proven superior in terms of either tolerance or efficiency. This fact contrasts strongly with the results of experimental studies, which demonstrated that the cytotoxicity of such combinations is exceedingly schedule-dependent (50).

TRASTUZUMAB-VINORELBINE COMBINATION

The synergism observed in preclinical models of trastuzumab paired with VNB (51) and its properties, such as weekly schedule of administration, lack of cardiac toxicity, and minimal alopecia, made this combination attractive. Burstein et al. (52) recently reported impressive results in a population of 40 HER-2-positive women (+3 by immunohistochemistry, n = 30; +2, n = 10), 29 of whom had received anthracyclines (n = 8), taxanes (n = 6) or both (n = 15) as part of previous therapy. The principal endpoint for this study was the OR rate expressed as intent-to-treat results. Responses were observed in 30 of 40 patients (75%; 95% confidence interval 57% to 89%) with 24 of 30 in 3+ overexpressing patients (80%). Patients receiving this regimen as first-line therapy had longer TTP (34 weeks versus 16 weeks, $p = 0.06$) and overall survival (median not reached versus 77.5 weeks, $p = 0.005$) than did patients receiving this treatment as second- or third-line therapy. This combination was well tolerated, with its only grade 4 toxicity being neutropenia. No patient had symptomatic heart failure but grade 2 toxicity was reported in three patients, associated with prior cumulative dose of doxorubicin in excess of 240 mg/m^2 and borderline preexisting cardiac function. Weekly VNB may be a useful foundation for combination treatments with biologic agents when protracted exposure is needed.

CONCLUSION

The as yet unresolved question is whether VNB should be considered as salvage (i.e., second-line or later) CT for metastatic breast cancer or as a component of first-line combinations containing other relevant drugs or biologics.

From the results of published trials, it can be concluded that:

(i) VNB is one of the most active agents against breast cancer with a favorable tolerance profile, even in patients at risk of severe side effects such as the elderly or subjects with liver involvement (with the proviso of dose reduction in patients with raised bilirubin/high transaminases) (level of evidence: 2). When used as a single agent, the schedule of choice seems to be weekly administration at a starting dose of 30 mg/m^2 per week in pretreated patients. However, this dose does not appear to be feasible mainly because of delays in hematologic recovery (level of evidence: 3).

(ii) No cross resistance is observed with other major drugs (i.e., taxanes and anthracyclines), and VNB is valuable as salvage therapy even in taxane-refractory patients (level of evidence: 2) although it is less effective than docetaxel given as second-line therapy after failure with anthracyclines (level of evidence: 3). These facts, together with its tolerance profile, provide a clinical rationale for first-line combination regimens.

(iii) Regimens combining VNB and other agents are feasible and as effective as other standard CT combinations (level of evidence: 2). In such regimens, VNB was usually given at a dose of 20 mg to 30 mg/m^2 per week on days 1 and 3, 5 or 8 with optional growth factor (G-CSF) support. Whether one combination has any advantage over the others remains to be established.

Because of its convenient administration and favorable tolerance profile allowing long-term therapy, there is considerable opportunity for combination regimens with new biological agents such as trastuzumab.

Acknowledgment: The authors are grateful to Lorna Saint Ange for editing.

REFERENCES

1. Marty M, Extra JM, Dieras V, et al. In: Cvitkovic E, Droz JP, Armand JP, Khoury S, eds. *Handbook of chemotherapy in clinical oncology*. Scientific Communication International, Jersey, 1993;317–326.
2. Fumoleau P, Delgado FM, Delozier T, et al. Phase II trial of weekly intravenous vinorelbine in first-line advanced breast cancer chemotherapy. *J Clin Oncol* 1993; 11(7):1245–1252.
3. Garcia-Conde J, Lluch A, Martin M, et al. Phase II trial of weekly IV vinorelbine in first-line advanced breast cancer chemotherapy. *Ann Oncol* 1994;5(9):854–857.
4. Weber BL, Vogel C, Jones S, et al. Intravenous vinorelbine as first-line and second-line therapy in advanced breast cancer. *J Clin Oncol* 1995;13(11):2722–2730.
5. Toussaint C, Izzo J, Spielmann M, et al. Phase I/II trial of continuous infusion vinorelbine for advanced breast cancer. *J Clin Oncol* 1994;12(10):2102–2112.
6. Ibrahim NK, Rahman Z, Valero V, et al. Phase II study of vinorelbine administered by 96-hour infusion in patients with advanced breast carcinoma. *Cancer* 1999; 86(7):1251–1257.
7. Havlin KA, Ramirez MJ, Legler CM, et al. Inability to escalate vinorelbine dose intensity using a daily ×3 schedule with and without filgrastim in patients with metastatic breast cancer. *Cancer Chemother Pharmacol* 1999;43(1):68–72.
8. Bertsch LA, Donaldson G. Quality of life analyses from vinorelbine (Navelbine) clinical trials of women with metastatic breast cancer. *Semin Oncol* 1995;22(2 Suppl 5):45–53; discussion 53–54.
9. Sorio R, Robieux I, Galligioni E, et al. Pharmacokinetics and tolerance of vinorelbine in elderly patients with metastatic breast cancer. *Eur J Cancer* 1997;33(2): 301–303.
10. Vogel C, O'Rourke M, Winer E, et al. Vinorelbine as first-line chemotherapy for advanced breast cancer in women 60 years of age or older. *Ann Oncol* 1999; 10(4):397–402.
11. Robieux I, Sorio R, Borsatti E, et al. Pharmacokinetics of vinorelbine in patients with liver metastases. *Clin Pharmacol Ther* 1996;59(1):32–40.
12. Jones S, Winer E, Vogel C, et al. Randomized comparison of vinorelbine and melphalan in anthracycline-refractory advanced breast cancer. *J Clin Oncol* 1995; 13(10):2567–2574.
13. Livingston RB, Ellis GK, Gralow JR, et al. Dose-intensive vinorelbine with concurrent granulocyte colony-stimulating factor support in paclitaxel-refractory metastatic breast cancer. *J Clin Oncol* 1997;15(4):1395–1400.
14. Udom DI, Vigushin DM, Linardou H, et al. Two weekly vinorelbine: administration in patients who have received at least two prior chemotherapy regimens for advanced breast cancer. *Eur J Cancer* 2000; 36:177–182.
15. Zelek L, Barthier S, Riofrio M, et al. Weekly vinorelbine is an effective palliative regimen after failure with anthracyclines and taxanes in metsatatic breast cancer. *Cancer* 2001;92(9):62–72.
16. Fazeny B, Zifko U, Meryn S, et al. Vinorelbine-induced neurotoxicity in patients with advanced breast cancer pretreated with paclitaxel—a phase II study. *Cancer Chemother Pharmacol* 1996;39(1–2): 150–156.
17. Trillet-Lenoir V, Delozier T, Lichinister M, et al. A phase II study of oral Vinorelbine (NVBo) in first line locally advanced/breast cancer (ABC) chemotherapy, preliminary results. *Proc Annu Meet Am Soc Clin Oncol* 2001;20:A185.

18. Blajman C, Balbiani L, Block J, et al. A prospective, randomized phase III trial comparing combination chemotherapy with cyclophosphamide, doxorubicin, and 5-fluorouracil with vinorelbine plus doxorubicin in the treatment of advanced breast carcinoma. *Cancer* 1999; 85(5):1091–1097.
19. Bonadonna G, Valagussa P, Moliterni A, et al. Adjuvant cyclophosphamide, methotrexate, and fluorouracil in node-positive breast cancer: the results of 20 years of follow-up: *N Engl J Med* 1995;332(14):901–906.
20. Norris B, Pritchard K.I, James K, et al. Phase III comparative study of vinorelbine combined with doxorubicin versus doxorubicin alone in disseminated metastatic/recurrent breast cancer: National Cancer Institute of Canada Clinical Trials Group Study MA8. *J Clin Oncol* 2000;18:2385–2394.
21. Namer M, Sler-Michel P, Turpin F, et al. Results of a phase III prospective, randomised trial, comparing mitoxantrone and vinorelbine (MV) in combination with standard FAC/FEC in front-line therapy of metastatic breast cancer. *Eur J Cancer* 2001;37(9): 1132–1140.
22. Bonneterre J, Roche H, Monnier A, et al. Taxotere (TXT) versus 5-fluorouracil + navelbine (FUN) as second-line chemotherapy (CT) in patients (pts) with metastatic breast cancer (MBC) (preliminary results) (Meeting abstract). *Proc Annu Meet Am Soc Clin Oncol* 1997;16:A564.
23. Spielmann M, Dorval T, Turpin F, et al. Phase II trial of vinorelbine/doxorubicin as first-line therapy of advanced breast cancer. *J Clin Oncol* 1994;12(9): 1764–1770.
24. Blomqvist C, Hietanen P, Teerenhovi L, et al. Vinorelbine and epirubicin in metastatic breast cancer. A dose finding study. *Eur J Cancer* 1995;31A(13–14):2406–2408.
25. Adenis A, Vanlemmens L, Fournier C, et al. Does induction chemotherapy with a mitoxantrone/vinorelbine regimen allow a breast-conservative treatment in patients with operable locoregional breast cancer? A French Northern Oncology Group trial in 105 patients. French Northern Oncology Group. *Breast Cancer Res Treat* 1996;40(2):161–169.
26. Chollet P, Charrier S, Brain E, et al. Clinical and pathological response to primary chemotherapy in operable breast cancer. *Eur J Cancer* 1997;33(6):862–866.
27. Llombart-Cussac A, Pivot X, Rhor-Alvarado A, et al. First-line vinorelbine-mitoxantrone combination in metastatic breast cancer patients relapsing after an adjuvant anthracycline regimen: results of a phase II study. *Oncology* 1998;55(5):384–390.
28. Baldini E, Tibaldi C, Chiavacci F, et al. Epirubicin/vinorelbine as first line therapy in metastatic breast cancer. *Breast Cancer Res Treat* 1998;49(2):129–134.
29. Nistico C, Garufi C, Barni S, et al. Phase II study of epirubicin and vinorelbine with granulocyte colony-stimulating factor: a high-activity, dose-dense weekly regimen for advanced breast cancer. *Ann Oncol* 1999; 10(8):937–942.
30. Dieras V, Extra JM, Bellissant E, et al. Efficacy and tolerance of vinorelbine and fluorouracil combination as first-line chemotherapy of advanced breast cancer: results of a phase II study using a sequential group method. *J Clin Oncol* 1996;14(12):3097–3104.
31. Zambetti M, Demicheli R, De Candis D, et al. Five-day infusion fluorouracil plus vinorelbine i.v. in metastatic pretreated breast cancer patients. *Breast Cancer Res Treat* 1997;44(3):255–260.
32. Nole F, de Braud F, Aapro M, et al. Phase I-II study of vinorelbine in combination with 5-fluorouracil and folinic acid as first-line chemotherapy in metastatic breast cancer: a regimen with a low subjective toxic burden. *Ann Oncol* 1997;8(9):865–870.
33. Goss PE, Fine S, Gelmon K, et al. Phase I studies of fluorouracil, doxorubicin and vinorelbine without (FAN) and with (SUPERFAN) folinic acid in patients with advanced breast cancer. *Cancer Chemother Pharmacol* 1997;41(1):53–60.
34. Kornek GV, Haider K, Kwasny W, et al. Effective treatment of advanced breast cancer with vinorelbine, 5-fluorouracil and l-leucovorin plus human granulocyte colony-stimulating factor. *Br J Cancer* 1998;78 (5):673–678.
35. Fabi A, Tonachella R, Savarese A, et al. A phase II trial of vinorelbine and thiotepa in metastatic breast cancer. *Ann Oncol* 1995;6(2):187–189.
36. Campisi C, Fabi A, Papaldo P, et al. Ifosfamide given by continuous-intravenous infusion in association with vinorelbine in patients with anthracycline-resistant metastatic breast cancer: a phase I-II clinical trial. *Ann Oncol* 1998;9(5):565–567.
37. Scheithauer W, Kornek G, Haider K, et al. Effective second line chemotherapy of advanced breast cancer with navelbine and mitomycin C. *Breast Cancer Res Treat* 1993;26(1):49–53.
38. Vici P, Di Lauro L, Carpano S, et al. Vinorelbine and mitomycin C in anthracycline-pretreated patients with advanced breast cancer. *Oncology* 1996;53(1): 16–18.
39. Ray-Coquard I, Biron P, Bachelot T, et al. Vinorelbine and cisplatin (CIVIC regimen) for the treatment of metastatic breast carcinoma after failure of anthracycline- and/or paclitaxel-containing regimens. *Cancer* 1998;82(1):134–140.
40. Shamseddine AI, Taher A, Dabaja B, et al. Dandashi Combination cisplatin-vinorelbine for relapsed and chemotherapy-pretreated metastatic breast cancer. *Am J Clin Oncol* 1999;22(3):298–302.
41. Michelotti A, Gennari A, Salvadori B, et al. Paclitaxel and vinorelbine in anthracycline-pretreated breast cancer: a phase II study. *Ann Oncol* 1996;7(8):857–860.
42. Fumoleau P, Fety R, Delecroix V, et al. Docetaxel combined with vinorelbine: phase I results and new study designs. *Oncology* 1997 (Huntingt);11(6 suppl 6):29–31.
43. Tortoriello A, Facchini G, Caponigro F, et al. Phase I/II study of paclitaxel and vinorelbine in metastatic breast cancer. *Breast Cancer Res Treat* 1998;47(1): 91–97.
44. Romero Acuna L, Langhi M, Perez J, et al. Vinorelbine and paclitaxel as first-line chemotherapy in metastatic breast cancer. *J Clin Oncol* 1999;17(1):74–81.
45. Ellis GK, Gralow JR, Pierce HI, et al. Infusional paclitaxel and weekly vinorelbine chemotherapy with concurrent filgrastim for metastatic breast cancer: high complete response rate in a phase I-II study of doxorubicin-treated patients. *J Clin Oncol* 1999;17(5): 1407–1412.
46. Budman DR, Weiselberg L, O'Mara V, et al. A phase I study of sequential vinorelbine followed by paclitaxel. *Ann Oncol* 1999;10(7):861–863.

47. Lokich JJ, Anderson N, Bern M, et al. The multifractionated, twice-weekly dose schedule for a three-drug chemotherapy regimen: a phase I-II study of paclitaxel, cisplatin, and vinorelbine. *Cancer* 1999;85(2):499–503.
48. Cohen RB, Mueller SC, Haden K, et al. Phase I study of weekly vinorelbine in combination with weekly paclitaxel in adult patients with advanced refractory cancer. *Cancer Invest* 2000;18(5):422–428.
49. Freasci G, Comella P, D'Aiuto G, et al. Weekly docetaxel plus gemcitabine or vinorelbine in refractory advanced breast cancer patients a parallel dose-finding study. Southern Italy Cooperative Oncology Group (SICOG). *Ann Oncol* 2000;11:367–371.
50. Kano Y, Akutsu M, Suzuki K, et al. Schedule-dependent interactions between vinorelbine and paclitaxel in human carcinoma cell lines in vitro. *Breast Cancer Res Treat* 1999;56(1):79–90.
51. Pergram M, Hsu S, Lewis G, et al. Inhibitory effects of combinations of HER-2/neu antibody and chemotherapeutic agents used for treatment of human breast cancers. *Oncogene* 1999;18:2241–2251.
52. Burstein HJ, Kuter I, Campos SM, et al. Clinical activity of trastuzumab and vinorelbine in women with HER2-overexpressing metastatic breast cancer. *J Clin Oncol* 2001;19:2722–2730.

13

Liposomal Doxorubicin in the Treatment of Metastatic Breast Cancer

Michael Smylie

The chemotherapy agent doxorubicin has had a profound impact on breast cancer therapy for over 30 years. It was initially discovered and introduced into clinical practice in the late 1960s. It continues to be the most commonly used anthracycline and one of several active agents in metastatic breast cancer (MBC) (1). Single-agent response rates in MBC have been reported from 30% to 50%. When anthracycline versus non-anthracycline regimens are compared, the former have shown an increase in the response rate, duration of response, time to progression, and a significant improvement in survival (2). Overview analyses of randomized clinical trials in adjuvant breast cancer patients have shown that anthracycline-containing regimens produced a greater reduction of recurrence and mortality rates when compared to non–anthracycline-containing regimens (3).

The antitumor effects of doxorubicin are affected through various mechanisms, including intercalating with DNA, inhibition of topoisomerase I and II, membrane binding, metal chelation, and through the generation of free radicals (4).

The optimum schedule of doxorubicin has yet to be defined. The drug can be given as an i.v. bolus every 3 weeks, as a weekly bolus, or as a prolonged infusion. Theoretically, prolonged infusions of doxorubicin would be most effective; however, response rates in phase 2 trials have been disappointing. The only randomized trial comparing doxorubicin given as a 3-bolus, versus a weekly bolus, versus a prolonged infusion was closed due to poor accrual (5). There exists a clear dose response relationship with doxorubicin, albeit at the cost of significant toxicity (6). In addition, trials of prolonged infusion times of 48 to 96 hours have been shown to significantly reduce the incidence and severity of cardiac toxicity at equivalent dose levels (7).

The dose-limiting toxicity of anthracyclines is myelosuppression; however, other acute toxicities include nausea/vomiting, alopecia, mucositis, risk of extravasation injury, and both acute and chronic cardiac toxicity. Acute cardiac toxicity is rare but can manifest as arrythmias, pericarditis/myocarditis, and acute heart failure. The most worrisome toxicity is the cumulative dose-dependent cardiomyopathy that can lead to congestive heart failure. The risk can vary from 7% to 42% of patients receiving a total dose of 550 mg/m^2 and 900 mg/m^2 by bolus, respectively (4,8).

The cardiac toxicity is related to peak plasma levels of doxorubicin, and although the exact mechanism is unclear, it is hypothesized that the interaction of doxorubicin with ferric iron, which in turn reacts with oxygen, generates free radicals such as superoxide anions, hydroxyl radicals and hydrogen peroxide (9). Once formed, these free radicals cause a multitude of cellular effects such as lipid peroxidation of miochondrial membranes, and thus myocyte damage. Histological changes include various subcellular alterations such as loss of myofibrils, distension of the sarcoplasmic reticulum, and vacuolization of myocardial cells. Cardiac toxicity occurs in all patients with the first dose of anthracycline, although it remains subclinical in most patients below cumulative doses of 450 mg/m^2. Patients at increased risk of cardiac toxicity include the elderly and pediatric populations, those with preexisting heart disease, and those with prior anthracycline exposure.

Different approaches have been used in an attempt to reduce cardiac toxicity. Because cardiac toxicity is related to peak plasma levels, one approach is to use prolonged infusions, thereby decreasing the peak levels of drug. This shift in delivery has led to reduced incidence of cardiac toxicity and allows higher cumulative doses of doxorubicin.

An alternative possibility is to augment normal cellular defenses against free radical damage by using exogenous antioxidants such as alpha tocopherol or by using an iron chelator such as ADR-529, or amifostine (10).

Doxorubicin analogues such as epirubicin and the related anthracenedione, mitoxantrone, have clinical efficacy with less cardiotoxicity (11). In a randomized trial comparing doxorubicin to mitoxantrone, the response rate to mitoxantrone was 20.6% versus 29.3% for doxorubicin, with mitoxantrone proving less toxic (12).

A completely different approach is to use a carrier system such as a liposome. Liposomes, which form spontaneously when phospholipids are placed in water, can be loaded with a variety of drugs (13,14). There are three compartments in the liposome into which a drug can be loaded. The first is the aqueous core, which is the appropriate locus for water-soluble drugs; the second is the lipid-rich membrane, which is the desired locus for fat-soluble drugs; and the last is the interface between the lipid-soluble membrane and the adjacent water, where small molecules, such as peptides and small proteins, can be loaded. A complete spectrum of drug release rates can be engineered into these structures. As an example, selection of highly unsaturated fatty acids increases the rate of drug release, whereas saturated fatty acids and cholesterol slows the rate of drug release. With the advent of the commercial liposome industry in the early 1980s, two major problems were identified. The first was preparing stable drug-loaded liposomes reproducibly. The second major obstacle to overcome was pharmacologic. By virtue of the fact that liposomes are opsonized by plasma proteins, they are recognized as foreign and are rapidly broken down by cells of the reticuloenclothelial system (RES), thereby decreasing their plasma half-life. In order to overcome this problem, investigators began looking for ways to avoid liposome breakdown by cells of the RES. Allen and Chonn (15) demonstrated that coating liposomes with specialized glycolipids (GM1) prolonged circulation time. Scientists at Sequus Pharmaceuticals demonstrated that methoxypolyethylene glycol (MPEG), a hydrophilic polymer, could be engrafted onto the surface of the liposome and this resulted in prolonged longevity of the liposome in the circulation.

There are currently two liposomal preparations of doxorubicin, and one liposomal daunorubicin undergoing clinical development in breast cancer. A pegylated liposomal doxorubicin, known as Caelyx (Doxil), is approved for Kaposi sarcoma (KS) and platinum-refractory ovarian cancer, and a non-pegylated liposomal doxorubicin, known as TLC D-99 (Myocet) is being evaluated in metastatic breast cancer.

Preclinical studies with MPEG-coated doxorubicin containing liposomes showed more activity on a dose-equivalent basis than either free doxorubicin or non-pegylated doxorubicin containing liposomes. These new liposomes are remarkably stable in the circulation, and can circulate intact for many days. Ultimately the liposomes are removed by macrophages but at a relatively slow rate, and not by the blood vessel attached macrophages, but by macrophages residing in the tissues. MPEG liposomes are relatively small with a diameter of approximately 100 nm. This small size allows them to circulate freely in the blood and to extravasate through endothelial gaps in the capillary.

In a pilot pharmacokinetics trial using an early version of Caelyx, patients were crossed over from Caelyx 50 mg/m^2 to free doxorubicin. Caelyx showed a prolonged circulation time, with a half-life of approximately 50 hours. In the same study, investigators also showed that doxorubicin was not released from the liposome during the prolonged circulation time into the plasma. The volume of distribution at study state (VssL/m^2) was only slightly greater than the plasma volume, indicating that the liposomes were clearly confined during their plasma distribution to the central compartment. This is in contrast to conventional doxorubicin, which has a volume of distribution that includes virtually the entire body (approximately 1,000 liters in humans). The area under the curve (AUC) for Caelyx is hundreds of times greater than that of equivalent, conventional doses of doxorubicin.

Liposomal encapsulation of anthracyclines lowers peak plasma levels of free drugs, and a variety of animal models have demonstrated decreased cardiac toxicity. Non-invasive methods of monitoring cardiac toxicity such as left ventricular ejection fraction (LVEF) and clinical examination are most frequently used to monitor for signs of heart failure. However, considerable irreversible heart damage must occur prior to these tests becoming abnormal. The diagnostic test with the greatest specificity and sensitivity for doxorubicin-induced cardiomyopathy is endomyocardial biopsy. Histologic changes can be graded on a Billingham scale of 1 to 3 to quantify the amount of doxorubicin-induced damage (Table 13.1).

Berry et al. (16) reported reduced cardiotoxicity with pegylated liposomal doxorubicin. Myocardial biopsies from ten AIDS patients with KS who had received cumulative Caelyx doses of (20 mg/m^2 biweekly) 440 mg/m^2 to 840 mg/m^2 were compared to historical controls assembled from patients who had received cumulative doses of conventional doxorubicin of 174 mg/m^2 to 671 mg/m^2 in two earlier cardiac biopsy protocols. Two control groups were selected based upon both cumulative and peak doxorubicin dose (60 mg/m^2 or 20 mg/m^2, group one), and peak dose alone (20 mg/m^2, group two). Median biopsy scores for the pegylated liposomal doxorubicin and doxorubicin groups, respectively, were 0.3 versus 3.0 ($p = 0.002$) for group one and 1.25 for group two (p less than 0.001).

Due to their small size, MPEG liposomes can extravasate through capillary endothelial junctions. Tumor capillaries are leakier than their normal tissue counterparts. Therefore, more liposomes should extravasate into tumors, thereby giving increased drug concentration to the tumor tissue. Northfeld demonstrated that biopsies of AIDS-KS lesions where patients were pretreated with Caelyx had several fold higher concentrations in the tumor tissue than the normal skin. The difference was highest 46 hours after dosing. Conversely, tissues with tight endothelial junctions such as cardiac muscle and the gastrointestinal tract should have lower rates of extravasation and therefore less exposure to doxorubicin leading to less toxicity.

The results of two phase 1 trials of Caelyx in solid tumors have been reported (17). Antitumor activity was seen in breast cancer, prostate cancer, non-small cell lung cancer, renal cell carcinoma, head and neck cancer, and ovarian carcinoma. A phase 2 trial of Caelyx in metastatic breast cancer was recently reported by Ranson et al. (18). The objectives were to define the safety and tolerability of Caelyx and to obtain preliminary data on its anti-tumor activity in metastatic breast cancer.

Patients enrolled in the study had histologically confirmed metastatic breast cancer. They were also allowed to have had one prior chemotherapy regimen, providing it did not contain anthracyclines. Seven of the first thirteen patients developed palmar plantar erythrodysthesia of grade 3 or more after multiple cycles of treatment, and the dose was reduced to 45 mg/m^2 every 3 weeks. A subsequent detailed analysis of the phase 1 data suggested that the

TABLE 13.1. *Billingham scale for grading anthracycline-induced cardiomyopathy*

Biopsy grade	Morphology
0	No evidence of anthracycline-specific damage
0.5	Not completely normal but no evidence of anthracycline-specific damage
1.0	Isolated myocytes affected and/or early myofibrillar loss; damage to 5% of all cells
1.5	Changes similar to grade 1 except with damage to 6%–15% of all cells
2.0	Clusters of myocytes affected by myofibrillar loss and/or vacuolization, with damage to 16%–25% of all cells
2.5	Many myocytes, 26%–35% of all cells, affected by vacuolization and/or myofibrillar loss
3.0	Severe diffuse myocyte damage (>35% of all cells)

development of skin toxicity may be particularly influenced by dosing interval; thus a third cohort of patients were treated at a dose of 45 mg/m^2 every 4 weeks. Of the patients evaluable for response, 6% obtained a complete response and 25% a partial response, for an overall response rate of 31%. The median overall survival was 7 months, and median time to disease progression was 9 months in responding patients. Myelosuppression, alopecia, nausea, and vomiting were seen but were mild. The most significant toxicities were palmar plantar erythrodysthesia and mucositis. In all cases the skin toxicity was reversible.

Although this study was not designed to assess cardiac toxicity, extensive pre-clinical data support the notion that liposomal preparations are associated with reduced cardiac toxicity. Based on these encouraging results, a phase 3 trial was designed to compare Caelyx in advanced metastatic breast cancer patients who were refractory to taxanes to a standard comparator such as Navelbine or mitomycin-C/vinblastine sulfate. The primary endpoint was to compare progression-free survival with secondary endpoints of overall response rate, response duration, and overall survival and to compare tolerability. This study has completed accrual and results are pending.

The pivotal trial to assess the activity of Caelyx in metastatic breast cancer accrued a total of 400 patients worldwide and randomized them to either Caelyx (50 mg/m^2) or to single-agent doxorubicin (60 mg/m^2). Patients were randomized according to the following parameters: previous anthracycline therapy, WHO performance status (0 to 1 versus 2), and presence of bone metastases only. The primary objective of this trial is to compare time to disease progression of Caelyx versus doxorubicin. Secondary objectives are to compare response rate, overall survival time, time to treatment failure, toxicity, clinical benefit response, quality of life, and health care utilization of Caelyx versus doxorubicin. Results are expected in late 2002.

Several other phase trials are underway to assess Caelyx-containing regimens. Drugs that are currently being evaluated in combination with Caelyx include cyclophosphamide, vinorelbine, paclitaxel, and docetaxel (19–21).

The feasibility of combining Caelyx with herceptin is also currently being assessed.

Two other liposomal preparations of doxorubicin are also undergoing clinical development. TLC D-99 (Myocet), manufactured by Elan Pharmaceuticals, is a liposomal encapsulated form of doxorubicin that incorporates doxorubicin loading by generating an electropotential gradient across the liposome membrane. This mechanism for remote loading involves the generation of a pH gradient between the inside of the liposome and the extra liposomal buffer, which acts to pull the doxorubicin into the vesicle. TLC D-99 does not contain a polyethylene coating and has been shown to concentrate in organs rich in reticuloendothelial cells.

A phase 1 trial of TLC D-99 performed at Roswell Park Memorial Institute demonstrated that the dose-limiting toxicity was myelosuppression (22). Other toxicities, such as nausea and vomiting, diarrhea, alopecia, malaise, rigors, and fever, were mild. No cardiac toxicity was seen. An open-label, non-randomized trial of TLC D-99 (75 mg/m^2) in 32 patients showed an overall response rate of 56%. Toxicity was tolerable with ten patients (31%) having grade 4 leukopenia and 1 patient (3%) having grade 4 thrombocytopenia. Grade 3 mucositis occurred in 10% of the patients.

A subsequent phase 2 trial of TLC D-99 in combination with 5-fluorouracil, and cyclophosphamide has been reported (23). Forty-one patients were enrolled onto the study and were treated with TLC D-99 (60 mg/m^2), cyclophosphamide (500 mg/m^2, day 1 every 21 days), and 5-fluorouracil (500 mg/m^2 on day 1 and day 8 every 21 days). The overall objective response rate was 73% with a median overall survival duration of 19.4 months. Myelosuppression was the most common adverse event causing dose delays and dose reductions, and 17 patients developed neutropenic fever. Cardiac toxicity was low despite the high cumulative doxorubicin dose. No cases of congestive heart failure (CHF) were seen during the study, although one patient developed CHF during the follow-up period that was not felt to be anthracycline induced. Unlike liposomes with an MPEG coating, no cases of palmar plantar erythrodysthesia were encountered.

Two multicenter, randomized, parallel, open-label, phase 3 trials comparing Myocet to Adriamycin have been reported. In a monotherapy trial involving 224 patients, Myocet (75 mg/m^2) was compared with Adriamycin (75 mg/m^2) (24). Dose escalation or decreases due to toxicity were allowed in this trial. There was no significant difference in the response rates (26% versus 26%), time to disease progression (2.9 vs 3.1 months for Myocet and Adriamycin, respectively), and median overall survival (16 versus 20 months, respectively; $p = 0.09$). Cardiac toxicity was less frequent in the Myocet arm than the Adriamycin arm.

A recent phase 3 study published by Batist et al. (25) involving 297 patients compared the combination of Myocet (60 mg/m^2) and cyclophosphamide (MC) to the combination of Adriamycin (60 mg/m^2) and cyclophosphamide (AC). Myocet showed an improved safety profile with significantly less cardiotoxicity. No cases of congestive heart failure occurred in the Myocet arm, compared to 5 cases in the Adriamycin arm. Likewise the median cumulative dose of Adriamycin at the onset of cardiac toxicity in the MC arm was more than 1,800 mg/m^2. At the same time, anti-tumor efficacy was maintained with no significant differences in response rates (43% versus 43%), median time to tumor progression (5.1 versus 5.5 months), median time to treatment failure (4.6 versus 4.4 months), and overall survival (19 versus 16 months).

A similar trial reported by Erdkamp et al. (26) in 160 women with metastatic breast cancer compared Myocet (75 mg/m^2) and cyclophoshamide to Epirubicin (75 mg/m2) and cyclophosphamide. There was no significant difference in response rate (46% versus 39%) but there was a significant benefit in time-to-treatment failure (6.4 versus 4.9 months) and progression-free survival (7.6 versus 6.0 months) in favor of Myocet. There was no difference in the incidence of CHF (4% versus 4%).

Daunorubicin hydrochloride, a related anthracycline, has also been prepared as a liposomal preparation known as DaunoXome (daunorubicin citrate liposome) (27). Although daunorubicin is used primarily in hematologic malignancies, DaunoXome has been evaluated in metastatic breast cancer and has shown encouraging activity (28). Similar to Caelyx and TLC D-99, DaunoXome has shown no significant alopecia or cardiac toxicity. Nausea and vomiting were mild to moderate, as was hematologic toxicity.

In summary, liposome-encapsulated doxorubicin exhibits a very different toxicity profile than free doxorubicin. Whereas the dose-limiting toxicity of free doxorubicin is myelosuppression, the dose-limiting toxicity of Caelyx is mucositis and palmar plantar erythrodysthesia. Other distressing chemotherapy side effects such as alopecia and nausea and vomiting were also uncommon and when present tended to be mild. More importantly, cardiac toxicity was rarely seen, which was probably the result of minimal free doxorubicin released into the circulation. The phase 2 study of Caelyx reported by Ranson et al. yielded a response rate of 31% in patients with metastatic breast cancer. This response rate is on the low side of response rates reported in other phase 2 studies for free doxorubicin but is similar to the recent response rate reported by Chan et al. in their phase 3 study of doxorubicin versus docetaxel. The patient population in Ranson's study also included patients who had received prior non-anthracycline based chemotherapy for metastatic disease and two or more lines of hormonal therapy, and many patients had three or more sites of disease and a high incidence of visceral metastases. Unfortunately, mucositis and palmar plantar erythrodysthesia limit the ability to dose escalate Caelyx, and it is not clear if Caelyx, at its present recommended dose, is dose-equivalent to free doxorubicin. The current phase 3 trial comparing Caelyx to free doxorubicin should better define the true activity of Caelyx compared to doxorubicin, and thus its place in our armentarium of breast cancer chemotherapy drugs. If, indeed, Caelyx is dose equivalent to doxorubicin, then the potential of Caelyx to replace doxorubicin exists. This is particularly important in adjuvant patients, as a drug without the potential for cardiac toxicity would be attractive.

Likewise, both TLC D-99 and DaunoXome have also shown encouraging results in metastatic breast cancer, with a corresponding decrease in cardiac toxicity, but, like Caelyx, further studies are warranted to better define its activity.

Liposomes offer a unique carrier system for cytotoxic agents that drastically change their pharmacokinetic parameters and their toxicities. To date, however, their true efficacy is unproven and further studies are warranted in solid tumors such as breast cancer before their routine use can be advocated.

REFERENCES

1. Honing SF. Treatment of metastatic disease, hormonal therapy and chemotherapy. In: Harris JR, Lippman ME, Morrow M, Hellman S, ed. *Breast diseases.* Philadelphia: JB Lippincott, 1996:669–734.
2. A'Hern RP, Smith IE, Ebbs SR. Chemotherapy and survival in advanced breast cancer: The inclusion of doxorubicin in Cooper type regimens. *Br J Cancer* 1993; 67:801–805.
3. Early Breast Cancer Trialists' Collaborative Group. Polychemotherapy for early breast cancer: An overview of the randomised trials. *Lancet* 1998;352:930–942.
4. Shan K, Lincoff AM, Young JB. Anthracycline-induced cardiotoxicity. *Ann Intern Med* 1996;125:47–58.
5. Lokich J, Auerbach M, Smith L, et al. A comparative trial of three schedules for single-agent doxorubicin in advanced breast cancer: an aborted investigation. *Infusional Chemother* 1992;2(4):185–192.
6. Jones RB, Holland JF, Bhardwaj S, et al. A phase I-II study of intensive-dose adriamycin for advanced breast cancer. *J Clin Oncol* 1987;5(2):172–177.
7. Ewer MS, Benjamin RS. Cardiac complications. In: Holland JF, Frei III E, Bast RC Jr, et al., eds. *Cancer Medicine,* 3rd ed. Baltimore: Williams & Wilkins, 1997:3197–3215.
8. Legha SS, Benjamin RS, Mackay B, et al., Reduction of doxorubicin cardiotoxicity by prolonged continuous intravenous infusion. *Ann Intern Med* 1982;96:133–139.
9. Singal P, Iliskovic N. Doxorubicin-induced cardiomyopathy. *New Eng J Med* 1998;13(339):900–905.
10. Hochster H, Wasserheit C, Speyer J. Cardiotoxicity and cardioprotection during chemotherapy. *Curr Opin Oncol* 1995;7:304–309.
11. Von Hoff DD, Layard MW, Basa P, et al. Risk factors for doxorubicin-induced congestive heart failure. *Ann Intern Med* 1979; 91:710–717.
12. Henderson C, Allegra J, Woodcock T, et al. Randomized clinical trial comparing mitoxantrone with doxorubicin in previously treated patents with metastatic breast cancer. *J Clin Oncol* May 1989;7(5):560–571.
13. Martin FH. STEALTH® Liposome Technology: An Overview. *DOXIL Clinical Series* 1997;1:1–11.
14. Gabizon A, Goren D, Cohen R, Barenholz Y. Development of liposomal anthracyclines: from basics to clinical applications. *Controlled Release* 1998;53(1–3): 275–279.
15. Allen TM, Chonn A. Large unilmellar liposomes with low uptake by the reticuloendothelial system. *FEBS Lett* 1987;223(1):42–46.
16. Berry G, Billingham M, Alderman E, et al. The use of cardiac biopsy to demonstrate reduced cardiotoxicity in AIDS Kaposi's sarcoma patients treated with pegylated liposomal doxorubicin. *Ann Oncol* 1998;9: 711–716.
17. Uziely B, Jeffers S, Isacson R, et al. Liposomal doxorubicin: antitumor activity and unique toxicities during two complementary phase I studies. *J Clin Oncol* 1995; 13(7):1777–1785.
18. Ranson MR, Carmichael J, O'Byrne K, et al. Treatment of advanced breast cancer with sterically stabilized liposomal doxorubicin: results of a multicenter phase II trial. *J Clin Oncol* 1997;15(10):3185–3191.
19. Israel VK, Jeffers S, Gernal G, et al. Phase I study of Doxil® (liposomal doxorubicin) in combination with paclitaxel. *Proc ASCO* 1997;842:239a.
20. Burstein HJ, Ramirez MF, Petros WP, et al. Phase I study of Doxil and vinorelbine in metastatic breast cancer. *Ann Oncol* 1999;10(9):1113–1116.
21. Sparano JA, Wolffe A, Albert Einstein Cancer Center, Bronx, NY; Winship Cancer Center, Atlanta GA. Phase I trial of liposomal doxorubicin (Doxil) and docetaxel (Taxotere) in patients (pts) with advanced breast cancer (ABC). *Proc ASCO* 1998;672:175a.
22. Cowens JW, Creaven PJ, Greco WR, et al. Initial clinical (phase I) trial of TLC D-99 (doxorubicin encapsulated in liposomes). *Cancer Res* 1993;53:2796–2802.
23. Valero V, Buzdar A, Theriault R, et al. Phase II trial of liposome-encapsulated doxorubicin, cyclophosphamide and fluorouracil as first-line therapy in patients with metastatic breast cancer. *J Clin Oncol* 1999; 17(5):1425–1434.
24. Harris L, Batist G, Belt R, et al. Liposome-encapsulated doxorubicin compared with conventional doxorubicin in a randomized multicenter trial as first-line therapy of metastatic breast cancer. *Cancer* 2002;94, No. 1.
25. Batist G, Ramakrisnan G, Rao CS, et al. Reduced cardiotoxicity and preserved antitumor efficacy of liposome-encapsulated doxorubicin and cyclophosphamide compared with conventional doxorubicin and cyclophosphamide in a randomized multicenter trial of metastatic breast cancer. *J Clin Oncol* 2001;19: 1444–1454.
26. Erdkamp F, Chan C, Davidson, N, et al. Phase III study of TLC-99 plus cyclophosphamide vs. epirubicin plus cyclophosphamide in patients with metastatic breast cancer. *Proc ASCO* 1999;18:121a (abstr. 459).
27. Gill PS, Espina BM, Cabriales S, et al. Phase I/II clinical and pharmacokinetic evaluation of liposomal daunorubicin. *J Clin Oncol* 1995;13(4):996–1003.
28. Darskaia EI, Zubarovskaia LS, Afanas'ev BV. Administration of liposomal preparation of DaunoXome for breast cancer for breast cancer in patients with poor prognosis. *Vopr Onkol* 1999;45(4):440–444.

14
High-Dose Chemotherapy and Autologous Stem Cell Transplantation for Metastatic Breast Cancer

Edward A. Stadtmauer

No area of treatment for metastatic breast cancer has benefited from and been altered more by widely publicized results of clinical trials than high-dose chemotherapy and autologous stem cell transplantation. By the late 1990s, the use of high-dose chemotherapy and autologous stem cell transplantation had outstripped allogeneic transplantation because of the lack of a need of a donor and the decreased toxicity. The most rapid growth had been for solid tumors, particularly metastatic and high-risk breast cancer. Breast cancer became the number one disease indication for stem cell transplant of any kind, with more than 10,000 procedures conducted in North America over the past decade. However, after a number of randomized comparative trials failed to demonstrate a significant benefit for high-dose chemotherapy and autologous stem cell transplantation for breast cancer in 1999, the number of these procedures has fallen precipitously to the extent that few, at most, are conducted per year at an active center. This chapter reviews the outcomes of clinical trials of this procedure for metastatic breast cancer.

During the early 1980s, phase 1 and phase 2 trials of high-dose single-agent and combination chemotherapy with autologous stem cell rescue as salvage therapy for patients with relapsed and refractory metastatic breast cancer were performed (1–15). Response rates of approximately 70% were observed, with 20% to 30% of the patients achieving complete remission. The average duration of response, however, was short, with few, if any, long-term relapse-free survivors.

In an attempt to improve outcome, patients with newly diagnosed or relapsed metastatic breast cancer were first treated with a course of conventional dose induction chemotherapy to reduce tumor burden, improve performance status, and decrease the chance of stem cell tumor contamination; they then went on to a stem cell harvest, followed by a single course of high-dose chemotherapy and stem cell transplantation. A number of trials of this design suggested an approximate 80% response rate, with 10% to 30% of patients relapse free at 2 years (Table 14.1). The mortality rate in these early trials was substantial, however, ranging from 3% to 30% within the first 100 days of transplantation. The survival benefits were perceived to be superior to historical controls. To further improve on these results, cycles of high-dose chemotherapy with stem cell transplant were administered with or without an initial course of induction therapy, with further promising results. Registry data as reported to the Autologous Bone Marrow Transplant Registry (ABMTR) corroborated these results (16).

The most common high-dose chemotherapy treatment scenario became the use of a course of four to six cycles of conventional dose-induction chemotherapy, usually: cyclophosphamide, doxorubicin, and 5-FU (CAF); doxorubicin and cyclophosphamide (AC); or doxorubicin, 5-FU and methotrexate (AFM), followed by assessment of response. Patients achieving complete or partial response then proceeded to stem cell collection, followed by a single course of high-dose chemotherapy utilizing primarily one of three regimens—CBP (cyclophosphamide, carmustine, and cisplatinum), CTCb (cyclophosphamide, thiotepa and carboplatinum), or CT (cyclophosphamide and thiotepa)—and stem cell rescue. The ABMTR analyzed the factors associated with disease

TABLE 14.1. *Early pilot trials of high-dose chemotherapy and stem cell transplant in metastatic breast cancer*

Author	Yr	# Pts	HDC	RR (%)	OS (mo)	PFS	Toxic death	Ref
Peters	1988	22	CBP	73	10.1	14%	23%	1
Williams	1989	27	CT	86	15.1	7%	14%	2,4
Kennedy	1991	30	CT	100	22	10%	0	6
Antman	1992	29	CTCb	100	24	17%	3%	3

CBP, cyclophosphamide, carmustine, cis-platinum; CT, cyclophosphamide and thiotepa; CTCb, cyclophosphamide, thiotepa, and carboplatin; HDC, high-dose chemotherapy; OS, overall survival; PFS, progression-free survival; Pts, patients; Ref, reference; RR, response rate; Toxic death, death within 100 days of stem cell infusion.

progression or death in a total of 1,188 consecutive women age 18 to 70 years receiving autologous transplant for metastatic or locally recurrent breast cancer in this manner with a median follow-up of 29.5 months (16). Nine factors were associated with a significantly increased risk of treatment failure, including age older than 45 years, Karnofsky performance score less than 90%, hormone receptor-negative status, prior use of adjuvant chemotherapy, initial disease-free interval after adjuvant chemotherapy less than 18 months, liver metastases, central nervous system metastases, three or more sites of metastatic disease, and less-than-complete response to standard-dose chemotherapy. Tamoxifen treatment after transplant was associated with a reduced risk of treatment failure in women with hormone receptor-positive tumors. Women with no risk factors had a 3-year probability of progression-free survival of 43%, whereas women with more than three risk factors had a 3-year probability of progression-free survival of 4%. The 3-year probability of progression-free survival for the entire group was 13%. The group of patients with no risk factors (n = 38) accounted for only 3% of the entire population that was reported, whereas 84% of the patients registered had two or more risk factors and experienced worse outcomes.

Even if favorable prognostic factors for autologous stem cell transplant could be identified, the incremental benefit over conventional dose chemotherapy required comparative trials. A number of these trials have recently been reported.

COMPARISON TRIALS OF INDUCTION THERAPY FOLLOWED BY A SINGLE COURSE OF HIGH-DOSE CHEMOTHERAPY

The Philadelphia Bone Marrow Transplant Group (PBT) developed a randomized trial for patients with chemotherapy-untreated metastatic breast cancer that became a national intergroup trial, designated high priority by the National Cancer Institute. PBT-1 was designed to compare the time-to-progression and overall survival and toxicity of high-dose chemotherapy and stem cell transplantation to a prolonged course of maintenance chemotherapy for women with metastatic breast cancer responding to first-line chemotherapy. Eligibility required: locally recurrent or distant metastatic disease; premenopausal or postmenopausal status; age 60 years or less; no prior chemotherapy for metastatic disease; prior adjuvant chemotherapy more than 6 months before entry; at least one prior hormonal treatment if estrogen receptor positive, unless life threatening visceral disease presents; and performance status of zero or one. Patients then received induction chemotherapy with CAF for four to six cycles, or cyclophosphamide, methotrexate, and 5-FU (CMF) with optional prednisone, if the prior doxorubicin dose was 400 mg/m^2 or more. Patients achieving stable or progressive disease were taken off the study, and patients achieving partial or complete response went on to further therapy. To be eligible for randomization, patients could not have had bone marrow involvement with tumor, and normal hematopoietic, cardiac, pulmonary and hepatic function was required. Additionally, assigned therapy was to begin within 8 weeks of the last chemotherapy.

Eligible patients were randomized to a single autologous stem cell transplantation or to CMF maintenance chemotherapy for up to 2 years. Patients discontinued CMF early at time of progression, unacceptable toxicity, or removal of informed consent. Patients undergoing stem cell transplant underwent bone marrow harvest and granulocyte/macrophage colony stimulating factor (GM-CSF)–stimulated peripheral stem cell harvest followed by high-dose CTCb therapy with stem cell transplant and GM-CSF–stimulated marrow recovery. In 1995, the trial was amended to allow for G-CSF–stimulated stem cell harvest as the sole source of stem cells.

Five hundred fifty-three patients were enrolled in the trial (17); 296 achieved response and were therefore potentially eligible for randomization, and 199 proceeded to randomization. Of the 199 patients, 110 were assigned to transplant and 89 to maintenance therapy; of these, 15 (7.5%) were ineligible (9 ABMT and 6 CMF), leaving 184 eligible randomized patients (101 ABMT, 83 CMF). With a median follow-up of the entire group of 37 months, there was no difference in median survival between transplant and maintenance therapy (24 months versus 26 months), or 3-year survival (32% versus 38%; $p = 0.23$). Patients in complete remission at time of randomization fared better in terms of both overall survival and time-to-progression than patients who had obtained a partial response. There was also no difference in time-to-progression between ABMT and maintenance therapy (9.6 months versus 9 months) or 3-year progression-free survival (6% versus 12%; $p = 0.31$). No significant benefit for transplant was observed in any stratified subgroup, including response, hormone receptor status, age 42 years or less versus more than 42 years, or dominant metastatic site.

These data have recently been updated with a median follow-up of 70 months (18). There remains no difference in median survival or 5-year survival (15% versus 14%). The median time-to-progression remains 9.6 months versus 9.1 months, and the 5-year progression-free survival is 4% in both groups. No significant benefit for transplant was observed in any stratified subgroup except age, where women who received CMF and were 42 years old or younger were observed to have a higher hazard of dying, while women over 42 years old had a 28% reduction in the hazard of dying when receiving CMF rather than high-dose chemotherapy ($p = 0.03$).

A surprising finding was the low conversion rate of patients in partial response at time of randomization to complete response with the high-dose chemotherapy. One hundred thirty-nine patients were in partial response at time of randomization; eleven (8%) were converted to complete remission after consolidation therapy, five were converted by transplant, and six were converted by CMF. Another pleasantly surprising finding was the low incidence of lethal toxicity of transplant on this trial. No lethal toxicity was observed on the CMF arm, and only one patient died on the transplant arm of veno-occlusive disease. Nonlethal severe toxicities, however, were increased on the transplant arm, including hematologic toxicity, infection, nausea, vomiting, and diarrhea, as well as cardiac, pulmonary, and hepatic toxicities. Mucositis, however, was not substantially increased. This study demonstrated that high-dose chemotherapy with stem cell rescue did not confer incremental improvement and overall survival or time-to-progression to CMF; there were no substantial differences in lethal toxicity, although non-lethal grade serious toxicities were greater in the transplant arm.

A prospective analysis of quality of life by questionnaires was also conducted in this trial (19). Quality of life as measured primarily by mood disturbance was inferior for high-dose chemotherapy patients at 6 months after randomization but normalized by 12 months. Additionally, a retrospective analysis of resource utilization and cost was conducted (20). Overall, patients receiving high-dose chemotherapy had a mean $105,000 in costs from randomization, while patients on the CMF arm had a mean

$67,000 in costs with a mean difference in cost of $39,000. In this trial, high-dose chemotherapy with stem cell transplantation required somewhat more resources when compared to up to 24 months of CMF chemotherapy, but the difference in costs was less than anticipated.

A similar trial has been conducted in Canada by the National Cancer Institute of Canada Clinical Trials Group (21). Patients with chemotherapy-naive metastatic breast cancer were treated with four cycles of anthracycline- or taxane-based induction chemotherapy, and a partial or complete response was required. Patients then went on to two to four additional cycles of the induction chemotherapy or one to two cycles of this therapy followed by a single course of high-dose cyclophosphamide, mitoxantrone, and carboplatin with stem cell transplant. Three hundred seventy nine patients were enrolled, and 224 were randomized. One hundred twelve patients were assigned to each arm. Seven patients experienced toxic death on the transplant arm, while no patient died on the control arm of toxicity. At one year, the progression-free survival favored high-dose chemotherapy (41% versus 28%, $p = 0.014$), but at 2 years, survival was no different at 31% and 36%, respectively.

A French trial, PEGASE 3, was also a prospective multi-center phase 3 randomized trial for chemotherapy-naive metastatic breast cancer (22). Patients first received four cycles of 5-FU, epirubicin, and cyclophosphamide, and responding patients were randomized to either no further treatment or a course of high-dose cyclophosphamide and thiotepa with stem cell transplantation. Three hundred eight patients were enrolled on the trial, and 180 responding patients were randomized. Of those, 91 patients were assigned to no further therapy and 89 patients to stem cell transplantation, of whom 80 patients underwent transplant, with one toxic death. At one year, progression-free survival favored transplant (19% versus 46%), but by three years, overall survival was no different at 30% and 38%, respectively.

A similar smaller trial had also been conducted in France (PEGASE 4) (23). Patients with chemotherapy-naive metastatic breast cancer were treated with induction chemotherapy for six cycles, and a partial or complete response was required. Patients then went on to two to four additional cycles of induction chemotherapy or cyclophosphamide–plus-G-CSF–stimulated stem cell harvest followed by high-dose cyclophosphamide, melphalan and mitoxantrone (CMA) with stem cell transplantation. Thirty-two patients were assigned to transplant and twenty-nine to conventional dose therapy. At two years, there was a trend toward improved survival in the transplant arm, but by 5 years no significant difference in the two arms was observed.

Few patients in complete remission were transplanted on these comparative trials. Peters et al. (24) have made a preliminary report of a randomized trial examining the use of high-dose chemotherapy and stem cell transplant as consolidation treatment in patients who achieved a complete remission after intensive induction therapy. Four-hundred twenty three patients with hormone-insensitive metastatic breast cancer who had not been treated with any prior chemotherapy received two to four cycles of doxorubicin, 5-FU, and methotrexate (AFM) induction therapy. Twenty-five percent achieved complete remission (106 patients), and 98 of them were randomized to either immediate consolidation with CVP and stem cell transplant or observation. The randomization was balanced both for pretreatment patient characteristics and for site and extent of disease. The disease-free survival rate was significantly improved in the patients who received high-dose chemotherapy up front. With a median follow-up of 3.9 years, the event-free survival at 5 years was 25% for the high-dose arm versus 8% for the observation arm.

The Cancer and Leukemia Group B (CALGB) has conducted a retrospective database comparison utilizing historical data from the CALGB metastatic breast cancer trials and compared these data with high-dose chemotherapy and stem cell transplant for metastatic breast cancer as reported to the ABMTR (25). To be eligible, patients on the CALGB trials had to receive CAF induction chemotherapy, and although the induction chemotherapy was not reported in the

ABMTR data, a response was required. In the CALGB trials, the control arm was further courses of CAF with or without other chemotherapy regimens, whereas the experimental arm contained all transplants for metastatic breast cancer reported to the ABMTR from 1989 to 1995. Most patients had received a cyclophosphamide and thiotepa regimen with or without carboplatin. All patients were younger than 65 years. The resulting populations included 635 standard-dose patients and 441 high-dose patients. The high-dose chemotherapy group displayed better performance status, while the standard dose group had slightly better survival in the first year after treatment. The high-dose chemotherapy group did have a somewhat higher probability of 5-year survival (23% versus 15%, $p = 0.03$).

The combined analysis of the results of the five prospective comparison trials reported to date, as well as the large database analysis, give us at least level 2 evidence and category grade B to suggest that the incremental benefit of an added single cycle of high-dose chemotherapy with stem cell transplantation for responding metastatic breast cancer is low at best.

UP-FRONT TRANSPLANTATION AND TANDEM TRANSPLANTATION

Two randomized comparison trials of up-front high-dose chemotherapy have now been reported. One trial has been discredited owing to falsification of data (26). In the other trial, women without prior chemotherapy for metastatic cancer were randomly assigned to six to nine cycles of Adriamycin and paclitaxel, versus double, high-dose therapy with cyclophosphamide, mitoxantrone, and VP-16 with stem cell rescue (27). Ninety-two patients were randomized, 48 to high-dose chemotherapy and 44 to conventional dose therapy. The overall response rate was similar (67.4% versus 60.5%), as was the complete response rate (13% versus 11.6%). The median progression-free survival showed a mild advantage for high-dose therapy (14.3 versus 10 months), but median overall survival was no different at 28.4 versus 25.3 months.

Investigators from the Dana-Farber Cancer Institute have reported on 67 women with metastatic breast cancer receiving the sequence of high-dose melphalan followed by CTCb with stem cell transplantation (28). Patients initially received three or four cycles of doxorubicin and 5-FU, followed by G-CSF stimulated peripheral stem cell harvest. Patients subsequently received melphalan 140 mg/m^2 to 180 mg/m^2 with stem cell support, followed by CTCb with stem cell transplantation, and then went on to radiotherapy, surgery and hormonal therapy if they were estrogen receptor positive. Forty-four percent were progression-free a median of 16-months after high-dose therapy. The median progression-free survival and overall survival were 11 and 20 months, respectively. These results were not substantially improved from a historical cohort of single stem cell transplant, however. The sequence of dose-intensive therapy may play a role in these results. The same authors have recently reported on a group of 58 patients receiving two courses of induction chemotherapy with 90 mg/m^2 of doxorubicin followed by tandem transplant in the opposite sequence with CTCb, initially, and then a melphalan and paclitaxel combination. Preliminary results show that 78% can achieve complete or near-complete response with 60% event-free survival at 2 years (29).

A multiinstitutional trial investigating the role of induction chemotherapy as part of tandem sequential high-dose chemotherapy for metastatic breast cancer has been reported (30). Sixty-three patients were treated with four cycles of doxorubicin (50 mg/m^2) and docetaxel (75 mg/m^2), followed by a course of cyclophosphamide (5 g/m^2), VP-16 (1.5 g/m^2), and cisplatin (120 mg/m^2), with G-CSF-stimulated stem cell harvest; this was followed by a CTCb transplant. Patients subsequently went on to long-term anastrozole. Additionally, a group of 36 patients received the same sequential high-dose chemotherapy without the four cycles of induction therapy. A comparison of these two groups demonstrated a significantly greater complete response rate in the induction therapy group (42% versus 11%), as well as improved progression-free survival. There was a 2.3-fold

Table 14.2. Comparative trials of high-dose chemotherapy in metastatic breast cancer

Trial (ref)	Total	Randomized	Assignment		Toxic death		EFS (%)		OS (%)		p value
			ABMT	Control	ABMT	Control	ABMT	Control	ABMT	Control	
Philadelphia (17)	553	199	110	89	1	0	4[b]	4[b]	15[b]	14[b]	NS
Duke CR (24)	425	98	49	44	7.5%	0	24[b]	8[b]	40[b]	46[b]	<0.001
Pegase 3 (22)	308	180	89	91	1	0	19[c]	46[c]	30[a]	38[a]	NS
Pegase 4 (23)	61	61	32	29	0	0	49[a]	21[a]	55[a]	28[a]	0.06
Canada (21)	379	224	112	112	7	0	9[b]	9[b]	30[b]	18.5[b]	NS
CALGB (25)	1,706	—	441	635	—	—	—	—	23[b]	15[b]	0.03

ABMT, autologous bone marrow transplant; CR, complete response; EFS, event-free survival; OS, overall survival.
[a]3 years.
[b]5 years.
[c]1 year.

increase in risk of disease progression in the noninduction therapy group. This trial suggests a benefit for induction chemotherapy prior to high-dose chemotherapy and stem cell transplant for metastatic breast cancer.

CONCLUSIONS AND FUTURE DIRECTIONS

After almost two decades of clinical research investigating high-dose therapy and stem cell transplantation for metastatic breast cancer, the body of data, particularly in comparative trials and large registry analyses, has reached a critical mass to aid in clinical decision-making. Unfortunately, there is little evidence that induction chemotherapy followed by a single course of high-dose chemotherapy with stem cell transplant improves the outcome for women with metastatic breast cancer (Table 14.2). Toxicity, however, has been reduced substantially over the last decade, and a single course of high-dose therapy is at least equivalent to prolonged multiple cycles of conventional dose chemotherapy. Future investigations should focus on selection of patients who are most likely to benefit from high-dose therapy, therapy directed at elimination of minimal residual disease after high-dose therapy, and decreased stem cell breast cancer contamination. It will require a collaboration of physicians, patients, and insurers to investigate these newer approaches in a timely fashion and ensure optimal care for our patients with metastatic breast cancer.

REFERENCES

1. Peters WP, Shpall EJ, Jones RB, et al. High-dose combination alkylating agents with bone marrow support as initial treatment for metastatic breast cancer. *J Clin Oncol* 1988;6:1368–1376.
2. Williams SF, Mick R, Desser R, et al. High-dose consolidation therapy with autologous stem cell rescue in stage IV breast cancer. *J Clin Oncol* 1989;7:1824–1830.
3. Antman K, Ayash L, Elias A, et al. A phase II study of high-dose cyclophosphamide, thiotepa, and carboplatin with autologous marrow support in women with measurable advanced breast cancer responding to standard-dose therapy. *J Clin Oncol* 1991;10:102–110.
4. Williams SF, Gilewski T, Mick R, et al. High-dose consolidation therapy with autologous stem cell rescue in stage IV breast cancer: follow-up report. *J Clin Oncol* 1992;10:1743–1747.
5. Moonneier JA, Williams SF, Kamminer LS, et al. High-dose trialkylator chemotherapy with autologous stem cell rescue in patients with refractory malignancies. *J Natl Cancer Inst* 1990;82:29–34.
6. Kennedy MJ, Beveridge RA, Rowley SD, et al. High-dose chemotherapy with reinfusion of purged autologous bone marrow following dose intense induction as initial therapy for metastatic breast cancer. *J Natl Cancer Inst* 1991;83:920–926.
7. Eddy DM. Review article. High-dose chemotherapy with autologous bone marrow transplantation for the treatment of metastatic breast cancer. *J Clin Oncol* 1992;10:657–670.
8. Klumpp TR, Mangan KF, Glenn LD. Phase II pilot study of high-dose busulfan and CY followed by autologous BM or peripheral blood stem cell transplantation in patients with advanced chemosensitive breast cancer. *Bone Marrow Transplant* 1993;11:337–339.
9. Lazarus HM, Gray R, Ciobanu N, et al. A phase I trial of high-dose melphalan, high-dose etoposide, and autologous bone marrow reinfusion in solid tumors: An Eastern Cooperative Oncology Group (ECOG) study. *Bone Marrow Transplant* 1994;14:443–448.
10. Weaver CH, Bensinger WI, Appelbaum FR, et al. Phase I study of high-dose busulfan, melphalan, and thiotepa with autologous stem cell support in patients with refractory malignancies. *Bone Marrow Transplant* 1994;14:813–819.
11. Vaughan WP, Reed EC, Edwards B, et al. High-dose cyclophosphamide, thiotepa and hydroxyurea with autologous hematopoietic stem cell rescue: An effective consolidation chemotherapy regimen for early metastatic breast cancer. *Bone Marrow Transplant* 1994;13:619–624.
12. Fields KK, Elfenbein GJ, Lazarus HM, et al. Maximum tolerated doses of ifosfamide, carboplatin, and etoposide given over six days followed by autologous stem cell rescue: Toxicity profile. *J Clin Oncol* 1995;13:323–332.
13. Spitzer TR, Cirenza E, McAfee S, et al. Phase I-II trial of high-dose cyclophosphamide, carboplatin and autologous bone marrow or peripheral blood stem cell rescue. *Bone Marrow Transplant* 1995;15:537–542.
14. Gisselbrecht C, Extra JM, Lotz JP, et al. Cyclophosphamide/mitoxantrone/melphalan (CMA) regimen prior to autologous bone marrow transplantation (ABMT) in metastatic breast cancer. *Bone Marrow Transplant* 1996;18:857–863.
15. Stemmer SM, Cagnoni PJ, Shpall EJ, et al. High-dose paclitaxel, cyclophosophamide, and cisplatin with autologous hematopoietic progenitor-cell support: A phase I trial. *J Clin Oncol* 1996;14:1463–1472.
16. Rowlings PA, Williams SF, Antman KH, et al. Factors correlated with progression-free survival after high-dose chemotherapy and hematopoietic stem cell transplantation for metastatic breast cancer. *JAMA* 1999;282:1335–1343.
17. Stadtmauer EA, O'Neill A, Goldstein LJ, et al. Conventional dose chemotherapy compared with high-dose chemotherapy plus autologous hematopoietic stem cell transplantation for metastatic breast cancer. *New Eng J Med* 2000;342(15):1069–1076.
18. Stadtmauer EA, O'Neill A, Goldstein LJ, et al. Conventional-dose chemotherapy compared with high-dose chemotherapy (HDC) plus autologous stem-cell transplantation (SCT) for metastatic breast cancer: 5

year update of the 'Philadelphia Trial' (PBT-1). *Proc ASCO* 2002;21:43a.
19. Daly MB, Goldstein LJ, Topolsky D, et al. Quality of life experience in women randomized to high-dose chemotherapy (HDC) and stem cell support (SCT) or standard dose chemotherapy for responding metastatic breast cancer in Philadelphia Intergroup Study (PBT-1). *Proc ASCO* 2000;19:85a.
20. Schulman KA, Glick HA, Goldstein LJ, et al. Economic analysis of high-dose chemotherapy (HDC) and stem cell support (SCT) vs standard dose chemotherapy for women with responding metastatic breast cancer in the Philadelphia Intergroup Study (PBT-1). *Proc ASCO* 2000;19:85a.
21. Crump M, Gluck D, Stewart M, et al. A randomized trial of high-dose chemotherapy (HDC) with autologous peripheral blood stem cell support (ASCT) compared to standard therapy in women with metastatic breast cancer: A National Cancer Institute of Canada (NCIC) Clinical Trials Group Study. *Proc ASCO* 2001;20:21a.
22. Biron P, Durand M, Roche H, et al. High-dose thiotepa (TTP), cyclophosphamide (CPM) and stem cell transplantation after 4 FEC 100 compared with 4 FEC alone allowed a better disease free survival but the same overall survival in first line chemotherapy for metastatic breast cancer. Results of the PEGASE 3 French Protocole. *Proc ASCO* 2002;21:42a.
23. Lotz JP, Cure H, Janvier M, et al. High-dose chemotherapy with hematopoietic stem cells transplantation for metastatic breast cancer: results of the French protocol Pegase 04. *Proc ASCO* 1999;18:43A.
24. Peters W, Jones R, Vredenburgh J, et al. A large prospective randomized trial of high-dose combination alkylating agents (CPB) with autologous cellular support as consolidation for patients with metastatic breast cancer achieving complete remission after intensive doxorubicin-based induction therapy (AFM). *Proc ASCO* 1996;15:121.
25. Berry DA, Broadwater G, Perry MC, et al. High-dose versus standard chemotherapy in metastatic breast cancer: Comparison of Cancer and Leukemia Group B trials with data from the Autologous Blood and Marrow Transplant Registry. *J Clin Oncol* 2002;20:743–750.
26. Bezwoda W, Seymour L, Dansey R. High-dose chemotherapy with hematopoietic rescue as primary treatment for metastatic breast cancer: A randomized trial. *J Clin Oncol* 1995;13:2483–2489.
27. Schmid P, Samonigg H, Nitsch T, et al. Randomized trial of up front tandem high-dose chemotherapy (HD) compared to standard chemotherapy with doxorubicin and paclitaxel (AT) in metastatic breast cancer (MBC). *Proc ASCO* 2002;21:43a.
28. Ayash LJ, Elias A, Schwartz G, et al. Double dose-intensive chemotherapy with autologous stem-cell support for metastatic breast cancer: No improvement in progression-free survival by the sequence of high-dose melphalan followed by cyclophosphamide, thiotepa and carboplatin. *J Clin Oncol* 1996; 14:2984–2992.
29. Elias AD, Richardson P, Avigan D. et al. A short course of induction chemotherapy followed by 2 cycles of high-dose chemotherapy with stem cell rescue for chemotherapy naive metastatic breast cancer: sequential phase I/II studies. *Bone Marrow Transplant* 2001; 28:447–454.
30. Pecora A, Lazarus H, Stadtmauer E, et al. Effect of induction chemotherapy on outcomes in autologous stem cell transplant for metastatic breast cancer. *Bone Marrow Transplant* 2001;27:1245–1253.

SECTION 4

Metastatic Disease: Hormone Treatment

15

Aromatase Inhibitors in the Treatment of Breast Cancer

Kellie L. Jones, Aman U. Buzdar, and Gabriel N. Hortobagyi

For breast cancer patients with estrogen-receptor (ER)-positive and/or progesterone-receptor (PgR)-positive disease, hormonal or endocrine therapy provides a viable and effective treatment option. Several of these therapies are effective in treating 25% to 30% of unselected patients and in those with ER-positive disease, more than half of the them receive clinical benefit from hormonal therapy (1–3).

The main goal of endocrine therapy is to reduce the production of estrogen or block the action of estrogen at the receptor level in tumor cells. A complex cycle of feedback mechanisms is activated to initiate estrogen production involving the hypothalamus, pituitary, ovary, adrenal glands, and the breast. The hormones that are produced by these glands serve as regulators for the feedback loop. In premenopausal patients, the control mechanism is through the luteinizing hormone-releasing hormone (LHRH) produced by the hypothalamus. Subsequently, LHRH activates the anterior pituitary to produce gonadotropins, follicle-stimulating hormone (FSH), and luteinizing hormone (LH), ultimately acting on the ovaries. In addition to the numerous hormones released by the anterior pituitary gland, it also produces adrenocorticotropic hormone (ACTH) which in the end acts on the breast tissue. Androgens and corticosteroids are produced by the adrenal glands. At the final step of this complex feedback system, estrone and estradiol are converted from testosterone and androstenedione via the aromatase enzyme (4). In this chapter, we discuss aromatase inhibitors as treatment options for postmenopausal breast cancer patients.

The production of estrogens through this complex system is illustrated in Figure 15.1. These pathways entail numerous series of reactions with a common precursor, cholesterol. A sequence of related cytochrome P-450 enzymes controls these multiple reactions. The aromatase enzyme itself differs from other cytochrome P-450 enzymes in that it contains the usual cytochrome P-450 hemoprotein and flavoprotein components, but only the hemoprotein is specific for aromatase. This is unlike the cytochrome P-450 nicotinamide adenine dinucleotide phosphate (NADPH) reductase that is seen with other cytochrome P-450 enzymes. These reactions take place in numerous areas of the body including muscle, adipose tissue, and the breast tumor itself. This is important because about two-thirds of malignant breast tumors contain the aromatase enzyme, potentially leading to *in situ* production of estrogen and growth stimulation of the tumor (5,6). For premenopausal patients, the ovary serves as the main source of estrogen production; however, estrogen is also produced at a much lower level by peripheral aromatization. Even with these smaller amounts, it is sufficient to support the growth of estrogen-dependent tumors in women who are postmenopausal.

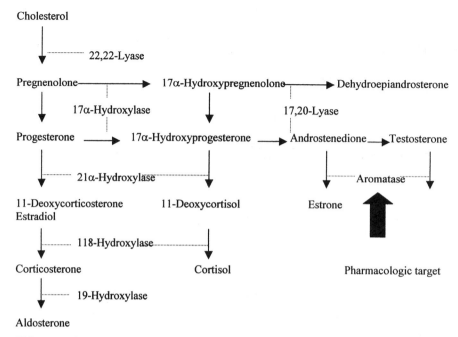

FIG. 15.1. Steroid and estrogen biosynthesis pathways.

Through this pathway, approximately 100 ng of estrone is produced, resulting in plasma estradiol levels of 10 pg to 20 pg per mL.

AROMATASE INHIBITORS

Numerous aromatase inhibitors have been evaluated in the treatment of breast cancer as seen in Table 15.1. The objective when developing these agents was to create drugs that were selective for the aromatase enzyme, while having minimal side effects and maintaining clinical efficacy. Various compounds have been studied and currently only five drugs are available for clinical use: anastrozole, letrozole, exemestane, fadrozole and formestane. Non-selective aromatase inhibitors are also available including: aminoglutethimide, testolactone, and trilostane. Two classifications or subtypes can be used when discussing the aromatase inhibitors: type I (suicide or noncom-

TABLE 15.1. *Aromatase inhibitors*

	Type	Selectivity	Potency
Non-selective			
Aminoglutethimide	Competitive	Low	Moderate
Testolactone	Noncompetitive	Low	Moderate
Trilostane	Competitive	Moderate	Moderate
Selective non-steroidal			
Fadrozole	Competitive	Moderate	Moderate
Vorozole	Competitive	High	High
Letrozole	Competitive	High	High
Anastrozole	Competitive	High	High
Selective steroidal			
Formestane	Noncompetitive	High	High
Exemestane	Noncompetitive	High	High

petitive) and type II (competitive) inhibitors. Type I inhibitors are all steroidal compounds while type II inhibitors can be either steroidal or non-steroidal. Both of these classes mimic the normal substrates (androgens), and compete for binding on the enzyme.

Once a noncompetitive inhibitor binds to the aromatase enzyme, a sequence of hydroxylation is activated which produces an irreversible covalent bond between the inhibitor and the enzyme protein. Aromatase activity is thus permanently blocked. This activity can only be restored by the production of new enzyme, even if all of the unattached inhibitor is removed. Competitive inhibitors reversibly bind to the active enzyme site allowing the inhibitors to remain or be disassociated from the binding site. This allows renewed competition between the inhibitor and substrate. The effectiveness of the type II inhibitors depends on both the relative concentration and affinity for the inhibitor and the substrate. Important structural features must be shared between both types of inhibitors to compete for binding to the active site. For noncompetitive inhibitors to be inherently selective, they must share androgenic features allowing them to interact with catalytic residues on the enzyme protein. On the other hand, most type I inhibitors interact with heme iron, a common feature of all cytochrome P-450 enzymes. Some of these inhibitors may also bind to both the highly conserved oxygen-binding sites in addition to the substrate-binding site. Other structural features reinforce the specificity of the competitive inhibitors, but it may also block the activity of a wide variety of cytochrome P-450 enzymes, similar to aminoglutethimide.

Aromatase inhibitors can only be used in women who are postmenopausal. When used in premenopausal women, the aromatase inhibition results in greater estrogen production due to the feedback mechanisms of the steroid biosynthesis pathway increasing the gonadotropin-releasing hormone levels. This in turn increases FSH levels, leading to increased aromatase production. Luteinizing hormone levels in response to the increased FSH lead to more ovarian steroidogenesis, particularly for androstenedione, and the substrate for aromatase.

NON-SELECTIVE AROMATASE INHIBITORS

This class of aromatase inhibitors were the first available agents of its kind for the treatment of metastatic breast cancer. However, these medications had numerous side effects. They did provide practical treatment options for patients who were otherwise considered to be poor surgical candidates for ablative procedures such as adrenalectomy or hypophysectomy (7,8).

Testolactone

Testolactone was the first non-selective aromatase inhibitor to become available (9,10). In the beginning, it was believed to be an androgen, although virilizing effects were almost completely nonexistent (11). This agent is no longer in use due to limited efficacy.

Aminoglutethimide

Aminoglutethimide was more extensively evaluated and became another treatment option to surgical ablative procedures. Initially, this agent was introduced as an anticonvulsant. Later, however, it was withdrawn due to its substantial morbidity as a result of adrenal insufficiency. Aminoglutethimide decreases circulating estrogen levels by 60% to 70% through competitively inhibiting aromatization. This aromatase inhibitor also blocks the cholesterol side-chain cleavage, thus blocking steroidal synthesis, resulting in a significant reduction in glucocorticoid and mineralocorticoid levels. Therefore, it is required to use concomitant hydrocortisone supplementation with aminoglutethimide therapy.

The initial half-life of aminoglutethimide is 12.3 ± 2.6 hours and decreases to 7.3 ± 2.4 hours with prolonged use because of induction of this enzyme, which catalyzes its own elimination (12).

Two major studies have demonstrated no significant differences in response rates when comparing aminoglutethimide with hypophysectomy and adrenalectomy in advanced breast cancer patients (5,7,8).

When used as initial therapy for metastatic breast cancer patients, aminoglutethimide demonstrated similar response rates and duration of remission when compared to tamoxifen (13–16). Aminoglutethimide has also been compared to progestins, illustrating similar efficacy between the two treatment arms (17).

Different doses of aminoglutethimide have been evaluated in four randomized studies. They have compared aminoglutethimide at doses of 500 mg and 1,000 mg per day, both with supplemental hydrocortisone. Response varied from 15% to 35% in the trials; however, the differences were not statistically significant (17–20). In phase 2 trials, lower doses (as low as 250 mg per day), with or without hydrocortisone, have been evaluated and have antitumor activity (21,22). Due to the number of side effects and less selectivity of this agent, the newer aromatase inhibitors are utilized before aminoglutethimide therapy.

Trilostane

Trilostane is another non-selective aromatase inhibitor. This agent inhibits 3β-hydroxysteroid dehydrogenase, thus decreasing the conversion of Δ^5-steroids to the estrogen precursor Δ^4-steroid. As with aminoglutethimide, this inhibition leads to depressed cortisone synthesis requiring supplemental replacement therapy. This compound did illustrate a 26% response rate in a phase 2 study; however, it was associated with significant side effects including: nausea, vomiting, lethargy, postural hypotension, rash, hot flashes, facial/tongue pain, Cushingoid features, and epigastric discomfort and diarrhea (4). This drug is no longer in clinical use.

SELECTIVE AROMATASE INHIBITORS

Steroidal Aromatase Inhibitors

Formestane

4-Hydroxyandrostenedione (formestane, a noncompetitive or suicide inhibitor) was one of the first of its class to be developed and was widely studied. Formestane is an irreversible inhibitor of both peripheral and breast tissue aromatase and has no estrogenic activity. Trials have demonstrated that this agent is highly selective for aromatase, therefore exerting no effect on serum levels of androstenedione, testosterone, dihydrotestosterone, aldosterone, cortisol or 17α-hydroxyprogesterone (23,24). After oral administration, formestane has demonstrated some weak androgenic activity. This is reflective in a 15% fall in serum levels of sex hormone-binding globulin (SHBG), but there is lack of androgen activity after intramuscular injection, probably reflecting a lack of first pass metabolism (23,26,35).

The injectable formulation of formestane also significantly suppresses estrogen concentrations, but to a lesser extent than the newer aromatase inhibitor, anastrozole (27). Inconsistent suppression of serum estradiol is evident in that estradiol levels begin to rise between the biweekly dosing of formestane (27,28). A small, randomized, comparative study evaluated formestane (250 mg i.m. every 2 weeks; n = 31) and anastrozole (1 mg by mouth daily; n = 29). The regimens were administered over a 4-week period in postmenopausal women with breast cancer (27). Estradiol suppression was identified to be more reliable and consistent with anastrozole versus formestane (79% versus 58%; $p = 0.0001$). In addition to estradiol, estrone and estrone sulfate levels were suppressed more significantly with anastrozole compared to formestane (estrone, 85% versus 67%; $p = 0.0043$; estrone sulfate 92% versus 67%, $p = 0.0007$) (27). Recent results also indicate that the steroidal aromatase inhibitor exemestane, when compared with formestane, suppresses estrogen concentrations to 6% to 15% of pretreatment levels (29–30).

Formestane needs to be given as an intramuscular injection, but few patients experience pain and inflammation at the injection site. Other side effects after injection include weakness, lethargy, hot flashes, spotting, and mild nausea and vomiting (31). The drug is well tolerated and 90% of the patients experience no side effects (32). Studies with different doses of this drug by intramuscular injection have shown no differences in response rates. However, side effects were less frequent at 250 mg i.m. every 2 weeks.

Second-line Therapy

A phase 3 prospective, randomized, crossover trial compared formestane (250 mg i.m. every 14 days) to megestrol acetate (160 mg by mouth daily) in postmenopausal patients with advanced breast cancer who had failed tamoxifen therapy (n = 179) (33). No significant differences were identified between formestane and megestrol acetate in regards to response rates, stable disease (SD) (6 months or more), or time to treatment failure (TTF) (3.9 versus 3.7 months, respectively). In this population, formestane was considered to be as effective as megestrol acetate. Another trial with the same treatment arms evaluated 547 postmenopausal patients with receptor-positive or receptor-unknown, tamoxifen resistant, advanced breast cancer. No significant differences were identified between the groups in terms of median TTF and overall survival (OS) (34).

First-line Therapy

Formestane was also tested in a comparative trial for first-line hormonal treatment in postmenopausal breast cancer patients. Tamoxifen (30 mg by mouth daily) was evaluated against formestane (250 mg i.m. every 2 weeks; n = 409). Study endpoints included safety and tolerability. Patient characteristics were well matched, except that more patients with soft tissue metastases were randomized to the formestane group. No statistically significant differences were found between the groups (overall response [OR], median duration of response, and survival), and tamoxifen resulted in significantly longer time to treatment progression (TTP) (9.7 months versus 7 months; $p = 0.003$) and TTF (9.7 months versus 6.5 months; $p = 0.001$) compared to formestane (35).

Conclusions

These data provide support for formestane as second-line therapy. Formestane was as effective as megestrol acetate in terms of SD and TTF. There is also evidence to support the use of formestane as first-line therapy. No statistically significant differences were identified between tamoxifen and formestane in regards to OR, median duration of response, and survival. Time to treatment progression and TTF were statistically longer with tamoxifen compared to formestane.

Exemestane

Exemestane is a type I steroidal inhibitor and is derived from steroidal androgens. Due to the similar androgen-like structures of these type I compounds, there is a potential for androgenic side effects. In early trials, patients with higher doses (up to 200 mg per day) reported androgenic symptoms including alopecia in 10% of patients and hoarseness in 5% of patients (n = 78) (36). The plasma level of SHBG is a sensitive guide to the androgenic side effects of this orally administered medication. At a dose of 25 mg per day, there was negligible change in SHBG levels, suggesting that it was associated with little androgenic side effects (29). When compared to anastrozole and letrozole, exemestane suppresses estradiol levels by 97.9% in similar assays (29).

Second-line Therapy

A phase 3 randomized, double-blind trial in postmenopausal, tamoxifen resistant, advanced breast cancer patients evaluated exemestane (25 mg by mouth daily; n = 366) and megestrol acetate (40 mg by mouth 4 times a day; n = 403) (36). At the time of analysis, the median duration of follow-up was 48.9 weeks. The median survival had not been achieved, and 143 patients were still participating in the study. Equivalency between the two treatment arms was the primary study objective. Both groups illustrated similar OR rates as well as overall clinical benefit (CR plus PR plus SD more than or equal to 24 weeks). Median survival ($p = 0.039$) and median TTP ($p = 0.037$), however, were significantly improved with exemestane (37). These data identified exemestane as an appropriate second-line option for tamoxifen-resistant, postmenopausal breast cancer patients.

First-line Therapy

Data using exemestane as first-line therapy in metastatic breast cancer patients are limited. Results from ongoing studies will be available soon. It is believed that these data will also illustrate the role of exemestane as a first-line therapy. In a small, phase 2 study comparing exemestane (25 mg by mouth daily) with tamoxifen (20 mg by mouth daily) as first-line therapy, the median TTP was 8.9 months with exemestane (n = 31) compared to 5.2 months with tamoxifen (n = 32). The overall response rate (CR plus PR) illustrated the superiority of exemestane over tamoxifen (42% versus 16%, respectively) (38). However, at the time of data analysis, no statistical information was presented. The general conclusions were that exemestane showed promise in the first-line treatment setting in metastatic breast cancer patients.

Adjuvant Therapy

Many studies are also currently accruing patients to identify the role of adjuvant exemestane. Examples of regimens include the International Collaboration Cancer Group (ICCG) trial where patients receive tamoxifen for 2 to 3 years and then either tamoxifen or exemestane for the remainder of the 5-year period. The National Surgical Adjuvant Breast and Bowel Project (NSABP) will have patients receive either exemestane or placebo for 2 years after they have completed their 5 years of standard tamoxifen therapy (39–42).

One question of concern is the effects of aromatase inhibitors on bone and lipid profiles of patients in the adjuvant setting. It is known that tamoxifen has beneficial effects on these factors (43). A recent abstract evaluated the role of exemestane on bone mineral density and lipid profile in ovariectomized rats (44). The study arms consisted of: (a) intact control; (b) ovariectomized rats; and (c) ovariectomized rats plus exemestane (biweekly administration of 100 mg per kg of intramuscular exemestane for 16 weeks). Bone mineral density (BMD) decreased to 11% of control in group two and 99% of control in group three ($p < 0.0001$). The addition of exemestane produced a 32.3% decrease in serum cholesterol levels ($p < 0.0001$) compared to no exemestane. Group three also decreased the level of low-density lipoproteins by 78% compared to group two ($p < 0.0001$) (44). These data will need to be verified in much larger human trials, but they do appear to demonstrate that exemestane may be a suitable therapeutic option for adjuvant treatment or chemoprevention.

Neoadjuvant Therapy

Using endocrine therapy in this setting is not a new concept. This was first described in 1957 by Kennedy et al. (45) using neoadjuvant diethylstilbestrol. A small phase 2 study (n = 12) has shown promising results using exemestane in the neoadjuvant setting. These results have only been published in abstract form. Prior to treatment, ten patients would have required mastectomy. With exemestane, 25 mg for 3 months, ten patients were able to undergo breast conservative surgery. However, to date, no randomized comparative trials have been reported with exemestane and tamoxifen (46).

Conclusions

There is data in support of using exemestane for second-line therapy of metastatic breast cancer. Exemestane was proven to be similar to megestrol acetate in OR and overall clinical benefit. Median survival and median TTP were significantly improved with exemestane compared to megestrol acetate. Data is also currently available for exemestane as first-line therapy for advanced disease. Results of definitive trials are still pending, and as new data become available, the level of evidence in support of this indication will likely increase.

Non-Steroidal Aromatase Inhibitors

Fadrozole

Fadrozole is also a competitive aromatase inhibitor. It is more selective than aminoglutethimide, but less so than anastrozole. This agent appears to have little or no effect on the enzyme desmolase. However, it does partially hinder 11-hydroxylase and 18-hydroxylase enzymes. The half-life of fadrozole is 10.5 hours and maximum effects have been seen with daily doses of 2 mg to 4 mg. Currently, this aromatase inhibitor is only available in Japan.

Second-line Therapy

Two double blind, placebo-controlled, prospective studies compared fadrozole and megestrol acetate in postmenopausal patients who had failed tamoxifen. The primary endpoints of both were ORR and, secondarily, TTP and survival. A total of 683 patients were included in these two trials. Both studies randomized patients to receive either fadrozole (1 mg twice daily) or megestrol acetate (40 mg four times daily). The first trial enrolled 380 patients and the second study enrolled 303 patients. No differences in response rates between the two trials were identified. The fadrozole arm in the first study had a longer median survival time than megestrol acetate (26.8 versus 22.8 months, respectively). The second trial, however, produced the opposite results with a longer median survival time with megestrol acetate compared to fadrozole (25.4 versus 22.8 months, respectively) (47). Both of these trials identified fadrozole as equivalent therapy in comparison to megestrol acetate in the second-line treatment of postmenopausal women with advanced breast cancer.

Conclusion

There are data to support the application of fadrozole as second-line therapy. However, due to the toxicities with the agent, other therapies are utilized in preference to fadrozole. In addition to this, fadrozole is currently only available in Japan.

Vorozole

Vorozole is the active isomer of R-76713. *In vitro,* this drug has a 10,000-fold more potent selectivity for aromatase compared with any other cytochrome P-450 enzyme. In experimental animal models, even at 200 times the normal dose for estrogen suppression, there was no effect of vorozole on the production of adrenal glucocorticoids or mineralocorticoids.

Second-line Therapy

Goss et al. (49) conducted an open-labeled, multicentered, parallel-grouped phase 3 trial with 452 postmenopausal patients whose disease had previously progressed on tamoxifen therapy. The treatment arms included vorozole (2.5 mg once daily) and megestrol acetate (40 mg four times a day). Overall response rate was the primary endpoint. No significant difference was demonstrated between the two treatment groups in terms of response rates and clinical benefit (CR plus PR plus NC [no change] in 6 months or more), TTP, or survival. In conclusion, the authors summarized that vorozole had similar efficacy to megestrol acetate in the second-line treatment of postmenopausal advanced breast cancer patients who had failed tamoxifen.

In a second trial by Houston and colleagues (49), postmenopausal women who had progressed on tamoxifen therapy were randomized to receive vorozole (2.5 mg daily) or aminoglutethimide (250 mg twice daily) until disease progression or death. This study was an open-labeled, centrally randomized, multicenter, phase 3 trial that included 424 patients. Patients in the aminoglutethimide group also received supplemental hydrocortisone (30 mg daily). Overall response rates in the vorozole group were higher than the aminoglutethimide arm; however, no statistical significance was demonstrated (24% versus 17%, $p = 0.07$). Also, there were no differences identified in terms of duration of response, TTP, TTF, or survival (49). It was concluded that vorozole and aminoglutethimide were equivalent with respect to clinical efficacy as second-line therapy in this patient population.

One last open-labeled, comparative trial illustrated superiority of vorozole over aminoglutethimide therapy in advanced breast cancer patients (CR plus PR plus NC more than or equal to 6 months; $p = 0.07$ and $p = 0.017$, respectively) (50). Although these were positive results, none of the previous studies had shown a significant advantage of vorozole over megestrol acetate or aminoglutethimide in terms of OS or TTP. Because of these results, vorozole is no longer in clinical development.

Anastrozole

In early 1996, anastrozole became available for clinical use in the United States. It is a competitive, nonsteroidal and highly selective aromatase inhibitor. Animal studies have demonstrated that anastrozole has no significant effect against desmolases or any other enzyme involved in steroid biosynthesis. The average plasma half-life is approximately 50 hours in postmenopausal women, and no significant differences between breast cancer patients and healthy postmenopausal women have been illustrated (4). At 10 mg daily for 14 days, anastrozole did not alter plasma cortisol or aldosterone levels or the response to ACTH stimulation (50).

Second-line Therapy

The antitumor activity and safety of anastrozole were compared with megestrol acetate in two large randomized phase 3 trials in postmenopausal women with breast cancer who had failed tamoxifen. These two studies were run in parallel and included three treatment arms consisting of anastrozole (1 mg or 10 mg once daily) and megestrol acetate (40 mg four times daily) (51,52). One was conducted in Europe with 378 participants while the other took place in North America and included 386 patients. The reason for this study design was to enable the data to be combined at the end of both trials (53). Each study was a multicentered, randomized, controlled, parallel group, double-blind schematic trial. The primary objectives were TTP and OR (CR plus PR) with secondary endpoints including survival, TTF, and response duration. At the time of median follow-up (6 months), there were no statistically significant differences in TTP or tumor response, and only one-third of patients in all categories had experienced any clinical benefit from their treatment (54).

After further follow-up of 31.2 months, an interim, intention-to-treat analysis was performed from the combined data (55). At that time, 62% of the patients had died. Both of the anastrozole groups demonstrated survival advantages over megestrol acetate. The median duration of survival with 10 mg anastrozole was increased (25.5 versus. 22.5 months for anastrozole and megestrol acetate, respectively); however, the difference was not statistically significant (HR = 0.83, p = 0.0951). The 1 mg anastrozole arm did illustrate a significant increase in the median duration of survival (26.7 vs. 22.5 months, respectively) (HR = 0.78, $p < 0.025$). The combined analysis showed two-year survival rates of 56.1%, 54.6%, and 46.3%, respectively, in patients who received 1 mg anastrozole, 10 mg anastrozole, and 160 mg megestrol acetate daily (Table 15.2). These results did not suggest any additional benefit when using the 10 mg dose of anastrozole (55). Anastrozole was well tolerated and its safety profile is summarized in Table 15.3. This confirmed the use of the 1 mg anastrozole dosing regimen and provided statistically significant data to support the use of anastrozole as second-line therapy in postmenopausal patients with advanced breast cancer.

First-line Therapy

In the development of a first-line trial for anastrozole, the same approach was taken as previously performed in the second-line studies. Two large-scale trials recruited patients concurrently to evaluate the role of anastrozole (1 mg daily) as first-line therapy compared with tamoxifen (20 mg daily) in postmenopausal women with advanced breast cancer in the North American trial [0030] and the European trial [0027]. A total of 1,021 patients were evaluated in two international, multicentered, randomized, double blind, double-dummy trials. These trials were designed to demonstrate equivalence in each of the primary endpoints: TTP and OR. Secondary endpoints included TTF and survival (56,57). Tolerability was also statistically evaluated. Included were patients

TABLE 15.2. *Efficacy of second-line phase 3 trials comparing anastrozole to megestrol acetate (MA) in postmenopausal, advanced breast cancer patients*

	OR = CR + PR (%)	Clinical benefit (%)	Median TTP (months)	Median survival (months)	2-year survival (%)
European (49)					
Anastrozole 1 mg (n = 135)	10.4	34.1	4.3		50.5
MA 40 mg qid (n = 118)	10.4	32.8	3.9		39.1
North American (51)					
Anastrozole 1 mg (n = 128)	10	37	5.6		62
MA 40 mg qid (n = 130)	6	36	4.7		53.1
Combined (31 months) (54)					
Anastrozole 1 mg (n = 263)	12.6	42.2	4.8	26.7	56.1
MA 40 mg qid (n = 253)	12.2	40.3	4.6	22.5	46.3
			(p = 0.49)	(p = 0.0248)	

CR, complete response; MA, megestrol acetate; OR, overall response; PR, partial response; TTP, time to treatment progression.

eligible for endocrine therapy with ER-positive and/or PgR-positive tumors or those with unknown hormone status. Patients could be newly diagnosed or could have received previous endocrine or chemotherapy in the adjuvant setting. However, patients had to have completed tamoxifen therapy at least one year before entering the trial.

In the North American trial, 353 patients were enrolled (n = 171 anastrozole, n = 182 tamoxifen) and an interim analysis was conducted at a median follow-up of 17.7 months (57). Patient characteristics were evenly distributed and 89% of patients demonstrated ER positivity. The median TTP was 11.1 months with anastrozole versus 5.6 months with tamoxifen (p = 0.005). Twenty-one percent of anastrozole patients achieved an OR, compared with 17% for those treated with tamoxifen. Statistically significant differences in clinical benefit rates were observed: anastrozole 59% versus 46% with tamoxifen (p = 0.0098). Toxicities were also less frequently seen with anastrozole compared to tamoxifen. Fewer thromboembolic events were reported with anastrozole (4.1%) versus tamoxifen (8.2%) and less vaginal bleeding (1.2% versus 3.8%, respectively). Nausea was less with anastrozole (30.6% versus 34.1%, respectively). However, more patients experienced hot flashes with anastrozole compared to tamoxifen (36.5% versus 24.2%). These results do show superior benefit with anastrozole (57). Survival was not evaluated at the time of the analysis because the data were considered to be immature.

One would presume to find similar results in the European trial; however, this was not the case. Six hundred and sixty-eight women were

TABLE 15.3. *Tolerability data of newer aromatase inhibitors versus megestrol acetate in second-line trials*

Side effects (%)	Anastrozole 1 mg (54)	Letrozole 2.5 mg (70)	Exemestane 25 mg (37)	Megestrol acetate 40 mg qid (37,54,70)
Headache	13	13	NR	7–9
Hot flashes	12	6	13	4–8
Nausea	16	11	9	5–11
Vomiting	9	8	3	1–6
Weight gain	2	2	NR	9–12
Asthenia	16	11	8	7–11

NR, not reported.

enrolled in the European trial (n = 340 anastrozole, n = 328 tamoxifen) (56). The same inclusion criteria were utilized with a similar median follow-up of 19 months. Once again, the groups were well balanced except in one area. Patients with known estrogen-receptor-positive tumors represented only 45% of the trial population compared to 89% in the partner study. The median TTP was 8.2 months with anastrozole and 8.3 months with tamoxifen, while the ORR were 32.9% and 32.6%, respectively. Overall clinical benefit rates were similar to the previous trial with 56.2% with anastrozole and 55.5% with tamoxifen. This study analyzed alone would suggest that anastrozole is equivalent to tamoxifen.

However, retrospective subgroup analysis of the ER-positive patients (45%) in the European trial showed a median TTP of 8.9 months with anastrozole versus 7.8 with tamoxifen. This difference in median TTP was statistically significant in the 611 patients with known ER/PR positive tumors ($p = 0.022$) (58).

A combined analysis of efficacy and tolerability was also performed including all patients (59). Anastrozole was found to be as effective as tamoxifen in terms of TTP. The median TTP was 8.5 months in the anastrozole group compared to 7 months with tamoxifen (hazard ratio [HR] = 1.12; lower 95% confidence interval [CI], 1.00 to 1.13). These data demonstrated equivalence because the confidence interval crossed 1.0 and lacked statistical significance.

Clinical benefit was greater in the anastrozole arm (57% versus 52%). This benefit appeared to improve with anastrozole compared to tamoxifen, but this was not statistically evaluated (Table 15.4).

A smaller, independent study also maintained the same results as previously demonstrated in the North American trial. This trial consisted of 238 postmenopausal breast cancer patients with ER-positive tumors who had not been administered previous therapy for their advanced cancer. Patients were randomized to receive 1 mg anastrozole (n = 121) or 40 mg tamoxifen daily (n = 117) (60). Median TTP of 10.6 months was demonstrated with anastrozole versus 5.3 months with tamoxifen (HR = 0.77, 95% CI, 0.56–0.91; $p < 0.05$) (38). By the cut-off date, 92% of the tamoxifen patients had died compared to only 61% in the anastrozole group (HR = 0.63; 95% CI 0.51–0.89; $p =$ less than 0.05). This information is promising, but median overall survival is a more reliable endpoint. With all of these data, anastrozole became the first aromatase inhibitor to be considered as an appropriate and better-tolerated treatment option for first-line therapy of hormone sensitive, metastatic breast cancer in postmenopausal women.

Adjuvant Therapy

Tamoxifen is currently considered the gold standard in hormonal adjuvant treatment for

TABLE 15.4. *Efficacy results from first-line phase 3 trials of newer aromatase inhibitors versus tamoxifen*

	Anastrozole (combination data) (58)		Letrozole (77,78)	
	Anastrozole 1 mg	Tamoxifen 20 mg	Letrozole 2.5 mg	Tamoxifen 20 mg
CBR (%)	57	52	49	38
		NR	OR: 1.62 (95% CI: 1.24–2.11)	
			$p = 0.0004$	
Median TTP (months)	8.5	7.0	9.4	6.0
	HR: 1.12 (lower 95% CI: 1.00)		$p = 0.0001$	
All receptor positive patients	N = 305	N = 306	N = 294	N = 305
Median TTP (months)	10.7	6.4	9.7	6.0
	$p = 0.022$		HR: 0.90, (95% CI: 0.77–1.06)	
			$p = 0.20$	

CBR, clinical benefit rate; CI, confidence interval; HR, hazard ratio; N, number of patients; NR, not reported; OR, odds ratio; TTP, time to treatment progression.

breast cancer. However, this medication has a higher frequency of serious side effects compared to the newer, more selective aromatase inhibitors. Tamoxifen is associated with increased risks of thromboembolic events as well as endometrial cancer (41,61). It is known that anastrozole, as well as letrozole, offer efficacy similar to tamoxifen in the first-line treatment of metastatic breast cancer (55,56). With fewer side effects and similar efficacy, aromatase inhibitors are a logical choice to evaluate in the adjuvant treatment setting.

Multiple trials are currently under investigation to assess anastrozole's role in the adjuvant setting (40,62–64). The largest trial to date is the Arimidex or Tamoxifen Alone or in Combination (ATAC) trial (65). This is a randomized, double blind, placebo-controlled, multicentered trial evaluating tolerability and efficacy of three treatment arms for 5 years: (a) anastrozole 1 mg daily plus placebo; (b) placebo plus tamoxifen 20 mg daily; and (c) anastrozole 1 mg daily plus tamoxifen 20 mg daily. Disease-free survival (DFS) and safety/tolerability were primary endpoints. Secondarily, OS, time to distant metastasis, and incidence of new breast primaries were evaluated. In addition to these endpoints, companion studies were conducted to evaluate quality of life, effects on bone and the endometrium, and pharmacokinetics. Preliminary results were presented at the San Antonio Breast Cancer Symposium in December 2001 (65).

A total of 9,366 patients were enrolled from 21 countries worldwide. Patient characteristics were equally balanced in all categories (Table 15.5). The first interim analysis was planned to take place when 1,056 events had occurred. A total of 1,079 events had been reported at the time of this analysis with most events occurring with combination therapy. The median duration of therapy was 30.7 months with a median follow-up of 33.3 months (Table 15.6). Disease-free survival was significantly longer with anastrozole compared to tamoxifen but not with the combination versus tamoxifen ($p = 0.0129$; $p = 0.7718$, respectively). A planned retrospective subgroup analysis of only ER-positive patients also illustrated similar results ($p = 0.0054$; $p = 0.7786$, respectively).

Anastrozole was better tolerated when compared to tamoxifen. Anastrozole patients had

TABLE 15.5. *ATAC trial patient characteristics*

	Anastrozole (n = 3,125)	Tamoxifen (n = 3,116)	Anastrozole + tamoxifen (n = 3,125)
Median age (years)	64.1	64.1	64.3
Receptor status (%)			
Positive	83.7	83.3	84.0
Negative	7.4	8.0	6.9
Other	8.9	8.7	9.1
Primary treatment (%)			
Mastectomy	47.8	47.3	48.1
Axillary Surgery	95.5	95.7	95.2
Radiotherapy	63.3	62.5	62.0
Chemotherapy	22.3	20.8	20.8
Prior tamoxifen	1.6	1.7	1.7
Primary tumor size (%)			
T1	63.9	62.9	64.1
T2	32.6	34.2	32.9
T3	2.7	2.2	2.3
Nodal status (%)			
Node positive	34.9	33.6	33.5

T, tumor size; T1, ≤ 2 cm; T2, > 2 cm and ≤ 5 cm; T3, > 5 cm.
Data from Baum et al. (65).

TABLE 15.6. *Disease free survival in ATAC trial*

	HR	95% CI	p
All patients			
A vs. T	0.83	0.71–0.96	0.0129
A + T vs. T	1.02	0.88–1.18	0.7718
ER (+) patients only			
A vs. T	0.78	0.65–0.93	0.0054
A + T vs. T	1.02	0.87–1.21	0.7786

A, anastrozole; CI, confidence interval; ER, estrogen receptor; HR, hazard ratio; T, tamoxifen.
From Baum et al. (65).

less toxicity in terms of endometrial cancer, thromboembolic events, hot flashes, and weight gain compared to tamoxifen. No absolute numbers were presented, and these data have not been fully published. Tamoxifen, on the other hand, was more beneficial in terms of reduction in fractures and musculoskeletal disorders. These data show superiority of anastrozole over tamoxifen in the adjuvant setting. However, these are preliminary results. Longer follow-up is needed to confirm these positive results. In addition, data regarding bone mineral density (BMD) and other toxicity profiles will need to be further evaluated.

Other adjuvant trials are also being conducted. The Arimidex-Nolvadex (ARNO) trial is underway with the German Breast Cancer Group. This study is evaluating tamoxifen for 2 years followed by randomization to either 3 years of anastrozole or 3 years of tamoxifen therapy for a total duration of therapy of 5 years. Endpoints include overall survival, relapse-free survival, tolerability, and quality of life (40,41,62,63). The Austrian Breast Cancer Study Group (ABCSG) is also conducting two trials (64). One involves the addition of aminoglutethimide to tamoxifen in stage I and II breast cancers. After patients receive 5 years of endocrine therapy in either arm, those who are recurrence-free will be randomized to anastrozole or placebo for another 3 years. A second study compares tamoxifen for 3 years to anastrozole for 3 years after the patient has received 2 years of tamoxifen therapy (65). All of this information will provide much needed data regarding the best endocrine management of breast cancer in the adjuvant setting.

Neoadjuvant Therapy

Studies are also currently underway to evaluate the role of anastrozole in the neoadjuvant setting. Currently, only phase 2 neoadjuvant studies are available with anastrozole. One small study by a group from Edinburgh included 24 patients in a randomized, double-blind fashion to compare 1 mg anastrozole or 10 mg anastrozole daily for three months. Ultrasound showed the average reduction in tumor volume with 1 mg of anastrozole was 80.5% compared to 69.6% with 10 mg of anastrozole. At the start of the study, 15 patients (63%) were expected to have undergone a mastectomy. However, with neoadjuvant therapy, these 15 patients were able to undergo breast-conserving surgery (66). With these promising results, a larger randomized study is underway to evaluate anastrozole compared to tamoxifen and compared to the combination of both agents in the preoperative setting (67).

A recent abstract presented at the San Antonio Breast Cancer Symposium in 2001 evaluated a phase 2, open-labeled trial of 89 postmenopausal, hormone-dependent, locally advanced breast cancer patients (68). The primary endpoints were clinical response rates (OR = CR plus PR). All patients received 1 mg anastrozole daily for 4 months. Those who did not show response went on to receive radiotherapy. Patients with a PR and/or CR went on to surgery followed by 2 years of therapy with anastrozole or until disease progression, whichever was sooner. At the time of analysis, data were only available on 74 of the 89 patients. The median age of the population was 64.7 years, and 61% of patients had stage IIIA or IIIB disease. Thirteen patients (18%) had no response and proceeded on to radiotherapy. Forty-two patients (57%) achieved a PR, 19 patients (26%) achieved CR, and an OR was observed in 61 patients (83%). These patients went on to surgery. Specimens from surgery identified a pathologic complete response (pCR) in 14 patients (23%) and a pathologic partial response (pPR) in 47 patients (64%) (68). These results are comparable to neoadjuvant chemotherapy, CR (47%–88%) and pCR (4%–30%) (69). From these results, anastrozole appears to be a highly effective neoadjuvant therapy for locally advanced breast cancer patients. However, larger confirmatory trials need to be conducted to assess benefit.

Conclusions

These data provide support for anastrozole as second-line therapy of metastatic breast cancer in tamoxifen-resistant patients in terms of OS and TTP. There are also data to support first-line therapy with anastrozole in advanced breast cancer patients. However, there are conflicting data from the two parallel trials. The North American trial illustrated significant advantage in TTP with 11.1 months with anastrozole versus 5.6 months with tamoxifen ($p = 0.005$), unlike the European trial, where the TTP was 8.2 months with anastrozole and 8.3 months with tamoxifen. When a subgroup analysis was performed from the combined analyses, ER-positive patients were found to have statistically significantly better TTP for anastrozole versus tamoxifen ($p = 0.022$). In addition to efficacy, anastrozole was proven to produce less toxicity. Retrospective subgroup analyses, however, are not reliable due to many compounding factors. With all of the data combined, anastrozole was FDA approved as an option for first-line therapy in the treatment of advanced breast cancer patients. Promising results are available for the use of anastrozole in the adjuvant and neoadjuvant settings; however, these are only preliminary results. The complete publication of these data, may change the current standard of endocrine therapy in postmenopausal women with hormone-receptor-positive disease in both of these settings.

Letrozole

Letrozole is a potent and selective non-steroidal competitive inhibitor. In postmenopausal patients with daily doses ranging from 0.1 mg to 5 mg, no clinically relevant changes in plasma levels of cortisol, aldosterone, 11-dexycortisol, 17-hydroxyprogesterone, ACTH or plasma renin activity are seen. Estradiol, estrone, and estrone sulfate plasma levels were suppressed by more than 95% within 2 weeks of starting therapy with 1 mg per day of letrozole. A recent study also identified significant reductions in ACTH-stimulated cortisol ($p = 0.015$) and aldosterone concentrations ($p = 0.04$) after 3 months of exposure to 2.5 mg letrozole daily (70). These changes in concentrations of ACTH levels question the specificity of letrozole for the aromatase enzyme. Trials are currently underway to assess the clinical efficacy of the degree of suppression of estrone, estradiol, and estrone sulfate. Geisler and colleagues have illustrated significant decreases *in vivo* of these estrogen levels with letrozole compared to anastrozole (71). Twelve patients each received letrozole 2.5 mg by mouth daily and anastrozole 1 mg by mouth daily for 6 weeks in a double-blind, cross-over study. Estrone and estrone sulfate levels were significantly reduced with letrozole versus anastrozole ($p = 0.05$ and $p = 0.12$, respectively). How this figures into the clinical setting is yet to be determined. A study is currently underway to evaluate the clinical role of this data in a trial of letrozole 2.5 mg versus anastrozole 1 mg as second-line therapy for metastatic breast cancer. This information will be instrumental in determining if the degree of estrogen suppression will play a role in efficacy and how aromatase inhibitors are selected in therapy.

Second-line Therapy

Letrozole has been compared to both megestrol acetate and aminoglutethimide as second-line hormonal therapy in postmenopausal, tamoxifen-resistant breast cancer patients. Dombernowsky et al. compared two doses of letrozole (2.5 mg or 0.5 mg daily) to megestrol acetate (160 mg daily) in a multicentered, randomized, double blind trial (71). Five hundred and fifty-one patients were randomized with a primary endpoint of OR (CR plus PR). Secondary endpoints included TTP, TTF, and OS. Higher overall OR was obtained with letrozole 2.5 mg versus letrozole 0.5 mg ($p = 0.004$) and megestrol acetate ($p = 0.04$). For TTP, however, letrozole 2.5 mg (5.6 months) was comparable to megestrol acetate (5.5 months; $p = 0.07$), while with the 0.5-mg dose of letrozole, the TTP was 5.1 months ($p = 0.02$). Overall survival (OS) was significantly longer with letrozole 2.5 mg compared to 0.5 mg (25.3 months versus 21.5 months, respectively, $p = 0.03$) (72). No survival advantage was identified with letrozole over megestrol acetate even at an extended follow-up of 51 months. Letrozole 2.5 mg exhibited a median overall survival of 25 months versus 21.5 months with letrozole 0.5 mg and megestrol acetate (HR = 0.86, 95% confidence interval 0.67–1.11). This trial concluded that the appropriate dose for letrozole was 2.5 mg and that this medication was more effective than megestrol acetate in the second-line treatment of advanced breast cancer. A similar trial conducted by Buzdar et al. (73) and colleagues only demonstrated equivalency between the letrozole (2.5 mg or 0.5 mg by mouth daily) and megesterol acetate (40 mg by mouth four times a day). Six hundred and two patients were randomized in this double blind, multicentered, multinational trial. No statistically significant difference was illustrated among treatment arms in terms of objective tumor response. (letrozole 0.5 mg/megesterol, odds ratio = 1.50, $p = 0.13$; letrozole 2.5 mg/megesterol, odds ratio = 1.09, $p = 0.75$; and letrozole 2.5 mg/0.5 mg, odds ratio = 0.73, $p = 0.22$) (73). Overall, letrozole was concluded to be equivalent to megestrol acetate in second-line therapy of advanced breast cancer patients. Another trial has also demonstrated equivalency. A subset analysis was performed on the duration of response and the TTP. Overall survival had not been reported. Compared to megestrol acetate, letrozole exhibited a significantly longer duration of response (33 months versus 18 months, respectively). The median TTP in predominantly soft tissue disease was 17 months for letrozole compared to only 8.6 months with megestrol acetate (74). Data from this trial have not been fully published and at the time of this abstract publication, no statistical analysis had been conducted. These conflicting data appear to indicate letrozole is as effective as megestrol acetate in this setting.

Letrozole has also been compared to aminoglutethimide in a similar setting. Letrozole 2.5 mg and 0.5 mg was compared to aminoglutethimide (250 mg twice daily) in one open-labeled, randomized trial (75). Supplemental glucocorticoids (hydrocortisone 30 mg, or cortisone acetate 37.5 mg) were given to those patients who were treated with aminoglutethimide. Five hundred and fifty five postmenopausal, advanced breast cancer patients were enrolled. As with previous studies, the primary endpoint was OR (CR plus PR) and secondary endpoints included TTP, TTF, and duration of survival. There was no significant difference in OR when all of the groups were compared (19.5%, 16.7%, 12.4%, respectively) (Table 15.7) (75). Overall survival and TTP were significantly longer with letrozole 2.5 mg versus the other two arms of the study ($p = 0.002$ and $p = 0.008$, respectively). Fewer side

TABLE 15.7. *Results of second-line therapy comparing letrozole to aminoglutethimide in advanced breast cancer patients (75)*

	Letrozole 0.5 mg (n = 192)	Letrozole 2.5 mg (n = 185)	Aminoglutethimide 250 mg p.o. b.i.d. (n = 178)
OR (CR + PR) (%)	16.7	19.5	12.4
95% CI	(11.4–21.9)	(13.8–25.2)	(7.5–17.2)
Median TTP (months)	3.3	3.4	3.2
		RR: 0.72 (95% CI: 0.57–0.92) $p = 0.008$	
OS (months)	21	28	20
		RR: 0.64 (95% CI: 0.49–0.85) $p = 0.002$	

CI, confidence interval; CR, complete response; OR, objective response; OS, overall survival; PR, partial response; RR, risk ratio; TTP, time to treatment progression.
From Gershanovich et al. (75).

effects were reported with letrozole compared to aminoglutethimide (AG). Nausea was the most common side effect with letrozole (2.5 mg = 10%, 0.5 mg = 7%, AG = 10%). Only hot flashes and fatigue were reported more with letrozole than AG (hot flashes: 2.5 mg = 4.9%, 0.5 mg = 3.1%, and AG = 3.4%) (fatigue: 2.5 mg = 3.2%, 0.5 mg = 2.6%, and AG = 2.8%). With these data, letrozole was found to be superior to aminoglutethimide in terms OS and TTP for the second-line therapy of advanced breast cancer patients.

The first head-to-head trial comparing letrozole to anastrozole has been completed in postmenopausal, advanced breast cancer patients. This information was presented at the 2002 American Society of Clinical Oncology meeting. Of the 713 patients enrolled, 48% had estrogen/progesterone receptor-positive breast cancer. The primary endpoint of the study was TTP. Secondary endpoints included: OR, duration of response, duration of clinical benefit, TTF, time to response, and OS. There were no statistically significant differences shown with TTP, TTF, duration of response, or duration of clinical benefit. Letrozole was shown to be superior to anastrozole in terms of OR (19.1% versus 12.3%, $p = 0.014$, odds ratio = 1.70). Overall, letrozole was not shown to be superior to anastrozole in the second-line treatment of postmenopausal advanced breast cancer patients (76).

First-line Therapy

As with anastrozole, letrozole has also been approved for first-line treatment of metastatic breast cancer in postmenopausal patients. This recommendation was based on data from Mouridsen and colleagues (77). This phase 3, randomized, double blind, double-dummy, international, parallel group study was originally designed to be a three-arm study comparing tamoxifen 20 mg daily, letrozole 2.5 mg daily, or the combination. The combination arm of the study was not pursued due to the pharmacokinetic interaction between tamoxifen and letrozole. When tamoxifen and letrozole are administered simultaneously, letrozole serum concentrations are decreased by 38%, resulting in an unacceptable level for clinical use. A total of 907 patients were randomized to letrozole 2.5 mg daily (n = 453) versus tamoxifen 20 mg daily (n = 454). The primary endpoint of the trial was TTP. Secondary endpoints included ORR, duration of response, rate and duration of clinical benefit, TTF, OS, and tolerability. This trial was powered to detect superiority over tamoxifen (5%, two-sided significance with 80% power: HR = 0.80), unlike the first-line anastrozole studies previously discussed.

Patients could be crossed over to the opposite treatment arm upon progression if deemed clinically appropriate. Letrozole was shown to be superior to tamoxifen in regards to TTP and TTF (HR = 0.72, $p < 0.0001$; HR = 0.73, $p < 0.0001$, respectively). Overall response and clinical benefit rate also were statistically better with letrozole (OR = 1.78 [95% CI: 1.30–2.40], $p = 0.0002$; OR = 1.62 [95% CI: 1.24–2.11], $p = 0.0004$, respectively) (Table 15.8) (78).

TABLE 15.8. *Efficacy rates of letrozole in first-line therapy of advanced breast cancer patients (78)*

	Letrozole (n = 453)	Tamoxifen (n = 454)	HR / OR (95% CI)	p value
Median TTP (months)	9.4	6.0	HR = 0.72 (0.62–0.83)	< 0.0001
Median TTF (months)	9.0	5.7	HR = 0.73 (0.64–0.84)	< 0.0001
ORR = (CR + PR)	32%	21%	OR = 1.78 (1.32–2.4)	0.0002
CBR = CR + PR + NC ≥ 24 weeks	50%	38%	OR = 1.62 (1.24–2.11)	0.0004

CBR, clinical benefit rate; CR, complete response; HR, hazard ratio; NC, no change; OR, odds ratio; ORR, objective response rate; PR, partial response; TTF, time to treatment failure; TTP, time to progression.

TABLE 15.9. *Survival analysis of letrozole in first-line therapy of advanced breast cancer patients (78)*

	Letrozole	Tamoxifen (log-rank test)	p value
Median survival (months)	34	30	0.53
1 year (%)	83	75	0.004
2 year (%)	64	58	0.02

At initial publication, the data were too immature to evaluate OS (77). Recently, this survival information was presented and discussed at the 2001 San Antonio Breast Cancer Symposium (78). No statistical difference was identified in the median OS between letrozole (34 months) and tamoxifen (30 months, $p = 0.53$). The first and second year survival analysis, however, did demonstrate superiority of letrozole over tamoxifen (first year, 83%, $p = 0.004$, and second year, 64%, $p = 0.02$) (Table 15.9). Closer scrutiny of the data suggests that the crossover design may explain why survival curves converged and a statistical advantage cannot be identified with letrozole. Tolerability and safety were also evaluated in this trial. Common side effects such as hot flashes, nausea, and alopecia/hair thinning were similar among treatment groups. Thromboembolic events were less with letrozole (less than 1%, or three patients) compared to tamoxifen (2%, nine patients) (78). Letrozole 2.5 mg daily is now FDA approved as a therapeutic option for first-line therapy in the treatment of metastatic, postmenopausal breast cancer patients.

Adjuvant Therapy

Two trials are currently underway to evaluate the use of letrozole in the adjuvant setting. The Femara-Tamoxifen Breast International Group (FEMTABIG) trial being conducted by the Breast International Group consists of four treatment arms: tamoxifen, letrozole, tamoxifen for 2 to 3 years followed by letrozole for 2 to 3 years, or letrozole for 2 to 3 years followed by tamoxifen for 2 to 3 years (39–41). The MA-17 trial being conducted by the National Cancer Institute of Canada Clinical Trials Group (NCIC CTG) randomizes patients who are disease-free after taking tamoxifen for 5 years, to either 5 years of placebo or 5 years of letrozole therapy. Also in this trial, bone mineral density and lipid profile measurements will be evaluated (39). Investigating the benefit of sequential treatment in the adjuvant setting is key to advancing the clinical utility of these agents.

Neoadjuvant Therapy

As with the other aromatase inhibitors, letrozole has been evaluated in the neoadjuvant setting. A phase 2 trial conducted by Dixon and colleagues led the way to a randomized, double-blind, multicentered study comparing neoadjuvant letrozole 2.5 mg daily to tamoxifen 20 mg daily over a 4 month period (79,80). A total of 337 postmenopausal patients with ER-positive tumors who were not candidates for initial surgery were enrolled. Tumor response and the impact of down-staging the tumor volume was the primary endpoint. Letrozole patients (n = 154) exhibited significant improvement in clinical OR rates compared to tamoxifen (n = 170; 55% versus 36%, respectively; $p < 0.001$). Ultrasound and mammographically determined responses were also significantly improved with letrozole compared to tamoxifen (35% versus 25%, $p = 0.042$; 34% versus 17%, $p = < 0.001$, respectively). After 4 months of treatment, 45% of letrozole patients underwent breast-conserving therapy compared to 35% with tamoxifen ($p = 0.022$) (80,81). A phase 3 study of 324 patients also evaluated the efficacy of letrozole 2.5 mg daily to tamoxifen 20 mg daily over a 4-month period in those patients who were ineligible for breast conservation surgery. This was a double-blind, randomized, multicentered trial. The primary endpoint was the overall objective response, which was evaluated by clinical response. Secondary endpoints included the number of patients to undergo breast-conserving surgery, RR (CR plus PR) determined by mammogram at 4 months and RR (CR plus PR) determined by ultrasound at 4 months. The overall RR to letrozole was 60%, compared to 41% with tamoxifen ($p = 0.004$). Sixty letrozole patients (48%) were able to undergo breast-conserving surgery versus only 45 patients (36%) with tamoxifen ($p = 0.36$) (82).

Two smaller studies have shown similar results. Letrozole has been evaluated to determine its effects on *in situ* estrogen synthesis. Eleven patients with primary ER-positive tumors were enrolled. In this study, nine of the ten tumors with *in situ* estrogen synthesis demonstrated significant decreases in activity after letrozole therapy ($p = 0.022$) (83). Dixon et al. (84) also conducted a comparative trial in 24 patients receiving letrozole 2.5 mg daily (n = 12) and letrozole 10 mg daily (n = 12) for 3 months. Response was evaluated by monthly ultrasounds and changes in tumor volume. Median reduction in tumor volume was 81%. After treatment, 15 patients (75%) were eligible for breast-conserving surgery. Neoadjuvant letrozole therapy has been demonstrated to be as effective as tamoxifen, but larger randomized trials need to be conducted.

Conclusion

These data provide evidence to support the use of letrozole as second-line therapy in advanced breast cancer patients. Letrozole demonstrated significantly better TTP compared to aminoglutethimide and megestrol acetate. However, survival was the same as megestrol acetate. Therefore, individual treatment needs to be based on risk factors and comorbid conditions. There are also data available for letrozole as first-line therapy in metastatic breast cancer, with TTP and TTF being significantly better with letrozole versus tamoxifen. Newer analysis of these data shows no significant improvement in OS compared to tamoxifen. The role of letrozole in the adjuvant setting is unknown at this time. As these data mature, recommendations may be forthcoming.

CONCLUSION

The role of aromatase inhibitors in the treatment of breast cancer has dramatically changed in the last few years. Anastrozole and letrozole have become FDA approved for first-line treatment of metastatic breast cancer. These agents are as effective as tamoxifen and are better tolerated. First-line data with exemestane will soon become available and will likely join the ranks of its counterparts. Exciting information concerning the role of aromatase inhibitors in the adjuvant setting is now becoming available. The ATAC trial, in its first analysis, demonstrated superiority of anastrozole compared to tamoxifen in this setting. Extended follow-up data will need to be collected to assess the long-term benefit/risk (efficacy, BMD, and cholesterol profiles) ratio of anastrozole in this population. Results from small, randomized trials in the neoadjuvant setting are also becoming available. Decreases in tumor volumes have led to increased rates of breast conservation surgeries in these trials. This is an exciting time in the world of endocrine therapy for breast cancer and many changes are likely to occur in terms of recommendations once larger trials with longer follow-up are evaluated.

REFERENCES

1. Jensen EV, Block GE, Smith Seal, Estrogen receptors and breast cancer response to adrenalectomy. In: *Prediction of response in cancer therapy*. Washington, DC: US Department of Health, Education and Welfare, 1971:55–70.
2. Sedlacek SM, Horowitz KB. The role of progestins and progesterone receptors in the treatment of breast cancer. *Steroids* 1984;44:467–484.
3. Beck WW. *Obstetrics and gynecology*. Baltimore: Williams & Wilkins, 1989:126.
4. Buzdar AU, Hortobagyi GN. Update on endocrine therapy for breast cancer. *Clin Cancer Res* 1998;4:527–534.
5. Longcope C, Pratt JH, Schneider SH, Fineberg SE. Aromatization of androgens by muscle and adipose tissue in vivo. *J Clin Endocrinol Metab* 1978;46:146–152.
6. Reed MJ, The role of aromatase in breast tumors. *Breast Cancer Res Treat* 1994;30:7–17.
7. Harvey HA, Santen RJ, Osterman J, et al. A comparative trial of transsphenoidal hypophysectomy with aminoglutethimide plus hydrocortisone in women with advanced breast cancer. *Cancer* 1979;43:2207–2214.
8. Santen RJ, Worgul TJ, Samojlik E, et al. A randomized trial comparing surgical adrenalectomy with aminoglutethimide plus hydrocortisone in women with advanced breast cancer. *N Engl J Med* 1981;305:545–551.
9. Segaloff A, Weeth JB, Meyer KK, et al. Hormonal therapy in cancer of the breast. XIX. Effect of oral administration of delta[1]-testololactone on clinical course and hormonal excretion. *Cancer* 1962;15:633–635.
10. Van Rymenant M, Coune A, Tagnon HJ, Somon S. Le traitement hormonal du cancer de sein en phase avancee. Methodes d'etudes—comparaison de la delta-1-testololactone avec le propionate de testostrone. *Acta Clin Belg* 1963;18:469–479.

11. Volk H, Deupree RH, Goldenberg IS, et al. A dose response evaluation of delta-1-testololactone in advanced breast cancer. *Cancer* 1974;33:9–13.
12. Swain SM, Lippman ME. Endocrine therapies of cancer. In: Chabner BA, Collins JM, eds. *Cancer chemotherapy: principles and practice*. Philadelphia: JB Lippincott, 1990:59–109.
13. Lipton A, Harvey HA, Santen RJ, et al. A randomized trial of aminoglutethimide versus tamoxifen in metastatic breast cancer. *Cancer* 1982;50:2265–2268.
14. Smith IE, Harris AL, Morgan M, et al. Tamoxifen versus aminoglutethimide in advanced breast carcinoma: A randomized cross-over trial. *BMJ* 1981;283:1432–1434.
15. Alonso-Munoz MC, Ojeda-Gonzalez MB, Beltran-Fabregat M, et al. Randomized trial of tamoxifen versus aminoglutethimide and versus combined tamoxifen and aminoglutethimide in advanced postmenopausal breast cancer. *Oncology* 1988;45:350–353.
16. Gale KE, Anderson JW, Tormey DC, et al. Hormonal treatment for metastatic breast cancer. An Eastern Co-operative Oncology Group Phase III trial comparing aminoglutethimide to tamoxifen. *Cancer* 1994;73:354–361.
17. Robustelli DCG. 500 mg versus 1000 mg aminoglutethimide in advanced breast cancer: 3 year results of an Italian multicentric trial. *Eur J Cancer* 1991;2:569.
18. Upright C, Ragaz J, Basco V, Grafton C. Double blind randomized trial of conventional versus low dose aminoglutethimide and hydrocortisone in patients with metastatic hormone responsive breast cancer. *Proc Am Soc Clin Oncol* 1991;9:45.
19. Illiger HJ, Caffier H, Carterier B, et al. Aminoglutethimide in advanced breast cancer low dose vs standard dose. *J Cancer Res Clin Oncol* 1986;3:569.
20. Bonneterre J, Pion JM, Demaille A. Low-dose aminoglutethimide (500 mg/day) and hydrocortisone (30 mg/day) in advanced cancer of breast. *Bull Cancer* 1987;74:241–247 (in French).
21. Harris AL, Cantwell BM, Carmichael J, et al. Phase II study of low dose aminoglutethimide 250 mg/day plus hydrocortisone in advanced postmenopausal breast cancer. *Eur J Cancer* 1989;25:1105–1111.
22. Willard EM, Carpenter JT, Low dose aminoglutethimide is active in metastatic breast cancer. *Proc Am Soc Clin Oncol* 1991;10:55.
23. Dowsett M, Cunningham DC, Stein RC, et al. Dose-related endocrine effects and pharmacokinetics of oral and intramuscular 4-hydroxyandrostenedione in postmenopausal breast cancer patients. *Cancer Res* 1989;49:1306–1312.
24. Dowsett M, Mehta A, King N, et al. An endocrine and pharmacokinetic study of four oral doses of formestane in postmenopausal breast cancer patients. *Eur J Cancer* 1992;28:415–420.
25. Brodie AM, Garrett WM, Hendrickson JR, Tsai-Morris CH. Effects of aromatase inhibitor 4-hydroxyandrostenedione and other compounds in the 7,12-dimethylbenz(a)anthracene-induced breast carcinoma model. *Cancer Res* 1982;42:3360s–3364s.
26. Brodie AM, Banks PK, Inkster SE, et al. Aromatase inhibitors and hormone-dependent cancers. *J Steroid Biochem Mol Biol* 1990;37:327–333.
27. Vorobiof DA, Kleeberg UR, Perez-Carrion R, et al. A randomized, open, parallel-group trial to compare the endocrine effects of oral anastrozole (Arimidex) with intramuscular formestane in postmenopausal women with advanced breast cancer. *Ann Oncol* 1999;10:1219–1225.
28. Coombes RC, Hughes SW, Dowsett M. 4-Hydroxyandrostenedione: a new treatment for postmenopausal patients with breast cancer. *Eur J Cancer* 1992;28A:1941–1945.
29. Plourde PV, Dyroff M, Dowsett M, et al. Arimidex. A new oral, once-a-day aromatase inhibitor. *J Steroid Biochem Mol Biol* 1995;53:175–179.
30. Johannessen DC, Engan T, di Salle E, et al. Endocrine and clinical effects of exemestane (PNU 155971), a novel steroidal aromatase inhibitor, in postmenopausal breast cancer patients: a phase 1 study. *Clin Cancer Res* 1997;3:1101–1108.
31. Jones S, Vogel C, Arkhipov A, et al. Multicenter Phase II trial of exemestane as hormonal therapy of postmenopausal women with breast cancer. *J Clin Oncol* 1999;17:3418–3425.
32. Dowsett M, Smithers D, Moore J, et al. Endocrine changes with the aromatase inhibitor fadrozole hydrochloride in breast cancer. *Eur J Cancer* 1994;30A:1453–1458.
33. Cunningham DC, Powels TJ, Dowsett M, et al. Oral 4-hydroxyandrostenedione, a new endocrine treatment for disseminated breast cancer. *Cancer Chemother Pharmacol* 1987;20:253–255.
34. Thurlimann B, Castiglione M, Hsu-Schmitz SF, et al. Formestane versus megestrol acetate in postmenopausal breast cancer patients after failure of tamoxifen: a Phase III prospective randomized cross over trial of second-line hormonal treatment (SAKK 20/90). *Eur J Cancer* 1997;33:1017–1024.
35. Freue M, Kjaer M, Boni C, et al. Open comparative trial of formestane versus megestrol acetate in postmenopausal patients with advanced breast cancer previously treated with tamoxifen. *Breast* 2000;9:9–16.
36. Perez-Carrion R, Candel VA, Calabresi F, et al. Comparison of the selective aromatase inhibitor formestane with tamoxifen as first-line hormonal therapy in postmenopausal women with advanced breast cancer. *Ann Oncol* 1994;5(suppl 7):S19–S24.
37. Thurlimann B, Paridaens R, Serin D, et al. Third-line hormonal treatment with exemestane in postmenopausal patients with advanced breast cancer progressing on aminoglutethimide: A phase 11 multicentre multinational study. Exemestane Study Group. *Eur J Cancer* 1997;33:1767–1773.
38. Kaufmann M, Bajetta E, Dirix LY, et al. Exemestane is superior to megestrol acetate after tamoxifen failure in postmenopausal women with advanced breast cancer: results of a phase III randomized double-blind study. *J Clin Oncol* 2000;18:1399–1411.
39. Paridaens R, Dirix LY, Beex L, et al. Exemestane (Aromasin) is active and well tolerated as first-line hormonal therapy (HT) of metastatic breast cancer (MBC) patients (Pts): results of a randomized phase II trial. *Proc Am Soc Clin Oncol* 2000;19:83a.
40. Goss PE. Risks versus benefits in the clinical application aromatase inhibitors. *Endocr Relat Cancer* 1999;6:325–332.
41. Goss PE, Strasser K. Aromatase inhibitors in the treatment and prevention of breast cancer. *J Clin Oncol* 2001;19:881–894.
42. Baum M. Use of aromatase inhibitors in the adjuvant treatment of breast cancer. *Endocr Relat Cancer* 1999;6:231–234.

43. Fisher B, Costantino J, Wickerham D, et al. Tamoxifen for prevention of breast cancer: report of the National Surgical Adjuvant Breast and Bowel Project P-1 Study. *J Natl Cancer Inst* 1998;90(18):1371–1388.
44. Goss P, Grynpas M, Qi S, et al. The effects of exemestane on bone and lipids in the ovariectomized rat. *Breast Cancer Res Treat* 2001;64(3):209–325.
45. Kennedy B, Kely R, White G, et al. Surgery as an adjunct to hormone therapy of breast cancer. *Cancer* 1957;10:1055–1075.
46. Dixon JM, Anderson T, Miller WR. Phase IIb study of neoadjuvant exemestane (EXE) in locally advanced breast cancer. *Proc Am Soc Clin Oncol* 2001;20:40b (Abstract 1908).
47. Buzdar AU, Smith R, Vogel C, et al. Fadrozole HCL (CGS-16949A) versus megestrol acetate treatment of postmenopausal patients with metastatic breast carcinoma: Results of two randomized double blind controlled multi-institutional trials. *Cancer* 1996;77:2503–2513.
48. Goss PE, Winer EP, Tannock IF, et al. Randomized Phase III trial comparing the new potent and selective third-generation aromatase inhibitor vorozole with megestrol acetate in postmenopausal advanced breast cancer patients. *J Clin Oncol* 1999;17:52–63.
49. Houston SJ, for the Rivizor Study Group. Rivizor versus aminoglutethimide (AG) in the second-line endocrine treatment of postmenopausal patients with advanced breast cancer (ABC) following tamoxifen failure. *Breast* 1997;6:244–245.
50. Bengtsson N-O, Focan C, Gudgeon A, et al. A phase III trial comparing vorozole (Rivizor) versus aminoglutethimide in the treatment of advanced postmenopausal breast cancer. *Eur J Cancer* 1997;33:S148.
51. Jonat W, Howell A, Blomqvist C, et al. A randomized trial comparing two doses of the new selective aromatase inhibitor anastrozole (Arimidex) with megestrol acetate in post-menopausal patients with advanced breast cancer. *Eur J Cancer* 1996;32A:404–412.
52. Buzdar A, Jones S, Vogel C, et al. A phase III trial comparing anastrozole (1 and 10 mg), a potent and selective aromatase inhibitor, with megestrol acetate in postmenopausal women with advanced breast cancer. *Cancer* (Phila) 1997;79:730–739.
53. Howell A. Clarification of anastrozole/megestrol acetate trial program design. *J Clin Oncol* 2000;18:4109.
54. Buzdar A, Jonat W, Howell A, et al. Anastrozole, a potent and selective aromatase inhibitor, versus megestrol acetate in post-menopausal women with advanced breast cancer: Results of overview analysis of two phase III trials. *J Clin Oncol* 1996;14:2000–2011.
55. Buzdar A, Jonat W, Howell A, et al. Anastrozole versus megestrol acetate in the treatment of postmenopausal women with advanced breast carcinoma. Results of a survival update based on a combined analysis of data from two mature Phase III trials. *Cancer* (Phila) 1998;83:1142–1152.
56. Bonneterre J, Thurlimann BJK, Robertson JFR. Anastrozole versus tamoxifen as first-line therapy for advanced breast cancer in 668 postmenopausal women: results of the tamoxifen or Arimidex randomized group efficacy and tolerability study. *J Clin Oncol* 2000;18:3748–3757.
57. Nabholtz J, Buzdar A, Pollak M, et al. Anastrozole is superior to tamoxifen as first-line therapy for advanced breast cancer in postmenopausal women: results of a North American multicenter randomized trial. *J Clin Oncol* 2000;18:3758–3767.
58. Bonneterre J, Buzdar A, Nabholtz J, et al. Anastrozole is superior to tamoxifen as first line therapy in hormone receptor positive advanced breast cancer. *Cancer* 2001;92(9):2247–2258.
59. Nabholtz J, Bonneterre J, Buzdar A, et al. Preliminary results of two multi-center trials comparing the efficacy and tolerability of "Arimidex" (anastrozole) and tamoxifen in postmenopausal women with advanced breast cancer. *Breast Cancer Res Treat* 1999;57:27.
60. Milla-Santos A, Milla L, Ralo L, et al. Anastrozole vs. tamoxifen in hormonedependent advanced breast cancer. A Phase II randomized trial. *Breast Cancer Res Treat* 2000;64:54.
61. Early Breast Cancer Trialist's Collaborative Group. Tamoxifen for early breast cancer: an overview of the randomized trials. *Lancet* 1998;351:1451–1467.
62. Baum M, Houghton J. "Arimidex", tamoxifen alone or in combination (ATAC) adjuvant trial in postmenopausal breast cancer. *Eur J Cancer* 1998;34 (suppl 1):S39.
63. Lonning P. Aromatase inhibitors and their future role in postmenopausal women with early breast cancer. *Br J Cancer* 1998;78(suppl 4):12–15.
64. Piccart M, Goldhirsch A. *An overview of recent and ongoing adjuvant clinical trials for breast cancer,* 2nd ed. Belgium: Moreau PCE 2000.
65. Baum M, et al. The ATAC (Arimidex, tamoxifen, alone or in combination) adjuvant breast cancer trial in postmenopausal (PM) women. *Breast Cancer Res Treat* 2001;(Abstract 8).
66. Dixon J, Renshaw L, Bellamy C, et al. The effects of neoadjuvant anastrozole (Arimidex) on tumor volume in postmenopausal women with breast cancer: a randomized, double blind, single-center study. *Clin Cancer Res* 2001;6:2229–2235.
67. Boeddinghaus I, Dowsett M, Smith I, et al. Neoadjuvant Arimidex or tamoxifen alone or in combined, for breast cancer (IMPACT): PgR-related reductions in proliferation marker Ki67. *Proc Am Soc Clin Oncol* 2000;94a:360.
68. Milla-Santos A, Milla I, Rallo L, et al. Anastrozole (A) as neoadjuvant (NEO) therapy for hormone-dependent locally advanced breast cancer (LABC) in postmenopausal (PM) patients (pts). *Breast Cancer Res Treat* 2001; (Abstract 302).
69. Mamounas E, Fisher B. Preoperative neoadjuvant chemotherapy in patients with breast cancer. *Semin Oncol* 2001;28(4):389–399.
70. Bajetta E, Zilembo N, Dowsett M, et al. Double blind, randomised, multicentre endocrine trial comparing two letrozole doses, in postmenopausal breast cancer patients. *Eur J Cancer* 1999;35:208–213.
71. Dombernowsky P, Smith I, Falkson G, et al. Letrozole, a new oral aromatase inhibitor for advanced breast cancer: Double-blind randomized trial showing a dose effect and improved efficacy and tolerability compared with megestrol acetate. *J Clin Oncol* 1999;16:453–461.
72. Chaudri H, Trunet P. Letrozole. Updated duration of response. *J Clin Oncol* 1999;17:3859–3860.
73. Buzdar A, Douma J, Davidson N, et al. Phase III, multicenter, double-blind, randomized study of letrozole, an aromatase inhibitor, for advanced breast cancer versus megestrol acetate. *J Clin Oncol* 2001;19(14):3357–3366.

74. Gardin G, Fornasiero A, et al. Long duration of response with letrozole 2.5 mg (Femara®) in two trials in postmenopausal women with advanced breast cancer after anti-estrogen therapy. *Eur J Cancer* 1998;34(suppl 5):S13.
75. Gershanovich M, Chaudri HA, Campos D, et al. Letrozole, a new oral aromatase inhibitor: Randomised trial comparing 2.5 mg daily, 0.5 mg daily and aminoglutethimide in post-menopausal women with advanced breast cancer. *Ann Oncol* 1998;9:639–645.
76. Rose C, Vtoraya A, Pluzanska F, et al. Letrozole (Femara) vs. anastrozole (Arimidex): second line treatment in postmenopausal women with advanced breast cancer. *Proc Am Soc Clin Oncol* 2002;34a:131.
77. Mouridsen H, Mikhail G, Sun Y, et al. Superior efficacy of letrozole (Femara) versus tamoxifen as first-line therapy for postmenopausal women with advanced breast cancer: results of a phase III study of the International Letrozole Breast Cancer Group. *J Clin Oncol* 2001;19(10):2596–2606.
78. Mouridsen H, Sun Y, Gershanovich M, et al. Final survival analysis of the double-blind, randomized, multinational phase III trial of letrozole (Femara®) compared to tamoxifen as first-line hormonal therapy for advanced breast cancer. *Breast Cancer Res Treat* 2001; 64(3).
79. Dixon J, Love C, Bellamy C, et al. Letrozole as primary medical therapy for locally advanced and large operable breast cancer. *Breast Cancer Res Treat* 2001; 66:191–199.
80. Eiermann W, Paepke S, Appffelstaedt J, et al. Preoperative treatment of postmenopausal breast cancer patients with letrozole: A randomized double blind multicenter study. *Ann Oncol* 2001;12(11) 1527–1532.
81. Paepke S, Apffelstaedt J, Eremin J, et al. Neo-adjuvant treatment of postmenopausal breast cancer patients with letrozole (Femara): a randomized study versus tamoxifen. *Eur J Cancer* 2000;36(suppl 5):S76.
82. Ellis M, Coop A, Singh B, et al. Letrozole is more effective neoadjuvant endocrine therapy than tamoxifen for ErbB-1- and/or ErbB-2-positive, estrogen receptor-positive primary breast cancer: evidence from a phase III randomized trial. *J Clin Oncol* 2001;19(18): 3808–3816.
83. Miller W, Telford J, Love C, et al. Effects of letrozole as primary medical therapy on *in situ* estrogen synthesis and endogenous levels within the breast. *Breast* 1998;7:273–276.
84. Dixon J, Love C, Tucker C, et al. Letrozole as primary medical therapy for locally advanced and large operable breast cancer. *Eur J Cancer* 1998;34(suppl 5):S13.

16
New Antiestrogens: Modulators of Estrogen Action

Anthony Howell and S.J. Howell

Breast cancer remains the most common cancer and a leading cause of cancer death in women in the United States and Europe (1). A substantial body of experimental, clinical, and epidemiological evidence indicates that steroid hormones play a major role in the aetiology of breast cancer. Endogenous estrogens not only support the development and growth of the breast and breast tumor cells but have profound beneficial and carefully regulated effects on other tissues such as the endometrium, vagina, bone, liver, and vessels of the cardiovascular system as summarised in Table 16.1.

The clinical responsiveness of the breast to estrogen deprivation was first demonstrated over 100 years ago (2). Pharmacological inhibition of the tumor stimulatory effects of physiological estrogen concentrations was first reported using high-dose stilboestrol, triphenylchlorethylene and triphenylbromoethylene (3,4). Antiestrogen therapy since the 1940s, and tamoxifen in particular, has revolutionized the treatment of breast cancer.

Today, tamoxifen (Nolvadex, ICI 147,741) is the antiestrogen of choice for adjuvant therapy after surgery (although early data suggest third-generation aromatase inhibitors may suprecede it). However, there are important general issues surrounding the health of perimenopausal and postmenopausal women associated with changes in their estrogen levels. Breast cancer occurs predominantly in postmenopausal women where reduced estrogen levels are associated with skeletal problems resulting from reduced bone density (osteoporosis) and increased cardiovascular risk. Many of the modulators of estrogen action, such as tamoxifen, have a beneficial effect on bone density and serum lipids but have adverse effects on the uterus. Thus, an antiestrogen breast cancer therapy which safely eliminates the negative effects of the menopause on womens' health in the absence of toxicity is the challenge for the new millennium.

The term "antiestrogen" refers to agents which block the effects of physiological concentrations of estrogen at the estrogen receptor (ER). Selective estrogen receptor modulator (SERM) was a term coined to describe the phenomenon of apparent blocking of the ER at one site (e.g., the tumor) and stimulatory activity at another site (e.g., bone). Thus, a single drug could have both agonist and antagonist activity depending on the cell type. SERMs were then divided into SERM 1 (tamoxifen), SERM 2 (raloxifene hydrochloride) and SERM 3 (now known as arzoxifene). However, nearly all estrogens or antiestrogens may have agonist or antagonist activity depending upon drug dose and target cell type. For example, the high-doses of synthetic estrogens used to inhibit breast tumors in the 1940s have agonist activity in normal tissues (4). They may also become agonists to the tumor with the passage of time as demonstrated by the phenomenon of withdrawal responses (5). An exception to the combined agonist/antagonist activity of most estrogens and antiestrogens may be the so-called steroidal pure antiestrogens, which are apparently devoid of agonist activity. The lack of agonist activity may be related to the fact that they appear to have a different mechanism of action with respect to their effect on ER. Since tumor ER levels decline markedly on treatment, this group of compounds have been called selective estrogen receptor down-regulators. The acronym SERM may have some uses, but we have used the term antiestrogen throughout this article for the sake of clarity.

TABLE 16.1. *Summary of the effects of estrogen (E_2, 17β-oestradiol) on target tissues*

Target organ/tissue	Pharmacological and physiological effects of estrogen
Breast	Promotes breast epithelial cell proliferation, development and growth of the breast together with other growth-stimulating factors, progesterone, corticosteroids, prolactin, and insulin. Associated with poor clinical outcome in ER+ breast cancer patients.
Endometrium and vagina	Stimulates proliferation of epithelial cells and regulates cyclical changes. Unopposed is associated with malignancy. Cornification of vaginal epithelium.
Cardiovascular system	Reduces risk factors associated with CVD, predominantly serum lipid and lipoprotein composition. Arterial smooth muscle relaxation via ER- and non–ER-mediated pathways.
Bone	ER found on both osteoclasts and osteoblasts. Regulates expression of bone cytokines. Increases bone density.
CNS (brain)	Feedback actions on the hypothalamus and limbic system. Controls mood swings and cognitive function, possibly delaying the onset and progression of Alzheimer disease.
Liver	Influences liver-derived coagulation factors and plasma proteins and regulation of lipids (see also CVD).

CVD, cardiovascular disease; ER, estrogen receptor.

TAMOXIFEN: ADVANTAGES AND DISADVANTAGES

Tamoxifen, a non-steroidal, triphenylethylene-based, antiestrogen (Fig. 16.1), with tissue-specific estrogenic (agonist) and antiestrogenic (antagonist) activity, has been the compound of choice in the clinic for over 25 years (6). Its biological effects are mediated primarily by inhibiting the actions of estrogen through its binding to the ER. The differential actions of tamoxifen occur by selective estrogen receptor modulation according to the cell and gene promoter type.

The antiestrogenic activity of tamoxifen in the breast established it as the gold standard for treatment in all stages of breast cancer. Tamoxifen given for 5 years in an adjuvant setting has been associated with the greatest reduction in the risk of both contralateral breast cancer and metastatic cancer (level of evidence: I) (7). These data supported the prospective evaluation of tamoxifen in the prevention of cancer in

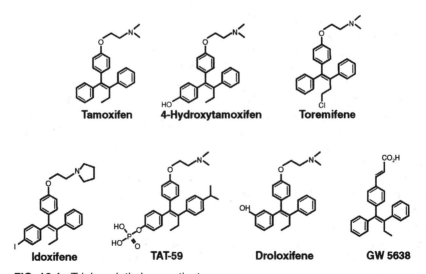

FIG. 16.1. Triphenylethylene antiestrogens.

women at high risk for the disease in the NSABP P-1 study (8). The positive results of this U.S. study led to approval of tamoxifen by the FDA for breast cancer prevention (9) (level of evidence: I); however, two further prevention trials have not confirmed this positive result in women with a low to moderate increase in breast cancer risk (level of evidence: I) (10,11).

The estrogenic activity of long-term tamoxifen treatment is associated with clinical benefits associated with premenopausal physiological estrogen concentrations (Table 16.1). Tamoxifen helps to maintain bone density (12) and lowers circulating low-density lipoprotein cholesterol (13) effects of importance to perimenopausal and postmenopausal women.

The most frequent side effect associated with tamoxifen therapy is the occurrence of hot flashes, thought to be related to the antagonistic action of tamoxifen on the hypothalamic pituitary axis. However, the side effect causing most concern is the increased risk of endometrial cancer related to estrogen agonist activity on the uterus (8,14,15). Other, but less serious, side effects on the uterus, in the form of endometrial polyps, and simple and complex hyperplasia, also occur. Antiestrogen therapy more importantly is associated with an increased incidence of thromboembolic phenomena, including deep-vein thrombosis, pulmonary embolism, and possibly cerebrovascular events (8). Finally, therapy is associated with the phenomenon of tamoxifen resistance, where tumor growth may actually be promoted by continuing treatment (5).

Despite negative aspects of tamoxifen therapy, the benefits for the treatment and prevention of breast cancer generally substantially outweigh the risks. The success of tamoxifen in the treatment of breast cancer has proved invaluable in the search for, and development of, new antiestrogens that selectively retain the favourable estrogenic and antiestrogenic properties of tamoxifen. It has been the standard against which all new hormone therapy has been measured in established preclinical models and clinical trials (Table 16.2). Although tamoxifen has revolutionized the treatment of breast cancer, the search continues for new agents which will confer increased response rate and duration of response in patients with advanced disease, increased cure rate and time to relapse in the adjuvant setting, reduce tumor burden in the neo-adjuvant setting, play a clearly defined role in disease prevention, and potentially improve the general health of postmenopausal women (16).

TABLE 16.2. *Preclinical and clinical assessment of new antiestrogens*

1. Preclinical *in vitro* and *in vivo* assessments
   - ERα and ERβ receptor binding
   - ERα and ERβ transcriptional activation
   - antiestrogenic activity in breast and uterus
   - tumor antagonism in animal models
   - activity in cell lines
   - estrogenic activity on bone and serum lipids
   - mechanism of ER activation (coactivators, corepressors and ligand-independent activity)
2. Clinical assessment
   - activity as first-line therapy in MBC
   - activity in tamoxifen resistant tumors
   - activity as neo-adjuvant and adjuvant therapy
   - activity in prevention
   - side-effect profile
   - effects on women's health

NEW ANTIESTROGENS

Since the mid 1990s (17), there has been a marked increase in preclinical and clinical information available on the new antiestrogens and in our understanding of their mechanisms of action via the ER.

Three main avenues have been followed in attempting to improve on tamoxifen. First, analogues of tamoxifen produced by chemically altering the triphenylethylene structure in an attempt to block the metabolic hydroxylation at the 4-position and to reduce metabolic inactivation by altering the side chain. Second, new non-steroidal fixed-ring structures derived from the stilbene structure of stilboestrol have been synthesised in order to prevent the isomerization that occurs around the double bond in the triphenylethylenes (hence the term *fixed-ring*). These structures include benzothiophenes (18,19), napthalenes (20), and benzopyrans (21,22). The third approach has been to

TABLE 16.3. *Antiestrogens with past or potential clinical value*

- Triphenylethylenes (tamoxifen derivatives)
  - Toremifene
  - Droloxifene
  - Idoxifene
  - TAT-59
  - GW 5638
- Fixed-ring compounds
  Benzothiophenes
    - Raloxifene (LY 156,758)
    - SERM 3 Arzoxifene (LY 353,381)
  Naphthalenes
    - Lasofoxifene (CP-336,156)
    - LY 326,315
  Benzopyrans
    - EM-800 (SCH 57050)
    - EM652 (SCH 57068)
    - ERA-923
- Steroidal compounds
  - ICI 164,384
  - ICI 182,780
  - RU 58668
  - SR 16234

synthesize steroidal analogues of estrogen with growth-inhibitory activity (23–25,16).

These three classes of antiestrogens (triphenylethylenes, fixed-ring and steroidal) (Table 16.3) are known to differ in their affinities for the ER, mechanisms of action in relation to the ER, and in effects on the key tissues as assessed in a whole range of *in vitro* and *in vivo,* preclinical assay systems (Table 16.2). Clarification of the clinical potential of these and future agents will, however, depend on improvements in understanding of the various mechanisms and molecular determinants of ER-mediated response in the breast and particularly other sites of activity such as bone and the cardiovascular system.

The newer triphenylethylenes include the tamoxifen analogues toremifene, idoxifene, droloxifene (3-hydroxytamoxifen), TAT-59, and GW 5638 (Fig. 16.1, Table 16.3) (26–30). The newer fixed-ring compounds include: benzothiophenes (raloxifene, LY 156,758) and arzoxifene (LY 353,381) (18,19); naphthalenes (lasofoxifene, CP-336,156, and LY326,315) (20,21); benzopyrans (EM 800, SCH 57050, and its metabolite EM652, SCH 57068) (22); and a novel fixed-ring antiestrogen, ERA-923. All these agents competitively inhibit estrogen binding to the ER and have mixed agonist/antagonist activity mediated by the ER.

The steroidal antiestrogens (Table 16.2) include ICI 164,384 and ICI 182,780, in which the addition of a side-chain at the 7a position of estradiol leads to the complete abrogation of the trophic/agonist action of estradiol on the uterus and also blocks the uterotropic action of tamoxifen (23). Another steroidal, pure antiestrogen devoid of any partial agonist activity is RU 58668 (25). It differs from ICI 182,780 in that its bulky side chain extends from the 11b carbon atom of estradiol, rather than from the 7a carbon. The orally active steroidal antiestrogen SR 16234 has a methyl group at the 7a position and a bulky side chain at the 17b position (Fig. 16.2).

Although some of the agents outlined above have already been withdrawn from clinical development (particularly many of the triphenylethylenes) for the treatment of breast cancer because they offer no advantage over tamoxifen, their preclinical and clinical characteristics are briefly reviewed in the following section in an attempt to provide an insight into the properties that might contribute to the development of optimally clinically effective antiestrogens.

Triphenylethylenes

These are the most extensively studied of all ER modulators and include the early antiestrogens: triphenylethylenes and bromoethylenes, chlomiphene, and tamoxifen. It was the concern over the effects of tamoxifen on the uterus and the desire for more active compounds that led to the development of the tamoxifen analogues described below.

Toremifene

Toremifene is a chlorinated analogue of tamoxifen (Fig. 16.1), with similar site-specific estrogenic and antiestrogenic activity (26). It has been shown in preclinical studies to have similar ER binding and antitumor activity to tamoxifen (23), but less DNA adduct formation in the endometrium (31). Toremifene has similar

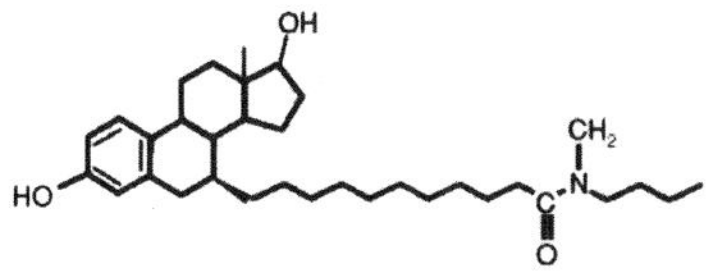

FIG. 16.2. Steroidal antiestrogens.

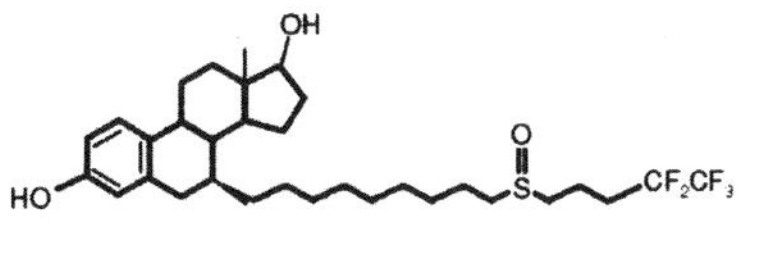

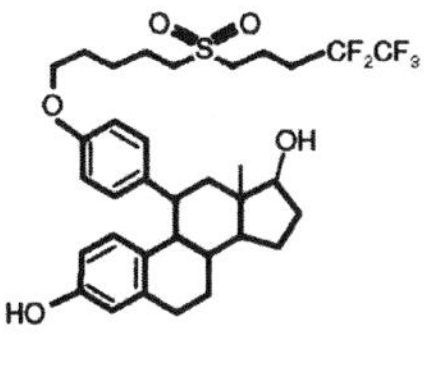

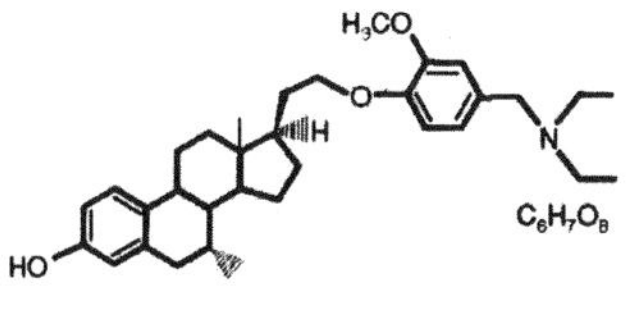

stimulatory effects to tamoxifen on the endometrium in athymic mice (26) and in postmenopausal patients receiving therapy for 12 months (32), which suggests that toremifene, like tamoxifen, might be associated with an increased risk of endometrial cancer. Five phase 3 trials (33–37) have demonstrated that toremifene is as effective as tamoxifen in the first-line treatment of metastatic breast cancer (MBC), with a similar side effect profile. As a result, toremifene has been approved for the first-line treatment of MBC in patients with ER-positive and ER-unknown disease. Use in an adjuvant setting also shows no difference in recurrence rates between it and tamoxifen (38), with a similar side effect profile. Low response rates in phase 2 studies in patients previously treated with tamoxifen suggest cross-resistance with tamoxifen (17,39). Meta-analysis of 1,421 patients in these trials showed similar response rates for toremifene and tamoxifen (24% versus 25.3%) with no significant difference in time to disease progression or overall survival (40). Thus, to date, toremifene shows no advantages over tamoxifen (level of evidence: I).

Idoxifene, Droloxifene and TAT-59

Unlike toremifene, all three agents bind to the ER more effectively than tamoxifen (17,27,29). Idoxifene has an iodine atom at the 4 position of tamoxifen (Fig. 16.1), which is associated with reduced carcinogenic potential (41). Preclinical and phase 1 and 2 studies(27,42) were moderately encouraging, although idoxifene showed little activity when used after tamoxifen failure (43).

The preclinical (28,44) and phase 2 data (45–48) for droloxifene (3-hydroxy tamoxifen) (Fig. 16.1), were encouraging. However, droloxifene did not appear to offer any advantages over tamoxifen for the treatment of breast cancer (level of evidence: II). TAT-59 is a prodrug developed in Japan that, after dephosphorylation, becomes the active metabolite of tamoxifen, 4-hydroxytamoxifen (Fig. 16.1). This agent has a high affinity for the ER (29,49). A phase 2 trial comparing TAT-59 with tamoxifen in the first-line treatment of MBC has been reported (level of evidence: II) (50). The overall response rates were 30% and 26.5%, respectively. The side effect profile was mild and similar to that of tamoxifen. There are no details of the effects of TAT-59 on bone density or serum lipid profile. All three drugs have been withdrawn from development for the treatment of breast cancer, although droloxifene remains in development for the prevention of osteoporosis.

GW 5638 is an acidic triphenylethylene in which the amino side chain has been replaced by a carboxylic acid moiety (Fig. 16.1). When assayed *in vitro,* it functions as an ER antagonist in a manner distinct from that of other known ER modulators (30). However, quite unexpectedly, it has the properties of a bone selective antiestrogen and exhibits decreased uterotropic activity relative to tamoxifen in preclinical studies (30). GW 5638 is currently in clinical development but no efficacy data are available.

FIXED-RING COMPOUNDS

Benzothiophenes

These were developed in an attempt to avoid the agonist problems associated with the triphenylethylenes on the uterus and to be more selective in their action on target tissues, namely breast and bone. Detailed structure activity studies (51) identified raloxifene (Fig. 16.3) as having a unique profile of biological activity. Currently, raloxifene and its derivative, arzoxifene, are undergoing clinical trials. Raloxifene is a proven agent for the treatment of osteoporosis and, in the populations treated for osteoporosis prevention, appears to decrease breast cancer incidence. Arzoxifene is being developed for the treatment of early and advanced breast cancer.

Raloxifene

Raloxifene (formerly called Keoxifene) is a non-steroidal benzothiophene derivative that binds to the ER with high affinity. It has been shown in preclinical studies to have antiestrogenic effects on both the breast and the uterus and estrogenic effects on the bone, cholesterol levels, and vascular smooth muscle cells (18,52–54). In fact, raloxifene was developed for, and most of its clinical evaluation has been for, the treatment of osteoporosis in postmenopausal women (55–57). Preliminary clinical studies showed raloxifene to decrease bone turnover and lower serum cholesterol levels without increasing serum triglyceride concentrations or causing endometrial proliferation (55). These observations were confirmed by a 2-year osteoporosis prevention trial (57), and raloxifene has already been approved for the prevention of osteoporosis in postmenopausal women in the United States.

Evidence of the potential of raloxifene as a breast cancer therapy came from the Multiple Outcomes of Raloxifene Evaluation (MORE) trial (58) which showed that the incidence of ER-positive breast cancer was 74% lower in the raloxifene group than in the placebo group. As in the tamoxifen breast cancer prevention trial (8), the effect was seen exclusively in patients who developed ER-positive breast cancers. Significantly, the incidence of endometrial cancer was not increased but was, in fact, slightly lower in the raloxifene treatment groups when compared with placebo.

There have been two clinical reports of raloxifene use in MBC involving a total of 32 postmenopausal women. In the first study (59), no objective tumor response was observed in 14 patients with tamoxifen-resistant disease. In the second, more recent study, three objective responses were reported in 18 patients with ER-positive breast cancer (Table 16.4) (level of

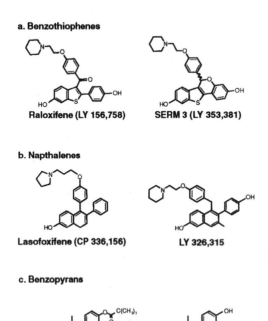

FIG. 16.3. Fixed ring antiestrogens.

TABLE 16.4. *Response to new antiestrogens as first- or second-line treatments for MBC compared with tamoxifen (as first line)*

	Response to SERMs and SERDS in advanced breast cancer			
	n	CR + PR (%)	SD	Total (%)
Tamoxifen	500+	27	25	52
Raloxifene	18	17	28	45
SERM3	88	32	19	51
SCH 57050[a]	43	14	23	37
ICI 182780[a] (Faslodex)	19	37	32	69

[a]Denotes previous treatment with tamoxifen for advanced disease.

evidence: III) (60). The American Society for Clinical Oncology (ASCO) evidence-based technology assessment to determine whether tamoxifen and raloxifene were appropriate as breast cancer risk-reduction therapies in clinical practice suggested that raloxifene use should currently be reserved for its approved indication, i.e., to prevent bone loss in postmenopausal women (9). A Study of Tamoxifen Against Raloxifene (STAR) is ongoing in postmenopausal women at high risk of developing breast cancer (61,62), and the results are awaited with interest.

Arzoxifene

Modification of the carbonyl hinge which attaches the side chain of raloxifene to the ER-binding benzothiophene nucleus (Fig. 16.3) resulted in the production of LY353,381 (arzoxifene, previously SERM 3), which in preclinical breast cancer models is one of the most potent oral estrogen antagonists produced to date (63). Estrogen antagonist effects were observed in the uterus, while estrogen agonist effects were observed in assays evaluating effects on bone, lipids, and the central nervous system (CNS). Overall, arzoxifene is a more potent estrogen antagonist than raloxifene and has better bone-preserving properties (19,64). Results have been reported from a phase 1 dose-finding study (65) and a phase 2 study in which arzoxifene was administered first-line to patients with MBC (Tables 16.4 and 16.5) (66). From the phase 1 study, two doses of arzoxifene were chosen for phase 2 evaluation and patients were randomized to receive either 20 mg or 50 mg. Only a small number (approximately 9%) were previously treated with endocrine therapy (all tamoxifen). Thirty nine percent of patients had locally advanced disease. The preliminary results of this study are shown in Table 16.5. The complete and partial remission rates were 32% and rose to 51% when stable disease for more than 6 months was included. Thus arzoxifene shows response rates equivalent or possibly superior to tamoxifen (level of evidence: II). More data are

TABLE 16.5. *Phase 1 and phase 2 studies with arzoxifene*

	Dose (mg)				
	Total	10	20	50	100
Phase 1					
Patients	32	8	8	8	8
CR/PR/SD	0/0/6	0/0/3	0/0/0	0/0/1	0/0/2
% response	19	38	0	13	25
Phase 2					
Patients	88	—	44	44	—
CR/PR/SD	0/28/17	—	0/14/8	0/14/9	—
% response	51	—	50	52	—

required to be certain of the appropriate dose. Based on the phase 2 data, 20 mg arzoxifene has been taken forward into a large multicentre phase 3 trial against tamoxifen as first line therapy in metastatic breast cancer.

Napthalenes

The naphthalene nucleus has provided a structural template for several ER modulators, including the antifertility agent, nafoxidene (67). Nafoxidene was shown to be equivalent to ethynylestradiol for the treatment of advanced breast cancer but was withdrawn because of severe skin phototoxicity. A reduced nafoxidine derivative, lasofoxifene (Fig. 16.3) has been shown in preclinical evaluations to have potent tissue selective estrogen action when administered orally (20). Recently, a hydroxynaphthalene ER modulator, LY 326,315, that exhibits fully differentiated agonist/antagonist activity in reproductive and nonreproductive tissues in preclinical assays and also has good oral bioavailability, has been reported (21). There are no data on its use in breast cancer to date.

Benzopyrans

Historically, several estrogen receptor modulators have been based upon a benzopyran molecule, including the contraceptive agent centchroman (68,69) and the osteoporosis/HRT agent levormeloxifene (70).

EM-800

EM-800 is a derivative of centchroman and was originally developed as an orally active pure antiestrogen. EM-800 is a prodrug that requires the removal of two carboxylic acids to produce its active metabolite, EM-652 (SCH 57068) (Fig. 16.3) (22). Comparison of the structure of EM-800 with centchroman shows that the antiestrogenic component of the centchroman molecule is moved to a position in the nonsteroidal skeleton equivalent to the 7α position of the steroidal antiestrogen, ICI 182 780 (Fig. 16.2). Both EM-800 and its active metabolite, EM-652, are potent antagonists of the ER subtypes α and β (71). Preclinical, in vitro data showed EM-800 and EM-652 to be the most potent antiestrogens known to date when tested in breast cancer cell lines. They were also devoid of any of the estrogen agonist activity: for example, stimulation of cell growth in ZR 75–1 and MCF-7 cell lines in the absence of estrogens (72). Mice treated with EM-800 developed uterine and vaginal atrophy that was greater than seen in ovariectomized animals. Also there was complete inhibition of mammary gland development (73,74). These studies confirmed the pure anti-estrogenic effect of EM-800 on the mammary gland, uterus, vagina, and hypothalamic-pituitary-gonadal axis (74). Recent data concerning its activity on bone have led to the reclassification of EM-800 as an antiestrogen with both antagonist and agonist activity.

EM-800 was assessed in a phase 2 study in patients who had failed tamoxifen treatment as an adjuvant or for advanced disease (Table 16.4). Of 43 evaluable patients treated, 14% had a complete or partial remission, and 23% had stable disease for more than 6 months. Encouraged by these results, a phase 3 second-line trial of EM-800 versus Arimidex was initiated but abandoned when the first interim analysis showed inferiority of the antiestrogen to Arimidex. EM-800 has been withdrawn from the clinic for the treatment of MBC. It continues to be developed for breast cancer prevention.

Era-923

This is a novel SERM which appears to have an improved preclinical profile compared with tamoxifen and raloxifene (75). ERA-923 is now being evaluated in a randomized dose-finding phase 2 trial (25 mg versus 100 mg) as second-line therapy in 100 ER-positive patients with tamoxifen-resistant metastatic breast cancer. A similar randomized phase 2 trial has been proposed in receptor-positive, hormone-sensitive metastatic breast cancer as first-line therapy.

Steroidal Antiestrogens

These compounds include the pure antiestrogens ICI 164,384, ICI 182,780 (fulvestrant,

Faslodex), RU 58668 (25,76,77), and the oral agent SR16234 (78), which has agonist activity with regard to bone density and serum cholesterol. Currently there are no clinical data for RU58668 or SR16234. ICI 164,384 has been extensively studied in the preclinical setting, but it is the more potent fulvestrant that is being actively studied in clinical trials in patients with breast cancer.

The preclinical characteristics of ICI 182,780 that define this compound as a pure antiestrogen devoid of estrogen-like activity have been extensively reviewed (79–81). These include ER affinity approximately a hundred times that of tamoxifen, the specific absence of estrogen-like activity on the uterus, and the capacity to block completely the stimulatory activities of estrogens and partial estrogen agonists like tamoxifen. Moreover, ICI 182,780 has been shown not to block the uptake of $_3$H estradiol in the brain, suggesting that ICI 182,780 does not cross the blood-brain barrier (82) and therefore may not cause hot flashes. The preclinical animal data on the effects of ICI 182,780 on bone density are conflicting with reports of reduced cancellous bone volume in one study (83) and no effect on overall density in another (84). The absence of estrogenic activity has important consequences for the development of resistance, which is of major concern during tamoxifen therapy. *In vitro* studies have demonstrated that tamoxifen-resistant cell lines remain sensitive to growth inhibition by ICI 182,780 (85,86), and that tamoxifen-resistant tumors remain sensitive to ICI 182,780 *in vivo* (87). Preclinical studies in nude mice showed ICI 182,780 to suppress the growth of established MCF-7 xenografts for twice as long as tamoxifen and to delay the onset of tumor growth for longer than tamoxifen (87). Preclinical animal studies have also confirmed the complete absence of uterine stimulatory activity and have shown ICI 182,780 to block the uterotropic action of tamoxifen (79). In ovariectomized, estrogen-treated monkeys, the extent of involution of the endometrium was similar in animals treated with ICI 182,780 and in animals in which estrogen treatment was withdrawn (80). Overall, these data indicate that the mode of action and the preclinical effects of ICI 182,780 (fulvestrant) are distinct from those of tamoxifen and the newer non-steroidal antiestrogens cited above.

In a phase 1 study, administration of fulvestrant to postmenopausal breast cancer patients prior to surgery resulted in a reduction in proliferation as measured by Ki67 labelling index (LI) (24). In ER-positive tumors, fulvestrant caused a profound decrease in ER expression whereas tamoxifen had no effect (88), leading to the suggestion that this type of drug be called a "selective estrogen receptor downregulator." Fulvestrant also significantly reduced the expression of two estrogen-related genes, progesterone receptor and pS2, whereas tamoxifen had no effect.

One small phase 2 trial in 19 patients with tamoxifen refractory disease demonstrated a partial response rate of 37% and a stable disease of 32% with a median duration of 25 months (Table 16.4) (16,89), confirming the lack of cross-resistance with tamoxifen predicted by the animal studies. This trial also suggested that ICI 182,780 might have fewer side effects in terms of menopausal symptoms than tamoxifen.

The phase 2 second-line and preoperative trials reported above provided the initiative for two phase 3 studies, one in North America and one in Europe, Australia and South Africa (ROW), which compared the efficacy and tolerability of fulvestrant (250 mg) administered once monthly with those of the third-generation aromatase inhibitor anastrozole (Arimidex 1 mg) administered orally once daily in postmenopausal women whose disease had progressed on or after prior endocrine therapy (90,91). The vast majority (more than 96%) of patients, across both trials, had received prior tamoxifen therapy. The North American trial was a double-blind trial and recruited patients from 83 cities in the United States and Canada, whilst the second trial was an open-label study, conducted principally in Europe, and recruited patients from 82 cities. Four hundred and fifty-one patients were analyzed for efficacy in the North American and ROW trials, respectively. In both trials, the primary endpoint was disease progression with secondary endpoints including objective response, duration of response, time to death, tolerability, quality of life, and pharmacokinetics.

The median time to disease progression was numerically longer with fulvestrant compared with anastrozole for both the North American (5.4 versus 3.4 months) and ROW (5.5 versus 5.1 months) trials, but was not statistically significant in either trial. The objective response rates were not significantly different in either trial: 17.5% for both arms in the North American trial and 20.7% versus 15.7% for fulvestrant and anastrozole, respectively, in the ROW trial. In those patients who responded, median duration of response to fulvestrant and anastrozole was 19.3 months and 10.5 months, respectively, in the North American trial, and 14.3 months and 14 months, respectively, in the ROW trial. The clinical benefit rate (defined as complete and partial responses and disease stabilization lasting 24 weeks or more) for fulvestrant versus anastrozole were 42.2% versus 36.1% for the North American trial and 44.6% versus 45.0% for the ROW trial. In both trials, the most frequently reported adverse events were gastrointestinal disturbances, e.g., nausea, vomiting, constipation, and diarrhea: 53.4% and 39.7% of patients suffered from at least one gastrointestinal disturbance in the North American and ROW trials, respectively. Overall, the incidence of adverse events was similar for the recipients of anastrozole and fulvrestrant in both trials (90,91). Thus, in both studies, fulvestrant was at least as effective as the aromatase inhibitor anastrozole, with a longer duration of response in the North American trial, confirming fulvestrant as an effective treatment in postmenopausal patients with advanced breast cancer recurring or progressing after tamoxifen therapy (level of evidence: 1). Fulvestrant was also well-tolerated and is the first antiestrogen reported to be at least as effective as a new generation aromatase inhibitor. This is of particular significance in light of the fact that two trials comparing anastrozole with tamoxifen in the first-line metastatic treatment of breast cancer have shown anastrozole to be superior to tamoxifen, both in terms of time to progression and in terms of a lower incidence of thromboembolic events and vaginal bleeding (92,93).

There are, therefore, several antiestrogens in preclinical and clinical development. A major question is, which will be the most useful clinically? Clinical utility may be decided by a trade off between the antitumor activity of the antiestrogen and its beneficial effects on normal tissues. In order to decide and also to determine how to develop even more selective agents, it is important to understand the mechanisms of interaction of antiestrogens with the estrogen receptor. We need to know if we can group antiestrogens into particular classes and the molecular determinants of their antagonist and/or agonist activity in specific tissues. The first step in this process is to understand the interaction of the natural ligand estrogen with the ER and the factors that influence its site-specific activity.

ESTROGEN AND THE ESTROGEN RECEPTOR

The direct effects of estrogens on estrogen responsive tissues are mediated via the ER. The ER is found in hormone-responsive tissues, in low levels in normal breast tissue, and in higher concentrations in approximately two-thirds of all human breast cancers (94). The ER mediates most of the biological effects of estrogen on the breast and all the compounds discussed above were designed to interfere with this process, although it should be remembered that the ER can be activated in the absence of ligand by growth factors that increase intracellular second messengers (95). It is only by understanding the complex interactions of estrogen with the ER and the regulation of its downstream effectors that we can hope to gain a meaningful insight it the mechanism of action of the antiestrogens.

Structure

The human ER is a member of the steroid hormone receptor superfamily that functions as ligand-inducible DNA transcription factors (94). In the absence of hormone, the ER is sequestered within the nuclei of the target cell, and maintained in an inactive or repressed state by association with heat shock proteins (HSPs) and /or corepressors in a multiprotein inhibitory complex (96). Estrogen signal transduction is now known to be mediated by at least two dif-

Two Estrogen Receptors

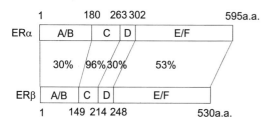

FIG. 16.4. Domain structure of the two estrogen receptors ERα and ERβ. ERα comprises 595 amino acids and ERβ 530. Percentages refer to the degree of amino acid homology between the two receptors. C is the DNA binding domain where there is a high degree of homology, whereas elsewhere in the molecules, homology is low.

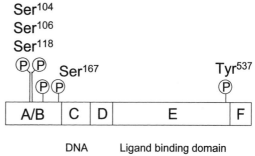

FIG. 16.5. Phosphorylation sites and sites for ligand and DNA binding in ERα. Activation function 1 is in the A/B domain and activation function 2 in the E domain.

ferent ERs, ER-α and the recently discovered ER-β (97–100). The two ERs (ERα and ERβ) have similar overall structures, exhibiting a high degree of amino acid conservation within the DNA binding domain (DBD), moderate amino acid conservation in the C-terminal, ligand binding domain (LBD), and considerable divergence at the amino terminus (Fig. 16.4). Estrogen binding induces an activating conformational change within the ER and the receptors dissociate from the HSP-inhibitory complex and the ER is phosphorylated (101). There are at least five phosphorylation sites on the ER, four serines at amino acids 104, 106, 118, and 167 of the A/B domain (Fig. 16.5), and another at tyrosine 537 in the LBD. Phosphorylation of tyrosine 537 is constitutive and is mediated by SRC kinases. Serine phosphorylation occurs in response to estrogen binding. The ligand-bound, phosphorylated ER then undergoes dimerization and binds as homodimers or heterodimers (102,103) to a specific DNA estrogen-responsive element (ERE). From this location on the DNA, the receptor enhances transcription from the nearby promoter.

Transcriptional Activation

Although the precise mechanism by which the ER regulates transcription remains to be determined, it is known that transcriptional activation by the ER is mediated by at least two different activating functions (AFs), AF-1 and AF-2 (Fig. 16.5). AF-1 is a weak constitutive AF that lies in the ER N-terminal A/B domain and AF-2 is a stronger estrogen-dependent AF that lies within the ER C-terminal LBD. Together AF-1 and AF-2 synergize strongly to give the final overall level of estrogen activation. These transactivating functions are thought to act by binding coactivators and bringing them to the promoter (104–107). The surface of AF-2 consists of helices 3, 5 and 12 of the estrogen receptor (108,109) which form a hydrophobic patch when estrogen binds to its specific site (110). This hydrophobic patch binds to a family of proteins, the p160s (111–118), which include the glucocorticoid receptor interacting protein (GRIP), its human homologue TIF2 (111–113), and the steroid receptor coactivator (SRC), SRC-1 (114). In each case, AF-2 recognizes a specific sequence, LXXLL (where L is leucine and X is any other amino acid) termed the "NR (nuclear receptor)-box," conserved across p160 coactivators and within the proteins that act as AF-2 repressors (corepressors) such as RIP140 (119–121). The p160s, in turn, interact with other coactivator proteins, and together this large coactivator complex is responsible for the ability of AF-2 to stimulate gene expression.

The activity of AF-1 is less well understood. AF-1 shows little independent activity and is responsible for the synergy with AF-2. The amino acid residues responsible for AF-1 activity lie between amino acids 41 and 120 to 150, dependent on cell type (108,122,123). Within this region, amino acid sequences that contribute to AF-1 independent activity (amino acids 41 to 64) and synergism with the LBD (amino acids 87 to 108) have been identified (Fig. 16.5) (124). AF-1 is also regulated by growth factors acting through the MAP kinase pathway (125–128). Several serine residues that are phosphorylated by MAP kinases or cyclin-dependent kinases have been identified (125, 126,129). Each phosphorylated serine contributes to AF-1 activity (125,126). Although the AF-1 coactivator complex is poorly defined, there is evidence that it shares features with the AF-2 coactivator complex. Webb et al. (96) provided evidence that the p160s are direct targets for both AF-1 and AF-2, and that the choice between AF-1/AF-2 synergism and independent AF-1 activity may be regulated by p160s. They demonstrated that the p160, GRIP1, enhances the independent activity of AF-1 and provided a hypothesis for why AF-1 synergizes with AF-2 in some cells, but works independently in others. They proposed that the ordinary weak AF-1/p160 contacts supported the stronger interaction of the ER-LBD with the p160s, and that this forms the basis of the synergy between AF-1 and AF-2. At increased p160 levels, however, AF-1/p160 contacts become sufficient to recruit p160s independently. The balance between AF-1/AF-2 synergy and AF-1 independent activity could therefore be regulated by the levels of p160s.

Interaction between ERα and ERβ

ERα and ERβ interact with the same DNA response elements and exhibit similar but nonidentical ligand binding characteristics. ERα and ERβ can also form heterodimers with each other. However, the experimental data clearly indicate that ERβ has biological functions that are distinct from those of ERα. Localization studies have indicated that there are several types of tissue that express both types of receptor (Table 16.6) (95,130), and recent evidence suggests that the relative levels of ERα and

TABLE 16.6. *Distribution of ERα and ERβ in different tissues*

Tissue	ERα	ERβ
Breast (normal)	+	+++
Breast (tumor)	+++	++
Uterus	+++	+
Bone	+	+
Cardiovascular system	+	+
CNS	+	+
GI tract	−	++
Liver	++	−
Urogenital tract	+	+++

+, expression; −, no expression.

ERβ within a tissue are important determinants of cellular sensitivity to estrogens.

Although ERα is a strong transcriptional activator, at physiological concentrations of estrogen, co-expression of ERβ results in suppression of both the potency and efficacy of the hormone-stimulated response (95). In ERα, the activating functions AF-1 and AF-2 act synergistically, whereas the AF-1 of ERβ is masked or replaced by an amino-terminal-suppressor domain. The absence of AF-1 in ERβ will clearly influence its ligand responsiveness, as the AF-1 of ERα is known to be essential for maximal transcriptional activation (131). Moreover, the AF-2 domain of ERβ functions as an independent activator domain, making it likely that ERα and ERβ will display differences in their preferences for coactivators and corepressors within their target cells. Furthermore, ERs α and β signal in opposite ways from their AP-1 site in the presence of the transcription factors fos and jun (Fig. 16.6) (132). When bound to ERα, estrogen activates transcription, whereas when bound to ERβ, it inhibits transcription when the receptors act via AP-1 sites.

Thus one can predict that knowledge of the patterns of colocalization and concentrations of both receptors within different tissues will provide an insight into the biological responses induced by them to estrogen. The observation that ERβ can act as a transcriptional activator or inhibitor dependent on agonist concentration suggests that it must play a significant role in the mechanism of estrogen action in the many tissues (breast, uterus, bone, and cardiovascular) in which it is expressed. It is becoming in-

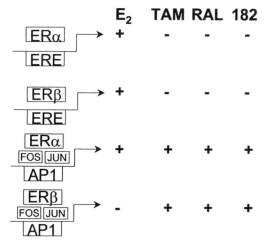

FIG. 16.6. Differential effects of estradiol (E_2) and antiestrogens (*TAM*, tamoxifen; *RAL*, raloxifene; 182, ICI 182780) on ERα and ERβ according to whether the receptors bind directly to the estrogen response element (ERE) or to an AP1 site via the transcription factors fos and jun.

creasingly obvious that our understanding of the tissue distribution of these receptors will be crucial to the development of new antiestrogen anticancer therapies and to the development of non–cancer-inducing hormone replacement therapies for postmenopausal women. The known distributions are shown in Table 16.6. The receptors are co-expressed in most tissues (although not necessarily in the same cell), with the exception that ERα is not found in the GI tract and ERβ is not found in the liver.

INTERACTION OF NEW ANTIESTROGENS WITH THE ESTROGEN RECEPTOR

Until very recently, all the studies on the elucidation of the molecular mechanisms of ER activity have involved ERα (133–135), although increasingly data are becoming available for ERβ.

Ligand Binding-induced Conformational Changes

The binding of agonists triggers AF-2 activity by directly affecting the structure of the LBD. Only the binding of agonists triggers the AF-2 activity, whilst the binding of antagonists does not (136).

Comparison of the structure of the LBD of ERα complexed with E_2 and raloxifene shows that, although both ligands bind at the same site within the core of the LBD (137), each ligand induces a different conformation of helix 12, the most C-terminal helix of the LBD. Helix 12 in the raloxifene-LBD complex is bound in a hydrophobic groove composed of residues from helices 3 and 5. This alternative orientation of helix 12 partially buries residues in the groove that are necessary for AF-2 activity, suggesting that raloxifene and possibly other antagonists block AF-2 functioning by disrupting the topography of the AF-2 surface.

Differences in secondary structure between the agonist complexes with estrogen and diethylstilbestrol (DES) and 4-OH-tamoxifen also arise from distinct arrangements of the packing interactions induced by the different ligands. 4-OH-tamoxifen binds to the AF-2 complex without directly interacting with helix 12 and occludes the coactivator recognition site (138–140). The binding mode of 4-OH tamoxifen has two distinct effects on the positioning of helix 12. First, helix 12 is prevented from positioning itself over the ligand-binding pocket by the 4-OH-tamoxifen side chain; and secondly, the alternative packing arrangement of ligand binding residues around 4-OH-tamoxifen stabilizes a conformation of the LBD that mimics bound coactivator (138). Raloxifene also sterically hinders the agonist-bound conformation of helix 12 (137), inducing a distinct ER conformation (141,142), which is dependent upon amino acid 351 (143). The differences in the effects on the uterus between tamoxifen and raloxifene have been attributed to distinct ligand conformations (51).

The ER-antagonist fulvestrant is also known to induce a distinct ER conformation (141,142), and specific peptide probes have demonstrated that ER ligands known to produce distinct biological effects induce distinct conformational changes in the receptors. This provides evidence of a strong correlation between ER conformation and biological activity (144). Furthermore, these ER modulators are able to induce distinct conformational changes in ERα and ERβ, suggesting that the biological effects of

ER-agonists and antagonists operating through these receptors are likely to be different (144).

Transcriptional Activation

Both pure antagonists and partial agonists deliver the ER to its DNA target within the cell; however, the ability of the DNA-bound receptor to activate transcription is dependent on the cell and promoter context (141). As stated previously, ERα and ERβ share high-sequence homology, especially in the regions responsible for specific binding to DNA and in their LBDs (98,99,145). Moreover, antiestrogen agonism via the ER is, for the most part, mediated by the A/B domain of ERα and is not supported by the AF-1 (A/B domain) of ERβ (131). The 24 amino acid residue domain of ERα required for antiestrogen agonism, but not E_2-stimulated transcription, is not found in ERβ (124), suggesting that these differences in sequence between the N-terminal domains of ERα and ERβ contribute to the cell and promoter specific transcriptional activity of these receptors and their ability to respond to different ligands.

Dose-dependent inhibition studies of E_2-induced ERα and ERβ activity show that the active metabolite of EM-800 and EM-652 was more potent at inhibiting ERα activity than the pure steroidal antiestrogen ICI 182,780 (fulvestrant), and that both antiestrogens were more potent inhibitors of ERβ than ERα. The inhibitory properties of the various antiestrogens with regard to AF-1 and AF-2 of ERα are summarized in Figure 16.6. EM-652 and ICI 182,780 (fulvestrant) both inhibit the AF-1 and AF-2 functions of both ERα and ERβ, acting as pure estrogen antagonists on ERα and ERβ transcriptional activities. 4-OH tamoxifen, however, only blocks the AF-2 activity of both ERs (145) which, coupled with the information about antiestrogen agonism being mediated by the AB domain of ERα (131), might explain the agonist activity of tamoxifen.

SRC-1 has been shown to stimulate ERα and ERβ activity in the absence of ligand. The ligand-independent activation of AF-1 is presumed to be closely linked to phosphorylation of the steroid receptors by cellular protein kinases (146). Enhancement of ERβ activation in the absence of ligand was found to be independent of AF-2. Significantly, 4-OH-tamoxifen had no appreciable effect on SRC-1-induced unliganded activity, while EM-652 completely abolished this effect. The absence of the inhibition of the ligand-independent, AF-2–independent, SRC-1 coactivator activity by 4-OH-tamoxifen could explain why the benefits of tamoxifen are lost after 5 years and why resistance develops.

Biological Effects

Estrogen, the natural ligand for the ER, acts as an agonist in all environments, regardless of whether or not AF-1 or AF-2 is the dominant activator. The steroidal, pure antiestrogen ICI 182, 780 (fulvestrant), which inhibits the activity of both AF-1 and AF-2, completely blocks the ability of ERα to activate transcription through the classical ERE-mediated pathways. Unlike fulvestrant, however, the relative agonist/antagonist activities of the other new antiestrogens are determined by the cell and promoter context and not solely by their ability to differentially regulate AF-1 and AF-2. For example, the antiestrogens raloxifene and GW 5638 function as estrogens on bone and the cardiovascular system but don't appear to act as AF-1 or AF-2 agonists. This suggests that the current theories of ER modulation are incomplete and, increasingly, the role of ERβ has to be considered. Tamoxifen, for example, is a more potent competitive antagonist of ERβ (97) and does not display ERβ agonist activity. This makes the authors wonder whether there is better response to tamoxifen in ERβ-positive tumors (147).

Estrogens and antiestrogens are also known to induce differential activation of ERα and ERβ to control the transcription of genes that are under the control of an AP-1 element (132). The ligand-bound ER binds to EREs as a homodimer, but the ER also mediates gene transcription from an AP-1 enhancer element that requires ligand and the AP-1 transcription factors fos and jun (132). ERα and ERβ were found to signal in opposite ways from the AP-1 site depending on the ligand (Fig. 16.6). This adds another potential control mechanism for the transcriptional regulation of estrogen-responsive genes. Recently, an isoform of human ERβ has been cloned that has the potential to inhibit human ERα-mediated estrogen activity, adding yet another layer of complexity to our attempts to understand the diverse biological effects of estrogens and antiestrogens (148).

Clinical Relevance of Knowledge of Estrogen Receptor Structure and Function

It is clear that interaction with ER with a ligand is a highly complex event. The ER may be regarded as an integrator of the functions of a mammary cell, including regulating the effects of growth factors such as EGF1 and IGF1 (insulin growth factor-1) through phosphorylation of the receptor. In the future, more knowledge of the complexity of the ER may allow the development of specific regulators of ERβ or inhibitors of specific coactivators. At present, the most appropriate synthesis in this complex area may be to recognize three classes of antiestrogen which affect ERα (at least) in distinctive ways. This is illustrated in Figure 16.7 with respect to binding of estrogen or antiestrogen to the ligand-binding domain of ERα. Estrogen binding allows helix 12 to cover the binding site and for coactivators to bind, whereas the three classes of antiestrogen with progressively larger side chains may block helix 12 movement to different degrees. Steroidal antiestrogens with the largest side chain may block all movement of helix 12, and thus coactivator binding and AF1 and AF2 are not activated. Such a model would account for the intermediate activity of raloxifene and arzoxifene, which have less partial agonist activity on the uterus than tamoxifen. It would also account for the lack of effect of fulvestrant on lipid concentrations or bone. It is of interest that mutations of a single amino acid (aspartate 351) in the LBD prevents binding of the side chains of raloxifene and EM-800, making them into estrogens, whereas this mutation does not affect the antiestrogenicity of fulvestrant, suggesting a differ-

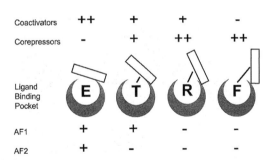

FIG. 16.7. Cartoon of the potential differences in mechanism of action of the three classes of antiestrogen (*T*, triphenylethylene [tamoxifen]; *R*, cyclic/fixed ring structures [raloxifene]; *F*, steroidal antiestrogens [ICI 182,780 faslodex]). The ligand-binding pocket of ERα is shown with helix 12 as a box. When estrogen occupies the binding site, helix 12 covers the pocket, whereas it is likely that the three classes of antiestrogen sterically hinder the action of helix 12 to differing degrees. Thus the steroidal antiestrogens, because of their bulky side chain, may maximally inhibit binding of coactivators resulting in inactivation of both activating functions 1 and 2.

ent mechanism of binding to the LBD of the ER (143).

Many antiestrogens have been withdrawn from development. None of the triphenylethylenes has been shown to have superior clinical activity to tamoxifen, while all have uterotropic effects which limit their clinical utility. Thus, we are left in the clinic with two equally active compounds, tamoxifen and toremifene.

At present, the sole fixed-ring structure being developed for the treatment of breast cancer is arzoxifene. Raloxifene and EM652, which appear to have lower anti-tumor activity, are being used for prevention only.

There is also only one steroidal compound in the clinic. Fulvestrant appears highly active, and in two recently published phase 3 trials was shown to be as effective as the third generation aromatase inhibitor anastrozole in metastatic breast cancer. It will be some time before we know whether the newer compounds in each of the three classes of antiestrogen (GW5638, LY325315 and SR 16234) will have superior activities to the agents already available.

TABLE 16.7. *Effects of the three different types of antiestrogen*

	Triphenylethylene	Fixed ring	Steroidal
Antitumor	+	++	+++
Tamoxifen-resistant growth	−	?	++
Bone density	+	++	?
Uterus	+	−	−
Hot flushes	+	+	−
Clotting factors	+	+	−
Serum lipids	+	+	−
Cardiovascular	?	?	?
Brain	?	?	?

+, expression; −, no expression.

We still have a lack of knowledge of many of the potential beneficial activities of the three groups of antiestrogens (Table 16.7). For example, there are few data on the effects of triphenylethylenes on the cardiovascular system (in contradiction to clotting or lipids) and brain, and similar considerations apply to the fixed-ring and the steroidal compounds. In addition, we do not know whether the fixed-ring or the steroidal compounds will have greater antitumor activity than the triphenylethylenes, although these data should be available in 2002.

REFERENCES

1. Landis SH, Murray T, Bolden S, Wingo PA. Cancer statistics. *CA Cancer J Clin* 1998;48:6–29.
2. Beatson G. On the treatment of inoperable cases of carcinoma of the mamma: with suggestions for a new method of treatment, with illustrative cases. *Lancet* 1896;2:104–107.
3. Haddow A, Watkinson JM, Patterson E. Influence of synthetic oestrogens upon advanced malignant disease. *Br Med J* 1944;2:393–398.
4. Walpole AE, Patterson E. Synthetic oestrogens in mammary cancer. *Lancet* 1949;ii:783–786.
5. Howell A, De Friend D, Anderson E. Clues to the mechanisms of endocrine resistance from clinical studies in advanced breast cancer. *Endocrinol-Rel Cancer* 1995;2:131–139.
6. Cole MP, Jones CTA, Todd IDH. A new antiestrogenic agent in late breast cancer : an early clinical appraisal of ICI 146474. *Br J Cancer* 1971;25:270–275.
7. Early Breast Cancer Trialist's Collaborative Group. Tamoxifen for early breast cancer: an overview of the randomised trials. *Lancet* 1998;851:1451–1467.
8. Fisher B, Constantino JP, Wickerham DL, et al. Tamoxifen for prevention of breast cancer: report of the National Surgical Adjuvant Breast and Bowel Project P-1 Study. *J Natl Cancer Inst* 1998;90:1371–1388.
9. Chlebowski R, Collyar DE, Somerfield MR, et al. American Society of Clinical Oncology Technology. Assessment of breast cancer risk reduction strategies: tamoxifen and raloxifene. *J Clin Oncol* 1999;17:1939–1955.
10. Veronesi U, Maisonneuve P, Costa A, et al. Prevention of breast cancer with tamoxifen: preliminary findings from the Italian randomised trial among hysterectomised women. Italian Tamoxifen Prevention Study. *Lancet* 1998;11:352:93–97.
11. Powles T, Eeles R, Ashley S, et al. Interim analysis of the incidence of breast cancer in the Royal Marsden Hospital tamoxifen randomised chemoprevention trial. *Lancet* 1998;11:352:98–101.
12. Love RR, Mazess RB, Barden HS, et al. Effects of tamoxifen on bone mineral density in postmenopausal women with breast cancer. *N Engl J Med* 1992;326:852–856.
13. Love RR, Newcomb PA, Wiebe DA, et al. Effects of tamoxifen therapy on lipid and lipoprotein levels in postmenopausal patients with node-negative breast cancer. *J Natl Cancer Inst* 1990;82:1327–1332.
14. Fisher B, Constantino JP, Redmond CK, et al. Endometrial cancer in tamoxifen treated breast cancer patients: findings from the National Surgical Adjuvant Breast and Bowel Project (NASBP) B-14 Study. *J Natl Cancer Inst* 1994;86:527.
15. Assirikis VJ, Neven P, Jordan VC, et al. A realistic clinical perspective of tamoxifen and endometrial carcinogenesis. *Eur J Cancer* 1996;32A(9):1464–1476.
16. Howell A, DeFriend DJ, Robertson JFR, et al. Pharmacokinetics, pharmacological and antitumor effects of the specific antioestrogen ICI 182780 in women with advanced breast cancer. *Br J Cancer* 1996;74:300–308.
17. Howell A, Downey S, Anderson E. New endocrine therapies for breast cancer. *Eur J Cancer* 1996;32A:576–588.
18. Clemens JA, Bennet DR, Black IJ, Jones CD. Effects of a new antiestrogen keoxifene (LY156758), on growth of carcinogen-induced mammary tumors and on LH and prolactin levels. *Life Sci* 1983;32:2869–2875.
19. Palkowitz AD, Glasebrook AL, Thresher KJ, et al. Discovery and synthesis of [6-hydroxy-3[4-[2-(1-piperidinyl)ethoxy]phenoxy]-2-(4-hydroxyphenyl)]benzo[β]thiophene: a novel highly potent selective estrogen receptor modulator. *J Med Chem* 1997;40:1407–1416.
20. Ke HZ, Paralkar VM, Grasser WA, et al. Effects of CP-336,156, a new, non steroidal estrogen agonist/antagonist, on bone serum cholesterol, uterus and

body composition in rat models. *Endocrinology* 1998; 139:2068–2076.
21. Grese TA, Dodge JA. Selective estrogen receptor modulators (SERMS). *Current Pharmaceutical Design* 1998;4:71–92.
22. Gauthier S, Caron B, Cloutier J, et al. (S)-(+)-4-[7-(2,2-dimethyl-1-oxopropoxy)-4-methyl-2-[4-[2-(1-piperidinyl)-ethoxy]phenyl]-2H-1-benzopyran-3-yl]-phenyl2,2-dimethyl-propanoate (EM-800): a highly potent, specific and orally active nonsteroidal antiestrogen. *J Med Chem* 1997;40:2117–2122.
23. Wakeling AE. Pharmacology of antiestrogens. In: Oettle M, Schillinger E, eds. *Estrogens and anti-estrogens II*. Vol 135. Berlin: Springer, 1999:179–194.
24. De Friend DJ, Howell A, Nicholson RT, et al. Investigation of a new pure antiestrogen (ICI 182780) in women with primary breast cancer. *Cancer Res* 1994;54:408–414.
25. Van de Velde P, Nique F, Bouchoux J, et al. RU 58668, a new pure antiestrogen inducing a regression of human mammary carcinoma implanted in nude mice. *J Steroid Biochem Mol Biol* 1994;48:187–196.
26. Kangas L, Nieminen A-L, Blanco G, et al. A new triphenylethylene compound Fc-1157a II. Antitumor effects. *Cancer Chemother Pharmacol* 1986;17:109–113.
27. Chander SK, McCague R, Luqmani Y, et al. Pyrrolidino-4-iodotamoxifen and 4-iodotamoxifen, new analogues of the anti-estrogen tamoxifen for the treatment of breast cancer. *Cancer Res* 1991;51:5851–5858.
28. Loser R, Seibel K, Roos W, Eppenberger U. In vivo and in vitro antioestrogenic action of 3-OH-tamoxifen, tamoxifen and 4-OH-tamoxifen. *Eur J Cancer Clin Oncol* 1985;21:985–990.
29. Toko T, Sugimoto Y, Matsuo E, et al. TAT-59, a new triphenylethylene derivative with antitumor activity against hormone-dependent tumors. *Eur J Cancer* 1990;26:397–404.
30. Willson TM, Norris JD, Wagner BL, et al. Dissection of the molecular mechanism of action of GW 5638, a novel estrogen receptor ligand, provides an insight into the role of the estrogen receptor in bone. *Endocrinology* 1997;138:3901–3911.
31. Hemminki K, Rajaniemi H, Lindahl B, et al. Tamoxifen-induced DNA adducts in endometrial samples from breast cancer patients. *Cancer Res* 1996;56:4374–4377.
32. Tomas E, Kauppila A, Blanco G, et al. Comparison between effects of tamoxifen, toremifene and ICI 182780 on the uterus in postmenopausal breast cancer patients. *Gynaecol Oncol* 1995;59(2):261–266.
33. Gershanovich M, Garin A, Baltina D, et al. A phase III comparison of two toremifene doses to tamoxifen in post menopausal women with advanced breast cancer. Eastern European Study Group. *Breast Cancer Res Treat* 1997;45:251–262.
34. Pyrhonen S, Valavaara R, Modig H, et al. Comparison of toremifene and tamoxifen in post-menopausal patients with advanced breast cancer: a randomised double-blind trial, the "Nordic" phase III study. *Br J Cancer* 1997;76:270–277.
35. Hayes DE, Van Zyl JA, Hacking A, et al. Randomised comparison of tamoxifen and two separate doses of toremifene in post-menopausal patients with metastatic breast cancer. *J Clin Oncol* 1995;13:2556–2566.
36. Nomura Y, Tominaga T, Abe O, et al. Clinical evaluation of NK622 (toremifene citrate) in advanced or recurrent breast cancer- a comparative study by a double blind method with tamoxifen. *Jpn J Cancer Chemotherapy* 1993;20:247–258.
37. Milla-Santos A, Milla A, Rallo L, et al. Anastrozole vs tamoxifen in hormonodependent advanced breast cancer. A phase II randomised trial. *Breast Cancer Res Treat* 2000;64:A173.
38. Holli K, Joensun H, Valavaara R, et al. Interim results of the Finnish toremifene versus tamoxifen adjuvant trial. *Breast Cancer Res Treat* 1998;50:283.
39. Pyrhonen S, Valavaara R, Vuorinen J, et al. High dose toremifene in advanced breast cancer resistant to or relapsed during tamoxifen treatment. *Breast Cancer Res Treat* 1994;29:223–228.
40. Pyrohnen S, Ellmen J, Vuorinen M, et al. Meta-analysis of trials comparing toremifene with tamoxifen and factors predicting outcome of antiestrogen therapy in postmenopausal women with breast cancer. *Breast Cancer Res Treat* 1999;56:133–143.
41. McCague R, Parr IB, Haynes BP. Metabolism of the 4-iodo-derivative of tamoxifen by isolated rat hepatocytes. Demonstration that the iodine atom reduces metabolic conversion and identification of four metabolites. *Biochem Pharmacol* 1990;40:2277–2283.
42. Nuttall ME, Bradbeer JN, Strorp GB, et al. Idoxifene a novel selective estrogen receptor modulator prevents bone loss and lowers cholesterol levels in ovariectomised rats and reduces uterine weight in intact rats. *Endocrinology* 1998;139:5224–5234.
43. Johnston SRD, Gumbrell L, Evans TRJ, et al. A phase II randomised double blind study of idoxifene (40mg/d) vs tamoxifen (40mg/d) in patients with locally advanced/metastatic breast cancer resistant to tamoxifen (920mg/d). *Proc Am Soc Clin Oncol* 1999;18:A413.
44. Ke HZ, Simmons HA, Pirie CM, et al. Droloxifene a new oestrogen antagonist/agonist prevents bone loss in ovariectomised rats. *Endocrinology* 1995;136: 2435–2441.
45. Abe O. Japanese early phase II study of droloxifene in the treatment of advanced breast cancer. Preliminary dose-finding study. *Am J Clin Oncol* 1991;14: S40–S45.
46. Bellmunt J, Sole L. European early phase II dose-finding study of droloxifene in advanced breast cancer. *Am J Clin Oncol* 1991;S36–S39.
47. Haarstad H, Gundersen S, Wist, et al. Droloxifene a new antioestrogen phase II study in advanced breast cancer. *Acta Oncol* 1992;31:425–428.
48. Rauschning W, Pritchard KI. Droloxifene a new antiestrogen its role in metastatic breast cancer. *Breast Cancer Res Treat* 1994;31:83–94.
49. Koh JR, Kubota T, Asanuma F, et al. Antitumor effect of triphenylethylene derivative (TAT-59) against human breast carcinoma xenografts in nude mice. *J Surg Oncol* 1992;51:254–258.
50. Noguchi S, Koyama H, Nomura Y, et al. Late phase II study of TAT-59 (new antiestrogen) in advanced or recurrent breast cancer patients: a double-blind comparative study with tamoxifen citrate. *Breast Cancer Res Treat* 1998;50:307.
51. Grese TA, Sluka JP, Bryant HU, et al. Molecular determinants of tissue selectivity in estrogen receptor modulators. *Proc Natl Acad Sci* 1997;94:14105–14110.
52. Anzano MA, Peer CW, Smith JM, et al. Chemoprevention of mammary carcinogenesis in the rat: combined use of raloxifene and 9-cis-retinoic acid. *J Natl Cancer Inst* 1996;88:123–125.

53. Black IJ, Sato M, Rowley ER, et al. Raloxifene (LY 139481-HCl) prevents bone loss and reduces serum cholesterol without causing uterine hypertrophy in ovariectomised rats. *J Clin Invest* 1994;93:63–69.
54. Turner CH, Sato M, Rowley ER, et al. Raloxifene preserves bone strength and bone mass in ovariectomised rats. *Endocrinology* 1994;135:2001–2005.
55. Draper MW, Flowers DE, Huster WJ, et al. A controlled trial of raloxifene (LY 39481) HCl: impact on bone turnover and serum lipid profile in healthy post-menopausal women. *J Bone Minor Res* 1996;11:835–842.
56. Walsh BW, Kuller LH, Wild RA, et al. Effects of raloxifene on serum lipids and coagulation factors in healthy post menopausal women. *JAMA* 1998;279:1445–1451.
57. Delmas PD, Bjarnason NH, Mitlak BH, et al. Effects of raloxifene on bone mineral density, serum cholesterol concentrations and uterine endometrium in post menopausal women. *N Engl J Med* 1997;337:1641–1647.
58. Cummings SR, Norton L, Eckert S, et al. Raloxifene reduces the risk of cancer and may decrease the risk of endometrial cancer in post menopausal women: two year findings from the Multiple Outcomes of Raloxifene Evaluation (MORE) trial. *Proc Am Soc Clin Oncol* 1998;17:2a.
59. Buzdar AV, Marcus C, Holmes F, et al. Phase II evaluation of LY 156758 in metastatic breast cancer. *Oncology* 1988;45:344–345.
60. Gradishar WJ, Glusman JE, Vogel CH, et al. Raloxifene HCl a new endocrine agent is active in estrogen receptor positive (ER+) metastatic breast cancer. *Breast Cancer Res Treat* (San Antonio Cancer Symposium Proc) 1997;20:53.
61. Jordon VC. Development of a new prevention maintenance therapy for postmenopausal women. *Recent Results Cancer Res* 1999;151:96–109.
62. Jordon VC, Morrow M. Raloxifene as a multifunctional medicine? *Br Med J* 1999;319:331–332.
63. Sato M, Turner CH, Wang T, et al. LY 353381.Hcl: a novel raloxifene analog with improved SERM potency and efficacy in vivo. *J Pharmacol Exp Ther* 1998;287:1–7.
64. Sato M, Glasebrook AL, Bryant HU. Raloxifene: A selective estrogen receptor modulator. *J Bone Miner Met* 1994;12:S9–S20.
65. Hudis C, Buzdar A, Munster P, et al. Phase I study of a third generation selective estrogen receptor modulator (SERM 3, LY 353381.HCl) in refractory metastatic breast cancer. *Breast Cancer Res Treat* 1998;50:306 (abstract 442).
66. Baselga J, Llombart-Cussac A, Bellet M, et al. Randomised double-blind phase 2 study of a selective estrogen receptor mobulator SERM (LY 353381) in patients (pts) with locally advanced or metastatic breast cancer. *Breast Cancer Res Treat* 1999;57:31 (abstract 35).
67. Tagnon HJ. Antiestrogens in treatment of breast cancer. *Cancer* 1977;39:2959–2964.
68. Ray S, Groves P, Kamboj VP, et al. Antifertility agent 12. Structure-activity relationship of 3,4-diphenylchromenes and chromans. *J Med Chem* 1976;19:276–279.
69. Kamboj VP, Ray S, Dhawan RB. Centchroman. *Drugs Today* 1992;227–232.
70. Holm P, Shalmi M, Korsgaard N, et al. A partial estrogen receptor antagonist with strong anti atherogenic properties without noticable effect on reproductive tissue in cholesterol-fed female and male rabbits. *Arterioscler Thromb Vasc Biol* 1997;17:2264–2272.
71. Martel C, Provencher I, Li X, et al. Binding characteristics of novel nonsteroidal antiestrogens to the rat uterine estrogen receptors. *J Steroid Biochem Mol Biol* 1998;64:199–205.
72. Simard J, Labrie C, Bélanger A, et al. Characterisation of the effects of the novel non-steroidal antiestrogen EM-800 on basal and estrogen-induced proliferation on T-47-D, 2R-75-1 and MCF-7 human cancer cells in vitro. *Int J Cancer* 1997;73:104–112.
73. Sourla A, Luo S, Labrie C, et al. Morphological changes induced by six-month treatment of intact and ovariectomised mice with tamoxifen and the pure antioestrogen EM-800. *Endocrinology* 1997;138:5605–5617.
74. Luo S, Sourla A, Gauthier S, et al. Effect of 24-week treatment with the antioestrogen EM-800 on estrogen-sensitive parameters in intact and ovariectomised mice. *Endocrinology* 1998;139:2645–2656.
75. Greenberger L, Komm B, Miller C, et al. Preclinical pharmacology profile of a new selective estrogen receptor modulator (SERM), ERA-923, for the treatment of ER positive breast cancer. *Breast Cancer Res Treat* 2000;64:52 (A166).
76. Van De Velde P, Nique F, Brémaud M-C, et al. Exploration of the therapeutic potential of the antiestrogen RU 58668 in breast cancer treatment. *Ann NY Acad Sci* 1995;761:164–175.
77. Van De Velde P, Nique F, Planchon P, et al. RU 58668: Further in vitro and in vivo pharmacological data related to its antitumoral activity. *J Steroid Biochem Mol Biol* 1996;59:449–457.
78. Tanabe M, Peters RH, Chao W-R, et al. SR 16234, a novel steroidal selective estrogen receptor modulator (SERM). *Breast Cancer Res Treat* 1999;57:52 (abstract 172).
79. Wakeling AE, Dukes M, Bowler J. A potent specific pure antiestrogen with clinical potential. *Cancer Res* 1991;51:3867–3873.
80. Dukes M, Miller D, Wakeling AE, Waterton JC. Antiuterotrophic effects of a pure antioestrogen, ICI 182780;magnetic resonance imaging of the uterus in ovariectomised monkeys. *J Endocrinol* 1992;135:239–247.
81. Dukes M, Waterton JC, Wakeling AE. Antiuterotrophic effects of the pure antioestrogen ICI 182780 in adult female monkeys (Macaca nemestrina): quantitative magnetic resonance imaging. *J Endocrinol* 1993;138:203–209.
82. Wade GN, Blaustein JD, Gray JM, Meredith JM. ICI 182780: a pure antiestrogen that affects behaviour and energy balance in rats without acting in the brain. *Am J Physiol* 1993;34:R1392–R1398.
83. Gallagher A, Chambers TJ, Tobias JH. The estrogen antagonist ICI 182780 reduces cancellous bone in female rats. *Endocrinology* 1993;133:2787–2791.
84. Wakeling AE. The future of pure antiestrogens in clinical breast cancer. *Breast Cancer Res Treat* 1993;25:1–9.
85. Coopman P, Garcia M, Brunner N, et al. Antiproliferative and anti-estrogenic effects of ICI 164, 384 and

ICI 182780 in 4-OH-tamoxifen resistant human breast cancer cells. *Int J Cancer* 1994;56:295–300.
86. Hu XF, Veroni M, De Luise M, et al. Circumvention of tamoxifen resistance by the pure anti-estrogen ICI 182780. *Int J Cancer* 1993;55:873–876.
87. Osborne CK, Coronado-Heinsohn ER, Hilsenbeck SG, et al. Comparison of the effects of a pure steroidal antiestrogen with those of tamoxifen in a model of human breast cancer. *J Natl Cancer Inst* 1995;87:746–750.
88. Robertson JFR, Dixon M, Bundred N, et al. A partially-blind, randomised, multi-centre study comparing the anti-tumor effects of single-doses (50, 125, 250mg) of long-acting (LA) "Faslodex" (ICI 182780) with tamoxifen in postmenopausal women with primary breast cancer prior to surgery. *Breast Cancer Res Treat* 1999;57:31 (abstract 28).
89. Howell A, Osborne K, Morris C, Wakeling A. Faslodex (ICI 182,780). Development of a novel 'pure' antiestrogen. *Cancer* 2000;89:817–825.
90. Howell A, Robertson JFR, Quaresma AJ, et al. Comparison of efficacy and tolerability of fulvestrant (Faslodex) with anastrozole (Arimidex) in postmenopausal women (PM) with advanced breast cancer (ABC)—preliminary results. *Breast Cancer Res Treat* 2000;64:A6.
91. Osborne CK, Pippen J, Jones SE, et al. Faslodex (ICI 182,780) shows longer duration of response compared with arimidex (anastrozole) in postmenopausal (PM) women with advanced breast cancer (ABC). Preliminary results of a phase III North American trial. *Breast Cancer Res Treat* 2001;65:261.
92. Nabholtz JM, Buzdar A, Pollack M, et al. Anastrozole is superior to tamoxifen as first-line therapy for advanced breast cancer in postmenopausal women: results of a North American multicenter randomized trial. Arimidex Study Group. *J Clin Oncol* 2000;18:3758–3767.
93. Bonneterre J, Thurlimann B, Robertson JF, et al. Anastrozole versus tamoxifen as first line therapy for advanced breast cancer in 668 postmenopausal women: results of the tamoxifen or Arimidex Randomised Group Efficacy and Tolerability Study. *J Clin Oncol* 2000;18:3748–3757.
94. Evans RM. The steroid and thyroid hormone receptor super family. *Science* 1988;240:889–895.
95. Hall JM, McDonnell DP. The estrogen receptor b-isoform (ER b) of the human estrogen receptor modulates Era transcriptional activity and is a key regulator of the cellular response to estrogens and antiestrogens. *Endocrinology* 1999;140:5566–5578.
96. Webb P, Nguyen P, Shinsako J, et al. Estrogen receptor activation function 1 works by binding p160 coactivator proteins. *Mol Endocrinol* 1998;12:1605–1618.
97. Kuiper GGJM, Enmark E, Pelto-Huikko M, et al. Cloning of a novel estrogen receptor expressed in rat prostate and ovary. *Proc Natl Acad Sci, USA* 1996;93:5925–5930.
98. Mosselman S, Polman J, Dijkema R. ERβ identification and characterisation of a novel human oestrogen receptor. *FEBS Letts* 1996;392:49–53.
99. Kuiper GGJM, Carlsson B, Grandien J, et al. A comparison of ligand binding specificity and transcript tissue distribution of estrogen receptors α and β. *Endocrinology* 1997;138:863–870.
100. Katzenellenbogen BS, Korach KS. Editorial—a new actor in the estrogen receptor drama—enter ERβ. *Endocrinology* 1997;138:861–862.
101. Lieberman BA. Estrogen receptor activity cycle: dependence on multiple protein-protein interactions. *Crit Rev Eukatyot Gene Expr* 1997;7:43–59.
102. Petersson K, Grandien K, Kuiper GG, et al. Mouse estrogen receptor beta forms estrogen response element binding heterodimers with estrogen receptor alpha. *Mol Endocrinol* 1997;11:1486–1496.
103. Cowley SM, Hoare S, Mosselman S, Parker MG. Estrogen receptors alpha and β form heterodimers on DNA. *J Biol Chem* 1997;272:19858–19862.
104. Le Douarin B, Vom Baur E, Zechel C, et al. Ligand-dependent interaction of nuclear receptors with potential transcriptional intermediary factors (mediators). *Philos Trans R Soc Lond Biol Sci* 1996;351:569–578.
105. Horowitz KB, Jackson TA, Bain DL, et al. Nuclear receptor coactivators and co-repressors. *Mol Endocrinol* 1996;10:1167–1177.
106. Glass CK, Rose DW, Rosenfeld MG. Nuclear receptor coactivators. *Curr Opinion Cell Biol* 1997;9:222–232.
107. Shibata H, Spencer TE, Onate SA, et al. Role of coactivators and co-repressors in the mechanism of steroid/thyroid receptor action. *Recent Prog Horm Res* 1997;52:141–164.
108. Danielian PS, White R, Lees JA, et al. Identification of a conserved region required for hormone dependent transcriptional activation by steroid hormone receptors. *EMBO J* 1992;11:1025–1033.
109. Henttu PM, Kalkhoven E, Parker MG. AF-2 activity and recruitment of steroid receptor coactivator 1 to the estrogen receptor depend on a lysine residue conserved in nuclear receptors. *Mol Cell Biol* 1997;17:1832–1839.
110. Feng WJ, Ribeiro RCJ, Wagner RL, et al. Hormone-dependent coactivator binding to a hydrophobic cleft on nuclear receptors. *Science* 1998;280:1747–1749.
111. Hong H, Kohli K, Trivedi A, et al. GRIP1, a novel mouse protein that serves as a transcriptional coactivator in yeast for the hormone binding domains of steroid receptors. *Proc Natl Acad Sci* 1996;93:4948–4952.
112. Hong H, Kohli K, Garabedian MJ, Stallcup MR. GRIP1, a transcriptional coactivator for the AF-2 transcriptional activation domain of steroid, thyroid, retinoid and vitamin D receptors. *Mol Cell Biol* 1997;17:2735–2744.
113. Voegel JJ, Heine MJS, Tini M, et al. The coactivator TIF2 contains three nuclear receptor-binding motifs and mediates transactivation through CBP binding Chen H dependent and independent pathways. *EMBO J* 1998;17:507–519.
114. Onate SA, Tsai SY, Tsai MJ, O'Malley BW. Sequence and characterisation of a co-activator for the steroid hormone receptor superfamily. *Science* 1995;270:1354–1357.
115. Li H, Gomes PJ, Chen JD. RAC3, a steroid/nuclear receptor-associated coactivator that is related to SRC-1 and TIF2. *Proc Natl Acad Sci USA* 1997;94:8479–8484.
116. Torchia J, Rose DW, Inostroza J, et al. The transcriptional co-activator p/CIP binds CBP and mediates nuclear receptor function. *Nature* 1997;387:677–684.

117. Chen H, Lin RJ, Schiltz RL, et al. Nuclear receptor coactivator ACTR is a novel histone acetyltransferase and forms a multimeric activation complex with p/CAF and CBP/p300. *Cell* 1997;90:569–580.
118. Anzick SL, Koonen J, Walker RL, et al. AIB1, a steroid receptor co-activator amplified in breast and ovarian cancer. *Science* 1997;277:965–968.
119. Heery DM, Kalkhoven E, Hoare S, Parker MG. A signature motif in transcriptional coactivators mediates binding to nuclear receptors. *Nature* 1997;387:733–736.
120. Horset F, Dauvois S, Heery DM, et al. RIP-140 interacts with multiple nuclear receptors by means of two distinct sites. *Mol Cell Biol* 1996;16:6029–6036.
121. Vom Baur E, Zechel C, Heery D, et al. Differential ligand dependent interaction between the AF-2 activating domain of nuclear receptors and the putative transcriptional intermediary factors MSUG1 and TIF1. *EMBO J* 1996;15:110–124.
122. Imakado S, Koike S, Kondo S, et al. The N-terminal transactivation domain of rat estrogen receptor is localized in a hydrophobic domain of eighty amino acids. *J Biochem (Tokyo)* 1991;109:684–689.
123. Metzger D, Ali S, Bornet JM, Chambon P. Characterization of the amino-terminal tarnscriptional activation function of the human estrogen receptor in animal and yeast cells. *J Biol Chem* 1995;270:9535–9542.
124. McInerney EM, Katzenellenbogen BS. Different regions in activation function 1 of the human estrogen receptor required for antiestrogen and estradiol dependent transcription activation. *J Biol Chem* 1996;271:24172–24178.
125. Ali S, Metzger D, Bornert JM, Chambon P. Modulation of transcriptional activation by ligand-dependent phosphorylation of the human oestrogen receptor A/B region. *EMBO J* 1993;12:1153–1160.
126. Le Goff P, Montano MM, Schodin DJ, Katzenellenbogen BS. Phosphorylation of the human estrogen receptor. Identification of hormone regulated sites and examination of their influence on transcriptional activity. *J Biol Chem* 1994;269:4458–4466.
127. Kato S, Endoh H, Masuhiro Y, et al. Activation of the oestrogen receptor through phosphorylation by mitogen-activated protein kinase. *Science* 1995;270:1491–1494.
128. Bunone G, Briand PA, Miksicek RJ, Picard D. Activation of the unliganded receptor by EGF involves the MAP kinase pathway and direct phosphorylation. *EMBO J* 1996;15:2174–2183.
129. Lahooti H, White R, Danielian PS, Parker MG. Characterization of the ligand-dependent phosphorylation of the estrogen receptor. *Mol Endocrinol* 1994;8:182–188.
130. Gustafsson JA. Estrogen receptor α—a new dimension in estrogen mechanism of action. *J Endocrinology* 1999;163:379–383.
131. McInerney EM, Weis KE, Sun J, et al. Transcription activation by the human estrogen receptor subtype β (ERβ) studied with ERβ and ERα receptor chimeras. *Endocrinology* 1998;139:4513–4522.
132. Paech K, Webb P, Kuiper GGJM, et al. Differential ligand activation of estrogen receptors ERα and ERβ at AP1 sites. *Science* 1997;277:1508–1510.
133. Green S, Walter P, Kumar V, et al. Human estrogen receptor cDNA sequence expression and homology to v-erb-A. *Nature* 1986;320:134–139.
134. Greene GL, Gilna P, Waterfield M, et al. Sequence and expression of human estrogen receptor complementary DNA. *Science* 1986;231:1150–1154.
135. White R, Lees JA, Needham M, et al. Structural organisation and expression of mouse estrogen receptor. *Mol Endocrinol* 1987;1:735–744.
136. Berry M, Metzger D, Chambon P. Role of the two activating domains of the oestrogen receptor in the cell type and promoter-context-dependent against activity of the antioestrogen 4-OH-tamoxifen. *EMBO J* 1990;9:2811–2818.
137. Brzozowski A, Pike A, Dauker Z, et al. Molecular basis of agonism and antagonism in the estrogen receptor. *Nature* 1997;389:753–758.
138. Shiau AK, Barstad D, Loria PM, et al. The structural basis of estrogen receptor/coactivator recognition and the antagonism of this interaction by tamoxifen. *Cell* 1998;95:927–937.
139. Jordan VC, Gosden B. Importance of the alkylaminoethoxy-sidechain for the estrogenic and antiestrogenic actions of tamoxifen and trioxifene in immature rat uterus. *Mol Cell Endocrinol* 1982;27:291–306.
140. Robertson DW, Katzenellenbogen JA, Hayes JR, Katzenellenbogen BS. Antiestrogen basicity activity relationships a comparison of the estrogen receptor binding and antiuterotrophic potencies of several analogues of (Z)1–2-diphenyl-1-[4-[2-dimethylamino) ethoxy]phenyl]-1-butene(tamoxifen, Noluadex) having altered basicity. *J Med Chem* 1982;25:167–171.
141. McDonell DP, Clemm DL, Hermann T, et al. Investigation of estrogen receptor function in vitro reveals three distinct classes of antiestrogens. *Mol Endocrinol* 1995;9:659–669.
142. Beekman JM, Allan GF, Tsai SY, et al. Transcriptional activation by the estrogen receptor requires a conformational change in the ligand binding domain. *Mol Endocrinol* 1993;1:1266–1274.
143. Levinson AS, Jordan VC. The key to the antiestrogenic mechanism of raloxifene is amino acid 351 (Aspartate) in the estrogen receptor. *Cancer Res* 1998;58:1872–1875.
144. Paige LA, Christensen DJ, Grøn H, et al. Estrogen receptor (ER) modulators each induce distinct conformational changes in ERα and ERβ. *Proc Natl Acad Sci* 1999;96:3999–4004.
145. Tremblay GB, Tremblay A, Copeland NG, et al. Cloning localisation and functional analysis of the murine estrogen receptor β. *Mol Endocrinol* 1997;11:353–365.
146. Weigel NL. Steroid hormone receptors and their regulation by phosphorylation. *Biochem J* 1996;319:657–667.
147. Speirs V, Malone C, Walton DS, et al. Increased expression of estrogen receptor β in tamoxifen resistant breast cancer patients. *Cancer Res* 1999;59:5421–5424.
148. Ogawa S, Inoue S, Watanabe T, et al. Molecular cloning and characterisation of human estrogen receptor βcx: a potential inhibitor of estrogen action in human. *Nucl Acid Res* 1998;26:3505–3512.

PART II

Translational Approaches: Current, Planned, and Most Promising

SECTION 1

Current

17
HER-2/*neu* and Trastuzumab

Mark D. Pegram and Dennis J. Slamon

HER-2/*neu* is an 185-kDα surface membrane protein encoded by the c-erb-B2 gene which has been assigned to chromosome 17q21 (1). The protein is expressed in a wide variety of tissues such as the breast, ovary, endometrium, lung, gastrointestinal tract, kidney, central nervous system, and, in low levels, the myocardium (2,3). The normal physiological role of HER-2/*neu* in these tissues is incompletely understood. However, in epithelial cells it is believed to play a signaling role in cellular proliferation and differentiation processes, and in the myocardium it may play a role in cardiac myocyte response to physiologic stress (4). Studies conducted in knock-out mice demonstrate that animals lacking murine *neu* die *in utero* due to neural tube developmental defects as well as abnormalities of the endomyocardium (5).

HER-2/*neu* belongs to the type I epithelial growth factor receptor family of cell surface receptors. It forms heterooligomers with other members of this receptor family (such as HER-3 and HER-4) in order to bind specific ligands called neuregulins/heregulins (Fig. 17.1) (6–9). Ligand activation of HER-2/*neu* results in an increase in HER-2/*neu* kinase activity, which in turn initiates signal transduction resulting in both cell proliferation and differentiation, depending on the experimental conditions (10–14).

In breast cancers, the c-erb-B2 gene is amplified in approximately 20% to 25% of all cases such that, instead of having two copies of the gene per cell (one on each chromosome 17), there may be as many as 50 or 100 c-erb-B2 gene copies per cell (15–17). This gene amplification event results in overexpression of p185$^{HER-2/neu}$ at both the transcript and protein levels; there can be as many as approximately 2,000,000 HER-2/*neu* molecules per cell in malignant tissues, instead of the normal compliment of approximately 20,000 to 50,000 molecules per cell. When HER-2/*neu* is overexpressed at these abnormally high levels, the kinase activity becomes constitutively activated, possibly due to autoactivation caused by crowding of adjacent HER-2/*neu* receptor molecules within the cell membrane (18). The net result is ligand-independent activation of p185$^{HER-2/neu}$, resulting in an increase in mitogenic cell signaling and increased cell proliferation.

The HER-2/*neu* molecular alteration is associated with a poor clinical prognosis in early stage breast cancer in terms of shortened time to relapse and shortened overall survival (15–17). Initially this finding was controversial, with many published studies failing to demonstrate an association between HER-2 gene amplification and clinical outcome; but, in retrospect, it is clear that most of these negative studies were statistically underpowered (small sample sizes), had too short a duration of clinical follow-up, or were doomed to failure from the start because the reagents used to detect HER-2 overexpression (usually antibodies) were insensitive (19). It is now clear from larger published cohorts, with long clinical follow-up (as much as 30 years) and suitable reagents, that HER-2 overexpression is an independent prognostic factor predicting poor clinical outcome (increasing the relative

The HER Family

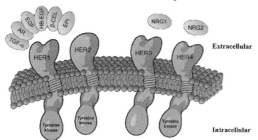

FIG. 17.1. The epidermal growth factor of receptors comprises 4 transmembrane proteins, each with different properties but all involved in the regulation of cell proliferation and differentiation. (Courtesy of Kenneth Bloom.)

risk of relapse by a factor of approximately 2) for both node-positive as well as node-negative breast cancers (20,21).

A significant body of laboratory and clinical data demonstrates that HER-2/*neu* overexpression, as a result of its effects on mitogenic cell signaling pathways, plays an important role in the pathophysiology of malignancies with the alteration. Cells with HER-2/*neu* overexpression have an increase in cell proliferation, an increase in anchorage-independent cell growth (a marker of transformation), an increase in tumorigenicity, and an increase in rate of metastasis compared to control cells lacking HER-2/*neu* overexpression (Fig. 17.2). Since HER-2/*neu* overexpression and coordinate increased kinase activity are at least in part directing these tumors to exhibit an aggressive biological behavior, it is an even more attractive target for therapeutic intervention using antibodies or other molecules which can oppose the effects of HER-2 kinase on cell signal transduction (22). The effects of the humanized monoclonal anti-HER-2 antibody trastuzumab (Herceptin) on downregulation of p185$^{HER-2/neu}$ expression levels and/or its effects on HER-2 mediated signaling are likely to be critical to the clinical activity of this therapeutic antibody.

HER-2 DETECTION IN CLINICAL TUMOR SPECIMENS

As a result of the availability and clinical efficacy of trastuzumab, clinicians are now faced with a dilemma with regard to accurate identification of patients with HER-2 overexpression. Multiple methodologies have been used to detect HER-2 gene amplification at the DNA level (slot blot or Southern blot, fluorescence *in situ* hybridization, PCR-based techniques), at the transcript level (Northern analysis, RT-PCR), and at the protein level (Western blot, immunohistochemistry, or enzyme-linked immunosorbent assay [ELISA] to detect soluble HER-2 protein). It is clear that the solid matrix blotting techniques suffer from dilutional artifacts resulting from admixture of normal stromal cells with tumor cells in clinical tumor samples (9,23). Therefore, *in situ* techniques are generally more sensitive in detecting HER-2 gene amplification or protein overexpression. The most widely used technique for detection of HER-2 overexpression at the protein level is immunohistochemistry. The problem with this technique is that multiple primary antibodies are currently in clinical use, each of which binds to a different epitope; these antibodies also have differing sensitivity and specificity, and as well have different cut-off values to distinguish overexpressing form non-overexpressing tumors (Fig. 17.3). Detection of HER-2/*neu* alteration is therefore not well standardized, and while immunohistochemical detection methods are widely com-

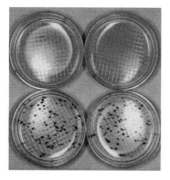

MCF7 controls

MDF7/HER2 - overexpressing cells

FIG. 17.2. Effect of HER2/*neu* transduction and overexpression in MCF7 breast carcinoma cells on colony formation in soft agar. [From Pegram M, Salmon D. *Semin Oncol* 2000 October 27; (suppl 9):13–9.] See color plate.

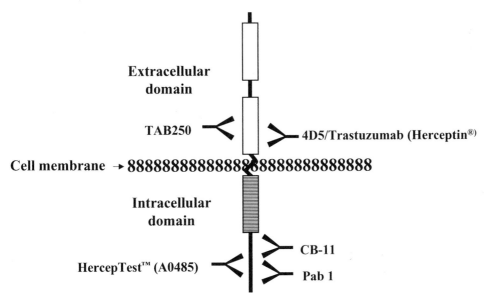

FIG. 17.3. HER2 receptor epitopes. (Adapted with permission from Seidman et al. *J Clin Oncol* 2001; 19:2587.)

mercially available, some of these assays may be suboptimal. Another concern is that the degree of immunohistochemical staining intensity for HER-2 is subjective and qualitative. As a consequence, it may be difficult to know whether a sample scored as HER-2 positive in one laboratory will be confirmed to be HER-2 positive by another laboratory.

It is clear that formalin fixation of tumor samples and storage in paraffin results in epitope degradation so that sensitivity is lost over time in archival clinical material. To combat this problem, some assays resort to a technique called antigen retrieval, which consists of boiling the tumor sample using heat or microwave radiation in order to rehabilitate epitopes that have been lost during tissue processing and storage. This can create new problems in that normal tissues and non-HER-2-overexpressing malignancies often have some constitutive physiologic level of HER-2 expression. Antigen retrieval can enhance the signal from this small amount of HER-2 protein resulting in a false-positive interpretation of HER-2 overexpression. Reports from the Mayo Clinic, the University of North Carolina, the NSABP, and others suggest a higher-than-expected false-positive rate using the FDA-approved HercepTest for detection of HER-2 overexpression (especially when it is performed in laboratories other than commercial reference laboratories), and it is interesting to note that this assay also employs an antigen retrieval step (24–26).

ELISA assays designed to detect soluble HER-2 protein in serum samples, while potentially useful clinically for monitoring disease course in patients with HER-2-positive advanced breast cancer, are not practical as diagnostic assays for early stage breast cancer, because soluble HER-2 protein is usually found only in the serum of patients with both high disease burden and high-level HER-2 overexpression, such as in cases of metastatic disease (27). For patients with small primary tumors, this assay is frequently negative even if tumor overexpression of HER-2 exists at the tissue level.

Perhaps the most accurate technique currently available for detection of HER-2 gene alteration is DNA-fluorescence *in situ* hybridization (FISH). In this assay, a fluorescently labeled genomic DNA probe containing the HER-2 gene and its flanking sequences is allowed to hybridize to tumor cell DNA within a thin tumor section mounted on a microscope slide. A second DNA probe, specific for chromosome 17 centromere and labeled with a different color than the HER-2 probe, is used to distinguish true HER-2 gene amplification from chromosome 17 ploidy. Using this technique, a quantitative copy number of HER-2 genes per chromosome 17 centromere can be ascertained (Fig. 17.4, see color plate). One theoretical disadvantage of this assay is the inability to detect the so-called "single copy overexpressors." In such cases, the HER-2 protein is overexpressed in absence of HER-2 gene amplification (28). However, the frequency of single copy HER-2 overexpression in breast cancers is estimated to be less than 5% of all overexpressing tumors; therefore the advantages of FISH in terms of sensitivity and specificity far outweigh this disadvantage in terms of diagnostic accuracy (28,29). The other potential problem with FISH methodology is availability and cost. These problems will become less pressing with the recent approval of FISH technology for HER-2 analysis by the U.S. Food and Drug Administration (FDA), both for prognosis and for patient selection for trastuzumab therapy. It is likely that costs for FISH analysis will decrease with the increased economy of scale of HER-2 testing utilizing this technique.

It is critical to remember that HER-2 overexpression correlates well with a number of other established prognostic factors and clinical parameters in breast cancer (Table 17.1). Therefore, a clinician can estimate the probability that a particular breast tumor will harbor HER-2 overexpression based on these clinical parameters. If the results of a particular HER-2 diagnostic assay are inconsistent with the clinical picture (particularly if an immunoassay was used for the HER-2 analysis), then a different assay methodology such as FISH should be used to retest the sample to confirm or refute the first result. For example, a high-grade, lymph-node-positive, ER-negative tumor with a high S-phase fraction and aneuploidy is consistent with a HER-2 positive phenotype, especially if the patient relapses quickly. By contrast, a node-negative, diploid, ER-positive, well differentiated, tubular breast carcinoma with low S-phase is not likely to be HER-2 positive. Another important clinical observation is that HER-2 overexpression is only rarely seen in lobular carcinomas. Thus, despite the availability of sophisticated molecular diagnostic tools, there still appears to be no substitute for good clinical judgment.

DEVELOPMENT OF TRASTUZUMAB

Soon after the HER-2 receptor subunit was shown to play a role in the pathogenesis of breast cancer, efforts were made in our laboratory to identify and characterize inhibitors of HER-2 which would interrupt mitogenic signaling. To date numerous agents have been identified which target HER-2, including tyrosine kinase inhibitors, inhibitors of various constituents of the ras-signaling pathway, neuregulin-toxin fusion proteins, single-chain antibodies, HER-2 antisense molecules, small molecule receptor antagonists, monoclonal antibodies, and bispecific antibodies. Of these agents, a particular murine monoclonal antibody, 4D5, was found to have dose-dependent antiproliferative activity specifically against HER-2-overexpressing cancer cells, while having no effect on cells expressing physiologic amounts of HER-2 (30).

Of course, murine monoclonal antibodies had been tested in clinical trials against numerous tumor targets in the past, but to no avail because of the development of human anti-murine antibodies (HAMA), which rapidly neutralized murine antibodies rendering them useless as far as antitumor activity is concerned. However, breakthroughs in biotechnology allowed

TABLE 17.1. *Association of HER-2 overexpression with other clinicopathologic variables*

HER-2 Overexpressions

- high S-phase fraction
- aneuploidy
- absence of ER/PR expression
- presence of nodal metastasis
- high nuclear grade
- short relapse-free interval
- ductal (as opposed to lobular) histology

Trastuzumab (Herceptin®) in Murine Xenograft Model

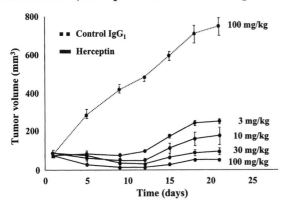

FIG. 17.5. Dose-dependent preclinical antitumor activity of trastuzumab. (From Pietras et al. *Oncogene* 1998;17:2235.)

the possibility of overcoming this limiting clinical problem. Murine monoclonal antibodies may be humanized by identifying the minimum set of amino acid residues in the complementarity determining region (CDR) of the murine antibody required for antigen specificity and antigen binding affinity, and substituting these regions into the CDRs of a consensus human IgG framework sequence. Maintaining both antigen specificity and binding affinity through this process is a painstaking exercise, but is essential in order to identify a humanized variant with desired specifications.

Ultimately, antibody humanization was achieved for the murine monoclonal antibody 4D5, resulting in a recombinant, humanized, monoclonal antibody directed against HER-2 (rhuMAb HER-2) known now as trastuzumab (31). The specificity of 4D5 for HER-2 was maintained, and the binding affinity (kD approximately 0.1 n*M*) of the humanized variant was actually slightly improved over that of 4D5 (Kd approximately 0.3 n*M*). In addition, trastuzumab is based on an IgG1 consensus sequence, thus allowing for the possibility of antibody-mediated cellular cytotoxicity against tumor target cells by immune effector cells expressing Fc receptors. Preclinical studies conducted in our laboratory for the first time demonstrated that the antiproliferative effects of 4D5 and dose-dependent antitumor efficacy against HER-2-overexpressing xenografts in athymic mice were maintained following antibody humanization (Fig. 17.5) (32).

Based on the demonstration of preclinical efficacy in our laboratory, a series of single-dose and multi-dose phase 1 clinical trials were conducted at the University of California Los Angeles in order to study tumor localization, toxicology, and pharmacokinetics of single-dose and multi-dose trastuzumab administered intravenously (i.v.) to patients with HER-2-positive, refractory, metastatic breast cancer (33). The conclusions from these studies are summarized in Table 17.2. Trastuzumab has a favorable pharmacokinetic profile, achieving trough serum concentrations above the concentration needed for maximal antiproliferative effects *in vitro*. Trastuzumab also has a unique toxicology profile, with fevers and/or chills during the first infusion, and pain at sites of metastasis as the most commonly reported side effects during the initial phase 1 studies. In most cases, these symptoms were described as mild or moderate. Furthermore, there was no evidence of human anti-humanized antibodies

TABLE 17.2. *Conclusions from phase 1 clinical trials of trastuzumab*

Conclusions
• defined pharmacokinetics with a long serum half-life in high dose, achieving desired serum trough concentrations
• favorable toxicology profile (low-grade fevers)
• no evidence of human anti-mouse antibodies (HAMA)
• demonstration of tumor localization with radio-iodinated 4D5

(HAHA) raised against trastuzumab following i.v. administration. This was in contrast to our phase 1 trial conducted with the murine antibody 4D5, in which HAMA developed rapidly, as expected, in treated patients.

MECHANISM(S) OF ACTION OF TRASTUZUMAB

The mechanism of action of trastuzumab against HER-2-overexpressing cells is complex and likely involves multiple cellular processes. Trastuzumab binds to a juxtamembrane epitope in the extracellular domain of the $p185^{HER-2}$ molecule (Fig. 17.3). On binding to the epitope, the tratuzumab/$p185^{HER-2}$ complex is internalized, resulting in net downregulation of $p185^{HER-2}$ protein on the cell surface (Fig. 17.6). Moreover, there is experimental evidence that internalized anti-HER-2 antibody–p185HER-2 complexes enter the endosomal compartment following internalization (34). In the acidified environment of the endosome, antibody-bound $p185^{HER-2}$ undergoes ubiquitination, a process which is directed by the ubiquitin ligase protein *cbl* (35). Ubiquitination of $p185^{HER-2}$ by *cbl* targets the $p185^{HER-2}$ protein for degradation, so that it cannot be recycled back to the cell surface for further participation in mitogenic signaling. In addition to its direct effects on $p185^{HER-2}$ cell surface expression, trastuzumab attenuates HER-2-mediated signal transduction through both the ras-raf-MAP kinase pathway, and through the PI3-kinase/AKT pathway, thus perturbing signaling processes ordinarily directed by the activation of the p185HER-2 tyrosine kinase (Fig. 17.6) (36).

In addition to its effects on signal transduction, there is now experimental evidence that trastuzumab may in fact be a true immunotherapeutic antibody through activation of antibody-dependent, cell-mediated cytotoxicity (ADCC) via the Fc domain. This evidence is based on experiments performed in Fc-receptor knock-out mice. Tumor-bearing mice lacking Fc receptors on immune effector cells have significantly less antitumor response to trastuzumab or 4D5 treatment compared to mice with intact Fc receptors. Moreover, if the Fc domain of trastuzumab is experimentally modified (mutated) so that it can no longer bind to Fc receptors, its *in vivo* antitumor activity against HER-2-positive xenografts is also significantly reduced (37). Taken together, these experiments support the hypothesis that a significant de-

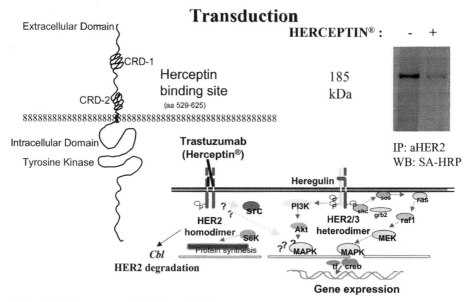

FIG. 17.6. Trastuzumab binding to HER2 epitope leads to receptor downregulation and effects on signal. (Data from L. Bald and B. Fendly). See color plate.

gree of the observed *in vivo* antitumor efficacy of trastuzumab results from an immune mechanism of action (37).

Recently, yet another potentially important potential mechanism of action of trastuzumab has been elucidated. Trastuzumab has antiangiogenic activity against HER-2-overexpressing xenografts, at least in part due to the effect of trastuzumab on expression of the vascular endothelial growth factor (VEGF) (38). VEGF is a secreted heparin-binding glycoprotein that has multiple effects on endothelial cells. It increases vascular permeability, induces alterations in ion flow, enhances cell proliferation and migration, and induces the release of proteinases involved in tumor invasion (39–43). Multiple studies have now examined tumor VEGF levels as a prognostic indicator in early breast cancer. Over 3,000 patient specimens have been evaluated for VEGF expression and outcome, using either immunohistochemistry or measurement of serum VEGF levels (44–53). A large majority of these studies have demonstrated a strong correlation between elevated VEGF expression and poor prognosis, in general revealing both decreased relapse-free survival and overall survival in the subset of patients with the highest levels of VEGF expression. When viewed in total, these data provide compelling evidence that VEGF overexpression contributes to the progression of breast cancer and is associated with inferior clinical outcome. These observations establish VEGF as perhaps the most important molecule regulating angiogenesis and subsequent invasion and metastasis in human cancer.

Recent laboratory studies indicate that, in addition to its effects on cell mitogenesis, heregulin also stimulates VEGF production. In human breast cancer cells growing both *in vitro* and *in vivo*, heregulin rapidly induces VEGF mRNA and protein expression; this increased VEGF production correlates with increased angiogenesis, enhanced motility, and a greater propensity to invasion in treated cells (54–57). Heregulin may mediate its effects on VEGF expression via upregulation of hypoxia-inducible factor 1 alpha or activation of p21-activated kinase (Pak), a transcriptional activator and intracellular signaling molecule, respectively, that help control VEGF gene expression (57,58). The observation that HER-2 activation induces VEGF expression raises the possibility that anti-HER-2 therapy might decrease VEGF production and inhibit angiogenesis. Indeed, treatment of SKBR-3 cells, which have high-level HER-2 overexpression, with trastuzumab results in a dose-dependent reduction of VEGF production (59). Moreover, trastuzumab treatment of SCID mice bearing HER-2-overexpressing xenografts significantly reduces the volume and diameter of tumor infiltrating blood vessels (Fig. 17.7), and also reduces

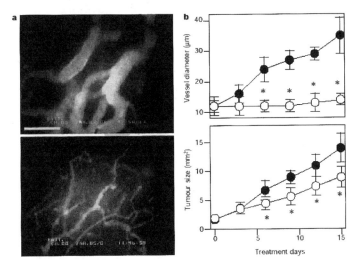

FIG. 17.7. Antiangiogenic effect of trastuzumab *in vivo*. (From Izumi et al., Brief communication. *Nature* 2002;416: 279–280.)

vascular permeability (38). The expression of VEGF mRNA was significantly reduced in the trastuzumab-treated xenografts compared to control (38).

In summary, a composite of a myriad of biological effects of trastuzumab on HER-2 expression, HER-2 degradation, signal transduction mediated by HER-2 kinase, ADCC, and anti-angiogenic effects probably contribute to the antitumor activity of trastuzumab.

COMBINING TRASTUZUMAB WITH CYTOTOXIC CHEMOTHERAPY: RECEPTOR-ENHANCED CHEMOSENSITIVITY

Trastuzumab is not cytotoxic to HER-2-overexpressing breast carcinoma cells *in vitro*. HER-2-positive cancer cells undergo cell cycle arrest with accumulation in the G0/G1 phase of the cell cycle on exposure to trastuzumab, but there is no evidence of apoptosis or cytotoxicity (unless immune effector cells are introduced along with trastuzumab) (60,61).

One popular method of rendering antibodies cytotoxic envisioned by researchers in the anticancer antibody field was to covalently conjugate cytotoxic drugs with therapeutic monoclonal antibodies. In one such effort, antiepidermal growth factor receptor (EGFR/HER-1) antibodies were coupled to cisplatin and tested against HER-1 expressing xenografts *in vivo* (62). As controls for this experiment, the investigators also tested uncoupled, free anti-HER-1 given concomitantly with free cisplatin. What resulted was surprising, in that free anti-HER-1 plus free cisplatin had more antitumor activity than the covalently linked species. Because of the close homology between HER-1 and HER-2, we conducted a similar experiment in our laboratory and found the same result with anti-HER-2 antibody plus cisplatin (Fig. 17.8) (63). Furthermore, we studied the nature of the interaction between anti-HER-2 and cisplatin using a mathematical computer model to test for two-drug interactions, and we found the combination to be highly synergistic (60,63). The mechanism of synergy in this case was antibody-mediated attenuation of DNA repair activity, resulting

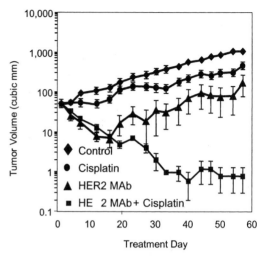

FIG. 17.8. A model for HER2 MAb combination with chemotherapy.

in the accumulation of platinum-DNA adducts in the nucleus and concomitant enhanced cytotoxicity of cisplatin. We have termed this effect "receptor enhanced chemosensitivity" (REC), as it applies to both the HER-1 and HER-2 systems.

We have now expanded our antibody/drug interaction studies to include combinations of trastuzumab with antimetabolites, alkylating agents, taxanes, topoisomerase II inhibitors, vinca alkaloids, and anthracyclines. Of these, we have found the platinum analogues, docetaxel, vinorelbine, etoposide, thiotepa, and ionizing radiation to have synergistic cytotoxicity with trastuzumab (Table 17.3) (60,64). One drug, 5-fluorouracil, is antagonistic with trastuzumab.

TABLE 17.3. *Synergistic cytotoxicity with trastuzumab*

Drug	Interaction with herceptin
Cisplatin/carboplatin	Synergistic
Docetaxel	Synergistic
Vinorelbine	Synergistic
Etoposide	Synergistic
Thiotepa	Synergistic
Ionizing radiation	Synergistic
Doxorubicin	Additive
Vinblastine	Additive
Paclitaxel	Additive
Methotrexate	Additive
5-Fluorouracil	Antagonistic

The mechanism of this antagonistic interaction remains unknown but is the subject of ongoing investigation.

PHASE 2 TRASTUZUMAB CLINICAL TRIALS

Four phase 2 clinical trials of single-agent trastuzumab or trastuzumab in combination with cisplatin have been conducted. In a pilot phase 2 study of single-agent trastuzumab for patients with HER-2-overexpressing breast cancer who were heavily pretreated but had failed prior chemotherapy for metastatic disease, an 11% response rate was observed (65). In an expanded phase 2 study of trastuzumab as a single agent for patients who had failed one or two prior chemotherapeutic regimens for metastatic disease, a 14% response rate was noted (66). More recently, results from single-agent trastuzumab given as first-line therapy for HER-2 positive metastatic breast cancer were reported (67). In this study, a higher response rate of 34% was observed (in the FISH positive subset), suggesting that single-agent trastuzumab may be more effective in patients less heavily pretreated with chemotherapy. In addition, this study randomized patients to two different dose levels of trastuzumab. The first dose level was standard 4 mg/kg loading dose followed by 2 mg/kg per week, and the second was double the standard dose (8 mg/kg load plus 4 mg/kg per week). No apparent difference in response rate was seen at the higher dose level, and the higher dose appeared to be associated with more frequent side effects.

A significant contribution from all of these studies is a better understanding of the toxicology of trastuzumab. In general, trastuzumab is very well tolerated when administered as a single agent. Approximately 30% to 40% of patients may experience fevers and/or chills, usually during the 4 mg/kg loading dose of trastuzumab. These reactions, though sometimes dramatic due to the rigors, can easily be managed by administration of acetaminophen, diphenhydramine hydrochloride, or meperidine hydrochloride, and/or by slowing the rate of trastuzumab infusion. Rare cases of severe anaphylactic reactions have been reported, especially in patients with underlying compromised pulmonary function (68). Other commonly reported side effects of single-agent trastuzumab are shown in Table 17.4.

TABLE 17.4. *Common side effects of single-agent trastuzumab at first infusion*

Common side effects, single-agent trastuzumab
Fever/chills
Nausea/vomiting
Pain at site of tumor
Asthenia
Diarrhea
Headache

We were the first to report combination of trastuzumab with chemotherapy in a clinical trial (27). A unique feature of this phase 2 trial was that, to gain entry into the study, all patients had to have chemoresistant breast cancer (defined as objective evidence of disease progression *during* active chemotherapy treatment). The study population consisted of extensively pretreated advanced breast cancer patients with HER-2 overexpression. Patients were treated with a loading dose of 250 mg i.v. herceptin, followed by weekly doses of 100 mg i.v. for 9 weeks. Chemotherapy consisted of cisplatin (75 mg/m^2) on days 1, 29 and 57. Clinical response data in this multicenter study were confirmed by an independent, blinded, response evaluation committee. Objective clinical responses were seen in 24% of patients and an additional 24% had either minor response or disease stabilization. This compares favorably to either single-agent cisplatin (reported response rate from five separate clinical trials = 7%, 95% confidence limits, 2% to 11%, or single-agent trastuzumab [response rate 11% to 14%]) in pretreated patients with metastatic disease (27). In this study, the concomitant administration of cisplatin chemotherapy had no effect on trastuzumab pharmacokinetics.

This protocol was also the first comprehensive analysis of the relationship between trastuzumab pharmacokinetics and serum levels of a soluble form of the HER-2 protein. The extracellular domain of p185^{HER-2} can be proteolytically cleaved from the surface of tumor cells and can then be measured by ELISA in serum. There is a clear inverse relationship between serum soluble HER-2 protein and trastuzumab trough concentration (27,65). It has been suggested that soluble HER-2 protein may be a marker of clinical response to trastuzumab. However, our data demonstrate that a decrease in HER-2 serum levels is not always associated with an objective clinical response. An increase in soluble HER-2 protein, however, was associated with disease progression in a majority of patients in our phase 2 program, suggesting that this may be a useful clinical marker to estimate probability of disease progression (27). Pretreatment serum HER-2 levels did not correlate with objective clinical response to trastuzumab in this study.

Finally, a notable conclusion of this study was that trastuzumab did not appear to increase toxicity of cisplatin chemotherapy over that expected for cisplatin alone in this patient population. This is important since renal epithelial cells are known to express HER-2 protein and therefore could have theoretically been at risk for cisplatin-induced renal damage.

FIRST-LINE CHEMOTHERAPY PLUS HERCEPTIN FOR HER-2-OVEREXPRESSING METASTATIC BREAST CANCER

A large, prospective, randomized controlled trial of chemotherapy alone or in combination with trastuzumab has been conducted (69). The study population consisted of 469 patients with HER-2-overexpressing metastatic breast cancer who had not previously been treated with chemotherapy for metastatic disease. Chemotherapy consisted of doxorubicin 60 mg/m^2 (or epirubicin 75 mg/m^2) plus cyclophosphamide 600 mg/m^2 i.v. every 21 days for anthracycline-naive patients (N = 281), and paclitaxel 175 mg/m^2 i.v. over 3 hours for those patients who had been previously treated with an anthracycline in the adjuvant setting (N = 188). A unique feature of the patient characteristics for this cohort was that the patients in the paclitaxel arm were more likely to have adverse prognostic features at diagnosis (hence their prior adjuvant treatment with an anthracycline). Patients on the paclitaxel arm were also more likely to be premenopausal, have negative ER/PR, had a greater number of positive lymph nodes, had a higher incidence of prior radiation treatment, were more likely to have been treated with myeloablative chemotherapy followed by peripheral blood or bone marrow-derived hematopoetic stem cells, and had a shorter time from diagnosis to relapse compared to patients treated on the doxorubicin-cyclophosphamide arm.

On the basis of these pretreatment characteristics alone, one would have expected that the response to treatment in the paclitaxel group would be lower than the response to doxorubicin-cyclophosphamide-treated group. This was, in fact, the case for the subgroups of patients randomized to treatment with chemotherapy alone, where the response rate for single-agent paclitaxel was 15% compared to 38% for the doxorubicin-containing arm. This does *not* necessarily mean that HER-2-overexpressing patients are resistant to paclitaxel. Rather, it merely confirms that patients with multiple adverse prognostic factors who have relapsed despite anthracycline-based adjuvant chemotherapy have a poor response rate to any chemotherapy, a fact which is already well documented in the breast cancer literature.

Patients randomized to receive trastuzumab in conjunction with conventional chemotherapy had a significantly longer time to disease progression, higher overall response rate, a longer median response duration, and higher one- and two-year survival rates (69). With a median follow-up of 29 months, trastuzumab combined with either chemotherapy regimen decreased the relative risk of death by 24% and increased median survival from 20.3 months to 25.1 months. This is especially noteworthy in light of the fact that approximately two-thirds of the women on the chemotherapy alone arms subsequently received trastuzumab on a companion study protocol at the time of disease progression following initial protocol treatment. It is also noteworthy that trastuzumab, the first biologic agent to be approved by the FDA for breast cancer treatment, prolongs survival of metastatic breast cancer patients, whereas high-

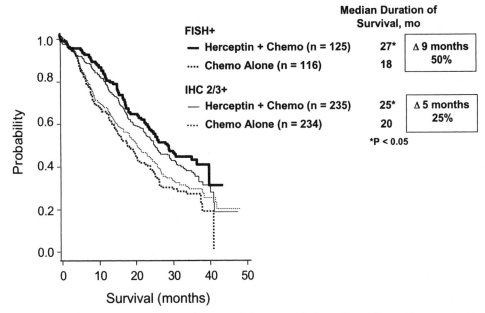

FIG. 17.9. Overall survival for 2+/3+ vs. FISH+ population. (Data from Slamon et al., *N Engl J Med* 2001;344:783–792 and Mass et al. *Proc ASCO* 2001;20:22a. Abstract 85.)

dose chemotherapy followed by reinfusion of autologous hematopoietic stem cells apparently does not (70).

Tumor samples, originally obtained for detection of HER-2 by IHC in this study, have recently been re-analyzed using FISH analysis to detect HER-2 gene amplification *in situ*. In this analysis, the subset of patients whose tumors contain amplified HER-2 appear to derive an even greater survival benefit than was apparent in the IHC analysis from combined chemotherapy-plus-trastuzumab treatment, compared to chemotherapy alone (Fig. 17.9). Of note in this analysis is the fact that the FISH-negative subset did not appear to benefit from the addition of trastuzumab to conventional chemotherapy (71).

Unfortunately, along with the clinical success of trastuzumab came an unfortunate and unexpected toxicity: congestive heart failure. This was most common in those patients who received concomitant trastuzumab and doxorubicin, and in the elderly. However, the incidence of trastuzumab-associated cardiotoxicity was also significantly increased in the paclitaxel-trastuzumab-treated group (69). The incidence and clinical course of trastuzumab-associated cardiotoxicity has recently been reviewed (72).

The mechanism(s) of this unique toxicity are currently unknown, but may involve cross-talk between HER-2 and the shared cytokine receptor gp130, a protein which is involved in the cardiac myocyte response to physiologic stress (4,73). Expression of HER-2 in adult myocardium was not previously well characterized, although it was presumed to be very low or absent on the basis of low-level HER-2 transcript expression by Northern analysis, and undetectable levels of protein expression by immunohistochemistry. Two patients at UCLA who developed clinically symptomatic congestive heart failure had endomyocardial biopsy performed as part of their diagnostic evaluation. Both of these patients had pathological findings consistent with doxorubicin-associated myocardial cell damage by either ordinary light microscopy or electron microscopy (unpublished observation).

Most of the patients with this syndrome have improvement in symptoms and/or an increase in left ventricular ejection fraction (LVEF) following treatment with ACE inhibitors, diuretics, or digitalis. Clearly, all patients receiving trastuzumab should undergo baseline assessment of cardiac function and periodic monitoring of LV function. If a significant decrease in LVEF is noted, the drug should probably be discontinued unless there is an eminent risk of dying from progressive cancer, which, in exceptional cases, could outweigh the risks of congestive failure. The drug should be used cautiously or even avoided altogether in cases of known underlying serious cardiac illness, at least until the mechanism of cardiotoxicity is better defined and until pretreatment risk factors for cardiotoxicity can be studied more completely.

FUTURE CLINICAL DEVELOPMENT OF TRASTUZUMAB

At the time of this writing, there are perhaps more unknown questions regarding the potential clinical applications of trastuzumab in cancer therapy than there are questions that have been answered. For example, the precise mechanisms of action of trastuzumab are still incompletely understood. To date there is still no direct experimental evidence from clinical studies that confirm that trastuzumab is a true immunotherapeutic. The optimum duration of trastuzumab therapy is also currently unknown. The clinical trials performed to date have been conducted with trastuzumab treatment until the time of disease progression. Would shorter duration of trastuzumab be as efficacious? Or, conversely, would continued trastuzumab treatment beyond the time of progression in fact slow the rate of progression? Whether or not trastuzumab will have activity in other malignancies is not yet known, but many trials designed to address this question are underway in multiple tumor types, including ovarian cancer, non-small cell lung cancer, prostate cancer, colon cancer, gastric cancer, bladder cancer, and others.

The integration of trastuzumab with standard chemotherapy, hormonal therapy, and radiation therapy remains an active area of research. Clinical trials of numerous chemotherapy drug combinations with trastuzumab are completed or underway (74–77). Especially promising among these is the synergistic, non-anthracycline combination of trastuzumab with docetaxel and platinums. Two pilot phase 2 studies have been completed by the UCLA Community Oncology Research Network (BCIRG 102) and the Breast Cancer International Research Group (BCIRG 101) (78). The former group utilized the combination of docetaxel, carboplatin, and trastuzumab, while the later group investigated the clinical activity of docetaxel, cisplatin, and trastuzumab. The objective clinical response rates among the FISH-positive patients treated first line with these combinations were 64% (BCIRG 102) and 77% (BCIRG 101), respectively. Especially remarkable in these two studies was the time to tumor progression (TTP) data. Among the FISH-positive patients, the TTP was 12.7 months (BCIRG 101) and 17 months (BCIRG 102) (78). These results compare favorably to the TTP of 7.1 months seen in the FISH-positive subset of patients (N = 69) treated with paclitaxel plus trastuzumab in the previously reported trastuzumab-chemotherapy randomized study (71). Importantly, there were just two reported cases of clinical CHF in these two trials, despite the fact that 32% (BCIRG 101) and 45% (BCIRG 102) of these patients were previously treated with anthracyclines (78). Therefore, the docetaxel-platinum-trastuzumab combination has been selected for advancement into clinical studies of trastuzumab in the adjuvant setting.

The use of adjuvant trastuzumab for early-stage breast cancer is a very attractive treatment approach from a theoretical point of view. As trastuzumab is a macromolecule with a molecular weight of nearly 150 kDa, penetration of the drug into bulky tumor deposits is hindered by the high interstitial oncotic pressure and poor vascularization within metastatic solid tumors. Therefore, the efficacy of trastuzumab would theoretically be maximal in a micrometastatic disease situation, where intratumoral pharmacokinetic boundaries are not pertinent.

Large-scale studies of adjuvant trastuzumab for breast cancer are now underway. The study being conducted by the BCIRG has been carefully designed to avoid the cardiotoxicity issue surrounding trastuzumab-anthracycline administration. This is a difficult problem in light of the fact that anthracyclines are of particular benefit in patients who have HER-2 amplification/overexpression (79–81). Most of the planned adjuvant studies (with one exception) will use one year of adjuvant trastuzumab, but the decision for this duration of trastuzumab administration, though entirely reasonable, was made empirically. We hypothesize that the synergistic, non-anthracycline adjuvant regimen consisting of docetaxel-platinum-trastuzumab will avoid anthracycline-associated cardiotoxicity issues, while at the same time, be able to take advantage of the observed synergy between these agents.

Whether or not trastuzumab has activity in non-HER-2 overexpressing breast cancers is an important issue which is being addressed in a number of ongoing clinical trials. The optimal dosing schedule and route of administration of trastuzumab are continuing to be studied. Because trastuzumab has a long serum half-life, it lends itself to less frequent administration such as using triple the standard dose every three weeks. Such a study has been conducted in advanced breast cancer patients with HER-2 amplification or overexpression. The study involved combination of trastuzumab (8 mg/kg i.v. loading dose, followed by 6 mg/kg i.v. every 3 weeks) with paclitaxel (175 mg/m^2). Preliminary results from this trial suggest that: (a) the serum trough concentrations of trastuzumab on this schedule are similar to those observed previously with standard doses of trastuzumab; (b) that every-3-week trastuzumab plus paclitaxel appears to be clinically active, with a response rate among the first 25 patients of 53%; and (c) the combination at these doses/schedules appears to be safe with no unexpected toxicities (82). In the future, formulations of trastuzumab may allow for subcutaneous administration of the drug. Data from our laboratory indicate that efficacy of trastuzumab is maintained when given subcutaneously in mouse models (unpublished observation).

Finally, very little is known about trastuzumab resistance, but clearly such mechanisms must exist since a majority of breast cancer patients treated with the drug do not, in fact, have an objective clinical response. One study suggests that signaling via the insulin-like growth factor-I receptor can alter response to trastuzumab in HER-2-overexpressing cells (83). A better understanding of such mechanisms might allow for improved treatment approaches for patients with HER-2-driven malignant disease.

The many unresolved clinical issues regarding HER-2 amplification/overexpression—its use as prognostic factor, its use as a predictive marker for response to conventional breast cancer therapies, and its use as a target for future drug development—provide a wealth of opportunities for future basic and clinical research. The fact that trastuzumab prolongs survival of patients with metastatic breast cancer is not only a clinical breakthrough in breast cancer therapy, but it also is the ultimate experimental proof from a scientific perspective that HER-2 does in fact play an important role in the pathophysiology of breast cancer. This fact has long been disputed by investigators who sharply criticized early laboratory investigations on HER-2 biology, and dismissed or rejected the concept of therapeutic targeting of HER-2 with monoclonal antibodies. The HER-2 paradigm of targeted cancer therapy is now a model for drug discovery and drug development in the biotechnology and pharmaceutical industries, and we believe that there will be other targets like HER-2 which will be the focus of future novel cancer treatments. New targets for cancer therapy must be validated through careful scientific studies conducted in the laboratory and through carefully designed clinical trials. Hopefully, identification of new targeted therapeutic approaches will result in meaningful clinical benefit for future patients suffering from breast cancer as well as other cancers.

REFERENCES

1. Shih C, Padhy L, Murray M, et al. Transforming genes of carcinomas and neuroblastomas introduced into mouse fibroblasts. *Nature* 1981;260:261–264.
2. Coussens L, Yang-Feng TL, Liao YC, et al. Tyrosine kinase receptor with extensive homology fo EGF receptor shares chromosomal location with neu oncogene. *Science* 1985;230:1132–1139.
3. King CR, Kraus MH, Aaronson SA. Amplification of a novel v-erb-B-2-related gene in human mammary carcinoma. *Science* 1985;229:974–976.

4. Chien KR. Myocyte survival pathways and cardiomyopathy: implications for trastuzumab cardiotoxicity. *Semin Oncol* 2000;27(6 suppl 11):9–14.
5. Lee KF, Simon H, Chen H, et al. Requirement for neuregulin receptor erbB2 in neural and cardiac development. *Nature* 1995;378:394–398.
6. Carraway K, Cantley L. A neu acquaintance for erbB3 and erbB4: a role for receptor heterodimerization in growth signaling. *Cell* 1994;78:5–8.
7. Sliwkowski M, Schaefer G, Akita R, et al. Coexpression of erB2 and erbB3 proteins reconstitutes a high affinity receptor for heregulin. *J Biol Chem* 1994;269:15661–15665.
8. Plowman G, Culouscou J-M, Whitney G, et al. Ligand-specific activiation of HER4/p180erB4, a fourth member of the epidermal growth factor receptor family. *Proc Natl Acad Sci USA* 1993;90:1746–1750.
9. Reese DM, Slamon DJ. HER-2/neu signal transduction in human breast and ovarian cancer. *Stem Cells* 1997;15:1–8.
10. Wen D, Suggs SV, Karunagaran D, et al. Structural and functional aspects of the multiplicity of neu differentiation factors. *Mol Cell Biol* 1994;14:1909–1919.
11. Wen D, Peles E, Cupples R, et al. Neu differentiation factor: a transmembrane glycoprotein containing and EGF domain and an immunoglobulin homology unit. *Cell* 1992;69:559–572.
12. Falls DL, Rosen KM, Corfas G, et al. ARIA, a protein that stimulates acetylcholine receptor synthesis, is a member of the neu ligand family. *Cell* 1993;72:801.
13. Marchionni M, Goodearl A, Chen M, et al. Glial growth factors are alternatively spliced erbB2 ligands expressed in the nervous system. *Nature* 1993;362:312.
14. Peles E, Ben-Levy R, Tzahor E, et al. Cell-type specific interaction of neu differentiation factor (NDF/heregulin) with neu/HER-2 suggests complex ligand-receptor relationships. *EMBO J* 1993;12:961–971.
15. Slamon DJ, Clark GM, Wong SG, et al. Human breast cancer: correlation of relapse and survival with amplification of the HER-2/neu oncogene. *Science* 1987;235:177–182.
16. Slamon DJ, Godolphin W, Jones LA, et al. Studies of HER-2/neu proto-oncogene in human breast and ovarian cancer. *Science* 1989;244:707–712.
17. Seshadri R, Firgaira FA, Horsfall DJ, et al. Clinical significance of HER-2/neu oncogene amplification in primary breast cancer. The South Australian Breast Cancer Study Group. *J Clin Oncol* 1993;11:1936–1942.
18. Sharpe S, Barber KR, Grant CW. Evidence of a tendency to self-association of the transmembrane domain of ErbB-2 in fluid phospholipid bilayers. *Biochemistry* 2002;41(7):2341–2352.
19. Press MF, Hung G, Godolphin W, et al. Sensitivity of HER-2/neu antibodies in archival tissue samples: potential source of error in immunohistochemical studies of oncogene expression. *Cancer Res* 1994;54:2771–2777.
20. Toikkanen S, Helin H, Isola J, Joensuu H. Prognostic significance of HER-2 oncoprotein expression in breast cancer: a 30-year follow-up. *J Clin Oncol* 1992;10:1044–1048.
21. Andrulis IL, Bull SB, Blackstein ME, et al. for the Toronto Breast Cancer Study Group: neu/erbB-2 amplification identifies a poor-prognosis group of women with node-negative breast cancer. Toronto Breast Cancer Study Group. *J Clin Oncol* 1998;16:1340–1349.
22. Pegram M, Slamon D. Biological rationale for HER2/neu (c-erbB2) as a target for monoclonal antibody therapy. *Semin Oncol* 2000;27(5 suppl 9):13–19.
23. Pauletti G, Godolphin W, Press MF, Slamon DJ. Detection and quantitation of HER-2/neu gene amplification in human breast cancer archival material using fluorescence in situ hybridization. *Oncogene* 1996;13:63–72.
24. Roche, Ingle. Increased HER with U.S. FDA-approved antibody. *J Clin Oncol* 1999;17:434–435 (letter).
25. Diane M. Immunohistochemical assays for HER2 overexpression. *J Clin Oncol* 1999;17:434.
26. Personal Communication: Tan-Chiu, Elizabeth, NSABP B-31 Protocol Officer, National Surgical Adjuvant Breast and Bowel Project Operations Center, March 14, 2001.
27. Pegram M, Lipton A, Hayes D, et al. Phase II study of receptor-enhanced chemosensitivity using recombinant humanized anti-p185HER-2/neu monoclonal antibody plus cisplatin in patients with HER-2/neu-overexpressing metastatic breast cancer Refractory to Chemotherapy Treatment. *J Clin Oncol* 1998;16:2659–2671.
28. Pauletti G, Godolphin W, Press MF, Slamon DJ. Detection and quantitation of HER-2/neu gene amplification in human breast cancer archival material using fluorescence in situ hybridization. *Oncogene* 1996;13(1):63–72.
29. Pauletti G, Dandekar S, Rong H, et al. Assessment of methods for tissue-based detection of the HER-2/neu alteration in human breast cancer: a direct comparison of fluorescence in situ hybridization and immunohistochemistry. *J Clin Oncol* 2000;18(21):3651–3664.
30. Lewis GD, Figari I, Fendly B, et al. Differential responses of human tumor cell lines to anti-p185[HER-2] monoclonal antibodies. *Cancer Immunol Immunother* 1993;37:255–263.
31. Carter P, Presta L, Gorman CM, et al. Humanization of an anti-p185HER-2 antibody for human cancer therapy. *Proc Natl Acad Sci* 1992;89(10):4285–4289.
32. Pietras RJ, Pegram MD, Finn RS, et al. Remission of human breast cancer xenografts on therapy with humanized monoclonal antibody to HER-2 receptor and DNA-reactive drugs. *Oncogene* 1998;17:2235–2249.
33. Pegram MD, Konecny G, Slamon DJ. The molecular and cellular biology of HER-2/neu gene amplification/overexpression and the clinical development of herceptin (trastuzumab) therapy for breast cancer. *Cancer Treat Res* 2000;103:57–75.
34. Klapper LN, Waterman H, Sela M, Yarden Y. Tumor-inhibitory antibodies to HER-2/ErbB-2 may act by recruiting c-Cbl and enhancing ubiquitination of HER-2. *Cancer Res* 2000;60(13):3384–3388.
35. Levkowitz G, Oved S, Klapper LN, et al. c-Cbl is a suppressor of the neu oncogene. *J Biol Chem* 2000;275(45):35532–35539.
36. Baselga J, Albanell J, Molina MA, Arribas J. Mechanism of action of trastuzumab and scientific update. *Semin Oncol* 2001;28(5 suppl 16):4–11.
37. Clynes RA, Towers TL, Presta LG, Ravetch JV. Inhibitory Fc receptors modulate in vivo cytoxicity against tumor targets. *Nat Med* 2000;6(4):443–446.
38. Izumi Y, Xu L, di Tomaso E, et al. Tumour biology: herceptin acts as an anti-angiogenic cocktail. *Nature* 2002;416(6878):279–280.
39. Senger DR, Galli SJ, Dvorak AM, et al. Tumor cells secrete a vascular permeability factor that promotes accumulation of ascites fluid. *Science* 1983;219:983–985.

40. Dvorak HF. Tumours: Wounds that do not heal—Similarity between tumour stroma generation and wound healing. *N Engl J Med* 1983;315:1650–1658.
41. Ferrara N, Henzel WJ. Pituitary follicular cells secrete a novel heparin-binding growth factor specific for vascular endothelial cells. *Biochem Biophys Res Commun* 1989;161:851–859.
42. Unemori EN, Ferrara N, Bauer EA, et al. Vascular endothelial growth factor induces interstitial collagenase expression in human endothelial cells. *J Cell Physiol* 1992;153:557–562.
43. Lindgren M, Johansson M, Sandström J, et al. VEGF and tPA co-expressed in malignant glioma. *Acta Oncologica* 1997;6:615–618.
44. Toi M, Inada K, Suzuki H, et al. Tumor angiogenesis in breast cancer: its importance as a prognostic indicator and the association with vascular endothelial growth factor expression. *Breast Cancer Res Treat* 1995;36:193–204.
45. Gasparini G, Toi M, Gion M, et al. Prognostic significance of vascular endothelial growth factor protein in node-negative breast carcinoma. *J Natl Cancer Inst* 1997;89:139–147.
46. Eppenberger U, Kueng W, Schlaeppi JM, et al. Markers of tumor angiogenesis and proteolysis independently define high- and low-risk subsets of node-negative breast cancer patients. *J Clin Oncol* 1998;16:129–136.
47. Linderholm B, Tavelin B, Grankvist K, et al. Does vascular endothelial growth factor (VEGF) predict local relapse and survival in radiotherapy-treated node-negative breast cancer? *Br J Cancer* 1999;81:727–732.
48. Obermair A, Kucera E, Mayerhofer K, et al. Vascular endothelial growth factor (VEGF) in human breast cancer: correlation with disease-free survival. *Int J Cancer* 1997;74:455–458.
49. Linderholm B, Lindh B, Tavelin B, et al. p53 and vascular-endothelial-growth-factor (VEGF) expression predicts outcome in 833 patients with primary breast carcinoma. *Int J Cancer* 2000;89:51–62.
50. Kinoshita J, Kitamura K, Kabashima A, et al. Clinical significance of vascular endothelial growth factor-C (VEGF-C) in breast cancer. *Breast Cancer Res Treat* 2001;66:159–164.
51. Gasparini G, Toi M, Miceli R, et al. Clinical relevance of vascular endothelial growth factor and thymidine phosphorylase in patients with node-positive breast cancer treated with either adjuvant chemotherapy or hormone therapy. *Cancer J Sci Am* 1999;5:101–111.
52. Linderholm B, Grankvist K, Wilking N, et al. Correlation of vascular endothelial growth factor content with recurrences, survival, and first relapse site in primary node-positive breast carcinoma after adjuvant treatment. *J Clin Oncol* 2000;18:1423–1431.
53. Gown AM, Rivkin SE, Hunt HN, et al. Prognostic factor of vascular endothelial growth factor (VEGF) expression in node-positive breast cancer. *Proc Am Soc Clin Oncol* 2001;20:427a (abstract 1703).
54. Russell KS, Stern DF, Polverini PJ, et al. Neuregulin activation of ErbB receptors in vascular endothelium leads to angiogenesis. *Am J Physiol* 1999;277:H2205–H2211.
55. Yen L, You XL, Al Moustafa AE, et al. Heregulin selectively upregulates vascular endothelial growth factor secretion in cancer cells and stimulates angiogenesis. *Oncogene* 2000;19:3460–3469.
56. Xiong S, Grijalva R, Zhang L, et al. Up-regulation of vascular endothelial growth factor in breast cancer cells by the heregulin-beta1-activated p38 signaling pathway enhances endothelial cell migration. *Cancer Res* 2001;61:1727–1732.
57. Bagheri-Yarmand R, Vadlamudi RK, Wang RA, et al. Vascular endothelial growth factor up-regulation via p21-activated kinase-1 signaling regulates heregulin-beta1-mediated angiogenesis. *J Biol Chem* 2000;275:39451–39457.
58. Laughner E, Taghavi P, Chiles K, et al. HER-2 (neu) signaling increase the rate of hypoxia-inducible factor 1alpha (HIF-1alpha) synthesis: novel mechanism for HIF-1alpha mediated vascular endothelial growth factor expression. *Mol Cell Biol* 2001;21:3995–4004.
59. Petit AM, Rak J, Hung MC, et al. Neutralizing antibodies against epidermal growth factor and ErbB-2/neu receptor tyrosine kinases down-regulate vascular endothelial growth factor production by tumor cells in vitro and in vivo: angiogenic implications for signal transduction therapy of solid tumors. *Am J Pathol* 1997;151:1523–1530.
60. Pegram M, Hsu S, Lewis G, et al. Inhibitory effects of combinations of HER-2/*neu* antibody and chemotherapeutic agents used for treatment of human breast cancers. *Oncogene* 1999;18(13):2241–2251.
61. Pegram MD, Baly D, Wirth C, et al. Antibody dependent cell-mediated cytotoxicity in breast cancer patients in phase III clinical trials of a humanized anti-HER-2 antibody. *Proc Am Assoc Cancer Res* 1997;38:602 (abstract 4044).
62. Aboud-Pirak E, Hurwitz E, Pirak ME, et al. Efficacy of antibodies to epidermal growth factor receptor against KB carcinoma in vitro and in nude mice. *J Natl Cancer Inst* 1988;80:1605–1611.
63. Pietras RJ, Fendly BM, Chazin VR, et al. Antibody to HER-2/neu receptor blocks DNA repair after cisplatin in human breast and ovarian cancer cells. *Oncogene* 1994;9:1829–1838.
64. Konecny G, Pegram MD, Beryt M, et al. Therapeutic advantage of chemotherapy drugs in combination with Herceptin against human breast cancer cells with HER-2/neu overexpression. *Breast Cancer Res Treat* 1999;57:114a.
65. Baselga J, Tripathy D, Mendelsohn J, et al. Phase II study of weekly intravenous recombinant humanized anti-p185HER-2 monoclonal antibody in patients with HER-2/neu-overexpressing metastatic breast cancer. *J Clin Oncol* 1996;14(3):737–744.
66. Cobleigh MA, Vogel CL, Tripathy D, et al. Multinational study of the efficacy and safety of humanized anti-HER-2 antibody in women who have HER-2-overexpressing breast cancer that has progressed after therapy for metastatic disease. *J Clin Oncol* 1999;17:2639–2648.
67. Vogel CL, Cobleigh MA, Tripathy D, et al. Efficacy and safety of trastuzumab as a single agent in first-line treatment of HER-2-overexpressing metastatic breast cancer. *J Clin Oncol* 2002;20(3):719–726.
68. Herceptin® (Trastuzumab) anti-HER-2 monoclonal antibody: product package insert, Genentech, Inc. South San Francisco, CA, copyright September, 1998.
69. Slamon DJ, Leyland-Jones B, Shak S, et al. Use of chemotherapy plus a monoclonal antibody against HER-2

for metastatic breast cancer that overexpresses HER-2. *N Engl J Med* 2001;344(11):783–792.
70. Montemurro F, Ueno NT, Rondon G, et al. High-dose chemotherapy with hematopoietic stem-cell transplantation for breast cancer: current status, future trends. *Clin Breast Cancer* 2000;1(3):197–209.
71. Mass, et al. *Proc Am Soc Clin Oncol* 2001;20:22a. Abstract 85.
72. Seidman A, Hudis C, Pierri MK, et al. Cardiac dysfunction in the trastuzumab clinical trials experience. *J Clin Oncol* 2002;20(5):1215–1221.
73. Sawyer DB, Zuppinger C, Miller TA, et al. Modulation of anthracycline-induced myofibrillar disarray in rat ventricular myocytes by neuregulin-1beta and anti-erbB2: potential mechanism for trastuzumab-induced cardiotoxicity. *Circulation* 2002;105(13):1551–1554.
74. Pegram MD, O'Callaghan C. Combining the anti-HER-2 antibody trastuzumab with taxanes in breast cancer: results and trial considerations. *Clin Breast Cancer* 2001;2(suppl 1):S15–19.
75. Esteva FJ, Valero V, Booser D, et al. Phase II study of weekly docetaxel and trastuzumab for patients with HER-2-overexpressing metastatic breast cancer. *J Clin Oncol* 2002;20(7):1800–1808.
76. Fountzilas G, Tsavdaridis D, Kalogera-Fountzila A, et al. Weekly paclitaxel as first-line chemotherapy and trastuzumab in patients with advanced breast cancer. A Hellenic Cooperative Oncology Group phase II study. *Ann Oncol* 2001;12(11):1545–1551.
77. Burstein HJ, Kuter I, Campos SM, et al. Clinical activity of trastuzumab and vinorelbine in women with HER-2-overexpressing metastatic breast cancer. *J Clin Oncol* 2001;19(10):2722–2730.
78. Nabholtz J-M, Pienkowski T, Nothfelt D, et al. Results of two open label multicentre phase II pilot studies with Herceptin in combination with docetaxel and platinum salts (Cis or carboplatin) (TCH) as therapy for advanced breast cancer (ABC) in women with tumors over-expressing the HER-2-neu proto-oncogene. *Eur J Cancer* 2001;37:190. Abstract 695 and poster presented at: The Twentieth Annual Meeting of the European Society for Therapeutic Radiology and Oncology and The Eleventh European Cancer Conference; October 21–25, 2001; Lisbon, Portugal.
79. Muss HB, Thor AD, Berry DA, et al. c-erbB-2 expression and response to adjuvant therapy in women with node-positive early breast cancer. *N Engl J Med* 1994; 330:1260–1266.
80. Thor AD, Berry DA, Budman DR, et al. erbB-2, p53, and efficacy of adjuvant therapy in lymph node-positive breast cancer. *J Natl Cancer Inst* 1998;90: 1346–1360.
81. Paik S, Bryant J, Park C, et al. erbB-2 and response to doxorubicin in patients with axillary lymph node-positive, hormone receptor-negative breast cancer. *J Natl Cancer Inst* 1998;90:1361–1370.
82. Leyland-Jones B. Dose scheduling—Herceptin. *Oncology* 2001;61(suppl 2):31–36.
83. Lu Y, Zi X, Zhao Y, et al. Insulin-like growth factor-I receptor signaling and resistance to trastuzumab (Herceptin). *J Natl Cancer Inst* 2001;93(24):1852–1857.

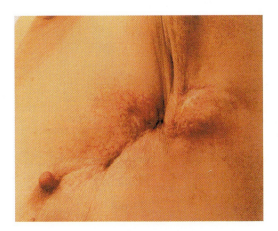

FIG. 1.1. Severe skin fibrosis and telangectasia 10 years after treatment for an early-stage breast cancer. Two main factors contributed to the poor cosmetic outcome in this patient: (a) Lumpectomy and axillary dissection were performed through the same incision; (b) A 14-Gy boost was given at a 3-cm depth with a direct ^{60}Co field, giving a high dose per fraction to the skin surface.

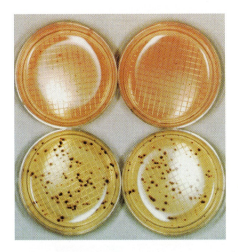

FIG. 17.2. Effect of HER2/neu transduction and overexpression in MCF7 breast carcinoma cells on colony formation in soft agar. [From Pegram M, Salmon D. *Semin Oncol* 2000 October 27; (suppl 9):13–9.]

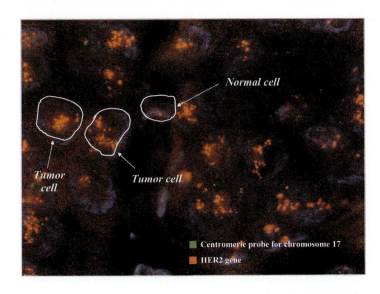

FIG. 17.4. HER2/neu and chromosome 17 detected by FISH. (Courtesy of Kenneth Bloom).

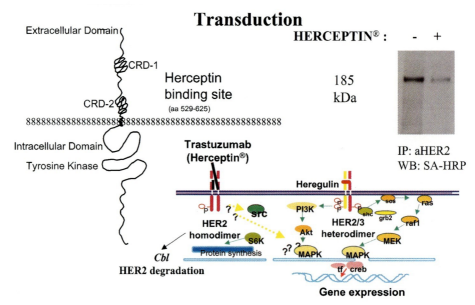

FIG. 17.6. Trastuzumab binding to HER2 epitope leads to receptor downregulation and effects on signal. (Data from L. Bald and B. Fendly).

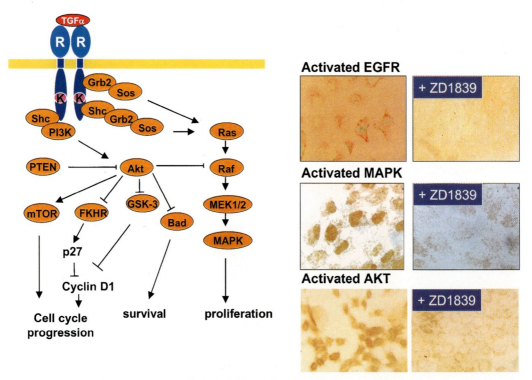

FIG. 19.2. The MAP-Kinase and PI3K/AKT signaling pathways. **A:** A major signaling route of EGFR is the Ras-Raf-MAP-kinase pathway. Activation of Ras initiates a multistep phosphorylation cascade that leads to the activation of MAPKs. Another important pathway in EGF receptor signaling is constituted by phosphatidylinositol 3-kinase (PI3K) and the downstream protein-serine/threonine kinase Akt. After activation, Akt transduces signals that fall into two main classes: regulators of apoptosis, or regulators of cell growth, including protein synthesis and cell-cycle regulation. **B:** Signal transduction via these pathways is efficiently blocked by anti-EGFR therapies, as shown here with the cell line A431 treated with the EGFR tyrosine kinase inhbitor ZD1839 second- and third-line therapy for non-small cell lung cancer (IDEAL 1 study).

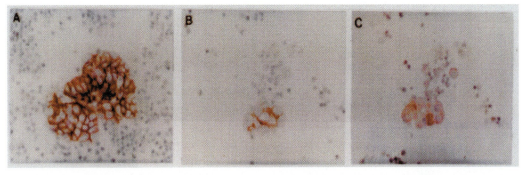

FIG. 21.2. HER-2/*neu* downregulation is observed in the same cells that express *E1A*. Breast cancer cells are immunohistochemically stained for *E1A* and HER-2/*neu* 22 days after administration of the *E1A*/DC-Chol complex. **A:** Before treatment (on day 0), staining intensity is 3+. **B:** On day 22 after treatment, staining intensity is 1+. **C:** *E1A* is expressed in both the cytoplasm and the nucleus.

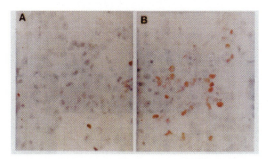

FIG. 21.3. TUNEL assay shows increased numbers of apoptotic tumor cells after administration of *E1A*/DC-Chol complex. **A:** Before treatment. **B:** After treatment.

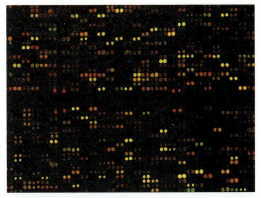

FIG. 22.1. Portion of a hybridized oligonucleotide array containing a total of 14,000 genes. Each spot is printed in duplicate. Red dye corresponds to the reference RNA (10 pooled cell lines). Green corresponds to the breast tumor RNA.

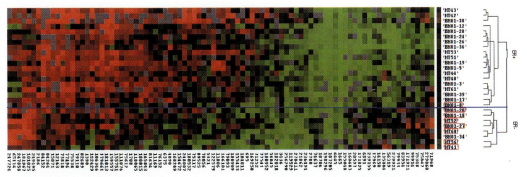

FIG. 22.2. Two-way hierarchical clustering of ER+ vs. ER− patients using Eisen's Cluster and TreeView. Unigene code for genes are shown on the horizontal axis. The vertical axis shows a clustering of 27 patient tumor samples (each is an average over 3 microarray slides). Sample names with a red rectangle were found to be ER− by immunohistochemical assay. Those without a red rectangle were found to be ER+ by immunohistochemical assay. The clustering was instructed to use the 90 genes that correlate best with ER status on an individual basis, weighted by a missing value penalty. The overall concordance rate between the immunohistochemical classification and the cluster-induced partition is 92%. Grey squares are missing values.

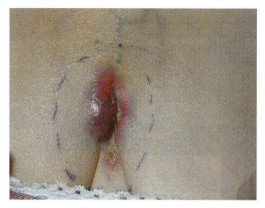

FIG. 35.1. Breast cancer with a suprasternal subcutaneous nodule.

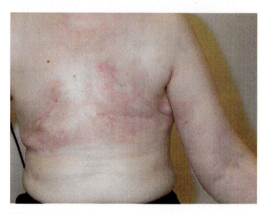

FIG. 35.2. Breast cancer with early subcutaneous metastasis presenting as inflammation known as carcinoma erysipeloides.

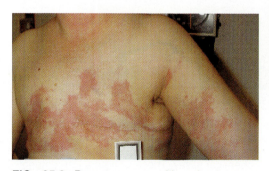

FIG. 35.3. Breast cancer with subcutaneous metastasis with induration of the skin called carcinoma en cuirasse.

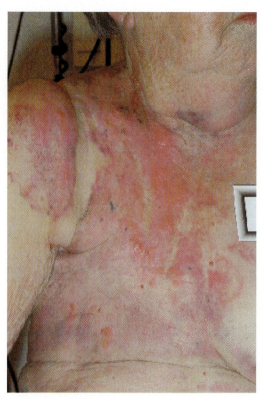

FIG. 35.4. Breast cancer with subcutaneous metastasis presenting as carcinoma en cuirasse with elephantiasic skin changes in the thickened tissue. This patient experienced lymphedema of the head and neck and upper extremity.

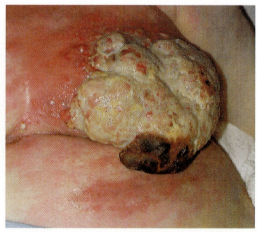

FIG. 35.5. Fungating malignant wound with surrounding carcinoma en cuirasse from breast carcinoma.

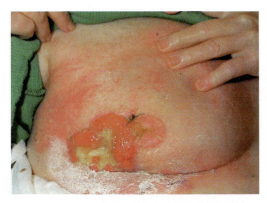

FIG. 35.6. Ulcerating malignant wound from carcinoma of the breast.

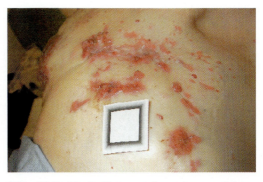

FIG. 35.7. Zosteriform malignant wound from carcinoma of the breast; this is the patient's left lateral chest wall.

18

Low-Dose Metronomic Antiangiogenic Chemotherapy: Preclinical and Clinical Applications in Breast Cancer

Robert S. Kerbel and Giannoula Klement

For decades, treatment of cancer patients using chemotherapy, including those with breast cancer, has been dominated by the "more is better" concept in which such drugs are often administered at maximum tolerated doses in a pulsed fashion with long breaks between cycles. The most extreme form of this type of therapeutic approach is, of course, the use of high-dose chemotherapy with a stem cell transplant. These methods of administering chemotherapy have had very limited success in inducing significant prolongations of survival or cures in advanced metastatic disease settings, and, moreover, they are often associated with unpleasant or serious toxic side effects which compromise quality of life. Recently, however, the beginning of what may turn out to be a paradigm shift has emerged in which the use of continuous, relatively non-toxic, low-dose chemotherapy regimens are being investigated, particularly in combination with new molecularly targeted therapies aimed at inhibiting endothelial cell functions relevant to tumor angiogenesis. The rationale for this therapeutic concept, sometimes called "metronomic" or "antiangiogenic chemotherapy," is to use chemotherapy in such a way so as to avoid or at least significantly delay acquired drug resistance, and hence prolong survival, as explained in this chapter. Not only might this be the case, but the approach may increase quality of life by reducing the morbidities often associated with conventional or high-dose chemotherapy.

LOW-DOSE CONTINUOUS CHEMOTHERAPY: AN APPROACH TO CIRCUMVENT OR DELAY ACQUIRED DRUG RESISTANCE?

The major contributing factor behind acquired resistance to both conventional chemotherapeutic and hormonal antagonist drugs is the extensive genetic instabilities of cancer cells (1,2). Enormous effort has been devoted to devising strategies to circumvent acquired drug resistance in cancer, e.g., the use of combination chemotherapy treatment regimens or the use of drug resistance reversal agents such as P-glycoprotein antagonists (3). These strategies have had only very limited success (4), and, moreover, they are frequently associated with increased cost and morbidities.

In 1991 we put forward the hypothesis that antiangiogenic drugs might represent a therapy that is potentially capable of circumventing drug resistance (5). The rationale is that the cellular target of such drugs in many cases is the normal and hence genetically stable endothelial cell of a newly formed, or forming, tumor blood vessel, rather than the genetically unstable tumor cell population per se. The relative inability of genetically stable, normal host cells to acquire stable drug resistance phenotypes is implicated, or suggested, by such clinical observations as the unchanged maximum levels of myelosuppression in cancer patients after multiple cycles of chemotherapy (6), and the cures achieved in treating nonmalignant (i.e., relatively genetically stable) tumors such as giant cell tumors of the mandible or life-threatening pediatric hemangiomas in children, using chronic (year-long) low-dose, daily, interferon alpha treatment (7,8).

There is also some very limited preclinical support for the hypothesis that antiangiogenic therapy may be resistance free (9). However, there is also evidence that tumor cell genetic mutations, such as p53 tumor suppressor gene inactivation, can have a negative impact over time on the antitumor effects of antiangiogenic therapy in preclinical models (10). This may be due to the induction of increased tumor hypoxia by the antiangiogenic therapy and the subsequent selection/overgrowth of tumor cell mutants that can survive under relatively hypoxic conditions (10). By definition, such mutants or variants would be less vessel dependent. Indeed, we recently published evidence to show that tumor cells are heterogeneous in terms of their relative vascular dependence. These results, if corroborated, make a stronger case for use of combination antiangiogenic therapies. An example of this is described below, in which conventional chemotherapy drugs are used as antiangiogenics in combination with newer, investigational molecularly targeted antiangiogenic agents.

ON THE ORIGINS OF THE CONCEPT OF METRONOMIC ANTIANGIOGENIC CHEMOTHERAPY

In 1991 we also raised a conundrum about conventional anticancer chemotherapy agents (5), namely, that such drugs, in theory, should be significantly antiangiogenic and, if so, capable of causing durable responses in patients, even when tumor cells comprising a tumor are themselves highly drug resistant. This is because, unlike normal mature vessels, the endothelial cells of newly forming vessels are not quiescent: Depending on the type of tumor and stage of progression, moderately high fractions of proliferating endothelial cells can be detected during tumor angiogenesis (11,12). Such cells, like any dividing host cell, should be vulnerable to the cytotoxic effects of chemotherapeutic drugs, virtually all of which were designed to target proliferating cells. However, since it is known that the majority of cancers are intrinsically drug resistant, or acquire resistance over time, the hypothetical antiangiogenic side effect of most chemotherapy drugs and/or regimens are presumably negligible. This is all the more perplexing given that the majority of known chemotherapeutic drugs have been shown to suppress angiogenesis *in vivo* in various short-term assays, and sometimes impressively so, as reviewed in depth recently by Miller et al. (13), as well as by Gately and Kerbel (14).

A possible solution to this conundrum was recently reported by Folkman's laboratory. Browder et al. (15) found that a chemotherapeutic drug such as cyclophosphamide, when administered to tumor-bearing mice at the maximum tolerated dose (MTD), can cause detectable levels of endothelial cell death in the microvessels of the tumor-associated microvasculature. However, this potentially desirable side effect of chemotherapy does not translate into a therapeutic benefit because the damage to the tumor's vasculature is largely repaired during the long (2 to 3 weeks) rest periods between successive cycles of MTD-based therapy. Such breaks are required to allow recovery of the animals (as in patients) from the harmful myelosuppressive side effects of MTD chemotherapy. It was reasoned, therefore, that if cyclophosphamide was instead given more frequently, e.g., once a week (on a chronic basis with no breaks), there would be less opportunity for repair of the damage inflicted upon the tumor endothelium. This of course necessitates using drug doses much lower than the MTD. It was found that such frequent, lower dose therapy (one-third the MTD for mice) caused impressive antitumor effects (15). Indeed, such a schedule was even capable of causing tumors, previously selected *in vivo* for acquired cyclophosphamide resistance, using a conventional MTD regimen, to regain responsiveness to the same drug. In other words, a state of acquired drug resistance could be reversed simply by altering drug dose and frequency of administration and shifting the main focus of the treatment from the drug-resistant tumor cell population to the drug-sensitive tumor endothelium.

These preclinical results actually have many intriguing clinical precedents, as reviewed recently by Gately and Kerbel (14). For example, 40% of patients with non-small cell lung cancer who showed no response to standard doses of intravenous etoposide administered intermittently responded to the same drug given orally at a much lower dose using a much more frequent (e.g., every day or every other day) basis, with a 1-week break every month (16). However, some of the best clinical examples or precedents for the preclinical results of Browder et al. come from studies of weekly versus every-3-week taxane treatment in women with breast or ovarian cancer, or patients with lung cancer (17–21). The original rationale for weekly administration of lower doses of a taxane (approximately one-third the MTD), instead of using the conventional once-every-3-week MTD schedule, was to minimize the severity of the toxic side effects associated with the latter dosing regimen (in particular myelosuppression). Given the long-held view that host toxicity may be a surrogate for antitumor activity and that "more is better" when it comes to chemotherapy, it perhaps came as a surprise that the less toxic, weekly, lower-dose taxane schedules were sometimes associated with high response rates, even in patients who had previously been treated with the same drug at the MTD given once every three weeks, and who had apparently stopped responding to this treatment (18). Thus, reversal of an apparent state of clinical drug resistance could be achieved by altering the dosing and frequency of the drug to a more metronomic-like schedule. Does this actually lead to a prolongation of survival, and are the responses observed in resistant patients due to antiangiogenic side effect? Recent clinical trial results appear to indicate an affirmative to the former question, on the basis of head-to-head comparisons of standard, once-every-3-week versus weekly metronomic-like regimens in breast cancer, as well as other types of cancer, e.g., non-small cell cancer (20,21).

Despite these encouraging preliminary clinical results, most patients on the weekly lower-dose taxane schedule will eventually relapse, as with other lower-dose metronomic chemotherapy protocols. It was for this reason that we decided to modify the lower-dose chemotherapy protocol of Browder et al. by combining it with another drug, specifically, an angiogenesis inhibitor such as anti-vascular endothelial growth factor (VEGF) receptor 2 antibodies (22) with the aim of significantly improving efficacy of the treatment, but without necessarily significantly increasing host toxicity (23). The rationale for this was based on the following considerations: (a) VEGF is now thought to be a major survival (i.e., antiapoptotic) factor for endothelial cells of newly formed vessels (24,25), and is the most important and ubiquitous known tumor angiogenic growth factor (26–29); (b) the pro-survival function of VEGF is mediated through VEGF type 2 receptors (flk-1/KDR), which are highly expressed by activated vascular endothelial cells, a property shared by few other cell types in the body, and appears to involve the downstream induction of several antiapoptotic genes such as bcl-2 (30,31), X-linked inhibitor of apoptosis proteins (XIAP) (32) and survivin (32,33), as well as activation of the PI3 kinase-Akt/PKB survival pathway (33,34); (c) high local concentrations of VEGF in the tumor microenvironment, bound to VEGF receptors expressed by tumor endothelium, could exert an epigenetic form of resistance (i.e., a chemo-protective effect) comprising the action of cytotoxic drugs on such cells; indeed there is evidence that the anti-proliferative (35) or proapoptotic actions of taxol (33), vinblastine, cisplatin or doxorubicin (Adriamycin) (33) on human endothelial cells in culture are reduced in the presence of VEGF (33,35); (d) therefore, combining a chemotherapy agent with a drug which blocks VEGF or flk-1/KDR should selectively amplify the proapoptotic effects of chemotherapy on activated endothelial cells, but not other host cells (23), i.e., an improved antiangiogenic therapeutic ratio would be obtained. It is already well known that antiangiogenic drugs can improve the effects of standard regimens of chemotherapy (36,37). We wanted to determine if the same would hold for continuous low-dose chemotherapy, where the side effects would be much more tolerable. In addition, because antiangiogenic therapy will probably work best as a chronic treatment, integration of antiangiogenic drugs with continuous low-dose/metronomic chemotherapy regimens would seen a more feasible way to combine the two therapies compared to standard MTD-based chemotherapy schedules, especially if orally bioavailable chemotherapy drugs are used.

RECENT PRECLINICAL RESULTS USING LOW-DOSE METRONOMIC CHEMOTHERAPY REGIMENS IN COMBINATION WITH AN ANTIANGIOGENIC DRUG

We initiated experiments to validate this combination treatment concept using childhood neuroblastoma xenografts (23), and, subsequently, human breast cancer (38). In the case of the breast cancer cell lines used, all were preselected for very high levels of resistance to the drug used for the low-dose therapy studies (38). The neuroblastoma results were published in 2000 (23) and, together with the results of Browder et al., stimulated considerable interest among both basic research scientists and medical oncologists (39–43). Indeed, the term "metronomic" dosing was coined by Hanahan et al. in one such editorial (39) to describe this type of therapeutic approach involving more regular and frequent "beats" of chemotherapy. In our initial neuroblastoma studies, an empirical regimen of very frequent and low-dose vinblastine treatment (1.5 mg/m^2 twice weekly, which is about 1/10 to 1/20 the MTD for mice [44,45]) used in combination with an anti-flk-1/VEGFR2 blocking monoclonal antibody, called DC101 (46), could cause complete and sustained regressions of large (0.75 cm^3) established (subcutaneous) neuroblastoma xenografts in SCID mice (Fig. 18.1). The combination treatment (in which the drugs were

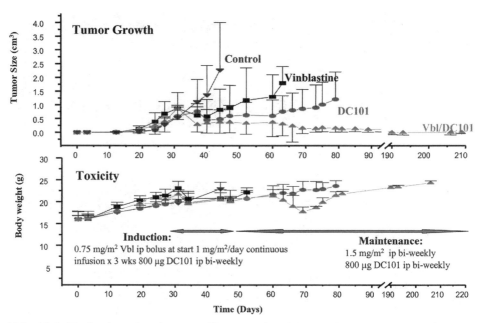

FIG. 18.1. Evaluation of anti-tumor efficacy and toxicity continuous low dose ("metronomic") vinblastine and anti-VEGFR2 (anti-flk1) monoclonal antibody (DC101) treatment of large (0.75 cm^3) established subcutaneous human neuroblastoma xenografts in SCID mice. The dose of vinblastine used is approximately 1/10–1/20 the MTD for mice, and was administered twice a week. Thus, the total drug dose was still less than the MTD. Long-term regression and survival was observed only in the combination treatment group. No overt toxicity (e.g., loss in body weight) was detected in any group. (From Klement G, Baruchel S, Rak J, et al. Continuous low-dose therapy with vinblastine and VEGF receptor-2 antibody induces sustained tumor regression without overt toxicity. *J Clin Invest* 2000;105:R15-R24,2000, with permission.)

given every three days with no breaks) could be maintained for exceptionally long periods, e.g., for 7 months (about one-third the life span of mice), since they were not toxic to the mice (47). In marked contrast, treatment with either vinblastine or DC101 alone, though non-toxic, resulted in growth delays followed by relapses and death of the animals within 1 to 2 months after initiation of treatment. Thus, apparent lack of drug resistance was noted only in the combination treatment group. Somewhat similar results have been obtained using the drug-resistant human breast cancer cell lines as shown in Figure 18.2 (38). In these experiments, the tumor cell lines were injected orthotopically into the mammary fat pads of SCID mice. An unexpected finding in these experiments is that the various empirical metronomic low-dose chemotherapy regimens had little antitumor effect on their own. But when combined with DC101 (given twice a week), the effect in tumor growth and survival was generally superior than DC101 alone. This was seen for all drugs tested, including cisplatin, vinblastine, doxorubicin, and taxol (38). In addition, host toxicity was not observed with taxol or vin-

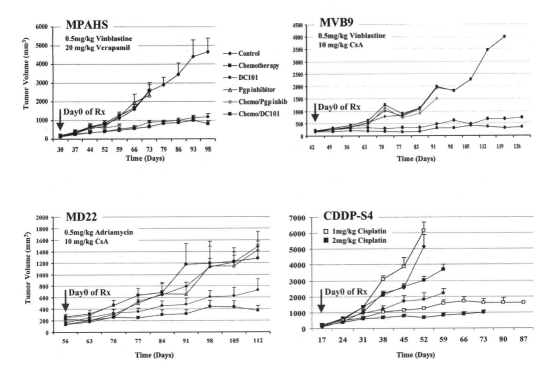

FIG. 18.2. Treatment of orthotopic human breast cancer tumor xenografts in SCID mice using metronomic chemotherapy regimens in combination with the DC101 anti-VEGFR-2 antibody. Drug-resistant variants were injected in the mammary fat pad of 4- to 6-week-old SCID mice, grown to approximately 300 mm^3 and treated two to three times per week with low doses of the chemotherapeutic drug to which they were resistant. There is no evidence of significant tumor growth suppression in the mice treated by the low-dose chemotherapeutic regimens alone, and a partial regression by the DC101 antibody alone. However, the combination of the two agents causes a reliable and reproducible tumor growth suppression or even regression in all treated cell lines. Each point on the graphs is presented as mean ± SE and represents an average of two different experiments with five mice per group in each experiment. (From Klement G, Huang P, Mayer B, et al. Differences in therapeutic indexes of combination metronomic chemotherapy and an anti-VEGFR-2 antibody in multidrug-resistant human breast cancer xenografts. *Clin Cancer Res* 2002; 8(1):221–232, with permission)

blastine, whereas significant body weight loss was seen after protracted cisplatin or doxorubucin treatment (38). The superiority of combination low-dose/continuous chemotherapy combined with an antiangiogenic drug compared to the respective monotherapies has been confirmed by several laboratories (48–50). In addition, head-to-head comparisons of standard MTD chemotherapy versus continuous low-dose chemotherapy regimens in this experimental context have shown the superiority of the latter (51,52). Indeed, some preclinical studies clearly show that host toxicity is inversely related to treatment efficacy, i.e., the less toxic, the more efficacious as an antitumor treatment strategy (51).

EXPLOITING ORAL CHEMOTHERAPY DRUGS FOR METRONOMIC ANTIANGIOGENIC CHEMOTHERAPY: PRECLINICAL AND CLINICAL STUDIES

Chronic administration of chemotherapeutic drugs given on a frequent (e.g., daily) basis is made more practical by the availability of several chemotherapeutic drugs which can be taken orally (14,53). These include, among others, cyclophosphamide, methotrexate, etoposide, and capecitabine. We therefore decided to test the antitumor effects of low-dose continuous cyclophosphamide in mice where the drug is administered in the drinking water. This has never been done before. Months of continuous, daily treatment at a dose of approximately 20 mg to 25 mg/kg per day (based on a mouse drinking, on average, 4 mL to 5 mL per day) resulted in growth delays of established human colon or breast cancer xenografts, implanted ectopically in the skin (colon cancer) or orthotopically, in the mammary fat pads (breast cancer). When established PC3 prostate tumors in nude mice were tested, the results were surprisingly dramatic (52). Thus, the subcutaneous tumors regressed and remained largely dormant for 2 months of continuous therapy, which was followed by relapses. The basis for these tumor relapses is unknown, but it is not due to acquired tumor cell cyclophosphamide resistance since, if such tumors are removed and grown in secondary hosts, they respond to the regimen exactly as before (52).

Figure 18.3 shows the results of an experiment in which SCID mice with an orthotopically implanted human breast cancer xenograft were treated with either the oral cyclophosphamide protocol, the DC101 antibody, or a combination of the two (52). The combination treatment was clearly superior in prolonging survival compared to the monotherapies. Also of considerable importance is the fact that SCID mice given the MTD of cyclophosphamide for most other mouse strains died within a week or two of treatment—such mice are extremely sensitive to cyclophosphamide, and yet, when exposed to this drug continuously for months at low dose, there was no obvious toxicity, as measured by weight loss or general appearance. This seems to mirror results in humans where daily oral low-dose (50 mg) cyclophosphamide can be given for years without serious side effects, even to elderly patients (54,55). Indeed, a phase 2 clinical trial demonstrating the relative safety of continuous low-dose metronomic chemotherapy employing cyclophosphamide (and methotrexate) in advanced breast cancer patients was recently reported (55,56). Specifically, Colleoni et al. (55) treated a total of 64 women with advanced metastatic cancer using a combination of oral low-dose methotrexate (MTX) and oral cyclophosphamide (CTX). The dose of CTX was 50 mg per day, continuously (with no breaks), while MTX was administered orally at 2.5 mg twice a day, on days 1 and 2 every week. Fifty of the patients had two or more sites of metastatic disease, and 51 had progressive disease at study entry. All patients had prior chemotherapy, 41 as adjuvant or neoadjuvant therapy and 52 for metastatic disease. Among 63 evaluable patients, there were two complete remissions (CR) and ten partial remissions (PR) for an overall response rate of 19%. In view of the palliative goal of the treatment in this setting, the investigators felt it was reasonable to consider disease stabilization (i.e., no change for 24 weeks or longer) as an appropriate clinical outcome, thus raising the overall success rate (i.e., CR plus PR plus NC for at least 24 weeks) to 32%. A total of 26% patients were still responding after 23

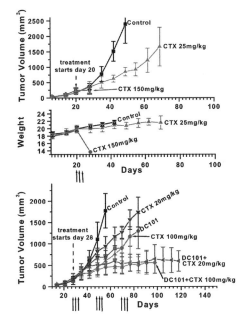

FIG. 18.3. Top Panel: The response of established human MDA-MB-231 breast tumor xenografts to contrasting cyclophosphamide (CTX) therapy regimens. CTX 25 mg/kg refers to a continuous low-dose oral (administered via the drinking water) regimen. Mice were sacrificed at day 70. CTX 150 mg/kg refers to a "maximum tolerated dose" regimen in which CTX was injected intraperitoneally every other day (150 mg/kg) over six days for a total dose of 450 mg/kg per cycle of therapy. The vertical arrows below the middle panel indicate the time of injections. This panel also shows body weight of tumor-bearing control and CTX treated mice. Note the rapid decline in body weight is the group treated with the 450 mg/kg cycle (150 mg/kg per injection) of CTX. The bottom panel shows the effects of an oral low-dose CTX regimen at approximately 20 mg/kg per day (estimated dose) versus an MTD regimen consisting of 100 mg/kg per injection (300 mg/kg per cycle) of MTD CTX therapy. Three injections (*vertical arrowheads*) comprised one cycle of therapy, which was followed by a 2-week rest period. DC 101 refers to the DC101 anti-VEGFR2 antibody treatment, which was administered twice a week at a dose of 800 μg/mouse. All mice in the MTD CTX + DC101 group died between day 82 and 100. In contrast, all mice in the low-dose-plus DC101 treatment group were alive at day 120. Thus, prolongation of survival was maximal in the low-dose CTX plus DC101 treatment group. These mice were also found to be largely free of lymph node, lung and liver metastases, in contrast to the other treatment groups, and control mice (52).

months of continuous treatment. Remarkably, this was achieved in the absence of any serious toxicity or adverse events. Grade 2 or more leukopenia was observed in only 13 patients. Alopecia, nausea/vomiting, and mucositis of grade 2 or more were very rare, occurring in 0% to 5% of patients.

Clearly, these encouraging preliminary results will lead to further future confirmation of this concept in randomized, controlled clinical trials, including head-to-head comparisons to standard versus continuous low-dose chemotherapy regimens such as the trial by Engelsman et al. (57), which compared "classical" CMF versus a 3-weekly intravenous CMF schedule in advanced breast cancer, and reported a small but statistically significant improvement in survival using the classic (more continuous, lower-dose) regimen. Such results add to a small but growing body of evidence which challenge the dogma that more is better when it comes to chemotherapy (39,41) or that host toxicity is a surrogate marker of simultaneous antitumor drug activity. Colleoni et al. (55) also drew attention to the personal and economic advantages of their treatment regimen. The low toxicity of the regimen and the oral bioavailability of the drugs make it particularly suitable for outpatient therapy, significantly enhancing the quality of life of patients. The decrease of hospital admissions for febrile neutropenias, mucositis, and necrotizing inflammation of the colon in neutropenic patients is likely to translate into a significant economic benefit, considering the cost of the treatment, which was estimated to be at a rate of $10 per month.

As a result of the findings of Colleoni et al., combined with the preclinical results summarized above, and confirmed by others (48–50), a number of phase 2 clinical trials have been initiated assessing the effects of combination treatment regimens involving continuous low-dose oral cyclophosphamide, sometimes combined with methotrexate, as described by Colleoni et al., combined with a commercially available drug considered to have antiangiogenic effects, such as the selective inhibitor of cyclooxygenase-2 (COX-2), Celebrex (58,59), or low molecular weight heparins such as Fragmin (60,61).

TABLE 18.1. *Summary of phase II clinical trials or pilot studies of low-dose metronomic anti-angiogenic chemotherapy in Ontario*

Trial/Study	Investigators	Sites
1. "Treatment of relapsed and refractory non-Hodgkin's lymphoma with continuous low-dose cyclophosphamide and Celebrex: A multicentre phase II study"	Rena Buckstein (P.I.); Michael Crump; Robert S. Kerbel	T-SRCC; PMH/OCI; SWCHSC
2. "Phase II trial of continuous low-dose cyclophosphamide and celecoxib in patients with progressive advanced renal cell carcinoma"	Ian Tannock (P.I.); Georg Bjarnason; Monika Krzyzanowska; Robert S. Kerbel	PMH; T-SRCC; SWCHSC
3. "Pilot study of low-dose chemotherapy and cyclo-oxygenase-2 inhibitor as anti-angiogenic therapy in children with progressive or recurrent solid tumors" (initiated)	Sylvain Baruchel (P.I.); Giannoula Klement; Sheila Weitzman; Mike Noseworthy; Benjamin Gesunheit; Mark Greenberg; Robert S. Kerbel	HSC; SWCHSC
4. "Low molecular weight heparin combined with low-dose continuous cyclophosphamide, and prednisone and weekly methotrexate (FraCM-P) for metastatic breast carcinoma: case reports"	Rob Buckman, Don Sutherland, Robert S. Kerbel, Joyce Slingerland	T-SRCC; SWCHSC

HSC, Hospital for Sick Children; OCI, Ontario Cancer Institute; PMH, Prince Margaret Hospital; SWCHSC, Sunnybrook and Women's College Health Sciences Centre; T-SRCC, Toronto-Sunnybrook Regional Cancer Centre.

Table 18.1 provides a summary of some of these trials or pilot studies that are currently underway.

CONCLUDING REMARKS

The notion of using seemingly nonaggressive palliative care-type or chemoprevention-like treatment strategies involving chemotherapy to treat aggressive, advanced metastatic disease would seem counterintuitive. But the successful preclinical studies, especially those involving continuous low-dose chemotherapy used in combination with an antiangiogenic drug, combined with some preliminary encouraging results of such low-dose chemotherapy regimens in the clinical setting, make a reasonably strong case for adopting a more proactive stance for undertaking clinical trials to evaluate the merit and impact of this combination treatment concept. The potential benefits of moving to the "left" of the chemotherapy dosing spectrum (already established by pediatric oncology study results [42]) include: reduced severity of host toxicity; potentially longer responses (including stable disease) due to delay, or avoidance, of acquired drug resistance; easier integration of this type of chemotherapeutic drug therapeutic approach with antiangiogenic drugs; and, perhaps, other types of new anticancer drugs, when the new therapies are designed to be chronic in nature. Of course, there are numerous problems which must be overcome, such as the difficulty in determining optimal low-dose levels and schedules, and the probability of obtaining fewer objective responses over short periods of time in comparison to standard maximum tolerated dose therapies. It is probable that tumor dormancy/stable disease will be a more likely outcome of such therapies, when they are successful. But it has been argued that this may be a more valid endpoint, or surrogate, for prolongation of survival than tumor shrinkage (62,65). Continuous low-dose chemotherapy regimens should not be viewed as necessarily replacing standard chemotherapy regimens, but rather as being used with them. For example, if particular standard therapies are known to cause major reductions in tumor burden in certain disease settings, such as ovarian cancer, it may be prudent to consider using the metronomic low-dose regimens once evidence of resistance to such standard therapies emerges—or perhaps even before, in a proactive manner. Indeed, upfront "loading" injections of a chemotherapeutic drug such as vinblastine or CPT-11/Camptosar can significantly improve the subsequent effects of continuous low-dose chemotherapy regimens using these drugs (51). In addition, we must stress again the probable necessity of integrating metronomic low-dose chemotherapy regimens with other drugs such as VEGF or VEGF receptor inhibitors in order to obtain optimal results.

REFERENCES

1. Folkman J, Hahnfeldt P, Hlatky L. Cancer: looking outside the genome. *Nature Reviews* 2000;1:76–79.
2. Stoler DL, Chen N, Basik M, et al. The onset and extent of genomic instability in sporadic colorectal tumor progression. *Proc Natl Acad Sci USA* 1999;96:15121–15126.
3. Sikic BI, Fisher GA, Lum BL, et al. Modulation and prevention of multidrug resistance by inhibitors of P-glycoprotein. *Cancer Chemother Pharmacol* 1997;40 (suppl):S13–S19.
4. Houghton PJ, Kaye SB. Multidrug resistance is not an important factor in therapeutic outcome in human malignancies. *J NIH Res* 1994;6:55.
5. Kerbel RS. Inhibition of tumor angiogenesis as a strategy to circumvent acquired resistance to anti-cancer therapeutic agents. *BioEssays* 1991;13:31–36.
6. Crawford J, Ozer H, Stoller R, et al. Reduction by granulocyte colony-stimulating factor of fever and neutropenia induced by chemotherapy in patients with small-cell lung cancer. *N Engl J Med* 1991;325:164–170.
7. Ezekowitz RA, Mulliken JB, Folkman J. Interferon alfa-2a therapy for life-threatening hemangiomas of infancy. *N Engl J Med* 1992;326:1456–1463.
8. Kaban LB, Mulliken JB, Ezekowitz RA, et al. Antiangiogenic therapy of a recurrent giant cell tumor of the mandible with interferon alpha-2a. *Pediatrics* 1999;103:1145–1149.
9. Boehm T, Folkman J, Browder T, O'Reilly MS. Antiangiogenic therapy of experimental cancer does not induce acquired drug resistance. *Nature* 1997;390:404–407.
10. Yu J, Rak J, Coomber BL, et al. Effect of p53 status on tumor response to anti-angiogenic therapy. *Science* 2002;295:1526–1528.
11. Eberhard A, Kahlert S, Goede V, et al. Heterogeneity of angiogenesis and blood vessel maturation in human tumors: implications for antiangiogenic tumor therapies. *Cancer Res* 2000;60:1388–1393.
12. Folkman J, Hahnfeldt P, Hlatky L. The logic of antiangiogenic gene therapy. In: Friedmann T, ed. The development of gene therapy. Cold Spring Harbor, NY: Cold Spring Harbor Laboratory Press, 1998:1–17.
13. Miller KD, Sweeney CJ, Sledge GW. Redefining the target: chemotherapeutics as antiangiogenics. *J Clin Oncol* 2001;19:1195–1206.
14. Gately S, Kerbel R. Antiangiogenic scheduling of lower dose cancer chemotherapy. *Cancer J* 2001;7:427–436.
15. Browder T, Butterfield CE, et al. Antiangiogenic scheduling of chemotherapy improves efficacy against experimental drug-resistant cancer. *Cancer Res* 2000;60:1878–1886.
16. Kakolyris S, Samonis G, Koukourakis M, et al. Treatment of non-small-cell lung cancer with prolonged oral etoposide. *Am J Clin Oncol* 1998;21:505–508.
17. Burstein HJ, Manola J, Younger J, et al. Docetaxel administered on a weekly basis for metastatic breast cancer. *J Clin Oncol* 2000;18:1212–1219.
18. Alvarez A, Mickiewicz E, Brosio C, et al. Weekly taxol (T) in patients who had relapsed or remained stable with T in a 21 day schedule. *Proc Am Soc of Clin Oncol* 1998;17:188a (Abstract).
19. Fennelly D, Aghajanian C, Shapiro F, et al. Phase I and pharmacologic study of paclitaxel administered weekly in patients with relapsed ovarian cancer. *J Clin Oncol* 1997;15:187–192.
20. Green MC, Buzdar AU, Smith T, et al. Weekly (wkly) paclitaxel (P) followed by FAC as primary systemic chemotherapy (PSC) of operable breast cancer improves pathologic complete remission (pCR) rates when compared to every 3-week (Q 3 wk) P therapy (tx) followed by FAX-final results of a prospective phase III randomized trial. *Proc Am Soc Clin Oncol* 2002;21:Abstract No 135.
21. Schutte W, Nagel S, Lautenschlager C, et al. Randomized phase III study of weekly versus three-weekly docetaxel as second-line chemotherapy for advanced non-small cell lung cancer (NSCLC). *Proc Am Soc Clin Oncol* 2002;21:Abstract 1228.
22. Witte L, Hicklin DJ, Zhu Z, et al. Monoclonal antibodies targeting the VEGF receptor-2 (Flk1/KDR) as an anti-angiogenic therapeutic strategy. *Cancer Metastasis Rev* 1998;17:155–161.
23. Klement G, Baruchel S, Rak J, et al. Continuous low-dose therapy with vinblastine and VEGF receptor-2 antibody induces sustained tumor regression without overt toxicity. *J Clin Invest* 2000;105:R15–R24.
24. Alon T, Hemo I, Itin A, et al. Vascular endothelial growth factor acts as a survival factor for newly formed retinal vessels and has implications for retinopathy of prematurity. *Nature Med* 1995;1:1024–1028.
25. Benjamin LE, Golijanin D, Itin A, et al. Selective ablation of immature blood vessels in established human tumors follows vascular endothelial growth factor withdrawal. *J Clin Invest* 1999;103:159–165.
26. Joseph IBJK, Nelson J, Denmeade SR, Isaacs JT. Androgens regulate vascular endothlelial growth factor content in normal and malignant prostatic tissue. *Clin Cancer Res* 1999;3:2507–2511.
27. Melnyk O, Zimmerman M, Kim KJ, Shuman M. Neutralizing anti-vascular endothelial growth factor antibody inhibits further growth of established prostate cancer and metastases in a pre-clinical model. *J Urol* 1999;161:960–963.
28. Balbay MD, Pettaway CA, Kuniyasu H, et al. Highly metastatic human prostate cancer growing within the prostate of athymic mice overexpresses vascular endothelial growth factor. *Clin Cancer Res* 1999;5:783–789.
29. Jain RK, Safabakhsh N, Sckell A, et al. Endothelial cell death, angiogenesis, and microvascular function after

castration in an androgen-dependent tumor: role of vascular endothelial growth factor. *Proc Natl Acad Sci USA* 1998;95:10820–10825.
30. Morales DE, McGowan KA, Grant DS, et al. Estrogen promotes angiogenic activity in human umbilical vein endothelial cells in vitro and in a murine model. *Circulation* 1995;91:755–763.
31. Gerber HP, Dixit V, Ferrara N. Vascular endothelial growth factor induces expression of the antiapoptotic proteins Bcl-2 and A1 in vascular endothelial cells. *J Biol Chem* 1998;273:13313–13316.
32. Tran J, Rak J, Sheehan C, et al. Marked induction of the IAP family anti-apoptotic proteins survivin and XIAP by VEGF in vascular endothelial cells. *Biochem Biophys Res Commun* 1999;264:781–788.
33. Tran J, Master Z, Yu J, et al. Induction of endothelial cell resistance to chemotherapy by VEGF mediated upregulation of survivin. *Proc Natl Acad Sci USA* 2002; 99:4349–4354.
34. Gerber HP, McMurtrey A, Kowalski J, et al. Vascular endothelial growth factor regulates endothelial cell survival through the phosphatidylinositol 3′-kinase/Akt signal transduction pathway. Requirement for Flk-1/KDR activation. *J Biol Chem* 1998;273:30336–30343.
35. Sweeney CJ, Miller KD, Sissons SE, et al. The antiangiogenic property of docetaxel is synergistic with a recombinant humanized monoclonal antibody against vascular endothelial growth factor or 2-methoxyestradiol but antagonized by endothelial growth factors. *Cancer Res* 2001;61:3369–3372.
36. Teicher BA, Sotomayor EA, Huang ZD. Antiangiogenic agents potentiate cytotoxic cancer therapies against primary and metastatic disease. *Cancer Res* 1992;52: 6702–6704.
37. Kakeji Y, Teicher BA. Preclinical studies of the combination of angiogenic inhibitors with cytotoxic agents. *Invest New Drugs* 1997;15:39–48.
38. Klement G, Mayer B, Huang P, et al. Differences in therapeutic indexes of combination metronomic chemotherapy and an anti-VEGFR-2 antibody in multidrug resistant human breast cancer xenograft. *Clin Cancer Res* 2002;8:221–232.
39. Hanahan D, Bergers G, Bergsland E. Less is more, regularly: metronomic dosing of cytotoxic drugs can target tumor angiogenesis in mice. *J Clin Invest* 2000; 105:1045–1047.
40. Baringa M. Angiogenesis research: cancer drugs found to work in new way. *Science* 2000;288:245.
41. Fidler IJ, Ellis LM. Chemotherapeutic drugs—more really is not better. *Nat Med* 2000;6:500–502.
42. Kamen BA, Rubin E, Aisner J, Glatstein E. High-time chemotherapy or high time for low dose. *J Clin Oncol* 2000;18:2935–2937.
43. Gasparini G. Metronomic scheduling: the future of chemotherapy? *Lancet Oncology* 2001;2:733–740.
44. Tashiro T, Inaba M, Kobayashi T, et al. Responsiveness of human lung cancer/nude mouse to antitumor agents in a model using clinically equivalent doses. *Cancer Chemother Pharmacol* 1989;24:187–192.
45. Inaba M, Kobayashi T, Tashiro T, et al. Evaluation of antitumor activity in a human breast tumor/nude mouse model with a special emphasis on treatment dose. *Cancer* 1989;64:1577–1582.
46. Prewett M, Huber J, Li Y, et al. Antivascular endothelial growth factor receptor (fetal liver kinase 1) monoclonal antibody inhibits tumor angiogenesis and growth of several mouse and human tumors. *Cancer Res* 1999;59:5209–5218.
47. Williams CS, Mann M, DuBois RN. The role of cyclooxygenases in inflammation, cancer, and development. *Oncogene* 1999;18:7908–7916.
48. Bello L, Carrabba G, Giussani C, et al. A. Low-dose chemotherapy combined with an antiangiogenic drug reduces human glioma growth in vivo. *Cancer Res* 2001;61:7501–7506.
49. Soffer SZ, Moore JT, Kim E, et al. Combination antiangiogenic therapy: increased efficacy in a murine model of Wilms tumor. *J Pediatr Surg* 2001;36:1177–1181.
50. Takahashi N, Haba A, Matsuno F, Seon BK. Antiangiogenic therapy of established tumors in human skin/severe combined immunodeficiency mouse chimeras by anti-endoglin (CD105) monoclonal antibodies, and synergy between anti-endoglin antibody and cyclophosphamide. *Cancer Res* 2001;61:7846–7854.
51. Wodarz D, Krakauer DC. Genetic instability and the evolution of angiogenic tumor cell lines (Review). *Oncol Rep* 2001;8:1195–1201.
52. Man S, Bocci G, Francia G, et al. Anti-tumor and antiangiogenic effects in mice of low-dose (metronomic) cyclophosphamide administered continuously through the drinking water. *Cancer Res* 2002;62(10):2731–2735.
53. Machein MR, Kullmer J, Ronicke V, et al. Differential downregulation of vascular endothelial growth factor by dexamethasone in normoxic and hypoxic rat glioma cells. *Neuropathol Appl Neurobiol* 1999; 25:104–112.
54. Asou N, Suzushima H, Nishimura S, et al. Long-term remission in an elderly patient with mantle cell leukemia treated with low-dose cyclophosphamide. *Am J Hematol* 2000;63:35–37.
55. Colleoni M, Rocca A, Sandri MT, et al. A. Low dose oral methotrexate and cyclophosphamide in metastatic breast cancer: antitumor activity and correlation with vascular endothelial growth factor levels. *Ann Oncol* 2002;13:73–80.
56. Kerbel RS, Klement G, Pritchard KI, Kamen BA. Continuous low-dose anti-angiogenic (metronomic) chemotherapy: from the research laboratory into the oncology clinic. *Ann Oncol* 2002;13:12–15.
57. Engelsman E, Klijn JC, Rubens RD, et al. "Classical" CMF versus a 3-weekly intravenous CMF schedule in postmenopausal patients with advanced breast cancer. An EORTC Breast Cancer Co-operative Group Phase III Trial (10808). *Eur J Cancer* 1991;27:966–970.
58. Masferrer JL, Leahy KM, Koki AT, et al. Antiangiogenic and antitumor activities of cyclooxygenase-2 inhibitors. *Cancer Res* 2000;60:1306–1311.
59. Sawaoka H, Tsuji S, Tsujii M, et al. Cyclooxygenase inhibitors suppress angiogenesis and reduce tumor growth in vivo. *Lab Invest* 1999;79:1469–1477.
60. Zacharski LR, Costantini V, Wojtukiewicz MZ, Memoli VA, Kudryk BJ. Anticoagulants as cancer therapy. *Semin Oncol* 1990;17:217–227.
61. Zacharski LR, Ornstein DL, Mamourian AC. Low-molecular-weight heparin and cancer. *Semin Thromb Hemost* 2000;26 (suppl 1):69–77.

62. Schipper H, Goh CR, Wang TL. Editorial: Shifting the cancer paradigm: must we kill to cure? *J Clin Oncol* 1995;13:801–807.
63. Eisenhauer EA. Phase I and II trials of novel anti-cancer agents: endpoints, efficacy and existentialism. The Michel Clavel Lecture. *Ann Oncol* 1998;9:1047–1052.
64. Takahashi Y, Nishioka K. Survival without tumor shrinkage: re-evaluation of survival gain by cytostatic effect of chemotherapy. *J Natl Cancer Inst* 1995;87:1262–1263.
65. Takahashi Y, Mai M, Taguchi T, et al. Prolonged stable disease effects survival in patients with solid gastric tumor: analysis of phase II studies of doxifluridine. *Int J Oncol* 2000;17:285–289.
66. Klement G, Huang P, Mayer B, et al. Differences in therapeutic indexes of combination metronomic chemotherapy and an anti-VEGFR-2 antibody in multidrug-resistant human breast cancer xenografts. *Clin Cancer Res* 2002;8(1):221–232.

19
Epidermal Growth Factor Receptor: Biology and New Therapeutics

Sonia González and Jose Baselga

BIOLOGY OF THE EPIDERMAL GROWTH FACTOR RECEPTOR (EGFR)

The EGF receptor is a tyrosine kinase receptor that is frequently overexpressed in epithelial tumors. It is a plasma membrane glycoprotein composed of an extracellular ligand-binding domain, a transmembrane lipophilic segment, and an intracellular protein kinase domain with a regulatory carboxyl terminal segment. EGFR was the first identified of a family of receptors known as the type-I receptor tyrosine kinase, or Erb-B tyrosine kinase receptors. This receptor family is comprised of four homologue receptors: the EGFR itself (Erb-B1/EGF receptor/HER-1), Erb-B2 (HER-2/*neu*), Erb-B3 (HER-3), and Erb-B4 (HER-4) (1–3). Since EGFR was the first molecule identified, this family is also collectively described as the EGF receptor family. The receptors of the EGF receptor family are activated by dimerization between two identical receptors (homodimerization) or between different receptors of the same family (heterodimerization) (Fig. 19.1) (4). There is a multiplicity of EGF receptor family ligands that drive the formation of homodimeric or heterodimeric complexes among the four ErbB receptors, which provides for signal amplification and diversification (1). Interestingly, Erb-B3 (HER-3) is different from the others because it lacks intrinsic tyrosine kinase activity. Following receptor dimerization, activation of the intrinsic protein tyrosine kinase activity of the receptor and tyrosine autophosphorylation occur. These events result in the recruitment and phosphorylation of several intracellular substrates, leading to mitogenic signaling and other cellular activities (5–7).

A major signaling route of the Erb-B family is the Ras-Raf-MAP-kinase pathway (6). Activation of Ras initiates a multistep phosphorylation cascade that leads to the activation of MAPKs (8).

Another important pathway in EGF receptor signaling is constituted by phosphatidylinositol 3-kinase (PI3K) and the downstream protein serine/threonine kinase, Akt (9–11). After its activation, Akt transduces signals that fall into two main classes: regulators of apoptosis, on one hand, and of cell growth, including protein synthesis and cell-cycle regulation, on the other (12,13). The Akt substrates involved in cell death regulation include Forkhead transcription factors, the BCL-2 family member BAD (14), the cell-death pathway enzyme caspase-9 (15), and the cyclic AMP response element-binding protein (CREB). Akt also has a prominent role in regulation of cell cycle progression (12).

EGFR was identified almost 20 years ago as a promising target for cancer therapy, for a variety of reasons. First, EGFR is frequently overexpressed in human tumors, including breast, lung, glioblastoma, head and neck, bladder, colorectal, ovarian, and prostate cancer, among others (16). In the case of glioblastomas and breast cancer, mutant EGF receptors have been described. In some of these tumors, a specific variant, denominated EGFR VIII, contains a deletion of the extracellular domain, and its tyrosine kinase activity is constitutively activated. An inverse correlation between EGFR and estrogen receptor expression has also been noted in breast cancer (17,18).

Second, increased EGFR expression correlates with a poorer clinical outcome in malignancies of the bladder, breast, and lung (16). The level of increased expression can reach an order of magnitude or greater compared with normal tissue expression levels. Increased receptor content is often associated with increased production of the ligand TGF-α by the

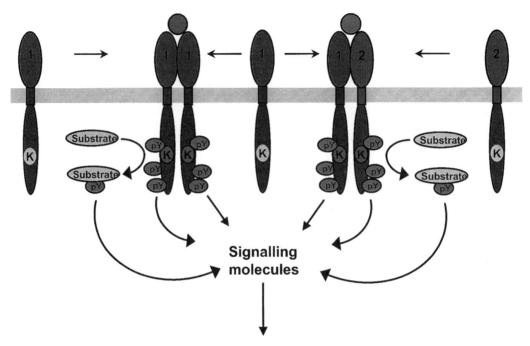

FIG. 19.1. Mechanisms of receptor activation. EGFR and members of its receptor family (HER-2, HER-3, and HER-4) are activated by dimerization. Mechanisms that promote the formation of receptor dimers include ligand binding, receptor overexpression, and transactivation (heterodimerization). Following receptor dimerization, activation of the intrinsic protein tyrosine kinase activity, of the receptor and tyrosine autophosphorylation occur. These events result in the recruitment and phosphorylation of several intracellular substrates, leading to mitogenic signaling and other cellular activities.

same tumor cells. This establishes conditions conducive to receptor activation by an autocrine stimulatory pathway.

Third, in early studies performed almost 20 years ago, a series of monoclonal antibodies directed at EGFR were shown to inhibit the growth of cancer cells bearing the receptor (19–22). In addition, potential qualitative differences in the response to disrupted receptor function in cancer cells versus normal cells were observed, predicting the feasibility of antireceptor therapy in the clinic (23,24). The promise of EGF receptor blockade has been further confirmed by the preclinical activity of receptor tyrosine kinase inhibitors (25,26).

Several strategies have been designed to target the epidermal growth factor receptor. The two that have been most extensively tested are monoclonal antibodies against the extracellular domain of the receptor and inhibitors of the receptor tyrosine kinase (Fig. 19.2).

ANTI-EGFR MONOCLONAL ANTIBODIES

The demonstration that anti-EGFR monoclonal antibodies inhibited the growth of cancer cells expressing the EGF receptor (19–22) led to a series of clinical trials in patients with EGFR-positive tumors. Among these antibodies, the one furthest ahead in clinical development is IMC-C225 (Cetuximab). IMC-C225 is a chimeric human-murine monoconal antibody derived from murine MAb 225 (27). This antibody is a potent inhibitor of growth of cancer cells that have an active EGFR signaling loop, and it is capable of inducing complete regressions of well established tumor xenografts overexpressing EGFR.

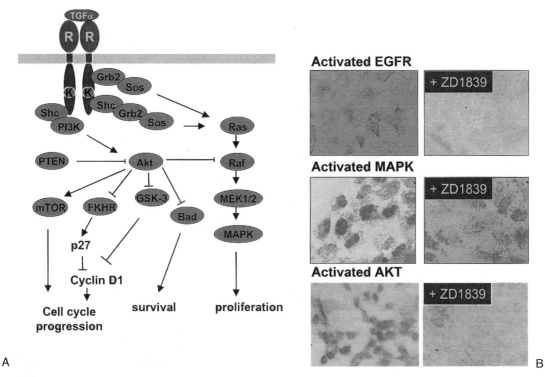

FIG. 19.2. The MAP-Kinase and PI3K/AKT signaling pathways. **A:** A major signaling route of EGFR is the Ras-Raf-MAP-kinase pathway. Activation of Ras initiates a multistep phosphorylation cascade that leads to the activation of MAPKs. Another important pathway in EGF receptor signaling is constituted by phosphatidylinositol 3-kinase (PI3K) and the downstream protein-serine/threonine kinase Akt. After activation, Akt transduces signals that fall into two main classes: regulators of apoptosis, or regulators of cell growth, including protein synthesis and cell-cycle regulation. **B:** Signal transduction via these pathways is efficiently blocked by anti-EGFR therapies, as shown here with the cell line A431 treated with the EGFR tyrosine kinase inhbitor ZD1839 second- and third-line therapy for non-small cell lung cancer (IDEAL 1 study). See color plate.

IMC-C225 binds to the EGF receptor with high affinity (Kd = 0.39 nM); it competes with ligand binding and blocks activation of receptor tyrosine kinase activity by EGF or TGF-α (19,20, 28). In addition, MAb 225/IMC-C225 induces antibody-mediated receptor dimerization, resulting in receptor downregulation. This effect appears to be important for its growth inhibitory capacity (29). As a consequence of this receptor inhibition/downregulation, the antibody inhibits molecules involved in the EGFR downstream signaling pathway, such as mitogen-activated protein kinase (MAPK) (30). The end result includes a series of events that are felt to be responsible for its antitumor effects:

1. *Cell cycle arrest and apoptosis.* MAb 225/IMC-C225 induces G1 phase arrest that is accompanied by elevated levels of the p27[kip1] inhibitor of cyclin dependent kinases (31,32). In some cases, the antibody induces irreversible G1 arrest followed by apoptosis (33).
2. *Inhibition of angiogenesis.* MAb 225/IMC-C225 induces suppression of angiogenesis by inhibition of vascular endothelial growth factor (VEGF), IL-8 and bFGF production (34,35). In addition, IMC-C225 can elicit antibody-dependent cellular cytotoxicity (ADCC) (36).
3. *Inhibition of tumor cell invasion and metastasis.* IMC-C225 inhibits lung metastasis in mice with established human tumor xenografts (35).

IMC-C225 and similar antibodies directed against the external region of the EGFR have also been shown to inhibit the expression and activity of several matrix metalloproteinases (MMPs) that play a key role in tumor-cell adhesion (37–39).

4. *Augmentation of the antitumor effects of chemotherapy and radiation therapy.* MAb 225/IMC-C225 markedly augments the antitumor effects of conventional chemotherapeutic agents (22,40–43). The positive interaction with chemotherapy and anti-EGFR antibodies has been reported in various tumor types and with different classes of chemotherapy agents, including cisplatin, doxorubicin, topotecan, and paclitaxel. As with chemotherapy, preclinical studies have also shown that anti-EGFR monoclonal antibodies enhance the antitumor effects of radiation therapy (44).

The inhibitory effects of the antibody on invasion, metastasis and angiogenesis may explain why IMC-C225 treatment is often more effective *in vivo* than *in vitro*.

A series of phase 1 and 2 studies of IMC-C225 given alone or in combination with either chemotherapy or radiation have now been completed. IMC-C225 in these early studies was found to be safe, the most common side effects, including skin toxicity and allergic reactions, occurring in up to 7% of patients; these allergic reactions occur only after the first infusion and respond well to standard therapy (45). Human antibodies against chimeric antibodies (HACAs) were detected in 4% of patients and were not related to allergic or anaphylactic reactions; these HACA responses had no clinically limiting effect following repeated weekly infusions of IMC-C225 (46). The optimal biological dose, as determined by saturation of antibody clearance, was found to be in the range of 200 mg to 400 mg/m^2 per week (47). In patients, these doses have been confirmed to block *in vivo* EGFR activation and downstream signaling (30).

In phase 2 studies, IMC-C225 has been shown to have the ability to reverse chemotherapy resistance to CPT-11 in colorectal cancer and cisplatin-based treatment in head and neck tumors. Following a striking clinical observation that the addition of IMC-C225 induced responses in CPT-11-refractory patients with advanced colorectal carcinoma (48), a phase 2 study in patients with advanced colorectal carcinoma and documented progression on CPT-11 was performed. In this study, 120 patients continued on the same dose and schedule of CPT-11, and IMC-C225 was added on a full-dose weekly schedule (Fig. 19.3). The combination was found to be safe, and the response rate, determined by an independent review board, was 22.5% with a median duration of response of 186 days (49). In a recent update of this trial (50), a median survival of 232 days was reported. Interestingly, response was

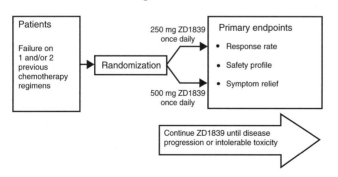

FIG. 19.3 Trial design and results of the phase 2 study of ZD1839 as randomized, double-blind, parallel-group, international, multicenter trial conducted at centers in Europe, Australia, South Africa and Japan. Two hundred and eight (of 209 treated) patients were evaluable for response with a minimum follow-up of 4 months. There was no difference between the two ZD1839 doses for the efficacy endpoints.

highly correlated with the presence of the acne-like rash, with 30% of patients with rash responding compared to 3% of those who did not report a rash. In patients with advanced head and neck tumors, a phase 2 study evaluated the addition of IMC-C225 to patients who had received two cycles of cisplatin-based therapy and who had either stable or progressive disease. In the subgroup with progressive disease, five responses were seen out of 22 treated patients for a response rate of 23% (51).

A third chemotherapeutic agent, gemcitabine, has been studied in combination with IMC-C225 in a phase 2 study in 40 patients with advanced pancreatic carcinoma (52). IMC-C225 plus gemcitabine achieved a median time to progressive disease of 3.5 months (105 days), median overall survival of 6.75 months (202.5 days), and 1-year overall survival of 32.5%.

Promising results have also been observed with the addition of IMC-C225 to radiation therapy. In a phase 1 study, escalating doses of IMC-C225 were added to conventional radiation therapy in patients with unresectable head and neck carcinomas (53). The study population had adverse predictive features of response, including a high proportion of patients with carcinoma of the oropharynx, and all had unresectable disease. Of 15 evaluable patients, all responded (100% response rate), and 13 out of 15 patients achieved a complete remission. Further, the median duration of response has not been reached at a median follow-up time of 17 months (53). These results are highly encouraging, since the expected response rate in this patient population with radiation alone would have been in the 20% to 50% range. These data have led to the initiation of a phase 3 study of radiation with or without IMC-C225 that is being conducted in the United States and Europe.

Other anti-EGFR monoclonal antibodies are also being investigated. ABX-EGF is a fully humanized anti-human EGFR monoclonal antibody that effectively inhibits the growth of various human tumor xenografts (54). Recently, clinical results of a phase 1 study have been reported (55), and biological activity was observed at the 1 mg/kg dose. One patient with esophageal cancer had stable disease for 7 months, and one patient with prostate cancer had a minor response. EMD-7200, another humanized anti-EGFR monoclonal antibody, is currently in phase 1 studies (56).

Bispecific antibodies directed against EGFR are also being studied as potential therapeutic tools. These antibodies have two different antigen binding regions and therefore dual specificity. One site is specific for EGFR while the other binds to an immunological effector cell. The result is an antibody that binds to EGFR and concomitantly enhances the host's antitumor immune response. Data have been published on three bispecific antibodies: M26.1 F(ab')2 targets EGFR and CD3 and reduces tumor cell growth when coated with human lymphocytes (57). MDX-447 targets EGFR and CD64 (IgG receptor); preliminary data from an ongoing phase 1 and 2 trial show immunological activity, good tolerability, and some biological response in treatment-refractory patients (58,59). H22-EGF targets EGFR and CD64; treatment with this antibody reduces tumor cell growth and enhances immunologically mediated cellular cytotoxicity (60).

EGFR TYROSINE KINASE INHIBITORS

As noted above, the tyrosine kinase activity of EGFR is required to initiate the biochemical responses that lead to cell growth and proliferation (5,61). Over the last decade, drug discovery efforts have produced a variety of chemical structures that inhibit the EGFR tyrosine kinase (62,63) and several of these agents are currently under clinical development (Table 19.1).

The mechanisms responsible for the antitumor activity of these compounds are under investigation. Tyrosine kinase inhibitors share some of their mechanisms of action with anti-EGFR monoclonal antibodies, suggesting that blocking ligand binding with antibodies or preventing kinase activation with specific inhibitors results in a similar, but not identical, inhibition of EGFR-dependent processes. The suggestion that the antitumor effects of monoclonal antibodies and tyrosine kinase inhibitors

TABLE 19.1. Anti-EGF receptor family tyrosine kinase inhibitors

	Agent	EGFR IC_{50}	HER2 IC_{50}	Irreversible	Clinical activity	Development stage
EGF receptor Specific and reversible	ZD1839	0.02	3.7	No	✓ NSCLC, prostate	Phase 2 and 3 completed
	OSI-774	0.02	3.5	No	✓ NSCLC, H&N, ovarian	Phase 2 completed
	PKI-166	0.02	NR	No		Phase 1
EGF receptor Specific and irreversible	EKB-569	0.038	1.2	Yes		Phase 1
Pan-HER Reversible	GW-2016	0.011	0.009	No		Phase 1
Pan-HER Irreversible	CI-1033	0.0008	0.019	Yes	✓ SCC skin	Phase 1

IC_{50}, Concentrations required to inhibit 50% the receptor kinase (μM); NR, not reported.

do not completely overlap stems from the observation that, in cancer cells maximally inhibited by EGFR tyrosine kinase inhibitors, the addition of anti-EGF receptor monoclonal antibodies results in further antitumor activity (64). This finding also provides a rationale for combining anti-EGFR monoclonal antibodies and tyrosine kinase inhibitors in the clinic. The known mechanisms of antitumor activity of EGFR tyrosine kinase inhibitors include:

1. *Blockade of EGF receptor downstream signal transduction pathways,* including the MAPK and the PI3K/AKT pathways (30,65–69).
2. *Prevention of activation of other receptors of the EGF receptor family.* The selectivity for EGFR inhibition varies for every compound and some agents under clinical development block the *in vitro* kinase activity of all catalytically active members of the EGF receptor family (70). However, there is evidence that some selective EGFR inhibitors are also potent inhibitors of HER-2 in intact cells. HER-2-overexpressing breast cancer cells are exquisitely sensitive to ZD1839, a specific EGFR inhibitor (66,67,69). Further, ZD1839 prevents constitutive- and heregulin-induced HER-2 signaling (66). These data support the concept that the EGF receptor is a key regulator of the erb-B family of receptors, and that inhibition of the EGF receptor tyrosine kinase prevents *in vivo* activation of other members of the EGF receptor family.
3. *Cell cycle arrest.* Inhibition of EGFR signaling leads to an accumulation of the CDK2 inhibitor p27^{KIP1} and a marked accumulation of hypophosphorylated Rb protein that leads to a G1 arrest (65,71,72).
4. *Inhibition of angiogenesis.* Blockade of EGFR activation by tyrosine kinase inhibitors results in a significant decrease in tumor cell production of angiogenic growth factors such as bFGF, VEGF and IL-8 (73,74). This decrease in angiogenic growth factors in turn correlates with a significant decrease in microvessel density and an increase in apoptotic endothelial cells in human tumor xenografts (73).
5. *Augmentation of the antitumor effects of chemotherapy, hormonotherapy and radiation therapy.* EGFR tyrosine kinase inhibitors enhance the antitumor activity of conventional chemotherapeutic agents both in cell culture and in human tumor xenografts (75,76). Similar findings are observed when these agents are given in combination with radiation therapy (77). In breast carcinoma cell lines, the EGFR tyrosine kinase inhibitor ZD-1839 (Iressa) has been shown to augment the antitumor effects of tamoxifen (78). Further, this combination may prevent tamoxifen resistance.

As noted in Table 19.1, there are a number of EGF receptor compounds that are under clinical development, and we will review the salient points of some of them briefly. These agents may be classified by their degree of reversibility or irreversibility of action:

Class 1: Reversible EGF Receptor Specific Tyrosine Kinase Inhibitors

These compounds are the ones further ahead in clinical development and can be exemplified by ZD1839 and OSI-774. ZD1839 inhibits the EGFR kinase *in vitro* with an IC_{50} of 0.02 µ*M* and requires a dose almost 200-fold higher to inhibit HER-2 (79). Preclinical studies with ZD1839 have shown antitumor activity in a variety of cell lines in tissue culture and in human tumor xenografts, both as a single agent and in combination with chemotherapy and radiation therapy (74–77,79,80). An intriguing finding has been that breast cancer cells that express high levels of HER-2, even in the presence of a low number of EGFR, are exquisitely sensitive to ZD1839 (66–69). Since growth inhibition in these HER-2-overexpressing cells occurs at ZD1839 concentrations that do not suppress *in vitro* HER-2 tyrosine kinase activity, a working hypothesis is that, in intact breast cancer cells, HER-2 transactivation occurs via the formation of heterodimers with EGFR. ZD1839, preventing EGF receptor activation may, in turn, prevent transactivation of the ligandless receptor HER-2.

Phase 1 studies have demonstrated that daily administration of ZD1839 is safe. The drug has dose-dependent pharmacokinetics, albeit with a high degree of interpatient variability (81–83). The most common side effects were an acneiform skin rash and diarrhea, both generally mild and reversible on cessation of treatment. The dose-limiting toxicity was diarrhea, which was observed at a dose level of 1,000 mg per day, well above the doses used in phase 2 and 3 studies. In these early studies, the pharmacodynamic effects of ZD1839 on EGFR activation and receptor-dependent events in the skin, an EGFR-dependent tissue, were analyzed (30). ZD1839 significantly suppressed EGFR phosphorylation, inhibited MAPK activation, reduced keratinocyte proliferation, and increased $p27^{KIP1}$ levels and apoptosis. These effects on EGFR phosphorylation were profound at doses well below the one producing unacceptable toxicity, a finding that strongly supports pharmacodynamic assessments, instead of identification of a maximum tolerated dose, to select the optimal clinical doses (84). Clinical responses were observed in patients with non-small cell lung cancer (NSCLC) and prostate carcinoma (81–83).

Phase 2 studies with two dose levels of ZD1839 (250 mg and 500 mg) have been completed in patients with advanced NSCLC that had progressed after first- or second-line chemotherapy. The results of the first trial, the IDEAL 1 study, have recently been reported (85). We randomized 210 patients who had previously received platinum-based chemotherapy to receive once-daily oral doses of ZD1839, either 250 mg or 500 mg, as second- or third-line therapy. The overall response rate was 18.7% (95% CI: 13.7% to 24.7%) and the overall disease control rate was 52.9% (95% CI: 45.9% to 59.8%). There was no difference between the two ZD1839 doses for any of the efficacy endpoints. The median progression-free survival was 84 days, with 34% of patients progression-free after 4 months (Fig. 19.3). The Functional Assessment of Cancer Therapy-Lung scale (FACT-L) was completed by patients to assess quality of life every month. Disease-related symptoms were also assessed by patients using the previously validated 7-item lung cancer subscale (LCS). Overall there was a high degree of concordance between tumor response and symptom improvement. Of the responding patients, 78% also showed symptom improvement by LCS, and 52% showed improved quality of life by FACT-L. The median time to symptom improvement was 8 days, a very short period of time. Adverse events at both dose levels were generally mild (grade 1/2), consisting mainly of skin reactions and diarrhea. Fewer patients receiving the 250 mg per day dose experienced severe (grade 3/4), adverse reactions, therapy interruptions, or withdrawal than those receiving the 500 mg per day dose (85). The level of activity seen in this setting compares favorably with accepted second-line treatments such as docetaxel (5.5% to 6.7% RR). This trial supports a role of ZD1839 as a second- or third-line treatment in NSCLC. A similar U.S. study has been conducted in patients previously treated with two or more prior regimens, including platinum and docetaxel. These studies will correlate EGFR expression with tumor response.

In phase 1 trials of ZD1839, myelosuppression was not observed, and objective responses were seen in heavily pretreated patients with NSCLC. These clinical observations, together with the potentiated antitumor effects of ZD1839 when combined with platins and taxanes in human lung tumor xenograft models, led to the design of pilot NSCLC trials of chemotherapy and ZD1839. In patients with advanced solid tumors, Giaconne et al. (86) evaluated combination therapy with ZD1839 (250 mg or 500 mg daily), gemcitabine (1,250 mg/m^2 days 1 and 8) and cisplatin (80 mg/m^2 day 1), given on a 21-day cycle. There were no dose-limiting toxicities or drug-related deaths, and partial responses were seen in patients with NSCLC (4 PRs). There were no significant pharmacokinetic interactions, and the toxicity profile was predictable. In another trial, Miller et al. (87) assessed the safety and pharmacokinetics of escalating doses of ZD1839 (250 mg or 500 mg daily) given concurrently with carboplatin (AUC = 6) and paclitaxel (200 mg/m^2) in chemo-naive patients with stage IIIB/IV NSCLC (87). When all three agents were given concomitantly, there was no change in the exposures to carboplatin-paclitaxel compared with administration of chemotherapy alone; however, the exposure of ZD1839 was increased by approximately 50% and 25% for the 250 mg and 500 mg dose levels, respectively. Radiographic responses included 7 PRs, and the combination was well tolerated.

Two multicenter, multinational, phase 3 trials have been conducted using combination therapy as first-line treatment in nonoperable stage 3 and stage 4 NSCLC. Patients received ZD1839 (250 mg or 500 mg daily) in combination with standard regimens of gemcitabine-cisplatin (INTACT 1 trial) or paclitaxel-carboplatin (INTACT 2 trial). Both trials are randomized, parallel-group, double-blind, placebo-controlled studies in more than 1,000 chemotherapy-naive patients with advanced NSCLC. The primary objective of these studies is to demonstrate an increase in overall survival in patients receiving ZD1839 compared with those receiving placebo. Secondary endpoints include improvement in disease-related symptoms, quality of life, safety, and correlations between EGFR expression and survival. For both studies, accrual (1,030 patients in each trial) was completed in March 2001.

Additional ongoing studies with ZD1839 include single-agent phase 2 studies in breast, gastric and prostate cancer. Combination studies with 5-fluorouracil and leucovorin in colorectal carcinoma (88) and with mitroxantone-prednisone and docetaxel-estramustine in hormone-refractory prostate carcinoma are also underway.

OSI-774 (Tarceva) (formerly known as CP-358,774) is an orally available quinazoline that is a selective inhibitor of EGFR. A phase 1 study with increasing daily doses of OSI-774 demonstrated that the MTD was 150 mg per day. At this recommended dose level, OSI-774 treatment resulted in a steady state serum concentration (Css) higher than that required in preclinical nodels to achieve full receptor inhibition. Similar to ZD1839, OSI-774 inhibited EGFR-dependent processes in skin and tumor biopsies, although it should be noted these assays were performed in a small number of patients (89). Clinical responses were also seen.

The clinical activity of OSI-774 has also been demonstrated in phase 2 studies conducted in patients with NSCLC, head and neck tumors, and ovarian carcinoma (Table 19.1) (90,91). Ongoing efforts include phase 3 first-line combination therapy in stage 3B/4 NSCLC, as well as phase 3 studies in pancreatic and refractory NSCLC. Concurrently, phase 2 studies are underway in other tumor types such as breast cancer, and phase 1B studies are exploring the feasibility of combining OSI-774 with a variety of conventional chemotherapeutic agents.

Another specific tyrosine kinase inhibitor, PKI-166, has been tested in oral squamous cancer cell lines (93). This molecule promotes the formation of desmosomes and induces increased intercellular adhesion *in vivo*, thus reducing invasiveness and metastatic potential. In a phase 1 study (94), this oral inhibitor is being tested in an intermittent dosing regimen due to reversible transaminase elevation with a continuous daily scheme.

Class 2: Irreversible EGFR-Specific Tyrosine Kinase Inhibitors

This class is represented by EKB-569, a tyrosine kinase inhibitor that binds covalently and irreversibly to EGFR and has an IC_{50} of 38.5 nM *in vitro* (95). To demonstrate that EKB-569 bound covalently and irreversibly to the EGFR, ^{14}C-labeled EKB-569 was synthesized and incubated *in vitro* with cellular membranes from cell lines expressing the receptor; it terminated the reaction under reducing conditions, and demonstrated continued binding of labeled EKB-569 to the EGF receptor. EKB-569 does not significantly inhibit other members of the EGF receptor family *in vitro* and has an IC_{50} 30 times higher for HER-2 than for EGFR.

Class 3: Reversible PAN-HER (EGF Receptor Family) Tyrosine Kinase Inhibitors

Coexpression of EGFR and HER-2 occurs in human tumors (16), a situation that leads to receptor heterodimerization and activation of downstream signaling pathways. Under these circumstances, a dual EGFR and HER-2 inhibitor may have potential advantages by simultaneously targeting the two receptors. GW2016 is a dual-specificity, reversible inhibitor of EGFR and HER-2 that is currently undergoing clinical development (96,97). This compound inhibits the kinase activity of the two receptors with an IC_{50} of 10 nM for the EGF receptor and of 9 nM for HER-2. GW2016, however, does not substantially inhibit HER-4, for which it has an IC_{50} more than 30-fold higher.

A relevant question is whether a dual inhibitor will be of greater efficacy than a receptor-specific tyrosine kinase inhibitor, taking into consideration the observation that EGFR-specific tyrosine kinase inhibitors prevent activation of HER-2 *in vivo*. In the A431 human tumor xenograft model, a single dose of EKB-569 resulted in a 50% inhibition of receptor phosphorylation at 24 hours despite a serum half life of 2 hours, a finding consistent with its reported irreversibility (95).

Class 4: Irreversible Pan-HER (EGF Receptor Family) Tyrosine Kinase Inhibitors

CI-1033 is a 4-anilinoquinazoline that irreversibly inhibits *in vitro* the three catalytically active members of the EGF receptor family: EGFR, HER-2 and HER-4 (70). Irreversibility is achieved by virtue of the compound's ability to covalently modify a specific cysteine residue in the ATP binding site of these receptors (cys-773) (70). CI-1033 is currently undergoing phase 1 evaluation (98). Reported adverse events include acneiform rash, diarrhea, thrombocytopenia, and one episode of reversible hypersensitivity reaction. One clinical response has been reported in a patient with an advanced squamous cell carcinoma (98).

CHALLENGES IN THE DEVELOPMENT OF ANTI-EGFR COMPOUNDS

The clinical activity observed with anti-EGF receptor therapies has validated the receptor as a target for cancer therapy. However, as with any new class of agents, a series of questions remains unanswered.

First, the level of EGFR expression required in the tumor in order to obtain clinical benefit from these therapies is not known at the present time. Although it may be tempting to postulate an analogy between trastuzumab and the required amplification of the target receptor HER-2, the biology of EGFR is different than that of the HER-2 receptor. EGFR has a number of well known ligands, and ligand binding to the receptor triggers homodimer and heterodimer formation; in contrast, HER-2 is a ligand less receptor, and receptor overexpression may be required to activate downstream signaling. In addition, the data with IMC-C225 in colorectal carcinoma showed that response rates were comparable in patients expressing 1+, 2+ and 3+ levels of EGFR (49). Further, in cell lines there is not a linear correlation between EGFR expression and response to tyrosine kinase inhibitors (75); there is a very linear relationship between HER-2 receptor number and growth inhibition in breast cancer cell lines treated with trastuzumab (99). Therefore, it will be critical in the new series of clinical trials to analyze the level of EGFR expression in the tumor and, if possible, the level of expression of selected ligands such as TGFα, which are felt to be required for the maintenance of an active EGFR autocrine signaling loop.

Second, the observed responses in colorectal carcinoma, head and neck tumors, and NSCLC provide a strong rationale to further study anti-EGFR agents against these tumor types. In addition, it will be important to initiate studies or to extend prior limited phase 2 studies to other tumor types such as breast, ovarian, prostate, pancreatic, and bladder cancer.

Third, the combination of these agents with conventional chemotherapy, radiation therapy and new targeted agents has to be explored further in order to identify the best available combinations. Whether any particular combination of chemotherapy and anti-EGFR agents provides a synergistic interaction ultimately will need to be established in the clinic; such synergism may be tumor specific.

Fourth, there is a need to study the mechanisms of intrinsic and acquired resistance to anti-EGFR agents. This resistance could be due to multiple factors, varying from receptor mutations to rescue by other receptors. It has been recently observed that the insulin-like growth factor receptor I mediates resistance in primary human glioblastoma cells through continued activation of phosphoinositide 3-kinase signaling (100). It has also been observed in tumor xenografts of the human A431 squamous cell carcinoma cell line that acquired resistance to anti-EGFR antibodies can emerge *in vivo* and can do so, at least in part, by mechanisms involving the selection of tumor cell subpopulations with increased angiogenic potential (101).

The fundamental observation, however, is that these compounds have shown activity in several tumor types, including NSCLC, prostate carcinoma, colorectal carcinoma, ovarian carcinoma, renal cell carcinoma, and head and neck cancers. These findings—observed with different agents and in different tumor types—validate the EGF receptor as a target for cancer therapy. The results of ongoing studies with these agents in diverse indications and tumor types will hopefully establish their role in the treatment of human cancer.

Acknowledgments: This work was supported in part by Spanish Health Ministry grant "Fondo de Investigación Sanitaria" (99/ 0020–01).

REFERENCES

1. Yarden Y, Sliwkowski M. Untangling the ErbB signalling network. *Nat Rev Mol Cell Biol* 2001;2:127–137.
2. Klapper L, Waterman H, Sela M, Yarden Y. Tumor-inhibitory antibodies to HER-2/ErbB-2 may act by recruiting c-Cbl and enhancing ubiquitination of HER-2. *Cancer Res* 2000;60(13):3384–3388.
3. Olayioye M, Neve R, Lane H, Hynes N. The ErbB signaling network: receptor heterodimerization in development and cancer. *EMBO J* 2000;19(13):3159–3167.
4. Lemmon MA, Schlessinger J. Regulation of signal transduction and signal diversity by receptor oligomerization. *TIBS* 1994;19:459–463.
5. Pawson T, Schlessinger J. SH2 and SH3 domains. *Curr Biol* 1993;3(7):434–442.
6. Alroy I, Yarden Y. The ErbB signaling network in embryogenesis and oncogenesis: signal diversification through combinatorial ligand-receptor interactions. *FEBS Lett* 1997;410(1):83–86.
7. Riese DJ, Stern DF. Specificity within the EGF family/erbB receptor family signaling network. *Bioessays* 1998;20:41–48.
8. Lewis TS, Shapiro PS, Ahn NG. Signal transduction through MAP kinase cascades. *Adv Cancer Res* 1998; 74:49–139.
9. Burgering BM, Coffer PJ. Protein kinase B (c-Akt) in phosphatidylinositol-3-OH kinase signal transduction. *Nature* 1995;376:599–602.
10. Muthuswamy SK, Gilman M, Brugge JS. Controlled Dimerization of erbB receptors provides evidence for differential signalling by homo- and heterodimers. *Mol Cell Biol* 1999;19(10):6845–6857.
11. Liu W, Li J, Roth RA. Heregulin regulation of Akt/protein kinase B in breast cancer cells. *Biochem Biophys Res Comm* 1999;261(3):897–903.
12. Chan TO, Rittenhouse SE, Tsichlis PN. AKT/PKB and other D3 phosphoinositide-regulated kinases: kinase activation by phosphoinositide-dependent phosphorylation. *Annu Rev Biochem* 1999;68:965–1014.
13. Blume-Jensen P, Hunter T. Oncogenic kinase signalling. *Nature* 2001;411:355–365.

14. Datta SR, Dudek H, Tao X, et al. Akt phosphorylation of BAD couples survival signals to the cell-intrinsic death machinery. *Cell* 1997;91:231–241.
15. Cardone MH, Roy N, Stennicke HR, et al. Regulation of cell death protease caspase-9 by phosphorylation. *Science* 1998;282:1318–1321.
16. Salomon D, Brandt R, Ciardiello F, Normanno N. Epidermal growth factor-related peptides and their receptors in human malignancies. *Crit Rev Oncol Hematol* 1995;19(3):183–232.
17. Sainsbury JRC, Sherbet GV, Farndon JR, Harris AL. Epidermal growth factor and oestrogen receptors in human breast cancer. *Lancet* 1985;1(8425):364–366.
18. Koenders PG, Beex LV. EGFR-negative tumors are predominantly confined to the subgroup of estradiol-receptor positive human primary breast cancers. *Cancer Research* 1991;51(17):4544–4548.
19. Kawamoto T, Sato JD, Le A, et al. Growth stimulation of A431 cells by EGF: Identification of high affinity receptors for epidermal growth factor by an anti-receptor monoclonal antibody. *Proc Natl Acad Sci USA* 1983;80:1337–1341.
20. Sato JD, Kawamoto T, Le AD, et al. Biological effect in vitro of monoclonal antibodies to human EGF receptors. *Mol Biol Med* 1983;1:511–529.
21. Rodeck U, Herlyn M, Herlyn D, et al. Tumor growth modulation by a monoclonal antibody to the epidermal growth factor receptor: immunologically mediated and effector cell-independent effects. *Cancer Res* 1987;47:3692–3696.
22. Aboud-Pirak E, Hurwitz E, Pirak ME, et al. Efficacy of antibodies to epidermal growth factor receptor against KB carcinoma in vitro and in nude mice. *J Natl Cancer Inst* 1988;80:1605–1611.
23. Baselga J, Mendelsohn J. Receptor blockade with monoclonal antibodies as anti-cancer therapy. *Pharmacol Ther* 1994;64(1):127–154.
24. Mendelsohn J. Epidermal growth factor receptor inhibition by a monoclonal antibody as anticancer therapy. *Clin Cancer Res* 1997;3:2703–2707.
25. Mendelsohn J, Baselga J. The EGF receptor family as targets for cancer therapy. *Oncogene* 2000;19:6550–6565.
26. Baselga J, Averbuch SD. ZD1839 ('Iressa') as an anti-cancer agent. *Drugs* 2000;60(suppl 1):33–40.
27. Goldstein NI, Prewett M, Zuklys K, et al. Biological efficacy of a chimeric antibody to the epidermal growth factor receptor in a human tumor xenograft model. *Clin Cancer Res* 1995; 1(11):1311–1318.
28. Gill GN, Kawamoto T, Cochet C, et al. Monoclonal anti-epidermal growth factor receptor antibodies which are inhibitors of epidermal growth factor binding and antagonists of epidermal growth factor-stimulated tyrosine protein kinase activity. *J Biol Chem* 1984;259:7755–7760.
29. Fan Z, Lu Y, Wu X, Mendelsohn J. Antibody-induced epidermal growth factor dimerization mediates inhibition of autocrine proliferation of A431 squamous carcinoma cells. *J Biol Chem* 1994;269:27595–27602.
30. Albanell J, Codony-Servat J, Rojo F, et al. Activated extracellular signal-regulated kinases: association with epidermal growth factor receptor/transforming growth factor alpha expression in head and neck squamous carcinoma and inhibition by anti-EGF receptor treatments. *Cancer Res* 2001;61(17):6500–6510.
31. Fan Z, Shang BY, Lu Y, et al. Reciprocal changes in p27(Kip1) and p21(Cip1) in growth inhibition mediated by blockade or overstimulation of epidermal growth factor receptors. *Clin Cancer Res* 1997;3(11):1943–1948.
32. Peng D, Fan Z, Lu YTD, et al. Anti-epidermal growth factor receptor monoclonal antibody 225 up-regulates p27KIP1 and induces G1 arrest in prostatic cancer cell line DU145. *Cancer Res* 1996;56(16):3666–3669.
33. Wu X, Fan Z, Masui H, et al. Apoptosis induced by an anti-epidermal growth factor receptor monoclonal antibody in a human colorectal carcinoma cell line and its delay by insulin. *J Clin Invest* 1995;95(4):1897–1905.
34. Petit AM, Rak J, Hung MC, et al. Neutralizing antibodies against epidermal growth factor and ErbB-2/neu receptor tyrosine kinases down-regulate vascular endothelial growth factor production by tumor cells in vitro and in vivo: angiogenic implications for signal transduction therapy of solid tumors. *American Journal of Pathology* 1997;151(6):1523–1530.
35. Perrotte P, Matsumoto T, Inoue K, et al. Anti-epidermal growth factor receptor antibody C225 inhibits angiogenesis in human transitional cell carcinoma growing orthotopically in nude mice. *Clin Cancer Res* 1999;5:257–264.
36. Naramura M, Gillies SD, Mendelsohn J, et al. Therapeutic potential of chimeric and murine anti-(epidermal growth factor receptor) antibodies in a metastasis model for human melanoma. *Cancer Immunol Immunother* 1993;37(5):343–349.
37. O-charoenrat P, Modjtahedi H, Rhys-Evans P, et al. Epidermal growth factor-like ligands differentially up-regulate matrix metalloproteinase 9 in head and neck squamous carcinoma cells. *Cancer Research* 2000;60:1121–1128.
38. O-charoenrat P, Rhys-Evans P, Court W, et al. Differential modulation of proliferation, matrix metalloproteinase expression and invasion of human head and neck squamous carcinoma cells by c-erbB ligands. *Clin Exp Metastasis* 1999;17(7):631–639.
39. Matsumoto T, Perrotte P, Bar-Eli M, et al. Blockade of EGF-R signaling with anti-EGFR monoclonal antibody (Mab) C225 inhibits matrix metalloproteinase-9 (MMP-9) expression and invasion of human transitional cell carcinoma (TCC) in vitro and in vivo. *Proc Am Assoc Cancer Res* 1998;39:83.
40. Baselga J, Norton L, Masui H, et al. Antitumor effects of doxorubicin in combination with anti-epidermal growth factor receptor monoclonal antibodies. *J Natl Cancer Inst* 1993;85(16):1327–1333.
41. Baselga J, Norton L, Coplan K, et al. Antitumor activity of pacitaxel in combination with anti-growth factor receptor monoclonal antibodies in breast cancer xenografts. *Proc Am Assoc Cancer Res* 1994;35:2262 (abstract).
42. Fan Z, Baselga J, Masui H, Mendelsohn J. Antitumor effect of anti-EGF receptor monclonal antibodies plus cis-Diaminnedichloroplatinum (cis-DDP) on well established A431 cell xenografts. *Cancer Res* 1993;53(19):4637–4642.
43. Ciardiello FRB, Damiano V, De Lorenzo S, et al. Antitumor activity of sequential treatment with topotecan and anti-epidermal growth factor receptor antibody. *Clin Cancer Res* 1999;5:909–916.
44. Milas L, Mason K, Hunter N, et al. *In vivo* enhancement of tumor radioresponse by C225 antiepidermal

growth factor receptor antibody. *Clin Cancer Res* 2000;6:701–708.
45. Cohen R, Falcey JW, Paulter VJ, et al. Safety profile of the monoclonal antibody (MOAB) IMC-C225, an anti-epidermal growth factor receptor (EGFR) used in the treatment of EGFR-positive tumors. *Proc Am Soc Clin Oncol* 2000;19:474a (A1862).
46. Khazaeli MB, LoBuglio AF, Falcey JW, et al. Low immunogenicity of a chimeric monoclonal antibody (MOAB), IMC-C225, used to treat epidermal growth factor receptor-positive tumors. *Proc ASCO* 2000;19:207a (A808).
47. Baselga J, Pfister D, Cooper MR, et al. Phase I studies of anti-epidermal growth factor receptor chimeric antibody C225 alone and in combination with cisplatin. *J Clin Oncol* 2000;18:904–914.
48. Rubin M, Shin D, Pasmantier M, et al. Monoclonal antibody (MoAb) IMC-C225, an anti-epidermal growth factor receptor (EGFR), for patients with EGFR-positive tumors refractory to or in relapse from previous therapeutic regimens (meeting abstract). *Proc ASCO* 2000;19:474a (A1860).
49. Saltz L, Rubin M, Hochster H, et al. Cetuximab (IMC-C225) plus irinotecan (CPT-11) is active in CPT-11-refractory colorectal cancer (CRC) that expresses epidermal growth factor receptor (EGFR). *Proc ASCO* 2001;20:3a (A7).
50. Saltz L, RM. Acne-like rash predicts response in patients treated with Cetuximab (IMC-225) plus Irinotecan (CPT-11) in CPT-11 refractory colorectal cancer that expresses EGFR. *Clin Cancer Res* 2001;7 (suppl):3766s(A559).
51. Hong WK, Arquette M, Nabell L, et al. Efficacy and safety of the anti-epidermal growth factor antibody IMC-C225 in combination with cisplatin in patients with recurrent squamous cell carcinoma of the head and neck refractory to cisplatin containing chemotherapy. *Proc ASCO* 2001;20(part 1):224a (A895).
52. Abbruzzese JL, Rosenberg A, Xiong Q, et al. Phase II study of anti-epidermal growth factor receptor (EGFr) antibody cetuximab (IMC-C225) in combination with gemcitabine in patients with advanced pancreatic cancer. *Proc ASCO* 2001;20:130a(A518).
53. Bonner J, Ezequiel MP, Robert F, et al. Continued response following treatment with IMC-C225, an EGFr MoAb, combined with RT in advanced head and neck carcinoma. *Proc ASCO* 2000;19:4a(A5F).
54. Yang XD, Jia XC, Corvalan JRF, et al. Erradication of established tumors by a fully human monoclonal antibody to the epidermal growth factor receptor without concomitant chemotherapy. *Cancer Res* 1999;59:1236–1243.
55. Figlin R, Belldegrun A, Crawford J, et al. Clinical results of the fully humanized anti-EGFR antibody in patients with advanced cancer. *Clin Cancer Res* 2001;7(suppl):3785s(A654).
56. Bier H, Hoffmann T, Hauser U, et al. Clinical trial with escalating doses of the antiepidermal growth factor receptor humanized monoclonal antibody EMD 72 000 in patients with advanced squamous cell carcinoma of the larynx and hypopharynx. *Cancer Chemother Pharmacol* 2001;47(6):519–524.
57. Negri DR, Tosi E, Valota O, et al. In vitro and in vivo stability and anti-tumour efficacy of an anti-EGFR/anti-CD3 F(ab')2 bispecific monoclonal antibody. *Br J Cancer* 1995;72(4):928–933.
58. Curnow RT. Clinical experience with CD64-directed immunotherapy. An overview. *Cancer Immunol Immunother* 1997;45(3–4):210–215.
59. Pfister DG, Lipton A, Belt R, et al. A phase I trial of the epidermal growth factor receptor (EGFR)-directed bispecific antibody (BsAB) MDX-447 in patients with solid tumors. *Proc ASCO* 1999;18:433a (A1667).
60. Goldstein J, Graziano RF, Sundarapandiyan K, et al. Cytolytic and cytostatic properties of an anti-human Fc gammaRI (CD64) x epidermal growth factor bispecific fusion protein. *J Immunol* 1997;158(2):872–879.
61. Chen WS, Lazar CS, Poenie M, et al. Requirement for intrinsic protein tyrosine kinase in the immediate and late actions of the EGF receptor. *Nature* 1987;328:820–823.
62. Levitzki A, Gazit A. Tyrosine kinase inhibition: an approach to drug development. *Science* 1995;267:1782–1785.
63. Fry DW, Kraker AJ, McMichael A, et al. A specific inhibitor of the epidermal growth factor receptor tyrosine kinase. *Science* 1994;265:1093–1095.
64. Bos M, Mendelsohn J, Kim YM, et al. PD153035, a tyrosine kinase inhibitor, prevents epidermal growth factor receptor activation and inhibits growth of cancer cells in a receptor number-dependent manner. *Clin Cancer Res* 1997;3(11):2099–2106.
65. Busse D, Doughty R, Ramsey T, et al. Reversible G(1) arrest induced by inhibition of the epidermal growth factor receptor tyrosine kinase requires up-regulation of p27(KIP1) independent of MAPK activity. *J Biol Chem* 2000;275(10):6987–6995.
66. Anido J, Albanell J, Rojo F, et al. Inhibition by ZD1839 (Iressa) of epidermal growth factor (EGF) and heregulin induced signaling pathways in human breast cancer cells. *Proc ASCO* 2001;20(part 1):429a(A1712).
67. Moasser MM, Basso A, Averbuch SD, Rosen N. The tyrosine kinase inhibitor ZD1839 ("Iressa") inhibits HER2-driven signaling and suppresses the growth of HER2-overexpressing tumor cells. *Cancer Res* 2001;61(19):7184–7188.
68. Normanno N, Bianco C, De Luca A, Salomon DS. The role of EGF-related peptides in tumor growth. *Front Biosci* 2001;6:D685–707.
69. Moulder SL, Yakes M, Muthuswamy SK, et al. Epidermal growth factor receptor (HER1) tyrosine kinase inhibitor ZD1839 (Iressa) inhibits HER2/Neu (erb-2)-overexpressing breast cancer cells in vitro and in vivo. *Cancer Res* 2001;61:8887–8895.
70. Fry DW, Bridges AJ, Denny WA, et al. Specific, irreversible inactivation of the epidermal growth factor receptor and erbB2, by a new class of tyrosine kinase inhibitor. *Proc Natl Acad Sci* 1998;95(20):12022–12027.
71. Moyer JD, Barbacci ES, Iwata KT, et al. Induction of apoptosis and cell cycle arrest by CP-358,774, an inhibitor of epidermal growth factor receptor tysosine kinase. *Cancer Res* 1997;57:4838–4848.
72. Budillon A, Di Gennaro E, Barbarino M, et al. ZD1839, an epidermal growth factor receptor tyrosine kinase

inhibitor, upregulates p27Kip1 inducing G1 arrest and enhancing the antitumor effect of Interferon a. *Proc Amer Assoc Cancer Res* 2000;41:59(A4910).
73. Bruns CJ, Solorzano CC, Harbison MT, et al. Blockade of the epidermal growth factor receptor signaling by a novel tyrosine kinase inhibitor leads to apoptosis of endothelial cells and therapy of human pancreatic carcinoma. *Cancer Res* 2000;60:2926–2935.
74. Ciardiello F, Caputo R, Bianco R, et al. Inhibition of growth factor production and angiogenesis in human cancer cells by ZD1839 ('Iressa'), a selective epidermal growth factor receptor tyrosine kinase inhibitor. *Clin Cancer Res* 2001;7(5):1459–1465.
75. Ciardiello F, Caputo R, Bianco R, et al. Antitumor effect and potentiation of cytotoxic drugs activity in human cancer cells by ZD-1839 (Iressa), an epidermal growth factor receptor-selective tyrosine kinase inhibitor. *Clin Cancer Res* 2000;6(5):2053–2063.
76. Sirotnak FM, Zakowsky MF, Miller VA, et al. Efficacy of cytotoxic agents against human tumor xenografts is markedly enhanced by coadministration of ZD1839 ('Iressa') an inhibitor of tyrosine kinase. *Clin Cancer Res* 2000;6:4885–4892.
77. Williams K, Telfer B, Stratford I, Wedge S. Combination of ZD1839 ('Iressa'), an EGFR tyrosine kinase inhibitor, and radiotherapy increases antitumour efficacy in a human colon cancer xenograft model. *Proc Am Assoc Cancer Res* 2001;42:Abstract 3840.
78. Nicholson RI, Harper ME, Hutcheson IR, et al. ZD1839 (Iressa) improves the antitumor activity of tamoxifen in anti-hormone-responsive breast cancer. *Clinical Cancer Research* 2001;7(suppl):3766s (A557).
79. Woodburn JR, Barker AJ, Gibson KH, et al. ZD1839, an epidermal growth factor tyrosine kinase inhibitor selected for clinical development (Meeting abstract). *Proc Am Assoc Cancer Res* 1997;38:A4521.
80. Woodburn J, Kendrew J, Fennell M, et al. ZD1839 ('Iressa') a selective epidermal growth factor tyrosine kinase inhibitor (EGFR-TKI): inhibition of c-fos mRNA, an intermediate marker of EGFR activation, correlates with tumor growth inhibition. *Proc Am Assoc Cancer Res* 2000;41:402(A2552).
81. Ferry D, Hammond L, Ranson M, et al. Intermittent oral ZD1839 (Iressa), a novel epidermal growth factor receptor tyrosine kinase inhibitor (EGFR-TKI), shows evidence of good tolerability and activity: final results from a Phase I study. *Proc ASCO* 2000; 19:3a(A5E).
82. Nakagawa K, Yamamoto N, Kudoh S, et al. A phase I intermittent dose-escalation trial of ZD1839 (Iressa) in Japanese patients with solid malignant tumours. *Proc Am Soc Clin Oncol* 2000;19:183a(A711).
83. Baselga J, Herbst R, LoRusso P, et al. Continuous administration of ZD1839 (Iressa), a novel oral epidermal growth factor receptor tyrosine kinase inhibitor (EGFR-TKI), in patients with five selected tumor types: evidence of activity and good tolerability. *Proc ASCO* 2000;19:177a(A686).
84. Albanell J, Rojo F, Averbuch S, et al. Pharmacodynamic studies of the EGF receptor inhibitor ZD1839 ('Iressa') in skin from cancer patients: histopathological and molecular consequences of receptor inhibition. *J Clin Oncol* 2002;20:110–124.
85. Baselga J, Yano S, Giaccone G, et al. Initial results from a phase II trial of ZD1839 ('Iressa') as second- and third-line monotherapy for patients with advanced non-small-cell lung cancer (IDEAL 1). AACR-NCI-EORTC, Miami Beach, FL, USA. 2001, pp. 630A.
86. Giaccone G, Gonzales-Larriba J, Smit E, et al. ZD1839 ('Iressa'), an orally-active, selective, epidermal growth factor receptor tyrosine kinase inhibitor (EGFR-TKI), is well tolerated in combination with gemcitabine and cisplatin, in patients with advanced solid tumours: preliminary tolerability, efficacy and pharmacokinetic results. *Eur J Cancer* 2001;37(suppl 6):S30(A102).
87. Miller V, Johnson D, Heelan R, et al. A pilot trial demonstrates the safety of ZD1839 ('Iressa'), an oral epidermal growth factor receptor tyrosine kinase inhibitor (EGFR-TKI), in combination with carboplatin (C) and paclitaxel (P) in previously untreated advanced non-small cell lung cancer (NSCLC). *Proc ASCO* 2001;20:326a (A1301).
88. Hammond LA, Figueroa J, Schwartzberg L, et al. Feasibility and pharmacokinetic (PK) trial of ZD1839 ('Iressa'), an epidermal growth factor receptor tyrosine kinase inhibitor (EGFR-TKI), in combination with 5-fluorouracil (5-FU) and leucovorin (LV) in patients with advanced colorectal cancer (aCRC). *Proc ASCO* 2001;20:137a(A544).
89. Hidalgo M, Siu LL, Nemunaitis J, et al. Phase I and pharmacologic study of OSI-774, an epidermal growth factor receptor tyrosine kinase inhibitor, in patients with advanced solid malignancies. *J Clin Oncol* 2001;19:3267–79.
90. Perez-Soler R, Chachoua A, Huberman M, et al. A phase II trial of the epidermal growth factor receptor (EGFR) tyrosine kinase inhibitor OSI-774, following platinum-based chemotherapy, in patients (pts) with advanced, EGFR-expressing, non-small cell lung cancer (NSCLC). *Proc ASCO* 2001;20:310a (A1235).
91. Senzer NN, Soulieres D, Siu L, et al. Phase 2 evaluation of OSI-774, a potent oral antagonist of the EGFR-TK in patients with advanced squamous cell carcinoma of the head and neck. *Proc ASCO* 2001; 20:2a(A6).
92. Finkler N, Gordon A, Crozier M, et al. Phase 2 evaluation of OSI-774, a potent oral antagonist of the EGFR-TK in patients with advanced ovarian carcinoma. *Proc ASCO* 2001;20:208a(A831).
93. Lorch JH, Huen A, Dusek R, et al. The EGF specific tyrosine kinase inhibitor PKI166 promotes desmosome formation in oral squamous cell cancer. *Clinical Cancer Research* 2001;7(suppl):3770s(A578).
94. Hoeskstra R, Dumez H, Eskens F, et al. A phase I and pharmacological study of intermitent dosing of PKI 166, a novel EGFR tyrosine kinase inhibitor administered orally to patients with advanced cancer. *Clin Cancer Res* 2001;7(suppl):3771s(A585).
95. Torrance CJ, Jackson PE, Montgomery E, et al. Combinatorial chemoprevention of intestinal neoplasia. *Nature Medicine* 2000;6:1024–1028.
96. Keith BR, Allen PP, Alligood KJ, et al. Anti-tumor activity of GW2016 in the ErbB-2 positive human breast cancer xenograft, BT-474. *Proc AACR* 2001;42:41 (A4308).

97. Rusnak DW, Affleck K, Gilmer TM, et al. The effects of the novel EGFR/ErbB-2 tyrosine kinase inhibitor, GW2016, on the growth of human normal and transformed cell lined. *Proc AACR* 2001;42:A 4309.
98. Zinner RG, Nemunaitis JJ, Donato NJ, et al. A phase I clinical and biomarker study of the novel pan-erbB tyrosine kinase inhibitor, CI-1033, in patients with solid tumors. *Clin Cancer Res* 2001;7(suppl):3767s (A566).
99. Lewis GD, Figari I, Fendly B, et al. Differential responses of human tumor cell lines to anti-p185HER2 monoclonal antibodies. *Cancer Immunol Immunother* 1993;37(4):255–263.
100. Chakravarti A, Loeffler JS, Dyson NJ. Insulin-like growth factor receptor I mediates resistance to anti-EGFR therapy in primary human glioblastoma cells trough continued activation of phosphoinositide 3-kinase signaling. *Cancer Res* 2002;62(1):200–207.
101. Viloria-Petit A, Crombet T, Jothy S, et al. Acquired resistance to the antitumor effect of EGFR-blocking antibodies in vivo: a role for altered tumor angiogenesis. *Cancer Res* 2001;61(13):5090–5101.

20
Dimming the Blood Tide: Angiogenesis, Antiangiogenic Therapy and Breast Cancer

Kathy D. Miller and George W. Sledge, Jr.

Angiogenesis, the process of new blood vessel formation, plays a central role in both local tumor growth and distant metastasis. Angiogenesis is a tightly regulated, multiply redundant process required only for wound healing, endometrial proliferation, and pregnancy in healthy adults. Thus the inhibition of angiogenesis offers an attractive therapeutic target with little expected (at least theoretically) toxicity. This chapter will explore the mechanisms underlying angiogenesis, its specific role in breast cancer, and recent attempts to quantify angiogenesis and tumor vasculature. It will also discuss early clinical trial results, potential mechanism of resistance and the specific challenges posed by the development of antiangiogenic agents.

ANGIOGENESIS

Growth of solid tumors in both primary and metastatic sites depends on angiogenesis, the formation of new blood vessels, to nourish the tumor. In pioneering work by Folkman, cancer cells implanted in vascular sites in animals grew rapidly and formed large tumors. In contrast, cells implanted in avascular sites were unable to form tumor masses more than 1 mm to 2 mm in size (1). This work led Folkman to hypothesize that angiogenesis was obligatory for tumor growth.

Under physiologic conditions, angiogenesis involves initial activation, including sequential basement membrane degradation, cell migration, extracellular matrix invasion, endothelial cell proliferation, and capillary lumen formation. The newly formed microvasculature matures through the process of resolution, which includes inhibition of proliferation, basement membrane reconstitution, pericyte investment and junctional complex formation (2). Both activation and resolution are tightly regulated processes, governed by specific stimulatory and inhibitory factors, many of which have been identified (Table 20.1).

In contrast to physiologic angiogenesis, tumor-associated angiogenesis is often a disordered and disorganized process. Tumor microvessels frequently lack complete endothelial linings and basement membranes. They tend to be highly irregular and tortuous, with arteriovenous shunts and commonly have blind ends. Blood flow through tumors tends to be sluggish, and the tumor-associated vessels leakier than normal (3).

Role of Angiogenesis in Breast Cancer

Preclinical Evidence

Extensive laboratory data suggest that angiogenesis plays an essential role in breast cancer development, invasion and metastasis. Hyperplastic murine breast papillomas (4) and histologically normal lobules adjacent to cancerous breast tissue (5) support angiogenesis in preclinical models, suggesting that angiogenesis precedes transformation of mammary hyperplasia to malignancy. Transfection of tumor cells with an angiogenic stimulatory peptide such as fibroblast growth factor-1 or -4 (6,7), vascular

TABLE 20.1. *Positive and negative regulators of angiogenesis*

Positive regulators
  VEGF
  bFGF
  TGF-β1
  PDGF
  Angiogenin
  Thymidine phosphorylase
  Angiopoietin-1

Negative regulators
  Angiostatin
  Endostatin
  2-Methoxyestradiol
  Thrombospondin-1
  Platelet factor IV
  TIMPs
  IFN-α
  Angiopoietin-2
  Prostate Specific Antigen

endothelial growth factor (VEGF) (8,9), or progelatinase-B (matrix metalloproteinase-9, MMP-9) (10), increases tumor growth, invasiveness, microvasculature, and metastasis (11). Conversely, transfection of tumor cells with inhibitors of angiogenesis, including thrombospondin-1 (12) or tissue inhibitor of metaloproteinase-4 (TIMP-4) (13) decreases growth and metastasis (14).

The matrix metalloproteinase (MMP) family of enzymes degrades the basement membrane and extracellular matrix and is associated with a family of endogenous inhibitors, TIMPs. Under normal physiologic conditions the MMPs and TIMPs exist in an exquisite balance—a balance that is upset during active angiogenesis. Expression of MMPs increases with the progression from benign to *in situ*, invasive, and metastatic breast cancer (15) and is associated with increasing histologic tumor grade (16). Microscopic metastases are growth restricted and remain dormant until they undergo an "angiogenic switch," presumably a result of further mutation (17,18). This angiogenic switch often results in increased expression of MMPs (19).

Hypoxia is a key signal for the induction of angiogenesis. Hypoxia-inducible factors (HIF-1 and HIF-2) are heterodymeric transcription factors consisting of alpha and beta subunits. The beta subunit is constitutively expressed while the alpha subunit is protected from degradation only under hypoxic conditions (20–22). HIF-2α shares sequence homology with HIF-1α (23), though expression patterns differ (24–26). HIF-1α expression progressively increases from normal breast tissue to usual ductal hyperplasia to ductal carcinoma *in situ* to invasive ductal carcinoma. HIF-1α expression is higher in poorly differentiated than in well differentiated lesions and is associated with increased proliferation and expression of the estrogen receptor and VEGF (27). Similarly, expression of carbonic anhydrase IX, an HIF-1α dependent enzyme important in pH regulation, is associated with worse relapse-free and overall survival in patients with invasive breast cancer (28,29).

Clinical Evidence

Clinicopathologic correlations also confirm the central role of angiogenesis in breast cancer progression. Fibrocystic lesions with the highest vascular density are associated with a greater risk of breast cancer (30). Two distinct vascular patterns have been described in association with ductal carcinoma *in situ*: a diffuse increase in stromal vascularity between duct lesions and a dense rim of microvessels adjacent to the basement membrane of individual ducts (31,32). Microvessel density was shown to be highest with histopathologically aggressive DCIS lesions (32) and associated with increased VEGF expression (33).

Weidner et al. (34) and colleagues assessed tumor vasculature in primary breast tumors by specifically staining endothelial cells with antibodies directed against factor VIII-associated antigen, scanning to identify the area with the greatest microvessel density and meticulously counting microvessels in a single 200× field. In a preliminary study of 49 unselected patients, mean microvessel density (MVD) was 101 in patients who developed metastases, compared to 45 in those who remained disease free ($p = 0.003$ in univariate analysis). The prognostic significance of tumor MVD was then confirmed in a blinded study of 165 consecutive patients by the same investiga-

TABLE 20.2. *Negative prognostic value of tumor microvessel density*

Investigator	Pts.	Nodal status	Antibody	Counting method	High vs. low MVD (p value) RFS	OS
Weidner 1991 (34)	49	N-/N+	FVIII	"hot spot"	0.003	NR
Weidner 1992 (35)	165	N-/N+	FVIII	"hot spot"	0.001	0.001
Hall 1992 (233)	87	N-/N+	FVIII	"hot spot"	NS	NS
Bosari 1992 (243)	88	N-	FVIII	"hot spot"	0.01	NR
	32	N+			NS	NR
Van Hoef 1993 (244)	93	N-	FVIII	"hot spot"	NS	NS
Obermair 1994 (234)	106	N-/N+	FVIII	"hot spot"	0.0002	NR
Toi 1995	328	N-/N+	FVIII	"hot spot"	0.00001	NR
Ogawa 1995 (236)	155	N-/N+	FVIII	"hot spot"	0.025	0.01
Axelsson 1995 (237)	220	N-/N+	FVIII	"hot spot"	NS	NS
Obermair 1995 (234)	230	N-	FVIII	"hot spot"	<0.05	NR
Inada 1995 (248)	110	N-	FVIII	"hot spot"	<0.05	<0.05
Costello 1995 (249)	87	N-	FVIII	"hot spot"	NS	NS
Morphopoulas 1996 (238)	160	N-/N+	FVIII	"hot spot"	NS	NS
Karaiossifidi 1996 (250)	52	N-	FVIII	"hot spot"	<0.05	NR
Ozer 1997 (252)	35	N-	FVIII	"hot spot"	0.034	NR
Tynninen 1999 (240)	84	N-/N+	FVIII	"hot spot"	NS	NR
Medri 2000 (253)	378	N-	FVIII	"hot spot"	NS	NS
Vincent-Salomon 2001 (242)	685	N-/N+	FVIII	"hot spot"	NS	NS
Fox 1994 (245)	109	N-	CD31	Chalkley	0.01	0.028
Gasparini 1994 (246)	254	N-	CD31	"hot spot"	0.0004	0.047
Bevilacqua 1995 (247)	211	N-	CD31	"hot spot"	0.0001	0.044
Fox 1995 (235)	211	N-/N+	CD31	Chalkley	NR	<0.05
Gasparini 1998 (239)	531	N-/N+	CD31	"hot spot"	<0.05	<0.05
Heimann 1996 (251)	167	N-	CD34	"hot spot"	0.018	NR
Kumar 1997(93)	106	N-/N+	CD105	"hot spot"	0.0362	0.0029
			CD34		NS	NS
Hansen 2000 (241)	836	N-/N+	CD34	Chalkley	<0.05	NR

Chalkley, Chalkley counting as a measure of angiogenesis; FVIII, factor VIII related antigen; N+, lymph node positive; N-, lymph node negative; NR, not reported; NS, not significant; OS, overall survival; Pts, patients; RFS, relapse free survival.

tors (35). Tumor MVD was the only significant predictor of overall and relapse free survival among the node-negative subset in this follow-up study.

Investigation in this area has flourished, with other groups modifying the technique to use different endothelial antibodies (36,37) and counting strategies (38). These studies have generally, though not uniformly, validated the poor prognosis and early relapse associated with increasing MVD (Table 20.2). Differences in sample size, technique, methods and interobserver variability likely account for the discrepancies (37,39–42). The extent of primary tumor vascularization has also been associated with tumor shedding at the time of surgery (43) and the probability of bone marrow micrometastases (44).

Multiple angiogenic factors are commonly expressed by invasive human breast cancers; at least six different pro-angiogenic factors were identified in each of 64 primary breast tumors studied by Relf and colleagues (45) with the 121-amino acid isoform of VEGF predominating. Several studies have found an inverse correlation between VEGF expression and overall survival in both node-positive and node-negative patients (Table 20.3). Increased VEGF expression has also associated with impaired response to tamoxifen or chemotherapy in patients with advanced disease (45).

Membrane-associated factors such as urokinase-type plasminogen activator (uPA) expression (47,48), the ratio of uPA to plasminogen activator inhibitor-1 (PAI-1) (49), integrin $\alpha_n b_3$, (50) and collagenase IV (51) have also been

TABLE 20.3. Negative prognostic value of VEGF

Investigator	Pts.	Status	Nodal Method	High vs. low VEGF (p value)	
				RFS	OS
Toi 1994 (254)	103	N-/N+	IHC	0.039	NR
Toi 1995 (255)	328	N-/N+	IHC	0.01	NR
Gasparini 1997 (260)	260	N-	IMA	<0.001	<0.001
Obermair 1997 (256)	89	N-/N+	IMA	NS	NR
Relf 1997 (45)	64	N-/N+	RNase	0.03	NR
Eppenberger 1998 (47)	305	N-/N+	ICMA	<0.001	NR
Eppenberger 1998 (47)	190	N-	ICMA	0.04	NR
Gasparini 1999 (258)	301	N+	IMA	<0.05	<0.05
Linderholm 2001 (257)	1,307	N-/N+	ELISA	0.034	0.0017
Gown 2001 (259)	123	N+ ≥4	IHC	NR	0.006
Toi 1994 (254)	103	N-/N+	IHC	0.039	NR
Toi 1995 (255)	328	N-/N+	IHC	0.01	NR
Obermair 1997 (256)	89	N-/N+	IMA	NS	NR
Relf 1997 (45)	64	N-/N+	RNase	0.03	NR
Linderholm 2001 (257)	1,307	N-/N+	ELISA	0.034	0.0017
Eppenberger 1998 (47)	305	N-/N+	ICMA	<0.001	NR
Gasparini 1999 (258)	301	N+	IMA	<0.05	<0.05
Gown 2001 (259)	123	N+ ≥4	IHC	NR	0.006
Gasparini (260)	260	N-	IMA	<0.001	<0.001
Eppenberger 1998 (47)	190	N-	ICMA	0.04	NR

ELISA, enzyme-linked immunosorbent assay; ICMA, chemiluminescence immunosorbent assay; IHC, immunohistochemistry; IMA, chemiluminescence immunoassay; N+, lymph node positive; N-, lymph node negative; NR, not reported; NS, not significant; OS, overall survival; Pts, patients; RFS, relapse-free survival; RNase, ribonucleotide protection assay.

associated with impaired survival or local relapse. In contrast, expression of many inhibitors of angiogenesis is lost or down-regulated in tumors (16,52).

ANGIOGENESIS: THE POTENTIAL AND PITFALLS OF A NEW THERAPEUTIC TARGET

Normal vasculature is quiescent in healthy adults with each endothelial cell dividing once every 10 years; active angiogenesis is required only for wound healing, endometrial proliferation, postlactational mammary gland involution, and pregnancy. In contrast, tissue remodeling and angiogenesis are crucial for the growth and metastasis of breast cancer. Redundancy in the angiogenic cascade offers both potential and problem. It may be possible to interrupt the process of angiogenesis at several different levels with the potential for synergy. Unfortunately, it may also be naïve to expect inhibition of only one angiogenic factor to alter the clinical course.

Antiangiogenic agents may be conceptually divided into two general categories (53). What might be called "vasculotoxins" has a direct toxic effect on proliferating endothelium, inducing endothelial apoptosis and cell death. Assuming that a given number of endothelial cells are required to support a population of tumor cells, and that some more-or-less fixed ratio between the two exists, the vasculotoxins might be expected to have a multiplier effect in human tumors. As such, they may produce clinical responses similar to traditional antineoplastics; standard drug development and clinical trials may be appropriate.

Conversely, we might term "vasculostatins" agents that merely prevent further new blood vessel formation without directly damaging the existing microvasculature. Such vasculostatins may require prolonged administration to induce and maintain tumor dormancy. Classic phase 2 trials of the vasculostatins in patients with well-established tumors may result in few (if any) objective responses without refuting the theoretical basis for their use. As such, delayed responses would be expected; prolonged stable disease might well be considered a win for such agents.

Successful development of antiangiogenic therapy, particularly the vasculostatins, will require a new conceptual approach to clinical research; biologically active rather than maximal tolerated dose, chronic rather than intermittent therapy, induction of tumor dormancy rather than tumor cell kill. Current testing of new clinical agents in the phase 2 setting regularly focuses on overall response rate; agents failing to pass some level of response determined *a priori* are frequently discarded. This may represent a strategic error for biological therapy that only prevent further tumor growth; progression-free survival may represent the preferred endpoint for such agents. In addition, it may be necessary and appropriate for some compounds to move quickly into a randomized trial once appropriate safety concerns have been met using a phase 1 study design (54).

Hahnfeldt et al. (55) have explored a model of tumor growth under angiogenic signaling. This model considers growth of the tumor vasculature to be explicitly time dependent (rather than dependent on tumor volume) and to be under the control of distinct positive and negative signals arising from the tumor. Overall the model parallels Gompertzian kinetics with tumor growth slowing as tumor size increases. Tumor growth eventually reaches a plateau as the action of stimulators of vascular growth are offset by the increasing production of vascular inhibitors by the primary tumor. Antiangiogenic therapies act to lower this plateau tumor size, hopefully to a level compatible with asymptomatic host survival. Importantly, the final tumor size is dependent only on the balance of positive and negative angiogenic factors and is independent of tumor size at the start of treatment. The model also predicts initial tumor growth with some inhibitors of angiogenesis (particularly angiostatin) before stabilization at the plateau size is achieved. This early growth could easily be interpreted (perhaps misinterpreted) as treatment failure unless surrogate markers of angiogenesis are used to guide therapy. If such a model is a correct approximation of clinical reality, then clinical trialists (and their patients) will need to learn to tolerate the prospect of initial disease progression. This will not be a comfortable prospect for many.

Surrogate Endpoints of Angiogenesis

Correlative laboratory studies assessing biologically meaningful intermediate endpoints of angiogenesis are a necessity. Unfortunately, the correlation between intermediate endpoints, angiogenesis and biological activity remains unproven. Despite the wealth of laboratory data, direct clinical evidence linking antiangiogenic activity, changes in tumor microvessel density and objective tumor response is lacking. In addition to the need to establish the clinical relevance of antiangiogenic activity, the development of reliable surrogate markers of angiogenesis that could guide therapy without repeated tissue samples is urgently needed. Though as yet no clear standard has emerged, the search for reliable surrogates of antiangiogenic activity has focused on two main areas: soluble factors and imaging of the tumor vasculature.

Soluble Measures of Angiogenesis

VEGF is a highly conserved, homodimeric, secreted, heparin-binding glycoprotein whose dominant isoform has a molecular weight of approximately 45,000 (56,57). VEGF produces a number of biologic effects, including endothelial cell mitogenesis and migration, induction of proteinases leading to remodeling of the extracellular matrix, increased vascular permeability and vasodilation, immune modulation via inhibition of antigen-presenting dendritic cells, and maintenance of survival for newly formed blood vessels by inhibiting endothelial cell apoptosis. VEGF expression is regulated by hypoxia via molecular pathways similar to those regulating erythropoietin gene expression (26). The biologic effects of VEGF are mediated through binding and stimulation of two receptors on the surface of endothelial cells: Flt-1 (fms-like tyrosine kinase) and KDR (kinase domain region). Though invasive human breast cancers commonly express multiple angiogenic factors, the 121-amino acid isoform of VEGF predominates (45).

VEGF has been measured in sera and is typically detected at higher levels in patients with breast cancer than in healthy volunteers (58,59). Higher serum concentrations have also been found in those patients with stage III compared to stage I or II breast cancer (60). Serum concentrations of VEGF may primarily reflect platelet count rather than tumor burden, limiting interpretation of these results (61–63). VEGF can also be easily measured in urine with urinary levels unaffected by platelet count (64). Elevated urinary VEGF concentrations in one reported study predicted recurrence of bladder cancer (65). Additionally, urine VEGF levels increased in patients with progressive disease during treatment with thalidomide (66). As urine VEGF excretion may be affected by renal function, normalization based on urine creatinine has been suggested (67,68). Though previous attempts to correlate single pretreatment plasma VEGF levels with response to therapy (69) and the ability of serial measurements to predict response (70) in patients with metastatic breast cancer have been disappointing, neither of these preliminary studies directly assessed angiogenesis.

Tumorigenesis and progression to metastatic disease are accompanied by changes in the expression of cell adhesion molecules (71). Though the major physiologic role of vascular cell adhesion molecule-1 (VCAM-1) appears to be in the adhesion of leukocytes to endothelium during acute inflammatory states, a role in the adhesion of malignant cells during the process of metastasis has been demonstrated (72,73). VCAM-1 is transiently expressed on endothelial cells in response to stimulation by various cytokines, including VEGF (74), IL-3, IL-4 (75), and TNF-alpha (76–78). VCAM-1 plays an integral role in angiogenesis. Human recombinant soluble VCAM-1 induces chemotaxis of human endothelial cells *in vitro* and angiogenesis *in vivo* in the rat corneal micropocket assay. Antibodies to soluble VCAM-1 have been shown to block both the *in vitro* chemotactic activity and the *in vivo* angiogenic activity of rheumatoid synovial fluid (79). Messenger RNA for VCAM-1 has been identified in juvenile rheumatoid arthritis synovium; the level of expression was significantly higher than in synovium from patients with osteoarthritis (80). Human dermal microvascular endothelial cells transplanted into severe combined immunodeficient (SCID) mice on biodegradable polymer matrices differentiate into functional microvessels that anastomose with the mouse vasculature. The newly formed microvessels express multiple markers of angiogenesis including CD31, CD34, intercellular adhesion molecule 1 and VCAM-1 (81).

Soluble VCAM-1 has been detected in the sera patients with rheumatoid arthritis (82), pancreatic, colon, prostate, and renal cell cancers (83–85). Increased concentrations of serum soluble VCAM-1 were detected in patients with breast cancer compared to patients with benign breast disease, further supporting its role (86,87). In a recently reported pilot study, serum VCAM-1 levels were more tightly correlated with breast cancer microvessel density than serum VEGF levels. Though initial levels in patients with known metastatic disease were not predictive of response, levels quickly rose in patients whose disease progressed but decreased or remained stable in responding patients (70). Similar results were found in a phase 2 study evaluating razoxane, an antiangiogenic topoisomerase II inhibitor, in patients with metastatic renal cell carcinoma. Serum VCAM-1 levels and urinary VEGF levels rose significantly after one cycle in patients with progressive disease but not in those with stable disease (64).

Endoglin (CD105), a receptor for transforming growth factor β1 and β3 in vascular endothelial cells, is significantly upregulated in areas of active angiogenesis (88,89). Endoglin and endothelial mesenchymal signaling is required for normal vascular development (90). Antiendoglin antibodies have produced complete remissions in xenograft models (91,92).

Endoglin expression in breast tumors is associated with a poor prognosis (93); plasma levels of soluble endoglin correlate with metastasis in many solid tumors including breast cancer (94,95). Changes in endoglin levels with antiangiogenic therapy has not been reported.

The matrix metalloproteinase (MMP) family of enzymes degrades molecules of the basement membrane and extracellular matrix and are critical for the process of cellular movement and invasion (96). The gelatinases (MMP-2 and MMP-9) have received particular attention due to their ability to degrade type IV collagen and the correlation of expression with tumor angiogenesis (97). Overall expression of the gelatinases has been associated with grade and stage of breast cancer (15,16); increased serum levels are found in patients with metastatic disease. Given the central role of these peptides in the angiogenic process, decreases in serum levels should theoretically correlate with changes in tumor MVD and may predict response to antiangiogenic therapy. This hypothesis has not yet been tested prospectively.

Fibroblast growth factor (FGF) is also commonly produced by breast cancers and can be measured in tumor cytosols (98), serum, and urine. Similar to VEGF, FGF levels are increased in patients with breast cancer (99,100) and may predict survival (101,102). The correlation of serial FGF measurements with changes in tumor microvasculature has not been reported but was not predictive of response to other systemic treatments in one pilot study (103). Other soluble factors including interleukin-6 (IL-6) (104) and tumor necrosis factor alpha (TNFα) remain under investigation (105).

IMAGING TUMOR VASCULATURE

Assessment of tumor blood flow by color Doppler ultrasonography (CDUS) did not correlate with tumor microvessel density in one small study (106), but nonetheless was an independent predictor of survival (107). Other investigators, however, found a significant correlation between CDUS images and microvessel density; increased blood flow as detected by CDUS was predictive of lymph node metastasis in this pilot study (108). The potential of this technique to monitor the effect of therapy was shown by investigators at the Royal Marsden Hospital. Thirty-four patients with large or centrally located breast tumors were followed with clinical examination, B-mode ultrasound, and CDUS. Changes in vascularity as measured by CDUS images were concordant with changes in tumor size at more than 75% of the time points assessed. Perhaps more striking, changes were apparent using CDUS in 40% of patients at least 4 weeks before any change in tumor size was detected by physical examination or B-mode ultrasound (109).

Use of ultrasound to measure breast tumor vasculature has been hampered by the technical limitations of traditional clinical ultrasound (2 MHz to 10 MHz) (110). Low-velocity flow within the central region of a tumor and increased peripheral perfusion is common. Traditional ultrasound cannot readily distinguish these regional variations because the low-velocity flow approximates the tissue motion velocity. Modifications to clinical ultrasound including laser Doppler flow measurements (111), use of encapsulated microbubbles as contrast agents (112), and high-frequency Doppler (20 MHz to 100 MHz) (110) to improve quantitative measurement of the tumor microvasculature are intriguing but as yet unproven in the clinic.

Positron emission tomography (PET) uses small doses of radiopharmaceuticals to depict and quantify biochemistry rather than measure static anatomic structures. The most commonly used agent in clinical PET imaging is 2-(^{18}F) fluoro-2-deoxyglucose (FDG). As a glucose analogue, FDG measures the uptake and phosphorylation of glucose as an indicator of metabolic activity. Sequential PET imaging using FDG predicted response to primary chemotherapy in three small pilot trials (113–115).

Popular tracers to quantify blood flow include ^{99m}technetium sestamibi, ^{201}thallium (TL) and ^{15}O water. ^{99m}Tc sestamibi and ^{201}TL are taken up so avidly by most tissues that levels predominantly reflect relative blood flow. While ^{99m}Tc sestamibi and ^{201}TL have gained widespread acceptance for assessment of myocardial perfusion, markedly increased uptake in tumors has also been demonstrated (116,117). Yoon et al. (118) evaluated ^{99m}Tc sestamibi uptake and washout in 31 patients with untreated primary breast cancer. Both early and late tumor-to-normal breast ratios correlated well with tumor MVD. ^{15}O-labeled water has a short half-life (2 minutes) mandating cyclotron production near the PET facility. However, ^{15}O-labeled water can quantify perfusion (milliliters/gram/minute) in all body tissues, including breast cancer. A small pilot study in breast cancer patients using ^{15}O-labeled water found increased blood flow associated with the tumor compared to surrounding normal breast tissue but didn't attempt any correlation with histology or MVD (119). Absolute tumor-associated blood volume can be calculated using ^{11}C carbon monoxide, either as an inhaled gas or mixed with whole blood *ex vivo* (120). ^{15}O-labeled oxygen has been used to measure changes in tumor oxygen metabolism during therapy (121). Several novel PET imaging strategies are currently in development to quantify tumor hypoxia, proliferation index, apoptosis, receptor/ligand interactions, and angiogenesis-related gene expression (122).

Magnetic resonance imaging (MRI) has been used to evaluate tumor-associated vasculature with either intrinsic or contrast-enhanced methods. Intrinsic methods use pulse sequences that detect the motion of water in the vascular bed (123,134) or the distortion of the magnetic field by deoxyhemoglobin (125,126). Intrinsic contrast methods rely solely on intravascular red blood cells and are not effected by changes in vascular permeability but have a lower contrast-to-noise ratio limiting resolution. Dynamic contrast enhanced MR using small molecular contrast media that equilibrate quickly between blood and the extracellular space is dependent on the tumor MVD, vascular permeability (K_{21}) and the transfer constant (K^{trans} = permeability-surface area product per unit volume of tissue). Such quantitative MRI parameters have been correlated with tumor MVD and VEGF expression in several studies (Table 20.4).

Macromolecular contrast agents quantitatively assay microvascular hyperpermeability and therefore produce an increased signal-to-noise ratio. In a pilot study of 32 patients, tumors with the most intense early signal enhancement and rapid contrast washout (high-signal enhancement ratio) had the highest MVD (127). A similar contrast-enhanced method correlated well with changes in tumor necrosis and increasing vascular permeability after treatment with ta-

TABLE 20.4. *Contrast enhanced MR parameters compared to angiogenesis in breast cancer*

Investigator	No. tumors (B:M)	MR parameter	VEGF	MVD	Comparisons with MVD (unless otherwise noted)	
					r	p
Buada (261)	20:51	Steepest slope	—	CD34	0.83	0.001
Stomper (262)	23:25	Max. amplitude	—	FVIII	NR	0.02
Buckley (263)	0:40	Enhancement at 1 minute	—	FVIII	0.47	0.002
Hulka (264)	36:21	Extraction flow product	—	FVIII	0.36	<0.01
Ikeda (265)	29:61	K^{trans}	—	NR	0.89	<0.01
Knopp (266)	20:7	K_{21}	IHC	CD31	K_{21}/VEGF, 0.52	0.05
					MVD/VEGF(+)	NS
					MVD/VEGF(−), 0.71	0.07
Matsubayashi (267)	4:31	Rim enhancement	IHC	ND	VEGF, NR	0.008

B, benign; IHC, immunohistochemistry; K^{trans}, permeability surface area product per unit volume of tissue; K_{21}, vascular permeability; M, malignant; MVD, microvessel density; ND, not done; NR, not reported; NS, not significant; *p,* level of statistical significance; *r,* correlation coefficient; VEGF, vascular endothelial growth factor.

moxifen (128) or a monoclonal antibody directed against VEGF (129).

ANTIANGIOGENIC ACTIVITY OF EXISTING AGENTS: OLD DOGS WITH NEW TRICKS?

Oncologists may have been unknowingly administering antiangiogenic therapy for years (130). Tamoxifen, initially thought to be merely a competitive inhibitor of estradiol, may have estrogen-independent mechanisms of action (131). Tamoxifen inhibits VEGF- and FGF-stimulated embryonic angiogenesis in the chick chorioallantoic membrane (CAM) model. This effect was not reversed by excess estradiol, suggesting that the antiangiogenic mechanism is not dependent on estradiol concentration or estrogen receptor content (132,133). Treatment with tamoxifen resulted in a more than 50% decrease in the endothelial density of viable tumor and an increase in the extent of necrosis in MCF-7 tumors growing in nude mice (134). The inhibition of angiogenesis was detected before measurable effects on tumor volume (135). Using differential display technology to assess gene expression in tumor and normal breast tissue from two patients, Silva et al. (136) reported that brief treatment with tamoxifen resulted in down-regulation of CD36, a glycoprotein receptor for matrix proteins thrombospondin-1 and collagen types I and IV. Thrombospondin-1 is involved in hematogenous tumor dissemination, invasion, and angiogenesis, thus down-regulation of CD36 represents a potential mechanism for the observed antiangiogenic effect.

Several chemotherapeutic agents used routinely in breast cancer treatment have known antiangiogenic activity (137–143). Maximal antiangiogenic therapy typically requires prolonged exposure to low drug concentrations, exactly counter to the maximum tolerated doses administered when optimal tumor cell kill is the goal (144). Three recent reports confirm the importance of dose and schedule. In all three, the combination of low, frequent dose chemotherapy plus an agent that specifically targets the endothelial cell compartment controlled tumor growth much more effectively than the cytotoxic agent alone. An "antiangiogenic schedule" (170 mg/kg every 6 days) of cyclophosphamide was more effective than the conventional maximum tolerated dose (150 mg/kg every other day for three doses every 21 days) in Lewis lung carcinoma and L1210 leukemia models; the antiangiogenic schedule was three times more effective in controlling growth of chemotherapy-resistant Lewis lung carcinoma and EMT-6 breast cancer cell lines (145). The addition of the angiogenesis inhibitor, TNP-470, to the antiangiogenic cyclophosphamide schedule induced endothelial cell apoptosis within tumors, an effect that preceded apoptosis of drug-resistant Lewis lung carcinomas. Low-dose vinblastine (0.75 mg/m^2 intraperitoneal with 1 mg/m^2 per day continuous infusion for three weeks followed by 1.5 mg/m^2 intraperitoneal twice per week) plus an antibody against the VEGF-receptor-2 controlled growth of neuroblastoma xenografts during 210 days of therapy (146). Similar findings have been reported with carboplatin plus a VEGF neutralizing antibody (147).

Thus far, only few clinical trials have tested antiangiogenic schedules of chemotherapy, so-called "metronomic therapy" (148). Nonetheless, the limited clinical evidence available is intriguing. Remissions can be induced, albeit infrequently, in patients resistant to taxane therapy administered on an every-3-week basis by altering the drug schedule. Specifically, Fennelly et al. (149) reported that 4 of 13 patients with ovarian cancer who had received and subsequently relapsed from prior paclitaxel therapy responded when treated with increasing doses of paclitaxel administered weekly (149). Moreover, 2 of these patients had progressed while receiving paclitaxel. Prolonged infusion paclitaxel (140 mg/m^2 over 96 hours) induced responses in 7 of 26 patients who had relapsed within a median of one month from prior short taxane infusions (150).

The European Organization for Research and Treatment of Cancer studied two CMF regimens: a classic 28-day regimen incorporating daily oral cyclophosphamide for 14 days and a modified intravenous schedule with bolus cyclophosphamide every 3 weeks. Overall response rate and survival clearly favored the classic regimen (151). Though generally viewed as a test of dose intensity (the classic regimen delivered higher total doses of both cyclophosphamide and 5-fluorouracil), this study may also be considered as a test of an antiangiogenic versus bolus schedule. A phase 2 study of low-dose methotrexate (2.5 mg twice daily for 2 days each week) and cyclophosphamide (50 mg daily) in patients with previously treated metastatic breast cancer found an overall response rate of 19% (an additional 13% of patients were stable for 6 months or more). Serum VEGF levels decreased in all patients remaining on therapy for at least 2 months but did not correlate with response (152).

ANGIOGENESIS INHIBITION IN THE CLINIC: PRELIMINARY DATA

Our burgeoning understanding of angiogenesis has fostered the development of agents targeting specific steps in the angiogeneic cascade, many of which have entered the clinic (Table 20.5). A detailed list of agents in clinical development can be obtained from the Angiogenesis Foundation (http://www.angiogenesis.org) or from the National Cancer Institute (http://cancernet.nci.nih.gov). While the number of ongoing phase 1 and 2 trials has grown rapidly, few have been reported in the peer-reviewed literature; no phase 3 trials in breast cancer have been completed. Rather than an exhaustive review of all agents currently in clinical testing, we have conceptually grouped agents into several categories: protease inhibitors, which either directly inhibit or otherwise interfere with the action of proteases critical for invasion; growth factor/receptor antagonists, which thwart signaling of proangiogenic growth factors; endothelial toxins, which specifically target endothelial antigens and natural inhibitors, which stimulate or mimic substances known to naturally inhibit angiogenesis. The clinical experience with representative agents in each category will be reviewed.

Protease Inhibitors

Degradation of the basement membrane and surrounding stroma by the MMPs is crucial for direct tissue invasion and angiogenesis. Inhibition of the MMPs decreases angiogenesis in preclinical systems and mouse xenografts (97, 153–158). Marimastat is a low molecular weight peptide mimetic containing a hydroxyamate group that chelates the zinc atom of the active site of the MMPs. Marimastat inhibits a broad spectrum of the MMPs and has activity in multiple human tumor xenograft models (159). Phase 1 trials identified musculoskeletal syndromes including arthralgia/arthritis, tendonitis, and bursitis as the dose-limiting toxicity with biologically active levels achieved in patients with advanced malignancy at doses ranging from 5 mg to 10 mg b.i.d. (160).

Though not predicted to induce substantial clinical response in patients with well-established bulky tumors, chronic therapy with an MMP inhibitor may delay or eliminate tumor regrowth after initial surgical excision or systemic chemotherapy. Two recently completed trials evaluated marimastat in breast cancer. ECOG-2196 measured time to progression in metastatic patients who were responding or stable after initial chemotherapy randomized to treatment with either marimastat or placebo. ECOG-2196 recently closed to accrual; preliminary results were expected in late 2001. In a limited institution phase 2 pilot study, 63 patients with early-stage breast cancer received marimastat at one of two dose levels either following doxorubicin-based chemotherapy or concomitantly with tamoxifen. Musculoskeletal toxicity resulted in significant dose reductions and limited chronic administration to doses yielding plasma levels below the target range (161).

BMS-275291 is a peptidimimetic MMP inhibitor that contains a chemically novel mercaptoacyl zinc-binding group. BMS-275291 inhibits a broad spectrum of MMPs without inhibiting the sheddases, related metalloproteinases which regulate pro-inflammatory cytokine and cytokine receptor shedding from the cell surface. BMS-275291 preserves the homeostasis of TNF-α and other proinflammatory cytokine and cytokine receptors hypothesized to play a role in the dose-limiting arthritis/arthralgia seen with other MMP inhibitors. A similar adjuvant pilot trial to

TABLE 20.5. *Representative antiangiogenic agents currently in clinical trials*

Agent	Phase	Pt. population	Combination therapy
Æ-941 (Neovastat)	II	Myeloma	
	III	Renal cell	
	III	IIIa/IIIb NSCLC	Platinum-based chemotherapy + RT
Angiostatin	I	All solid tumors	
	I	All solid tumors	RT
Avastin (rhuMab VEGF)	I	Advanced head and neck	5-fluorouracil + hydroxyurea + RT
	II	Relapsed myeloma	Thalidomide
	II	Colorectal	5-fluorouracil + leukovorin
	II	Renal cell, cervical, ovarian, lymphoma,	
	II	Hormone-refractory prostate	Docetaxel, estramustine
	II	Hematologic malignancies	Cytarabine, mitoxantrone
	II	Breast	Vinorelbine
	II	Ib-IIIa resectable NSCLC	Neoadjuvant paclitaxel + carboplatin
	II	Inflammatory breast	Neoadjuvant docetaxel + doxorubicin
	II/III	Colorectal	5-fluorouracil + leukovorin + CPT-11
	II/III	NSCLC	Paclitaxel + carboplatin
	II/III	Breast	Paclitaxel
	III	Breast	Capectabine
	III	Advanced colorectal	Oxaliplatin + 5-fluorouracil + leukovorin
BMS-275291	I/II	HIV-related Kaposi sarcoma	
	II	Ia-IIIa breast	Chemotherapy or tamoxifen
	II/III	NSCLC	Paclitaxel + carboplatin
Carboxyamodotriazole (CAI)	I	All solid tumor and lymphoma	Paclitaxel
	II	Renal cell, ovarian	
COL-3	I/II	Advanced solid tumors, glioma	
	II	HIV-related Kaposi sarcoma	
Celecoxib	I/II	Cervical	Cisplatin + 5-fluorouracil + RT
	II	Colorectal	5-fluorouracil + leukovorin + CPT-11
EMD-121974	I	All solid tumors	
	I/II	Glioma	
Endostatin	I/II	All solid tumors	
IM-862	II	Ovarian	Paclitaxel + carboplatin
	II	Colorectal	5-fluorouracil
Interleukin-12	I/II	HIV-related Kaposi sarcoma	Liposomal doxorubicin
Marimastat	III	Small cell lung	
2-methoxyestradiol	I	Breast, all solid tumors	
	I	Breast	Docetaxel
	II	Hormone-refractory prostate, myeloma	
RPI-4610	II	Renal cell	
Soy isoflavone	II	Breast	
Squalamine	II	Ovarian	Carboplatin
	II	Glioma	RT
SU-5416	I/II	All solid tumors, glioma, hematologic malignancies	
	I	All solid tumors	Paclitaxel
	I/II	Soft tissue sarcoma	Neoadjuvant RT
	I/II	Colorectal	CPT-11
	II	Renal cell	Interferon alfa-2b
	II	Hormone-refractory prostate	Dexamethasone
	III	Colorectal	5-fluorouracil + leukovorin + CPT-11
Suramin	II	Myeloma	
Thalidomide	I	Glioma	Topotecan
	I/II	Melanoma	Temozolomide
	II	Myelodysplastic syndromes, colorectal, ovarian, uterine sarcoma, endometrial, chronic lymphocytic leukemia, low-grade lymphoma, hepatocellular	

continued

TABLE 20.5. Continued

Agent	Phase	Pt. population	Combination therapy
Thalidomide (cont.)	II	Ovarian	Carboplatin
		Hormone-refractory prostate	Docetaxel
	II	Myeloma	Prednisone
	II	Chronic lymphocytic leukemia	Fludarabine
	II	NSCLC	Carboplatin + CPT-11
	II	Low-grade lymphoma, hepatocellular	Interferon-alfa
	II	Hepatocellular	Doxorubicin chemoembolization
	III	NSCLC	Carboplatin + paclitaxel + RT
	III	Myeloma	Dexamethasone + cyclophosphamide + etoposide + cisplatin
	III	Renal cell	Interferon alfa-2b
	III	Prostate	Hormone ablation

NSCLC, nonsmall cell lung carcinoma; RT, radiation therapy.
From http://cancernet.nci.nih.gov, with permission.

that with marimastat is ongoing with this agent.

Pro-Angiogenic Growth Factor/Receptor Antagonists

Angiogenesis requires stimulation of vascular endothelial cells through the release of angiogenic peptides, including VEGF. An antibody directed against VEGF inhibited the growth of several human tumors in animal models (162,163); a humanized recombinant version of this antibody has entered clinical trials. RhuMAb-VEGF was well tolerated and produced the expected decrease in free plasma VEGF levels in a multicenter phase 1 trial of 25 patients. Three patients had tumor-related bleeding episodes, including an intracranial hemorrhage into an unrecognized cerebral metastasis in a patient with hepatocellular carcinoma. Though no objective responses were seen, 14 patients had stable disease at evaluation on day 72 (164). A dual-institution phase 2 study of rhuMAb-VEGF in patients with previously treated metastatic breast cancer has recently been completed with 75 patients in three successive dose cohorts: 3 mg/kg (n = 18), 10 mg/kg (n = 41), and 20 mg/kg (n = 16) every other week. Overall, 17% of patients were responding or stable at 22 weeks; three patients continued therapy without progression for over 12 months. Therapy was generally well tolerated with mild hypertension and proteinuria in several patients; no significant bleeding episodes were noted (165).

Inhibition of the VEGF receptor tyrosine kinase domain (Flk-1 and Flt-1) also represents a fruitful therapeutic target. The critical role of Flk-1 in tumor angiogenesis was demonstrated using a dominant-negative Flk-1 transfectant. Eight of nine tumor cell lines with dominant negative Flk-1 showed growth inhibition and reduced MVD in athymic mice (166). A synthetic inhibitor of the Flk-1 kinase has been developed (SU-5416) that inhibits VEGF-dependent growth of endothelial cells without altering tumor growth *in vitro*. Systemic administration of SU-5416 inhibited the growth of human tumors in mice without apparent toxicity (167,168). SU-5416 was well tolerated in a phase 1 clinical trial with dose-limiting toxicity being a severe migraine syndrome with headache and projectile vomiting (169,170). Co-administration of SU-5416 and doxorubicin did not alter pharmacokinetics of either agent and produced no unexpected toxicity (171). A phase 3 trial in colorectal cancer as well as multiple disease-specific phase 2 trials are ongoing. ZD6474, an oral inhibitor of the Flk-1 tyrosine kinase that also inhibits the epidermal growth factor receptor tyrosine kinase, has also entered clinical development (172).

Ribozymes are small RNA elements with specific catalytic activity. Angiozyme is a synthetic ribozyme designed to cleave the messenger RNA for the VEGF Flt-1 receptor. Preclinical studies confirmed inhibition of both primary tumor growth and metastasis (173–175). A phase 1 study in patients with refractory solid tumors found limited toxicity and no evidence of drug accumulation. Immunohistochemical staining of accessible tumor samples found variable VEGF Flk-1 and Flt-1 expression with Angiozyme localized to tumor endothelial cells. Multiple disease-specific phase 2 studies are underway.

PNU-145156E (formerly FCE26644), a sulfonated distamycin A derivative, is a noncytotoxic molecule whose antitumor activity is exerted through the formation of a reversible complex with growth/angiogenic factors (177, 178). In vitro PNU-145156E did not modify the cytotoxicity induced by several chemotherapeutic agents. However, in vivo, at the optimal dose of each compound, the antitumor activity was significantly increased in all combinations, with no associated increase in general toxicity. In healthy mice treated with cyclophosphamide or doxorubicin the addition of PNU-145156E did not enhance the myelotoxic effect (179,180). In phase 1 testing, PNU-145156E induced an unpredictable and short-lasting decrease in antithrombin III levels without effects on serum FGF or VEGF concentrations (181).

Endothelial Toxins

The antibiotic-like antiangiogenic TNP-470 (AGM-1470) inhibits endothelial cell proliferation and entered clinical trials nearly a decade ago (182–184). Phase 1 studies found reversible dose-dependent neurological toxicity; only one transient objective response was reported though several patients had stabilization of disease (185,186). The half-life of TNP-470 was extremely short with practically no drug detectable an hour after treatment, suggesting alternate treatment schedules might be required for maximal activity (187,188).

Disruption of endothelial cell chemotaxis and migration interferes with angiogenesis. The integrins, particularly $\alpha_v\beta_3$, provide critical attachment between the migrating endothelial cell and the extracellular matrix (189); $\alpha_v\beta_3$ also localizes MMP-2 to the membrane of endothelial cells in the leading podosomes of new vessels providing carefully targeted matrix destruction (190). Moreover, immunohistochemical studies of clinical specimens from ocular pathologies suggest that both $\alpha_v\beta_3$ and $\alpha_v\beta_5$ are of importance for endothelial cell function in angiogenic neovascular disease (191). Antibodies which block $\alpha_v\beta_3$ inhibit angiogenesis and tumor growth in vitro (192) and in vivo (193). A humanized monoclonal antibody against $\alpha_v\beta_3$, vitaxin, was well tolerated and showed some activity in a phase 1 trial (194). Phase 2 trials are ongoing.

Specific antibodies used to characterize the vitronectin receptors $\alpha_v\beta_3$ and $\alpha_v\beta_5$ in vitro were employed to study the function of these integrins in vivo (195). The RGD (arg-gly-asp) epitope is critical for the function of many β_1 integrins and is the same epitope that $\alpha_v\beta_3$ recognizes in its extracellular matrix ligands. This has led to the development of a family of RGD-containing peptides that can serve as potent and selective inhibitors of the vitronectin receptors. EMD 121,974 is the inner salt of a cyclized pentapeptide c [Arg-Asp-DPhe-(NMeVal)], with significant antiangiogenic activity in a variety of preclinical in vitro and in vivo models. Phase 1 trials of EMD 121,974 are ongoing.

Resting endothelial cells are normally quiescent; proliferation increases dramatically in the leading podosomes of new capillaries. The protein endoglin is expressed much more strongly in growing tumor microvasculature than in the vasculature of surrounding normal tissues. Antibodies directed against endoglin decreased tumor growth in mice xenografts (88,196). Antiendoglin antibodies complexed to deglycosylated ricin A chain produced long-lasting complete remission of preformed tumors in immunocompromised mice (91,92).

Natural Inhibitors

The exact mechanism of action of angiostatin remains unclear; however, angiostatin binds ATP-synthase on the surface of endothelial cells inducing endothelial cell apoptosis (197–199). A phase 1 study of recombinant human angiostatin-treated patients with refractory solid tumors with doses ranging from 15 mg to 240 mg/m² as a daily 10-minute intravenous infusion. No dose-limiting toxicity or changes in coagulation factors were identified. Pharmocokinetics were linear with dose-proportionate increases in both peak concentration and total exposure. Antibodies to rhu-angiostatin were identified in 2 of 15 patients and did not appear clinically significant. No objective responses were reported, though some patients had measurable decreases in urine bFGF and VEGF levels (200). Treatment with angiostatin increased sensitivity to radiation in preclinical models (201,202), providing support for an ongoing phase 1 trial of angiostatin with radiation.

Endostatin, a 20-kD proteolytic fragment of collagen XVIII, has antiangiogenic activity similar to angiostatin (203). Endostatin has a highly basic region with significant affinity for heparin, suggesting that binding to heparin sulphate proteoglycans involved in growth factor signaling may be partly responsible for its activity (204). In addition, endostatin binds to tropomyosin *in vitro* and to tropomyosin-associated microfilaments in endothelial cells; a peptide that mimics the endostatin-binding epitope of tropomyosin and blocks endostatin anti-tumor activity. Thus disruption of microfilament integrity seems central to endostatin activity (205).

Phase 1 studies of endostatin have recently been reported (206–208). Patients with refractory solid tumors received daily bolus infusions ranging from 15 mg to 300 mg/m² with no apparent toxicity. Pharmacokinetics were linear (209); endostatin treatment had no effect on physiologic wound healing (210). Correlative studies found dose-dependent decreases in tumor associated blood flow with ^{15}O PET scanning and dynamic CT imaging, increased tumor apoptosis, and decreases in peripheral blood endothelial cell colony forming precursors.

A naturally occurring metabolite of estradiol, 2-methoxyestradiol (2ME2), has a dual mechanism of action: (a) as an antiproliferative drug acting directly on the tumor cell compartment; and (b) as an antiangiogenic drug acting on tumor vasculature. *In vitro*, 2ME2 exhibits antiproliferative activity in tumor cell lines with IC_{50} values generally in the submicromolar to low micromolar range independent of the estrogen responsiveness of the cell line. *In vivo*, 2ME2 is effective in xenograft and metastatic disease models (142,211,212). The antiangiogenic activity of 2ME2 has been demonstrated *in vivo* in corneal micropocket (142) and CAM systems (213), as well as by the observation of reduced tumor vasculature in 2ME2-treated mice. *In vitro*, 2ME2 inhibits tubule formation in bovine microvascular endothelial cells stimulated by basic fibroblast growth factor (bFGF) (211) and the proliferation of human umbilical vein endothelial cells (214). Several mechanisms of action of 2ME2 treatment in certain cell lines have been suggested including: (a) induction of apoptosis, possibly through the activation of p53 (215); and (b) slowing the rate, but not the degree, of tubulin depolymerization (216) and inhibition of superoxide dismutase resulting in increased oxidative stress (217).

Preliminary results of an ongoing phase 1 study of 2ME2 in patients with previously treated metastatic breast cancer have been reported (218). No dose-limiting toxicity was identified with doses ranging from 200 mg to 1,000 mg once daily. Metabolism was variable with a half-life was approximately 10 to 12 hours. Conversion to 2-methoxyestrone, an inactive metabolite, was significant with 2ME1 concentrations generally 10-fold higher than 2ME2 levels. No objective responses were produced though prolonged disease stabilization was achieved in several patients. Changes in VEGF and bFGF levels were inconsistent. Accrual continues with a twice daily dosing schedule. A phase 1 study of 2ME2 in combination with docetaxel in patients with newly diagnosed metastatic breast cancer completed accrual in late 2001 but has not yet been reported.

CONCLUSION

Initial laboratory studies and assertions of a "therapy resistant to resistance" produced enthusiasm almost unparalleled in the history of cancer treatments. The lessons of history seem likely to repeat—antiangiogenic therapy is neither devoid of toxicity nor resistance (130,219). The theoretical basis is strong, the laboratory and preclinical data persuasive. Nonetheless, only in carefully conducted prospective clinical trials will the role of angiogenesis inhibition be proven. While the early rampant enthusiasm has damped, cautious optimism remains appropriate. Unless we have completely misunderstood the biology of the disease, antiangiogenic agents will expand our therapeutic arsenal. Dimming cancer's blood tide should go far to controlling the mere anarchy of the disease. With the clinical trials currently underway, the next several years should see us measurably closer to that goal.

REFERENCES

1. Folkman J. What is the evidence that tumors are angiogenesis dependent? *J Natl Cancer Inst* 1990;82:4–6.
2. Pepper MS, Mandriota SJ, Vassalli JD, et al. Angiogenesis-regulating cytokines: activities and interactions. *Curr Top Microbiol Immunol* 1996;213:31–67.
3. Brown JM, Giaccia AJ. The unique physiology of solid tumors: opportunities (and problems) for cancer therapy. *Cancer Res* 1998;58:1408–1416.
4. Brem SS, Gullino PM, Medina D. Angiogenesis: a marker for neoplastic transformation of mammary papillary hyperplasia. *Science* 1977;195:880–882.
5. Jensen HM, Chen I, DeVault MR, et al. Angiogenesis induced by "normal" human breast tissue: a probable marker for precancer. *Science* 1982;218:293–295.
6. Kurebayashi J, McLeskey SW, Johnson MD, et al. Quantitative demonstration of spontaneous metastasis by MCF-7 human breast cancer cells cotransfected with fibroblast growth factor 4 and LacZ. *Cancer Res* 1993;53:2178–2187.
7. McLeskey SW, Zhang L, Kharbanda S, et al. Fibroblast growth factor overexpressing breast carcinoma cells as models of angiogenesis and metastasis. *Breast Cancer Res Treat* 1996;39:103–117.
8. Zhang HT, Craft P, Scott PA, et al. Enhancement of tumor growth and vascular density by transfection of vascular endothelial cell growth factor into MCF-7 human breast carcinoma cells. *J Natl Cancer Inst* 1995;87:213–219.
9. McLeskey SW, Tobias CA, Vezza PR, et al. Tumor growth of FGF or VEGF transfected MCF-7 breast carcinoma cells correlates with density of specific microvessels independent of the transfected angiogenic factor. *Am J Pathol* 1998;153:1993–2006.
10. Nakajima M, Welch DR, Wynn DM, et al. Serum and plasma M(r) 92,000 progelatinase levels correlate with spontaneous metastasis of rat 13762NF mammary adenocarcinoma. *Cancer Res* 1993;53:5802–5807.
11. Giunciuglio D, Culty M, Fassina G, et al. Invasive phenotype of MCF10A cells overexpressing c-Ha-ras and c-erbB-2 oncogenes. *Int J Cancer* 1995;63:815–822.
12. Weinstat-Saslow DL, Zabrenetzky VS, VanHoutte K, et al. Transfection of thrombospondin 1 complementary DNA into a human breast carcinoma cell line reduces primary tumor growth, metastatic potential, and angiogenesis. *Cancer Res* 1994;54:6504–6511.
13. Wang M, Liu YE, Greene J, et al. Inhibition of tumor growth and metastasis of human breast cancer cells transfected with tissue inhibitor of metalloproteinase 4. *Oncogene* 1997;14:2767–2774.
14. Liotta LA, Steeg PS, Stetler-Stevenson WG. Cancer metastasis and angiogenesis: an imbalance of positive and negative regulation. *Cell* 1991;64:327–336.
15. Monteagudo C, Merino MJ, San-Juan J, et al. Immunohistochemical distribution of type IV collagenase in normal, benign, and malignant breast tissue. *Am J Pathol* 1990;136:585–592.
16. Kossakowska AE, Huchcroft SA, Urbanski SJ, et al. Comparative analysis of the expression patterns of metalloproteinases and their inhibitors in breast neoplasia, sporadic colorectal neoplasia, pulmonary carcinomas and malignant non-Hodgkin's lymphomas in humans. *Br J Cancer* 1996;73:1401–1408.
17. Folkman J, Hanahan D. Switch to the angiogenic phenotype during tumorigenesis. *Princess Takamatsu Symp* 1991;22:339–347.
18. Holmgren L, O'Reilly MS, Folkman J. Dormancy of micrometastases: balanced proliferation and apoptosis in the presence of angiogenesis suppression [see comments]. *Nat Med* 1995;1:149–153.
19. Azzam HS, Arand G, Lippman ME, et al. Association of MMP-2 activation potential with metastatic progression in human breast cancer cell lines independent of MMP-2 production. *J Natl Cancer Inst* 1993;85:1758–1764.
20. Wang GL, Jiang BH, Rue EA, et al. Hypoxia-inducible factor 1 is a basic-helix-loop-helix-PAS heterodimer regulated by cellular O_2 tension. *Proc Natl Acad Sci USA* 1995;92:5510–5514.
21. Salceda S, Caro J. Hypoxia-inducible factor 1alpha (HIF-1alpha) protein is rapidly degraded by the ubiquitin-proteasome system under normoxic conditions. Its stabilization by hypoxia depends on redox-induced changes. *J Biol Chem* 1997;272:22642–22647.
22. Jewell UR, Kvietikova I, Scheid A, et al. Induction of HIF-1alpha in response to hypoxia is instantaneous. *FASEB J* 2001;15:1312–1314.
23. Wenger RH, Gassmann M. Oxygen(es) and the hypoxia-inducible factor-1. *Biol Chem* 1997;378:609–616.
24. Peng J, Zhang L, Drysdale L, et al. The transcription factor EPAS-1/hypoxia-inducible factor 2alpha plays an important role in vascular remodeling. *Proc Natl Acad Sci USA* 2000;97:8386–8391.
25. Ema M, Taya S, Yokotani N, et al. A novel bHLH-PAS factor with close sequence similarity to hypoxia-inducible factor 1alpha regulates the VEGF expression and is potentially involved in lung and vascular development. *Proc Natl Acad Sci USA* 1997;94:4273–4278.
26. Blancher C, Moore J, Talks K, et al. Relationship of hypoxia-inducible factor (HIF)-1alpha and HIF-2alpha expression to vascular endothelial growth factor induction and hypoxia survival in human breast cancer cell lines. *Cancer Res* 2000;60:7106–7113.
27. Bos R, Zhong H, Hanrahan CF, et al. Levels of hypoxia-inducible factor-1 alpha during breast carcinogenesis. *J Natl Cancer Inst* 2001;93:309–314.

28. Chia SK, Wykoff CC, Watson PH, et al. Prognostic significance of a novel hypoxia-regulated marker, carbonic anhydrase IX, in invasive breast carcinoma. *J Clin Oncol* 2001;19:3660–3668.
29. Wykoff CC, Beasley NJ, Watson PH, et al. Hypoxia-inducible expression of tumor-associated carbonic anhydrases. *Cancer Res* 2000;60:7075–7083.
30. Guinebretiere JM, Le Monique G, Gavoille A, et al. Angiogenesis and risk of breast cancer in women with fibrocystic disease [letter; comment]. *J Natl Cancer Inst* 1994;86:635–636.
31. Engels K, Fox SB, Whitehouse RM, et al. Distinct angiogenic patterns are associated with high-grade in situ ductal carcinomas of the breast. *J Pathol* 1997;181:207–212.
32. Guidi AJ, Fischer L, Harris JR, et al. Microvessel density and distribution in ductal carcinoma in situ of the breast. *J Natl Cancer Inst* 1994;86:614–619.
33. Guidi AJ, Schnitt SJ, Fischer L, et al. Vascular permeability factor (vascular endothelial growth factor) expression and angiogenesis in patients with ductal carcinoma in situ of the breast. *Cancer* 1997;80:1945–1953.
34. Weidner N, Semple J, Welch W, et al. Tumor angiogenesis and metastasis—correlation in invasive breast cancer. *N Engl J Med* 1991;324:1–8.
35. Weidner N, Folkman J, Pozza F, et al. Tumor angiogenesis: a new significant and independent prognostic indicator in early stage brest carcinoma. *J Natl Cancer Inst* 1992;84:1875–1887.
36. Horak E, Leek R, Klenk N. Angiogenesis, assessed by platelet/endothelial cell adhesion molecule antibodies, as indicator of node metastasis and survival in breast cancer. *Lancet* 1992;340:1120–1124.
37. Martin L, Green B, Renshaw C, et al. Examining the technique of angiogenesis assessment in invasive breast cancer. *Br J Cancer* 1997;76:40–43.
38. Simpson J, Ahn C, Battifora H, et al. Endothelial area as a prognostic indicator for invasive for invasive breast carcinoma. *Cancer* 1996;77:2077–2085.
39. Vermeulen PB, Libura M, Libura J, et al. Influence of investigator experience and microscopic field size on microvessel density in node-negative breast carcinoma. *Breast Cancer Res Treat* 1997;42:165–172.
40. Weidner N. Current pathologic methods for measuring intratumoral microvessel density within breast carcinoma and other solid tumors. *Breast Cancer Treat Res* 1995;36:169–180.
41. Fox SB, Leek RD, Weekes MP, et al. Quantitation and prognostic value of breast cancer angiogenesis: comparison of microvessel density, Chalkley count, and computer image analysis. *J Pathol* 1995;177:275–283.
42. de Jong JS, van Diest PJ, Baak JP. Heterogeneity and reproducibility of microvessel counts in breast cancer. *Lab Invest* 1995;73:922–926.
43. McCulloch P, Choy A, Martin L. Association between tumour angiogenesis and tumour cell shedding into effluent venous blood during breast cancer surgery [see comments]. *Lancet* 1995;346:1334–1335.
44. Fox S, Leek R, Bliss J, et al. Association of tumor angiogenesis with bone marrow micrometastases in breast cancer patients. *J Natl Cancer Inst* 1997;89:1044–1049.
45. Relf M, LeJeune S, Scott PA, et al. Expression of the angiogenic factors vascular endothelial cell growth factor, acidic and basic fibroblast growth factor, tumor growth factor beta-1, platelet-derived endothelial cell growth factor, placenta growth factor, and pleiotrophin in human primary breast cancer and its relation to angiogenesis. *Cancer Res* 1997;57:963–969.
46. Foekens JA, Peters HA, Grebenchtchikov N, et al. High tumor levels of vascular endothelial growth factor predict poor response to systemic therapy in advanced breast cancer. *Cancer Res* 2001;61:5407–5414.
47. Eppenberger U, Kueng W, Schlaeppi JM, et al. Markers of tumor angiogenesis and proteolysis independently define high- and low-risk subsets of node-negative breast cancer patients. *J Clin Oncol* 1998;16:3129–3136.
48. Malmstrom P, Bendahl PO, Boiesen P, et al. S-phase fraction and urokinase plasminogen activator are better markers for distant recurrences than Nottingham Prognostic Index and histologic grade in a prospective study of premenopausal lymph node-negative breast cancer. *J Clin Oncol* 2001;19:2010–2019.
49. Thomssen C, Prechtl A, Polcher M, et al. Interim analysis of a randomized trial of risk-adapted adjuvant chemotherapy in node-negative breast cancer patients guided by the prognostic factors uPA and PAI-1. *Breast Care Res Treat* 1999;57:25.
50. Gasparini G, Brooks PC, Biganzoli E, et al. Vascular integrin alpha(v)beta3: a new prognostic indicator in breast cancer. *Clin Cancer Res* 1998;4:2625–2634.
51. Daidone MG, Silvestrini R, D'Errico A, et al. Laminin receptors, collagenase IV and prognosis in node-negative breast cancers. *Int J Cancer* 1991;48:529–532.
52. Zajchowski DA, Band V, Trask DK, et al. Suppression of tumor-forming ability and related traits in MCF-7 human breast cancer cells by fusion with immortal mammary epithelial cells. *Proc Natl Acad Sci USA* 1990;87:2314–2318.
53. Sledge G, Gordon M. Therapeutic implications of angiogenesis inhibition. *Sem Oncol* 1998;25:59–65.
54. Korn EL, Arbuck SG, Pluda JM, et al. Clinical trial designs for cytostatic agents: are new approaches needed? *J Clin Oncol* 2001;19:265–272.
55. Hahnfeldt P, Panigrahy D, Folkman J, et al. Tumor development under angiogenic signaling: A dynamic theory of tumor growth, treatment response, and postvascular dormancy. *Cancer Res* 1999;59:4770–4775.
56. Dvorak HF, Detmar M, Claffey KP, et al. Vascular permeability factor/vascular endothelial growth factor: an important mediator of angiogenesis in malignancy and inflammation. *Int Arch Allergy Immunol* 1995;107:233–235.
57. Ferrara N, Davis-Smyth T. The biology of vascular endothelial growth factor. *Endocrinol Rev* 1997, 1997.
58. Dirix L, Vermeulen P, Pawinski A, et al. elevated levels of the angiogenic cytokines basic fibroblast growth factor and vascular endothelial growth factor in the sera of cancer patients. *Br J Cancer* 1997;76:238–243.
59. Salven P, Perhoniemi V, Tykka H, et al. Serum VEGF levels in women with a benign breast tumor or breast cancer. *Breast Cancer Res Treat* 1999;53:161–166.
60. Yamamoto Y, Toi M, Kondo S, et al. Concentrations of vascular endothelial growth factor in the sera of normal controls and cancer patients. *Clin Cancer Res* 1996;2:821–826.

61. Verheul H, Hoekman K, Luykx-de Bakker S, et al. Platelet: Transporter of vascular endothelial growth factor. *Clin Cancer Res* 1997;3:2187–2190.
62. Wynendaele W, Derua R, Hoylaerts M, et al. Vascular endothelial growth factor measured in platelet poor plasma allows optimal separation between cancer patients and volunteers: A key to study an angiogenic marker in vivo? *Ann Oncol* 1999;10:965–971.
63. Adams J, Carder P, Downey S, et al. Vascular endothelial growth factor (VEGF) in breast cancer: comparison of plasma, serum, and tissue VEGF and microvessel density and effects of tamoxifen. *Cancer Res* 2000;60:2898–2905.
64. Braybrooke JP, O'Byrne KJ, Propper DJ, et al. A phase II study of razoxane, an antiangiogenic topoisomerase II inhibitor, in renal cell cancer with assessment of potential surrogate markers of angiogenesis. *Clin Cancer Res* 2000;6:4697–4704.
65. Crew JP, O'Brien T, Bicknell R, et al. Urinary vascular endothelial growth factor and its correlation with bladder cancer recurrence rates [see comments]. *J Urol* 1999;161:799–804.
66. Eisen T, Boshoff C, Mak I, et al. Continuous low dose Thalidomide: a phase II study in advanced melanoma, renal cell, ovarian and breast cancer. *Br J Cancer* 2000;82:812–817.
67. Honkanen EO, Teppo AM, Gronhagen-Riska C. Decreased urinary excretion of vascular endothelial growth factor in idiopathic membranous glomerulonephritis. *Kidney Int* 2000;57:2343–2349.
68. Kitamoto Y, Matsuo K, Tomita K. Different response of urinary excretion of VEGF in patients with chronic and acute renal failure. *Kidney Int* 2001;59:385–386.
69. Zon R, Neuberg D, Wood W, et al. Correlation of plasma VEGF with clinical outcome in patients with metastatic breast cancer. *Proc Am Soc Clin Oncol* 1998;17:185.
70. Byrne G, Blann A, Venizelos J, et al. Serum soluble VCAM: A surrogate marker of angiogenesis. *Breast Cancer Treat Res* 1998;50:330.
71. Zelinski DP, Zantek ND, Stewart JC, et al. EphA2 overexpression causes tumorigenesis of mammary epithelial cells. *Cancer Res* 2001;61:2301–2306.
72. Rice GE, Bevilacqua MP. An inducible endothelial cell surface glycoprotein mediates melanoma adhesion. *Science* 1989;246:1303–1306.
73. Zetter BR. Adhesion molecules in tumor metastasis [see comments]. *Semin Cancer Biol* 1993;4:219–229.
74. Kim II, Moon SO, Kim SH, et al. VEGF stimulates expression of ICAM-1, VCAM-1 and E-selectin through nuclear factor-kappaB activation in endothelial cells. *J Biol Chem* 2000;6:6.
75. Fukushi J, Ono M, Morikawa W, et al. The activity of soluble VCAM-1 in angiogenesis stimulated by IL-4 and IL-13. *J Immunol* 2000;165:2818–2823.
76. Osborn L, Hession C, Tizard R, et al. Direct expression cloning of vascular cell adhesion molecule 1, a cytokine-induced endothelial protein that binds to lymphocytes. *Cell* 1989;59:1203–1211.
77. Ali S, Kaur J, Patel KD. Intercellular cell adhesion molecule-1, vascular cell adhesion molecule-1, and regulated on activation normal T cell expressed and secreted are expressed by human breast carcinoma cells and support eosinophil adhesion and activation. *Am J Pathol* 2000;157:313–321.
78. Gnant MF, Turner EM, Alexander HR. Effects of hyperthermia and tumour necrosis factor on inflammatory cytokine secretion and procoagulant activity in endothelial cells. *Cytokine* 2000;12:339–347.
79. Koch AE, Halloran MM, Haskell CJ, et al. Angiogenesis mediated by soluble forms of E-selectin and vascular cell adhesion molecule-1. *Nature* 1995;376:517–519.
80. Scola MP, Imagawa T, Boivin GP, et al. Expression of angiogenic factors in juvenile rheumatoid arthritis: correlation with revascularization of human synovium engrafted into SCID mice. *Arthritis Rheum* 2001;44:794–801.
81. Nor JE, Peters MC, Christensen JB, et al. Engineering and characterization of functional human microvessels in immunodeficient mice. *Lab Invest* 2001;81:453–463.
82. Kolopp-Sarda MN, Guillemin F, Chary-Valckenaere I, et al. Longitudinal study of rheumatoid arthritis patients discloses sustained elevated serum levels of soluble CD106 (V-CAM). *Clin Exp Rheumatol* 2001;19:165–170.
83. Kuehn R, Lelkes PI, Bloechle C, et al. Angiogenesis, angiogenic growth factors, and cell adhesion molecules are upregulated in chronic pancreatic diseases: angiogenesis in chronic pancreatitis and in pancreatic cancer. *Pancreas* 1999;18:96–103.
84. Dosquet C, Coudert MC, Lepage E, et al. Are angiogenic factors, cytokines, and soluble adhesion molecules prognostic factors in patients with renal cell carcinoma? *Clin Cancer Res* 1997;3:2451–2458.
85. Lynch DF Jr, Hassen W, Clements MA, et al. Serum levels of endothelial and neural cell adhesion molecules in prostate cancer. *Prostate* 1997;32:214–220.
86. Banks RE, Gearing AJ, Hemingway IK, et al. Circulating intercellular adhesion molecule-1 (ICAM-1), E-selectin and vascular cell adhesion molecule-1 (VCAM-1) in human malignancies. *Br J Cancer* 1993;68:122–124.
87. Regidor PA, Callies R, Regidor M, et al. Expression of the cell adhesion molecules ICAM-1 and VCAM-1 in the cytosol of breast cancer tissue, benign breast tissue and corresponding sera. *Eur J Gynaecol Oncol* 1998;19:377–383.
88. Burrows FJ, Derbyshire EJ, Tazzari PL, et al. Upregulation of endoglin on vascular endothelial cells in human solid tumors: implications for diagnosis and therapy. *Clin Cancer Res* 1995;1:1623–1634.
89. Bodey B, Bodey B Jr, Siegel SE, et al. Overexpression of endoglin (CD105): a marker of breast carcinoma-induced neo-vascularization. *Anticancer Res* 1998;18:3621–3628.
90. Li D, Sorensen L, Brook B, et al. Defective angiogenesis in mice lacking endoglin. *Science* 1999;284:1534–1537.
91. Matsuno F, Haruto Y, Kondo M, et al. Induction of lasting complete regression of preformed distinct solid tumors by targeting the tumor vasculature using two new anti-endoglin monoclonal antibodies. *Clin Cancer Res* 1999;5:371–382.
92. Seon B, Matsuno F, Haruto Y, et al. Long-lasting complete inhibition of human solid tumors in SCID mice by targeting endothelial cells of tumor vasculature with antihuman endoglin immunotoxin. *Clin Cancer Res* 1997;3:1031–1044.

93. Kumar S, Ghellal A, Li C, et al. Breast carcinoma: vascular density determined using CD105 antibody correlates with tumor prognosis. *Cancer Res* 1999;59: 856–861.
94. Li C, Guo B, Wilson PB, et al. Plasma levels of soluble CD105 correlate with metastasis in patients with breast cancer. *Int J Cancer* 2000;89:122–126.
95. Takahashi N, Kawanishi-Tabata R, Haba A, et al. Association of serum endoglin with metastasis in patients with colorectal, breast, and other solid tumors, and suppressive effect of chemotherapy on the serum endoglin. *Clin Cancer Res* 2001;7:524–532.
96. Matrisian LM. Metalloproteinases and their inhibitors in matrix remodeling. *Trends Genet* 1990;6:121–125.
97. Kurizaki T, Toi M, Tominaga T. Relationship between matrix metalloproteinase expression and tumor angiogenesis in human breast carcinoma. *Oncol Rep* 1998; 5:673–677.
98. Colomer R, Aparicio J, Montero S, et al. Low levels of nasic fibroblast growth factor (bFGF) are associated with prognosis in breast cancer. *Br J Cancer* 1997;76:1215–1220.
99. Dirix LY, Vermeulen PB, Pawinski A, et al. Elevated levels of the angiogenic cytokines basic fibroblast growth factor and vascular endothelial growth factor in sera of cancer patients. *Br J Cancer* 1997;76: 238–243.
100. Nguyen M, Watanabe H, Budson A, et al. Elevated levels of an angiogenic peptide, basic fibroblast growth factor, in the urine of patients with a wide spectrum of cancers. *J Natl Cancer Inst* 1994;86: 356–361.
101. Folkman J. Tumour angiogenesis: Diagnostic and therapeutic implications. *Am Assoc Cancer Res* 1993; 34:571–572.
102. Sliutz G, Tempfer C, Obermair A, et al. Serum evaluation of basic FGF in breast cancer patients. *Anticancer Res* 1995;15:2675–2677.
103. Pichon M, Moulin G, Pallud C, et al. Serum bFGF (basic fibroblast growth factor) and CA15.3 in the follow-up of breast cancer patients. *Anticancer Res* 2000;10:1189–1194.
104. Nishimura R, Nagao K, Miyayama H, et al. An analysis of serum interleukin-6 levels to predict benefits of medroxyprogesterone acetate in advanced or recurrent breast cancer. *Oncology* 2000;59:166–173.
105. Poon RT, Fan ST, Wong J. Clinical implications of circulating angiogenic factors in cancer patients. *J Clin Oncol* 2001;19:1207–1225.
106. Peters-Engl C, Medl M, Mirau M, et al. Color-coded and spectral Doppler flow in breast carcinomas—relationship with the tumor microvasculature. *Breast Cancer Res Treat* 1998;47:83–89.
107. Peters-Engl C, Frank W, Medl M. Tumor flow in malignant breast tumors measured by Doppler ultrasound: An independent predictor of survival. *Breast Cancer Treat Res* 1998;50:228.
108. Bhlomer J, Gohlke A, Hufnagel P, et al. Correlation between morphologic parameters of vascularization, color Doppler image features and lymph node metastasis in breast cancer. *Breast Cancer Res Treat* 1998; 50:331.
109. Kedar RP, Cosgrove DO, Smith IE, et al. Breast carcinoma: measurement of tumor response to primary medical therapy with color Doppler flow imaging. *Radiology* 1994;190:825–830.
110. Ferrara KW, Merritt CR, Burns PN, et al. Evaluation of tumor angiogenesis with US: imaging, Doppler, and contrast agents. *Acad Radiol* 2000;7:824–839.
111. Foltz RM, McLendon RE, Friedman HS, et al. A pial window model for the intracranial study of human glioma microvascular function. *Neurosurgery* 1995; 36:976–984; discussion 984–985.
112. Chaudhari MH, Forsberg F, Voodarla A, et al. Breast tumor vascularity identified by contrast enhanced ultrasound and pathology: initial results. *Ultrasonics* 2000;38:105–109.
113. Jansson T, Westlin JE, Ahlstrom H, et al. Positron emission tomography studies in patients with locally advanced and/or metastatic breast cancer: a method for early therapy evaluation? *J Clin Oncol* 1995;13: 1470–1477.
114. Bassa P, Kim EE, Inoue T, et al. Evaluation of preoperative chemotherapy using PET with fluorine-18-fluorodeoxyglucose in breast cancer. *J Nucl Med* 1996;37:931–938.
115. Wahl RL, Zasadny K, Helvie M, et al. Metabolic monitoring of breast cancer chemohormonotherapy using positron emission tomography: initial evaluation. *J Clin Oncol* 1993;11:2101–2111.
116. Arslan N, Ozturk E, Ilgan S, et al. 99Tcm-MIBI scintimammography in the evaluation of breast lesions and axillary involvement: a comparison with mammography and histopathological diagnosis. *Nucl Med Commun* 1999;20:317–325.
117. Mankoff D, Dunnwald L, Gralow J, et al. Monitoring the response of patients with locally advanced breast carcinoma to neoadjuvant chemotherapy using technetium 99m-sestamibi scintimammography. *Cancer* 1999;85:2410–2423.
118. Yoon J-H, Bom H-S, Song H-C, et al. Double-phase Tc-99m sestamibi scintimammography to assess angiogenesis with P-glycoprotein expression in patients with untreated breast cancer. *Clin Nuc Med* 1999;24: 314–318.
119. Wilson CB, Lammertsma AA, McKenzie CG, et al. Measurements of blood flow and exchanging water space in breast tumors using positron emission tomography: a rapid and noninvasive dynamic method. *Cancer Res* 1992;52:1592–1597.
120. Martin G, Caldwell J, Graham M, et al. Noninvasive detection of hypoxic myocardium using fluorine-18-fluoromisonidazole and positron emission tomography. *J Nucl Med* 1992;33:2202–2208.
121. Ogawa T, Uemura K, Shishido F, et al. Changes of cerebral blood flow and oxygen and glucose metabolism following radiochemotherapy of gliomas: a PET study. *J Comput Assist Tomog* 1988;12:290–297.
122. Blankenberg FG, Eckelman WC, Strauss HW, et al. Role of radionuclide imaging in trials of antiangiogenic therapy. *Acad Radiol* 2000;7:851–867.
123. Stejskal E. Use of spin echos in a pulsed magnetic-field gradient to study anisotropic, restricted diffusion and flow. *J Chem Phys* 1965;43:3597–3603.
124. Yamada I, Aung W, Himeno Y, et al. Diffusion coefficients in abdominal organs and hepatic lesions: evaluation with intravoxel incoherent motion echo-planar MR imaging. *Radiology* 1999;210:617–623.

125. Van Ziji P, Eleff S, Ulatowski J, et al. Quantitative assessment of blood flow, bloof volume and blood oxygenation effects in functional megnetic resonance imaging. *Nat Med* 1998;4:159–167.
126. Abramovitch R, Frenkiel D, Neeman M. Analysis of subcutaneous angiogenesis by gradient echo magnetic resonance imaging. *Magn Reson Med* 1998;39:813–824.
127. Esserman L, Hylton N, George T, et al. Contrast-enhanced magnetic resonance imaging to assess tumor histopathology and angiogenesis in breast carcinoma. *Breast Journal* 1999;5:13–21.
128. Furman-Haran E, Grobgeld D, Margalit R, et al. Response of MCF7 human breast cancer to tamoxifen: evaluation by the three-time point, contrast-enhanced magnetic resonance imaging method. *Clin Cancer Res* 1998;4:2299–2304.
129. Pham C, Roberts T, van Bruggen N, et al. Magnetic resonance imaging detects suppression of tumor vascular permeability after administrationof antibody to vascular endothelial growth factor. *Cancer Invest* 1998;16:225–230.
130. Miller K, Sweeney C, Sledge G. Redefining the target: chemotherpeutics as antiangiogenics. *J Clin Oncol* 2001;19:1195–1206.
131. Wiseman H. Tamoxifen: new membrane-mediated mechanisms of action and therapeutic advances. *Trends Pharmacol Sci* 1994;15:83–89.
132. Gagliardi A, Collins DC. Inhibition of angiogenesis by antiestrogens. *Cancer Res* 1993;53:533–535.
133. Gagliardi AR, Hennig B, Collins DC. Antiestrogens inhibit endothelial cell growth stimulated by angiogenic growth factors. *Anticancer Res* 1996;16:1101–1106.
134. Haran EF, Maretzek AF, Goldberg I, et al. Tamoxifen enhances cell death in implanted MCF7 breast cancer by inhibiting endothelium growth. *Cancer Res* 1994;54:5511–5514.
135. Lindner DJ, Borden EC. Effects of tamoxifen and interferon-beta or the combination on tumor-induced angiogenesis. *Int J Cancer* 1997;71:456–461.
136. Silva ID, Salicioni AM, Russo IH, et al. Tamoxifen down-regulates CD36 messenger RNA levels in normal and neoplastic human breast tissues. *Cancer Res* 1997;57:378–381.
137. Sweeney C, Sledge GJ. Chemotherapy agents as antiangiogenic therapy. *Cancer Conference Highlights* 1999;3:2–4.
138. Belotti D, Vergani V, Drudis T, et al. The microtubule-affecting drug paclitaxel has antiangiogenic activity. *Clin Cancer Res* 1996;2:1843–1849.
139. Schirner M, Hoffmann J, Menrad A, et al. Antiangiogenic chemotherapeutic agents: characterization in comparison to their tumor growth inhibition in human renal cell carcinoma models. *Clin Cancer Res* 1998;4:1331–1336.
140. Benbow U, Maitra R, Hamilton J, et al. Selective modulation of collagenase 1 gene expression by the chemotherapeutic agent doxorubicin. *Clin Cancer Res* 1999;5:203–208.
141. Lau D, Young L, Xue L, et al. Paclitaxel: an angiogenesis antagonist in a metastatic breast cancer model. *Proc Am Soc Clin Oncol* 1998;17:107.
142. Klauber N, Parangi S, Flynn E, et al. Inhibition of angiogenesis and breast cancer in mice by the microtubule inhibitors 2-methoxyestradiol and Taxol. *Cancer Res* 1997;57:81–86.
143. Iigo M, Shimamura M, Sagawa K, et al. Characteristics of the inhibitory effect of mitoxantrone and pirarubicin on lung metastases of colon carcinoma 26. *Jpn J Cancer Res* 1995;86:867–872.
144. Slaton JW, Perrotte P, Inoue K, et al. Interferon-alpha-mediated down-regulation of angiogenesis-related genes and therapy of bladder cancer are dependent on optimization of biological dose and schedule. *Clin Cancer Res* 1999;5:2726–2734.
145. Browder T, Butterfield CE, Kraling BM, et al. Antiangiogenic scheduling of chemotherapy improves efficacy against experimental drug-resistant cancer [In Process Citation]. *Cancer Res* 2000;60:1878–1886.
146. Klement G, Baruchel S, Rak J, et al. Continuous low-dose therapy with vinblastine and VEGF receptor-2 antibody induces sustained tumor regression without overt toxicity. *J Clin Invest* 2000;105:R15–R24.
147. Wild R, Ghosh K, Dings R, et al. Carboplatin differentially induces the VEGF stress response in endothelial cells: potentiation of anti-tumor effects by combination treatment with antibody to VEGF. *Proc Am Assoc Canc Res* 2000;41:307.
148. Hanahan D, Bergers G, Bergsland E. Less is more, regularly: metronomic dosing of cytotoxic drugs can target tumor angiogenesis in mice. *J Clin Invest* 2000;105:1045–1047.
149. Fennelly D, Aghajanian C, Shapiro F, et al. Phase I and pharmacologic study of paclitaxel administered weekly in patients with relapsed ovarian cancer. *J Clin Oncol* 1997;15:187–192.
150. Seidman AD, Hochhauser D, Gollub M, et al. Ninety-six-hour paclitaxel infusion after progression during short taxane exposure: a phase II pharmacokinetic and pharmacodynamic study in metastatic breast cancer. *J Clin Oncol* 1996;14:1877–1884.
151. Engelsman E, Klijn J, Rubens R, et al. "Classical" CMF versus a 3-weekly intravenous CMF schedule in postmenopausal patients with advanced breast cancer. *Eur J Cancer* 1991;27:966–970.
152. Rocca A, Colleoni M, Masci G, et al. Low dose oral methotrexate and cyclophosphamide in metastatic breast cancer: an attempt to exploit the antiangiogenic activity of common chemotherapeutics. *Proc Am Soc Clin Oncol* 2001;20:30a.
153. Fisher C, Gilbertson-Beadling S, Powers EA, et al. Interstitial collagenase is required for angiogenesis in vitro. *Dev Biol* 1994;162:499–510.
154. Low JA, Johnson MD, Bone EA, et al. The matrix metalloproteinase inhibitor batimastat (BB-94) retards human breast cancer solid tumor growth but not ascites formation in nude mice. *Clin Cancer Res* 1996;2:1207–1214.
155. Taraboletti G, Garofalo A, Belotti D, et al. Inhibition of angiogenesis and murine hemangioma growth by batimastat, a synthetic inhibitor of matrix metalloproteinases. *J Natl Cancer Inst* 1995;87:293–298.
156. Tamargo RJ, Bok RA, Brem H. Angiogenesis inhibition by minocycline. *Cancer Res* 1991;51:672–675.
157. Fife RS, Sledge GW Jr. Effects of doxycycline on in vitro growth, migration, and gelatinase activity of breast carcinoma cells. *J Lab Clin Med* 1995;125:407–411.

158. Sledge GW Jr, Qulali M, Goulet R, et al. Effect of matrix metalloproteinase inhibitor batimastat on breast cancer regrowth and metastasis in athymic mice. *J Natl Cancer Inst* 1995;87:1546–1550.
159. Steward WP, Thomas AL. Marimastat: the clinical development of a matrix metalloproteinase inhibitor. *Expert Opin Investig Drugs* 2000;9:2913–2922.
160. Wojtowicz-Praga S, Torri J, Johnson M, et al. Phase I trial of Marimastat, a novel matrix metalloproteinase inhibitor, administered orally to patients with advanced lung cancer. *J Clin Oncol* 1998;16:2150–2156.
161. Miller K, Gradishar W, Schuchter L, et al. A randomized phase II pilot trial of adjuvant marimastat in patients with early stage breast cancer. *Proc Am Soc Clin Oncol* 2000;in press.
162. Warren RS, Yuan H, Matli MR, et al. Regulation by vascular endothelial growth factor of human colon cancer tumorigenesis in a mouse model of experimental liver metastasis. *J Clin Invest* 1995;95:1789–1797.
163. Kim KJ, Li B, Winer J, et al. Inhibition of vascular endothelial growth factor-induced angiogenesis suppresses tumour growth in vivo. *Nature* 1993;362:841–844.
164. Gordon MS, Margolin K, Talpaz M, et al. Phase I safety and pharmacokinetic study of recombinant human anti-vascular endothelial growth factor in patients with advanced cancer. *J Clin Oncol* 2001;19:843–850.
165. Sledge G, Miller K, Novotny W, et al. A phase II trial of single-agent rhuMAb VEGF (recombinant humanized monoclonal antibody to vascular endothelial cell growth factor) in patients with relapsed metastatic breast cancer. *Proc Am Soc Clin Oncol* 2000;19:3a.
166. Millauer B, Longhi MP, Plate KH, et al. Dominant-negative inhibition of Flk-1 suppresses the growth of many tumor types in vivo. *Cancer Res* 1996;56:1615–1620.
167. Fong TA, Shawver LK, Sun L, et al. SU5416 is a potent and selective inhibitor of the vascular endothelial growth factor receptor (Flk-1/KDR) that inhibits tyrosine kinase catalysis, tumor vascularization, and growth of multiple tumor types. *Cancer Res* 1999;59:99–106.
168. Shaheen R, Davis D, Liu W, et al. Antiangiogenic therapy targeting the tyrosine kinase receptor for vascualr endothelial growth factor receptor inhibits the growth of liver metastasis and induces tumor and endothelial cell apoptosis. *Cancer Res* 1999;59:5412–5416.
169. Rosen L, KabbinaF, Rosen P, et al. Phase I trial of SU5416, a novel angiogenesis inhibitor in patients with advanced maliganacies. *Proc Am Soc Clin Oncol* 1998;17:218a.
170. Rosen L, Mulay M, Mayers A, et al. Phase I dose-escalating trial of SU5416, a novel angiogenesis inhibitor in patients with advanced malignancies. *Proc Am Soc Clin Oncol* 1999;18:161a.
171. Overmoyer B, Robertson K, Persons M, et al. A phase I pharmacokinetic and pharmacodynamic study of SU5416 and doxorubicin in inflammatory breast cancer. *Proc Am Soc Clin Oncol* 2001;20:99a.
172. Basser R, Hurwitz H, Barge A, et al. Phase I pharmacokinetic and biological study of the angiogenesis inhibitor ZD6474 in patients with solid tumors. *Proc Am Soc Clin Oncol* 2001;20:100a.
173. Sandberg JA, Sproul CD, Blanchard KS, et al. Acute toxicology and pharmacokinetic assessment of a ribozyme (ANGIOZYME) targeting vascular endothelial growth factor receptor mRNA in the cynomolgus monkey. *Antisense Nucleic Acid Drug Dev* 2000;10:153–162.
174. Sandberg JA, Bouhana KS, Gallegos AM, et al. Pharmacokinetics of an antiangiogenic ribozyme (ANGIOZYME) in the mouse. *Antisense Nucleic Acid Drug Dev* 1999;9:271–277.
175. Weng DE, Usman N. Angiozyme: a novel angiogenesis inhibitor. *Curr Oncol Rep* 2001;3:141–146.
176. Weng D, Weiss P, Kellackey C, et al. Angiozyme pharmacokinetic and safety results: a phase I/II study in patients with refractory solid tumors. *Proc Am Soc Clin Oncol* 2001;20:99a.
177. Ciomei M, Pastori W, Mariani M, et al. New sulfonated distamycin A derivatives with bFGF complexing activity. *Biochem Pharmacol* 1994;47:295–302.
178. Zamai M, Caiolfa VR, Pines D, et al. Nature of interaction between basic fibroblast growth factor and the antiangiogenic drug 7,7-(Carbonyl-bis[imino-N-methyl-4, 2- pyrrolecarbonylimino[N-methyl-4,2-pyrrole]-carbonylimino])bis-(1, 3- naphthalene disulfonate). *Biophys J* 1998;75:672–682.
179. Possati L, Campioni D, Sola F, et al. Antiangiogenic, antitumoural and antimetastatic effects of two distamycin A derivatives with anti-HIV-1 Tat activity in a Kaposi's sarcoma-like murine model. *Clin Exp Metastasis* 1999;17:575–582.
180. Sola F, Capolongo L, Moneta D, et al. The antitumor efficacy of cytotoxic drugs is potentiated by treatment with PNU 145156E, a growth-factor-complexing molecule. *Cancer Chemother Pharmacol* 1999;43:241–246.
181. deVries E, Groen H, Wynendaele W, et al. PNU-145156E—a novel angiogenesis inhibitor in patients with soldi tumors: an update of a phase I and pharmacokinetic study. *Proc Am Soc Clin Oncol* 1999;18:161a.
182. McLeskey SW, Zhang L, Trock BJ, et al. Effects of AGM-1470 and pentosan polysulphate on tumorigenicity and metastasis of FGF-transfected MCF-7 cells. *Br J Cancer* 1996;73:1053–1062.
183. Sasaki A, Alcalde RE, Nishiyama A, et al. Angiogenesis inhibitor TNP-470 inhibits human breast cancer osteolytic bone metastasis in nude mice through the reduction of bone resorption. *Cancer Res* 1998;58:462–467.
184. Singh Y, Shikata N, Kiyozuka Y, et al. Inhibition of tumor growth and metastasis by angiogenesis inhibitor TNP- 470 on breast cancer cell lines in vitro and in vivo. *Breast Cancer Res Treat* 1997;45:15–27.
185. Bhargava P, Marshall JL, Rizvi N, et al. A phase I and pharmacokinetic study of TNP-470 administered weekly to patients with advanced cancer. *Clin Cancer Res* 1999;5:1989–1995.
186. Stadler WM, Kuzel T, Shapiro C, et al. Multi-institutional study of the angiogenesis inhibitor TNP-470 in metastatic renal carcinoma. *J Clin Oncol* 1999;17:2541–2545.
187. Logothetis CJ, Wu KK, Finn LD, et al. Phase I trial of the angiogenesis inhibitor TNP-470 for progressive androgen-independent prostate cancer. *Clin Cancer Res* 2001;7:1198–1203.
188. Dezube BJ, Von Roenn JH, Holden-Wiltse J, et al. Fumagillin analog in the treatment of Kaposi's sarcoma:

a phase I AIDS Clinical Trial Group study. AIDS Clinical Trial Group No. 215 Team. *J Clin Oncol* 1998; 16:1444–1449.
189. Brooks PC, Clark RA, Cheresh DA. Requirement of vascular integrin alpha v beta 3 for angiogenesis. *Science* 1994;264:569–571.
190. Brooks PC, Silletti S, von Schalscha TL, et al. Disruption of angiogenesis by PEX, a noncatalytic metalloproteinase fragment with integrin binding activity. *Cell* 1998;92:391–400.
191. Friedlander M, Theesfeld C, Sugita M, et al. Involvement of integrins avb3 and avb5 in ocular neovascular disease. *Proc Natl Acad Sci USA* 1996;93:9764–9769.
192. Brooks PC, Montgomery AM, Rosenfeld M, et al. Integrin alpha v beta 3 antagonists promote tumor regression by inducing apoptosis of angiogenic blood vessels. *Cell* 1994;79:1157–1164.
193. Brooks PC, Stromblad S, Klemke R, et al. Antiintegrin alpha v beta 3 blocks human breast cancer growth and angiogenesis in human skin [see comments]. *J Clin Invest* 1995;96:1815–1822.
194. Gutheil J, Campbell T, Pierce J, et al. Phase I study of vitaxin, an antiangiogenic humanized monoclonal antibody to vascular integrin avb3. *Proc Am Soc Clin Oncol* 1998;17:215a.
195. Cheresh D, Spiro R. Biosynthetic and functional properties of an Arg-Gly-Asp directed receptor involved in human melanoma cell attachment to vitronectin. *J Biol Chem* 1987;262:17703–17711.
196. Thorpe PE, Burrows FJ. Antibody-directed targeting of the vasculature of solid tumors [see comments]. *Breast Cancer Res Treat* 1995;36:237–251.
197. Griscelli F, Li H, Bennaceur-Griscelli A, et al. Angiostatin gene transfer: inhibition of tumor growth in vivo by blockage of endothelial cell proliferation associated with a mitosis arrest. *Proc Natl Acad Sci USA* 1998;95:6367–6372.
198. Moser TL, Stack MS, Asplin I, et al. Angiostatin binds ATP synthase on the surface of human endothelial cells. *Proc Natl Acad Sci USA* 1999;96:2811–2816.
199. Moser TL, Kenan DJ, Ashley TA, et al. Endothelial cell surface F1-F0 ATP synthase is active in ATP synthesis and is inhibited by angiostatin. *Proc Natl Acad Sci USA* 2001;98:6656–6661.
200. DeMoraes E, Fogler W, Grant D, et al. Recombinant human angiostatin: a phase I clinical trial assessing safety, pharmacokinetics and pharmacodynamics. *Proc Am Soc Clin Oncol* 2001;20:3a.
201. Mauceri HJ, Hanna NN, Beckett MA, et al. Combined effects of angiostatin and ionizing radiation in antitumour therapy. *Nature* 1998;394:287–291.
202. Gorski DH, Mauceri HJ, Salloum RM, et al. Potentiation of the antitumor effect of ionizing radiation by brief concomitant exposures to angiostatin. *Cancer Res* 1998;58:5686–5689.
203. O'Reilly MS, Boehm T, Shing Y, et al. Endostatin: an endogenous inhibitor of angiogenesis and tumor growth. *Cell* 1997;88:277–285.
204. Hohenester E, Sasaki T, Olsen BR, et al. Crystal structure of the angiogenesis inhibitor endostatin at 1.5 A resolution. *EMBO J* 1998;17:1656–1664.
205. MacDonald NJ, Shivers WY, Narum DL, et al. Endostatin binds tropomyosin. A potential modulator of the antitumor activity of endostatin. *J Biol Chem* 2001; 276:25190–25196.
206. Eder J, Clark J, Supko J, et al. A phase I pharmacokinetic and pharmacodynamic trial of recombinant endostatin. *Proc Am Soc Clin Oncol* 2001;20:70a.
207. Thomas J, Schiller J, Lee F, et al. A phase I pharmacokinetic and pharmacodynamic study of recombinant human endostatin. *Proc Am Soc Clin Oncol* 2001; 20:70a.
208. Herbst R, Tran H, Mullani N, et al. Phase I clinical trial of recombinant human endostatin in patients with solid tumors: pharmcokinetic, safety and efficacy analysis using surrogate endpoints of tissue and radiologic response. *Proc ASCO* 2001;20:3a.
209. Fogler W, Song M, Supko J, et al. Recombinant human endostatin demonstrates consistent and predictable pharmacokinetics following intravenous bolus administration to cancer patients. *Proc ASCO* 2001;20:69a.
210. Mundhenke C, Thomas J, Neider R, et al. Endothelial cell kinetics in skin wounds and tumors of patients receiving endostatin. *Proc ASCO* 2001;20:70a.
211. Fotsis T, Zhang Y, Pepper MS, et al. The endogenous oestrogen metabolite 2-methoxyoestradiol inhibits angiogenesis and suppresses tumour growth. *Nature* 1994;368:237–239.
212. Schumacher G, Kataoka M, Roth J, et al. Potent antitumor activity of 2-methoxyestradiol in human pancreatic cancer cell lines. *Clin Cancer Res* 1999;5: 493–499.
213. Yue TL, Wang X, Louden CS, et al. 2-Methoxyestradiol, an endogenous estrogen metabolite, induces apoptosis in endothelial cells and inhibits angiogenesis: possible role for stress-activated protein kinase signaling pathway and Fas expression. *Mol Pharmacol* 1997;51:951–962.
214. Reiser F, Way D, Bernas M, et al. Inhibition of normal and experimental angiotumor endothelial cell proliferation and cell cycle progression by 2-methoxyestradiol. *Proc Soc Exp Biol Med* 1998; 219:211–216.
215. Seegers JC, Lottering ML, Grobler CJ, et al. The mammalian metabolite, 2-methoxyestradiol, affects P53 levels and apoptosis induction in transformed cells but not in normal cells. *J Steroid Biochem Mol Biol* 1997;62:253–267.
216. Attalla H, Makela TP, Adlercreutz H, et al. 2-Methoxyestradiol arrests cells in mitosis without depolymerizing tubulin. *Biochem Biophys Res Commun* 1996;228:467–473.
217. Huang P, Feng L, Oldham EA, et al. Superoxide dismutase as a target for the selective killing of cancer cells. *Nature* 2000;407:390–5.
218. Miller K, Haney L, Pribluda V, et al. A phase I safety, pharmacokinetic and pharmacodynamic study of 2-methoxyestradiol in patients with refractory metastatic breast cancer. *Proc Am Soc Clin Oncol* 2001; 20:43a.
219. Kerbel R, Yu J, Tran J, et al. Possible mechanisms of acquired resistance to antiangiogenic drugs: implications for combination therapy. *Cancer and Metastasis Reviews* 2001;in press.
220. Walker RA, Dearing SJ. Transforming growth factor beta 1 in ductal carcinoma in situ and invasive carcinomas of the breast. *Eur J Cancer* 1992;28:641–644.
221. de Jong JS, van Diest PJ, van der Valk P, et al. Expression of growth factors, growth-inhibiting factors, and

their receptors in invasive breast cancer. II: Correlations with proliferation and angiogenesis. *J Pathol* 1998;184:53–57.
222. Piccoli R, Olson KA, Vallee BL, et al. Chimeric antiangiogenin antibody cAb 26–2F inhibits the formation of human breast cancer xenografts in athymic mice. *Proc Natl Acad Sci USA* 1998;95:4579–4583.
223. Fox SB, Engels K, Comley M, et al. Relationship of elevated tumour thymidine phosphorylase in node-positive breast carcinomas to the effects of adjuvant CMF. *Ann Oncol* 1997;8:271–275.
224. Engels K, Fox SB, Whitehouse RM, et al. Up-regulation of thymidine phosphorylase expression is associated with a discrete pattern of angiogenesis in ductal carcinomas in situ of the breast. *J Pathol* 1997;182:414–420.
225. Koblizek TI, Weiss C, Yancopoulos GD, et al. Angiopoietin-1 induces sprouting angiogenesis in vitro. *Curr Biol* 1998;8:529–532.
226. Suri C, Jones PF, Patan S, et al. Requisite role of angiopoietin-1, a ligand for the TIE2 receptor, during embryonic angiogenesis [see comments]. *Cell* 1996;87:1171–1180.
227. Guo NH, Krutzsch HC, Inman JK, et al. Antiproliferative and antitumor activities of D-reverse peptides derived from the second type-1 repeat of thrombospondin-1. *J Pept Res* 1997;50:210–221.
228. Wang TN, Qian XH, Granick MS, et al. Inhibition of breast cancer progression by an antibody to a thrombospondin-1 receptor. *Surgery* 1996;120:449–454.
229. Soncin F, Shapiro R, Fett JW. A cell-surface proteoglycan mediates human adenocarcinoma HT-29 cell adhesion to human angiogenin. *J Biol Chem* 1994;269:8999–9005.
230. Maisonpierre PC, Suri C, Jones PF, et al. Angiopoietin-2, a natural antagonist for Tie2 that disrupts in vivo angiogenesis [see comments]. *Science* 1997;277:55–60.
231. Fortier AH, Nelson BJ, Grella DK, et al. Antiangiogenic activity of prostate-specific antigen. *J Natl Cancer Inst* 1999;91:1635–1640.
232. Heidtmann HH, Nettelbeck DM, Mingels A, et al. Generation of angiostatin-like fragments from plasminogen by prostate-specific antigen. *Br J Cancer* 1999;81:1269–1273.
233. Hall N, Fish D, Hunt N, et al. Is the relationship between angiogenesis and metastasis in breast cancer real? *Surg Oncol* 1992;1:223–229.
234. Obermair A, Kurz C, Czerwenka K, et al. Microvessel density and vessel invasion in lymph-node-negative breast cancer: effect on recurrence-free survival. *Int J Cancer* 1995;62:126–131.
235. Fox SB, Turner GD, Leek RD, et al. The prognostic value of quantitative angiogenesis in breast cancer and role of adhesion molecule expression in tumor endothelium. *Breast Cancer Res Treat* 1995;36:219–226.
236. Ogawa Y, Chung YS, Nakata B, et al. Microvessel quantitation in invasive breast cancer by staining for factor VIII-related antigen. *Br J Cancer* 1995;71:1297–1301.
237. Axelsson K, Ljung BM, Moore DH, 2nd, et al. Tumor angiogenesis as a prognostic assay for invasive ductal breast carcinoma [see comments]. *J Natl Cancer Inst* 1995;87:997–1008.
238. Morphopoulos G, Pearson M, Ryder WD, et al. Tumour angiogenesis as a prognostic marker in infiltrating lobular carcinoma of the breast. *J Pathol* 1996;180:44–49.
239. Gasparini G, Toi M, Verderio P, et al. Prognostic significance of p53, angiogenesis, and other conventional features in operable breast cancer: subanalysis in node-positive and node-negative patients. *Int J Oncol* 1998;12:1117–1125.
240. Tynninen O, von Boguslawski K, Aronen HJ, et al. Prognostic value of vascular density and cell proliferation in breast cancer patients. *Pathol Res Pract* 1999;195:31–37.
241. Hansen S, Grabau DA, Sorensen FB, et al. The prognostic value of angiogenesis by Chalkley counting in a confirmatory study design on 836 breast cancer patients. *Clin Cancer Res* 2000;6:139–146.
242. Vincent-Salomon A, Carton M, Zafrani B, et al. Long term outcome of small size invasive breast carcinomas independent from angiogenesis in a series of 685 cases. *Cancer* 2001;92:249–256.
243. Bosari S, Lee A, DeLellis R, et al. Microvessel quantitation and prognosis in invasive breast carcinoma. *Hum Pathol* 1992;23:755–761.
244. Van Hoef M, Knox W, Dhesi S, et al. Assessment of tumor vascularity as a prognostic factor in lymph node negative invasive breast cancer. *Eur J Cancer* 1993;29A:1141–1145.
245. Fox SB, Leek RD, Smith K, et al. Tumor angiogenesis in node-negative breast carcinomas—relationship with epidermal growth factor receptor, estrogen receptor, and survival. *Breast Cancer Res Treat* 1994;29:109–116.
246. Gasparini G, Weidner N, Bevilacqua P, et al. Tumor microvessel density, p53 expression, tumor size, and peritumoral lymphatic vessel invasion are relevant prognostic markers in node-negative breast carcinoma. *J Clin Oncol* 1994;12:454–466.
247. Bevilacqua P, Barbareschi M, Verderio P, et al. Prognostic value of intratumoral microvessel density, a measure of tumor angiogenesis, in node-negative breast carcinoma—results of a multiparametric study. *Breast Cancer Res Treat* 1995;36:205–217.
248. Inada K, Toi M, Hoshina S, et al. [Significance of tumor angiogenesis as an independent prognostic factor in axillary node-negative breast cancer]. *Gan To Kagaku Ryoho* 1995;22(suppl 1):59–65.
249. Costello P, McCann A, Carney DN, et al. Prognostic significance of microvessel density in lymph node negative breast carcinoma. *Hum Pathol* 1995;26:1181–1184.
250. Karaiossifidi H, Kouri E, Arvaniti H, et al. Tumor angiogenesis in node-negative breast cancer: relationship with relapse free survival. *Anticancer Res* 1996;16:4001–4002.
251. Heimann R, Ferguson D, Powers C, et al. Angiogenesis as a predictor of long-term survival for patients with node-negative breast cancer. *J Natl Cancer Inst* 1996;88:1764–1769.
252. Ozer E, Canda T, Kurtodlu B. The role of angiogenesis, laminin and CD44 expression in metastatic behavior of early-stage low-grade invasive breast carcinomas. *Cancer Lett* 1997;121:119–123.
253. Medri L, Nanni O, Volpi A, et al. Tumor microvessel density and prognosis in node-negative breast cancer. *Int J Cancer* 2000;89:74–80.

254. Toi M, Hoshina S, Takayanagi T, et al. Association of vascular endothelial growth factor expression with tumor angiogenesis and with early relapse in primary breast cancer. *Jpn J Cancer Res* 1994;85:1045–1049.
255. Toi M, Inada K, Suzuki H, et al. Tumor angiogenesis in breast cancer: its importance as a prognostic indicator and the association with vascular endothelial growth factor expression. *Breast Cancer Res Treat* 1995;36:193–204.
256. Obermair A, Kucera E, Mayerhofer K, et al. Vascular endothelial growth factor (VEGF) in human breast cancer: correlation with disease-free survival. *Int J Cancer* 1997;74:455–458.
257. Linderholm B, Lindh B, Beckman L, et al. The prognostic value of vascular endothelial growth factor (VEGF) and basic fibroblast growth factor (bFGF) and associations to first metastases site in 1307 patients with primary breast cancer. *Proc Am Soc Clin Oncol* 2001;20:24a.
258. Gasparini G, Toi M, Miceli R, et al. Clinical relevance of vascular endothelial growth factor and thymidine phosphorylase in patients with node-positive breast cancer treated with either adjuvant chemotherapy or hormone therapy. *Cancer J Sci Am* 1999;5:101–111.
259. Gown A, Rivkin S, Hunt H, et al. Prognostic factor of vascular endothelial growth factor (VEGF) expression in node-positive breast cancer. *Proc ASCO* 2001; 20:427a.
260. Gasparini G, Toi M, Gion M, et al. Prognostic significance of vascular endothelial growth factor protein in node-negative breast carcinoma. *J Natl Cancer Inst* 1997;89:139–147.
261. Buadu L, Murakami J, Murayama S, et al. Breast lesions: correlation of contrast medium enhancement patterns on MR images with histopathologic findings and tumor angiogenesis. *Radiology* 1996;200: 639–649.
262. Stomper P, Winston J, Klippenstein D, et al. Angiogenesis and dynamic MR imaging gadolinium enhancement of malignant and benign breast lesions. *Breast Cancer Res Treat* 1997;45:39–46.
263. Buckley D, Drew P, Mussurakis S, et al. Microvessel density of invasive breast cancer assessed by dynamic Gd-DTPA enhanced MRI. *J Magn Reson Imaging* 1997; 7:461–464.
264. Hulka C, Edmister W, Smith B, et al. Dynamic echoplanar imaging of the breast: experience in diagnosing breast carcinoma and correlation with tumor angiogenesis. *Radiology* 1997;1997:837–842.
265. Ikeda O, Yamashita Y, Takahashi M. Gd-enhanced dynamic magnetic resonance imaging of breast masses. *Top Magn Reson Inaging* 1999;10:143–151.
266. Knopp M, Weiss E, Sinn H, et al. Pathophysiologic basis of contrast enhancement in breast tumors. *J Magn Reson Imaging* 1999;10:260–266.
267. Matsubayashi R, Matsuo Y, Edakuni G, et al. Breast masses with peripheral rim enhancement on dynamic contrast-enhanced MR images: correlation of MR findings with histologic features and expression of growth factors. *Radiology* 2000;217:841–848.

21
Results from a Phase 1 Trial of *E1A* Gene Therapy in Breast and Ovarian Cancer: What's Next?

Naoto T. Ueno, Gabriel N. Hortobagyi, and Mien-Chie Hung

The use of gene therapy for treating cancer is undergoing tremendous scrutiny after an 18-year-old patient with an inherited enzyme deficiency died while participating in a clinical trial of human gene therapy in 1999. The scientific technology underlying human cancer gene therapy continues to improve through advances in basic and translational research. Clinical trials also continue to produce valuable information on the safety and efficacy of gene therapy. However, information on the long-term effects of gene therapy, its efficacy, and its adverse effects in comparison with those of conventional forms of therapy is lacking.

At the University of Texas M.D. Anderson Cancer Center, we have been investigating the adenovirus type 5 *E1A* gene for its therapeutic potential in breast and ovarian cancer since 1995. In the late 1980s, the *E1A* gene was shown to downregulate HER-2/*neu* overexpression, thus reversing the tumorigenic and metastatic phenotype associated with the expression of this protein. *E1A* can also function as a tumor suppressor gene by inducing apoptosis and inhibiting metastasis. We recently completed a phase 1 trial of *E1A* gene therapy, and we now need to confirm its antitumor properties in phase 2 studies, either as a single agent or in combination with conventional approaches such as chemotherapy. In this chapter, we provide a brief review of cancer gene therapy, recount our experience with developing *E1A* as a therapeutic gene, discuss the outcome of our phase 1 study, and note some implications for future studies.

CANCER GENE THERAPY: A BRIEF SUMMARY

Because cancer is a product of genetic changes (mutation, deletion, or overexpression), the underlying concept of cancer gene therapy is to reverse these genetic changes and consequently achieve a therapeutic effect by introducing—in most cases—a single gene. The simplicity of this concept has attracted a great deal of interest in clinical, translational, and basic research since the late 1980s. However, in its current form, cancer gene therapy is clearly not a "home run." The U.S. Food and Drug Association (FDA) has yet to approve a pharmaceutical product based on cancer gene therapy. Three major issues need to be addressed to promote the rapid clinical development of cancer gene therapy: identification of effective genes; identification of cancer-specific genes; and identification of an efficient, nontoxic gene delivery system.

Cancer gene therapy can be considered as one of two types—immunologic and nonimmunologic (Table 21.1). Immunologic approaches involve the transfection of genes that will enhance the host's immune response to cancer; examples include transfecting genes into dendritic cells or tumor cells that induce the expression of cytokines (such as interleukin [IL]-2 or interleukin-12, granulocyte-macrophage colony-stimulating factor [GM-CSF], interferon [IFN]-γ, or co-stimulatory molecules B7, beta 2 microglobulin). Nonimmunologic approaches are of five basic types. The first is based on conversion of a nontoxic prodrug into a toxic one by means of exposing a transferred gene to an enzyme that catalyzes this conversion. The genes for such enzymes are incorporated into the cancer cells by transfection, and those cancer cells (and sometimes the surrounding cells) are thus made susceptible to the prodrug through its conversion to cytotoxic products. Examples of such genes, called "suicide genes," include cytosine deaminase and

TABLE 21.1. *Classification of cancer gene therapy*

Immunologic approaches	Nonimmunologic approaches
Cytokine Costimulatory molecules	Prodrug Antisense Drug resistance genes (MDR, DHFR) Replacement or addition of gene (p53, E1A) Cancer-specific replication viruses (ONYX-015,)

herpes simplex virus thymidine kinase (HSV-tk) (1). The suicide-gene approach has been used in a phase 1 study of HER-2/*neu*-overexpressing breast cancer in which cytosine deaminase was linked to the HER-2/*neu* promoter so that cytosine deaminase was specifically expressed by the tumor cells that overexpressed the HER-2/*neu* protein (2). HSV-tk, another commonly used enzyme in suicide-gene therapy, converts the prodrug ganciclovir to the phosphorylated ganciclovir triphosphate form, which inhibits DNA replication in cancer cells. The gene for HSV-tk has been used in a variety of cancer clinical trials (3).

The second nonimmunologic approach is the use of antisense constructs to reduce the amount of mRNA produced by oncogenes, thereby inhibiting translation of the oncogene protein product. This approach has been explored in preclinical models targeting the expression of Bcl-XL, Bcl-2, insulin-like growth factor (IGF), basic fibroblast growth factor (bFGF), and HER-2/*neu*, all of which can be overexpressed in breast carcinoma (4–9). The third approach is to insert a gene that confers drug resistance (MDR, DHFR) into hematopoietic stem cells to prevent bone marrow suppression during chemotherapy (10,11). The fourth approach involves gene replacement or supplementation; in most cases, this approach explores the therapeutic modulation of cancer-cell apoptosis by manipulating the expression of genes, chiefly *p53, BRCA1,* and *E1A* (12–16). This approach is being evaluated for the treatment of breast cancer in several ways, i.e., by injecting an adenoviral vector that contains cDNA of wild-type *p53* directly into the tumor, by purging contaminated bone marrow with the adenoviral p53 vector, or by injecting the *E1A* gene into the tumor or the peritoneal/ thoracic cavity (13,17). The last approach is the use of cancer-specific replication viruses to kill cancer cells. One such example is the ONYX-015 virus, which, owing to deletion of the E1B gene, can replicate only in cells with mutated or deleted p53 (18,19); the E1B gene is the wild-type *p53* binding site. Viral replication in cells in which p53 is mutated or deleted kills those cells, but not normal cells that express wild-type p53.

Regardless of which approach is to be used, the question of whether gene therapy has a role in cancer treatment awaits the results of ongoing randomized trials, such as those involving the combination of p53 adenovirus or ONYX-015 virus with chemotherapy. Many nonimmunologic forms of gene therapy for cancer are being used in combination with conventional chemotherapy or radiation therapy, probably because none of the therapeutic genes tested to date have been particularly effective as single-agent therapy. Most likely this reflects the existence of redundant signaling pathways in humans, pathways that normally protect us against possible health hazards resulting from a single genetic defect or overexpression of a single gene. Combination therapy also seems to be more effective than single-agent treatment in preclinical models.

We also have yet to identify the most efficient gene delivery system (Table 21.2). Since there is currently no effective means of systemic gene delivery that allows treatment of metastatic disease, anticancer gene therapy at present is limited to treating lesions in the skin, tumor, muscle or accessible body cavities. In general, genes can be delivered in one of two ways: by viral or by nonviral vectors. The commonly used adenoviral vector allows the delivery of cDNA constructs, and it can efficiently transfect even nondividing cells in a transient manner. Retroviral vectors, in contrast, transfect only dividing cells; although this process is quite inefficient, the genes to be delivered in a retroviral vector can be integrated into the DNA of the transfected cells (stable transfec-

TABLE 21.2. Gene delivery systems

Viral vectors	Nonviral vectors
Adenovirus (transient expression, good transfection into non-dividing cells): local, immunogenic	Naked DNA (plasmid alone) (transient expression, transfection into nondividing cells)
Retrovirus (stable expression, transfection into dividing cells): local, overall poor transfection	Cationic liposome (transient/stable expression, transfection into nondividing cells): local, overall poor transfection, less immunogenicity?
Adeno-associated virus (stable/transient expression, good transfection into nondividing cells): more difficult for scale up production	
Other, e.g., vaccina virus, herpesvirus	Other, e.g., polymers, synthetic peptides

Vector	Expression	Advantages	Disadvantages
Viral			
Adenovirus	Transient	Good transfection into nondividing cells	Local therapy Immunogenic
Retrovirus	Stable	Transfection into dividing cells	Local therapy Overall poor transfection
Adeno-associated virus	Stable/transient	Good transfection into nondividing cells	Difficult to scale up production
Vaccinia virus	Unk	Unk	Unk
Herpesvirus	Unk	Unk	Unk
Nonviral			
Naked DNA (plasmid alone)	Transient	Transfection into nondividing cells	Local therapy
Cationic liposome	Transient/stable	Transfection into nondividing cells Less immunogenicity?	Local therapy Overall poor transfection
Polymers	Unk	Unk	Unk
Synthetic peptides	Unk	Unk	Unk

Unk, unknown.

tion). Another viral vector, adeno-associated virus, can transfect cells and become integrated into the host DNA, but achieving sufficiently high concentration titers has not been easy.

Nonviral vectors include the use of plasmids themselves and other synthetic delivery systems. The use of nonviral vector delivery systems was recently reviewed (20,21). Nonviral vectors have the advantage of possibly less immunogenicity, but they have low transfection efficiency in general. All vectors, viral or nonviral, have advantages and disadvantages (Table 21.3); none to date has been completely satisfactory.

Gene therapy now faces fierce competition from other new approaches for targeting cancer-specific molecules, in which the therapeutic molecule can be delivered efficiently with good safety profiles. One example is the recently FDA approved tyrosine-kinase inhibitor STI-571, which targets the abnormal tyrosine kinase bcr-abl in chronic myelogenous leukemia or c-kit in gastrointestinal stromal tumors. This drug has produced relatively high rates of complete response in both diseases (22,23) and seems to have minimal toxicity. Unlike STI-571, current forms of cancer gene therapy lack a simple, efficient means of delivery, are not particularly specific, and are not particularly effective relative to conventional forms of therapy. Nevertheless, cancer gene therapy can be a

TABLE 21.3. Issues involved in gene expression

Efficiency	Percentage of gene expression in the target tissue: low vs. high. Distribution of gene expression in a cell: central vs. periphery How to determine the gene expression efficiency?
Distribution	Expression at the injection site (local) vs. distant organ sites (systemic) Expression in tumor cells vs. non-tumor cells
Duration	Transient expression Stable expression: Does it integrate into host DNA?

powerful tool for understanding cancer genetics and immunology. Unfortunately, the reality of cancer treatment continues to be complicated. Cancer cells can develop resistance to STI-571 (24), and perhaps to the anti-HER-2/*neu* antibody (trastuzumab), which has shown promising activity in combination with chemotherapy. The activity of both drugs remains low when they are given as single agents, and even disease that responds initially will eventually progress.

At the M.D. Anderson Cancer Center, the adenoviral gene *E1A* was developed initially as a means of suppressing HER-2/*neu* overexpression and then later as a means of inducing apoptosis by delivering it to cancer cells. Below follows a brief review of the biology of *E1A,* after which findings from a phase 1 study of *E1A* to treat metastatic breast or ovarian cancer are presented; the chapter concludes with a discussion of outstanding issues that must be addressed.

ADENOVIRUS TYPE 5 *E1A* AS A TUMOR SUPPRESSOR GENE

Part of an adenovirus genome, the 36-kb *E1A* gene encodes proline-rich nuclear-localized phosphoproteins that regulate the replication of adenovirus (25). The primary function of *E1A* is to activate other adenoviral genes to allow efficient replication of the adenovirus (25). The oncogenicity of various adenoviruses varies considerably; the *E1A* protein produced by adenovirus type 12 is strongly oncogenic and induces tumors at high frequency (26). In contrast, *E1A* proteins produced by adenovirus type 5 and the closely related adenovirus type 2 are nononcogenic (27). Because *E1A* proteins can transcriptionally transactivate proteins that can "immortalize" transformed cells, *E1A* was originally considered to be an "immortalization oncogene" (28–30). In fact, *E1A* proteins can either stimulate transcription or repress the activity of certain viral and cellular transcriptional enhancers.

We found that *E1A* gene products inhibit HER-2/*neu* overexpression in both rodent fibroblasts and human cancer cells, through transcriptional repression at the HER-2/*neu* promoter (31). This finding prompted us to investigate whether *E1A* could function as a tumor suppressor in HER-2/*neu*-overexpressing cancer cells by repressing HER-2/*neu* overexpression. Initially, when we introduced the *E1A* gene into genomic HER-2/*neu*-transformed mouse fibroblasts, the *E1A* gene products did indeed suppress the transformed phenotype and inhibited metastatic potential (32,33). Interestingly, when these *E1A*-expressing HER-2/*neu*-transformed mouse fibroblasts were forced to overexpress HER-2/*neu,* their tumorigenicity was restored, but their ability to form metastatic tumors was still significantly inhibited by *E1A* (34). We then examined whether *E1A* could reverse tumorigenicity in HER-2/*neu*-overexpressing human ovarian cancer cells by transfecting the *E1A* gene into such cells. The *E1A*-expressing ovarian cancer cell lines expressed less HER-2/*neu* protein, had fewer malignant characteristics and were less able to induce tumors in immunocompetent mice (35).

In addition to having suppressive activity in HER-2/*neu*-overexpressing tumors, *E1A* also seems to be associated with tumor-suppression activities independent of HER-2/*neu*. For instance, *E1A* repressed transcription of various proteases involved in tumor cell invasion and metastasis, including type IV collagenase (33, 36), plasminogen activator (37), stromelysin (38,39), interstitial collagenase (36), and urokinase (36). *E1A* also inhibited metastasis by increasing the expression of the metastasis suppressor gene *Nm23* (40–42). In another study, *E1A* reduced anchorage-independent growth and tumorigenic growth of a variety of tumor cell lines, including human melanoma, fibrosarcoma (43), the A204 and RD rhabdomyosarcoma cell lines, the Saos-2 osteosarcoma cell line, the NCI-H23 non-small cell lung carcinoma cell line, the MDA-MB-435s breast carcinoma cell line, *ras*-transformed MDCK kidney epithelial cells (44), and murine melanoma (45). *E1A* has also been shown to induce apoptosis in various types of cells when *E1B* is absent (46–48). Further, *E1A* increases the cytotoxic activity of tumor necrosis factor (TNF)-α in *E1A*-transfected cells (49,50) and affects the susceptibility of target cells to TNF-α-independent cytolytic mechanisms by activated natural killer cells and macrophages (51). *E1A* also controls cell proliferation by repressing the expression of growth factor-inducible genes (39). *E1A* was also recently found to suppress at least one other tyrosine kinase besides HER-2/*neu,* namely Axl, which is the prototype of a family of transmembrane receptors called UFO that includes Sky and Eyk (52,53).

Thus, previous findings clearly demonstrate that *E1A* can function as a tumor suppressor gene through several different mechanisms, including transcriptional repression of HER-2/*neu,* inhibition of metastasis-related genes, activation of metastasis-suppressor genes, induction of apoptosis, induction of host immune responses, repression of growth factor-inducible genes, and induction of differentiation. The function of *E1A* as a tumor suppressor may depend on the individual oncogenic backgrounds of cancer cells. Recently, it was reported that *E1A* might induce the EWS-Fl11 rearrangement specific to Ewing sarcoma (54); however, other groups, including ourselves, could not confirm an association between *E1A* expression and oncogenicity in Ewing sarcoma (55–57). Indeed, when we introduced *E1A* into mouse fibroblasts, we did not detect any transforming phenotype (33). Further, there is no epidemiologic evidence to suggest that adenovirus type 5 can cause tumors in human subjects. Therefore, the bulk of the evidence suggests that *E1A* is a tumor suppressor gene and not an oncogene.

E1A GENE THERAPY FOR HUMAN BREAST AND OVARIAN CANCER

Preclinical Findings in a Murine Xenograft Model

As noted earlier, genes can be delivered by viral or nonviral means. Viral delivery of DNA plasmids is efficient but has disadvantages; for example, retroviral vectors cannot transfect nondividing cells, and adenoviral vectors can be strongly immunogenic (58). Nonviral delivery systems may allow repeated DNA transfections with minimum toxicity and immunogenicity; however, the transfection efficiency of nonviral vectors is limited compared with that of viral vectors (59).

One of the best-known nonviral delivery systems is the cationic liposome. The first cationic liposome was developed for *in vitro* gene transfer in the late 1980s by Felgner et al. (60). The system is designed so that even though the positive charge of the liposome interacts with the negative charge of the DNA, the overall charge remains positive even after the DNA/cationic liposome complex is formed. This positive charge promotes the interaction of the complex with the negatively charged cell membrane and thus aids transfection of the target cells.

The DC-Chol cationic liposome, which was developed by Leaf et al. at the University of Pittsburgh, can facilitate gene delivery into mammalian cells both *in vitro* and *in vivo,* without major toxic effects. It is also known for its biodegradable, nonmutagenic, and nonimmunogenic properties (61–65). These properties, along with the advantage of allowing multiple injections of a therapeutic gene, led us to select DC-Chol as the gene delivery system in a preclinical phase 1 trial of *E1A* gene therapy in models of ovarian and breast cancer. First, human breast cancer xenografts were established by injecting human HER-2/*neu*-overexpressing breast cancer cells (MDA-MB-361) into the mammary fat pads of nude mice. After tumor formation was confirmed, *E1A* genes complexed with DC-Chol cationic liposomes (*E1A*/DC-Chol complex) were injected intratumorally (66). This procedure inhibited the growth of the HER-2/*neu*-overexpressing breast cancer cell xenografts. Similar results were observed in a human ovarian cancer xenograft model. In this model, human HER-2/*neu*-overexpressing ovarian cancer cells (SKOV-3) were injected intraperitoneally into mice, and the *E1A*/DC-Chol complex was subsequently delivered into the peritoneal cavity of the tumor-bearing mice. The growth and dissemination of HER-2/*neu*-overexpressing ovarian cancer cells were inhibited. About 70% of the treated mice survived at least 365 days, whereas all untreated controls developed severe tumor-induced symptoms and died within 160 days (63).

Preclinical Toxicity Studies of the E1A Gene

Before beginning the phase 1 clinical trial, we evaluated the safety and toxicity of the *E1A*/DC-Chol complex by injecting it intraperitoneally into normal nude mice. In the short term, the cumulative dose, which was up to 40 times that proposed for use in the phase 1 trial, had no adverse effects on renal, hepatic, or hematologic function. No major changes were observed in any organ on pathologic examination. Further analyses were done to determine whether the *E1A* gene was still present in normal cells after the treatment had ceased and the mice had survived for a certain time. Nine months after treatment with the *E1A*/DC-Chol complex had been discontinued, the mice were analyzed for the effect of treatment on major organs, including the genitals (uterus, fallopian tube, and ovary in female mice), liver, lung, heart, kidney, spleen, and brain. No macroscopic or microscopic effects were evident. However, at 18 months after the last injection of *E1A*, *E1A* DNA was still present in lung and kidney but not in liver, heart, spleen, brain, uterus, or ovary. Therefore, we concluded that the DC-Chol cationic liposome gene delivery system might allow us to repeatedly inject the *E1A*/DC-Chol complex in human subjects without inducing any major toxic effects; nevertheless, long-term follow-up is needed to determine the ultimate effect of *E1A* (64,65). On the basis of these results, an Investigational New Drug application was filed with the U.S. FDA, and approved. In 1996, a phase 1 trial of *E1A* gene therapy for breast and ovarian cancer was opened at the University of Texas M.D. Anderson Cancer Center.

Phase 1 Trial of *E1A* Gene Therapy in Breast and Ovarian Cancer

A phase 1 study of *E1A* gene therapy for patients with metastatic breast or ovarian cancer that overexpressed HER-2/*neu* was initiated at M.D. Anderson Cancer Center in 1996 (Fig.

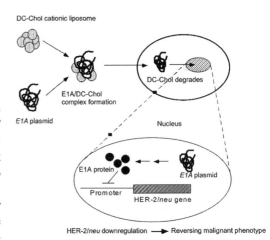

FIG. 21.1. Phase 1 study of *E1A* gene therapy for patients with metastatic breast or ovarian cancer that overexpressed HER-2/*neu*.

21.1) (67). At first, only patients with breast or ovarian tumors that overexpressed HER-2/*neu* were eligible; later, patients with tumors expressing low levels of HER-2/*neu* became eligible as well. A tumor was considered to overexpress HER-2/*neu* if more than 10% of tumor cells had an HER-2/*neu* signal intensity stronger than 1+ (68). In the trial, each patient was given weekly injections of the *E1A*/DC-Chol complex through a Tenckhoff catheter placed in either the pleural cavity (for patients with breast cancer) or the peritoneal cavity (for patients with ovarian cancer). After three consecutive weekly injections, patients were given a 1-week treatment break; these 4 weeks constituted one treatment cycle. The starting dose of the *E1A*/DC-Chol complex, derived from the effective dose established in the preclinical animal studies, was 1.8 mg/m^2 (63,66). The *E1A* was given at one of three doses: 1.8 mg, 3.6 mg, or 7.2 mg/m^2 per injection. The objective of this phase 1 trial was to determine the maximum tolerated dose and the maximum biologically active dose of the *E1A* plasmid. In other words, our goal was to demonstrate the feasibility of delivering *E1A*/DC-Chol complexes in this way in terms of transducing *E1A* into tumor cells and thus downregulating HER-2/*neu* overexpression in the tumor. Because no toxicity had been detected during the preclinical toxicity study, the dose of *E1A* plasmid was escalated in 100% increments instead of according to the Fibonacci dose-escalation method. Adverse events were monitored weekly and assigned a grade according to the National Cancer Institute Common Toxicity Criteria. Because certain toxic effects may not have been easily distinguished from other effects related to disease progression or other factors, all adverse events were recorded. These events were further graded on a scale of 1 to 5 to help determine whether there was a true cause-and-effect relationship between the treatment and the adverse event.

Outcome of Phase 1 Trial

A total of 18 heavily pretreated women who had either breast cancer (n = 6) or ovarian cancer (n = 12) were included in this trial. The median age of the patients was 55 years (range, 34 to 73 years) and the median Zubrod performance status was 2 (range, 0 to 3). All 18 patients had either metastatic or recurrent disease that had progressed despite multiple treatments (surgery, chemotherapy, hormonal therapy) before administration of the *E1A*/DC-Chol complex. The median number of previous chemotherapy regimens per patient was 3 (range, 1 to 6); five patients had undergone high-dose chemotherapy with autologous stem-cell transplantation. Tumors in 12 patients (six with breast cancer and six with ovarian cancer) overexpressed HER-2/*neu*. The *E1A* plasmid was given at 3 doses to consecutive cohorts of patients: 1.8 mg/m^2 (to six patients), 3.6 mg/m^2 (to seven patients), and 7.2 mg/m^2 (to five patients). A median of six injections (range, 1 to 8) was given over 2 treatment cycles, and the median cumulative dose of *E1A* plasmid was 10.8 mg/m^2 (range, 5.4 mg to 32.4 mg/m^2).

Toxicity

No patients died as a result of the treatment. However, all five patients who received the highest dose of *E1A* plasmid (7.2 mg/m^2) developed moderate to severe nausea, vomiting, and discomfort (pain or burning) at the injection site (the area in which the catheter had been inserted). In most patients (77.8%), self-limited fever (temperature up to 103°F) developed 3 to 48 hours after injection of the *E1A*/DC-Chol complex, regardless of dose. In most of those cases, however, the fever responded to acetaminophen or nonsteroidal anti-inflammatory agents. Thus, the maximum tolerated dose of the *E1A*/DC-Chol complex was fixed at 3.6 mg/m^2.

Expression of E1A and Suppression of HER-2/neu

To confirm our findings from the preclinical animal studies (63,66), we first examined whether HER-2/*neu* expression levels were downregulated in HER-2/*neu*-overexpressing cancer cells after administration of *E1A*/DC-Chol complex. An immunohistochemical staining technique was used to stain HER-2/*neu* in serial samples of tumor cells collected from the intracavitary fluids (5 pleural effusions, 1 ascites) of six patients (five of whom had breast cancer, and the sixth had ovarian cancer). To allay concerns about quantifying HER-2/*neu* downregulation in the presence of a heterogeneous collection of tumor and non-tumor cells, we also used a cell image analysis system to obtain a quantitative estimate of HER-2/*neu* expression (i.e., the signal intensity of HER-2/*neu* at the cell membrane of tumor cells without interference from the heterogeneous cell group) (69). In our six sets of serial samples taken from patients, the HER-2/*neu* signal-intensity ratio decreased significantly (by 39% to 98% from the original intensity measurement) after *E1A*/DC-Chol complex delivery, thus indicating a downregulation of HER-2/*neu* expression. After injection of *E1A*/DC-Chol complex, adjoining sections of tumor tissue were immunohistochemically stained to reveal HER-2/*neu* and *E1A* and then analyzed for the distribution of *E1A* gene expression in those HER-2/*neu*-overexpressing tumor cells. Although HER-2/*neu* downregulation was indeed seen in tumor cells that expressed *E1A* (Fig. 21.2), *E1A* gene expression was detected in both the cytoplasm and nucleus of tumor cells even after just a single injection of the *E1A*/DC-Chol complex. Further, the *E1A* signal was detected both in tumor cells and in

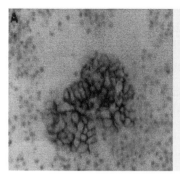 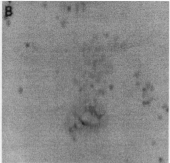 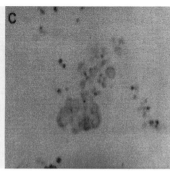

FIG. 21.2. HER-2/*neu* downregulation is observed in the same cells that express *E1A*. Breast cancer cells are immunohistochemically stained for *E1A* and HER-2/*neu* 22 days after administration of the *E1A*/DC-Chol complex. **A:** Before treatment (on day 0), staining intensity is 3+. **B:** On day 22 after treatment, staining intensity is 1+. **C:** *E1A* is expressed in both the cytoplasm and the nucleus. See color plate.

non-tumor cells such as mesothelial cells, macrophages, and lymphocytes.

We also analyzed the distribution of *E1A* gene expression in one patient with breast cancer after her death by using reverse transcriptase polymerase chain reaction (RT-PCR) with two different sets of primers. We extracted RNA for these analyses from several organs at autopsy, 2 weeks after the final injection of the *E1A*/DC-Chol complex had been given into the right thoracic cavity (cumulative dose, 5.4 mg/m^2). *E1A* mRNA was detected in the lung, liver, and kidney, and in metastatic tumors, but not in the brain, ovaries, or primary breast tumor. The absence of *E1A* mRNA in the ovary was consistent with the results of our previous preclinical experiments in nude mice (65).

apoptosis of tumor cells by conducting terminal deoxynucleotidyl transferase nick-end labeling (TUNEL) assays. We looked for a decrease in DNA replication (proliferation) in these tumor cells by examining Ki-67 expression. The percentage of apoptotic cells increased after treatment with *E1A*/DC-Chol (Fig. 21.3), and Ki-67 expression decreased within 15 days after the first dose.

To further address whether an immunologic mechanism might have contributed to the decrease in cell proliferation or the increase in percentage of apoptotic cells, we measured different immunologic markers (lymphocyte subsets [CD3, CD4, CD8, CD56] and the levels of IFN-γ and TNF-α) in the supernatants of the intracavitary fluids before and after treatment.

Enhanced Apoptosis and Reduced DNA Replication (Proliferation)

We also looked for any decreases in the number of tumor clumps in the intracavitary fluid over the course of the *E1A*/DC-Chol complex administration. When fluid samples (ascites or pleural) collected before and after treatment from six patients were compared, the percentage of tumor clumps decreased dramatically after administration of the *E1A*/DC-Chol complex. Because *E1A* itself is known to induce apoptosis and may contribute to reductions in the number of viable tumor cells, we examined

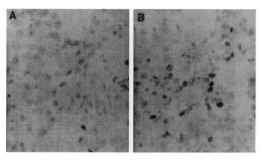

FIG. 21.3. TUNEL assay shows increased numbers of apoptotic tumor cells after administration of *E1A*/DC-Chol complex. **A:** Before treatment. **B:** After treatment. See color plate.

TNF-α was examined because it is known to sensitize *E1A*-transfected cells to apoptotic signals (50,51,70,71). Analysis revealed some increase in IFN-γ levels after delivery of the *E1A*/DC-Chol complex, but no correlation was found between this apparent increase and suppression of proliferation.

FINAL THOUGHTS

In conclusion, the findings from our phase 1 trial have generated new hypotheses to test in both preclinical and clinical experiments. To improve the efficacy, specificity, and safety of *E1A* cancer gene therapy, the molecular effects that can trigger antitumor activity or side effects should be investigated prospectively. Simply performing a clinical trial will not help in this regard, since the field of cancer gene therapy is evolving so rapidly in terms of both technology and gene delivery. Thus, flexibility in assessing and analyzing samples during phase 2 or phase 3 trials will be very important for designing future clinical trials.

The preclinical studies of *E1A* gene expression showed that local injection of the *E1A*/DC-Chol complex led to systemic expression of the gene in distant organs. This finding may suggest that systemic gene delivery is feasible by intravenous injection of a nonviral cationic liposome delivery system. We are currently exploring another liposomal delivery system, the liposome/polycation/DNA (LPD) system, for this purpose. LPD was formulated to overcome the serum stability issues noted by Leaf and colleagues at the University of Pittsburgh; the intent is to circumvent the inherent sensitivity of cationic liposome complexes to serum (72,77). Early studies with the LPD complexes demonstrated that intravenous administration through the tail vein of nude mice facilitates the delivery of DNA to distant organ sites such as lung or liver (72,73). Thus, the LPD system is an attractive candidate for the systemic delivery of therapeutic genes to treat advanced or metastatic cancer. We are currently studying the transfection capabilities and antitumor effects of systemically delivered *E1A*/LPD in tumor xenograft models for breast and head and neck cancer. Our preliminary findings indicate that LPD is effective for the delivery and subsequent expression of *E1A* at the tumor site, as well as reducing HER-2/*neu* protein expression and inducing apoptosis. These results, in our opinion, justify continuing the preclinical and clinical development of *E1A*/LPD as a novel therapeutic approach for the treatment of both primary and metastatic cancers.

Further, we are also attempting to improve the anticancer efficacy of *E1A* gene therapy by combining it with radiation (78) or chemotherapy. Recent reports indicate that *E1A* can sensitize cancer cell lines to chemotherapeutic agents. One group has reported sensitization to the alkylating agent cisplatin, through p53-dependent apoptosis induced by *E1A* (79). Other groups have reported sensitization to cisplatin through a mechanism independent of *p53* (80,81) or that *E1A* sensitized low-HER-2/*neu*-expressing cancer cell lines to cisplatin and VP-16 (44). We previously showed that downregulation of HER-2/*neu* expression is critical for *E1A* sensitization to paclitaxel both *in vitro* and *in vivo* (82,83); therefore, we are currently conducting a phase 1 trial in which *E1A* is combined with paclitaxel and other chemotherapeutic agents.

Another unique aspect of gene therapy that needs to be addressed is the fever that occurred at all dose levels during the phase 1 study. We speculate that the DNA/cationic liposome complex may be immunogenic and prompts the release of inflammatory cytokines such as TNF-α and interferon-γ, which can cause fever. However, evidence from preclinical animal studies and other studies of liposomal drug delivery systems indicates that the DC-Chol cationic liposome alone does not induce these cytokines. Because *E1A* can sensitize cancer cells to TNF-α, another approach might be to take advantage of endogenous TNF-α production.

The next immediate step is to conduct a phase 2 trial to determine the antitumor activity of *E1A*. The design of such a trial will benefit from what we have learned in the phase 1 trial. The phase 1 trial was difficult to conduct and complete for two reasons. First, the patients enrolled in this study had received many other treatments before *E1A* gene therapy for bulky disease. In addition, HER-2/*neu* overexpression, a known marker of poor prognosis, probably contributed to rapid disease progression. Therefore, the phase 2 trial should be limited to patients who have minimal residual disease after appropriate cytoreductive measures have been taken, or should involve combination therapy with chemotherapeutic agents. In this way, we will be more likely to obtain the high *E1A* transfection efficiency that is needed to induce effective antitumor activity.

REFERENCES

1. Niculescu-Duvaz I, Cooper RG, Stribbling, et al. Recent developments in gene-directed enzyme prodrug therapy (GDEPT) for cancer. *Curr Opin Mol Ther* 1999;1:480–486.
2. Pandha HS. Genetic prodrug activation therapy for breast cancer: A phase I clinical trial of erbB-2-directed suicide gene expression. *J Clin Oncol* 1999;17:2180–2189.
3. Ram Z. Therapy of malignant brain tumors by intratumoral implantation of retroviral vector-producing cells. [see comments.] *Nature Medicine* 1997;3:1354–1361.
4. Lopes D, Mayer LD. Pharmacokinetics of Bcl-2 antisense oligonucleotide (G3139) combined with doxorubicin in SCID mice bearing human breast cancer solid tumor xenografts. *Cancer Chemother Pharmacol* 2002;49:57–68.
5. Fenig E, Kanfi Y, Wang Q, et al. Role of transforming growth factor beta in the growth inhibition of human breast cancer cells by basic fibroblast growth factor. *Breast Cancer Res Treat* 2001;70:27–37.
6. Jackson JG, Zhang X, Yoneda T, et al. Regulation of breast cancer cell motility by insulin receptor substrate-2 (IRS-2) in metastatic variants of human breast cancer cell lines. *Oncogene* 2001;20:7318–7325.
7. Li Z, Xia W, Fang B, et al. Targeting HER-2/neu-overexpressing breast cancer cells by an antisense iron responsive element-directed gene expression. *Cancer Lett* 2001;174:151–158.
8. Simoes-Wust AP, Olie RA, Gautschi O, et al. Bcl-xl antisense treatment induces apoptosis in breast carcinoma cells. *Int J Cancer* 2000;87:582–590.
9. Roh H, Pippin DW, Boswell CB, et al. HER2/neu antisense targeting of human breast carcinoma. *Oncogene* 2000;19:6138–6143.
10. Hanania EG, Deisseroth AB. Simultaneous genetic chemoprotection of normal marrow cells and genetic chemosensitization of breast cancer cells in a mouse cancer gene therapy model *Clin Cancer Res* 1997;3:281–286.
11. Rahman Z, Kavanagh J, Champlin R, et al. Chemotherapy immediately following autologous stem-cell transplantation in patients with advanced breast cancer. *Clin Cancer Res* 1998;4:2717–2721.
12. Roth JA, Nguyen D, Lawrence DD, et al. Retrovirus-mediated wild-type p53 gene transfer to tumors of patients with lung cancer. [see comments] *Nat Med* 1996;2:985–991.
13. Hortobagyi GN, Ueno NT, Xia WY, et al. Cationic liposome-mediated E1A gene transfer to human breast and ovarian cancer cells and its biologic effects: A phase I clinical trial. *J Clin Oncol* 2001;19:3422–3433.
14. Tait DL, Obermiller PS, Hatmaker, et al. Ovarian cancer BRCA1 gene therapy: Phase I and II trial differences in immune response and vector stability. *Clin Cancer Res* 1999;5:1708–1714.
15. Tait DL, Obermiller PS, Redlin-Frazier S, et al. A phase I trial of retroviral BRCA1sv gene therapy in ovarian cancer. *Clin Cancer Res* 1997;3:1959–1968.
16. Holt JT, Thompson ME, Szabo C, et al. Growth retardation and tumour inhibition by BRCA1. *Nat Genet* 1996;12:298–302.
17. Murray JL, Yoo GH, Lopez-Berestein G, et al. Phase I trial of intratumoral liposomal-E1A gene therapy in patients with recurrent/refractory breast (BC) and head and neck (H&N) cancer. *Proc ASCO* 1998, pp. 431a.
18. Bischoff JR, Kirn DH, Williams A, et al. An adenovirus mutant that replicates selectively in p53-deficient human tumor cells. *Science* 1996;274:373–376.
19. Khuri FR, Nemunaitis J, Ganly I, et al. A controlled trial of intratumoral ONYX-015, a selectively-replicating adenovirus, in combination with cisplatin and 5-fluorouracil in patients with recurrent head and neck cancer. *Nat Med* 2000;6:879–885.
20. Pouton CW, Seymour LW. Key issues in non-viral gene delivery. *Adv Drug Deliv Rev* 2001;46:187–203.
21. Schatzlein AG. Non-viral vectors in cancer gene therapy: principles and progress. *Anticancer Drugs* 2001;12:275–304.
22. Druker BJ, Sawyers CL, Kantarjian H, et al. Activity of a specific inhibitor of the BCR-ABL tyrosine kinase in the blast crisis of chronic myeloid leukemia and acute lymphoblastic leukemia with the Philadelphia chromosome. *N Engl J Med* 2001;344:1038–1042.
23. Druker BJ, Talpaz M, Resta DJ, et al. Efficacy and safety of a specific inhibitor of the BCR-ABL tyrosine kinase in chronic myeloid leukemia. *N Engl J Med* 2001;344:1031–1037.
24. Gorre ME, Mohammed M, Ellwood K, et al. Clinical resistance to STI-571 cancer therapy caused by BCR-ABL gene mutation or amplification, *Science* 2001;293:876–880.
25. Berk AJ. Adenovirus promoters and E1A transactivation, *Annu Rev Genet* 1986;20:45–79.
26. Berk AJ. Functions of adenovirus E1A. *Cancer Surveys* 1986;5:367–387.
27. Schrier PI, Bernards R, Vaessen RT, et al. Expression of class I major histocompatibility antigens switched off by highly oncogenic adenovirus 12 in transformed rat cells. *Nature* 1983;305:771–775.
28. Ruley HE. Adenovirus early region 1A enables viral and cellular transforming genes to transform primary cells in culture. *Nature* 1983;304:602–606.
29. Byrd PJ, Grand RJ, Gallimore PH. Differential transformation of primary human embryo retinal cells by adenovirus E1 regions and combinations of E1A + Ras. *Oncogene* 1988;2:477–484.
30. Montell C, Courtois G, Eng C, Berk A. Complete transformation by adenovirus 2 requires both E1A proteins. *Cell* 1984;36:951–961.
31. Yu D, Suen TC, Yan DH, et al. Transcriptional repression of the neu protooncogene by the adenovirus 5 E1A gene products. *Proc Natl Acad Sci USA* 1990;87:4499–4503.
32. Yu DH, Scorsone K, Hung MC. Adenovirus type 5 E1A gene products act as transformation suppressors of the neu oncogene. *Mol Cell Biol* 1991;11:1745–1750.

33. Yu D, Hamada J, Zhang H, et al. Mechanisms of c-erbB2/neu oncogene-induced metastasis and repression of metastatic properties by adenovirus 5 E1A gene products. *Oncogene* 1992;7:2263–2270.
34. Yu D, Shi D, Scanlon M, et al. Reexpression of neu-encoded oncoprotein counteracts the tumor-suppressing but not the metastasis-suppressing function of E1A. *Cancer Res* 1993;53:5784–5790.
35. Yu D, Wolf JK, Scanlon M, et al. Enhanced c-erbB-2/neu expression in human ovarian cancer cells correlates with more severe malignancy that can be suppressed by E1A. *Cancer Res* 1993;53:891–898.
36. Frisch SM, Reich R, Collier IE, et al. Adenovirus E1A represses protease gene expression and inhibits metastasis of human tumor cells. *Oncogene* 1990;5:75–83.
37. Young KS, Weigel R, Hiebert S, Nevins JR. Adenovirus E1A-mediated negative control of genes activated during F9 differentiation. *Mol Cell Biol* 1989;9:3109–3113.
38. Timmers HT, van Dam H, Pronk GJ, et al. Adenovirus E1A represses transcription of the cellular JE gene. *J Virol* 1989;63:1470–1473.
39. van Dam H, Offringa R, Smits AM, et al. The repression of the growth factor-inducible genes JE, c-myc and stromelysin by adenovirus E1A is mediated by conserved region 1. *Oncogene* 1989;4:1207–1212.
40. Pozzatti R, McCormick M, Thompson MA, Khoury G. The *E1A* gene of adenovirus type 2 reduces the metastatic potential of ras-transformed rat embryo cells. *Mol Cell Biol* 1988;8:2984–2988.
41. Steeg PS, Bevilacqua G, Pozzatti R, et al. Altered expression of NM23, a gene associated with low tumor metastatic potential, during adenovirus 2 E1a inhibition of experimental metastasis. *Cancer Res* 1988;48:6550–6554.
42. Rosengard AM, Krutzsch HC, Shearn A, et al. Reduced Nm23/Awd protein in tumour metastasis and aberrant Drosophila development. *Nature* 1989;342:177–180.
43. Frisch SM. Antioncogenic effect of adenovirus E1A in human tumor cells. *Proc Natl Acad Sci USA* 1991;88:9077–9081.
44. Frisch SM, Dolter KE. Adenovirus E1A-mediated tumor suppression by a c-erbB-2/neu-independent mechanism. *Cancer Res* 1995;55:5551–5555.
45. Deng J, Xia W, Hung MC. Adenovirus 5 E1A-mediated tumor suppression associated with E1A-mediated apoptosis in vivo. *Oncogene* 1998;17:2167–2175.
46. Rao L, Debbas M, Sabbatini P, et al. The adenovirus E1A proteins induce apoptosis, which is inhibited by the E1B 19-kDa and Bcl-2 proteins. *Proc Natl Acad Sci USA* 1992;89:7742–7746.
47. Lowe SW, Ruley HE. Stabilization of the p53 tumor suppressor is induced by adenovirus 5 E1A and accompanies apoptosis. *Genes Dev* 1993;7:535–545.
48. Debbas M, White E. Wild-type p53 mediates apoptosis by E1A, which is inhibited by E1B. *Genes Dev* 1993;7:546–554.
49. Chen MJ, Holskin B, Strickler J, et al. Induction by E1A oncogene expression of cellular susceptibility to lysis by TNF. *Nature* 1987;330:581–583.
50. Shao R, Hu MC, Zhou BP, et al. E1A sensitizes cells to tumor necrosis factor-induced apoptosis through inhibition of IkappaB kinases and nuclear factor kappaB activities. *J Biol Chem* 1999;274:21495–21498.
51. Cook JL, May DL, Wilson BA, et al. Role of tumor necrosis factor-alpha in E1A oncogene-induced susceptibility of neoplastic cells to lysis by natural killer cells and activated macrophages. *J Immunol* 1989;142:4527–4534.
52. Lee WP, Liao Y, Robinson D, et al. Axl-Gas6 interaction counteracts E1A-mediated cell growth suppression and proapoptotic activity. *Mol Cell Biol* 1999;19:8075–8082.
53. Lee WP, Wen Y, Varnum B, Hung MC. Akt is required for Axl-Gas6 signaling to protect cells from E1A-mediated apoptosis. *Oncogene* 2002;21:329–336.
54. Sanchez-Prieto R, de Alava E, Palomino T, et al. An association between viral genes and human oncogenic alterations: the adenovirus E1A induces the Ewing tumor fusion transcript EWS-FLI1 [see comments]. *Nat Med* 1999;5:1076–1079.
55. Kovar H. E1A and the Ewing tumor translocation. *Nat Med* 1999;5:1331.
56. Melot T, Delattre O. E1A and the Ewing tumor translocation. *Nat Med* 1999;5:1331.
57. Meric F, Liao Y, Lee WP, et al. Adenovirus 5 early region 1A does not induce expression of the ewing sarcoma fusion product EWS-FLI1 in breast and ovarian cancer cell lines. *Clin Cancer Res* 2000;6:3832–3836.
58. Friedmann T. Overcoming the obstacles to gene therapy. *Sci Am* 1997;276:96–101.
59. Felgner PL. Nonviral strategies for gene therapy. *Sci Am* 1997;276:102–106.
60. Felgner PL, Ringold GM. Cationic liposome-mediated transfection. *Nature* 1989;337:387–388.
61. Nabel EG, Gordon D, Yang ZY, et al. Gene transfer in vivo with DNA-liposome complexes: lack of autoimmunity and gonadal localization. *Hum Gene Ther* 1992;3:649–656.
62. Nabel GJ, Nabel EG, Yang ZY, et al. Direct gene transfer with DNA-liposome complexes in melanoma: expression, biologic activity, and lack of toxicity in humans. *Proc Natl Acad Sci USA* 1993;90:11307–11311.
63. Yu D, Matin A, Xia W, et al. Liposome-mediated in vivo E1A gene transfer suppressed dissemination of ovarian cancer cells that overexpress HER-2/neu. *Oncogene* 1995;11:1383–1388.
64. Xing X, Liu V, Xia W, et al. Safety studies of the intraperitoneal injection of E1A—liposome complex in mice. *Gene Ther* 1997;4:238–243.
65. Xing X, Zhang S, Chang JY, et al. Safety study and characterization of E1A-liposome complex gene delivery in an ovarian cancer model. *Gene Ther* 1998;5:1538–1544.
66. Chang JY, Xia W, Shao R, et al. The tumor suppression activity of E1A in HER-2/neu-overexpressing breast cancer. *Oncogene* 1997;14:561–568.
67. Hortobagyi GN, Hung MC, Lopez-Berestein G. A phase I multicenter study of E1A gene therapy for patients with metastatic breast cancer and epithelial ovarian cancer that overexpresses HER-2/neu or epithelial ovarian cancer [In Process Citation]. *Hum Gene Ther* 1998;9:1775–1798.
68. Xia WY, Lau YK, Zhang HZ, et al. Strong correlation between c-Erbb-2 overexpression and overall survival of patients with oral squamous cell carcinoma. *Clin Cancer Res* 1997;3:3–9.
69. Ueno NT, Xia W, Tucker SD, et al. Issues in the development of gene therapy: preclinical experiments in E1A gene delivery. *Oncol Rep* 1999;6:257–262.

70. Rodrigues M, Dion P, Sircar S, Weber JM. Tumor necrosis factor mediated cytolysis requires the adenovirus E1a protein but not the transformed phenotype. *Virus Res* 1990;15:231–236.
71. Shisler J, Duerksen HP, Hermiston TM, et al. Induction of susceptibility to tumor necrosis factor by E1A is dependent on binding to either p300 or p105-Rb and induction of DNA synthesis. *J Virol* 1996;70:68–77.
72. Li S, Huang L. In vivo gene transfer via intravenous administration of cationic lipid-protamine-DNA (LPD) complexes. *Gene Ther* 1997;4:891–900.
73. Li S, Rizzo MA, Bhattacharya S, Huang L. Characterization of cationic lipid-protamine-DNA (LPD) complexes for intravenous gene delivery. *Gene Ther* 1998;5:930–937.
74. Li S, Wu SP, Whitmore M, et al. Effect of immune response on gene transfer to the lung via systemic administration of cationic lipidic vectors. *Am J Physiol* 1999;276:796–804.
75. Nikitin AY, Juarez-Perez MI, Li S, et al. RB-mediated suppression of spontaneous multiple neuroendocrine neoplasia and lung metastases in Rb+/− mice. *Proc Natl Acad Sci USA* 1999;96:3916–3921.
76. Tan Y, Li S, Pitt BR, Huang L. The inhibitory role of CpG immunostimulatory motifs in cationic lipid vector-mediated transgene expression in vivo. *Hum Gene Ther* 1999;10:2153–2161.
77. Whitmore M, Li S, Huang L. LPD lipopolyplex initiates a potent cytokine response and inhibits tumor growth. *Gene Ther* 1999;6:1867–1875.
78. Shao R, Tsai EM, Wei K, et al. E1A inhibition of radiation-induced NF-kappaB activity through suppression of IKK activity and IkappaB degradation, independent of Akt activation. *Cancer Res* 2001;61:7413–7416.
79. Lowe SW, Ruley HE, Jacks T, Housman DE. p53-dependent apoptosis modulates the cytotoxicity of anticancer agents. *Cell* 1993;74:957–967.
80. Sanchez-Prieto R, Lleonart M, Ramon Y, Cajal SR. Lack of correlation between p53 protein level and sensitivity of DNA-damaging agents in keratinocytes carrying adenovirus E1a mutants. *Oncogene* 1995;11:675–682.
81. Sanchez-Prieto R, Quintanilla M, Cano A, et al. Carcinoma cell lines become sensitive to DNA-damaging agents by the expression of the adenovirus E1A gene. *Oncogene* 1996;13:1083–1092.
82. Ueno NT, Bartholomeusz C, Herrmann JL, et al. E E1A-mediated paclitaxel sensitization in HER-2/neu-overexpressing ovarian cancer SKOV3.ip1 through apoptosis involving the caspase-3 pathway. *Clin Cancer Res* 2000;6:250–259.
83. Ueno NT, Yu D, Hung MC. Chemosensitization of HER-2/*neu*-overexpressing human breast cancer cells to paclitaxel (Taxol) by adenovirus type 5 *E1A*. *Oncogene* 1997;15:953–960.

SECTION 2

Early Clinical and Preclinical

22

DNA Microarray Analysis of Breast Cancer: Toward Customized Anti-cancer Drug Therapy and Rational Drug Design

John R. Mackey and Brent Zanke

Cancer is a genetic disease, due in large part to acquired mutations and epigenetic changes that affect gene expression. Early efforts to dissect these genetic changes identified single genes within functional classes involved in tumor formation and drug sensitivity—oncogenes, tumor suppressor genes, and genes associated with apoptosis, membrane transporters, DNA repair enzymes and drug target enzymes. However, breast cancers display marked aneuploidy, multiple gene amplifications and deletions, and genetic instability, complicating the study of the downstream effects of these genetic changes. Although the marked variability of the genetic changes among breast cancers probably accounts for the different clinical behaviors of histologically similar tumors, the complexity of cancer genetic changes has frustrated attempts to relate complex phenotypes to simple changes. More detailed pictures are now available as the identification of single-gene products has been superseded by high throughput and genome-wide analysis of breast cancers.

DNA MICROARRAY-BASED BREAST CANCER GENE EXPRESSION PROFILING

DNA Microarray Technology

The initial sequencing of the human genome identified approximately 30,000 different genes (1,2). Gene transcripts have been isolated through transcript sequencing and are catalogued, with commercial availability as isolated transcripts, at *www.ncbi.nlm.nih.gov/dbEST/dbEST access.html* or (*http://image.llnl.gov*). Recently, synthetic oligonucleotides corresponding to identified human gene transcripts have become available, providing another representation of the human "transcriptosome," at *www.operon.com.*

A microarray is an orderly arrangement of known or unknown DNA samples attached to a solid support. DNA microarrays are typically constructed using oligonucleotide probes, synthesized *in situ* using the techniques of masked photolithography and solid-phase chemical synthesis (*www.affymetrix.com/*) or by mechanical spotting of cDNA or oligonucleotides onto glass microscope slides (3). Each DNA spot on the microarray is usually less than 200 μm in diameter and a typical array contains thousands of spots. To detect global gene expression in tissues these arrays are hybridized to fluorescently labeled gene transcripts and detected after laser excitation by analysis of emission energy (Fig. 22.1; see color plate). Typically, dynamic ranges on the order of 10^5 are observed, allowing the comprehensive, sensitive and specific evaluation of gene expression.

Tumor Handling and Sampling

Microarray experiments usually require between 10 μg and 40 μg of high-quality RNA, which requires approximately 100 mm³ of tissue. Biopsy and surgical specimens must be snap-frozen in liquid nitrogen within 30 minutes of devitalization and stored in liquid nitrogen to prevent RNA degradation. To date, formalin-fixed tissues do not yield sufficient high-quality RNA for these experiments. Optimally, these tissues should be linked to a clinical database of information concerning each patient, her treatment and outcome.

Breast cancers are heterogenous mixtures of several cell types, including stromal elements, blood vessels, and tumor-associated lymphocytes. Tumors also vary markedly in the proportion of malignant cells comprising the tumor. Potentially, the signal derived from non-breast cancer cells might complicate the accurate assessment of the cancer transcriptosome. Alternatively, the expression signatures from stroma, endothelial cells, and immune cells may be informative markers of interactions that may play a critical role in tumor progression. Most breast cancer studies to date have used whole-tumor analysis, and although the signatures of other cell lineages are detectable, the microarray output is nonetheless informative for tumor classification and prognostication. Although it is possible to perform laser capture microdissection for microarray studies (4), this is technically challenging and precludes high-throughput analysis of breast tumors.

Data Analysis

Gene expression profiling of human tumors typically yields tens of thousands of data points for each sample analyzed. This abundance of data poses challenges for data organisation, storage and analysis. While new techniques for analyzing array data such as neural networks, Bayesian belief nets, classification and regression trees, discriminate analysis and logistic regression are in development, to date, two approaches have been most commonly applied to the analysis of breast cancer microarray data.

Unsupervised learning (also known as clustering analysis) aggregates data into clusters based on different features in a data set. Samples are grouped according to the similarity of their expression profiles. The output of cluster analysis is typically displayed as a dendrogram, where closely related samples cluster together and distantly related samples are separated (Fig. 22.2; see color plate). Such unsupervised analyses are unbiased and do not require prior assumptions about which genes or expression patterns are most important, nor are patterns selected for their associations with non-array data (such as histologic features or clinical outcomes).

Supervised learning incorporates non-microarray derived data to make distinctions of interest. Usually, a training data set is used to select the gene expression features that best make a distinction (for example, ER-positive versus ER-negative status derived by tumor immunohistochemistry). Often small numbers of genes can be identified that maximally distinguish these groups. These gene expression signatures must then be applied to an independent data set to determine whether or not the observed relationship occurred by chance.

CLINICAL APPLICATIONS

Diagnosis and Classification

The current standard for breast cancer diagnosis and classification relies on the assessment of tumor histology, assisted by a handful of immunohistochemical assays. Because the overall behavior of a breast cancer must be determined by the expression of the genes within it, it should be possible to identify sets of genes whose expression or lack thereof defines each individual property of a tumor, including its biologic behavior. Through comprehensive microarray-based gene expression profiles, distinct breast cancer classifications with potential prognostic relevance have been identified.

Perou et al. (20) first used microarray to systematically classify breast cancers. Samples were derived from 42 individuals; 20 of these patients had locally advanced breast cancers treated with pre-surgical doxorubicin therapy, providing pretreatment and post-treatment paired samples. Cluster analysis of 63 samples revealed that, despite the fact that most of the cases were histologically invasive ductal carcinomas, there was tremendous diversity of gene expression between cases. However, each of the "paired" samples derived from a given individual (whether pre-and post-doxorubicin treatment, or primary tumor and lymph node metastases) were strikingly similar. This suggested that microarray fingerprinting was a stable feature of breast cancer, independent of intervening treatment or metastatic spread to axillary lymph nodes. Once genes characteristic of contaminating endothelial cells, stromal cells, adipocytes and inflammatory cells had been excluded, the authors then selected a subset of 496 genes that showed the greatest variation in expression between patients. Reclustering identified five breast cancer classes: (a) ER-positive with luminal epithelial cell expression; (b) ER-negative with basal epithelial expression; (c) ER-negative/ER-poor; (d) HER-2 overexpressing; and (e) normal breast-like with basal epithelial and adipose cell expression. The potential prognostic value of these classifications is discussed below.

Several independent studies, including our own experiments, have confirmed that the ER status of primary breast cancers can be readily distinguished by microarray analysis (Fig. 22.2) (5–7).

Microarray analysis can aid the diagnosis of tumor clonality in an individual with multiple adjacent breast tumors. Two physically distinct foci of invasive ductal carcinoma within a single breast were analyzed and found to be essentially indistinguishable by microarray analysis, but markedly different from tumors matched for grade, stage, and hormone receptor status derived from other individuals (8). Additionally, microarray analysis of primary breast cancer shows some promise in the prediction of axillary lymph node status. Should this be validated, those patients with node-negative expression profiles would not require axillary lymph node dissection, avoiding its well known and significant morbidity (9).

The diagnosis of BRCA-1 and BRCA-2 associated breast cancers is critically important, because, unlike sporadic breast cancers, patients and physicians must consider the potential benefits of prophylactic mastectomy, prophylactic oophorectomy, and genetic screening of at-risk family members. Transcriptional profiling identifies distinct molecular signatures of BRCA-1– and BRCA-2–associated breast cancers, which differ both from each other and from sporadic breast cancers (10). However, the sample size of this study was very small, with only seven cases analyzed in each category; clearly these results require confirmation by analysis of larger series of hereditary and sporadic cancers.

Prognosis

Microarray analysis holds great promise as a marker of disease prognosis. This has been best defined as "capable of predicting relapse or progression independent of future treatment effects" (11). So far, two studies have supported microarray analysis as a meaningful prognostic marker (6,12).

In an extension of the initial study by Perou et al. (13), 78 invasive carcinomas were assessed by microarray methods, including the cancers previously described (6). Cluster analysis of 456 genes showed significantly greater expression between different tumors than between paired samples from the same cancer. Tumors could be classified into a basal epithelial-like group, a HER-2 overexpressing group, a normal breast-like group, and two subtypes of luminal cancers. Fifty-one of these patients participated in a prospective study on locally advanced breast cancer treated with doxorubicin monotherapy. Using this subset of 51 patients who received uniform therapy, the HER-2 overexpressing and basal epithelial-like groups had significantly shorter disease-free and overall survival, while the luminal A group had a markedly better outcome than other subtypes.

The study thus far providing the strongest evidence of prognostic utility for microarrays in early-stage breast cancer analyzed node negative invasive carcinomas from 97 patients younger than 55 years, not known to be BRCA-1 or BRCA-2 positive (12). None of these patients received adjuvant systemic therapy. Unsupervised clustering analysis of the 5,000 genes showing variability separated two groups with slightly different prognoses. However, using a supervised classification method, 231 genes with correlations to disease outcome were identified, rank-ordered on the basis of the correlation strength, then mathematically pared down to the 70 genes that most accurately reflected prognosis. The genes upregulated in the poor prognosis signature predominantly involved cell cycle regulation, invasion and metastasis, angiogenesis and signal transduction. This 70 signature-gene profile was validated with an independent tumor set and correctly prognosticated 5-year disease-free status in 17 of 19 patients. The authors suggest that signature-gene profile selects those high-risk, node-negative patients who would benefit from adjuvant therapy, but would substantially reduce the number of patients receiving potentially unnecessary treatments recommended by either using the St. Galen's (14) or NIH (15) consensus criteria. Although the authors state that microarray "provides a strategy to select patients who would benefit from adjuvant therapy," this study only reveals poor prognosis patients. It is not able to predict benefit from adjuvant therapy as patients were not randomized to therapeutic interventions based on microarray signature-gene profiling.

Microarray does not yet meet the highest level of evidence (level I) for prognostic factor utility (11), and will require high-powered prospective, controlled studies with specified follow-up to determine the independent value of expression analysis when compared to standard prognostic factors. However, the identification of novel molecular subclasses of breast cancer with apparent prognostic value, which may lead to individualized treatment, undoubtedly justifies the effort and expense of these studies.

Prediction of Therapeutic Benefit

Microarray analysis also shows promise as a predictive marker, defined as "capable of predicting response or resistance to a specific therapy" (11). Currently, there are only two well-validated predictive markers to guide systemic therapy: estrogen receptor status predicts benefit from hormonal therapy, while HER-2 amplification predicts benefit from trastuzumab treatment. Currently we lack predictive markers for the use of chemotherapy, the most toxic of the available breast cancer treatment modalities. Microarray analysis has the potential to be able to guide clinicians and patients in decisions regarding adjuvant and/or metastatic chemotherapy. However, the ultimate proof of the value of microarray as a predictive factor requires its prospective assessment in randomized trials.

DRUG DEVELOPMENT

Microarray analysis could, in principle, provide several types of information to assist in drug discovery and development. Microarray is now being applied to breast cancer target identification, target validation (demonstrating that affecting the enzyme or biochemical entity has therapeutic effects), optimizing efficacy, and reducing toxicity. DNA microarray analysis may also facilitate identification of clinical trial participants who are most likely to respond or to adversely react to treatment.

Drug Target Identification

Traditional anticancer drug discovery has included large-scale screening of compounds for *in vitro* anticancer effects, even when the mechanisms of action of such compounds might be unknown. Expression profiling of cells treated with a pharmacological agent can now be used to identify the target of an empirically identified drug (16).

The development of molecular-based breast cancer therapy requires a detailed molecular and genetic understanding of clinical cancers. Microarray analysis can define the genetic differences (and thereby potential drug targets) acquired during the process of breast carcinogenesis. In an elegant study, purified normal, primary invasive and lymph node metastatic breast cell populations were obtained from a single patient by laser capture microdissection. These cells were successfully subjected to cDNA microarray analysis to identify differentially expresses genes with potential roles in breast cancer pathogenesis (4). Similarly, a unique *ras* superfamily gene, *RERG* (*ras*-related and estrogen-regulated growth inhibitor) was identified after expression analysis linked low or absent expression in primary human breast tumors with poor prognosis (17). The functional analysis of *RERG* suggests that loss of *RERG* expression may contribute to breast tumorigenesis, and in addition has identified a novel signal transduction pathway for drug targeting.

The Use of DNA Microarrays in the Evaluation of Anti-cancer Drug Sensitivity

Cancer researchers have longed for a reliable assay to accurately predict tumor sensitivity to antineoplastic agents. While drug response is likely a composite of patient factors (such as performance status and metabolism capacity), and tumor factors (such as intrinsic sensitivity and tumor oxygenation) genome-based methodologies have focused on tumor gene expression as a predictor of clinical outcome.

As proof of principle, the drug sensitivity of 60 human tumor cell lines was related to global gene expression (18). For this study, the cell lines used by the National Cancer Institute for *in vitro* drug testing were subjected to cDNA expression analysis. For each cell line, *in vitro* sensitivity data to over 70,000 compounds was available, facilitating comparisons between gene expression and drug sensitivity. Of 8,000 total gene spots on the microarrays, 1,376 were identified as having the most variation among cell lines. While the overall correlation between grouping cells on the basis of gene expression and on the basis of drug activity was rather low ($r = 0.21$), several interesting relationships between individual compounds and genes were detected.

Microarray-determined gene expression in the breast carcinoma cell line MCF-7 was related to doxorubicin sensitivity. Acute exposure of MCF-7 cells to doxorubicin induced a subset of genes that tended to be overexpressed in lines with known constitutive drug resistance (20). The conclusion from these studies was that specific gene products, when expressed at the time of drug exposure, may modulate lethal effects and that their measurement may predict *in vitro* drug sensitivity.

Microarray will undoubtedly prove useful in the evaluation of the biological determinants of response to newer, molecularly targeted, therapies. One pragmatic and promising approach is to apply microarray to the evaluation of early stage primary breast cancers treated with neoadjuvant therapy. After an initial biopsy is obtained, a targeted therapy could be administered for a few weeks prior to definitive tumor resection. The pre- and post-therapy samples could then be compared to determine: (a) treatment-related changes in relevant drug targets or target pathways; and (b) pre-treatment correlates of drug response. This would facilitate the rapid screening of novel compounds for evidence of their intended biological effects *in vivo,* their efficacy in tumor control, and the identification of predictive assays to guide appropriate selection of subsequent clinical trial candidates.

THE FUTURE OF BREAST CANCER MICROARRAY

Although technical and analytical improvements will undoubtedly develop to increase the utility of breast cancer gene expression, the most promising changes will likely occur through the integration of gene expression with proteomics.

One approach to the integration of gene expression data with protein analysis is to subject gene expression data to data enrichment. Data enrichment adds layers of external data or "prior knowledge" to raw bioprofile data. For example, various bioanalytical tools can assign, derive or predict meta-information (information about the information) associated with microarray data. Identification of clusters of genes which are upregulated will not, however, necessarily indicate which signaling or metabolic pathways are being affected, which genes work together, or what genes act as repressors on others. Such insight could be gained by including, with the raw microarray data, additional protein interaction data (Biomolecular Interaction Database (BIND) *www.bind.ca* or signaling pathway data (Cancer Genome Anatomy Project (CGAP database at *http://cgap.nci.nih.gov*).

Dozens of bioinformatics databases are available, including:

- human genome sequence data (GenBank at *www.ncbi.nlm.nih.gov/Genbank*)
- Federated 2D gel data (Swiss 2D PAGE database at *www.expasy.ch/ch2d*)
- human mutation data (P53 mutation database *http://p53.genome.ad.jp*)
- KMDB (Human disease mutation database at *http://mutview.dmb.med.keio.ac.jp*)
- human disease information (OMIM at *www3.ncbi.nlm.nih.gov/Omim*)
- and a wide range of tumor-specific data (Cancer Chromosome Aberration project at *www.ncbi.nlm.nih.gov/CCAP/*, the Atlas of Genetics & Cytogenetics in Oncology at *www.infobiogen.fr/services/chromcancer*, and the Breast Cancer Gene Database *http://condor.bcm.tmc.edu/ermb/bcgd/bcgd.html*).

Such data add quantitative or relational information about protein-protein and protein-ligand interactions, homologs, paralogs, functional assignment, gene abundance, tertiary structure, quaternary structure, protein location, disease-causing mutations, protein and RNA turnover rates, chromosomal aberrations, chromosomal location, and karyotypic data. Because genomic and proteomic data are constantly changing (due to ongoing changes to the databases and improvements to algorithms), self-updating tools are required to automatically update this meta-information on a regular basis.

Another approach to integrating gene expression and protein abundance information is to perform paired DNA microarray and proteomic analysis on breast tumors. Analysis of linked relational databases would be expected to provide a more accurate impression of the biology of each tumor, reveal previously unsuspected relationships between genes and their protein products, and would be expected to further refine the utility of a cancer bioprofile.

Such methods have the power to explain complex biological phenomena of tumor progression and direct the development of prognosticators and new therapeutic targets. It is highly likely that this understanding will facilitate predictive markers and treatment based on the unique genetic aspects of individual tumors. Rational drug development designed to address specific genetic abnormalities means that molecular diagnosis will inevitably be followed by targeted drug therapy. Additionally, as the key molecular indicators of prognosis and therapeutic response to standard drugs are determined, array-based diagnosis, perhaps limited to those few signature-genes of highest relevance, may well become a routine study performed on each new breast cancer.

CONCLUSION

DNA microarray analysis is an extremely important new technology that allows genome-wide assessment of breast cancer biology. It appears capable of assisting in several unique diagnostic roles and has the potential to be an indicator of breast cancer prognosis that might well out-perform our current tools. Most importantly, gene expression analysis is poised to speed the discovery of novel, predictive assays and new targeted breast cancer therapeutics.

REFERENCES

1. Subramanian G, et al. Implications of the human genome for understanding human biology and medicine. *JAMA* 2001;286(18):2296–2307.
2. Venter JC, et al. The sequence of the human genome. *Science* 2001;291(5507):1304–1351.
3. Pollack JR, et al. Genome-wide analysis of DNA copy-number changes using cDNA microarrys. *Nature Genetics* 1999;23:41–46.
4. Sgroi DC, et al. In vivo gene expression profile analysis of human breast cancer progression. *Cancer Research* 1999;59:5656–5661.
5. Gruvberger S, et al. Estrogen receptor status in breast cancer is associated with remarkably distinct gene expression patterns. *Cancer Research* 2001;61:5979–5984.
6. Sorlie T, et al. Gene expression patterns of breast carcinomas distinguish tumor subclasses with clinical implications. *Proc Natl Acad Sci USA* 2001;98(19):10869–10874.

7. Mackey J, Zanke B. Unpublished observations.
8. Unger MA, et al. Characterization of adjacent breast tumors using oligonucleotide microarrays. *Breast Cancer Research* 2001;3:336–341.
9. West M, et al. Predicting the clinical status of human breast cancer by using gene expression profiles. *Proc Natl Acad Sci USA* 2001;98(20):11462–11467.
10. Hedenfalk I, et al. Gene-expression profiles in hereditary breast cancer. *N Engl J Med* 2001;344(8):539–548.
11. Hayes DF, et al. Tumor marker utility grading system: a framework to evaluate clinical utility of tumor markers. *J Natl Cancer Inst* 1996;88(20):1456–1466.
12. van't Veer LJ, et al. Gene expression profiling predicts clinical outcome of breast cancer. *Nature* 2002;415:530–536.
13. Perou CM, et al. Molecular portraits of human breast tumours. *Nature* 2000;406(6797):747–752.
14. Goldhirsch A, et al. Meeting highlights: International Consensus Panel on the Treatment of Primary Breast Cancer. Seventh International Conference on Adjuvant Therapy of Primary Breast Cancer. *J Clin Oncol* 2001;19(18):3817–3827.
15. Authors M. The National Institutes of Health Consensus Development Conference: Adjuvant therapy for breast cancer. *J Natl Cancer Inst Monogr* 2001;30:1–152.
16. Hughes TR, et al. Functional discovery via a compendium of expression profiles. *Cell* 2000;102(1):109–126.
17. Finlin B, et al. RERG is a novel ras-related, estrogen-regulated and growth-inhibitory gene in breast cancer. *J Biol Chem* 2001;276(45):42259–42267.
18. Scherf U, et al. A gene expression database for the molecular pharmacology of cancer. *Nat Genet* 2000;24(3):236–244.
19. Kudoh K, et al. Monitoring the expression profiles of doxorubicin-induced and doxorubicin-resistant cancer cells by cDNA microarry. *Cancer Research* 2000;60:4161–4166.
20. Perou CM, et al. Distinctive gene expression patterns in human mammary epithelial cells and breast cancers. *Proc Natl Acad Sci USA* 1999;3;96(16):9212–9217.

23

Proteomics of Breast Cancer: Marker Discovery and Signal Pathway Profiling

Hubert Hondermarck, Anne-Sophie Vercoutter-Edouart,
Françoise Révillion, Jérôme Lemoine, Ikram El Yazidi-Belkoura,
Victor Nurcombe, and Jean-Philippe Peyrat

The progressive completion of human genome sequencing and the introduction of mass spectrometry combined with advanced bioinformatics for protein identification, have led to the emergence of proteomics as a powerful tool for characterizing new markers and therapeutic targets. Breast cancer proteomics has already identified markers of potential clinical interest (such as the molecular chaperone 14-3-3 sigma) and technological innovations such as large-scale and high-throughput analysis are now driving the field. Methods in functional proteomics have also been developed to study the intracellular signaling pathways that underlie the development of breast cancer. As illustrated with fibroblast growth factor 2, a mitogen and scatter factor for breast cancer cells, proteomics is a powerful approach to identify signaling proteins and to decipher the complex signaling circuitry involved in tumor growth. Together with genomics, proteomics is opening new perspectives for the definition of new therapeutic targets.

BACKGROUND

Complementing the field of genomics, proteomics is designed to elucidate both protein levels and post-translational modifications in different cell types under different physiological conditions. This approach is now a powerful tool for the study of changes in protein expression inherent to the developing pathophysiology of any cell type, tissue, or whole organism (1,2).

Proteomic analysis encompasses different methodologies (Fig. 23.1). After protein extraction from cells in tissue culture or from biopsies, protein separation is usually performed using two-dimensional electrophoresis (2DE) which allows the separation of thousands of proteins from a single mixture. Mass spectrometry is now the most sensitive method for the characterization of picoquantities of polypeptides from 2DE gels and for the characterization of posttranslational modifications. The possibility of performing large-scale proteomic analysis of human protein profiles has finally become a reality due to the progressive sequencing of the human genome and the concomitant development of bioinformatics, allowing the compilation of searchable genomic and proteomic databases accessible via the Internet.

There are two main goals for the use of proteomic analysis in breast cancer. The first is to discover new molecular markers for the profiling of breast tumors. The second is to decipher the intracellular signaling pathways that lead to breast cancer cell development. Such data would provide the knowledge base for the identification of therapeutic targets and the development of new strategies against breast cancer.

PROTEOMICS FOR IDENTIFYING MOLECULAR MARKERS OF BREAST CANCER

The technology most commonly used for proteomic analysis is 2DE, which allows the separation and display of thousands of proteins from a complex mixture. The use of 2DE to resolve cancer patient serum proteins was reported as early as 1974, with differences being noted in the protein patterns of individuals suffering from cancer (3). However, this first study was essentially descriptive, and no protein identification, other than albumin, was made. In contrast, a few years later,

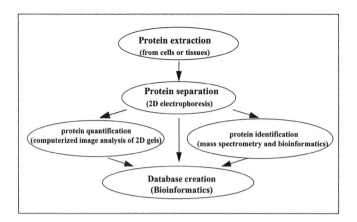

FIG. 23.1. Proteomic analysis.

Westley and Rochefort (4) detected, in human breast cancer cell lines, a secreted 46 kDa glycoprotein induced by estrogens which proved, with specific antibodies, to be the protease cathepsin D. The production of the protease inhibitor α1-antichymotrypsin was also shown in breast cancer cells (5), indicating the potential importance of the extracellular protease/anti-protease balance in the development of breast cancer. Interestingly, large-scale 2DE analysis has also been carried out and reveals the subtle nature of the protein differences observed between normal versus cancer samples. The overall profiles were globally quite similar, and only a very small proportion of proteins differed in expression levels between normal and cancer tissues. Stastny et al. (6), in 1984, found that most polypeptides were consistently present in both malignant and nonmalignant tissue, as only ten polypeptides differed out of 350. Using higher level resolution, Wirth et al. in 1987 (7), and in 1989 (8), and Worland et al. (9) have demonstrated that of approximately 1,000 silver-stained polypeptides in the cytosol, the 2DE patterns from normal and malignant tissue differed qualitatively in only six places, and only 22 places quantitatively. Similarly, Maloney et al. in 1989 (10) reported, after computer-based analyses of 2DE gels, a total of eight polypeptide differences between cancerous and normal breast epithelial cells in tissue culture. The fact that only a few differences are reported between cancer and normal breast epithelial cells emphasizes the need for using sensitive specific and reproducible protocols. More precise characterization of such polypeptide differences was published in the early 1990s. Trask et al. (11) demonstrated that normal cells produce keratins K5, K6, K7 and K17, whereas tumor cells produce mainly keratins K8, K18, and K19. This distribution was confirmed in tumor samples (12,13), and cytokeratin immunodetection is now used in histopathology to highlight epithelial cells versus other cell lineages and to help discriminate benign from malignant cells on slides. Another cytoskeletal family of proteins, the tropomyosins, have been shown by comigration and antibody labeling to be differentially expressed in normal and cancerous breast cells. In 1990, Bhattacharya et al. (14) detected a consistent defect of tropomyosin 1 expression in mammary carcinoma cell lines, which has been confirmed by other research groups for tropomyosin 2 and 3 (15), suggesting that such abnormalities might play a role in breast neoplasia.

From 1995, the possibility of performing large-scale proteomic analysis of human protein profiles become a reality due to three new major events in the biological sciences: (a) the progressive sequencing of the human genome; (b) the development of sensitive mass spectrometry-based strategies for protein characterization allowing the identification of even low-intensity spots on 2DE gels; and (c) the concomitant development of bioinformatics, allowing the compilation of searchable genomic and proteomic databases, accessible via the Internet. In the work of Bini et al. (16) 2DE gels from breast carcinomas were compared to normal breast tissue, leading to the detection of 32 highly expressed spots present in all the carcinomas. Spot identity was established mainly by matching to the Swiss-2DPAGE human liver, hepatoma, lymphoma, and erythroleukemia reference maps. Assignment was obtained for GRP94, GRP78, GRP75, mitochondrial HSP60 (heat-shock protein), calreticulin, protein disulfide isomerase, peptidyl-prolyl cistrans isomerase, collagen-binding protein 2, fructose bisphosphate aldolase, glyceraldehyde-3-phosphate deshydrogenase, thioredoxin, the cytochrome-C oxidase VA subunit, tubulin, and macrophage inhibitory factor. Differential distribution of heat-shock proteins (HSP) family members has also been described by Franzen et al. (17,18) and by Williams et al. (19) who have also reported elevated levels of metabolic enzyme inosine-5-monophosphate dehydrogenase, annexin V, elongation initiation factor 5A, Rho GDP dissociation inhibitor, and prohibitin. Finally, the first characterization of normal breast epithelial and myoepithelial cell proteins (20) and of breast cancer cells (21) using mass spectrometry exclusively was published recently. This last study of breast cancer cell 2DE protein profiles highlighted 20 proteins of potential importance as markers of tumor proliferation. In addition, these authors also highlighted the importance of truncated forms of previously identified proteins (for cytokeratin 6 and 8 as well as cathepsin D) as potential markers in breast cancer.

So, it is clear that proteomics has generated a considerable amount of valuable data for breast cancer research (Table 23.1). However, the relevance of these data for clinical practice has still to be established. Indeed, none of the potential markers thrown up so far by proteomics is routinely used by clinicians for diagnosis, treatment choice, or prognosis. Before large-scale proteomic analysis, the problem was to

TABLE 23.1 *Some markers identified by proteomics*

Protein name (Swiss-Prot accession number)	Function	Method of identification	Regulation in breast cancer	Reference
Cathepsin D (P07339)	Protease	Antibody	Induced by estrogens	Westley et Rochefort, *Cell*, 1980
Breast carbonic anhydrase (mouse, P16015)	Metabolic enzyme	Antibody	Up-regulated	Ring et al, *Cancer Res*, 1989
Cytokeratins K8 (P05787), K18 (P05783), K19 (P08727)	Cytoskeleton	Antibody	Up-regulated	Trask et al, *Proc Natl Acad Sci*, 1990
Cytokeratin K5	Cytoskeleton	Antibody	Down-regulated	Trask et al, *Proc Natl Acad Sci*, 1990
Tropomyosin 1 (P09494)	Cytoskeleton	Antibody	Down-regulated	Bhattacharya et al, *Cancer Res*, 1990
Tropomyosins 2 and 3 (P 12324)	Cytoskeleton	Comigration	Down-regulated	Franzen et al, *Br J Cancer*, 1996
PCNA (P12004)	DNA replication and reparation	Antibody	Up-regulated in rapidly proliferating cancer cells	Franzen et al, *Br J Cancer*, 1996
Heat Shock Proteins HSP60 (P10809), HSP90 (P08238), calreticulin (P27797)	Molecular chaperones	Matching with published maps	Up-regulated	Franzen et al, *Br J Cancer*, 1996 Giometti et al, *Electrophoresis*, 1997
Inosine-5' monophosphate dehydrogenase	Enzyme	Comigration antibody	Up-regulated	Williams et al, *Electrophoresis*, 1998
14-3-3-sigma (P31947)	Molecular chaperone	Mass spectrometry	Down-regulated	Vercoutter-Edouart et al, *Cancer Res*, 2001

detect molecular markers; now however, because of the efficiency of proteomics, many potential markers have been catalogued and the challenge has shifted towards the identification of markers that will prove clinically useful.

STRATEGY FOR IDENTIFICATION OF PROTEINS WITH CLINICAL INTEREST

Here, we review our own approach towards the identification of proteins of clinical interest in breast cancer. In delineating our strategy, we have considered the following points: (a) high-resolution 2DE technologies have already been developed for breast cancer analysis by experienced research teams; (b) 2DE databases of breast cancer have already been established, although they contain only a limited number of identified proteins; (c) results have been obtained from various cell types and from tumors with limited clinical data, but under different experimental conditions; and (d) proteomics has not been used for the functional analysis of breast cancer cell growth. Therefore, we have developed a strategy (Fig. 23.2) with the following parameters:

1. 2DE analysis of a limited number of breast cancer cell lines. Breast cancer cells are derived from epithelial origin, but breast tumors are not exclusively composed of these cells. They also contain normal cells, endothelial cells, or fibroblasts, each species of which will have its own characteristic proteomic profile. Therefore, studying breast cancer cells in culture primarily will allow for the selective identification of polypeptides regulated in the cancer cells only. In addition, we have limited the number of breast cancer cell lines studied to the two most representative lines available: MCF-7 (estrogen-sensitive and non-metastatic) and MDA-MB-231 (estrogen-insensitive and metastatic). Their profile is being compared to normal phenotype breast epithelial cells in primary culture. As a first approach, only major modifications in polypeptide levels are being taken into consideration.

2. Mass spectrometric identification of the most abundant polypeptides present in cells, as well as of the polypeptides whose level is different between normal and cancer cells. Two spectrometry methods have been used: MALDI-TOF (matrix-assisted laser desorption/ionization-time of flight) for the definition of mass fingerprints, and ESI-MS-MS (Electrospray ionization-tandem mass spectrometry MS-MS) for micro-sequencing.

3. 2DE analysis of a sufficient number of tumor biopsies to be representative of the different types of breast cancer. All tumors are obtained from the specialist Cancer Hospital of Lille (Centre Oscar Lambret) and undergo a standardized protocol for resection and protein solubilization. Attention is primarily focused on proteins already identified from breast cancer cells in culture, levels of which are quantified by computer analysis. Full clinical data (histoprognostic grading of the tumor, estrogen receptor assay, BRCA mutation, node invasion, survival of the patient) are accessible and statistical analyses are run to establish correlations between classical clinical parameters and individual polypeptide levels.

A protein profile of a ductal breast carcinoma is shown in Figure 23.3. More than 1,500 polypeptides were detected and localized between pI (Isoelectric point) 4 to 8 and molecular mass range 20 kDa to 200 kDa. Computer analysis

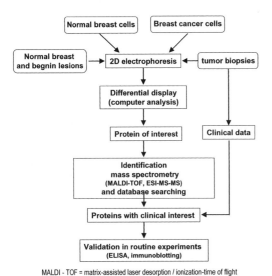

FIG. 23.2. Strategy for the identification of proteins with clinical interest

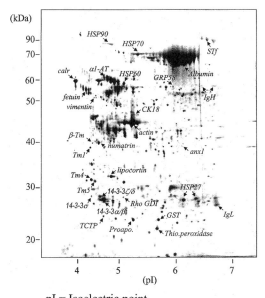

pI = Isoelectric point

kDa = kiloDaltons (molecular mass range)

FIG. 23.3. Silver-stained 2DE gel of a breast tumor sample. The major proteins were determined by MALDI-TOF and MS-MS after trypsin digestion. *Anx,* annexin; *CK,* cytokeratins; *crtc,* calreticulin; *GRP,* glucose-regulated protein; *GST,* glutathione S-transferase; *HSP,* heat-shock proteins; *Ig,* Immunoglobulins; *PCNA,* proliferating cell nuclear antigen; *PGM,* phosphoglycerate mutase; *RhoGDI,* Rho GTP-dissociation inhibitor 1; *SODM,* superoxide dismutase; *STf,* serotransferrine, *TCTP,* transcriptionaly controlled tumor protein; *thio. peroxidase,* thioredoxin peroxidase; *TM,* tropomyosin; *vim,* vimentin.

been reported before. For example, we were able to confirm a differential distribution of cytokeratins between normal and cancer cells: cancer cells produced mainly keratin 19 whereas keratins 7, 14, and 17 were found mostly in the noncancerous cells. We were not able to identify keratins 8 and 19 in normal breast epithelial cells, confirming that they are not likely present in high quantity in these cells. Another cytoskeletal protein, vimentin, is known to have higher levels in estrogen receptor-negative cells (such as MDA-MB-231 cells) than in estrogen receptor-positive breast cancer cells (such as MCF-7 cells) (22), and we found that vimentin is also expressed in normal cells. Other cytoskeletal proteins of the tropomyosin (Tm) family have been identified: Tm3 and Tm30. Tm3 has already been reported to be downregulated in malignant breast tumors as compared to benign lesions (22). Stress proteins HSP27, HSP60, HSP71, HSP90, calreticulin, and calnexin have also been previously detected in breast cancer cells as well as in breast tumor biopsies (16–19). The levels of HSP60 and HSP90 are higher in carcinomas than in fibroadenomas, and HSP27 is also known to be higher in estrogen receptor-positive cells, correlating with the growth- and drug-resistance characteristic of breast cancer. However, all of these stress proteins are present in large amounts in normal breast epithelial cells, suggesting their negligible potential for use as clinical markers.

of the autoradiograms allowed a determination of molecular masses and isoelectric points after comparison with standard 2DE gels of the Swiss-2DPAGE (polyacrylamide gel electrophoresis) database. Using mass spectrometry, we were able to identify about 80 spots: the positions of some of the identified proteins are indicated. Most of the identified proteins, such as the cytoskeletal elements actin, alpha-actinin, β-tubulin, vimentin, and tropomyosins have already been described in breast cancer cells. Some signal-related proteins (annexins, numatrin, *rho* GDI) were also detected. Interestingly, most of the variations in individual polypeptide levels that we were able to detect have already

14-3-3 SIGMA AS A POTENTIAL CLINICAL MARKER

14-3-3 is a family of highly conserved protein forms (alpha, beta, delta, sigma, zeta) of 25 kDa to 30 kDa expressed in all eukaryotic cells that play a role in the regulation of signal transduction pathways implicated in the control of cell proliferation, differentiation, and survival (23). 14-3-3 proteins are known to associate directly or indirectly with signaling proteins such as the IGF-1 (insulin growth factor) receptor, Raf, MEK kinases (MAP-kinase-kinase), and PI3-kinase, but the precise molecular mechanism by which they activate or inhibit these elements remains unclear (23).

Although most of the proteins that we initially identified in breast cancer cells and tumor biopsies were already identified using 2DE/proteomic technologies, this was not true for 14-3-3 sigma (24). Indeed, 14-3-3 sigma was easily detectable in 2DE gels of normal breast epithelial cells using Coomassie staining, although the spot was undetectable (under the same experimental conditions) in breast cancer protein profiles. Indeed, much more sensitive silver staining was necessary to reveal 14-3-3 sigma in breast cancer cells. It is important to note that this situation was observed only for 14-3-3 sigma, suggesting that it is a strong marker for the noncancerous state of breast epithelial cells. Figure 23.4 shows silver staining of the 14-3-3 sigma in breast cancer cells and tumor biopsies; it can be clearly observed that this protein is also downregulated in breast cancer biopsies.

Interestingly, we have shown that the amounts of the alpha, beta, zeta, and delta forms of 14-3-3 do not significantly vary between normal and cancer cells, suggesting that it is only the regulation of the sigma form of 14-3-3 that is related to breast neoplastic transformation. In keratinocytes and in the bladder, the expression of 14-3-3 sigma is lower in transformed cells than in normal cells (25,26), although other forms of 14-3-3 have not been reported in the literature. Transcription analysis has confirmed that gene expression of 14-3-3 sigma is seven- to tenfold lower in breast cancer cells than in normal breast cells due to the high frequency of hypermethylation of the 14-3-3 sigma locus (27). We found that the 14-3-3 sigma protein is present in breast cancer biopsies at levels which average tenfold lower than normal breast epithelial cells. Interestingly, Fergusson et al. (27) reported that the mRNA for 14-3-3 sigma was undetectable by Northern blot analysis in 45 of 48 primary breast carcinomas studied; in contrast, we have detected the 14-3-3 sigma protein in 30 of 35 primary tumor samples, indicating the higher sensitivity provided by proteomic analysis, compared to Northern blot analysis, as well as the complementarity of both strategies for identifying cancer markers.

Our data show that 14-3-3 sigma can be used to discriminate cancer from noncancerous breast epithelial cells. We are now investigating its potential clinical utility by first extending our study to a larger number of biopsies, both benign and invasive. A total of 400 biopsies are prospectively being assayed for their 14-3-3 sigma levels and the results of this quantification will be analyzed to test any relationship with classical clinical parameters.

PROTEOMICS FOR DECIPHERING GROWTH-SIGNALING PATHWAYS

Proteomics was first mooted as a method to map all cellular proteins. This aspect, designated expression proteomics, is now complemented by an emerging field dubbed functional proteomics. This latter field concerns itself with protein interactions and activations within functional contexts (28). Recent publications have demonstrated the value of proteomics for the study of intracellular signaling, especially in the case of growth-factor stimulation, opening a way of understanding the molecular mechanisms involved in tumor growth.

Deciphering the signaling pathways involved in cellular growth is of primary importance for an understanding of tumor growth and metastasis. Growth factors, essential polypeptides required for eukaryotic cell growth, initiate their stimulation through specific, tyrosine kinase-membrane receptors, which in turn induce intracellular protein-phosphorylation cascades. These activate a variety of signaling proteins such as the mitogen-

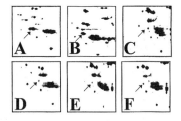

A-B = Normal breast epithelial cells
C = MCF-7 cells
D = MDA-MB-231 cells
E - F = representative primary breast tumors

FIG. 23.4. 2D-patterns showing the down-regulation of 14-3-3 sigma (indicated by an arrow) in 7 representative breast tumor samples **(C–F)** as compared to 2 normal breast samples **(A, B)**.

activated protein-kinases (MAP-kinases). This cascade of protein phosphorylation ultimately induces changes in gene expression, with consequent changes in protein synthesis, leading to cell proliferation, differentiation, or migration. Classical methods to study these processes were based on the use of specific antibodies to purify known signaling proteins, followed by SDS-PAGE (sodium dodecyl sulfate-polyacrylamide gel electrophoresis) separation and Western blot analysis of tyrosine phosphorylation. Alternatively, phosphotyrosine-containing proteins were purified and signaling proteins immunodetected. Similarly, early changes in gene expression are usually studied by Northern blotting or quantitative RT-PCR (reverse transcriptase-polymerase chain reaction) assays for specific mRNAs after cell stimulation. The great drawback of these traditional protocols is their difficulty in identifying proteins with no previously described function in signal transduction.

The use of 2DE for studying the mechanism of action of growth factors in cancer cells was initiated for pheochromocytoma PC12 cells (29). In these cells, early protein synthesis induced by the differentiating activity of NGF (nerve growth factor) and FGF-2 (fibroblast growth factor-2) has been compared to the mitogenic activity of epidermal growth factor (EGF) using 2DE separation of ^{35}S metabolically labeled amino acids. The results revealed an initial modulation of protein synthesis induced by the three growth factors, and provided evidence for a specificity of the differentiative versus proliferative pathways induced by these growth factors. This study demonstrated the value of 2DE technologies to investigate changes in protein synthesis induced by growth factors, revealing new methods for the detection of signaling involved in cellular growth. More recently, proteomics has been successfully used for the study of protein phosphorylation cascades. This has been demonstrated for platelet-derived growth factor (PDGF) and EGF stimulation of mouse fibroblasts (30,31). NIH 3T3 cells were exposed to the growth factors and the phosphotyrosine containing proteins immunoprecipitated before separation either on SDS-PAGE or 2DE. Mass spectrometry analysis allowed the identification of several known signaling proteins and of other proteins not previously reported to be activated with such stimuli, including a plexin-like protein and the guanine nucleotide exchange factor Vav-2. Proteomic analysis of growth factor signaling in breast cancer cells was only employed once we initiated a program to investigate the mechanism of action of FGF-2.

PROTEOMIC ANALYSIS OF FGF-2 SIGNALING PATHWAY IN BREAST CANCER CELLS

In addition to estrogenic hormones, the development of breast cancer cells can be regulated by various growth factors that control proliferation, migration, and apoptosis (32,33). For example, insulin-like growth factor I (IGF-I) or epidermal growth factor (EGF) stimulates proliferation of breast cancer cells, whereas other factors like mammary-derived growth factor inhibitor or transforming growth factor beta (TGF-β) inhibit their growth. Hepatocyte growth factor/scatter factor (HGF/SF) has been shown to stimulate the migration of breast cancer cells and, thus, metastasis (34). Interestingly, fibroblast growth factor-2 (FGF-2) has been shown to stimulate both proliferation and migration of breast cancer cells (35). Recently, we have demonstrated that nerve growth factor (NGF), better known as the archetypal neurotrophin, is able to stimulate both proliferation and survival of breast cancer cells (36,37). Most growth factor receptors such as IGFR-I (38), FGFR (39), EGFR (40), and NGFR (41) have a prognostic value in breast cancer. Altogether, the mechanism of action of these growth regulators is crucial for the process of breast tumor development and is yielding potential new strategies for prevention, detection, and treatment (42).

Fibroblast growth factors are pleiotropic polypeptides involved in the control of cell proliferation, differentiation, and survival (43) whose signaling pathway has been described (44). The prototypic FGF family member, FGF-2, has been shown to be involved in many forms of cancer cell growth and metastasis. In breast cancer, the over-expression of FGF-2, as well as its receptors, has been reported in a significant percentage of breast tumors (39,45,46). Moreover, high amounts of FGF-2 have been detected in sera from patients with breast cancer (47). We and others have found that FGF-2 is a strong activator of breast cancer cell proliferation and migration (35,48), indicating a key role for this growth factor in breast tumor growth and metastasis. Classical methods to study intracellular signaling have been applied to FGF-2 activation of breast cancer cells; they have uncovered a complex signaling network involving activation of the FGF-receptor tyrosine kinase and MAP kinase, as well as the signaling proteins FAK (focal adhesion kinase), Src, Rac-1 and Nck (35,49).

Using proteomics, we studied both the rapid changes (occurring during the first minutes) in protein tyrosine phosphorylation, and the modifications in protein synthesis induced by FGF-2 (50). Using phosphotyrosine immunoprecipitation and SDS-PAGE, we were able to detect an increase in tyrosine phosphorylation of several proteins which have been characterized by mass spectrometry as being the FGF receptor, the FGF receptor substrate (FRS2), the oncogenic protein Src and the MAP kinases (p42/p44) (Fig. 23.5). Interestingly, we also showed that FGF-2 stimulation induces the tyrosine phosphorylation of cyclin D2 (50). Phosphorylation of cyclin D2 was not previously described in growth-factor signaling, although it is known that progression through the cell cycle is strictly under the control of cyclins and their catalytic subunits Cdks (cyclin-dependent kinases). We showed, using pharmacological inhibition of the activities of the oncoprotein Src and of p42/p44, that Src activity is required for the FGF-2-induced phosphorylation of cyclin D2, whereas MAP-kinases are not.

After metabolic labeling of MCF-7 cells with ^{35}S-amino-acid proteins and using computerized analysis of 2DE autoradiograms, several proteins were found upregulated during FGF-2 stimulation (51). Two of the FGF-2 regulated proteins belong to the heat-shock protein family (HSP). Previous studies using mammalian cells have shown that mitogens such as insulin-like growth factor and epidermal growth factor increase cellular synthesis and accumulation of HSP90 and HSP70 (52). We demonstrated (51) that synthesis of HSP90 and HSP70 are both upregulated after FGF-2 stimulation in breast cancer cells, suggesting that appropriate protein folding and trafficking are essential processes for the regulation of breast cancer cell growth. In addition, we have shown that geldanamycin, an inhibitor of HSP90 activity, totally blocks the FGF-2-induced proliferation and general growth of breast cancer cells.

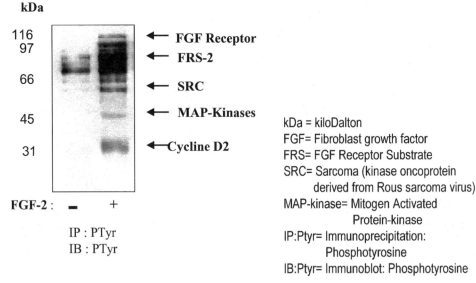

FIG. 23.5. Protein tyrosine phosphorylation induced by FGF-2 in breast cancer cells. The arrows indicates protein identification.

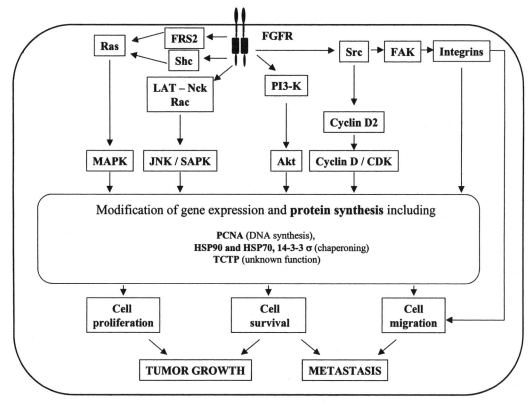

FIG. 23.6. Signaling pathways for FGF-2 in breast cancer cells. CDK, cyclin dependent kinase; FAK, focal adhesion kinase; FRS, FGF receptor substrate; JNK, c-jun N-terminal kinase; HSP, heat shock protein; Nck, novel cytoplasmic kinase; PCNA, proliferating cell nuclear antigen; PI3K, phosphatidylinositol-3-kinase; Ras, rat sarcoma (oncoprotein derived from rat sarcoma virus); SAPK, stress-activated protein kinase; Shc, Src-homology and collagen protein; Srk, kinase derived from rous sarcoma virus; TCTP, transcriptionally controlled tumor protein.

HSP90 can exist in a complex with many components of the growth-factor signaling pathway: tyrosine kinase receptors, Src, Raf or MAP-kinase-kinase (53), and its interaction with these signaling proteins allows for their protection and correct conformational folding. These data suggest that the expression of this protein is part of breast epithelial cell tumorigenesis, and thus HSP90 constitutes a potential therapeutic target for breast cancer treatment. Finally, we also found that the transcriptionally controlled tumor protein (TCTP) is upregulated by FGF-2. TCTP was initially described as a tumor-related polypeptide, but it has more recently been found in normal human cells. Despite its ubiquity and high level of conservation, the physiological role of TCTP remains to be determined, but the upregulation that we observed in breast cancer cells suggests a role in breast tumorigenesis.

Altogether, the proteomic analysis of FGF-2 signaling in breast cancer cells has allowed the identification of rapid changes in protein phosphorylation and synthesis, providing new information about the molecular basis of breast cancer cell growth. An overview of FGF-2 signaling pathways in breast cancer cells is presented in Figure 23.6.

DEFINING THERAPEUTIC TARGETS

Practical consequences for treatment derived from a better understanding of the molecular basis of breast cancer cell growth are now emerging as evidenced by the development of therapeutic strategies based, for example, on the inhibition of tyrosine kinase receptors. This is well illustrated with human epidermal growth factor 2 (HER-2 or *erb*-B2), an orphan tyrosine kinase receptor. HER-2/*erb*-B2 overexpression in breast cancer cells has been shown at both the mRNA and protein levels (54). Specific inhibition of HER-2/*erb*-B2 using monoclonal antibodies leads to a decreased level of cellular proliferation. Based on these *in vitro* experiments, trastuzumab (Herceptin), a truncated blocking-antibody directed against HER-2/*erb*-B2, has been successfully developed and is used in clinical practice and in recent clinical trials, especially in the adjuvant setting (55). Since proteomics is now providing global identification of protein regulation during pathological processes, the discovery of new therapeutic targets is a highly awaited outcome.

Drug development is generally based around the possibility of upregulating or downregulating a specific pathogenic activity. As we and others have described several proteins which are upregulated or downregulated in breast cancer, the next major challenge is to determine if such regulation is causal or simply the consequence of tumorigenesis. If causal, any observed regulation can only be used as a biomarker for diagnosis; if a consequence, the identified protein is a potential therapeutic target, and a strategy to inhibit its activity can be developed. Determining the potential function of a protein in pathogenesis can be achieved using known pharmacological inhibitors, specific antibodies or anti-sense messenger RNA (mRNA) approaches, although the multifactorial origin of cancer can be a source of difficulty in interpreting the experimental results. However, in the case of HSP90, we have been able to show that geldanamycin, an inhibitor of HSP90 activity, completely blocks the FGF-2-induced proliferation and general growth of breast cancer cells. HSP90 can exist in a complex with many components of the growth factor signaling pathway: tyrosine kinase receptors, Src, Raf or MAP-kinase-kinase (53), and its interaction with these signaling proteins allows for their protection and correct conformational folding. These data suggest that the expression of this protein is part of breast epithelial cell tumorigenesis, and thus constitutes a potential therapeutic target for breast cancer treatment.

The demonstration that the molecular chaperone 14-3-3 sigma is downregulated in breast cancer cells also aroused interest in it as a biomarker (24). It could also be pursued for new anticancer strategies. Similar to breast cancer cells, normal breast epithelial cells express specific tyrosine kinase receptors for NGF and FGF-2. Both NGF and FGF-2 activate the Ras/Raf/MAP-kinase pathway in breast cancer cells, resulting in stimulation of the cell proliferation (35,36). However, neither NGF nor FGF-2 has a mitogenic effect on normal breast epithelial cells (36,56). Paradoxically, therefore, normal breast epithelial cells express both NGF and FGF receptors but do not proliferate in response to either cognate factor. The reason for the lack of sensitivity to these mitogens for normal breast epithelial cells is not understood, but the growing body of evidence implicating 14-3-3 sigma in cell cycle progression suggests that its high level in normal cells may block the mitogenic effect of growth factors. The sigma form of 14-3-3 is a p53-regulated inhibitor of G2/M progression, and its overexpression can cause cell cycle arrest (57). In addition, 14-3-3 is able to regulate cdc phosphorylation and activities, so controlling cell proliferation (23). Importantly, in breast cancer cells it was shown that 14-3-3 sigma directly associates with cyclin-dependent kinases to negatively regulate cell growth (58). The higher level of 14-3-3 sigma in normal breast epithelial cells may therefore contribute to the blocking of high cellular proliferation. It can thus be reasonably proposed that restoring higher levels of 14-3-3 sigma to breast cancer cells might lead to their decreased proliferation. This proteomically generated hypothesis, which awaits further experimentation, certainly opens new avenues for breast cancer therapy.

PERSPECTIVES

The proteomic data obtained to date, in searching molecular markers and therapeutic targets for breast cancer, are clearly only the first step. Future developments in the field are likely to depend on further technological innovations. Proteomic technologies are constantly improving, not only on the "separation" side, but also on the "characterization" side, especially in the study of posttranslational modifications and biological activity.

Based on a concept developed for the study of nucleic acids, the possibility of using protein chip technologies has emerged as a way for bypassing the intensive, time-consuming method of 2DE. The principle of using protein chips for the identification of new markers depends on being able to flush potential ligands over arrays impregnated with different types of affinity probes, and perform subsequent analysis of any differential protein binding (59,60). Mass spectrometry would then allow for the identification of differentially expressed proteins. However, this approach still has two important drawbacks: it does not allow reliable quantification, and it does not offer the possibility of cataloguing proteins from a biological sample. One can argue that detecting a cancer marker does not necessarily require that all proteins be analyzed; however, the more systematic the study, the greater will be the probability of detecting a complete set of markers. Despite the limitation of protein chip technology for biomarker identification, the use of protein arrays has great potential for diagnostics. Indeed, once a specific set of biomarkers is determined to characterize a particular tumor type, its use for diagnosis would require a large-scale routine analysis of the protein profile of tumors which could not be achieved by 2DE. Then, automated chip-based technologies for analyzing hundreds or thousands of proteins simultaneously, similar to the cDNA-based technologies, would provide a powerful tool for cancer diagnosis, as well as to have the potential to determine treatment choice and monitoring.

To date, most of the proteomic-based strategies to discover new markers have focused on the study of individual protein levels, although post-translational modifications could equally be used as cancer markers. There have been about 200 cotranslational and posttranslational modifications described to date, among which phosphorylation and glycosylation have been most definitively shown to be essential for the regulation of protein function. Nearly all modifications change the molecular mass of the protein. Therefore, mass spectrometry has, due to its high mass accuracy and sensitivity, proven to be a method of choice for characterization of post-translational modifications (61–63). However, its implementation for proteins in 2DE gels has still not become routine, and there is as yet no methodology for dealing with posttranslational modifications in a high-throughput way. In addition, a major difficulty with cancer biopsies will be to maintain the stability of any posttranslational modification during the processes of sample preparation and 2DE analysis. For example, protein phosphorylation has been shown to be a very unstable and labile modification, making its analysis in a large number of breast tumor biopsies uncertain. Finally, mass spectrometry now offers the possibility to study directly the noncovalent interactions of proteins with other proteins, or with drug molecules, thus opening a methodology to study intracellular signaling networks.

Complementing improvements in proteomic technologies, new possibilities for the selection of specific biological targets by microdissection are also emerging prior to proteomic analysis. Breast tumor biopsies are composed mainly of cancer cells, but they also contain other cell types that complicate proteomic profiling. Techniques such as laser capture microdissection (64) could be used for the isolation of malignant cells prior to sample preparation and would facilitate downstream discovery. However, it should be noted that a major difficulty is in making the choice of which cells to select; morphology alone is unreliable. In addition, it should be noted that interesting markers could also emerge from the other cells present in tumors. For example, it is now established that tumor angiogenesis is a crucial arbiter of breast cancer growth/metastasis. In addition, the presence of endothelial proteins in breast cancer could be an interesting diagnostic parameter. However, obtaining sufficient material for proteomic analysis is time consuming, especially for the study of cell types present only in small numbers. Therefore, although microdissection has intrinsic limits, it may provide an alternative to the study of whole tumor biopsies, as well as offer the possibility to investigate the proteomic profile of virtually all cell types present in breast tumors.

CONCLUSION

During the 1980s and early 1990s one had to be a little provocative to sustain the idea that looking globally at proteins could be a productive way to understand fundamental mechanisms of cancer cell growth or be used to discover relevant markers. Indeed, those times were dominated by the concepts and methods—the panacea—of molecular genetics. With the progressive completion of the sequencing of the human genome, associated with its limited number of practical outcomes for cancer, and with the technical progress made in protein identification, it gradually became reasonable to believe that looking directly at proteins could be fruitful. Today, it has become common to read that as proteins are the main functional output of genes, proteomics could drive biology and medicine beyond genomics. However, we are still at a pioneer stage, as proteomics proposals have started to be financed to a significant degree only in the last few years and are relatively recently entering into a phase of data generation. Nevertheless, we have already entered into the next era, dominated by the idea of large-scale proteomic analyses, which will require high levels of standardization, automation, and massive funding from public as well as private sectors. There is no doubt that an integrated program of genomics and proteomics will be essential to progress towards any fundamental understanding of breast, and other cancers, and for the correlative development of new treatments.

Acknowledgments: Our work is supported by the Association pour la Recherche Contre le Cancer (Contart 4339), The Ligue Nationale Contre le Cancer (Comité du Pas-de-Calais), the Ministère de la Recherche et de l'Education Nationale, The Genopole de Lille and the Région Nord-Pas-de-Calais.

REFERENCES

1. Pandey A, Mann M. Proteomics to study genes and genomes. *Nature* 2000;405:837–846.
2. Banks RE, Dunn MJ, Hochstrasser DF, et al. Proteomics: new perspectives, new biomedical opportunities. *Lancet* 2000;356:1749–1756.
3. Wright GL Jr. Two-dimensional acrylamide gel electrophoresis of cancer-patient serum proteins. *Ann Clin Lab Sci* 1974;4:281–293.
4. Westley B, Rochefort H. A secreted glycoprotein induced by estrogen in human breast cancer cell lines. *Cell* 1980;20:353–362.
5. Gendler SJ, Dermer GB, Silverman LM, Tokes ZA. Synthesis of alpha 1-antichymotrypsin and alpha 1-acid glycoprotein by human breast epithelial cells. *Cancer Res* 1982;42:4567–4573.
6. Stastny J, Prasad R, Fosslien E. Tissue proteins in breast cancer, as studied by use of two-dimensional electrophoresis. *Clin Chem* 1984;30:1914–1918.
7. Wirth PJ, Egilsson V, Gudnason V, et al. Specific polypeptide differences in normal versus malignant human breast tissues by two-dimensional electrophoresis. *Breast Cancer Res Treat* 1987;10:177–189.
8. Wirth PJ. Specific polypeptide differences in normal versus malignant breast tissue bytwo-dimensional electrophoresis. *Electrophoresis* 1989;10:543–554.
9. Worland PJ, Bronzert D, Dickson RB, et al. Secreted and cellular polypeptide patterns of MCF-7 human breast cancer cells following either estrogen stimulation or v-H-ras transfection. *Cancer Res* 1989;49:51–57.
10. Maloney TM, Paine PL, Russo J. Polypeptide composition of normal and neoplastic human breast tissues and cells analyzed by two-dimensional gel electrophoresis. *Breast Cancer Res Treat* 1989;14:337–348.
11. Trask DK, Band V, Zajchowski DA, et al. Keratins as markers that distinguish normal and tumor-derived mammary epithelial cells. *Proc Natl Acad Sci USA* 1990;87:2319–2323.
12. Giometti CS, Tollaksen SL, Chubb C, et al. Analysis of proteins from human breast epithelial cells using two-dimensional gel electrophoresis. *Electrophoresis* 1995;16:1215–1224.
13. Giometti CS, Williams K, Tollaksen SL. A two-dimensional electrophoresis database of human breast epithelial cell proteins. *Electrophoresis* 1997;18:573–581.
14. Bhattacharya B, Prasad GL, Valverius EM, et al. Tropomyosins of human mammary epithelial cells: consistent defects of expression in mammary carcinoma cell lines. *Cancer Res* 1990;50:2105–2112.
15. Franzen B, Linder S, Okuzawa K, et al. Non enzymatic extraction of cells from clinical tumor material for analysis of gene expression by two-dimensional polyacrylamide gel electrophoresis. *Electrophoresis* 1993;14:1045–1053.
16. Bini L, Magi B, Marzocchi B, et al. Protein expression profiles in human breast ductal carcinoma and histologically normal tissue. *Electrophoresis* 1997;18:2832–2841.

17. Franzen B, Linder S, Alaiya AA, et al. Analysis of polypeptide expression in benign and malignant human breast lesions: down-regulation of cytokeratins. *Br J Cancer* 1996;74:1632–1638.
18. Franzen B, Linder S, Alaiya AA, et al. Analysis of polypeptide expression in benign and malignant human breast lesions. *Electrophoresis* 1997;18:582–587.
19. Williams K, Chubb C, Huberman E, Giometti CS. Analysis of differential protein expression in normal and neoplastic human breast epithelial cell lines. *Electrophoresis* 1998;19:333–343.
20. Page MJ, Amess B, Townsend RR, et al. Proteomic definition of normal human luminal and myoepithelial breast cells purified from reduction mammoplasties. *Proc Natl Acad Sci USA* 1999;96:12589–12594.
21. Bergman AC, Benjamin T, Alaiya A, et al. Identification of gel-separated tumor marker proteins by mass spectrometry. *Electrophoresis* 2000;21:679–686.
22. Thompson EW, Paik S, Brunner N, et al. Association of increased basement membrane invasiveness with absence of estrogen receptor and expression of vimentin in human breast cancer cell lines. *J Cell Physiol* 1992;150:534–544.
23. Fu H, Subramanian RR, Masters SC. 14-3-3 proteins: structure, function, and regulation. *Annu Rev Pharmacol Toxicol* 2000;40:617–647.
24. Vercoutter-Edouart AS, Lemoine J, Le Bourhis X, et al. Proteomic analysis reveals that 14-3-3sigma is down-regulated in human breast cancer cells. *Cancer Res* 2001;61:76–80.
25. Leffers H, Madsen P, Rasmussen HH, et al. Molecular cloning and expression of the transformation sensitive epithelial marker stratifin. *J Mol Biol* 1993;231:982–998.
26. Ostergaard M, Rasmussen HH, Nielsen HV, et al. Proteome profiling of bladder squamous cell carcinomas: identification of markers that define their degree of differentiation. *Cancer Res* 1997;57:4111–4117.
27. Ferguson AT, Evron E, Umbricht CB, et al. High frequency of hypermethylation at the 14-3-3 sigma locus leads to gene silencing in breast cancer. *Proc Natl Acad Sci USA* 2000;97:6049–6054.
28. Miklos GL, Maleszka R. Protein functions and biological contexts. *Proteomics* 2001;1:169–78.
29. Hondermarck H, McLaughlin CS, Patterson SD, et al. Early changes in protein synthesis induced by basic fibroblast growth factor, nerve growth factor, and epidermal growth factor in PC12 pheochromocytoma cells. *Proc Natl Acad Sci USA* 1994;91:9377–9381.
30. Soskic V, Gorlach M, Poznanovic S, et al. Functional proteomics analysis of signal transduction pathways of the platelet-derived growth factor beta receptor. *Biochemistry* 1999;38:1757–1764.
31. Pandey A, Podtelejnikov AV, Blagoev B, et al. Analysis of receptor signaling pathways by mass spectrometry: identification of vav-2 as a substrate of the epidermal and platelet-derived growth factor receptors. *Proc Natl Acad Sci USA* 2000;97:179–184.
32. Ethier SP. Growth factor synthesis and human breast cancer progression. *J Natl Cancer Inst* 1995;87:964–973.
33. Le Bourhis X, Toillon RA, Boilly B, Hondermarck H. Autocrine and paracrine growth inhibition of breast cancer cells. *Breast Cancer Res Treat* 2000;1722:1–8.
34. Rahimi N, Hung W, Tremblay E, et al. c-Src kinase activity is required for hepatocyte growth factor-induced motility and anchorage-independent growth of mammary carcinoma cells. *J Biol Chem* 1998;273:33714–33721.
35. Nurcombe V, Smart CE, Chipperfield H, et al. The proliferative and migratory activities of breast cancer cells can be differentially regulated by heparan sulfates. *J Biol Chem* 2000; 275:30009–30018.
36. Descamps S, Lebourhis X, Delehedde M, et al. Nerve growth factor is mitogenic for cancerous but not normal human breast epithelial cells. *J Biol Chem* 1998; 273:16659–16662.
37. Descamps S, Toillon RA, Adriaenssens E, et al. Nerve growth factor stimulates proliferation and survival of human breast cells through two distinct signaling pathways. *J Biol Chem* 2001a;276:17864–17870.
38. Bonneterre J, Peyrat JP, Beuscart R, Demaille A. Prognostic significance of insulin-like growth factor 1 receptors in human breast cancer. *Cancer Res* 1990;50:6931–6935.
39. Blanckaert VD, Hebbar M, Louchez MM, et al. Basic fibroblast growth factor receptors and their prognostic value in human breast cancer. *Clin Cancer Res* 1998; 4:2939–2947.
40. Pawlowski V, Revillion F, Hebbar M, et al. Prognostic value of the type I growth factor receptors in a large series of human primary breast cancers quantified with a real-time reverse transcription-polymerase chain reaction assay. *Clin Cancer Res* 2000;6:4217–4225.
41. Descamps S, Pawlowski V, Révillion F, et al. Expression of nerve growth factor receptors and their prognostic value in human breast cancer. *Cancer Research* 2001b;in press.
42. Nass SJ, Hahm HA, Davidson NE. Breast cancer biology blossoms in the clinic. *Nat Med* 1998;4:761–762.
43. McKeehan WL, Wang F, Kan M. The heparan sulfate-fibroblast growth factor family: diversity of structure and function. *Prog Nucleic Acid Res Mol Biol* 1998; 59:135–176.
44. Boilly B, Vercoutter-Edouart AS, Hondermarck H, et al. FGF signals for cell proliferation and migration through different pathways. *Cytokine Growth Factor Rev* 2000;11:295–302.
45. Adnane J, Gaudray P, Dionne CA, et al. BEK and FLG, two receptors to members of the FGF family, are amplified in subsets of human breast cancers. *Oncogene* 1991;6:659–662.
46. Marsh SK, Bansal GS, Zammit C, et al. Increased expression of fibroblast growth factor 8 in human breast cancer. *Oncogene* 1999;18:1053–1060.
47. Takei Y, Kurobe M, Uchida A, et al. Serum concentrations of basic fibroblast growth factor in breast cancers. *Clinical Chem* 1994;40:1980–1981.
48. Rahmoune H, Chen HL, Gallagher JT, et al. Interaction of heparan sulfate from mammary cells with acidic fibroblast growth factor (FGF) and basic FGF. Regulation of the activity of basic FGF by high and low affinity binding sites in heparan sulfate. *J Biol Chem* 1998;273:7303–7310.
49. Liu JF, Chevet E, Kebache S, et al. Functional Rac-1 and Nck signaling networks are required for FGF-2-induced DNA synthesis in MCF-7 cells. *Oncogene* 1999; 18:6425–6433.
50. Vercoutter-Edouart AS, Lemoine J, Smart CE, et al. The mitogenic signaling pathway for fibroblast growth factor-2 involves the tyrosine phosphorylation of cyclin D2 in MCF-7 human breast cancer cells. *FEBS Lett* 2000;478:209–215.

51. Vercoutter-Edouart AS, Czeszak X, Crepin M, et al. Proteomic detection of changes in protein synthesis induced by fibroblast growth factor-2 in MCF-7 human breast cancer cells. *Exp Cell Res* 2001;262:59–68.
52. Jolly C, Morimoto RI. Role of the heat shock response and molecular chaperones in oncogenesis and cell death. *J Natl Cancer Inst* 2000;92:1564–1572.
53. Pearl LH, Prodromou C. Structure and in vivo function of Hsp90. *Curr Opin Struct Biol* 2000;10:46–51.
54. Revillion F, Bonneterre J, Peyrat JP. ERBB2 oncogene in human breast cancer and its clinical significance. *Eur J Cancer* 1998;34:791–808.
55. Colomer R, Shamon LA, Tsai MS, Lupu R. Herceptin: from the bench to the clinic. *Cancer Invest* 2001;19:49–56.
56. Li S, Shipley GD. Expression of multiple species of basic fibroblast growth factor mRNA and protein in normal and tumor-derived mammary epithelial cells in culture. *Cell Growth Diff* 1991;2:195–202.
57. Hermeking H, Lengauer C, Polyak K, et al. 14-3-3 sigma is a p53-regulated inhibitor of G2/M progression. *Mol Cell* 1997;1:3–11.
58. Laronga C, Yang HY, Neal C, et al. Association of the cyclin-dependent kinases and 14-3-3 sigma negatively regulates cell cycle progression. *J Biol Chem* 2000;275:23106–23112.
59. Nelson RW, Nedelkov D, Tubbs KA. Biosensor chip mass spectrometry: a chip-based proteomics approach. *Electrophoresis* 2000;21:1155–1163.
60. Fung ET, Thulasiraman V, Weinberger SR, Dalmasso EA. Protein biochips for differential profiling. *Curr Opin Biotechnol* 2001;12:65–69.
61. Gygi SP, Aebersold R. Mass spectrometry and proteomics. *Curr Opin Chem Biol* 2000;4:489–494.
62. Gygi SP, Rist B, Gerber SA, et al. Quantitative analysis of complex protein mixtures using isotope-coded affinity tags. *Nat Biotechnol* 1999;17:994–999.
63. Patterson SD. Mass spectrometry and proteomics. *Physiol Genomics* 2000;2:59–65.
64. Banks RE, Dunn MJ, Forbes MA, et al. The potential use of laser capture microdissection to selectively obtain distinct populations of cells for proteomic analysis-preliminary findings. *Electrophoresis* 1999;20:689–700.

24

Steroid and Growth Factor Receptors: Cross-Talk and Clinical Implications

Richard J. Pietras

Growth of normal and malignant human breast tissue is closely regulated by steroid hormones such as estrogens, as well as by peptide growth factors that interact with epidermal growth factor and HER-2 receptors (1,2). At diagnosis, approximately 75% of human breast cancers are found to be estrogen receptor (ER)-positive, while 25% to 30% exhibit overexpression of the HER-2 receptor. Both the presence of ER (3) and the overexpression of HER-2 (4–6) are known to be important prognostic factors in human breast cancers. Findings from several studies evaluating HER-2 and ER expression in the same human breast cancer specimens consistently demonstrate an inverse relationship between HER-2 and ER expression levels, with about 50% to 65% of HER-2-positive samples showing absence of ER (7–9). Correlation with clinical outcome suggests that tumors with overexpression of HER-2 respond poorly to endocrine therapy with antiestrogens regardless of ER phenotype (10–12). These data imply a biologic interaction between ER and HER-2 receptors in human breast cancer, and significant cross-communication between the HER-2 receptor pathway and ER has been reported (8,13,14).

The estrogen receptor (ER) is a member of a large family of nuclear receptors that share a common structural and functional organization. These receptors are generally considered to function as ligand-activated transcription factors (15,16). However, accumulating evidence shows significant cross-communication between steroid hormone receptors and peptide growth factor signaling pathways, with some reports suggesting that growth factors may promote activation of steroid receptors even in the absence of natural ligand (Table 24.1). Agents capable of exerting such ligand-independent activation of ER include epidermal growth factor (EGF) (17–20), TGF-α (21), heregulin (14), insulin (22), IGF-I (18,21,23–25), and dopamine (26). Under estrogen-free conditions, *in vivo* administration of EGF alone mimics the effects of estrogen in the mouse reproductive tract (27,28). In gene knockout mice lacking ER-α expression, both estrogen- and EGF-stimulated uterine growth is blocked (27). Thus, ER and co-activator partners may mediate the transcription of target genes by integrating signals from growth factor-activated pathways as well as from steroid hormone binding (29).

Subversion of growth factor receptor function often occurs in malignant progression with members of the *erb*-B family most frequently implicated in human cancer (1). The EGF receptor (EGFR/HER-1) is a 170-kD transmembrane glycoprotein that consists of an extracellular ligand-binding domain, a transmembrane spanning region and a cytoplasmic EGF-stimulated protein tyrosine kinase in its C-terminus. Upon binding of growth factor with the extracellular domain of its receptor and dimerization, the receptor undergoes autophosphorylation on tyrosine residues. EGFR activation results, in turn, in phosphorylation of downstream protein kinases, such as MAP kinase and PI3 kinase/Akt kinase, and the subsequent activation of specific transcription factors. The EGF receptor family also includes the HER-2 (*erb*-B2) protein, a 185-kD transmembrane tyrosine kinase encoded by the HER-2 oncogene; the HER-3 protein, a 180-kD membrane receptor tyrosine kinase; and HER-4, a 180-kD tyrosine kinase.

The HER-2 tyrosine kinase receptor functions in a fashion similar to EGFR (30). In addition, upon binding of ligands to EGFR, HER-3 or HER-4, the HER-2 receptor is often recruited as a preferred partner of these ligand-bound receptors to form active, phosphorylated

TABLE 24.1. *Cross-communication between estrogen receptor and growth factor receptor signaling pathways*

Year	Selected observations
1975	Parallels in membrane-initiated signaling by estrogen and peptide growth factors (73,74)
1985	Estrogen-induced growth factors of breast cancer cells (99)
1989	Cooperative interactions between *erb*-A and *erb*-B receptors in malignant transformation (31)
1992	EGF action in uterus involves estrogen receptor (19)
1995	Activation of ER by MAP kinase phosphorylation cascade (18)
1996	Estrogen receptor knockout mice lack estrogen-like responses to EGF treatment (27)
1999	Non-transcriptional action of estradiol on Src/Ras/MAPK pathway triggers DNA synthesis (100)
2000	PI3 kinase/Akt kinase regulate estrogen receptor activation (32,33)
2001	Hyperactivation of MAPK in EGFR or HER-2-overexpressing cells promotes downregulation of ER, with reversal by inhibition of signaling pathways (101)
2002	Direct interactions between growth factor receptor tyrosine kinases and estrogen receptor-α (57)

EGF, epidermal growth factor; ER, estrogen receptor.

heterodimeric complexes that, in turn, activate downstream signaling pathways involved in the growth and survival of tumors. It is notable that cooperative interactions between *erb*-B and *erb*-A (such as estrogen receptor) receptor were first reported more than a decade ago (31). With emerging evidence for estrogen receptor-stimulated activation of MAP kinase (18) and PI3 kinase/Akt kinase (32,33) signaling pathways, growth factor and steroid hormone-dependent mitogenic cascades may well have significant interactions.

ESTROGEN RECEPTOR STRUCTURE AND FUNCTION

Estrogen receptor-α functions in the nucleus as a transcription factor. The nuclear actions of estrogen are determined by the structure of the ligand, the subtype (ER-α, ER-β) or isoform (transcriptional splice variants, post-translational modifications) of the ER, the characteristics of the gene promoter, and the balance of coactivator and corepressor molecules that modulate the transcriptional response to the estrogen-ER complex (34). ER-α is characterized by six major functional domains often termed A through F (Fig. 24.1). The A/B region contains an N-terminal transactivation domain, AF-1; the C region harbors the DNA-binding domain, while the D region is involved in nuclear localization signaling; and E/F contains the C-terminal portion of the receptor and is involved in hormone-binding, dimerization and the function of a second transactivation domain, AF-2 (16,35). AF-1 and AF-2 appear to contribute synergistically to the transcription of ER-regulated target genes, but they have different mechanisms of activation.

On binding estradiol, ER-α undergoes an alteration in the conformation of the ligand-binding domain to form a novel surface in the region of the C-terminal helix, helix 12 (36). This conformational shift appears to allow the binding of coactivators and other regulatory proteins (34). Ligand-bound estrogen receptors function directly as transcription factors by binding DNA as homodimers to specific sequences called estrogen-responsive elements (ERE), generally comprising short palindromic sequences in the vicinity of target genes (37,38). Activation of ER ultimately leads to its downregulation in those

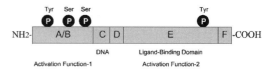

Fig. 24.1. Functional domains of human estrogen receptor-α. Full-length ER is composed of 595 amino acids. Locations of the DNA-binding domain (domain C) and the ligand-binding domain (domain E) are shown (38,63). Positions of the amino-terminal activation function 1 and the carboxy-terminal activation function 2 transactivation domains are also indicated. The general location of the six known phosphorylation sites in ER-α are represented by the letter P, with notation of serine (*Ser*) or tyrosine (*Tyr*) sites.

cells expressing it. Blockade of this ER-signaling pathway by interfering with binding of estrogen to its receptors is the basis of the major hormone treatment modality, tamoxifen, a partial agonist well-known to limit the proliferative effects of estrogen in the breast. In some tissues, estrogens may also indirectly regulate the transcription of genes that lack functional estrogen-responsive elements by modulating the activity of other transcription factors, such as activating protein-1 (AP-1) (34,38).

LIGAND-INDEPENDENT ACTIVATION OF ESTROGEN RECEPTOR

Growth factors, such as EGF (39–41) and estrogens (42) are known mitogens for breast cancer cells (Fig. 24.2). Activation of ER by growth factors in the absence of estrogen is a well-documented phenomenon that may play a critical role in steroid receptor signaling and breast cancer development (1,14,18,27,43,44).

Several studies document significant interactions between ER and the HER-2 receptor signaling complex (Table 24.2). The common inverse association between ER and HER-2 expression in invasive human breast cancers is poorly understood. Earlier studies of interactions between estrogen and HER-2 in breast cancer cells have shown that estrogen can transiently decrease the expression of HER-2 receptor (45,46). With regard to the problem of development of hormone resistance, it is notable that some experimental data show that long-term treatment *in vitro* with antihormone drugs, including tamoxifen, elicits enhanced expression of HER-2 and EGF receptors in tumor cells (47). Independent studies suggest that long-term suppression of ER may, in turn, be mediated by HER-2 signaling pathways (14). In laboratory studies, introduction in breast cancer cells of additional copies of the HER-2 gene, with the attendant increase in expression of its protein, leads to a significant reduction in the sensitivity of these cells to both estrogen and antiestrogens (13,14). ER-positive and HER-2-overexpressing primary breast cancers also show evidence of a deficient antiproliferative response to endocrine therapy using an antiestrogen or an aromatase inhibitor (48).

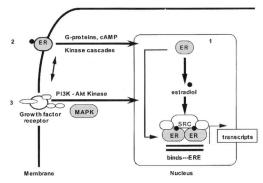

Fig. 24.2. Molecular mechanisms of estrogen action and potential pathways for cross-talk with growth factor receptor signaling. In the most common model of steroid hormone action (34), estrogen (*black circles*) binding to estrogen receptor (*ER*) promotes alterations in receptor conformation favoring enhanced association with coactivator proteins (*SRC*) and with specific estrogen-responsive elements (*ERE*) in the nucleus, leading, in turn, to initiation of selective gene transcription (see pathway 1). In some tissues, estrogens may also regulate the transcription of genes lacking a functional ERE by interacting with other transcription factors such as AP-1 (pathway not shown). Nonetheless, the genomic model alone fails to account for rapid cell responses to estrogen treatment or cross-communication with other cell signaling networks (see pathways 2 and 3) (34,112). The genomic model of hormone action requires integration with alternative pathways of estrogen action. For example, growth factor receptor-induced signaling may interact with ER or other components in the signaling network such as coactivator proteins (pathway 3). In addition, estrogens may bind a membrane-associated ER, with potential for promotion of responses via a complementary pathway that may cross-talk or interact directly with the genomic mechanism (pathway 2). Membrane-associated ER may affect one or more of several pathways, including interaction with transmembrane growth factor receptors; activation of G-proteins, nucleotide cyclases, and/or MAP kinase, with resultant increases in their catalytic products. These interactions may promote phosphorylation of ER itself via steroid-induced or ligand-independent pathways.

The exact mechanism(s) linking the HER-2 and ER systems, however, are as yet incompletely defined. The estrogen receptor is a phosphoprotein, and phosphorylation of ER occurs early in its activation by ligand binding (49).

TABLE 24.2. *Estrogen receptor and HER-2 receptor interactions*

Year	Selected observations[a]
1986	Tyrosine phosphorylation of estrogen receptor (55)
1989	HER-2 overexpression correlates inversely with ER-/PR-phenotype in breast cancers (5–7,9)
1990	HER-2/ER cross-talk: estrogen receptor downregulates HER-2 (45)
	HER-2 overexpressing breast cancers are tamoxifen-resistant (102)
1990	Tyrosine kinase inhibitors block estrogen-dependent cancer growth (56)
1991	Tamoxifen resistance with overexpressed HER-2 *in vitro* (13)
1995	HER-2-induced phosphorylation and activation of ER (14)
	HER-2/ER cross-talk : HER-2 downregulates estrogen receptor (14)
	HER-2 overexpressing cells with reduced estrogen dependence and tamoxifen sensitivity (103)
1997	HER-2 antibody enhances antitumor effects of tamoxifen (14,68)
1999	Overexpression of steroid receptor coactivator AIB1 correlates with HER-2 overexpression in breast cancer (29,104)
	HER-2 amplification impedes antiproliferative effects of hormonal therapy (48)
	Inhibition of HER-2 tyrosine kinase and MAPK enhances tamoxifen activity (53)
2002	Resistance to tamoxifen-induced apoptosis associated with ER-HER-2 interaction (78)

[a]See text for additional details.
ER, estrogen receptor; MAPK, mitogen-activated protein kinase.

Some studies suggest that ER phosphorylation at serine and tyrosine residues contributes to receptor activation and, possibly, binding to DNA (16,22,38,50,51). The transcriptional activity of AF-2 is activated by binding estrogens, but transcription mediated by the AF-1 domain of ER appears to require phosphorylation of serine-118 by mitogen-activated protein kinase (MAPK) signaling pathways (18,52). Thus, growth factor-stimulated activation of ER appears to be regulated, in part, by the AF-1 domain of ER. MAPK-induced phosphorylation of ER may lead to ligand-independent ER activation with loss of the inhibitory effect of tamoxifen on ER-mediated transcription, providing a potential mechanism for the association of growth factor signal transduction with tamoxifen resistance (17,18,53). Additional serine phosphorylation sites in ER that may participate in the transcriptional activation of ER include serine-167, a major estradiol-induced phosphorylation site on ER (50), as well as serine-104 and serine-106 (54).

Although MAP kinase-mediated phosphorylation of serine residues plays a role in the activation of AF-1 in the absence of estrogen, full activation of the AF-1 domain appears to require that other residues, as yet undetermined, must also be phosphorylated (18). Phosphorylation of ER at tyrosine residues occurs (55), and previous data have demonstrated enhanced tyrosine phosphorylation of ER after stimulation of tyrosine kinase signaling in MCF-7 cells by heregulin, a ligand for EGFR, HER-2, and HER-3 (14). Blockade of estrogen-induced growth of human breast cancer cells by tyrosine kinase inhibitors provides further evidence of the importance of tyrosine kinase pathways in ER signaling (56).

One phosphorylated tyrosine residue in human ER-α, tyrosine-537, is located at the N-terminus of helix 12 in the hormone-binding domain. Although several recent studies show that phosphorylation of estrogen receptor at tyrosine-537 is not an absolute requirement for hormone binding to ER or for activation of ER-dependent transcription (38,51,57–59), phosphorylation at this site may disrupt hydrophobic interactions that normally maintain the receptor in an inactive state. Thus, it could represent an alternative mechanism for ligand-independent activation of ER, possibly by forming an interacting surface for recruitment of coactivators (38). However, identification of a growth factor-signaling pathway that phosphorylates and activates the receptor at tyrosine-537 has been elusive. One new study suggests that EGFR tyrosine kinase interacts directly with ER in solution and in intact cells, leading to phosphorylation of ER at tyrosine-537 and tyrosine-43, and these alterations in ER may then contribute to promotion of estrogen-independent activation of ER-mediated transcription and cell proliferation (57). It remains to be determined what contribution tyrosine phosphorylation may make in regulating the activation of AF-1 or the interactions between AF-1 and AF-2 domains of ER.

RESISTANCE TO HORMONAL THERAPY AND GROWTH FACTOR SIGNALING

It is noteworthy that there is precedent for cross-communication between growth-factor receptor signaling and the activity of other steroid hormone receptors. In advanced stage breast cancers, progesterone may selectively enhance the sensitivity of key kinase cascades to growth factors, thereby priming cells for stimulation by latent growth signals and allowing a switch from steroid hormone to growth factor dependence (60). The progression of human prostate cancer from a hormone-sensitive, androgen-dependent stage to a hormone-refractory, androgen-independent tumor may occur, in part, by modulation of androgen receptor signaling by HER-2 tyrosine kinase (61,62).

The resistance or insensitivity of some breast tumors to hormonal therapy, such as tamoxifen, may be due, in part, to the activity of growth-factor signaling pathways that converge with ER. Although the structural features of ER required for its activation by growth-factor signaling are not completely understood, some data suggest that growth factor pathways may target different regions of ER depending on the presence or absence of estrogen, potentially as a result of different conformations of the receptor induced by estrogen (38,63). Growth factor signaling appears to stimulate ER transcriptional activity even in the absence of estrogen, albeit to levels significantly less than that of estrogen, and it may also increase the magnitude of target gene expression of ligand-occupied ER. New evidence suggests that estrogen receptor coactivators, such as AIB1, may also serve as substrates and conduits for kinase-mediated growth-factor signaling to the estrogen receptor (29). Convergence between growth factor and estrogen-signaling pathways may thus elicit a synergistic feed-forward circuit, leading to a stronger or more sustained proliferative response in breast cancer cells.

Structural alterations in ER elicited by growth factor receptor signaling may sensitize the steroid receptor to ligand or to coactivator interactions, thereby activating biologic responses even at suboptimal levels of estrogens. In this context, partial agonists, such as tamoxifen, may not provide effective therapy, but tumors may remain sensitive to alternative endocrine treatments. Thus, blockade of estrogen production using aromatase inhibitors may have utility in the treatment of growth factor-overexpressing tumors (64,65). Therapies that elicit downregulation of ER, such as ICI 182,780 (66) and some aromatase inhibitors (67), may also be efficacious as alternative antitumor agents.

Another approach to treatment of patients with ER-positive, growth-factor receptor-positive tumors may be to simultaneously block both growth-factor- and ER-dependent signaling pathways. Enhanced antiproliferative effects in HER-2-overexpressing cells with ER are found by combined treatment with antibody to HER-2 receptor and tamoxifen (14,68). Similarly, combination of the anti-HER-2 receptor antibody trastuzumab with the estrogen receptor downregulator ICI 182,780 is active in blocking *in vitro* growth of breast cancer cells expressing both HER-2 and estrogen receptors (69). There may also be considerable potential for use of growth-factor-selective tyrosine kinase inhibitors, alone or combined with antihormone agents, to treat and possibly prevent endocrine-resistant breast cancer (47,53). An autocrine growth-factor stimulatory loop involving EGFR and HER-2 may be critical to the growth and survival of endocrine-resistant cells (14,47). In this context, it is important to note that increased signaling through the EGFR pathway also results from overexpression of HER-2, an important signaling partner for EGFR in human breast cancers (70).

ALTERNATIVE PATHWAYS OF ESTROGEN ACTION

Although the estrogen receptor is generally considered to function exclusively as a nuclear transcription factor, numerous reports document rapid effects of estradiol that appear to be mediated by a membrane-associated form of ER (Fig. 24.2) (34,71–77). These membrane-associated receptors have not yet been isolated in pure form, but several lines of evidence suggest that they may derive from the same transcript as nuclear ER (71) and play a role in cross-communication with other membrane-initiated signaling pathways.

New studies provide evidence for direct interactions between transmembrane tyrosine kinase receptors and ER, and suggest that such acute cross-talk between growth factor and estrogen receptors may contribute to modulation of estrogen-induced growth (57,78). One potential cellular site for interaction between ER and growth factor receptors may be caveolae, specialized microdomains in plasma membrane. Caveolae are thought to occur in most cell types (79), although with reduced expression in breast cancer cells (80). Caveolae are enriched in several growth factor receptors, including members of the EGF receptor family (79,81), and a portion of estrogen receptors in target cells also localize in caveolar membrane fractions (82–85). It is clear that further work is now required to determine whether membrane-associated estrogen receptors are classical forms of ER complexed with other membrane-associated proteins, new isoforms of ER in membranes, known molecules (kinases, ion channels, other receptors) with previously unrecognized binding-sites for steroid, truly novel membrane proteins, or a combination of these (75,76).

CLINICAL SIGNIFICANCE OF CROSS-TALK BETWEEN ESTROGEN RECEPTOR AND GROWTH-FACTOR RECEPTOR PATHWAYS

One major problem in breast cancer management is the conversion of estrogen-sensitive to hormone-resistant malignancies after initiation of antiestrogen therapy (86). The molecular basis for this hormone-independent progression of breast cancer is not clear. However, as noted above, enhanced cross-communication between growth-factor receptor pathways and ER during cancer progression could contribute to ER activation in the absence of hormone. This development could then result in a reduced response

TABLE 24.3. *Endocrine therapy and the predictive value of HER-2 receptor expression in human breast cancer*

Study	Correlation with HER-2 overexpression
Wright et al. (1992) (12)	Yes
Borg et al. (1994) (10)	Yes
Tetu and Brisson (1994) (105)	Yes
Berns et al. (1995) (106)	Yes
Leitzel et al. (1995) (11)	Yes
Archer et al. (1995) (107)	No
Carlomagno et al. (1996) (108)	Yes
Elledge et al. (1998) (92)	No
Sjogren et al. (1998) (109)	Yes
Houston et al. (1999) (110)	Yes
Bianco et al. (2000) (89)	Yes
Berry et al. (2000) (111)	No
De Laurentis et al. (2000) (95)	Yes
Ellis et al. (2001) (64)	Yes

See text for details and discussion.

to antiestrogens (43). Current findings indicate that HER-2, and possibly EGFR, plays a leading role in breast tumor progression (1,4–6,47). In patients with breast cancer, prognosis is inversely correlated with overexpression and/or amplification of HER-2 or EGFR. In addition, an inverse correlation in the expression of ER and HER-2 or EGFR in breast cancers correlates with aggressiveness of the disease and with the response to endocrine treatment (14,43,87).

Some recent clinical studies suggest that measurement of EGFR and HER-2 levels in breast tumors may be used to select the most effective endocrine therapy (Table 24.3) (64,88). Several studies offer evidence that ER- or PR-positive, HER-2-overexpressing tumors are less likely to respond to endocrine therapy, primarily tamoxifen (11,12,89–91), while other trials have presented contradictory findings (Table 24.3) (92,93). Among those studies demonstrating that traditional hormonal treatments are less able to elicit responses in patients with HER-2-overexpressing as compared with non-overexpressing tumors, there are further differences with regard to the most effective form of alternative therapy (64,65,94). A recent meta-analysis of seven clinical studies concluded that metastatic breast cancers overexpressing HER-2 were resistant to tamoxifen (estimated odds ratio of disease progression was 2.46) (95,96).

However, the relative benefit of adjuvant tamoxifen in early breast cancers with HER-2 overexpression remains controversial.

The difficulty in comparing results from different clinical data sets is likely due to several factors. These studies were essentially all retrospective and standard methods for the assay of biologic factors were not employed. A wide variety of reagents and technologies are in use to detect HER-2 amplification/overexpression in clinical specimens (immunohistochemistry, fluorescence *in situ* hybridization, ELISA for HER-2 protein in plasma, Southern blot), with differing sensitivity and specificity for each approach (87). It is well known that HER-2 measurements have been plagued with problems of reproducibility (97). Similarly, measurements of steroid hormone receptors are not uniformly standardized (98). ER/PR measurements in routine practice are often not as reliable as required for rational management decisions (98). Further, the significance of subtypes and isoforms of estrogen receptors and their assay in clinical specimens still remains to be considered (34). Moreover, the generally negative correlation between HER-2 and ER expression in breast tumors is sometimes not considered in data analysis. As noted before (8), different endpoints associated with different disease settings (for example, metastatic, neoadjuvant) and the combination of endocrine therapy with chemotherapy in the reported studies tends to further compromise interpretation of the clinical data.

Although experimental systems indicate that overexpression of HER-2 leads to tamoxifen resistance or insensitivity in breast cancers bearing estrogen receptor, the data from the clinic are less definitive. A randomized prospective trial assigning patients with reliable HER-2 and ER/PR determinations to endocrine treatment or control groups would be ideal to answer this important question (96). However, in lieu of the latter approach, retrospective evaluation of a large cohort of clinical tumor specimens using more reliable and sensitive measures of HER-2 and estrogen receptors could be conducted to evaluate the true utility of HER-2 and estrogen receptors in predicting responsiveness to hormonal therapy and in the choice of different endocrine therapies. Further delineation of these complex pathways in breast cancer cells will, hopefully, lead to the design of novel therapies that combine anti-growth factor signaling strategies with more beneficial anti-hormone measures.

Acknowledgments: Drs. D. Marquez, D.J. Slamon, C.M. Szego, I. Dimery, and A. Wakeling provided useful discussions, and Cary Freeny provided expert editorial assistance. This work was supported by grants from the National Institutes of Health, U.S. Army Breast Cancer Research Program (DAMD17-99-1-9099, DAMD17-00-1-0177), Susan G. Komen Breast Cancer Research Foundation (99-3305), California Breast Cancer Research Program (5JB-0105), and the Stiles Program in Integrative Oncology.

REFERENCES

1. Bange J, Zwick E, Ullrich A. Molecular targets for breast cancer therapy and prevention. *Nat Med* 2001; 7:548–552.
2. Carpenter G, Cohen S. Epidermal growth factor. *Ann Rev Biochem* 1979;48:193–208.
3. McGuire WL, Clark G. Prognostic factors and treatment decisions in axillary-node-negative breast cancer. *N Engl J Med* 1992;326:1756–1762.
4. Slamon DJ, GM Clark, SG Wong, et al. Human breast cancer: Correlation of relapse and survival with amplification of the HER-2/neu oncogene. *Science* 1987; 235:177–181.
5. Slamon DJ, Godolphin W, Jones LA, et al. Studies of the HER-2/neu proto-oncogene in human breast and ovarian cancer. *Science* 1989;244:707–711.
6. Slamon D, Press M, Godolphin W, et al. Studies of the HER-2/neu oncogene in human breast cancer. *Cancer Cells* 1989;7:371–378.
7. Adnane J, Guadray P, Simon M-P, et al. Proto-oncogene amplification and human breast tumor phenotype. *Oncogene* 1989;4:1389–1395.
8. Dowsett M. Overexpression of HER-2 as a resistance mechanism to hormonal therapy for breast cancer. *Endocrine-Related Cancer* 2001;8:191–195.
9. Zeillinger R, Kury F, Cserwenka K, et al. HER-2 amplification, steroid receptors and EGF receptor in primary breast cancer. *Oncogene* 1989;4:109–113.
10. Borg A, Baldetorp B, Ferno M, et al. ErbB2 amplification is associated with tamoxifen resistance in steroid-receptor positive breast cancer. *Cancer Letters* 1994; 81:137–143.
11. Leitzel K, Teramoto Y, Konrad K, et al. Elevated serum c-erbB-2 antigen levels and decreased response to hormone therapy of breast cancer. *J Clin Oncol* 1995;13:1129–1135.
12. Wright C, Nicholson S, Angus B, et al. Relationship between c-erbB-2 protein product expression and response to endocrine therapy in advanced breast cancer. *Brit J Cancer* 1992;118–124.
13. Benz C, Scott G, Sarup J, et al. Estrogen-dependent, tamoxifen-resistant tumori-genic growth of MCF-7 cells

transfected with HER2/neu. *Breast Cancer Res Treatment* 1993;24:85–92.
14. Pietras RJ, Arboleda J, Reese D, et al. HER-2 tyrosine kinase pathway targets estrogen receptor and promotes hormone-independent growth in human breast cancer cells. *Oncogene* 1995;10:2435–2446.
15. Enmark E, Gustafsson JA. Oestrogen receptors—an overview. *J Intern Med* 1999;246:133–138.
16. Katzenellenbogen BS. Estrogen receptors: bioactivities and interactions with cell signaling pathways. *Biol Reprod* 1996;54:287–293.
17. Bunone G, Briand P, Miksicek R, Picard D. Activation of unliganded estrogen receptor by EGF involves the MAP kinase pathway and direct phosphorylation. *EMBO J* 1996;15:2174–2183.
18. Kato S, Endoh H, Masuhiro Y, et al. Activation of the estrogen receptor through phosphorylation by mitogen-activated protein kinase. *Science* 1995;270:1491–1494.
19. Ignar-Trowbridge DM, Nelson K, Bidwell M, et al. Coupling of dual signaling pathways: epidermal growth factor action involves the estrogen receptor. *Proc Natl Acad Sci USA* 1992;89:4658–4666.
20. Ignar-Trowbridge D, Pimentel M, Teng CT, et al. Cross talk between peptide growth factor and estrogen receptor signaling systems. *Environ Health Perspect* 1995;103 (suppl 7):35–38.
21. Ignar-Trowbridge DM, Pimentel M, Parker M, et al. Peptide growth factor cross-talk with the estrogen receptor requires the A/B domain and occurs independently of protein kinase C or estradiol. *Endocrinology* 1996;137:1735–1744.
22. Patrone C, Gianazza E, Santagati S, et al. Divergent pathways regulate ligand-independent activation of ER alpha in SK-N-BE neuroblastoma and COS-1 renal carcinoma cells. *Mol Endocrinol* 1998;12:835–841.
23. Lee AV, Weng CN, Jackson JG, Yee D. Activation of estrogen receptor-mediated gene transcription by IGF-I in human breast cancer cells. *J Endocrinol* 1997;152:39–47.
24. Newton CJ, Buric R, Trapp T, et al. The unliganded estrogen receptor (ER) transduces growth factor signals. *J Steroid Biochem Mol Biol* 1994;48:481–486.
25. Stewart AJ, Johnson MD, May FE, Westley BR. Role of insulin-like growth factors and the type-I insulin-like growth-factor receptor in the estrogen-stimulated proliferation of human breast cancer cells. *J Biol Chem* 1990;265:1172–1178.
26. Power RF, Mani SK, Codina J, et al. Dopaminergic and ligand-independent activation of steroid hormone receptors. *Science* 1991;254:1636–1639.
27. Curtis SW, Washburn T, Sewall C, et al. Physiological coupling of growth-factor and steroid-receptor signaling pathways: estrogen receptor knockout mice lack estrogen-like response to epidermal growth factor. *Proc Natl Acad Sci USA* 1996;93:12626–12630.
28. Nelson KG, Takahashi T, Bossert NL, et al. Epidermal growth factor replaces estrogen in the stimulation of female genital-tract growth and differentiation. *Proc Natl Acad Sci USA* 1991;88:21–25.
29. Font de Mora J, Brown M. AIB1 is a conduit for kinase-mediated growth factor signaling to the estrogen receptor. *Mol Cell Biol* 2000;20:5041–5047.
30. Zwick E, Bange J, Ullrich A. Receptor tyrosine kinase signaling as a target for cancer intervention strategies. *Endocrine-Related Cancer* 2001;8:161–173.
31. Beug H, Graf T. Cooperation between viral oncogenes in avian erythroid and myeloid leukaemia. *Eur J Clin Invest* 1989;19:491–501.
32. Marquez D, Pietras RJ. Membrane-associated binding sites for estrogen contribute to growth regulation in human breast cancer cells. *Oncogene* 2001;20:5420–5430.
33. Simoncini T, Hafezi-Moghadam A, Brazil DP, et al. Interaction of oestrogen receptor with the regulatory subunit of phosphatidylinositol-3-OH kinase. *Nature* 2000;407:538–541.
34. Gruber CJ, Tschugguel W, Schneeberger C, Huber JC. Mechanisms of disease: Production and actions of estrogens. *N Engl J Med* 2002;346:340–352.
35. Tora L, White J, Brou C, et al. The human estrogen receptor has two independent nonacidic transcriptional activation functions. *Cell* 1989;59:477–487.
36. Brzozowski A, Pike A, Dauter Z, et al. Molecular basis of agonism and antagonism in the oestrogen receptor. *Nature* 1997;389:753–758.
37. Green S, Chambon P. Nuclear receptors enhance our understanding of transcription regulation. *Trends Genet* 1988;4:309–314.
38. White R, Parker MG. Molecular mechanisms of steroid hormone action. *Endocrine-Related Cancer* 1998;5:1–14.
39. Das SK, Tsukamura H, Paria BC, et al. Differential expression of epidermal growth-factor receptor (EGF-R) gene and regulation of EGF-R bioactivity by progesterone and estrogen in the adult mouse uterus. *Endocrinology* 1994;134:971–981.
40. Gabelman BM, Emerman JT. Effects of estrogen, epidermal growth factor, and transforming growth factor-α on the growth of human breast epithelial cells in primary culture. *Exp Cell Res* 1992;201:113–118.
41. Nickell KA, Halper J, Moses HL. Transforming growth factors in solid human malignant neoplasms. *Cancer Res* 1983;43:1966–1971.
42. Harris J, Lippman M, Veronesi U, Willett W. Breast cancer. *N Engl J Med* 1992;327:473–451.
43. Nicholson RI, McClelland RA, Robertson JF, Gee JM. Involvement of steroid-hormone and growth-factor cross-talk in endocrine response in breast cancer. *Endocr Relat Cancer* 1999;6:373–387.
44. Smith C, Conneely O, O'Malley BW. Oestrogen receptor activation in the absence of ligand. *Biochem Soc Trans* 1995;935–939.
45. Read L, Keith D, Slamon D, Katzenellenbogen B. Hormonal modulation of HER-2/neu protooncogene messenger ribonucleic acid and p185 protein expression in human breast cancer cell lines. *Cancer Res* 1990;50:3947–3955.
46. Russell K, Hung M-C. Transcriptional repression of the neu protooncogene by estrogen stimulated estrogen receptor. *Cancer Res* 1992;52:6624–6632.
47. Nicholson RI, Hutcheson IR, Harper ME, et al. Modulation of epidermal growth-factor receptor in endocrine-resistant, oestrogen receptor-positive breast cancer. *Endocr Relat Cancer* 2001;8:175–182.
48. Dowsett M, Harper-Wynne C, Boeddinghaus I, et al. HER-2 amplification impedes the antiproliferative effects of hormone therapy in estrogen receptor-positive primary breast cancer. *Cancer Res* 2001;61:8452–8458.
49. Weigel NL. Steroid hormone receptors and their regulation by phosphorylation. *Biochem J* 1996;319:657–667.

50. Arnold SF, Obourn JD, Jaffe H, Notides AC. Serine 167 is the major estradiol-induced phosphorylation site on the human estrogen receptor. *Mol Endocrinol* 1994;8:1208–1214.
51. Yudt MR, Vorojeikina D, Zhong L, et al. Function of estrogen receptor tyrosine 537 in hormone binding, DNA binding, and transactivation. *Biochemistry* 1999;38:14146–14156.
52. Ali S, Metzger D, Bornert JM, Chambon P. Modulation of transcriptional activation by ligand-dependent phosphorylation of the human oestrogen receptor A/B region. *EMBO J* 1993;12:1153–1160.
53. Kurokawa H, Lenferink A, Simpson J, et al. Inhibition of HER2/neu (erbB-2) and mitogen-activated protein kinases enhances tamoxifen action against HER2-overexpressing, tamoxifen-resistant breast cancer cells. *Cancer Res* 2000;60:5887–5894.
54. Le Goff P, Montano MM, Schodin DJ, Katzenellenbogen BS. Phosphorylation of the human estrogen receptor. Identification of hormone-regulated sites and examination of their influence on transcriptional activity. *J Biol Chem* 1994;269:4458–4466.
55. Migliaccio A, Rotondi A, Auricchio F. Estradiol receptor: phosphorylation on tyrosine in uterus and interaction with antiphosphotyrosine antibody. *EMBO J* 1986;5:2867–2872.
56. Reddy K, Mangold G, Tandon A, et al. Inhibition of breast cancer cell growth in vitro by a tyrosine kinase inhibitor. *Cancer Res* 1992;52:3636–3644.
57. Marquez D, Lee J, Lin T, Pietras RJ. Epidermal growth factor receptor and tyrosine phosphorylation of estrogen receptor. *Endocrine* 2002; in press.
58. Weis K, Ekena K, Thomas J, et al. Constitutively active human estrogen receptors containing amino acid substitutions for tyrosine 537 in the receptor protein. *Mol Endocrinol* 1996;10:1388–1398.
59. Zhang Q, Borg A, Wolf D, et al. An estrogen receptor mutant with strong hormone-independent activity from a metastatic breast cancer. *Cancer Res* 1997;57:1244–1249.
60. Lange C, Richer J, Shen T, Horwitz K. Convergence of progesterone and epidermal growth factor signaling in breast cancer. *J Biol Chem* 1998;273:31308–31316.
61. Craft N, Shostak Y, Carey M, Sawyers C. A mechanism for hormone-independent prostate cancer through modulation of androgen receptor signaling by the HER-2/neu tyrosine kinase. *Nature Med* 1999;5:280–285.
62. Yeh S, Lin H-K, Kang H-Y, et al. From HER2/neu signal cascade to androgen receptor and its coactivators: A novel pathway by induction of androgen target genes through MAP kinase in prostate cancer cells. *Proc Natl Acad Sci USA* 1999;96:5458–5463.
63. Smith C. Cross-talk between peptide growth factor and estrogen receptor signaling pathways. *Biol Reprod* 1998;58:627–632.
64. Ellis MJ, Coop A, Singh B, et al. Letrozole is more effective neoadjuvant endocrine therapy than tamoxifen for erbB-1 and/or erbB-2-positive, estrogen receptor-positive primary breast cancer: Evidence from a phase III randomized trial. *J Clin Oncol* 2001;19:3808–3816.
65. Lipton A, Ali S, Leitzel K, et al. Elevated serum HER-2/neu levels predict decreased response to hormone therapy in metastatic breast cancer. *Proc Am Soc Clin Oncol* 2000;19:71a.
66. Howell A, Osborne CK, Morris C, Wakeling A. ICI 182,780 (Faslodex): development of a novel, pure antiestrogen. *Cancer* 2000;89:817–825.
67. Zhou JL, Brodie A. The effect of aromatase inhibitor 4-hydroxyandrostenedione on steroid receptors in hormone-dependent tissues of the rat. *J Steroid Biochem Mol Biol* 1995;52:71–76.
68. Witters I, Kumar R, Chinchilli V, Lipton A. Enhanced antiproliferative activity of the combination of tamoxifen plus HER-2-neu antibody. *Breast Cancer Res Trtmt* 1997;42:1–5.
69. Kunisue H, Kurebayashi J, Otsuki T, et al. Anti-HER-2 antibody enhances the growth inhibitory effect of anti-oestrogen on breast cancer cells expressing both oestrogen receptors and HER-2. *Brit J Cancer* 2000;82:46–51.
70. Worthylake R, Opresko L, Wiley H. ErbB-2 amplification inhibits down-regulation and induces constitutive activation of both ErbB-2 and epidermal growth factor receptors. *J Biol Chem* 1999;274:8865–8874.
71. Levin E. Cellular functions of the plasma membrane estrogen receptor. *Trends Endocrinol Metab* 1999;10:374–377.
72. Mendelsohn ME, Karas RH. The protective effects of estrogen on the cardiovascular system. *N Engl J Med* 1999;340:1801–1811.
73. Pietras RJ, Szego C. Endometrial cell calcium and oestrogen action. *Nature* 1975;253:357–359.
74. Pietras RJ, Szego CM. Specific binding sites for oestrogen at the outer surfaces of isolated endometrial cells. *Nature* 1977;265:69–72.
75. Pietras RJ, Szego CM. Cell membrane estrogen receptors resurface. *Nature Med* 1999;5:1330–1331.
76. Pietras RJ, Nemere I, Szego CM. Steroid hormone receptors in target cell membranes. *Endocrine* 2001;14:417–427.
77. Watson CS, Gametchu B. Membrane-initiated steroid actions and the proteins that mediate them. *Proc Soc Exp Biol Med* 1999;220:9–19.
78. Chung YL, Sheu ML, Yang SC, et al. Resistance to tamoxifen-induced apoptosis is associated with direct interaction between HER-2/neu and cell membrane estrogen receptor in breast cancer. *Int J Cancer* 2002;97:306–312.
79. Anderson RG. The caveolae membrane system. *Annu Rev Biochem* 1998;67:199–225.
80. Koleske AJ, Baltimore D, Lisanti MP. Reduction of caveolin and caveolae in oncogenically transformed cells. *Proc Natl Acad Sci USA* 1995;92:1381–1385.
81. Mineo C, James GL, Smart EJ, Anderson RG. Localization of epidermal growth factor-stimulated Ras/Raf-1 interaction to caveolae membrane. *J Biol Chem* 1996;271:11930–11935.
82. Chambliss KL, Yuhanna IS, Mineo C, et al. Estrogen receptor alpha and endothelial nitric oxide synthase are organized into a functional signaling module in caveolae. *Circ Res* 2000;87:E44–52.
83. Kim HP, Lee JY, Jeong JK, et al. Nongenomic stimulation of nitric oxide release by estrogen is mediated by estrogen receptor alpha localized in caveolae. *Biochem Biophys Res Commun* 1999;263:257–262.
84. Pietras RJ, Szego CM. Specific internalization of estrogen and binding to nuclear matrix in isolated uterine cells. *Biochem Biophys Res Comun* 1984;123:84–91.

85. Schlegel A, Wang C, Katzenellenbogen BS, et al. Caveolin-1 potentiates estrogen receptor alpha (ERalpha) signaling. Caveolin-1 drives ligand-independent nuclear translocation and activation of ERalpha. *J Biol Chem* 1999;274:33551–33556.
86. Katzenellenbogen BS, Montano MM, Ekena K, et al. William L. McGuire Memorial Lecture. Antiestrogens: mechanisms of action and resistance in breast cancer. *Breast Cancer Res Treat* 1997;44:23–38.
87. Pegram MD, Pauletti G, Slamon DJ. HER-2/neu as a predictive marker of response to breast cancer therapy. *Breast Cancer Res* 1998;52:65–77.
88. Pritchard K. Use of erbB-1 and erbB-2 to select endocrine therapy for breast cancer: Will it play in Peoria? *J Clin Oncol* 2001;19:3795–3797.
89. Bianco A, De Laurentis M, Carlomagno C, et al. HER-2 overexpression predicts adjuvant tamoxifen (TAM) failure for early breast cancer: Complete data at 20 yr of the Naples GUN randomized trial. *Proc Am Soc Clin Oncol* 2000;19:289.
90. Plunkett T, Houston S, Barnes D, et al. C-erbB-2 is a marker of resistance to endocrine therapy in advanced breast cancer. *Proc Am Soc Clin Oncol* 1998; 17:103a.
91. Yamauchi H, O'Neill A, Gelman R, et al. Prediction of response to antiestrogen therapy in advanced breast cancer patients by pretreatment circulating levels of extracellular domain of the HER-2/c-neu protein 386. *J Clin Oncol* 1997;15:2518–2525.
92. Elledge R, Green S, Ciocca D, et al. HER-2 expression and response to tamoxifen in estrogen receptor-positive breast cancer: A Southwest Oncology Group Study 385. *Clin Cancer Res* 1998;4:7–12.
93. Paik S, Bryant J, Park C, et al. ErbB-2 and response to doxorubicin in patients with axillary lymph node positive, hormone receptor negative breast cancer. *J Natl Cancer Inst* 1998;90:1361–1370.
94. Ali S, Leitzel K, Chinchilli V, et al. Serum HER-2/neu and response to Megace vs an aromatase inhibitor. *Proc Am Soc Clin Oncol* 2001;20:23a.
95. De Laurentis M, Arpino G, Massarelli E, et al. A meta-analysis of the interaction between HER2 and the response to endocrine therapy in metastatic breast cancer. *Am Soc Clin Oncol* 2000;19:301.
96. Hu JC, Mokbel K. Does c-erbB2/HER2 overexpression predict adjuvant tamoxifen failure in patients with early breast cancer? *Eur J Surg Oncol* 2001; 27:335–337.
97. Jacobs T, Gown A, Yaziji H, et al. Specificity of HercepTest in determining HER-2/neu status of breast cancers using the United States Food and Drug Administration-approved scoring system. *J Clin Oncol* 1999;17:1983–1987.
98. Allred C, Harvey JM, Berardo M, et al. Prognostic and predictive factors in breast cancer by immunohistochemical analysis. *Modern Pathol* 1998;11:155–168.
99. Dickson RB, McManaway M, Lippman M. Estrogen-induced factors of breast cancer cells partially replace estrogen to promote tumor growth. *Science* 1986; 232:1540–1543.
100. Castoria G, Barone N, Di Domenico M, et al. Non-transcriptional action of oestradiol and progestin triggers DNA synthesis. *EMBO J* 1999;18:2500–2510.
101. Oh A, Lorant L, Holloway J, et al. Hyperactivation of MAPK induces loss of ER-α expression in breast cancer cells. *Mol Endocrinol* 2001;15:1344–1359.
102. Nicholson S, Wright C, Sainsbury JR, et al. Epidermal growth factor receptor (EGFr) as a marker for poor prognosis in node-negative breast cancer patients: neu and tamoxifen failure. *J Steroid Biochem Mol Biol* 1990;37:811–814.
103. Liu Y, El-Ashry D, Chen D, et al. MCF-7 breast cancer cells overexpressing trans-fected c-erbB-2 have an in vitro growth advantage in estrogen-depleted conditions and reduced estrogen-dependence and tamoxifen-sensitivity in vivo. *Breast Cancer Res Trtmt* 1995;34: 97–117.
104. Bouras T, Southey MC, Venter DJ. Overexpression of the steroid receptor coactivator AIB1 in breast cancer correlates with the absence of estrogen and progesterone receptors and positivity for p53 and HER-2/neu. *Cancer Res* 2001;61:903–907.
105. Tetu B, Brisson J. Prognostic significance of HER-2/neu oncoprotein expression in node-positive breast cancer. *Cancer* 1994;73:2359–2365.
106. Berns E, Foekens J, van Staveren I, et al. Oncogene amplification and prognosis in breast cancer: relationship with systemic treatment. *Gene* 1995;159:11–18.
107. Archer S, Eliopoulos A, Spandidos D, et al. Expression of ras p21, p53 and c-erbB-2 in advanced breast cancer and response to first line hormonal therapy. *Brit J Cancer* 1995;72:1259–1266.
108. Carlomagno C, Perrone F, Gallo C, et al. c-erbB2 overexpression decreases the benefit of adjuvant tamoxifen in early-stage breast cancer without axillary lymph node metastases. *J Clin Oncol* 1996;14:2702–2708.
109. Sjogren S, Inganas M, Lindgren A, et al. Prognostic and predictive value of c-erbB-2 overexpression in primary breast cancer, alone and in combination with other prognostic markers. *J Clin Oncol* 1998;16:462–469.
110. Houston SJ, Plunkett T, Barnes D, et al. Overexpression of c-erbB2 is an independent marker of resistance to endocrine therapy in advanced breast cancer. *Brit J Cancer* 1999;79:1220–1226.
111. Berry D, Muss H, Thor A, et al. HER-2/neu and p53 expression versus tamoxifen resistance in estrogen receptor-positive, node-positive breast cancer. *J Clin Oncol* 2000;18:3471–3479.
112. Szego CM, Pietras RJ. Membrane recognition and effector sites in steriod hormone action. In: Litwack G, ed. *Biochemical actions of hormones,* Vol. VIII. New York: Academic Press, 1981:307–464.

25

Cell Cycle Inhibitors in the Treatment of Breast Cancer

Carolyn D. Britten

The cell cycle (Fig. 25.1) is the process by which proliferating cells duplicate the genome and divide into genetically identical daughter cells. During the first phase of the cell cycle, termed G_1 (gap), cells prepare for the DNA duplication that occurs during the S (synthesis) phase. This is followed by a second gap phase, termed G_2, which allows cells to repair errors that may have occurred during DNA synthesis. Finally, DNA is condensed into chromatids that separate between two daughter cells during the M (mitosis) phase. The daughter cells subsequently enter G_1 where they either commit to further replication or cross into the quiescent G_0 phase. Cells in G_0 may permanently relinquish their proliferative potential through the process of differentiation, or, alternatively, they may re-enter the cell cycle in response to extra-cellular signals.

A series of serine/threonine kinases called cyclin-dependent kinases (cdk-1 through cdk-9) govern cell cycle progression (1–4). Cdk activation is mediated by phosphorylation of the T-loop threonine by cdk-activating kinase (cdk7/cyclin H), dephosphorylation of threonine 14/tyrosine 15 mediated by cdc25 phosphatase, and association with cyclin cofactors, which are periodically expressed during the cell cycle due to phase-specific synthesis (1,2,4–7). The G_1 cyclins, D_1, D_2, and D_3, are produced in response to extra-cellular growth factors and activate cdk-4 and cdk-6 (2,4,8). Cdk-4/cyclin D_1 and cdk-6/cyclin D_3 complexes subsequently phosphorylate the retinoblastoma gene product, Rb. In quiescent cells, Rb functions as a transcriptional suppressor by associating with the transcription factor E2F. Once phosphorylated by cdk, Rb dissociates from E2F, allowing E2F to activate transcription of a set of genes required for entry into S phase, including thymidylate synthase, dihydrofolate reductase, and cyclin E (2,4,8,9). Cyclin E subsequently complexes with cdk-2 to complete phosphorylation of Rb, and this shift in Rb phosphorylation from a mitogen-dependent (cyclin D-driven) process to mitogen-independent (cyclin E-driven) process coincides with the irreversible commitment to enter S phase at the restriction point (2,8). During S phase, cyclin A replaces cyclin E in activating cdk-2, resulting in a change in substrate specificity for cdk-2 (2,4). Cdk-2/cyclin A phosphorylates a heterodimeric component of E2F, called DP-1, which disables E2F promoter activity and allows transition into G_2 (2). Thereafter, both entry into and exit from mitosis is controlled by cdk-1 (also called cdc2) in complexes with cyclin A and cyclin B (4).

Cdk/cyclin complexes are subjected to negative mechanisms of regulation, including association with cdk inhibitors, phosphorylation of threonine 14/tyrosine 15 residues mediated by Wee1 and Myt1 protein kinases, and selective proteolysis (2,4,6,10). Specific inhibitors of cdk-4 and cdk-6, the INK4 proteins (p16[INK4a], p15[INK4b], p18[INK4c], and p19[INK4d]) can directly block cyclin D-dependent kinase activity, resulting in G_1 arrest. Members of the Cip/Kip family of cdk inhibitors (p21[Cip1], p27[Kip1], and p57[Kip2]) have broader activity, inhibiting the activity of cyclin E- and A-dependent kinases, and promoting the assembly of active cyclin D-dependent kinases (2,4,10). Further cell cycle control is provided by the rapid and temporal destruction of regulatory proteins through the ubiquitin-proteasome pathway. Cyclins A and B, cdk inhibitors p27[Kip1] and p21[Cip1], and the G_1 cell cycle checkpoint protein p53 (discussed below) are targeted for degradation by the addition of a poly-ubiquitin chain. Ubiquinated proteins are subsequently captured within the

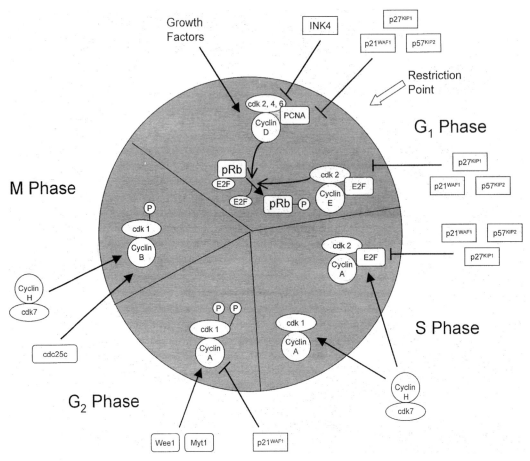

FIG. 25.1. The cell cycle (adapted from Senderowicz AM, Sausville EA. Preclinical and clinical development of cyclin-dependent kinase modulators. *J Natl Cancer Inst* 2000;92:376–387, with permission.)

26S proteosome where they undergo ATP-dependent proteolysis (10,11). Proteolysis and cdk inhibition downregulate cdk/cyclin activity, ensuring sequential and unidirectional cell cycle transitions.

Eukaryotic cells have developed a series of biochemically defined checkpoints that can be activated to prevent transition across certain cell-cycle phases. These checkpoints detect DNA damage, DNA replication errors, and chromosome segregation errors in order to ensure the integrity of the genome (3). DNA damage from ionizing radiation, for example, may induce cell cycle arrest before entry into S phase, within S phase, or before entry into M phase. At the G_1 to S phase checkpoint, DNA damage increases p53 activity, resulting in increased levels of the cdk inhibitor p21^{Cip1}, decreased Rb phosphorylation, and G_1 arrest. In certain cells, rather than inducing G_1 arrest, increased p53 activity initiates apoptosis through cellular programs that do not depend on p21^{Cip1} (2,12). The molecular pathways activated in response to DNA damage at the S phase and G_2 to M phase checkpoints are less clearly defined, although the ataxia-telangiectasia gene appears to be involved (12). Separate from the DNA damage checkpoint to prevent

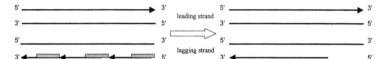

FIG. 25.2. The end-replication problem. DNA is replicated from the leading strand continuously in the 5' to 3' direction, whereas DNA is replicated from the lagging strand discontinuously. Without a mechanism to fill the gap, DNA is lost at the 3' end with every round of replication. Telomeres provide an elongated template, preventing the loss of genomic DNA during replication. (Adapted from Davis AJ, Siu LL. Telomerase: Therapeutic potential in cancer. *Cancer Invest* 2000; 18:269–277, with permission.)

entry into M phase, the mitotic spindle checkpoint recognizes chromosome segregation errors and prevents the progression of M phase if the spindle is not properly assembled, or if chromosomes are not properly aligned or attached to the spindle (3).

Cellular senescence has been proposed as an additional checkpoint that may be activated by the erosion of telomeres at the ends of chromosomes (13). Under normal conditions, telomeric DNA is lost during every cell cycle because DNA polymerases cannot completely replicate the 3' ends of DNA during S phase (Fig. 25.2). The progressive shortening of telomeres through successive cycles of replication eventually results in chromosome instability that may trigger cell-cycle arrest (13,14). Overall, cell cycle checkpoints verify that the events of one phase are properly executed before allowing progression to the next phase.

Aberrant cdk control and loss of cell cycle checkpoints have been linked to the molecular pathogenesis of cancer. Under normal conditions, environmental cues trigger cells transiting G_1 to either become quiescent, differentiate, or proliferate. Cancer cells have escaped these controls, demonstrating limitless replicative potential (13). Among the abnormalities demonstrated by cancer cells are inappropriate overexpression of cyclins, loss of endogenous cdk inhibitors, changes in cdk/cyclin substrates, and/or checkpoint failure. This chapter focuses on cell cycle deregulation in breast cancer, and the novel therapies being employed to counterbalance the related molecular abnormalities.

DEREGULATION OF THE CELL CYCLE IN BREAST CANCER

Breast cancer cells demonstrate defective G_1 to S phase transitions, modulated in part by abnormalities in cyclin D_1, cyclin E, and the cdk/cyclin substrate Rb (15,16). Transgenic mice that overexpress cyclin D_1 develop mammary carcinomas, suggesting that cyclin D_1 is important in breast tumorigenesis (17). Consistent with this, amplification of the cyclin D_1 gene, *ccnd1*, has been identified in 15% to 20% of human breast cancers, and appears to confer an unfavorable prognosis. In contrast, overexpression of the cyclin D_1 protein, identified in up to 50% of human breast cancers, appears to reflect a favorable prognosis. The contradictory data from gene amplification and protein expression studies may be explained by the fact that estrogens up-regulate cyclin D_1, and more favorable estrogen receptor positive tumors have been associated with cyclin D_1 overexpression (15,16,18). Interestingly, cyclin D_1 binds to estrogen receptors and regulates estrogen-dependent transcription, indicating a complex interaction between cyclin D_1 and estrogen receptors (15).

Like cyclin D_1, cyclin E has been linked to breast tumorigenesis in transgenic mice (19). Cyclin E gene amplification is relatively rare in human breast cancer, while cyclin E protein overexpression is more common and has been associated with loss of Rb function and poor prognosis (15,16). Changes in the cdk/cyclin substrate Rb are common in breast cancer, although no correlation between abnormal Rb and survival has been established to date (16).

Reduced expression of endogenous cdk inhibitors p16^{INK4}, p21^{Cip1}, and p27^{Kip1} has also been described in breast cancer. Studies of p16^{INK4} have revealed infrequent gene mutations, yet low p16^{INK4} expression has been described in some series (15,16). This discrepancy may be explained by the fact that the *cdkn2* gene encoding p16^{INK4} is inactivated by hypermethylation in 30% of primary breast cancers (16). In regards to p21^{Cip1}, both high- and low-protein expression has been related to decreased survival in breast cancer (15). Studies with p27^{Kip1} have been more consistent, with reduced expression of p27^{Kip1} being associated with a more aggressive phenotype and a poor prognosis (15,20), and increased expression of p27^{Kip1} being associated with a better overall survival (18).

Checkpoint failure due to mutated p53, present in 30% to 40% of breast cancers, is associated with high tumor grade, chemotherapy resistance, and reduced disease-free and overall survival (16,21,22). While the majority of p53 studies have employed immunohistochemistry, the relationship between protein function, protein expression, and gene mutation is complicated, and mutational analysis studies may provide more consistent results (16). In a prospective mutational analysis study in 90 patients, p53 status was the single most important predictor of recurrence ($p = 0.0032$) and death ($p = 0.001$) (22).

CELL CYCLE-BASED STRATEGIES FOR THE TREATMENT OF BREAST CANCER

Given the prevalence of cell cycle abnormalities in breast cancer, cell cycle modulation has been studied using currently available anticancer agents. Chemotherapeutic agents affect the cell cycle at the level of DNA replication, by damaging DNA, inhibiting DNA synthesis and repair, and disrupting chromosome segregation (23). Although clinically validated, chemotherapeutic agents have poor therapeutic indices and impact the cell cycle in a relatively non-specific manner (23). Antiestrogens affect the cell cycle in a more specific manner, owing to interactions between the estrogen receptor and cell cycle modulators, particularly cyclin D_1 (24). Antiestrogens induce G_1 arrest, decrease cyclin D_1 and cyclin A expression, suppress cdk-4 and cdk-2 activity, and increase p21^{Cip1} and p27^{Kip1} expression (25). Trastuzumab also alters the expression of cell cycle regulators, inducing p27^{Kip1} and Rb in HER-2-overexpressing breast cancer cell lines, and reducing the number of cells in S phase (26,27). While antiestrogens and trastuzumab perturb the cell cycle, the contribution of cell-cycle effects to their antitumor activity is unclear.

Contemporary agents are being developed to selectively target the cell cycle by direct and indirect inhibition of cdk. Direct inhibitors include compounds that inhibit a variety of cdk enzymes, such as flavopiridol, and newer compounds that specifically inhibit certain cdk enzymes. Indirect inhibitors include compounds that upregulate endogenous cdk inhibitors, exemplified by the induction of p21^{Cip1} and p27^{Kip1} by lovastatin; small peptides that mimic endogenous cdk inhibitors or cdk substrates; antisense ribonucleotides that deplete cdk/cyclin subunits; and proteosome inhibitors that prevent turnover of certain cell cycle modulators (4). The remainder of this chapter will concentrate on compounds currently in the clinic, including cdk inhibitors and proteosome inhibitors (Table 25.1).

DIRECT INHIBITOR OF MULTIPLE CDKS: FLAVOPIRIDOL

Flavopiridol, a semi-synthetic flavonoid, interferes with a number of cell cycle regulators to induce cell cycle arrest in G_1 and at the G_2/M boundary (4,28). Flavopiridol inhibits cdk activity directly, by inhibiting ATP-binding to cdk-1, cdk-2, cdk-4, cdk-6, and cdk-7, and indirectly, by preventing cdk-activating kinase (cdk-7/cyclin H) from phosphorylating other cdks (4). The effects of flavopiridol on the cell cycle

TABLE 25.1. *Examples of agents targeting the cell cycle*

Agent	Mechanism of action	Stage of development
Flavopiridol	Direct inhibition of cdk-1, -2, -3, -4, -6, -7 Inhibition of cdk-activating kinase Inhibition of transcription of cyclin D_1 Induction of apoptosis Inhibition of angiogenesis Inhibition of other kinases	Phase 1 combination studies Disease-specific studies
UCN-01	Direct or indirect inhibition of cdk-2 Regulation of kinases "upstream" of cdk-2 Abrogation of G_2/M checkpoint	Phase 1 combination studies Disease-specific studies
NU 6102	Inhibition of cdk-1 and -2	Preclinical studies
CYC 202	Inhibition of cdk-2	Phase 1 studies
CINK4	Inhibition of cdk-4	Preclinical studies
PS-341	Stabilization of multiple cell-cycle proteins	Phase 1 combination studies Disease-specific studies
CCI-779	Decreased translation of cyclin D_1	Phase 1 combination studies Disease-specific studies
E7070	Unknown	Disease-specific studies
Ro 31–7453	Unknown	Disease-specific studies

have been demonstrated in the human MCF-7 breast cancer model, where exposure to flavopiridol results in G_1 arrest, an associated loss of cdk-4 and cdk-2 activity, and decreased cyclin D_1 protein levels (29). In the MCF-7 model, rather than altering the half-life of cyclin D_1, flavopiridol specifically represses the activity of the full-length cyclin D_1 promoter linked to a luciferase reporter gene, decreasing intracellular concentrations of cyclin D_1 through transcriptional repression (30). Although flavopiridol is being developed as a first-generation cell cycle inhibitor, its activity appears to extend beyond that of cell cycle inhibition. Flavopiridol induces apoptosis, inhibits angiogenesis, and inhibits a number of kinases in addition to the cdks (4).

Flavopiridol has demonstrated both *in vitro* and *in vivo* activity against breast cancer. In MCF-7 breast cancer cells with an intact G_1 checkpoint, the IC_{99} (the dose that inhibits 99% of cell growth) is 1 μM, whereas in MDA-MB-468 breast cancer cells with a defective G_1 checkpoint, the IC_{99} is 1.6 μM. In contrast, flavopiridol 10 mg/kg administered daily for 5 days a week for 3 weeks to mice bearing MCF-7 and MDA-MB-468 xenografts results in tumor growth delay of 6.2 and 10.9 days, respectively (31). In MDA-MB435 parental breast cancer cell lines and MDA-MB435.eB cells transfected with c-*erb*B-2 cDNA, flavopiridol inhibits cell growth, regulates expression of apoptosis-related genes, and induces apoptosis. Flavopiridol also inhibits the expression of c-*erb*B-2, the secretion of matrix metalloproteinases, and cell invasion, suggesting that flavopiridol may inhibit breast cancer metastasis (32). These findings suggest that flavopiridol may be an effective therapy for breast cancer, but the molecular mechanism of this activity remains to be further defined.

In the initial phase 1 clinical trials of flavopiridol, the agent was administered as a 72-hour continuous infusion every 2 weeks, based on preclinical studies in colorectal and prostate cancer xenograft models in which flavopiridol was cytostatic when administered using protracted schedules (4). In the National Cancer Institute (NCI) phase 1 trial, 76 patients with refractory solid malignancies received doses ranging from 4 mg to 122.5 mg/m^2 per day for 3 days (33). Secretory diarrhea was dose-limiting at 62.5 mg/m^2 per day, but subsequent antidiarrheal prophylaxis allowed further dose escalation to 98 mg/m^2 per day and beyond, at which point hypotension became dose-limiting. Other toxicities included a proinflammatory syndrome characterized by flu-like symptoms, local tumor pain in some patients, and alterations in acute-phase reactants.

None of the five breast cancer patients enrolled in the NCI phase 1 trial responded, but one partial response was observed in a patient with renal cancer and minor responses were observed in one patient each with non-Hodgkin lymphoma, colon cancer, and renal cancer. Based on chronic tolerability, the recommended phase 2 dose was 50 mg/m² per day for 3 days without antidiarrheal prophylaxis (33). In another phase 1 trial exploring the same schedule, the dose-limiting toxicity of diarrhea was confirmed, and one patient with gastric cancer experienced a complete response (34). Subsequent phase 2 clinical trials employing the 72-hour infusion schedule in the treatment of renal cell cancer, non-small cell lung cancer, and gastric cancer all failed to demonstrate antitumor activity (35–37). Given the disappointing results with this schedule of single-agent flavopiridol, alternative schedules and combinations with chemotherapy are currently being explored. Preclinical data in human gastric and breast cancer cells have demonstrated that the activity of flavopiridol and paclitaxel is sequence-dependent. In MCF-7 cells, single agent paclitaxel induces transient mitotic arrest with the activation of cdk-1, followed by an exit from mitosis without cytokinesis, and subsequent arrest in G_1 with 4n DNA content (tetraploid cells). The addition of flavopiridol after paclitaxel accelerates the exit from mitotic arrest and potentiates paclitaxel-induced apoptosis by enhancing caspase activation (38). In MDA-MB-468 cells that lack a normal G_1 checkpoint, incubation with single-agent paclitaxel results in tetraploid cells that enter the S phase rather than arrest in G_1, in a process called endoreduplication. The administration of flavopiridol after paclitaxel to G_1 checkpoint-deficient cells prevents endoreduplication and the subsequent development of polyploidy (39). In contrast to the enhanced activity demonstrated by paclitaxel followed by flavopiridol, pretreatment of cancer cells with flavopiridol prevents mitotic entry by inhibiting cdk-1, thereby antagonizing the effect of paclitaxel (38).

On the basis of these preclinical data, a phase 1 study was recently completed in which 3- to 24-hour infusions of paclitaxel were followed by 24-hour infusions of flavopiridol administered once every 21 days. When doses of 100 mg or 135 mg/m² of paclitaxel were administered over 24 hours, the dose of flavopiridol could not be escalated to 20 mg/m² without dose-limiting neutropenia. At a dose of 135 mg/m² of paclitaxel administered over 3 hours, dose-limiting pulmonary and hematologic toxicity was observed with flavopiridol 94 mg/m² (40). One patient with esophageal cancer developed a complete response. The recommended phase 2 dose level was paclitaxel 135 mg/m² administered over 3 hours followed by flavopiridol 80 mg/m² administered over 24 hours (40).

CELL CYCLE INHIBITOR AND G_2 CHECKPOINT ABROGATOR: UCN-01

UCN-01 (7-hydroxystaurosporine), a staurosporine analogue that was initially developed as a protein kinase C (PKC) inhibitor, has demonstrated antiproliferative activity unrelated to its effects on PKC (4,41–43). As a single agent, UCN-01 induces apoptosis and G_1 arrest through mechanisms that may involve direct or indirect inhibition of cdk-2, or regulation of kinases upstream of cdks (4,44). When five breast cancer cell lines were continuously exposed to UCN-01 for 6 days, the IC_{50} values, or the concentrations required to inhibit 50% of cell growth, ranged from 30 nM to 100 nM (45). In vivo, UCN-01 demonstrated antitumor activity against MCF-7 breast cancer, A-498 renal cancer, and MOLT-4 and HL-60 leukemia xenografts, particularly when the agent was administered over prolonged periods (4).

Based on preclinical studies demonstrating increased activity with prolonged exposure, a single-agent phase 1 trial was performed in which UCN-01 was administered as a 36- to 72-hour continuous infusion every 2 to 4 weeks in patients with refractory malignancies (43). Nine patients received UCN-01 as a 72-hour infusion every 2 weeks, but extensive binding of UCN-01 to α_1-acid glycoprotein resulted in a prolonged half-life, dictating that the other 38 patients on the study receive the agent at 4-week intervals (43,46). Dose-limiting toxicity included nausea and vomiting, insulin-resistant hyperglycemia, and pulmonary toxicity characterized by hypoxia without radiographic changes. One patient with melanoma experienced a partial response, and one patient with non-Hodgkin lymphoma experienced stabilization of disease for more than 2.5 years. The recommended phase 2 dose was 42.5 mg/m^2 per day for 3 days, with subsequent courses administered at 4-week intervals for $1\frac{1}{2}$ days (43).

More exciting than the single-agent activity of UCN-01 is the potential for this agent to enhance the activity of traditional chemotherapy drugs in p53-deficient cells. In combination with certain DNA-damaging agents, UCN-01 abrogates the G_2/M checkpoint by inducing activation of cdk-1 through direct inhibition of Chk-1 kinase, a negative regulator of cdk-1 (47–49). Inappropriate activation of cdk-1/cyclin B subsequently results in premature mitosis and apoptosis (4), as illustrated by studies in human breast cancer models. Following treatment with cisplatin, MDA-MB-231 and T-47D breast cancer cells with deficient p53 accumulate in G_2, but subsequent treatment with non-cytotoxic doses of UCN-01 drives the cells through M phase, resulting in apoptosis (50). The combination of UCN-01 with DNA-damaging agents such as thiotepa, mitomycin-C, cisplatin, and melphalan results in synergistic antitumor activity in human MDA-MB-435 breast cancer cells with non-functional p53, but not in human MCF-7 breast cancer cells with intact p53 (51). Likewise, UCN-01 enhances the activity of topotecan and camptothecin in p53-deficient breast cancer cells (51–53). Future trials utilizing UCN-01 administered in combination with DNA-damaging agents are being explored (4).

DIRECT INHIBITORS OF SPECIFIC CDKS

In an effort to improve upon the poor target selectivity demonstrated by flavopiridol and UCN-01, second-generation cdk inhibitors are being designed to specifically inhibit only certain cdk enzymes (23). The new cdk inhibitors are broadly categorized into agents that inhibit cdk-1 and cdk-2 and agents that inhibit cdk-4 (54). The guanine- and pyrimidine-based compounds NU 2058 and NU 6027 inhibit cdk-1 and -2 (55), and a more potent compound, NU 6102, has recently been identified and is currently in preclinical development (56). Further along in development is CYC 202, a tri-substituted purine that competes with ATP for the active site of cdk 2. CYC 202 has demonstrated activity against a wide variety of human tumor cells and xenografts, and is currently in phase 1 clinical trials (23). Among the emerging class of small molecule inhibitors selective for cdk-4 is CINK4 (chemical inhibitor of cdk-4), a triaminopyrimidine derivative that causes growth arrest in tumor cells, prevents Rb phosphorylation, and slows tumor growth *in vivo* (57). Overall, only a few second-generation cdk inhibitors have entered the clinic, and results from phase 1 trials of these agents are not yet available.

PROTEOSOME INHIBITOR: PS-341

PS-341 is a dipeptide boronic acid that selectively inhibits the 26S proteasome, stabilizing the short-lived regulatory molecules driving the cell cycle (58). In cell culture, PS-341 increases intracellular levels of p21^{Cip1} and p27^{Kip1} and causes cell cycle arrest (58–60). In human non-small cell lung cancer cells, treatment with PS-341 results in a simultaneous cell cycle blockade at both S and G_2/M by inhibiting degradation of cyclins A and B (61). Unrelated to effects on the cell cycle, PS-341 also inhibits nuclear factor NF-κB through stabilization of the inhibitor protein IκB, thereby prohibiting the transcription of cell adhesion molecules and vascular cell adhesion molecules involved in tumor metastasis and angiogenesis (60,62).

The initial phase 1 trial of PS-341 employed a conservative starting dose and schedule, with patients receiving the agent once-weekly for 4 weeks followed by a 2-week break (63). More recent trials have implemented twice-weekly dosing, reflective of the more intensive regimens used in preclinical toxicology studies (64–66). Toxicities observed with PS-341 include low-grade fever and/or fatigue, mild to moderate transient thrombocytopenia, and peripheral neuropathy. Antitumor activity has been demonstrated in non-small cell lung cancer,

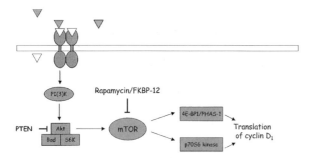

FIG. 25.3. Rapamycin-sensitive signal transduction pathway. Rapamycin and CCI-779 bind FKBP12, and subsequently block the kinase activity of mTOR. This interferes with downstream translational regulators, resulting in decreased cyclin D_1. (Adapted from Hidalgo M. and Rowinsky E.K. The rapamycin-sensitive signal transduction pathway as a target for cancer therapy. *Oncogene* 2000; 19:6680–6686, with permission.)

prostate cancer, melanoma, and multiple myeloma, and dose-related proteosome inhibition has been observed in peripheral mononuclear cells (63–66). To date, there have been no data published from breast cancer patients.

INHIBITOR OF TRANSLATION OF CYCLIN D MRNA: CCI-779

Rapamycin and its ester analogue, CCI-779, block cell cycle progression in response to proliferative stimuli by inhibiting the translation of specific mRNA sequences involved in the G_1 to S phase transition (67). As illustrated in Figure 25.3, rapamycin blocks the kinase activity of mTOR (mammalian target of rapamycin), thereby inhibiting downstream regulators, resulting in decreased translation of mRNA of proteins such as cyclin D_1 (68). *In vitro,* breast cancer cell lines that are estrogen-dependent, or lack expression of the tumor suppressor PTEN, and/or over-express HER-2/neu, are sensitive to CCI-779, whereas breast cancer cell lines that lack these properties are resistant. Treatment of sensitive breast cancer cell lines with CCI-779 results in decreased levels of cyclin D and c-myc, and increased levels of p27^{Kip1}. This suggests that mTOR may be a candidate for targeted therapy in breast cancers with Akt activation resulting from either growth factor dependency or loss of PTEN function (69).

Two phase 1 clinical trials of single-agent CCI-779 have been performed, both employing the frequent administration of 30-minute intravenous infusions. The principal toxicities have included dermatologic toxicity, myelosuppression, reversible elevations in liver function tests, and asymptomatic hypocalcemia. Partial responses have been observed in non-small cell lung cancer and renal cell cancer, and minor responses have been observed in a number of malignancies, including breast cancer (68,70,71). Disease-specific trials and phase 1 combination trials are planned.

CELL CYCLE INHIBITORS WITH UNKNOWN MOLECULAR TARGETS

At least two cell cycle inhibitors with unknown molecular targets are of interest for patients with breast cancer. The first compound, E7070, is a sulfonamide which blocks progression through G1 (72). In a recent phase 1 trial of E7070, dose-limiting toxicities included myelosuppression, diarrhea, folliculitis, asthenia, and stomatitis, and the recommended phase 2 dose was 130 mg/m^2 per day administered intravenously daily for 5 days every 3 weeks. A partial response was observed in a patient with heavily pretreated breast cancer (73). The second compound, Ro 31-7453, is an orally bioavailable cell cycle inhibitor that inhibits mitotic spindle formation and leads to M-phase arrest, although the precise molecular mechanism remains to be defined. In two single-agent phase 1 trials, the major toxicities were myelosuppression and mucositis, and phase 2 trials in breast cancer are currently underway employing a dose of 125 mg/m^2 every 12 hours (74,75).

CONCLUSION

The disregulated cell growth observed in breast cancer is at least in part due to interference with the coordinated activities of cdks and their regulators. A number of compounds are being developed to target the cell cycle, and the first-generation cdk inhibitors flavopiridol and UCN-01 are currently being investigated for the treatment of a number of malignancies. Second generation cdk inhibitors targeting specific cdks are entering phase 1 clinical trials. Other strategies, including the inhibition of proteasomes and mTOR have also led to the rational development of new anticancer agents. Although there is considerable preclinical evidence to suggest that these compounds will be promising in breast cancer, their role in the armamentarium against this disease remains to be defined.

REFERENCES

1. Morgan DO. Principles of CDK regulation. *Nature* 1995;374:131–134.
2. Sherr CJ. Cancer cell cycles. *Science* 1996;274:1672–1677.
3. Nurse P. A long twentieth century of the cell cycle and beyond. *Cell* 2000;100:71–78.
4. Senderowicz AM, Sausville EA. Preclinical and clinical development of cyclin-dependent kinase modulators. *J Natl Cancer Inst* 2000;92:376–387.
5. Kaldis P. The cdk-activating kinase (CAK): from yeast to mammals. *Cell Mol Life Sci* 1999;55:284–296.
6. Nurse P. Universal control mechanism regulating onset of M-phase. *Nature* 1990;344:503–508.
7. Yang J, Kornbluth S. All aboard the cyclin train: subcellular trafficking of cyclins and their CDK partners. *Trends Cell Biol* 1999;9:207–210.
8. Kato J. Induction of S phase by G1 regulatory factors. *Front Biosci* 1999;4:787–792.
9. Weinberg RA. The retinoblastoma protein and cell cycle control. *Cell* 1995;81:323–330.
10. Lee MH, Yang HY. Negative regulators of cyclin-dependent kinases and their roles in cancers. *Cell Mol Life Sci* 2001;58:1907–1922.
11. Shah SA, Potter MW, Callery MP. Ubiquitin proteasome pathway: implications and advances in cancer therapy. *Surg Oncol* 2001;10:43–52.
12. Morgan SE, Kastan MB. p53 and ATM: cell cycle, cell death, and cancer. *Adv Cancer Res* 1997;71:1–25.
13. Hanahan D, Weinberg RA. The hallmarks of cancer. *Cell* 2000;100:57–70.
14. Davis AJ, Siu LL. Telomerase: Therapeutic potential in cancer. *Cancer Invest* 2000;18:269–277.
15. Fernandez PL, Jares P, Rey MJ, et al. Cell cycle regulators and their abnormalities in breast cancer. *J Clin Pathol: Mol Pathol* 1998;51:305–309.
16. Landberg G, Roos G. The cell cycle in breast cancer. *APMIS* 1997;105:575–589.
17. Wang T, Cardiff R, Zukerberg L, et al. Mammary hyperplasia and carcinoma in MMTV-cyclin D1 transgenic mice. *Nature* 1994;369:669–671.
18. Barnes D, Gillet CE. Cyclin D1 and breast cancer. *Breast Cancer Res Treat* 1998;52:1–15.
19. Bortner DM, Rosenberg MP. Induction of mammary gland hyperplasia and carcinomas in transgenic mice expressing human cyclin E. *Mol Cell Biol* 1997;17:453–459.
20. Catzavelos C, Bhattacharya N, Ung YC, et al. *Nat Med* 1997;3:227–230.
21. Hartmann A, Blaszyk H, Kovach JS, Sommer SS. The molecular epidemiology of p53 gene mutations in human breast cancer. *Trends Genet* 1997;13:27–33.
22. Blaszyk H, Hartmann A, Cunningham JM, et al. A prospective trial of Midwest breast cancer patients: a p53 gene mutation is the most important predictor of adverse outcome. *Int J Cancer* 2000;89:32–38.
23. Newell DR. Review of clinical trials with cell cycle based strategies. *Proc 2001 AACR-NCI-EORTC Int Conf* #P825.
24. Zafonte BT, Hulit J, Amanatullah DF, et al. Cell-cycle dysregulation in breast cancer: Breast cancer therapies targeting the cell cycle. *Front Biosci* 2000;5:938–961.
25. Foster JS, Henley DC, Ahamed S, Wimalasena J. Estrogens and cell-cycle regulation in breast cancer. *Trends Endocrinol Metab* 2001;12:320–327.
26. Lane HA, Motoyama AB, Beuvink I, Hynes NE. Modulation of p27/Cdk2 complex formation through 4D5-mediated inhibition of HER2 receptor signaling. *Ann Oncol* 2001;12(suppl 1):S21–S22.
27. Sliwkowski MX, Lofgren JA, Lewis GD, et al. Nonclinical studies addressing the mechanism of action of trastuzumab (Herceptin). *Semin Oncol* 1999;26(4 suppl 12):60–70.
28. Kaur G, Stetler-Stevenson M, Sebers S, et al. Growth inhibition with reversible cell cycle arrest of carcinoma cells by flavone L86–8275. *J Natl Cancer Inst* 1992;84:1736–1740.
29. Carlson BA, Dubay MM, Sausville EA, et al. Flavopiridol induces G1 arrest with inhibition of CDK2 and CDK4 in human breast carcinoma cells. *Cancer Res* 1996;56:2973–2978.
30. Carlson B, Lahusen T, Singh S, et al. Down-regulation of cyclin D1 by transcriptional repression in MCF-7 human breast carcinoma cells induced by flavopiridol. *Cancer Res* 1999;59:4634–4641.
31. Lu K, Shih C, Teicher BA. Expression of pRB, cyclin/cyclin-dependent kinases and E2F1/DP-1 in human tumor lines in cell culture and in xenograft tissues and response to cell cycle agents. *Cancer Chemother Pharmacol* 2000;46:293–304.
32. Li Y, Bhuiyan M, Alhasan S, Senderowicz AM, Sarkar FH. Induction of apoptosis and inhibition of c-erbB-2 in breast cancer cells by flavopiridol. *Clin Cancer Res* 2000;5:223–229.
33. Senderowicz AM, Headlee D, Stinson SF, et al. Phase I trial of continuous infusion of flavopiridol, a novel cyclin-dependent kinase inhibitor, in patients with refractory neoplasms. *J Clin Oncol* 1998;16:2986–2999.
34. Thomas J, Cleary J, Tutsch K, et al. Phase I clinical and pharmacokinetic trial of flavopiridol. *Proc Am Assoc Cancer Res* 1997;38:A1496.
35. Stadler WM, Vogelzang NJ, Amato R, et al. Flavopiridol, a novel cyclin-dependent kinase inhibitor, in metastatic renal cancer: A University of Chicago Phase II Consortium Study. *J Clin Oncol* 2000;18:371–375.
36. Shapiro GI, Supko JG, Patterson A, et al. A phase II trial of the cyclin-dependent kinase inhibitor flavopiridol in

patients with previously untreated stage IV non-small cell lung cancer. *Clin Cancer Res* 2001;7:1590–1599.
37. Schwartz GK, Ilson D, Saltz L, et al. Phase II study of the cyclin-dependent kinase inhibitor flavopiridol administered to patients with advanced gastric carcinoma. *J Clin Oncol* 2001;19:1985–1992.
38. Motwani M, Delohery TM, Schwartz GK. Sequential dependent enhancement of caspase activation and apoptosis by flavopiridol on paclitaxel-treated human gastric and breast cancer cells. *Clin Cancer Res* 1999; 5:1876–1883.
39. Motwani M, Li X, Schwartz GK. Flavopiridol, a cyclin-dependent kinase inhibitor, prevents spindle inhibitor-induced endoreduplication in human cancer cells. *Clin Cancer Res* 2000;6:924–932.
40. Schwartz GK, Kaubisch A, Saltz L, et al. Phase I trial of sequential paclitaxel and the cyclin dependent kinase inhibitor flavopiridol. *Proc Am Soc Clin Oncol* 1999; 18:A614.
41. Takahashi I, Saitoh Y, Yoshida M, et al. UCN-01 and UCN-02, new selective inhibitors of protein kinase C. II. Purification, physicochemical properties, structural determinations, and biological activities. *J Antibiot (Tokyo)* 1989;42:571–576.
42. Seynaeve CM, Kazanietz MG, Blumberg PM, et al. Differential inhibition of protein kinase C isozymes by UCN-01, a staurosporine analogue. *Mol Pharmacol* 1994;45:1207–1214.
43. Sausville EA, Arbuck SG, Messmann R, et al. Phase I trial of 72-hour continuous infusion of UCN-01 in patients with refractory neoplasms. *J Clin Oncol* 2001; 19:2319–2333.
44. Akiyama T, Yoshida T, Tsujita T, et al. GI phase accumulation induced by UCN-01 is associated with dephosphorylation of Rb and CDK2 proteins as well as induction of CDK inhibitor p21/Cip1/WAF1/Sdi1 in p53-mutated human epidermoid carcinoma A341 cells. *Cancer Res* 1997;57:1495–1501.
45. Seynaeve CM, Stetler-Stevenson M, Sebers S, et al. Cell cycle arrest and growth inhibition by the protein kinase antagonist UCN-01 in human breast carcinoma cells. *Cancer Res* 1993;53:2081–2086.
46. Fuse E, Tanii H, Kurata N, et al. Unpredicted clinical pharmacology of UCN-01 cause by specific binding to human alpha 1-acid glycoprotein. *Cancer Res* 1998;58: 3248–3253.
47. Graves PR, Yu L, Schwarz JK, et al. The Chk1 protein kinase and the Cdc25C regulatory pathways are targets of the anticancer agent UCN-01. *J Biol Chem* 2000; 275:5600–5605.
48. Yu L, Orlandi L, Wang P, et al. UCN-01 abrogates G2 arrest through a Cdc2-dependent pathway that is associated with inactivation of the Wee1Hu kinase and activation of the Cdc25C phosphatase. *J Biol Chem* 1998;273:33455–33464.
49. Busby EC, Leistritz DF, Abraham RT, et al. The radiosensitizing agent 7-hydroxystaurosporine inhibits the DNA damage checkpoint kinase hChk1. *Cancer Res* 2000;60:2108–2112.
50. Lee SI, Brown MK, Eastman A. Camparison of the efficacy of 7-hydroxystaurosporine and other staurosporine analogs to abrogate cisplatin-induced cell cycle arrest in human breast cancer cell lines. *Biochem Pharmacol* 1999;58:1713–1721.
51. Monks A, Harris ED, Vaigro-Wolff A, et al. UCN-01 enhances the *in vitro* toxicity of clinical agents in human tumor cell lines. *Invest New Drugs* 2000;18: 95–107.
52. Jones CB, Clements MK, Wasi S, Daoud SS. Enhancement of camptothecin-induced cytotoxicity with UCN-01 in breast cancer cells: abrogation of S/G2 arrest. *Cancer Chemother Pharmacol* 2000;45:252–258.
53. Jones CB, Clements MK, Rekar A, Daoud SS. UCN-01 and camptothecin induce DNA double-strand breaks in p53 mutant tumor cells, but not in normal or p53 negative epithelial cells. *Int J Oncol* 2000;17:1043–1051.
54. Toogood PL. Cyclin-dependent kinase inhibitors for treating cancer. *Med Res Rev* 2001;21:487–498.
55. Arris CE, Boyle T, Calvert AH, et al. Identification of novel purine and pyrimidine cyclin-dependent kinase inhibitors with distinct molecular interactions and tumor cell growth inhibition profiles. *J Med Chem* 2000;43:2797–2804.
56. Griffin RJ, Arris CE, Bently J, et al. Structure-based design of potent inhibitors of CDK1 and CDK2. *Proc Am Assoc Cancer Res* 2001;42:A2452.
57. Soni R, O'Reilly T, Furet P, et al. Selective *in vivo* and *in vitro* effects of a small molecule inhibitor of cyclin-dependent kinase 4. *J Natl Cancer Inst* 2001;93:436–446.
58. Adams J, Palombella VJ, Sausville EA, et al. Proteasome inhibitors: A novel class of potent and effective antitumor agents. *Cancer Res* 1999;59:2615–2622.
59. Shah SA, Potter MW, McDade TP, et al. 26S proteasome inhibition induces apoptosis and limits growth of human pancreatic cancer. *J Cell Biochem* 2001;82:110–122.
60. Hideshima T, Richardson P, Chauhan D, et al. The proteasome inhibitor PS-341 inhibits growth, induces apoptosis, and overcomes drug resistance inhuman multiple myeloma cells. *Cancer Res* 2001;61:3071–3076.
61. Perez-Soler R, Ling YH, Mendoza S, et al. Effect of the proteasome inhibitor PS341 on cell cycle progression and cell cycle-related events: Implications for combination therapy with cell cycle-dependent agents. *Proc Am Soc Clin Oncol* 2000;19:A740.
62. Cusack JC, Liu R, Houston M, et al. Enhanced chemosensitivity to CPT-11 with proteasome inhibitor PS-341: Implications for systemic nuclear factor-κB inhibition. *Cancer Res* 2001;61:3535–3540.
63. Papandreou C, Daliani D, Millikan RE, et al. Phase I study of intravenous proteasome inhibitor PS-341 in patients with advanced malignancies. *Proc Am Soc Clin Oncol* 2001;20:A340.
64. Aghajanian C, Soignet S, Dizon DS, et al. A phase I trial of the novel proteasome inhibitor PS341 in advanced solid tumor malignancies. *Proc Am Soc Clin Oncol* 2001;20:A338.
65. Hamilton AL, Eder JP, Pavlick AC, et al. PS-341: Phase I study of a novel proteasome inhibitor with pharmacodynamic endpoints. *Proc Am Soc Clin Oncol* 2001;20: A336.
66. Erlichman C, Adjei AA, Thomas JP, et al. A phase I trial of the proteasome inhibitor PS-341 in patients with advanced cancer. *Proc Am Soc Clin Oncol* 2001;20:A337.
67. Wiederrecht GJ, Sabers CJ, Brunn GJ, et al. Mechanism of action of rapamycin: new insights into the regulation of G1-phase progression in eukaryotic cells. *Prog Cell Cycle Res* 1995;1:53–71.
68. Hidalgo M, Rowinsky EK. The rapamycin-sensitive signal transduction pathway as a target for cancer therapy. *Oncogene* 2000;19:6680–6686.

69. Yu K, Toral-Barza L, Discafani C, et al. mTOR, a novel target in breast cancer: the effect of CCI-779, an mTOR inhibitor, in preclinical models of breast cancer. *Endocr Relat Cancer* 2001;8:249–258.
70. Hidalgo M, Rowinsky E, Erlichman C, et al. CCI-779, a rapamycin analog and multifaceted inhibitor of signal transduction: a phase I study. *Proc Am Assoc Clin Oncol* 2000;19:A726.
71. Raymond E, Alexandre J, Depenbrock H, et al. CCI-779, a rapamycin analog with antitumor activity: a phase I study utilizing a weekly schedule. *Proc Am Assoc Clin Oncol* 2000;19:A728.
72. Owa T, Yoshino H, Okauchi T, et al. Discovery of novel antitumor sulfonamides targeting G1 phase of the cell cycle. *J Med Chem* 1999;42:3789–3799.
73. Punt CJ, Fumoleau P, van de Walle B, et al. Phase I and pharmacokinetic study of E7070, a novel sulfonamide, given at a daily times five schedule in patients with solid tumors. *Ann Oncol* 2001;12:1289–1293.
74. Soignet S, Beinvenu B, Breimer L, et al. A novel cell cycle inhibitor (Ro31–7453): a clinical and pharmacokinetic study in patients with solid tumors: final report of a 4-day q 3 week schedule. *Proc ASCO* 2001;20:A347.
75. Cassidy J, Twelves C, Bissett D, et al. Phase I clinical and pharmacokinetic study of the novel cell cycle inhibitors Ro31–7453. *Proc ASCO* 2000;19:A731.

26

Predictive Molecular Markers: A New Window of Opportunity in the Adjuvant Therapy of Breast Cancer

Angelo Di Leo, Fatima Cardoso, Sophie Scohy, and Martine J. Piccart

The results of important and large randomized clinical trials and the conclusions of the Oxford meta-analysis have had a major impact on treatment recommendations for patients with early breast cancer (1–8). Today, adjuvant medical therapy is offered to the vast majority of node-negative breast cancer patients (evidence type I and category A) (1,4–6). Indeed, the international panel of experts on adjuvant therapy met again in St. Gallen in February 2001, and concluded that only node-negative patients aged 35 years or more, with tumors of low size (2 cm or less), well differentiated (histological grade 1) and positive for both the estrogen (ER) and the progesterone (PgR) receptors, might be spared adjuvant chemotherapy because of their minimal risk of relapse. Adjuvant chemotherapy should at least be offered to all other patients, particularly those with endocrine non-responsive disease (i.e., ER- and PgR-negative) (9). The Oxford Overview 2000, based on data from 56 trials and 28,000 women, concluded that, after standardization for age and time since randomization, with the use of polychemotherapy proportional reductions in risk of recurrence and death are similar for women with node-negative and node-positive disease (8).

According to these guidelines, most early breast cancer patients receive adjuvant treatment, and the main challenge has become the identification of predictive factors that may help in selecting the optimal therapeutic strategy for individual patients. The accomplishment of this ambitious aim could translate into a substantial increase in the absolute benefit associated with adjuvant therapy.

PREDICTIVE FACTORS: DEFINITION AND GENERAL CONCEPTS

The main differences between predictive and prognostic factors are illustrated in Figure 26.1. While a prognostic factor influences disease outcome whichever adjuvant therapy is used (Fig. 26.1A), a predictive factor will interfere with disease outcome only when a specific treatment is given (Fig 26.1B and 26.1C). Fig 26.1B shows how the outcome of treatment A is positively influenced by the predictive factor under study, which, in contrast, has no impact on the efficacy of treatment B. A predictive factor might also differentially influence the outcome of two different adjuvant therapies, as described in Figure 26.1C. This latter scenario would be the ideal situation, because a single factor might clearly select between two different forms of adjuvant therapy.

The identification of predictive factors requires great effort and thus far only a few parameters can be reliably defined. Prospective studies in which two different treatments are compared in two different subgroups of patients, identified according to the putative predictive factor, have not been reported as of yet. The main advantage of these studies would be that the predictive marker hypothesis and the anticipated benefit would be formulated before study initiation. The study sample size could then be calculated to include an adequate number of patients in the two different subgroups,

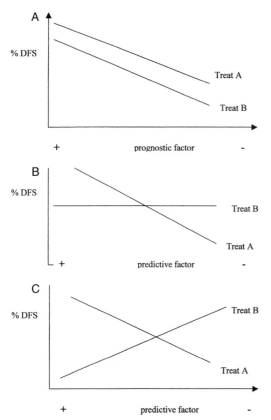

Fig. 26.1. Prognostic and predictive factors. **A:** Prognostic factors. **B:** Predictive factors interacting with only one treatment. **C:** Predictive factors interacting with two different treatments.

lems with the retrospective collection of tumor samples. Also, the quality of collected tumor tissue is often suboptimal for performing molecular markers analysis using immunohistochemistry (IHC), fluorescence *in situ* hybridization (FISH), or other techniques. In an effort to improve the reliability of data collected in such trials, investigators are trying to collect tumor samples from patients entered into a clinical trial on an ongoing basis, rather than at the end of the study, as previously done. This measure allows for the collection of tumor samples from the largest number of patients, leading to an improved quality and interpretation of the retrospective studies. Furthermore, prospective collection of samples enables the creation of extensive tissue banks that might contribute to the generation of new hypotheses regarding future predictive and prognostic factors. Nevertheless, the ultimate validation and transfer into clinical practice of potential predictive markers will require well-designed prospective studies, and it is now time to activate these trials.

In the following paragraphs, an overview of the different predictive markers already tested or under evaluation in patients with early breast cancer for both hormonal and chemotherapy will be presented. For each marker the level of evidence reached so far will be stated.

to statistically demonstrate the anticipated difference. To address these questions, two prospective studies have recently been initiated to evaluate the value of p53 (EORTC trial) and topoisomerase IIα (TOP trial, Jules Bordet Institute) as predictive markers of response to taxanes (EORTC trial) or to anthracycline-based chemotherapy (TOP trial), in locally advanced/inflammatory or large operable breast cancer patients.

The lack of prospective trials has led to a focus on retrospective studies. In addition to being limited by their retrospective nature, these studies have other difficulties, including the fact that the number of patients analyzed in the predictive marker study is often only a subset of the entire clinical trial population because of prob-

PREDICTIVE MARKERS FOR ADJUVANT HORMONAL THERAPY

The last meta-analysis performed by the Oxford group (8) provides data regarding the predictive power of ER when the efficacy of adjuvant tamoxifen given for approximately five years is evaluated. From these data it may be concluded that the activity of tamoxifen is strictly dependent on the ER status, and that there is a correlation between the level of ER positivity and the efficacy of tamoxifen. Although fewer patients had data available regarding PgR, its predictive role for the efficacy of tamoxifen has also been shown (10). To date, ER and PgR are the only firmly established factors known to predict the efficacy of adjuvant tamoxifen, with a level I/category A evidence. Nevertheless,

TABLE 26.1. *HER-2/neu and adjuvant tamoxifen*

Group (reference)	Study arms	No. of pts (in clinical trial)	% with HER-2 measured	Methods for HER-2 evaluation	Results
GUN (Bianco, 13)	TAM No TAM	433	57%	IHC	HER-2 is a strong predictor of adjuvant TAM failure, independently of ER
Swedish Group (Stal, 14)	TAM 2 years TAM 5 years	871	66%	DNA amplification assay (slot blot), Flow cytometry	HER-2 overexpression decreases the benefit from prolonged adjuvant TAM treatment
Spanish Group (Climent, 15)	Radical mastectomy Breast conserving surgery (TAM assignment not rando)	283	88%	IHC	Pts treated with adjuvant TAM had statistically longer DFS and OS when HER-2 was negative
CALGB 8541 (Berry, 16)	CAF 600/60/600 mg/m^2 CAF 400/40/400 mg/m^2 CAF 300/30/300 mg/m^2 (TAM assignment not rando)	999	65%	IHC, FISH, differential PCR	In ER+/Node positive patients, the efficacy of adjuvant TAM does not depend on HER-2 status
Danish Group (Knoop, 17)	TAM No TAM	1,716	88%	IHC	Does not support the hypothesis that HER-2 status could predict benefit from adjuvant TAM, in ER+ early stage BC

Rando, randomize.

about one third of ER and/or PgR positive tumors do not respond to endocrine therapy, clearly indicating the need for additional predictive markers.

With the exception of ER and PgR, the proto-oncogene HER-2 and its encoded protein have been the most extensively evaluated markers. Preclinical data suggest that HER-2 overexpression may be associated with decreased efficacy of tamoxifen, and even with a potential detrimental effect (11,12). Several clinical studies, both in the metastatic and adjuvant setting, have addressed this issue and provided contradictory results (Table 26.1). At the 1998 meeting of the American Society of Clinical Oncology (ASCO), Bianco et al. (13) presented the results of a retrospective study where the activity of adjuvant tamoxifen was correlated with the expression of HER-2. They concluded that tumors overexpressing the HER-2 protein, measured by IHC, are less responsive to tamoxifen. More recently, an update of the Swedish Breast Cancer Group study (14) and a study from a Spanish group (15) have been published, supporting the association between HER-2 overexpression and resistance to tamoxifen. On the other hand, both the Cancer and Leukemia Group B (CALGB) and the Danish Breast Cancer Cooperative Group reported, within the last 12 months, two trials in which no such association was found (16,17).

Several facts could account for these conflicting results: (a) all the studies are retrospective; (b) the actual number of HER-2 positive patients who received adjuvant tamoxifen is low in all the studies; and (c) there is lack of standardization of methods for assessing HER-2 overexpression across different laboratories. The level of evidence regarding HER-2 as a predictive marker for adjuvant tamoxifen is, therefore, of level II, category C.

Overexpression of the antiapoptotic molecule Bcl-2 is usually associated with high ER concentration and, contrary to expectation, has been associated with a higher likelihood of response to tamoxifen. In a total of 205 tumor samples from ER-positive metastatic breast cancer patients, high bcl-2 expression correlated with a better clinical response to tamoxifen (62% versus 49%; $p = 0.07$) and longer survival (18). In the adjuvant setting, in 81 patients treated with tamoxifen, a significantly better relapse-free survival was found among those with bcl-2-positive tumors than in those with bcl-2-negative disease ($p = 0.02$) (19). In another retrospective study, the interaction between bcl-2 and response to tamoxifen was evaluated in 289 ER and/or PgR positive early breast cancer patients. This is the only study in which a control group of patients who did not receive treatment with tamoxifen exists, although the assignment to each group was not randomized. Despite the relatively small number of patients in each subgroup, there was a trend towards a greater benefit of tamoxifen in ER-positive/bcl-2-positive patients, as opposed to ER-positive/bcl-2-negative patients (20).

The potential predictive role of other markers, such as the β isotype of ER, p53 mutations, the proliferation marker Ki67, and intratumoral aromatase activity (for aromatase inhibitors) is still under evaluation.

PREDICTIVE MARKERS FOR ADJUVANT CHEMOTHERAPY

Several trials have shown that chemotherapy combined with tamoxifen is superior to tamoxifen alone as adjuvant treatment of node-negative, ER-positive patients or of node-positive, ER-positive postmenopausal patients (3). Moreover, chemotherapy is, so far, the only adjuvant modality with proven efficacy in women with hormone receptor-negative tumors. Accordingly, the vast majority of early breast cancer patients currently receive adjuvant chemotherapy. In this setting, predictive markers should be able to identify the optimal chemotherapy regimen to be given to each individual patient. We describe below those putative predictive factors that have been the subject of a series of retrospective studies in patients with early breast cancer treated with adjuvant chemotherapy.

HER-2 as a Predictive Marker for CMF and Anthracycline-based Regimens

Only recently have trials convincingly shown the superiority of an anthracycline-based regimen over CMF in the adjuvant treatment of premenopausal node-positive breast cancer patients (21,22). The benefit is, however, modest and associated with a definite increase in toxicity. This is the typical clinical situation in which the use of a predictive marker might help in selecting those patients for whom the benefits of the more aggressive treatment might be substantial and justify the increased toxicity.

HER-2 has been investigated in this setting and its behavior as a predictive factor seems to be quite similar to the one presented in Figure 26.1C. Data suggesting that HER-2 positive tumors might be resistant to adjuvant treatment with CMF (with or without prednisone) comes from three retrospective studies (Table 26.2). In two of these trials, when patients were divided in two subgroups according to the expression of HER-2 as measured by IHC on primary tumor samples, it was observed that adjuvant CMF (plus prednisone) was more effective than no adjuvant treatment only in the subset of HER-2–negative patients (23,24). In the third trial, all patients benefited from adjuvant CMF, but the magnitude of the benefit was superior in HER-2–negative patients (25). However, in a study reported by the Milan group, HER-2 failed to show any predictive activity in a population of node-positive breast cancer patients randomly allocated to receive CMF or no treatment (26). Albeit based on a limited number of patients, this study is in contradiction with the previous ones. Therefore, regarding the predictive value of HER-2 for CMF-like chemotherapy regimens, the evidence is level II, category B.

Three retrospective studies (Table 26.3), performed by the NSABP, the Belgian Adjuvant Study Group and the Milan group (27–29), evaluated the predictive value of HER-2 in a population of node-positive breast cancer patients, randomly assigned to receive CMF or anthracycline-based chemotherapy. These reports suggest reduced CMF efficacy in patients overexpressing the HER-2 oncoprotein, and all three studies agree in defining the HER-2 positive subgroup as the most sensitive to anthracycline-based adjuvant chemotherapy. Two other retrospective studies (30,31) generated similar results regarding HER-2 overexpression and responsiveness to anthracyclines. Additionally, an Intergroup Study, presented at the 1998 ASCO meeting, showed that in tumors overexpressing HER-2, chemo-endocrine therapy with CAF plus tamoxifen seemed to yield better results than tamoxifen alone (32).

Taken together, these studies provide level II, category A evidence concerning clinical practice recommendations. But do these results indicate that the clinician should use HER-2 as a determinant factor for choosing between CMF and anthracycline-based chemotherapy? The answer is "no" for at least four reasons:

1. All six studies are retrospective, with all the limitations of retrospective studies.
2. The most suitable technique for HER-2 assessment remains unknown. In the six listed studies, IHC was used. However, in the NSABP studies, HER-2 oncoprotein was evaluated by a "cocktail technique" consisting of concomitant staining with two different antibodies (the monoclonal TAB-250 plus the polyclonal p-Ab1) (27,30). The Belgian study used two different monoclonal antibodies (CB11 and 4D5) directed towards two different epitopes of the HER-2 protein (28) while the CALGB (31) and the Milan group (29) used the CB11 monoclonal antibody. The cocktail technique used in the NSABP study allowed the identification of a higher percentage of HER-2 positive patients, compared to the monoclonal antibodies evaluated in the other studies. Along with the choice of antibody, another major technical issue of IHC is the use of antigen retrieval (i.e., a technical procedure designed to facilitate the interaction between the antibody and the corresponding antigen). A recent study investigated the degree of interlaboratory agreement when HER-2 was evaluated in two different laboratories by IHC on archival samples of 394 invasive primary breast cancer patients. Both laboratories used the primary antibody NCL-CB11 but different methods of immunostaining (antigen retrieval procedure and manual processing or no antigen retrieval and autostainer processing) as well as a different scoring system. Forty-eight of 394 analyzed tumors (12.2%) were scored as HER-2 positive in one laboratory, and 109 (27.7%) in the other laboratory

TABLE 26.2. *HER-2 and adjuvant CMF / CMF-like chemotherapy*

Group (reference)	Study arms	No. of pts (in clinical trial)	% with HER-2 measured	Methods for HER-2 evaluation	Results
Intergroup Group 0011 (Allred, 23)	Observation CMFP	677	100%	IHC	After CMFP, only HER-2 negative pts had longer DFS and OS, showing clear benefit from CT; no benefit in HER-2 positive pts
IBCSG trial V—Ludwig (Gusterson, 24)	N−: PeCT vs. Not N+: CMFp vs. Not	2,504	60%	IHC	Tumors that overexpress HER-2 are less responsive to CMF-containing adjuvant CT
ICRF study (Miles, 25)	Follow-up CMF	391	70%	IHC	All patients benefited from CMF, but benefit was greater in HER-2-negative [median OS: 7.3 (follow-up group) vs. 12.7 years (CMF group)] than HER-2-positive [median OS: 4.4 (follow-up group) vs. 6.1 years (CMF group)] pts
Milan trial (Menard, 26)	Follow-up CMF	386	87%	IHC	Clinical benefit of CMF in pts with HER-2-positive as well as HER-2-negative tumors

CMFp, postoperative CMF + prednisone; PeCT, perioperative CMF.

TABLE 26.3. *HER-2/neu and adjuvant anthracycline-based chemotherapy*

Group (ref.)	Study arms	No. of pts (clinical trial)	% pts-HER-2 measured	Methods-HER-2	Results
NSABP-B 15 (Paik-2000, 30)	AC CMF AC → CMF	2,295	89%	IHC	AC superior to CMF only in HER-2-positive pts (differences not statistically significant); both AC and CMF regimens may be considered for HER-2-negative pts
Belgian trial (Di Leo, 28)	CMF EC HEC	777	62%	IHC	Anthracycline-based CT better than CMF only in HER-2-positive tumors
Milan trial II (Moliterni, 29)	CMF CMF → A	552	92%	IHC	In the subset of HER-2-positive pts, doxorubicin-containing regimens are better than CMF alone (statistically borderline)
CALGB 8541 (Thor-JNCI, 31)	CAF 600/60/600 mg/m^2 CAF 400/40/400 mg/m^2 CAF 300/30/300 mg/m^2	1,549	64%	IHC	There was a significant dose-response effect of adjuvant CAF in patients with HER-2-positive tumors but not in patients with HER-2-negative tumors
NSABP-B 11 (Paik-JNCI98, 27)	PF PAF	682	94%	IHC	Clinical benefit from doxorubicin was statistically significant for pts with HER-2-positive tumors but not significant for patients with HER-2-negative tumors
US Intergroup (Elledge, 32)	TAM CAF + TAM CAF → TAM	1,470	40%	IHC	In patients with HER-2 overexpression CAF-TAM is superior to TAM alone, although not statistically significant

where antigen retrieval was performed. Furthermore, concordance between FISH and IHC was found in 211/248 cases (85.1%) and 220/248 cases (88.7%), when the CB11 antibody was used without and with antigen retrieval, respectively. In conclusion, both IHC methods generated similar error rates, but the positive predictive value was higher when antigen retrieval was not used (less false-positives) and, conversely, the negative predictive value improved with antigen retrieval (less false-negatives) (33). In recent years, there has been considerable controversy regarding the use of more sophisticated and reliable, but also more expensive techniques, such as FISH, instead of IHC, for HER-2 status determination (34,35). A reasonable approach would be to perform an initial evaluation by IHC using a monoclonal antibody with antigen retrieval, which would reduce the rate of false negatives to an acceptable level, and to confirm the positive results by FISH, eliminating therefore the false positive results (36).

3. The best cut-off value for defining a tumor as HER-2 positive or negative remains unknown. In most studies, all tumors with at least one percent of cells showing positivity for HER-2 were considered HER-2 positive. The rationale behind this policy relies on data indicating that, in snap-frozen sections, HER-2 expression is generally present in either none or in almost all cells. In formalin-fixed, paraffin-embedded tumor samples, the percentage of cells staining positively seems to correlate more with fixation defects, leading to a certain loss of HER-2 antigenicity (37). This phenomenon has already been well documented and a direct correlation has been found between loss of antigenicity and the time elapsed between preparation of the formalin-fixed, paraffin-embedded sample, and moment of marker assessment (38). According to these data, the selection of a cut-off different from 1% might be problematic, particularly in a retrospective study in which the quality of tumor samples, and therefore of HER-2 antigenicity, might be compromised. Along with the best cut-off value, another issue remains open and so far not entirely explored: the staining intensity. What would be the clinical behavior of those tumors with a high percentage of positive cells and low-intensity staining? So far intensity score has not been evaluated in any studies.

4. Another still-unresolved issue lies in the possible heterogeneity of HER-2 expression, as well as other markers, between the primary tumor and its metastases. This is particularly important since the control of these metastases is the main goal of adjuvant therapy. To date, five small retrospective studies have evaluated this problem through the comparison of HER-2 status between the primary tumor and its regional lymph node metastases (39–43). In all the studies, a high percentage of concordance between the primary and the metastatic sites was found but, however, it did not reach 100%. Therefore, until larger studies using standardized techniques are available, one should take into account that a difference in the expression of biological markers may exist between the primary tumor and its metastatic sites.

Markers Predicting the Activity of Anthracycline-based Regimens

Markers belonging to this category appear to have a behavior similar to the one illustrated in Figure 26.1B: they may predict the outcome of an anthracycline-based regimen, but they do not interfere with treatment efficacy when other chemotherapy regimens are evaluated.

Topoisomerase II alpha (topo II-α) is perhaps the most representative and promising marker in this category. The topo II-α gene is located next to the HER-2 gene on chromosome 17q12-q21, and its amplification leads to overexpression of the topo II-α protein. Since this enzyme is inhibited by anthracyclines and seems to be the main target of these drugs, its overexpression may render the cells more sensitive to these topo II-α inhibitors (44,45). Studies have shown that topo II-α amplification only occurs with concurrent HER-2 amplification, and it is possible that the predictive value of HER-2 regarding anthracycline-based chemotherapy is explained by the concomitant amplification of the topo II gene (44,46–48). Preclinical data also indicate that intratumoral topo II-α levels may explain some forms of resistance to anthracyclines observed in *in vitro* systems (49).

The Belgian group has evaluated topo II-α levels by IHC on 481 archival primary tumor samples from node-positive breast cancer patients randomly allocated to receive adjuvant therapy with CMF or epirubicin-plus-cyclophosphamide (28). The evaluation of this marker by IHC presented some technical difficulties (i.e., non-specific staining outside the nucleus of tumor cells), leading to a high rate of tumors with unknown topo II-α levels (27%). Interestingly, in those cases in which the topo II-α status was evaluable, it was observed that topo II-α-positive tumors had a better outcome with the anthracycline-based regimen than with CMF, while equivalence between the two regimens was found in the subgroup of topo II-α-negative tumors. Nevertheless, no formal statistical significance was noted when an interaction test was performed to evaluate the predictive role of topo II-α. Since this is a phase 2 study, its results must be confirmed in large prospective studies before a recommendation for clinical practice can be made. Accordingly, a randomized proof-of-principle trial, in which the predictive value of topo II-α and HER-2 will be tested prospectively, will soon start accrual at the Jules Bordet Institute in Brussels (TOP trial).

Two major studies evaluated the predictive value of p53 mutations for anthracycline-based chemotherapy in the adjuvant setting, and provide contradictory results. In the CALGB 8541 study, in which all patients received anthracycline-based adjuvant therapy, p53 expression seemed to have an important role only in those tumors overexpressing HER-2; HER-2-positive patients that also expressed p53 survived substantially longer than those with p53-negative tumors (31). However, these results must be considered preliminary and hypothesis generating only, due to the small number of patients (n = 101). In EORTC study 10854, premenopausal women with node-negative breast cancer were randomized between one cycle of perioperative FAC and no further treatment. Tumor samples from 441 patients were collected and p53 was assessed by IHC; p53 accumulation was found to be predictive of resistance to perioperative FAC (50). These two phase 2 studies, being discordant, provide only a category C evidence regarding the predictive value of p53 for anthracycline-based chemotherapy.

Drug-efflux pumps such as p-glycoprotein (PGP) and multidrug resistance-related protein (MRP) have been implicated in some forms of resistance to anthracyclines, taxanes, etoposide and vinblastine (51,52). While they might show predictive activity in clinical studies, the hypothesis has never been tested. Nevertheless these markers will not show any specificity for anthracyclines, given their involvement in multidrug resistance.

Markers Predicting the Activity of Taxane-based Regimens

Taxanes have been evaluated in the adjuvant setting only recently. Therefore, all available results regarding possible predictive factors were obtained in the context of metastatic or neo-adjuvant breast cancer studies. These retrospective studies have suggested that tumors overexpressing HER-2 might be more sensitive to a taxane-based than to an anthracycline-based regimen (53). Nevertheless, these observations are based on the analysis of response rates in phase 2 studies with few patients evaluated, and other reports from different trials have drawn opposite conclusions (54). Recently, at the 2001 ASCO meeting, the first results based on a phase 3 clinical trial were presented. HER-2 was retrospectively analyzed by FISH in 256 of 481 patients, previously randomized to receive either epirubicin-cyclophosphamide or epirubicin-paclitaxel. The addition of paclitaxel resulted in an improvement in response rate, progression-free survival and overall survival only in HER-2-positive patients, supporting the hypothesis of a higher benefit from taxanes in patients with HER-2-positive tumors (55). Once again, since this is a phase 2 study, its results must be confirmed in large prospective studies.

In a clinical study of neoadjuvant chemotherapy, p53 mutated tumors showed a high response rate when treated with taxanes, but a low response rate when treated with anthracyclines (56). This and other in vitro and in vivo studies have raised the hypothesis that p53 mutated tumors might be less sensitive to anthracyclines while retaining sensitivity to taxanes. To test this hypothesis, a large multicenter international prospective trial has recently been opened under the auspices of B.I.G. (Breast International Group) and coordinated by the EORTC.

The most attractive markers as far as taxane treatment is concerned are probably the microtubule-associated parameters (MTAP). The latter are a specific target for taxanes because these drugs interact with microtubules. Preclinical data suggest that mammary and pancreatic tumors with exquisite responsiveness to docetaxel in in vitro models have the highest expression of the Tau gene (MTAP-2 family) and of the α-tubulin protein (57). Assessment of MTAP-2 expression by IHC on paraffin embedded samples is feasible, making possible retrospective studies correlating MTAP-2 levels and docetaxel activity in both the metastatic and adjuvant settings. A pilot study was carried out at the Jules Bordet Institute correlating the clinical efficacy of docetaxel with the expression of MTAP in 41 patients with metastatic breast cancer. No association was found between expression of α-tublin and β-tubulin, class III and class IV β-tubulin isotypes, and docetaxel activity; an inverse correlation was seen between class II β-tubulin isotype expression and docetaxel activity, with patients defined as negative having a higher chance of responding to docetaxel than patients defined as positive ($p = 0.04$). On the other hand, Tau protein-negative tumors seemed to progress rapidly on docetaxel treatment, although the number of patients in this subgroup was too small to allow any definite conclusions (58). The results of this exploratory study are currently being tested in a large retrospective study that evaluates the expression of several potential predictive markers, such as MTAP, topo II-α, HER-2 and ER, in 326 metastatic breast cancer patients previously entered in a randomized phase 3 trial comparing docetaxel and doxorubicin as first- or second-line treatment (59). The Breast Cancer International research Group (BCIRG) is also testing the predictive value of MTAP in the context of an adjuvant trial comparing TAC (docetaxel plus doxorubicin plus cyclophosphamide) to FAC (5-FU plus doxorubicin plus cyclophosphamide) in node-positive breast cancer patients (TAX 316 trial).

Markers Predicting the Activity of Fluorouracil-based Regimens

The relevance of such markers for the clinician derives from two observations: Some regimens based on the administration of protracted fluorouracil infusion have shown an outstanding activity in the neo-adjuvant setting (60); and some fluorouracil pro-drugs such as capecitabine, administered orally to advanced breast cancer patients, retain an appreciable level of anti-tumor activity after anthracyclines and taxanes, with the obvious advantage of avoiding the protracted fluorouracil infusion (61).

Thymidylate synthase (TS) seems to be the most interesting predictive marker for fluorouracil and its derivatives. The enzyme is normally inhibited by fluorouracil and, in gastrointestinal malignancies, it has already been shown that high TS levels predict for a poor response rate to a fluorouracil-based regimen (62). At least three different techniques are available for TS assessment, although the polymerase chain reaction seems to be the most reliable (62). In breast cancer patients, TS levels have been investigated only as a prognostic factor (63), and no data are available regarding their potential predictive value for responsiveness to fluorouracil-based chemotherapy.

Implicated in the same metabolic pathway is another potential predictive marker: thymidine phosphorylase (TP). Its role has been evaluated by IHC in a series of 328 early breast cancer patients; the TP-positive patients showed a significant survival benefit when treated with CMF in the adjuvant setting (64). Further data are clearly needed to clarify the predictive role of both TS and TP in relation to the activity of fluorouracil-based regimens.

Markers Predicting the Activity of "High-dose" Chemotherapy

The CALGB group published the first predictive marker study in this area (65). This well-known study demonstrated that a dose-intensive CAF regimen was more effective that two other CAF regimens, of intermediate and low dose-intensity, only in the subgroup of node-positive breast cancer patients with HER-2 overexpression as measured by IHC on formalin-fixed, paraffin-embedded, primary tumor samples. The first results, presented with a 4-year median follow-up, have been confirmed by a second report with a 9-year median follow-up (31). This is the only trial suggesting that HER-2 positive tumors might be more sensitive to dose-intensive regimens. No other dose-intensive regimens have been evaluated in this manner to date, and therefore these data, although of considerable interest, cannot yet be translated into clinical practice.

Markers Predicting the Activity of Adjuvant Trastuzumab

Trastuzumab (Herceptin) is the first anti-HER-2 humanized recombinant monoclonal antibody with proven efficacy in advanced breast cancer patients, both as single agent and in combination with CT. Its value in the adjuvant setting is currently being evaluated in four randomized phase 3 trials. Since trastuzumab's target is the HER-2 protein (acting as a membrane receptor), its activity is highly dependent on the HER-2 status of the tumor, which is the only known predictive factor with level I, category A evidence. Nevertheless, in approximately 60% of patients with HER-2-positive tumors with high-level expression (3+ score by IHC or confirmed by FISH) who received single-agent trastuzumab as first-line therapy, no objective responses were observed, which suggests that other factors may be implicated in the prediction of response to trastuzumab. One such promising factor is the proportion of HER-2 receptors in an active state, i.e., the phosphorylated-HER-2 receptor (p-HER-2). Its prognostic value was suggested by a retrospective study of 816 primary breast cancer patients. HER-2-positive/p-HER-2-positive patients had a worse prognosis than HER-2-positive/p-HER-2-negative patients, and the presence of both markers was indicative of poor prognosis in both univariate and multivariate analysis (66). Since p-HER-2 seems to be an important downstream mediator in the HER-2 pathway, and may be associated with more aggressive tumor behavior, it may also be associated with a better response to trastuzumab. A pilot study evaluating this potential predictive value of p-HER-2 in metastatic breast cancer patients is ongoing at the Jules Bordet Institute.

CONCLUSIONS

In current clinical practice, the majority of early breast cancer patients receive some form of systemic adjuvant therapy. As a result, the main challenge for the oncology community has become the identification of predictive markers to assist the clinician in selecting the most suitable form of medical therapy for the individual patient. Hormone receptor (both ER and PgR) expression for adjuvant tamoxifen and HER-2 overexpression for trastuzumab's activity are the only predictive markers for which level I, category A evidence justifies their use in routine clinical practice. Regarding chemotherapy, a growing number of putative markers have been proposed to help in the selection of the best regimen. Among them, HER-2 is the one for which the largest amount of data has been gathered. The main difficulties with the published literature are the lack of prospective studies, needed to definitely clarify the merits of the investigated marker, and the loss of reproducibility of the assessment methods across different laboratories. Unfortunately, these pitfalls led to the non-recommendation for routine clinical practice of any predictive marker, including HER-2, by both the 2000 NIH (National Institutes of Health) Consensus (67) and the St. Gallen 2001 consensus (9) conferences. Nevertheless, the significant translational research efforts carried out in the last decade in this field have led to the generation of some fascinating hypotheses. New techniques now exist to test a number of these hypotheses. In particular, the use of cDNA microarrays will permit a better biologic characterization of breast cancer, and perhaps even a new classification of the disease, based on distinct molecular profiles, which may be of prognostic and/or predictive value. It is now time to test these hypotheses in a new generation of prospective predictive markers studies, some of which are already ongoing and the results of which are eagerly awaited. Their outcome may radically change the therapeutic approach to early breast cancer in the future.

REFERENCES

1. Fisher B, Dignam J, Wolmark N, et al. Tamoxifen and chemotherapy for lymph node-negative, estrogen receptor-positive breast cancer. *J Natl Cancer Inst* 1997;89:1673–1682.
2. International Breast Cancer Study Group. Effectiveness of adjuvant chemotherapy in combination with tamoxifen for node-positive postmenopausal breast cancer patients. *J Clin Oncol* 1997;15:1385–1394.
3. Wils J, Bliss JM, Coombes RC, et al. A multicentre randomized trial of tamoxifen vs. tamoxifen plus epirubicin in postmenopausal women with node-positive breast cancer. *Proc ASCO* 1996;15:109 (abstract 101).
4. Fisher B, Dignam J, Mamounas EP, et al. Sequential methotrexate and fluorouracil for the treatment of node-negative breast cancer patients with estrogen receptor-negative tumors: eight-year results from National Surgical Adjuvant Breast and Bowel Project (NSABP) B-13 and first report of findings from NSABP B-19 comparing methotrexate and fluorouracil with conventional cyclophosphamide, methotrexate, and fluorouracil. *J Clin Oncol* 1996;14:1982–1992.
5. Mansour EG, Gray R, Shatila AH, et al. Survival advantage of adjuvant chemotherapy in high-risk node-negative breast cancer: ten-year analysis. An Intergroup study. *J Clin Oncol* 1998;16:3486–3492.
6. Fisher B, Costantino J, Redmond C, et al. A randomized clinical trial evaluating tamoxifen in the treatment of patients with node-negative breast cancer who have estrogen receptor positive tumors. *N Engl J Med* 1989;320:479–484.
7. Early Breast Cancer Trialist's Collaborative Group. Polychemotherapy for early breast cancer: an overview of the randomized trials. *Lancet* 1998;352:930–942.
8. Peto R. Fifth main meeting of the Early Breast Cancer Trialist's Collaborative Group. Oxford, UK, September 2000
9. Goldhirsch A, Glick JH, Gelber RD, et al. Meeting highlights: international consensus panel on the treatment of primary cancer. *J Clin Oncol* 2001;19: 3817–3827.
10. Early Breast Cancer Trialist's Collaborative Group. Tamoxifen for early breast cancer: an overview of the randomized trials. *Lancet* 1998;351:1451–1467.
11. Heintz NH, Leslie KO, Rogers LA, et al. Amplification of the c-erb B2 oncogene in prognosis of breast adenocarcinoma. *Arch Pathol Lab Med* 1990;114:160–163.
12. Carlomagno C, Perrone F, Gallo C, et al. c-erb B2 overexpression decreases the benefit of adjuvant tamoxifen in early-stage breast cancer without axillary lymph node metastases. *J Clin Oncol* 1996;14(10):2702–2708.
13. Bianco AR, De Laurentis M, Carlomagno C, et al. 20 year update of the Naples GUN trial of adjuvant breast cancer therapy: evidence of interaction between c-erb B2 expression and tamoxifen efficacy. *Proc ASCO* 1998;17:97a (abstract 373).
14. Stal O, Borg A, Ferno M, et al. ErbB2 status and the benefit from two or five years of adjuvant tamoxifen in postmenopausal early stage breast cancer. *Annals Oncol* 2000;11:1545–1550.
15. Climent MA, Seguí MA, Peiró G, et al. Prognostic value of HER-2/*neu* and p53 expression in node-positive breast cancer. HER-2/*neu* effect on adjuvant tamoxifen treatment. *Breast* 2001;10:67–77.
16. Berry DA, Muss HB, Thor AD, et al. HER-2/*neu* and p53 expression versus tamoxifen resistance in estrogen receptor-positive, node-positive breast cancer. *J Clin Oncol* 2000;18:3471–3479.
17. Knoop AS, Bentzen SM, Nielsen MM, et al. Value of epidermal growth factor receptor, Her2, p53, and steroid receptors in predicting the efficacy of tamoxifen in high-risk postmenopausal breast cancer patients. *J Clin Oncol* 2001;19:3376–3384.
18. Elledge RM, Green S, Howes L, et al. bcl-2, p53, and response to tamoxifen in estrogen receptor-positive metastatic breast cancer: A Southwest Oncology Group Study. *J Clin Oncol* 1997;15:1916–1922.
19. Gasparini G, Barbareschi M, Doglioni C, et al. Expression of bcl-2 protein predicts efficacy of adjuvant treatments in operable node-positive breast cancer. *Clin Cancer Res* 1995;1:189–198.
20. Cardoso F, Di Leo A, Larsimont D, et al. Bcl-2 as a predictive marker for tamoxifen responsiveness in the adjuvant setting of node-positive breast cancer. *Breast Cancer Res Treat* 2001;69(3):243 (abstract 228).
21. Levine MN, Bramwell VH, Pritchard KI, et al. Randomized trial of intensive cyclophosphamide, epirubicin, and fluorouracil chemotherapy in premenopausal women with node-positive breast cancer. *J Clin Oncol* 1998;16:2651–2658.
22. Mouridsen HT, Andersen J, Andersson M, et al. Adjuvant anthracycline in breast cancer. Improved outcome in premenopausal patients following substitution of methotrexate in the CMF combination by epirubicin. *Proc ASCO* 1999;18:68a (Abstract 254).
23. Allred DC, Clarck GM, Tandon AK, et al. HER-2/neu node-negative breast cancer: prognostic significance of overexpression influenced by the presence of in-situ carcinoma. *J Clin Oncol* 1992;10:599–605.
24. Gusterson BA, Gelber RD, Goldhirsch A, et al. Prognostic importance of c-erb B2 expression in breast cancer. *J Clin Oncol* 1992;10:1049–1056.

25. Miles DW, Harris WH, Gillett CE, et al. Effect of c-erbB2 and estrogen receptor status on survival of women with primary breast cancer treated with adjuvant cyclophosphamide/methotrexate/fluorouracil. *Int J Cancer* 1999;84:354–359.
26. Menard S, Valagussa P, Pilotti S, et al. response to cyclophosphamide, methotrexate, and fluorouracil in lymph node-positive breast cancer according to HER2 overexpression and other tumor biological variables. *J Clin Oncol* 2001;19:329–335.
27. Paik S, Bryant J, Park C, et al. erb B2 and response to doxorubicin in patients with axillary lymph node-positive, hormone receptor-negative breast cancer. *J Natl Cancer Inst* 1998;90:1361–1370.
28. Di Leo A, Larsimont D, Gancberg D, et al. HER-2 and topoisomerase II α as predictive markers in a population of node-positive breast cancer patients randomly treated with adjuvant CMF or epirubicin plus cyclophosphamide. *Annals Oncol* 2001;12:1081–1089.
29. Moliterni A, Ménard S, Valagussa P, et al. Her2 overexpression and doxorubicin in the adjuvant chemotherapy of resectable breast cancer. *Proc ASCO* 2001;20:23a (abstract 89).
30. Paik S, Bryant, Tan-Chiu E, et al. HER2 and choice of adjuvant chemotherapy for invasive breast cancer: National Surgical Adjuvant Breast and Bowel Project Protocol B-15. *J Natl Cancer Inst* 2000;92:1991–1998.
31. Thor AD, Berry DA, Budman DR, et al. erb-B2, p-53, and efficacy of adjuvant therapy in lymph node-positive breast cancer. *J Natl Cancer Inst* 1998;90:1346–1360.
32. Elledge RM, Green S, Ciocca D, et al. HER-2 expression and response to tamoxifen in estrogen receptor-positive breast cancer: a Southwest Oncology Group Study. *Clin Cancer Research* 1998;4(1):7–12.
33. Gancberg D, Järvinen T, Di Leo A. Evaluation of HER2/neu protein expression in breast cancer by immunohistochemistry: an interlaboratory study assessing the reproducibility of HER2/neu testing. *Breast Cancer Res and Treat* 2002;in press.
34. Gancberg D, Lespagnard L, Rouas, G, et al. Sensitivity of HER-2/neu antibodies in archival tissue samples of invasive breast carcinomas. Correlation with oncogene amplification in 160 cases. *Am J Clin Pathol* 2000; 113:675–682.
35. Pauletti G, Dandekar S, Rong H, et al. Assessment of methods for tissue-based detection of the HER-2/neu alteration in human breast cancer: a direct comparison of fluorescence in situ hybridisation and immunohistochemistry. *J Clin Oncol* 2000;18:3651–3664.
36. Gancberg D, Di Leo A, Rouas G. Evaluation of HER-2/neu by different immunohistochemistry methods and fluorescence in situ hybridization in more than three hundreds archival primary breast cancer samples: implications for daily laboratory practice. Submitted for publication
37. Slamon DJ, Godolphin W, Jones LA, et al. Studies of the HER-2/neu proto-oncogene in human breast and ovarian cancer. *Science* 1989;244:707–712.
38. Jacobs TW, Prioleau JE, Stillman IE, et al. Loss of tumor marker-imunostaining intensity on stored paraffin slides of breast cancer. *J Natl Cancer Inst* 1996;88:1054–1059.
39. Cardoso F, Di Leo A, Larsimont D, et al. Evaluation of HER-2, p53, bcl-2, topoisomerase II-α, heat shock proteins 27 and 70 in primary breast cancer and metastatic ipsilateral axillary lymph nodes. *Annals Oncol* 2001; 12:615–620.
40. Simon R, Nocito A, Hübscher T, et al. Patters of HER-2/neu amplification and overexpression in primary and metastatic breast cancer. *J Natl Cancer Inst* 2001; 93:1141–1146.
41. Tanner M, Järvinen P, Isola J. Amplification of HER-2/neu and topoisomerase IIα in primary and metastatic breast cancer. *Cancer Res* 2001;61:5345–5348.
42. Iglehart JD, Kraus MH, Langton BC, et al. Increased erbB-2 gene copies and expression in multiple stages of breast cancer. *Cancer Res* 1990;50:6701–6707.
43. Nesland JM, Ottestad L, Borresen AL, et al. The c-erbB-2 protein in primary and metastatic breast carcinomas. *Ultrastruct Pathol* 1991;15:281–289.
44. Jarvinen TAH, Tanner M, Rantanen V, et al. Amplification and deletion of topoisomerase IIα associate with ErbB-2 amplification and affect sensitivity to topoisomerase II inhibitor doxorubicin in breast cancer. *Am J Pathol* 2000;156:839–847.
45. Smith K, Houlbrook S, Greenall M, et al. Topoisomerase IIα co-amplification with erbB2 in human primary breast cancer and breast cancer cell lines: relationship to m-AMSA and mitoxantrone sensitivity. *Oncogene* 1993; 8:933–938.
46. Jarvinen TAH, Kononen J, Pelto-Huikko M, et al. Expression of topoisomerase IIα is associated with rapid cell proliferation, aneuploidy, and c-erb B2 overexpression in breast cancer. *Am J Pathol* 1996;148: 2073–2082.
47. Jarvinen TAH, Tanner M, Barlund M, et al. Characterization of topoisomerase IIα gene amplification and deletion in breast cancer. *Genes Chromosomes Cancer* 1999;26:142–150.
48. Isola JJ, Tanner M, Holli K, et al. Amplification of topoisomerase IIα is a strong predictor of response to epirubicin-based chemotherapy in HER-2/neu positive breast cancer. *Breast Cancer Res Treat* 2000;64:31.
49. Nitiss JL, Beck WT. Anti-topoisomerase drug action and resistance. *Eur J Cancer* 1996;32A:958–966.
50. Clahsen PC, Van de Velde CJH, Duval C, et al. p53 protein accumulation and response to adjuvant chemotherapy in premenopausal women with node-negative early breast cancer. *J Clin Oncol* 1998;16:470–479.
51. Endicott JA, Ling V. The biochemistry of P-glycoprotein-mediated multidrug resistance. *Ann Rev Biochem* 1989; 58:137–171.
52. Loe DW, Deeley RG, Lole SPC. Biology of the multidrug resistance-associated protein, MRP. *Eur J Cancer* 1996;32A:945–957.
53. Gianni L, Capri G, Mezzelani A, et al. HER-2/neu amplification and response to doxorubicin/paclitaxel in women with metastatic breast cancer. *Proc ASCO* 1997;16:139a (abstract 491).
54. Stender MJ, Neuberg D, Wood W, et al. Correlation of circulating c-erb B2 extracellular domain (HER-2) with clinical outcome in patients with metastatic breast cancer. *Proc ASCO* 1997;16:154 a (abstract 541).
55. Konecny G, Thomssen C, Pegram M, et al. HER-2/neu gene amplification and response to paclitaxel in patients with metastatic breast cancer. *Proc ASCO* 2001; 20:23a (abstract 88).
56. Kandioler D, Taucher S, Steiner B, et al. p-53 genotype and major response to anthracycline or paclitaxel based neoadjuvant treatment in breast cancer patients. *Proc ASCO* 1998;17:102a (abstract 392).
57. Veitia R, Bissery MC, Martinez C, et al. Tau expression in model adenocarcinomas correlates with doc-

etaxel sensitivity in tumor-bearing mice. *British J Cancer* 1998;78:871–877.
58. Bernard C, Fellous A, Di Leo A, et al. Evaluation of microtubule associated parameters (MTAPs) as predictive markers for advanced breast cancer (ABC) patients treated with docetaxel. *Eur J Cancer* 2001;37(suppl 6): S182 (abstract 666).
59. Chan S, Friedrichs K, Noel D, et al. Prospective randomized trial of docetaxel versus doxorubicin in patients with metastatic breast cancer. *J Clin Oncol* 1999;17:2341–2354.
60. Smith IE, Walsh G, Jones A, et al. High complete remission rates with primary neoadjuvant infusional chemotherapy for large early breast cancer. *J Clin Oncol* 1995;13:424–429.
61. Blum JL, Buzdar AU, Lorusso PM, et al. A multicenter phase II trial of xeloda (capecitabine) in paclitaxel-refractory metastatic breast cancer. *Proc ASCO* 1998; 17:125a (abstract 476).
62. Lenz HJ, Leichman CG, Danenberg KD, et al. Thymidylate synthase m RNA level in adenocarcinoma of the stomach: a predictor for primary tumor response and overall survival. *J Clin Oncol* 1995;14: 176–182.
63. Pestalozzi BC, Peterson HF, Gelber RD, et al. Prognostic importance of thymidylate synthase expression in early breast cancer. *J Clin Oncol* 1997;15:1923–1931.
64. Fox SB, Engels K, Comley M, et al. Relationship of elevated tumor thymidine phosphorylase in node-positive breast carcinomas to the effects of adjuvant CMF. *Ann Oncol* 1997;8:271–275.
65. Muss HB, Thor AD, Berry DA, et al. C-erbB2 expression and response to adjuvant therapy in women with node-positive early breast cancer. *New Engl J Med* 1994;330:1260–1266.
66. Thor AD, Liu S, Edgerton S, et al. Activation (tyrosine phosphorylation) of erbB-2 (HER-2/neu): a study of incidence and correlation with outcome in breast cancer. *J Clin Oncol* 2000;18:3230–3239.
67. National Institutes of Health Consensus Development Panel. National Institutes of Health Consensus Development Conference Statement: Adjuvant therapy for breast cancer, November 1–3, 2000. *J Nat Cancer Inst* 2001;93:979–989.

PART III

Anatomapathology and the Metastatic Process

27
Basic Biology of the Metastatic Process: Clinical Implications

George N. Naumov, Ian C. MacDonald, Alan C. Groom, and Ann F. Chambers

Metastatic spread is responsible for most cancer deaths. However, clinical and experimental observations suggest that cancer metastasis is an inefficient process, in which many cancer cells may be shed from a primary tumor, but only a few grow to form clinically evident metastases. A better understanding of the biology and molecular events of the metastatic process is required for the development of effective anti-metastatic therapies. Using quantitative techniques, including *in vivo* videomicroscopy (IVVM) and cell accounting, we have been able to directly observe and quantify the fate of cancer cells at various steps of metastasis, as they occur *in vivo*. This approach has led to new insights into the metastatic process and new steps that result in metastatic inefficiency. As part of our experimental studies on mechanisms of metastasis, we have discovered that large numbers of disseminated solitary cells may persist dormant in secondary sites for extended time periods. Here we review these *in vivo* techniques and discuss the potential clinical implications of our experimental findings.

BACKGROUND

By the time a primary tumor is detected, cancer cells often have spread to distant sites. The growth of these cells in secondary sites is responsible for most deaths among cancer patients. Although clinically important, the metastatic process is poorly understood. Most current systemic cancer therapies target rapidly dividing cells, but also affect normal tissue and lead to undesirable side-effects and toxicity. Therapies that target specific molecular defects in cancer cells need to be developed in the context of the biology of the metastatic process.

TOOLS FOR STUDYING THE METASTATIC PROCESS

To clarify the biological basis of metastasis, we have developed methods to observe and quantify the fate of cancer cells at successive stages of the metastatic process in experimental animals. It is now possible to:

1. Directly observe metastatic progression as it occurs over time in a number of different organs and tissues by means of IVVM.
2. Monitor and quantify the fate of a population of individual cells (or metastases) over time following injection of cells using a cell "accounting" technique.
3. Detect and quantify the number of cancer cells within a tissue that have not divided since their injection.

Together, these approaches provide new insights into the steps involved in metastasis and their efficiency in relation to growth. Since these experimental methods have been described in detail previously (1,2), only a brief summary is given here.

IVVM for Detection of Cancer Cells in Secondary Sites

To study the mechanisms of metastasis, methods are needed to provide direct observations of the process as it occurs *in vivo* over time. High-resolution IVVM (Fig. 27.1A) has allowed us to directly observe and measure dynamic aspects of interactions between cancer cells and the host environment which were previously difficult to assess by commonly used *in vivo* and *in vitro* assays. With this technique, we have studied sequential steps in the metastatic process, using several experimental models (2).

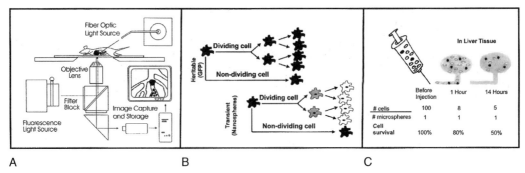

FIG. 27.1. Tools for studying the metastatic process. **A:** Schematic diagram of *in vivo* videomicroscopy (IVVM) technique. Using IVVM we can observe cancer cells in intact organs of a living animal. Organs are exposed and positioned in contact with a coverslip window overlying the objective lenses (×10–×100) of an inverted microscope. Using oblique fiberoptic light transillumination and/or episcopic fluorescence illumination with appropriate filter blocks, we can observe fluorescently labeled cancer cells. Images are viewed real-life using a video camera and monitor and can be recorded on videotape for subsequent analysis. **B:** Permanent versus transient cancer cell labeling techniques. Permanent cell markers (such as GFP) provide a heritable, stable cytoplasmic fluorescence that remains through generations of cell division. Thus, it is impossible to differentiate between originally injected cells that have not divided and those that have divided. In contrast, cancer cells labeled with transient markers (such as virus-sized fluorescent nanospheres) will lose their nanosphere content exponentially by dilution at each successive cell division. Thus, non-dividing cells retain their nanospheres over long periods and remain brightly fluorescent. **C:** Cell "accounting" procedure used for quantification of *in vivo* cell survival and metastatic efficiency. Inert plastic fluorescent microspheres (~10 μm) are included in a cell suspension in a known cell:microsphere ratio. The suspension is injected intravenously to target an organ. The microspheres remain indefinitely where they arrest in the microcirculation, providing a reference marker for the number of cells that originally reached that volume of tissue. The percentages of surviving cells at later time points can be calculated based on cell:microsphere ratios.

Visualization of cancer cells by IVVM requires that the cells carry a marker to distinguish them optically from the surrounding normal tissue. Although some cancer cells express natural markers (such as melanin) that can aid in their detection, most cell lines lack such identifying markers. Therefore, exogenously introduced fluorescent markers have been employed in many of our studies. Cytoplasmic labels such as Calcein-AM are very effective for cell detection during the initial period following injection, but can suffer from fluorescence fading due to bleaching when extended viewing periods are required (3). Alternatively, green fluorescent protein (GFP) is an endogenous marker that can be expressed in cancer cells by cDNA transfection, producing a heritable, stable cytoplasmic fluorescence that allows cells to be detected for long-term observations *in vivo* (4).

Although extremely useful for high-resolution detection of solitary cancer cells, GFP provides no indication of whether a cell has divided since injection. Due to the heritable expression of GFP, it is not possible to distinguish between a cell that has divided several times and a cell that has not undergone cell division (Fig. 27.1B). For example, if a solitary cancer cell is detected next to a rapidly growing metastasis, it would be impossible to determine if this cell had detached from the adjacent metastasis and invaded locally, or had remained undivided in the tissue following microvascular arrest and extravasation. Since we are interested in studying the fate of cancer cells in secondary organs it was imperative to develop a new strategy for labeling cells which would distinguish a population of non-dividing cancer cells from a background of actively proliferating cells.

Fluorescent Labeling of Cancer Cells for Detection of Non-dividing Cells

To identify non-dividing cancer cells, we have used fluorescent polystyrene nanospheres (0.05 μm to 0.07 μm diameter) which are spontaneously internalized when incubated with cancer cells *in vitro* prior to injection (3,5). Cells labeled in this fashion maintain their membrane integrity and their growth potential is undiminished (3). In contrast to GFP-labeled cancer cells, once in the organ dividing cells lose their nanosphere content exponentially by dilution at each successive cell division (Fig. 27.1B) (5). Non-dividing cells, however, retain nanospheres over long periods and remain brightly fluorescent. Such solitary cells may be readily observed both by IVVM and in formalin fixed 50-μm-thick histological sections.

Fluorescence labeling with either transient or heritable labels allows for high-resolution *in vivo* detection and follow-up of cancer cells; however, it does not allow for quantification of the fate of the cells over time. Thus, a new technique was needed that would introduce a reference point for the numbers of cancer cells that have arrived in a particular volume of tissue.

Cell Accounting Technique for Quantification of Solitary Cell Survival

To quantitatively study the fate of cancer cells at sequential steps in the metastatic process, we developed an accounting technique that allows measurement of cancer cell survival at various times after cells are injected into the circulation (Figure 27.1C) (2,3,6). Briefly, inert plastic microspheres of uniform size (10.2 ± 0.1 μm diameter) are added to cells prepared for injection at a known cell:microsphere ratio, e.g., 10 cells per microsphere. After injection of the suspension, both cells and microspheres are lodged by size restriction in the microcirculation of the first organ encountered. Because the microspheres remain permanently trapped within the vessels, the total number of microspheres present in an observed tissue volume, at any time following injection, provides a reference for the number of cancer cells that originally arrived in the same region. Percentage cell survival, at any stage of the metastatic process, can therefore be calculated by comparing the cell:microsphere ratio observed in the sampled volume of tissue to the corresponding ratio in the cell suspension originally injected. We have used this technique for quantification of the fate of both solitary undivided cells and cells that have begun to proliferate to form metastases, since metastases have been shown to be primarily clonal in origin (8,9).

FINDINGS FROM *IN VIVO* EXPERIMENTAL STUDIES

Collectively, the techniques described above allow for detection of cancer cells *in vivo* in experimental animals, and quantification of the fate of the cells over time during the metastatic process. A remarkably consistent picture of the early steps of the metastatic process has emerged from our studies using these techniques. These studies have been carried out using a variety of cancer cell types, injected into the circulation to target various organs. We have found that, regardless of metastatic potential, a high percentage of injected cancer cells survive while in the circulation, during arrest in the first encountered capillary bed, and as they extravasate from these vessels into the surrounding tissues. However, only a small subpopulation of these extravasated cells subsequently initiate growth and persist to form detectable macrometastases; the size of this subpopulation varies with the metastatic ability of the cells in end-point metastasis assays.

Cancer Cell Survival in the Circulation

Following vascularization of the primary tumor, a subpopulation of cancer cells may intravasate into the blood or lymphatic circulation and be carried to distant organs. It had been believed that the circulation represents a hostile environment for cancer cells, leading to their death. Thus, it would be reasonable to expect that the majority of the cells that successfully enter the circulation would be destroyed. However, by using IVVM and the cell accounting technique to assess the fate of cancer cells from the time of their injection into the circulation to their arrival and arrest in target organs, we have found that most cells are not destroyed in the circulation (2). These observations led us to conclude that the microcirculation is not a particularly hostile environment for cancer cells and that a larger population of cancer cells than previously appreciated may survive intact in the circulation and successfully reach secondary sites. If this holds true clinically, it becomes important to determine the fate of these cells.

Arrest of Cancer Cells in Secondary Sites

Using IVVM we are able to watch directly the arrival of blood-borne cancer cells in an organ and determine the way in which cells become arrested within the microvasculature in experimental animals. In the organs and tissues we have studied, the majority of injected cancer cells arrest in the first capillary bed they encounter. This initial arrest appears to be caused by physical size restriction. Many solid tumor cells are considerably larger (approximately 15 to 20 μm or more in diameter) than cells normally found in the circulation (e.g., red blood cells, leukocytes) and tumor cells become arrested when the vessels in which they are traveling simply become too small for their passage. Shortly after arrest, the cells undergo deformation in proportion to the blood pressure of the organ in which they arrest and conform to the boundary restrictions imposed by the vessel. The degree of deformation is modest in relatively low-pressure circulations such as chick embryo chorioallantoic membrane (CAM) and the liver in mice. However, under the higher hemodynamic pressures found in muscle, the arrested cells may reach length-to-width ratios of up to 8:1 (10). In spite of such severe deformations, the cells do not lyse but retain their membrane integrity, as shown by exclusion of ethidium bromide (11).

Based on extrapolation from *in vitro* studies, it had been suggested that the arrest of cancer cells in a secondary organ is determined primarily by specific adhesive interactions between cells and the endothelium of precapillary vessels. This concept appeared attractive since it would provide a rational basis for organ specificity of metastasis based on differential signature expression of vascular adhesive molecules to which specific populations of cancer cells might "home." However, we have not observed *in vivo* arrest of circulating cancer cells in vessels of diameters larger than that of the cancer cells. Scherbarth and Orr (12) obtained comparable results, but also found that when mice were pretreated with the cytokine interleukin 1α, circulating cancer cells could also be arrested in larger presinusoidal vessels (portal venules) based on adhesive interactions with the endothelium. Our findings suggest that adhesive interactions, which do indeed seem to contribute to metastasis (as measured by their effect in end point assays), must do so by an alternative mechanism, independent of the initial physical arrest of cancer cells in specific sites. One possibility includes the involvement of adhesion signaling in the stabilization of interactions between cancer cells and vessel walls during extravasation. Alternatively, signaling pathways stimulated by adhesion interactions might lead to preferential growth in specific sites or organs. In any case, studies from our group and others (13) suggest that adhesive interactions may not be required for the initial arrest of cancer cells in an organ. In addition, the location of initial arrest appears to be governed by patterns of blood flow from the primary tumor, which dictate which capillary bed will be first encountered, and size restriction of the cancer cells when they can no longer proceed through the microcirculation in that organ. Thus the blood flow patterns from a primary tumor to secondary organs, coupled with the relative diameters of cancer cells and capillaries, are factors that can determine the initial arrest of circulating cancer cells in secondary sites.

Successful Extravasation of Most Cells in Secondary Sites

It had generally been believed that the process of extravasation constitutes a barrier that few cancer cells successfully overcome, thus creating a rate-limiting step in metastasis. Furthermore, inhibition of extravasation was believed to represent an important clinical target for the development of antimetastatic therapeutics. However, our direct in vivo observations of cancer cell extravasation in chick CAM and mouse liver support the view that extravasation is a relatively efficient process which is independent of the metastatic status of the injected cells (14). For example, we compared the time course of extravasation in mouse liver for two murine mammary carcinoma cell lines, the first (D2A1) being highly invasive in matrigel invasion in vitro assays and highly metastatic in vivo, and the second (D2.0R), although tumorigenic, being noninvasive in vitro and poorly metastatic in vivo. Surprisingly, we found that both cell lines extravasated with the same time course in both CAM and murine liver (3).

Similar experiments in CAM and mouse liver showed that highly metastatic ras-transformed NIH-3T3 (PAP2) cells and non-transformed NIH 3T3 cells extravasated with the same kinetics (15,16). Nearly 90% of observed cells had completed the process of extravasation 24 hours after their injection and arrest in the microcirculation. Similarly, malignant melanoma cells engineered to overexpress the tissue inhibitor of matrix metalloproteinases (TIMP)-1 showed the same extravasation kinetics as control cells, despite clear inhibition of metastatic ability in the TIMP-1 overexpressing cells in endpoint assays. More than 80% of injected cells of both lines successfully extravasated. Other IVVM experiments that focused on the role of integrins in metastasis showed endpoint tumor inhibition due to effects on post-extravasation cell migration and growth, but not on the process of extravasation itself (2,17–19).

A consistent picture has thus emerged from our experimental IVVM studies. Contrary to previous belief, the process of extravasation does not appear to represent a major barrier for cancer cells. If these results apply to cancer patients, a large proportion of cells shed from human cancers may successfully extravasate in any organ to which the cells are carried by the circulation. Thus, extravasation can no longer be considered a rate-limiting step in metastasis and post-extravasational events will be of crucial importance.

Growth in Secondary Sites: A Key Regulator of Metastasis

The studies outlined above suggest that metastatic inefficiency must be due to postextravasation factors that affect the ability of cancer cells to grow to form metastases in the new organ. In 1889, Paget noted that metastases from breast cancers occurred preferentially in certain secondary sites (such as bone), but with limited success in others. This clinical observation led to the introduction of the "seed and soil" concept, suggesting that host factors (what he called "soil"), as well as intrinsic properties of the cancer cells (seed), would likely contribute to the formation of metastases. In Paget's own words, "When a plant goes to seed, its seeds are carried in all directions; but they can only live and grow if they fall on congenial soil" (20,21). To study the growth of cancer cells in secondary sites, we have thus used the above-described tools to quantify metastatic inefficiency after extravasation in experimental animals.

Initiation of Cancer Cell Growth to Form Preangiogenic Micrometastases

As a model to study metastatic inefficiency in the case of two seeds with different metastatic ability when introduced into a similar soil environment, we compared two murine mammary carcinoma cell lines, highly versus poorly metastatic (D2A1 versus D2.0R) (3,5). Both cell lines were separately injected into mice via a mesenteric vein to target them to the liver. The cell accounting technique allowed us to quantify the survival of solitary cells and metastases at various stages of the metastatic process. Cell proliferation (Ki-67) and apoptotic cell death (TUNEL: TdT dUTP nick end labeling) were quantified by immunohistochemistry. By day 10, approximately 64% of the injected highly metastatic D2A1 cells still remained in the tissue as undivided solitary cells, and only a small subpopulation of cells (0.62%) had begun to form preangiogenic micrometastases. In contrast, the poorly metastatic D2.0R cells remained as solitary cells with no evidence whatever of metastatic growth. Thus, only a very small subpopulation of the seeded, highly metastatic cancer cells initiated growth in the secondary site, and the majority of the cells (both highly and poorly metastatic) remained as solitary cells and did not die.

Other studies in which the postextravasation growth of melanoma cells in mouse liver was quantified yielded similar results (7). Although more than 80% of the cells had extravasated by day 3 after injection, only a small proportion (approximately 2%) began growth to form micrometastases. In another study comparing the survival of metastatic, *ras*-transformed (PAP2) versus control (NIH 3T3) cells in mouse liver, approximately 95% of both cell lines were fully extravascular by day 3 (16), although Ras had no effect on the proportion of cells that initiated proliferation to form micrometastases; however, by day 14 the majority of micrometastases formed by NIH 3T3 cells had completely disappeared. In contrast, in the same time period all of the mice injected with PAP2 cells had formed macroscopic metastases, and these were derived from the growth of a small subset (less than 1%) of the injected cells. Collectively these studies indicate that, although the majority of injected cancer cells survive and successfully extravasate, only a small subpopulation initiates growth to form micrometastases. Thus, a key factor limiting the growth of metastases is the fact that many extravasated cells simply remain in the tissue as solitary undivided cells, and only very few of them begin to divide.

Continued Growth of Micrometastases into Angiogenic Tumors

It had generally been believed that once a cancer cell reaches a favorable environment (i.e., soil) and starts to divide, it will continue to do so and form a highly vascularized macrometastasis. We were thus somewhat surprised to find that not all cells that initiated growth persisted in growth. In the mammary carcinoma metastasis model, there was an early loss of most micrometastases and only one in 100 of these micrometastases (corresponding to approximately 0.006% of the original cell inoculum) successfully continued growth to form large macrometastases by day 21 (5). In fact, the rate of loss of early micrometastases was almost two orders of magnitude greater than that for solitary cells. A similar 100-fold decrease in persistence of early metastases was documented in the case of melanoma cells (7). By day 3 after injection, 2% of the injected melanoma cells initiated growth to form micrometastases. However, only 1% of these micrometastases continued to grow to form macroscopic tumors by day 13. Taken together, our experimental studies using mammary carcinoma and melanoma cell lines have identified two key regulatory steps in the metastatic process: initiation of the growth of micrometastases from a subset of cells, and persistence of growth of a subset of micrometastases to form macroscopic tumors. If these observations hold true clinically, then the inefficiency of early metastatic growth may provide a useful therapeutic target.

Tumor Dormancy

In the study described above comparing poorly and highly metastatic mammary carcinoma cells, a surprisingly large population of solitary dormant cancer cells was also found. In this model, approximately 22% of the injected D2A1 cells remained dormant in the tissue as solitary cells, detected by their retention of fluorescent nanospheres both *in vivo* and in 50-µm-thick histological sections (5). A subpopulation of these dormant cells persisted through all stages of the metastatic process against a background of rapidly growing metastases. In our melanoma metastasis model similar results were obtained; even 2 weeks after injection, 36% of the injected cells still remained within the liver tissue as solitary undivided cells (7). In both models (carcinoma and melanoma), solitary cells were stained for apoptosis and proliferation. We found that more than 95% of the observed, highly fluorescent solitary cells were neither apoptosing nor proliferating, signifying that they were dormant.

We compared these results to the fate of the poorly metastatic (but tumorigenic) mammary carcinoma cell line (D2.0R). Surprisingly, approximately 80% of the originally injected cells remained as solitary undivided cells up to 21 days after injection. Even at 77 days after their injection, approximately 50% of the D2.0R cells remained within the liver tissue as undivided dormant cells. To determine whether the apparently dormant D2.0R cells were viable, liver tissue was dissociated and cancer cells were recovered based on drug resistance. At least some of these cells were shown to be viable, as defined by ability to grow in cell culture. When the recovered cells were reinjected in mammary fat pad (primary tumor site), they successfully formed primary tumors (5). This finding indicates that, despite their apparent dormancy at a secondary site, the recovered cells retain their tumorigenic phenotype. Such dormant cells would not have been detected by standard metastasis assays, in which only the endpoint of the process is assessed.

If our experimental observations hold true clinically, solitary dormant cells would be especially problematic, since they would be resistant to current treatment strategies based on the killing of actively dividing cells, as well being unaffected by anti-angiogenic therapies.

CLINICAL IMPLICATIONS OF EXPERIMENTAL STUDIES ON METASTASIS

Our experimental studies suggest that metastasis should be viewed as an ongoing process involving a number of sequential steps, all of which need to be successfully completed for macrometastases to become clinically relevant. A general pattern has emerged from our studies using IVVM and other quantitative techniques to assess the fate of cancer cells following their injection into the circulation of experimental animals. Our findings suggest that:

- cancer cells survive in high numbers in the circulation
- the majority of cells arrest in whatever organ they first encounter, based on blood flow patterns and size differences between the cells and the vessels
- the majority of the cells arrested in the microvasculature of an organ successfully extravasate
- only a small fraction of the extravasated cells proliferate, giving rise to preangiogenic micrometastases
- only a small fraction of the preangiogenic micrometastases persist in growth to form macroscopic tumors.

Thus, we have identified key post-extravasational determinants of metastatic progression. However, the factors that dictate what proportion of a population of cancer cells in a secondary site will initiate and persist in growth are not well understood. What is the difference between the small subpopulation that makes the decision to grow and the rest of the cells that do not? Are these differences a result of intrinsic properties of the cancer cell, the surrounding microenvironment, or both? These are some of the fundamental questions that need to be addressed in the future.

Any anti-metastatic therapy that prevents metastases from causing unfavorable clinical consequences to the patient would be of potential value. From a therapeutic standpoint, two key determinants of metastatic progression thus must be considered: (a) proliferation of solitary cells to form preangiogenic micrometastases; and (b) development of a blood supply within these micrometastases, permitting the development of macroscopic tumors. Most current therapeutic approaches would target either one (or both) of these determinants, resulting in delay or possibly destruction of metastatic growth. Control of metastatic growth by inducing dormancy, or prevention of growth, are clinically viable approaches that could impact on patient survival and quality of life. However, the source of metastatic growth (i.e., solitary cells seeded in various organs and tissues) in most cases would remain unaffected and could lead to growth after long latency periods following treatment. If our experimental observations hold true clinically, the population of dormant cells may greatly exceed in size the population of cancer cells that initiate and persist in growth. Solitary dormant cells would be especially problematic for treatment, since they would be inherently resistant to cytotoxic chemotherapies based on killing actively dividing cells, as well as to anti-angiogenic therapies. It is therefore imperative that the nature of clinical dormancy be better understood in order to learn how to prevent activation of dormant cells and/or micrometastases in cancer patients who are at risk of developing metastases.

Acknowledgments: This work was supported by a grant from the Canadian Institutes of Health Research (#42511), and an award from the Lloyd Carr-Harris Foundation. George Naumov is supported by a "Pre-doctoral Traineeship" Award from the U.S. Army Breast Cancer Research Program (DOD DAMD17-00-1-0501). The content of this article does not necessarily reflect the position or policy of the U.S. government, and no official endorsement should be inferred.

REFERENCES

1. Chambers AF, MacDonald IC, Schmidt EE, et al. Steps in tumor metastasis: new concepts from intravital videomicroscopy. *Cancer Met Rev* 1995;14:279–301.
2. Chambers AF, MacDonald IC, Schmidt EE, et al. Clinical targets for anti-metastasis therapy. *Adv Cancer Res* 2000;79:91–121.
3. Morris VL, Koop S, MacDonald IC, et al. Mammary carcinoma cell lines of high and low metastatic potential differ not in extravasation but in subsequent migration and growth. *Clin Exp Metastasis* 1994;12:357–367.
4. Naumov GN, Wilson SM, MacDonald IC, et al. Cellular expression of green fluorescent protein, coupled with high-resolution in vivo videomicroscopy, to monitor steps in tumor metastasis. *J Cell Sci* 1999;112:1835–1842.
5. Naumov GN, MacDonald IC, Weinmeister PM, et al. Persistence of solitary mammary carcinoma cells in a secondary site: A possible contributor to dormancy. *Cancer Res* 2002; in press.
6. Koop S, MacDonald IC, Luzzi K, et al. Fate of melanoma cells entering the microcirculation: over 80% survive and extravasate. *Cancer Res* 1995;55:2520–2523.
7. Luzzi KJ, MacDonald IC, Schmidt EE, et al. Multistep nature of metastatic inefficiency: dormancy of solitary cells after successful extravasation and limited survival of early micrometastases. *Am J Pathol* 1998;153:865–873.
8. Talmadge JE, Wolman SR, Fidler IJ. Evidence for the clonal origin of spontaneous metastases. *Science* 1982;217:361–363.
9. Chambers AF, Wilson S. Use of NeoR B16F1 murine melanoma cells to assess clonality of experimental metastases in the immune-deficient chick embryo. *Clin Exp Metastasis* 1988;6:171–182.
10. MacDonald IC, Schmidt EE, Morris VL, et al. In vivo videomicroscopy of experimental hematogenous metastasis: cancer cell arrest, extravasation, and migration. In: *Motion analysis of living cells*. New York: Wiley-Liss, 1998:263–288.
11. Morris VL, MacDonald IC, Koop S, et al. Early interactions of cancer cells with the microvasculature in mouse liver and muscle during hematogenous metastasis: videomicroscopic analysis. *Clin Exp Metastasis* 1993;11:377–390.
12. Scherbarth S, Orr FW. Intravital videomicroscopic evidence for regulation of metastasis by the hepatic microvasculature: Effects of interleukin-1α on metastasis and the location of B16F1 melanoma cell arrest. *Cancer Res* 1997;57:4105–4110.
13. Weiss L. Comments on hematogenous metastatic patterns in humans as revealed by autopsy. *Clin Exp Metastasis* 1992;10:191–199.
14. Chambers AF, Matrisian LM. Changing views of the role of matrix metalloproteinases in metastasis. *J Natl Cancer Inst* 1997;89:1260–1270.
15. Koop S, Schmidt EE, MacDonald IC, et al. Independence of metastatic ability and extravasation: metastatic *ras*-transformed and control fibroblasts extravasate equally well. *Proc Natl Acad Sci USA* 1996;93:11080–11084.
16. Varghese HJ, Davidson MTM, MacDonald IC, et al. Activated *ras* regulates the proliferation/apoptosis balance and early survival of developing micrometastases. *Cancer Res* 2002;62:887–891.
17. Morris VL, Schmidt EE, Koop S, et al. Effects of the disintegrin eristostatin on individual steps of hematogenous metastasis. *Exp Cell Res* 1995;219:571–578.
18. Hangan D, Uniyal S, Morris VL, et al. Integrin VLA-2 (alpha2beta1) function in postextravasation movement of human rhabdomyosarcoma RD cells in the liver. *Cancer Res* 1996;56:3142–3149.
19. Groom AC, MacDonald IC, Schmidt EE, et al. Tumor metastasis to the liver, and the role of proteinases and adhesion molecules: new concepts from in vivo videomicroscopy. *Can J Gastroenterol* 1999;13:733–743.
20. Paget S. The distribution of secondary growths in cancer of the breast. *Lancet* 1889;1:571–573.
21. Paget S. The distribution of secondary growths in cancer of the breast. 1889. *Cancer Met Rev* 1989;8:98–101 (re-publication of Paget's 1889 *Lancet* article).

28
Prognostic and Predictive Factors in Breast Cancer: An Evidence-Based Medicine Approach

Syed K. Mohsin, Valerie-Jean Bardou, Grazia Arpino, Gary C. Chamness, and D. Craig Allred

Prognosis for patients is defined as the prediction of future behavior of an established primary or metastatic cancer, either in the absence of or after application of local or systemic therapy. Clark (1) suggests that prognostic variables be divided into two categories, prognostic factors and predictive factors. A prognostic factor is defined as any measurement available at the time of diagnosis or surgery that is associated with alteration in disease-free or overall survival in the absence of systemic adjuvant therapy. Prognostic factors can be used to predict the natural history of the tumor. A predictive factor is defined as any measurement associated with response or lack of response to a particular therapy. The prototype predictive factor has been the presence of steroid hormone receptors, which influence the response to both adjuvant and metastatic endocrine therapy.

Today, prognostic and predictive factors are useful in at least three clinical situations (2). The first is to identify patients whose prognosis is so good after local surgery that the addition of systemic adjuvant therapy would not be cost-effective. The second is to identify patients whose prognosis is so poor with conventional treatment that other potentially more aggressive therapy might be warranted. The third is to ascertain which patients are or are not likely to benefit from specific therapies.

In primary breast cancer, the recognized prognostic factors generally include: axillary lymph node involvement, tumor size, histological grade, estrogen and progesterone receptor status, and measure of proliferation. However, none of these factors, alone or in combination, can completely separate patients cured by local therapy from those whose cancer will recur. Newer markers that have not yet been fully evaluated must be considered. Several guidelines have been published to determine if and/or when use of these tumor markers should become routine.

EVALUATION AND VALIDATION METHODOLOGIES

First, it is useful to consider the problem of how the reader should interpret results of published studies that have evaluated potential prognostic and predictive factors. Improper clinical decisions based on incorrectly interpreted tumor marker results will not only likely increase the cost of care but also expose patients to potentially adverse consequences. McGuire (3) proposed minimal criteria that must be considered for the design and conduct of prognostic factor studies. He classified studies as "pilot" to generate the hypothesis and provide estimates, so that a "definitive" study could be designed. He insisted on the requirement of an adequate sample size for meaningful calculations.

Gasparini et al. (4) gave more details on evaluation of these factors and suggested four distinct phases for a proper evaluation of a new potential prognostic or predictive factor in breast cancer. Hayes et al. (5) proposed a Tumor Marker Utility Grading System (TMUGS) to evaluate the clinical utility of tumor markers and to establish an investigational agenda for evaluation of new tumor markers. This system allows objective assessment to accept or to reject a marker for use in clinical practice. It is a standardized method

TABLE 28.1. *Criteria for recommendations using the principles of evidence-based medicine*

Level	Type of evidence for recommendation
I	Evidence obtained from meta-analysis of multiple well-designed controlled studies; randomized trials with low false-positive and low false-negative errors (high power)
II	Evidence obtained from at least one well-designed experimental study; randomized trials with low false-positive and/or low false-negative errors (low power)
III	Evidence obtained from well-designed quasi-experimental studies, such as nonrandomized controlled single-group pre-pot, cohort, time or matched case-control series.
IV	Evidence obtained from well-designed nonexperimental studies, such as comparative and correlation descriptive and case studies
V	Evidence from case reports and clinical examples
Category	Grade of evidence
A	There is evidence of type I or consistent findings from multiple studies of types II, III or IV
B	There is evidence of types II, III or IV and findings are generally consistent
C	There is evidence of types II, III or IV, but findings are inconsistent
D	There is little or no systemic evidence
NG	Grade not given

including semiquantitative utility scales (0, 3+) to assign a score, and to establish a hierarchy of five levels of evidence to support conclusions regarding the utility of a given markers for a given use. He also described a process for assessing the clinical impact of factors in terms of risk ratio for prognostic factors or benefit ratio for predictive factors (6).

EVIDENCE-BASED MEDICINE

The tremendous volume of literature makes it extremely challenging to keep oneself abreast of the medical literature. One approach to meeting these challenges and avoiding clinical entropy is to learn how to practice evidence-based medicine (EBM). EBM involves integrating clinical expertise with the best available clinical evidence derived from systematic research (7). The role of EBM is not to discount expert opinion, but whenever possible, to permit recommendations to be based on the results of rigorous, controlled scientific studies. When such studies have not been performed, and may never be done, this approach allows the recommendations to be much more circumspect. In the 1970s, the Canadian Task Force on Periodic Health Examination developed a set of standardized criteria for evaluating and grading scientific evidence (8) that was enhanced by the U.S. Preventive Services Task Force (9). For this review, the literature was reviewed to evaluate the status of validation of prognostic and predictive factors in breast cancer, particularly the newer ones, and recommendations are made using the guidelines of EBM (Table 28.1). A brief summary of established markers, such as tumor stage and histological types, is followed by detailed review of the newer biomarkers.

AXILLARY NODAL STATUS

Axillary lymph node status has been shown to be the most powerful prognostic factor of disease-free and overall survival for patients with primary breast cancer (10,11). Only 20% to 30% of node-negative patients will develop recurrence within 10 years, compared with about 70% of patients with axillary nodal involvement. Most clinical trials stratify patients into three nodal groups (negative nodes, one to three positive nodes, and four or more positive nodes), but the absolute number of involved nodes is also of prognostic importance (12).

Lymph node involvement is associated with larger tumors, but independent of other tumor markers such as presence of steroid receptors or measures of proliferation. A meta-analysis of published results on association between various prognostic factors is compatible with the hypothesis that the prognostic influence of node status and tumor size cannot be explained by an analysis of the biology of breast cancer, but is merely a reflection of the relative chronological age of breast cancer (13).

Even if axillary dissection in early breast cancer provides important prognostic information, its therapeutic use remains controversial because of substantial side effects and because its value with respect to recurrence or survival has not been unequivocally proven. Some studies have found a modest benefit. A prospective randomized comparison of lumpectomy alone versus lumpectomy-plus-axillary dissection shows that axillary dissection is justified for treatment of small breast cancers, although whether the better survival is due to axillary clearance itself or to adjuvant treatment for lymph node involvement is unclear (14). Several investigators have conducted studies to investigate the possibility of using other prognostic indicators to replace axillary dissection to predict axillary node status of patients with primary breast cancer. Using data from 26,683 patients from the National Breast Cancer Tissue Resource, randomly assigned to a training set (patient information used to construct predictive models) or a validation set (patient information used to prospectively evaluate predictive models), Ravdin et al. (15) showed that addition of prognostic indicator information (patient age, S phase, and ER concentration) to tumor size can refine estimates of whether a patient is likely to be node-positive. However, no patient subsets could be identified as having greater than 95% chance of being node-negative or node-positive. However, use of sentinel lymph node biopsy (SLNB) with extensive pathological examination may be a relatively well-tolerated and cost-effective way to predict the status of axillary lymph nodes (see below).

Evaluation of axillary lymph node status is also an established parameter (category A grade of evidence). The standard practice is to administer systemic adjuvant treatment to all patients with node-positive breast cancer, unless there is a contraindication. But there remains need to identify new prognostic factors for node-negative patients, and predictive factors for treatment response of both node-negative and -positive breast cancer individuals (1).

TUMOR SIZE

Tumor size is one of the most powerful predictors of tumor behavior in breast cancer. Data on 24,740 cases recorded in the Surveillance, Epidemiology, and End Results (SEER) Program of the National Cancer Institute confirm that as tumor size increases, survival decreases, regardless of lymph node status; and as lymph node involvement increases, survival status also decreases regardless of tumor size (16). A study from the National Surgical Adjuvant Breast and Bowel Project (NSABP) reported that the frequency of nodal metastases in patients with tumors smaller than 1 cm is 10% to 20% (17), and data from Memorial Sloan-Kettering Cancer Center indicated that node-negative patients with tumors smaller than 1 cm have a 10-year disease-free survival rate of about 90% (18). In fact, in the subset of node-negative breast cancer, tumor size is the most powerful and consistent predictor of recurrence.

A long-term follow-up study (19) has reported that patients with extremely large tumors tend to have better outcomes than those with intermediate size. This suggests that patients with large tumors, if not already metastatic at diagnosis, might have a lower subsequent potential for metastatic spread. However, the San Antonio Data Base suggests a plateau in the risk of recurrence between 3 cm and 6 cm, and a significant decrease in disease-free survival for node-negative patients with tumors larger than 6 cm (1).

A review by McGuire and Clark (20) suggested criteria for adjuvant therapy in node-negative breast cancer, including tumor size. The 25% of patients with tumors smaller than 1 cm and favorable histologic subtypes have a sufficiently low recurrence rate that few should be treated. The 25% of patients with tumors larger than 3 cm, usually associated with poor prognostic features, have a sufficiently high recurrence rate (over 50%) that most or all should be treated. The remaining 50% of patient with intermediate size tumors have an average overall recurrence rate of 30%. In these patients, the use of other prognostic factors will help to identify low-risk and high-risk groups so that adjuvant treatment efforts can be focused on those most likely to benefit.

Tumor size is an established parameter that can be documented as a category A grade of evidence marker in all breast cancers. In certain categories of tumor size, such as tumors less than 1 cm, other factors have to be measured to further refine the prognosis of such patients.

New Aspects of Tumor Staging

The immunocytologic detection of isolated tumor cells in bone marrow, termed micro-metastasis, has been considered as an optional factor in the tumor-node-metastasis (TNM) classification indicated as M1(i). A meta-analysis of 20 studies, which included 2,494 patients, concluded that the presence of epithelial cells in bone marrow was detectable in all carcinoma types. But only five of 20 studies confirmed positive micrometastasis status as an independent predictor of short disease-free survival, and only two studies confirmed it as an independent predictor of poor survival (21). Braun et al. (22) suggest that the prognostic impact of epithelial cells in bone marrow remains to be substantiated by further international studies using standardized methodology protocols, not meta-analyses, before its entrance into the TNM classification. At this time, the evidence on bone marrow micrometastases is inconsistent and no recommendation can be made based on the present evidence.

The sentinel lymph node (SLN) is defined as the first node draining the primary tumor in the regional lymphatic basin. A multicentric study, which enrolled 443 patients and 11 surgeons, confirmed the sensitivity and the specificity in predicting axillary status. Biopsy of sentinel nodes can predict the presence or absence of axillary node metastases in patients with breast cancer. However, the procedure can be technically challenging, and the success rate varies according to the surgeon and the characteristics of the patient (23). Nearly 25 studies have now compared the SLN biopsy to full axillary node dissection. These studies have shown that SLN is positive in 36% of the cases and in nearly 60% of the cases SLN is the only positive node. The false-negative rate (i.e., SLN negative but axillary node positive) is between 5% and 10%.

Other important issues involve the method of evaluation of SLN. One aspect is the intraoperative evaluation, with the intent that if SLN is positive, then the axillary node dissection can be completed in one surgical procedure. However, the combination of frozen section and touch imprint cytology has a false negative rate of >80% for metastases <2 mm in size, which represent 36% of the metastases in SLN. The other major issue is the use of serial hematoxylin and eosin (H&E)-stained sections and immunohistochemistry (IHC) with antibodies to keratin in postoperative evaluation. IHC can identify an additional 11% cases after serial H&E. Using exhaustive measures, Dowlatshahi et al. (24) reported an SLN-positive rate of 83% in pT1a breast cancers. This finding suggests that micrometastases, particularly single or isolated small clusters of cancer cells in SLN, may not be clinically important.

SLN biopsy without axillary dissection has not yet been shown to yield disease-free and overall survival rates equivalent to those of axillary dissection to endorse the newer procedure in routine practice. Some of these issues may be answered by the results of two large prospective clinical trials (ACSOG Z-0011 and NSABP B-31). At this time, the practice of SLN biopsy should be considered as an alternative procedure for some patients, and the use of special techniques to evaluate SLN should be restricted to research protocols. The technique of identifying SLN biopsy has been validated (category A) but there is too much inconsistency in the studies regarding pathological evaluation of SLN to make any recommendations about the use of SLN status as a prognostic factor.

Histological Subtype

Special types of invasive breast cancers were recognized nearly 100 years ago (25,26). Later studies have found that several of these are associated with favorable prognosis. Those types that have consistently been shown to have excellent prognosis include tubular and mucinous carcinomas (27,28)—the prognosis of women with T1N0 lesions and these two types of breast cancers is similar to that of general population (29). Two other special types (i.e., lobular and medullary carcinomas) have slightly better prognosis than breast cancer NOS (ductal) (11). However, strict diagnostic criteria need to be applied when diagnosing these special types of breast cancers, because the prognostic value is likely to be diminished without this exercise. Despite the fact that there are some reproducibility issues (30–32), subtyping of invasive breast cancer is recommended as a category A factor.

Histological Grading

Greenhough, working at the Massachusetts General Hospital in Boston in the 1920s, was the first to evaluate histological grading, and all modern methods stem from his original work (33). Histological grade is based on the evaluation of gland formation, cell and nuclear size, variation in the size both of cells and nuclei, nuclear hyperchromatism, and number of mitoses. Using these features, a number of grading systems have been proposed; some of the most important ones are Scarff, Black's nuclear grade, Fisher, Scarff-Bloom-Richardson, and the Nottingham combined histological grade (NCHG) (34–38). Nuclear grade and mitotic activity are the two most important components of these grading systems (39). The most widely used grading system for breast cancer is the Scarff-Bloom-Richardson (SBR) classification used in Europe and Australia, and recently in the United States. This system is often used in modified version, such as the Nottingham prognostic index, which combines histological grade with node status and tumor size.

Tumor grading is a subjective evaluation with issues of reproducibility (1). This is highlighted by the wide variation in the proportion of each grade in published series (40), as well as from the SEER Program, in which only 25.1% of breast tumors were graded (41). Nevertheless, a study using a modified Bloom-Richardson (B-R) scheme on a single slide from 10 invasive breast cancers submitted to 25 pathologists from six separate groups, indicated that reproducibility of grading breast cancers can probably be achieved when a histological grading scheme with specified guidelines is used (42,43). Interobserver reproducibility means that some clinicians are reluctant to use histological grading in patient management.

Irrespective of this problem, numerous studies have demonstrated the importance of tumor grade, especially high grades, in predicting disease-free interval (DFI) and long-term survival (OS) (35,37–39,41,44–47). Survival analysis of 22,616 cases of breast cancer listed in the SEER Program of the National Cancer Institute (48) revealed that histological grade in conjunction with stage of disease could improve the prediction of outcome. The College of American Pathologists has recommended Nottingham Combined Histological Grade (NCHG) (49) and some recent publications have indeed demonstrated that NCHG is an independent prognostic and predictive factor (50,51).

Based on evidence, histological grade is a category A factor, which should be documented in every breast cancer. NCHG is the recommended system.

Estrogen and Progesterone Receptors

Estrogen receptor (ER) is a nuclear transcription factor that regulates expression of genes, such as pS2, progesterone receptor (PgR), and bcl2 apoptosis inhibitor. For example, the presence of PgR in a tumor is an indicator of an intact estrogen-response pathway and suggests that ER is present and functional (52). ER and PgR levels are strongly inversely correlated with measures of proliferation (53), and directly related to histological grade. ER and PgR determinations are established prognostic and predictive factors in the routine management of patients with breast cancer, but today they are assessed primarily as predictive factors for response to therapeutic and adjuvant hormonal therapy (54,55).

Numerous studies and the EBCTCG (Early Breast Cancer Trialists Collaborative Group) overview of all tamoxifen trials have also correlated ER status with response to adjuvant hormonal therapy (56,57). Women with ER-positive tumors derive significant benefit from 5 years of tamoxifen treatment with reduction in the odds of recurrence (40% to 50% annual reduction) and death, whereas those with ER-negative tumors do not. The benefit is the greatest when the ER level is over 100 fmol/mg protein. The value of PgR in predicting benefit from tamoxifen in the adjuvant setting has been less well studied. Data from the last meta-analysis shows that PgR is not so powerful as ER in predicting benefit from adjuvant hormonal therapy and knowledge of its status does not provide much additional information (56).

Both ER and PgR status predict response to therapeutic hormonal therapy in metastatic breast cancer (58–62). Overall results indicate that 50% to 60% of all patients with ER-positive tumors benefit from first-line hormone therapy, compared to 5% to 10% of patients with ER-negative tumors. Among patients with ER-positive metastatic breast cancer, PgR provides additional predictive power for response to hormonal therapy (52,58,59,63,64).

As a prognostic factor, ER status may be a time-dependent variable; as follow-up time lengthens, the advantage of ER positivity in terms of relapse and death decreases and ultimately disappears (65–70). The value of PgR status as a prognostic factor is more doubtful. Some evidence supports its usefulness (46,71,72), whereas other data do not (73). In multivariate analysis of node-negative patients, ER and PgR are equal predictors of clinical outcomes. However, ER status is more closely associated with disease-free survival, and PgR is more associated with overall survival (1).

Most studies conducted during the past 2 decades used ligand-binding assay to detect ER or PgR in tumor specimens and have established this technique as a validated methodology. Recently IHC has been proposed as an alternative method to determine steroid receptor levels and in fact all North American laboratories offer only IHC testing. Several comparative studies have been performed. For ER, the reported correlation between the two methods ranges from 70% to 90% (59,73–79) while for PgR determination it is somewhat weaker, ranging from 70% to 80% (59,80–82). The clinical validation of ER by IHC is promising but at best mediocre for PgR (83).

The primary reason is lack of technical validation of IHC. With few exceptions (84,85), most studies that have evaluated the prognostic and predictive value of ER and PgR by IHC have used frozen tissue, primary antibodies of variable sensitivity and specificity, subjective interpretation, and variable cutoff to define positivity (83). This has resulted is a very high error rate (86,87) and it is nearly impossible to compare these studies to make recommendations (88).

Evaluation of receptor status by ligand-binding assay is an established parameter (category A). At least some studies that have used standardized IHC methodology suggest an equivalent or even better technique (84,89). Additional studies are needed to validate IHC for routine assay (1).

*c-erbB2 (HER-2/*neu)

The proto-oncogene HER-2/*neu* (c-erbB-2) has been localized to chromosome 17q and encodes a trans-membrane tyrosine kinase growth factor receptor. Amplification of HER-2/*neu* gene or overexpression of the HER-2/*neu* protein is found in 10% to 34% of breast cancers. High HER-2/*neu* in breast cancer is associated with high histological grade (90,91). Since protein expression of HER-2/*neu* correlates well with gene amplification (92–95), many studies measured expression of the Her-2/neu protein product rather than gene amplification. Both immunoblotting and IHC have been used to measure HER 2/*neu* protein levels. The two methods have been compared in a large series of patients with 95% concordance (96).

The first studies measured HER-2/*neu* gene amplification and found that it is predictive of poorer disease-free and overall survival in node positive patients but seldom in node-negative subgroups (94,97–104). Most recent studies assessed HER-2/*neu* protein expression by IHC

(1,83,105). The results were similar to those seen in gene amplification studies. Ravdin and Chamness reviewed the published literature and concluded that the interpretation of studies on the use of this gene and its protein product as prognostic and predictive test for breast cancer is complicated by multiple methods and inherent difficulties in many studies (106). Deficiencies in the design of the studies, different definitions for scoring HER2/*neu* positivity and lack of a widely accepted standard methodology for detection are largely responsible for unclear results (99,107).

Several reports, including those from cooperative group clinical trials (108–112), suggest that the prognostic significance of HER-2/*neu* protein levels is greatest in node-positive studies while little value is found in node-negative studies, suggesting that Her-2/*neu* may be a predictive factor. The general trend is that patients whose tumors have little or no detectable levels of HER-2/*neu* derive considerable benefit from CMF regimens, while patients whose tumors have amplified HER-2/*neu* genes or overexpress HER-2/*neu* protein do not benefit (110,113). Evidence is accumulating that an interaction exists between HER-2/neu expression and adjuvant doxorubicin (111,112,114, 115); patients with tumors negative for HER-2/*neu* had the same clinical outcome with or without the use of doxorubicin, but patients whose breast tumors expressed high c-erbB-2 benefited from dose-intensive CAF (114). The Southwest Oncology group study reported very similar results—CAF significantly improved disease-free survival in patient whose tumors overexpressed HER-2/*neu* (115). Some studies suggest that HER-2/*neu* overexpression may predict resistance to endocrine treatment (116–122) but two recently published studies of 1,716 patients and 1,611 patients, respectively, showed clearly that HER-2/*neu* status did not predict response to tamoxifen in ER-positive patients with early-stage breast cancer (123,124).

One of the most exciting areas in breast cancer treatment is the development of a humanized murine monoclonal antibody to Her-2/*neu*. Herceptin® alone or in combination is well tolerated and clinically active in patients with HER-2/*neu* overexpressing metastatic breast cancers. Herceptin® in these clinical trials has shown objective clinical response rates, which are higher in combination with chemotherapy (125,126), although attention to cardiac toxicity is necessary (127).

Lack of standardization of testing has led to conflicting results and controversy as to the value of HER-2/*neu* value in evaluating breast cancer patient prognosis and selection for therapeutic options. HER-2/*neu* testing is not yet routine for patients with newly diagnosed breast cancer and a conservative approach is warranted. Since Herceptin® has become available, the issue of reliable and reproducible methods to assess Her-2/*neu* status has become increasingly important. Recent approval of a few methods for both IHC and FISH by the U.S. FDA has further complicated this issue. These approvals are limited to prediction of response to Herceptin® in metastatic breast cancer and may not be applicable to other situations. In addition, this does not mean that other methodologies used in the previous studies are not valid. At this time, it is difficult to make any recommendations for this marker. It appears that the most important aspect of HER2/*neu* is the prediction of response to Herceptin® therapy, and results of larger clinical trials such as NSABP B-32, BCIRG 006 and EORTC/BIG studies are awaited to guide in identifying the predictive role of HER2/*neu* in early-stage breast cancer.

Proliferation Index

Assessment of proliferative activity is one of many promising prognostic factors. High proliferation rates have been found to be associated with poor clinical outcome (1). Several methods have been utilized, including mitotic index, S-phase fraction (SPF) by DNA flow cytometry, thymidine-labeling index, BrdU index, IHC using a variety of markers (antibodies include anti-Ki-67, MIB-1, Ki-S5, and Ki-S11), proliferating cell nuclear antigen (PCNA), topoisomerase II alpha (Ki-S1), mitosin, and Ki-S2 (1,83,128–131). Mitotic index,

SPF and IHC using Ki-67 and MIB-1, are the best characterized.

Mitotic Index

Mitotic index (MI), defined as the number of mitotic figures in a given area of tumor such as 10 microscope fields or 1,000 cells or a specified area, is an accepted means of estimating tumor cell proliferation. Combined with other histopathological features, it represents an integral part of the Nottingham combined histological grade (38,132).

In nearly 30 studies, looking at more than 12,000 patients, there is a unanimous correlation of high MI with decreased DFS and/or OS (39,47,50,51,133–154). Multivariate analysis has shown correlation of high mitotic rates with poor clinical outcomes. Clayton analyzed 378 node-negative breast carcinomas without and showed that high mitotic count was the best single predictor of poor outcome—patients with more than 4.5 mitotic figures per 10 high-power fields had 2.8 fold increased risk of death (135). MI has been evaluated in at least three randomized clinical trials with similar results (50,51,153).

A prospective study on the reproducibility of the mitotic activity index, which included 2,469 patients and 14 pathology laboratories throughout the Netherlands, provided correlation coefficients between 0.91 and 0.97 (mean, 0.96). The reproducibility was also fairly constant over time (155).

Although the methods of calculating MI and the cut-off to define low versus high MI may vary, it appears to be a simple and cost-effective method of measuring proliferation rate, and provides similar if not better information than other more costly and time demanding methods (50,149).

S-phase Fraction (SPF) by DNA Flow Cytometry

SPF is derived by DNA flow cytometry, measuring DNA content in each cell to produce a DNA histogram, from which DNA ploidy and the fraction of cells synthesizing DNA can be assessed.

DNA flow cytometry has shown consistent correlations between high SPF and poor clinical outcome. A consensus conference (156) that reviewed 43 published papers supported an association between high S-phase fraction and increased risk of recurrence and death for patients with node-negative and -positive invasive breast cancer. Wenger and Clark (157) reviewed 273 published articles on S-phase fraction determined by flow cytometry published in the past decade. They concluded that there was considerable variability among laboratories regarding assay methodology, cell-cycle analysis techniques, and cutpoints for classifying and interpreting SPF. However, correlations between SPF and other prognostic markers were relatively consistent across studies; higher SPF was generally associated with worse tumor grade, absence of steroid receptors, larger tumors, and positive axillary lymph nodes. Higher SPF was generally associated with worse disease-free and overall survival both in univariate and multivariate analyses. In large studies of node-negative patients with long-term follow-up (158–167), multivariate analyses confirm that SPF provides independent prognostic information.

Regarding the predictive value of SPF, Remkos et al. (168) reported that in 60 previously untreated, early-stage premenopausal patients, tumor responsiveness to neoadjuvant chemotherapy was directly related to SPF. However, Dressler et al. (163) analyzed tumors from node-negative patients enrolled in a large randomized intergroup study comparing CMF regimen and observation and found therapy was equally effective for patients with either low or high S-phase fraction.

Measurement of SPF has clinical utility for patients with breast cancer, but standardization and quality control needs to be improved. Recent advances in analysis of SPF data from different laboratories suggest that some of the technical issues can be resolved (169). SPF measured on frozen tissue, using optimized technique and cut-off, may potentially be a useful prognostic marker, at least in a subset of patients in which other factors are equivocal in defining risk of relapse or death (170).

Ki-67 Proliferation Index by IHC

Measurement of proliferation by IHC is mostly done on frozen sections using Ki-67 antibody, and on paraffin sections using MIB-1 antibody. Both antibodies appear to measure the same proliferation-related protein. For other IHC methods, readers are referred to studies in the introduction to "Proliferation Index." Several studies used Ki-67 on frozen sections and most reported a significant relationship (mostly by univariate analysis) between their results and clinical outcome (83). There is a suggestion that MIB-1 on paraffin sections may provide better results than Ki-67 on frozen sections (171,172) and since most laboratories assessing proliferation by IHC today use paraffin sections, the remaining discussion is focused on studies that have used MIB-1 antibody on fixed tissue. In 24 studies, looking at a total of more than 6,000 patients, 22 have shown a significant correlation between high MIB-1 index and shorter DFS or OS by univariate analysis (128,149, 152,153,171–190). Eighteen of the 22 studies performed multivariate analyses, but only 9 studies confirmed its significance (128,149, 173,175,176,180,184–186). However, the limitations of these studies are the technical variables leading to varied sensitivities and cut-offs ranging from >1% to 25%. Compared to SPF, there is still a relative lack of level 1 evidence for use of MIB-1 proliferation index for clinical prognosis. Use of this marker in randomized clinical trials, with a uniform cut-off, may replace flow cytometry SPF measurement, which requires relatively expensive equipment.

Proliferation index is a useful and potentially important prognostic and predictive factor. SPF on frozen sections is the most validated technique and is recommended as a category A factor. MI and MIB-1 index by IHC are not thoroughly validated and are recommended as category B factors.

Tumor Suppressor Gene p53

The p53 tumor suppressor gene is located on 17p13 and encodes a 53-kD nuclear phosphoprotein. Alterations in this gene are the most frequent genetic changes reported in many malignancies, including breast cancer (191). Nearly one third of breast cancers have mutation of the p53 gene (192–194). Techniques to measure p53 overexpression/mutation include IHC, based on the prolonged half-life of mutated p53, or PCR-based amplification with screening using single-strand conformation polymorphism assays (SSCP) and sequencing. Most p53 abnormalities occur as spontaneous somatic events, although recent evidence suggests a relationship between BRCA1 and p53 in hereditary breast cancer, with p53 acting as a cancer-inducing cofactor in these patients (195).

IHC is the most commonly employed method, and studies using this technique have shown that overexpression of p53 seems to be relatively independent of axillary node and menopausal status, weakly related to tumor size, and strongly associated with DNA ploidy, other measures of proliferation, steroid receptors and nuclear grade (192,194,196–198). All these studies included node-negative patients who received no systemic adjuvant therapy. Overall they suggest that p53 combined with other prognostic factors appears to be a modestly effective marker to identify node-negative breast cancer patients at high risk for early disease recurrence and/or death, for whom the use of adjuvant chemotherapy may thus be justified.

Elledge and Allred (199) reviewed 13,000 patients from 57 studies and concluded that the inactivation of p53 appears to lead to a more aggressive breast cancer phenotype and a worse clinical outcome, with risk of recurrence and death increasing by ≥50% if p53 is abnormal. Lack of unanimity of results may be due to differences in technique, study design and variety of treatment, or population. At least 13 different monoclonal antibodies induced by the product of the human p53 are available. Elledge et al. (200) evaluated five different antibodies and mutations detected by SSCP in 169 patients. The p53 staining rates for the different antibodies ranged from 18% to 36%.

Two studies provide evidence that radiation therapy may be more beneficial in preventing local breast cancer relapse, in patients with node-negative tumors that express elevated levels of p53 (201,202). However a randomized trial of 329 patients with breast cancer treated with neoadjuvant FAC chemotherapy or by radiotherapy prior to surgery found no correlation between p53 staining and response to treatment (203). Two clinical trials suggested that patients with overexpression of p53 may benefit from a CMF regimen (204,205), while another clinical trial concluded that, in a node-negative breast tumor population, alteration of p53 does not predict response to this chemotherapy (206). Thor et al. reported that both p53 and HER-2/neu overexpression might be associated with increased survival after high-dose CAF (114). No positive relationship between p53 abnormalities and response to other types of chemotherapy has been found.

There is category A evidence that p53 overexpression predicts poor clinical outcome in the untreated setting. The evidence about p53 as a predictive factor falls in level 2 and is controversial. Lack of consensus on the best methodology to assess p53 alterations and presence of other more useful factors has prevented the use of p53 in routine clinical practice.

Angiogenesis

Cancer requires an adequate blood supply to grow, invade, and develop metastases. Several reports have proposed that assessing microvessel density (MVD) in tumors might provide prognostic information for predicting distant disease recurrence (207). The most commonly employed method is IHC using antibodies to Factor VIII-related antigen (208), CD31 or CD34, type IV collagen, or laminin. These reagents have widely differing sensitivities and specificities (209,210).

Investigators have shown a strong association between high vascular density and poor clinical outcome (211–217). MVD seems to be an independent predictor of disease-free and overall survival in node-negative and -positive patients (198,209,216). Most studies, however, had small numbers of patients with mixed stage and treatment and relatively short follow-up (105). Axelsson et al. (218) also found that measurement of MVD was too variable to be clinically useful, and definitions of high vascularity have been largely arbitrary rather than determined by their relationship to clinical outcome.

At this time, assessment of angiogenesis by MVD is not an established marker (category B/C). Well-designed studies following recommended methodology from international consensus conference are needed (210). Techniques which focus on assessment of neovascularization, such as antibodies specific to proliferating vessels, pro- and anti-angiogenic factors, and methods assessing *in vivo* tumor blood flow, such as Doppler ultrasound, are areas of future research (219). An attractive feature of angiogenesis is that it may offer a target for novel therapeutic interventions. Several antiangiogenic agents, including enzymes that control the vascularization process, steroids and steroid-related substances, antibiotics and synthetic antibiotic derivatives and specific immunotherapies, have been tested in both animal models and human trials (220). Successful regimens may have their greatest efficacy early in the course of the disease, most likely in the adjuvant setting.

Epidermal Growth Factor Receptor (EGFR)

EGFR is a 170-kD transmembrane tyrosine kinase activated by both epidermal growth factor and transforming growth factor-α (221). EGFR has been measured by several methods, including radioligand-binding assays, autoradiography, IHC, immunoenzymatic assays, and measurement of EGFR transcripts; no clear difference is seen among the different assay techniques. EGFR has been reported to be overexpressed in 40% to 50% of breast carcinomas, particularly those with a poor prognostic phenotype (222,223).

Studies have generally reported a correlation between EGFR and absence of steroid receptor status, and worse tumor grade and high proliferation indices (224–230). Recent studies suggest EGFR positivity may be correlated with overexpression of abnormal p53 and angiogenesis. These studies have provided mixed results about the prognostic significance of EGFR overexpression, only some showing correlation with a poor disease-free survival (222,224,229,231–241).

Several groups have shown that tumors expressing EGFR are more like to be resistant to endocrine therapy. Conversely, EGFR-negative tumors, especially if they are also ER positive, tend to have higher response rates (242,243). In a clinical trial of 1,716 high-risk postmenopausal breast cancer patients randomly assigned to treatment with tamoxifen or to observation, Knoop et al. did not find support for the hypothesis that EGFR status predicts benefit from tamoxifen treatment in estrogen receptor-positive patients with early stage disease (123).

The prognostic and predictive value of EGFR is unclear and this factor falls in category C at present. The most exciting reason to measure EGFR in breast cancer today is its potential use as a target for new therapies (244–247). Several monoclonal antibodies directed against EGFR are under evaluation in breast cancer patients (246) as are clinical trials testing tyrosine kinase inhibitors such as ZD 1839 in metastatic breast cancer patients that are either ongoing or being planned (for more information go to http://cancertrials.nci.nih.gov).

SUMMARY

Early-Stage Breast Cancer

Selection of therapy should be based upon knowledge of an individual's risk of tumor recurrence balanced against the short-term and long-term risks of adjuvant treatment. This approach should help clinicians to aid individuals in determining whether the anticipated gains are reasonable for their particular situation. Treatment options need to be modified based upon both patient and tumor characteristics.

Nodal status and the number of nodes involved remain the strongest variables in estimating risk of relapse. Women with more than four positive lymph nodes are universally considered higher-risk patients. For patients with node-negative disease, tumor size, histological grade, and steroid hormone-receptor status are the main factors considered to define groups with differential prognosis for use in treatment selection. Traditionally, certain uncommon histological types (tubular, medullary, and mucinous)

TABLE 28.2. *Summary of recommendations for prognostic and predictive factors in breast cancer*

Factor	Recommendation category[a]	Comment
Lymph node status	A	Established factor
Tumor size	A	Established factor
Sentinel lymph node status	0	Surgical technique is validated but pathological evaluation is inconsistent
Histological subtype	A	
Histological grading	A	Nottingham combined histological grading system is recommended
Hormone receptors	A/B	As measured by ligand binding assay. The use of IHC needs more studies, particularly for PgR
c-erbB2 (HER-2/*neu*)	0	Inconsistent results, except for limited number of studies in patients treated with Herceptin. There are several technical validation issues about the techniques, i.e., IHC vs. FISH and appropriate cut-off
Mitotic index	B	
S-phase fraction	A	As assessed by flow cytometry on frozen tissue
Ki-67 proliferation index	B	Technical validation issues, particularly in regards to cut-off to define low vs. high index
p53	A	As a prognostic factor, however, it is not very useful
	0	As a predictive factor
Angiogenesis	B/C	Several technical validation issues. Potentially useful to predict response to targeted therapy
EGFR	C	Inconsistent results. Potentially useful to predict response to targeted therapy

[a]Based on guidelines for evidence based medicine (see text).
EGFR, epidermal growth factor receptor; FISH, florescent *in situ* hybridization; IHC, immunohistochemistry; PgR, progesterone receptor.

have also been associated with favorable prognosis and may be considered as low-risk factors. Some additional tumor characteristics that may eventually prove helpful in the prognosis of node-negative disease include tumor proliferative fraction (S-phase) and the level of HER-2/*neu* expression.

The level of evidence that exists for these factors is reviewed and the recommendations based on EBM criteria are summarized in Table 28.2.

Metastatic Breast Cancer

The most important prognostic factors for patients with metastatic disease are the extent of disease at time of recurrence, the site(s) of recurrence, disease-free interval, performance status, and response to prior metastatic therapy. Cytological or histological documentation of recurrent or metastatic disease should be obtained whenever required for certainty of diagnosis or when predictive factors can be identified that influence choice of therapy. ER/ PgR status, and HER2/*neu* overexpression/amplification in the primary tumor are factors for predicting the response to hormonal and Herceptin® therapies respectively. These two factors remain the only predictive factors widely available and used both routinely and for clinical research trials, in the therapy of breast cancer whatever the disease stage.

Acknowledgment: This work was supported by NIH Grants P01-CA30195 and P50-CA58183.

REFERENCES

1. Clark G. Prognostic and predictive factors. In: Harris JR LM, Morrow M, Hellman S, eds. *Diseases of the breast.* Philadelphia: Lippincott-Raven, 2000:489–514.
2. Clark GM. Do we really need prognostic factors for breast cancer? *Breast Cancer Res Treat* 1994;30(2):117–126.
3. McGuire WL. Breast cancer prognostic factors: evaluation guidelines. *J Natl Cancer Inst* 1991;83(3):154–155.
4. Gasparini G, Pozza F, Harris AL. Evaluating the potential usefulness of new prognostic and predictive indicators in node-negative breast cancer patients. *J Natl Cancer Inst* 1993;85(15):1206–1219.
5. Hayes DF, Bast RC, Desch CE, et al. Tumor marker utility grading system: a framework to evaluate clinical utility of tumor markers. *J Natl Cancer Inst* 1996;88(20):1456–1466.
6. Hayes DF, Trock B, Harris AL. Assessing the clinical impact of prognostic factors: when is "statistically significant" clinically useful? *Breast Cancer Res Treat* 1998;52(1–3):305–319.
7. Sackett DL, Rosenberg WM, Gray JA, et al. Evidence based medicine: what it is and what it isn't. *BMJ* 1996;312(7023):71–72.
8. Goldbloom R, Battista RN. The periodic health examination: 1. Introduction. *CMAJ* 1986;134(7):721–723.
9. Harris RP, Helfand M, Woolf SH, et al. Current methods of the U.S. Preventive Services Task Force. A review of the process. *Am J Prev Med* 2001;20(3 suppl):21–35.
10. Russo J, Frederick J, Ownby HE, et al. Predictors of recurrence and survival of patients with breast cancer. *Am J Clin Pathol* 1987;88(2):123–131.
11. Fisher ER, Anderson S, Redmond C, Fisher B. Pathologic findings from the National Surgical Adjuvant Breast Project protocol B-06. 10-year pathologic and clinical prognostic discriminants. *Cancer* 1993;71(8):2507–2514.
12. Saez RA, McGuire WL, Clark GM. Prognostic factors in breast cancer. *Semin Surg Oncol* 1989;5(2):102–110.
13. Mittra I, MacRae KD. A meta-analysis of reported correlations between prognostic factors in breast cancer: does axillary lymph node metastasis represent biology or chronology? *Eur J Cancer* 1991;27(12):1574–1583.
14. Cabanes PA, Salmon RJ, Vilcoq JR, et al. Value of axillary dissection in addition to lumpectomy and radiotherapy in early breast cancer. The Breast Carcinoma Collaborative Group of the Institut Curie. *Lancet* 1992;339(8804):1245–1248.
15. Ravdin PM, De Laurentiis M, Vendely T, Clark GM. Prediction of axillary lymph node status in breast cancer patients by use of prognostic indicators. *J Natl Cancer Inst* 1994;86(23):1771–1775.
16. Carter CL, Allen C, Henson DE. Relation of tumor size, lymph node status, and survival in 24,740 breast cancer cases. *Cancer* 1989;63(1):181–187.
17. Fisher ER, Costantino J, Fisher B, Redmond C. Pathologic findings from the National Surgical Adjuvant Breast Project (Protocol 4). Discriminants for 15-year survival. National Surgical Adjuvant Breast and Bowel Project Investigators. *Cancer* 1993;71(6 suppl):2141–2150.
18. Rosen PP, Groshen S, Kinne DW, Norton L. Factors influencing prognosis in node-negative breast carcinoma: analysis of 767 T1N0M0/T2N0M0 patients with long-term follow-up. *J Clin Oncol* 1993;11(11):2090–2100.
19. Adair F, Berg J, Joubert L, Robbins GF. Long-term followup of breast cancer patients: the 30-year report. *Cancer* 1974;33(4):1145–1150.
20. McGuire WL, Clark GM. Prognostic factors and treatment decisions in axillary-node-negative breast cancer. *N Engl J Med* 1992;326(26):1756–1761.
21. Funke I, Schraut W. Meta-analyses of studies on bone marrow micrometastases: an independent prognostic impact remains to be substantiated. *J Clin Oncol* 1998;16(2):557–566.
22. Braun S, Pantel K. Clinical significance of occult metastatic cells in bone marrow of breast cancer patients. *Oncologist* 2001;6(2):125–132.
23. Krag D, Weaver D, Ashikaga T, et al. The sentinel node in breast cancer—a multicenter validation study. *N Engl J Med* 1998;339(14):941–946.

24. Dowlatshahi K, Fan M, Bloom KJ, et al. Occult metastases in the sentinel lymph nodes of patients with early stage breast carcinoma: A preliminary study. *Cancer* 1999;86(6):990–996.
25. McDivitt RW, Boyce W, Gersell D. Tubular carcinoma of the breast. *Am J Surg Pathol* 1982;6:401–411.
26. Ewing J. *Neoplastic diseases,* 1st ed. Philadelphia: Saunders, 1919.
27. Pinder SE, Wlston CW, Ellis IO. Invasive carcinoma—usual histological types. In: Elston CW, Ellis IO, eds. *The breast,* 3rd ed. Edinburgh: Churchill Livingstone, 1998:283–337.
28. Schnitt SJ, Guidi AJ. Pathology and biological markers of invasive breast cancer. In: Harris JR, Lippman ME, Morrow M, Osborne CK, eds. *Diseases of the breast,* 2nd ed. Philadelphia: Lippincott Williams & Wilkins, 2000:425–449.
29. Diab SG, Clark GM, Osborne CK, et al. Tumor characteristics and clinical outcome of tubular and mucinous breast carcinomas. *J Clin Oncol* 1999;17(5):1442–1448.
30. Gaffey MJ, Mills SE, Frierson HF Jr, et al. Medullary carcinoma of the breast: interobserver variability in histopathologic diagnosis. *Mod Pathol* 1995;8(1):31–38.
31. Cutler SJ, Black MM, Friedell GH, et al. Prognostic factors in cancer of the female breast. II. Reproducibility of histopathologic classification. *Cancer* 1966;19(1):75–82.
32. Sloane JP, Ellman R, Anderson TJ, et al. Consistency of histopathological reporting of breast lesions detected by screening: findings of the U.K. National External Quality Assessment (EQA) Scheme. U. K. National Coordinating Group for Breast Screening Pathology. *Eur J Cancer* 1994;30A(10):1414–1419.
33. Greenhough RB. Varying degress of malignancy in cancer of the breast. *J Cancer Res* 1925;9:452–463.
34. Scarff RW, Torioni H. Histological typing of breast tumors. In: Organization WH, ed. *International histological classification of tumors.* Geneva: 1968:13–20.
35. Black MM, Opler SR, Speer FD. Survival in breast cancer cases in relation to structure of the primary tumor and regional lymph nodes. *Surg Gynecol Obstet* 1955;100:543–551.
36. Fisher ER, Gregorio RM, Fisher B, et al. The pathology of invasive breast cancer. A syllabus derived from findings of the National Surgical Adjuvant Breast Project (protocol no. 4). *Cancer* 1975;36(1):1–85.
37. Bloom HJG, Richardson WW. Histological grading and prognosis in breast cancer: a study of 1409 cases of which 359 have been followed for 15 years. *Br J Cancer* 1957;11:359.
38. Elston CW, Ellis IO. Pathological prognostic factors in breast cancer. I. The value of histological grade in breast cancer: experience from a large study with long-term follow-up. *Histopathology* 1991;19(5):403–410.
39. Le Doussal V, Tubiana-Hulin M, Friedman S, et al. Prognostic value of histologic grade nuclear components of Scarff-Bloom-Richardson (SBR). An improved score modification based on a multivariate analysis of 1262 invasive ductal breast carcinomas. *Cancer* 1989;64(9):1914–1921.
40. Elston CW, Ellis IO. Assessment of histological grade. In: *Systemic pathology. The breast.* Edinburgh: Churchill Livingstone, 1998:365–384.
41. Henson DE, Ries L, Freedman LS, Carriaga M. Relationship among outcome, stage of disease, and histologic grade for 22,616 cases of breast cancer. The basis for a prognostic index. *Cancer* 1991;68(10):2142–2149.
42. Dalton LW, Page DL, Dupont WD. Histologic grading of breast carcinoma. A reproducibility study. *Cancer* 1994;73(11):2765–2770.
43. Dalton LW, Pinder SE, Elston CE, et al. Histologic grading of breast cancer: linkage of patient outcome with level of pathologist agreement. *Mod Pathol* 2000;13(7):730–735.
44. Davis BW, Gelber RD, Goldhirsch A, et al. Prognostic significance of tumor grade in clinical trials of adjuvant therapy for breast cancer with axillary lymph node metastasis. *Cancer* 1986;58(12):2662–2670.
45. Contesso G, Mouriesse H, Friedman S, et al. The importance of histologic grade in long-term prognosis of breast cancer: a study of 1,010 patients, uniformly treated at the Institut Gustave-Roussy. *J Clin Oncol* 1987;5(9):1378–1386.
46. Fisher B, Redmond C, Fisher ER, Caplan R. Relative worth of estrogen or progesterone receptor and pathologic characteristics of differentiation as indicators of prognosis in node negative breast cancer patients: findings from National Surgical Adjuvant Breast and Bowel Project Protocol B-06. *J Clin Oncol* 1988;6(7):1076–1087.
47. Schumacher M, Schmoor C, Sauerbrei W, et al. The prognostic effect of histological tumor grade in node-negative breast cancer patients. *Breast Cancer Res Treat* 1993;25(3):235–245.
48. Henson DE. The histological grading of neoplasms. *Arch Pathol Lab Med* 1988;112(11):1091–1096.
49. Fitzgibbons PL, Page DL, Weaver D, et al. Prognostic factors in breast cancer. College of American Pathologists Consensus Statement 1999. *Arch Pathol Lab Med* 2000;124(7):966–978.
50. Page DL, Gray R, Allred DC, et al. Prediction of node-negative breast cancer outcome by histologic grading and S-phase analysis by flow cytometry: an Eastern Cooperative Oncology Group Study (2192). *Am J Clin Oncol* 2001;24(1):10–18.
51. Simpson JF, Gray R, Dressler LG, et al. Prognostic value of histologic grade and proliferative activity in axillary node-positive breast cancer: results from the Eastern Cooperative Oncology Group Companion Study, EST 4189. *J Clin Oncol* 2000;18(10):2059–2069.
52. Horwitz KB, McGuire WL, Pearson OH, et al. Predicting response to endocrine therapy in human breats cancer. *Science* 1975;189:726–727.
53. Wenger CR, Beardslee S, Owens MA, et al. DNA ploidy, S-phase, and steroid receptors in more than 127,000 breast cancer patients. *Breast Cancer Res Treat* 1993;28(1):9–20.
54. Pertschuk LP, Kim DS, Nayer K, et al. Immunocytochemical estrogen and progestin receptor assays in breast cancer with monoclonal antibodies. Histopathologic, demographic, and biochemical correlations and relationship to endocrine response and survival. *Cancer* 1990;66(8):1663–1670.
55. Pertschuk LP, Feldman JG, Kim YD, et al. Estrogen receptor immunocytochemistry in paraffin embedded tissues with ER1D5 predicts breast cancer endocrine response more accurately than H222Sp gamma in

frozen sections or cytosol-based ligand-binding assays. *Cancer* 1996;77(12):2514–2519.
56. Anonymous. Tamoxifen for early breast cancer: an overview of the randomised trials. Early Breast Cancer Trialists' Collaborative Group. *Lancet* 1998; 351(9114):1451–1467.
57. Anonymous. Adjuvant tamoxifen in the management of operable breast cancer: the Scottish Trial. Report from the Breast Cancer Trials Committee, Scottish Cancer Trials Office (MRC), Edinburgh. *Lancet* 1987; 2(8552):171–175.
58. Ravdin PM, Green S, Dorr TM, et al. Prognostic significance of progesterone receptor levels in estrogen receptor-positive patients with metastatic breast cancer treated with tamoxifen: results of a prospective Southwest Oncology Group study. *J Clin Oncol* 1992; 10(8):1284–1291.
59. Elledge RM, Green S, Pugh R, et al. Estrogen receptor (ER) and progesterone receptor (PgR), by ligand-binding assay compared with ER, PgR and pS2, by immuno-histochemistry in predicting response to tamoxifen in metastatic breast cancer: a Southwest Oncology Group Study. *Int J Cancer* 2000;89(2):111–117.
60. Bezwoda WR, Esser JD, Dansey R, et al. The value of estrogen and progesterone receptor determinations in advanced breast cancer. Estrogen receptor level but not progesterone receptor level correlates with response to tamoxifen. *Cancer* 1991;68(4):867–872.
61. Manni A, Arafah B, Pearson OH. Estrogen and progesterone receptors in the prediction of response of breast cancer to endocrine therapy. *Cancer* 1980; 46(12 suppl):2838–2841.
62. Robertson JF, Bates K, Pearson D, et al. Comparison of two oestrogen receptor assays in the prediction of the clinical course of patients with advanced breast cancer. *Br J Cancer* 1992;65(5):727–730.
63. Pertschuk LP, Feldman JG, Eisenberg KB, et al. Immunocytochemical detection of progesterone receptor in breast cancer with monoclonal antibody. Relation to biochemical assay, disease-free survival, and clinical endocrine response. *Cancer* 1988;62(2):342–349.
64. Gross GE, Clark GM, Chamness GC, McGuire WL. Multiple progesterone receptor assays in human breast cancer. *Cancer Res* 1984;44(2):836–840.
65. Adami HO, Graffman S, Lindgren A, Sallstrom J. Prognostic implication of estrogen receptor content in breast cancer. *Breast Cancer Res Treat* 1985;5(3):293–300.
66. Mason BH, Holdaway IM, Mullins PR, et al. Progesterone and estrogen receptors as prognostic variables in breast cancer. *Cancer Res* 1983;43(6):2985–2990.
67. Aamdal S, Bormer O, Jorgensen O, et al. Estrogen receptors and long-term prognosis in breast cancer. *Cancer* 1984;53(11):2525–2529.
68. Hahnel R, Woodings T, Vivian AB. Prognostic value of estrogen receptors in primary breast cancer. *Cancer* 1979;44(2):671–675.
69. Hilsenbeck SG, Ravdin PM, de Moor CA, et al. Time-dependence of hazard ratios for prognostic factors in primary breast cancer. *Breast Cancer Res Treat* 1998; 52(1–3):227–237.
70. Coradini D, Daidone MG, Boracchi P, et al. Time-dependent relevance of steroid receptors in breast cancer. *J Clin Oncol* 2000;18(14):2702–2709.
71. Clark GM, McGuire WL, Hubay CA, et al. Progesterone receptors as a prognostic factor in stage II breast cancer. *N Engl J Med* 1983;309(22):1343–1347.
72. Huseby RA, Ownby HE, Brooks S, Russo J. Evaluation of the predictive power of progesterone receptor levels in primary breast cancer: a comparison with other criteria in 559 cases with a mean follow-up of 74.8 months. The Breast Cancer Prognostic Study Associates. *Henry Ford Hosp Med J* 1990;38(1):79–84.
73. Stierer M, Rosen H, Weber R, et al. A prospective analysis of immunohistochemically determined hormone receptors and nuclear features as predictors of early recurrence in primary breast cancer. *Breast Cancer Res Treat* 1995;36(1):11–21.
74. Allred DC, Bustamante MA, Daniel CO, et al. Immunocytochemical analysis of estrogen receptors in human breast carcinomas. Evaluation of 130 cases and review of the literature regarding concordance with biochemical assay and clinical relevance. *Arch Surg* 1990;125(1):107–113.
75. Molino A, Micciolo R, Turazza M, et al. Prognostic significance of estrogen receptors in 405 primary breast cancers: a comparison of immunohistochemical and biochemical methods. *Breast Cancer Res Treat* 1997;45(3):241–249.
76. Remmele W, Hildebrand U, Hienz HA, et al. Comparative histological, histochemical, immunohistochemical and biochemical studies on oestrogen receptors, lectin receptors, and Barr bodies in human breast cancer. *Virchows Arch A Pathol Anat Histopathol* 1986; 409(2):127–147.
77. Reiner A, Spona J, Reiner G, et al. Estrogen receptor analysis on biopsies and fine-needle aspirates from human breast carcinoma. Correlation of biochemical and immunohistochemical methods using monoclonal antireceptor antibodies. *Am J Pathol* 1986;125(3): 443–449.
78. Charpin C, Martin PM, De Victor B, et al. Multiparametric study (SAMBA 200) of estrogen receptor immunocytochemical assay in 400 human breast carcinomas: analysis of estrogen receptor distribution heterogeneity in tissues and correlations with dextran coated charcoal assays and morphological data. *Cancer Res* 1988;48(6):1578–1586.
79. Hanna W, Mobbs BG. Comparative evaluation of ER-ICA and enzyme immunoassay for the quantitation of estrogen receptors in breast cancer. *Am J Clin Pathol* 1989;91(2):182–186.
80. Gasparini G, Pozza F, Dittadi R, et al. Progesterone receptor determined by immunocytochemical and biochemical methods in human breast cancer. *J Cancer Res Clin Oncol* 1992;118(7):557–563.
81. Helin H, Isola J, Helle M, Koivula T. Discordant results between radioligand and immunohistochemical assays for steroid receptors in breast carcinoma. *Br J Cancer* 1990;62(1):109–112.
82. Reiner A, Neumeister B, Spona J, et al. Immunocytochemical localization of estrogen and progesterone receptor and prognosis in human primary breast cancer. *Cancer Res* 1990;50(21):7057–7061.
83. Allred DC, Harvey JM, Berardo M, Clark GM. Prognostic and predictive factors in breast cancer by immunohistochemical analysis. *Mod Pathol* 1998;11(2): 155–168.
84. Harvey JM, Clark GM, Osborne CK, Allred DC. Estrogen receptor status by immunohistochemistry is superior to the ligand-binding assay for predicting response to adjuvant endocrine therapy in breast cancer. *J Clin Oncol* 1999;17(5):1474–1481.

85. Rhodes A, Jasani B, Balaton AJ, et al. Frequency of oestrogen and progesterone receptor positivity by immunohistochemical analysis in 7016 breast carcinomas: correlation with patient age, assay sensitivity, threshold value, and mammographic screening. *J Clin Pathol* 2000;53(9):688–696.
86. Rhodes A, Jasani B, Balaton AJ, Miller KD. Immunohistochemical demonstration of oestrogen and progesterone receptors: correlation of standards achieved on in house tumours with that achieved on external quality assessment material in over 150 laboratories from 26 countries. *J Clin Pathol* 2000;53(4):292–301.
87. Rhodes A, Jasani B, Balaton AJ, et al. Study of interlaboratory reliability and reproducibility of estrogen and progesterone receptor assays in Europe. Documentation of poor reliability and identification of insufficient microwave antigen retrieval time as a major contributory element of unreliable assays. *Am J Clin Pathol* 2001;115(1):44–58.
88. Layfield LJ, Gupta D, Mooney EE. Assessment of tissue estrogen and progesterone receptor levels: a survey of current practice, techniques, and quantitation methods. *Breast J* 2000;6(3):189–196.
89. Barnes DM, Millis RR, Beex LV, et al. Increased use of immunohistochemistry for oestrogen receptor measurement in mammary carcinoma: the need for quality assurance. *Eur J Cancer* 1998;34(11):1677–1682.
90. Berger MS, Locher GW, Saurer S, et al. Correlation of c-erbB-2 gene amplification and protein expression in human breast carcinoma with nodal status and nuclear grading. *Cancer Res* 1988;48(5):1238–1243.
91. Tsuda H, Hirohashi S, Shimosato Y, et al. Correlation between histologic grade of malignancy and copy number of c-erbB-2 gene in breast carcinoma. A retrospective analysis of 176 cases. *Cancer* 1990;65(8):1794–1800.
92. Slamon DJ, Godolphin W, Jones LA, et al. Studies of the HER-2/neu proto-oncogene in human breast and ovarian cancer. *Science* 1989;244(4905):707–712.
93. Thor AD, Schwartz LH, Koerner FC, et al. Analysis of c-erbB-2 expression in breast carcinomas with clinical follow-up. *Cancer Res* 1989;49(24 Pt 1):7147–7152.
94. Borg A, Tandon AK, Sigurdsson H, et al. HER-2/neu amplification predicts poor survival in node-positive breast cancer. *Cancer Res* 1990;50(14):4332–4337.
95. Ciocca DR, Fujimura FK, Tandon AK, et al. Correlation of HER-2/ neu amplification with expression and with other prognostic factors in 1103 breast cancers. *J Natl Cancer Inst* 1992;84(16):1279–1282.
96. Molina R, Ciocca DR, Tandon AK, et al. Expression of HER-2/neu oncoprotein in human breast cancer: a comparison of immunohistochemical and western blot techniques. *Anticancer Res* 1992;12(6B):1965–1971.
97. Slamon DJ, Clark GM, Wong SG, et al. Human breast cancer: correlation of relapse and survival with amplification of the HER-2/neu oncogene. *Science* 1987;235(4785):177–182.
98. Ali IU, Campbell G, Lidereau R, Callahan R. Lack of evidence for the prognostic significance of c-erbB-2 amplification in human breast carcinoma. *Oncogene Res* 1988;3(2):139–146.
99. Press MF, Pike MC, Chazin VR, et al. Her-2/neu expression in node-negative breast cancer: direct tissue quantitation by computerized image analysis and association of overexpression with increased risk of recurrent disease. *Cancer Res* 1993;53(20):4960–4970.
100. Berns EM, Klijn JG, van Putten WL, et al. c-myc amplification is a better prognostic factor than HER2/neu amplification in primary breast cancer. *Cancer Res* 1992;52(5):1107–1113.
101. Clark GM, McGuire WL. Follow-up study of HER-2/neu amplification in primary breast cancer. *Cancer Res* 1991;51(3):944–948.
102. Paterson MC, Dietrich KD, Danyluk J, et al. Correlation between c-erbB-2 amplification and risk of recurrent disease in node-negative breast cancer. *Cancer Res* 1991;51(2):556–567.
103. Winstanley J, Cooke T, Murray GD, et al. The long term prognostic significance of c-erbB-2 in primary breast cancer. *Br J Cancer* 1991;63(3):447–450.
104. Tsuda H, Hirohashi S, Shimosato Y, et al. Immunohistochemical study on overexpression of c-erbB-2 protein in human breast cancer: its correlation with gene amplification and long-term survival of patients. *Jpn J Cancer Res* 1990;81(4):327–332.
105. Mohsin SK, Allred DC. Immunohistochemical biomarkers in breast cancer. *J Histotechnol* 1999;22(3):249–261.
106. Ravdin PM, Chamness GC. The c-erbB-2 proto-oncogene as a prognostic and predictive marker in breast cancer: a paradigm for the development of other macromolecular markers—a review. *Gene* 1995;159(1):19–27.
107. Press MF, Hung G, Godolphin W, Slamon DJ. Sensitivity of HER-2/neu antibodies in archival tissue samples: potential source of error in immunohistochemical studies of oncogene expression. *Cancer Res* 1994;54(10):2771–2777.
108. Allred DC, Clark GM, Molina R, et al. Overexpression of HER-2/neu and its relationship with other prognostic factors change during the progression of in situ to invasive breast cancer. *Hum Pathol* 1992;23(9):974–979.
109. Anbazhagan R, Gelber RD, Bettelheim R, et al. Association of c-erbB-2 expression and S-phase fraction in the prognosis of node positive breast cancer. *Ann Oncol* 1991;2(1):47–53.
110. Gusterson BA, Gelber RD, Goldhirsch A, et al. Prognostic importance of c-erbB-2 expression in breast cancer. International (Ludwig) Breast Cancer Study Group. *J Clin Oncol* 1992;10(7):1049–1056.
111. Muss HB, Thor AD, Berry DA, et al. c-erbB-2 expression and response to adjuvant therapy in women with node-positive early breast cancer. *N Engl J Med* 1994;330(18):1260–1266.
112. Paik S, Bryant J, Park C, et al. erbB-2 and response to doxorubicin in patients with axillary lymph node-positive, hormone receptor-negative breast cancer. *J Natl Cancer Inst* 1998;90(18):1361–1370.
113. Allred DC, Clark GM, Tandon AK, et al. HER-2/neu in node-negative breast cancer: prognostic significance of overexpression influenced by the presence of in situ carcinoma. *J Clin Oncol* 1992;10(4):599–605.
114. Thor AD, Berry DA, Budman DR, et al. erbB-2, p53, and efficacy of adjuvant therapy in lymph node-positive breast cancer. *J Natl Cancer Inst* 1998;90(18):1346–1360.
115. Ravdin PM, Green S, Albain V. Initial report of the SWOG biological correlatine study of CerbB2 expression as a predictor of outcome in a trial comparing adjuvant CAFT with Tamoxifen (J) alone. *Proc ASCO* 1998;17.

116. De Placido S, Carlomagno C, De Laurentiis M, Bianco AR. c-erbB2 expression predicts tamoxifen efficacy in breast cancer patients. *Breast Cancer Res Treat* 1998;52(1–3):55–64.
117. Wright C, Nicholson S, Angus B, et al. Relationship between c-erbB-2 protein product expression and response to endocrine therapy in advanced breast cancer. *Br J Cancer* 1992;65(1):118–121.
118. Leitzel K, Teramoto Y, Konrad K, et al. Elevated serum c-erbB-2 antigen levels and decreased response to hormone therapy of breast cancer. *J Clin Oncol* 1995;13(5):1129–1135.
119. Elledge RM, Green S, Ciocca D, et al. HER-2 expression and response to tamoxifen in estrogen receptor-positive breast cancer: a Southwest Oncology Group Study. *Clin Cancer Res* 1998;4(1):7–12.
120. Yamauchi H, O'Neill A, Gelman R, et al. Prediction of response to antiestrogen therapy in advanced breast cancer patients by pretreatment circulating levels of extracellular domain of the HER-2/c-neu protein. *J Clin Oncol* 1997;15(7):2518–2525.
121. Sjogren S, Inganas M, Lindgren A, et al. Prognostic and predictive value of c-erbB-2 overexpression in primary breast cancer, alone and in combination with other prognostic markers. *J Clin Oncol* 1998;16(2): 462–469.
122. Borg A, Baldetorp B, Ferno M, et al. ERBB2 amplification is associated with tamoxifen resistance in steroid-receptor positive breast cancer. *Cancer Lett* 1994;81(2):137–144.
123. Knoop AS, Bentzen SM, Nielsen MM, et al. Value of epidermal growth factor receptor, HER2, p53, and steroid receptors in predicting the efficacy of tamoxifen in high-risk postmenopausal breast cancer patients. *J Clin Oncol* 2001;19(14):3376–3384.
124. Berry DA, Muss HB, Thor AD, et al. HER-2/neu and p53 expression versus tamoxifen resistance in estrogen receptor-positive, node-positive breast cancer. *J Clin Oncol* 2000;18(20):3471–3479.
125. Pegram MD, Slamon DJ. Combination therapy with trastuzumab (Herceptin) and cisplatin for chemoresistant metastatic breast cancer: evidence for receptor-enhanced chemosensitivity. *Semin Oncol* 1999;26(4 suppl 12):89–95.
126. Baselga J. Clinical trials of Herceptin(R) (trastuzumab). *Eur J Cancer* 2001;37 (suppl 1):18–24.
127. Vogel C, Cobleigh MA, Tripathy D, et al. First-line, single-agent Herceptin (trastuzumab) in metastatic breast cancer: a preliminary report. *Eur J Cancer* 2001;37 (suppl 1): S25–S29.
128. Rudolph P, MacGrogan G, Bonichon F, et al. Prognostic significance of Ki-67 and topoisomerase II alpha expression in infiltrating ductal carcinoma of the breast. A multivariate analysis of 863 cases. *Breast Cancer Res Treat* 1999;55(1):61–71.
129. Rudolph P, Alm P, Heidebrecht HJ, et al. Immunologic proliferation marker Ki-S2 as prognostic indicator for lymph node-negative breast cancer. *J Natl Cancer Inst* 1999;91(3):271–278.
130. Rudolph P, Alm P, Olsson H, et al. Concurrent overexpression of p53 and c-erbB-2 correlates with accelerated cycling and concomitant poor prognosis in node-negative breast cancer. *Hum Pathol* 2001;32(3):311–319.
131. Clark GM, Allred DC, Hilsenbeck SG, et al. Mitosin (a new proliferation marker) correlates with clinical outcome in node-negative breast cancer. *Cancer Res* 1997;57(24):5505–5508.
132. Galea MH, Blamey RW, Elston CE, Ellis IO. The Nottingham Prognostic Index in primary breast cancer. *Breast Cancer Res Treat* 1992;22(3):207–219.
133. Hatschek T, Grontoft O, Fagerberg G, et al. Cytometric and histopathologic features of tumors detected in a randomized mammography screening program: correlation and relative prognostic influence. *Breast Cancer Res Treat* 1990;15(3):149–160.
134. Aaltomaa S, Lipponen P, Eskelinen M, et al. Hormone receptor status and mitotic activity as risk factors for recurrence and death in female breast carcinoma. *Anticancer Res* 1991;11(5):1701–1706.
135. Clayton F. Pathologic correlates of survival in 378 lymph node-negative infiltrating ductal breast carcinomas. Mitotic count is the best single predictor. *Cancer* 1991;68(6):1309–1317.
136. Lipponen PK, Collan Y, Eskelinen MJ. Volume corrected mitotic index (M/V index), mitotic activity index (MAI), and histological grading in breast cancer. *Int Surg* 1991;76(4):245–249.
137. Aaltomaa S, Lipponen P, Eskelinen M, et al. Mitotic indexes as prognostic predictors in female breast cancer. *J Cancer Res Clin Oncol* 1992;118(1):75–81.
138. Aaltomaa S, Lipponen P, Eskelinen M, et al. Tumor size, nuclear morphometry, mitotic indices as prognostic factors in axillary-lymph-node-positive breast cancer. *Eur Surg Res* 1992;24(3):160–168.
139. Parham DM, Hagen N, Brown RA. Simplified method of grading primary carcinomas of the breast. *J Clin Pathol* 1992;45(6):517–520.
140. Eskelinen M, Lipponen P, Papinaho S, et al. DNA flow cytometry, nuclear morphometry, mitotic indices and steroid receptors as independent prognostic factors in female breast cancer. *Int J Cancer* 1992;51(4): 555–561.
141. Lipponen P, Papinaho S, Eskelinen M, et al. DNA ploidy, S-phase fraction and mitotic indices as prognostic predictors of female breast cancer. *Anticancer Res* 1992;12(5):1533–1538.
142. Collan YU, Eskelinen MJ, Nordling SA, et al. Prognostic studies in breast cancer. Multivariate combination of nodal status, proliferation index, tumor size, and DNA ploidy. *Acta Oncol* 1994;33(8):873–878.
143. Ladekarl M, Jensen V. Quantitative histopathology in lymph node-negative breast cancer. Prognostic significance of mitotic counts. *Virchows Arch* 1995;427(3): 265–270.
144. Biesterfeld S, Noll I, Noll E, Wohltmann D, Bocking A. Mitotic frequency as a prognostic factor in breast cancer. *Hum Pathol* 1995;26(1):47–52.
145. Jannink I, van Diest PJ, Baak JP. Comparison of the prognostic value of four methods to assess mitotic activity in 186 invasive breast cancer patients: classical and random mitotic activity assessments with correction for volume percentage of epithelium. *Hum Pathol* 1995;26(10):1086–1092.
146. Iwaya K, Tsuda H, Fukutomi T, et al. Histologic grade and p53 immunoreaction as indicators of early recurrence of node-negative breast cancer. *Jpn J Clin Oncol* 1997;27(1):6–12.
147. Genestie C, Zafrani B, Asselain B, et al. Comparison of the prognostic value of Scarff-Bloom-Richardson and Nottingham histological grades in a series of 825

cases of breast cancer: major importance of the mitotic count as a component of both grading systems. *Anticancer Res* 1998;18(1B):571–576.
148. Kronqvist P, Kuopio T, Collan Y. Morphometric grading in breast cancer: thresholds for mitotic counts. *Hum Pathol* 1998;29(12):1462–1468.
149. Thor AD, Liu S, Moore DH 2nd, Edgerton SM. Comparison of mitotic index, in vitro bromodeoxyuridine labeling, and MIB-1 assays to quantitate proliferation in breast cancer. *J Clin Oncol* 1999;17(2):470–477.
150. de Jong JS, van Diest PJ, Baak JP. Hot spot microvessel density and the mitotic activity index are strong additional prognostic indicators in invasive breast cancer. *Histopathology* 2000;36(4):306–312.
151. Biesterfeld S, Reitmaier M. Re-evaluation of prognostic mitotic figure counting in breast cancer: results of a prospective clinical follow-up study. *Anticancer Res* 2001;21(1B):589–594.
152. Clahsen PC, van de Velde CJ, Duval C, et al. The utility of mitotic index, oestrogen receptor and Ki-67 measurements in the creation of novel prognostic indices for node-negative breast cancer. *Eur J Surg Oncol* 1999;25(4):356–363.
153. Mandard AM, Denoux Y, Herlin P, et al. Prognostic value of DNA cytometry in 281 premenopausal patients with lymph node negative breast carcinoma randomized in a control trial: multivariate analysis with Ki-67 index, mitotic count, and microvessel density. *Cancer* 2000;89(8):1748–1757.
154. Baak JP, van Diest PJ, Benraadt T, et al. The Multi-Center Morphometric Mammary Carcinoma Project (MMMCP) in The Netherlands: value of morphometrically assessed proliferation and differentiation. *J Cell Biochem Suppl* 1993;17G:220–225.
155. van Diest PJ, Baak JP, Matze-Cok P, et al. Reproducibility of mitosis counting in 2,469 breast cancer specimens: results from the Multicenter Morphometric Mammary Carcinoma Project. *Hum Pathol* 1992; 23(6):603–607.
156. Hedley DW, Clark GM, Cornelisse CJ, et al. Consensus review of the clinical utility of DNA cytometry in carcinoma of the breast. Report of the DNA Cytometry Consensus Conference. *Cytometry* 1993;14(5):482–485.
157. Wenger CR, Clark GM. S-phase fraction and breast cancer—a decade of experience. *Breast Cancer Res Treat* 1998;51(3):255–265.
158. Peiro G, Lerma E, Climent MA, et al. Prognostic value of S-phase fraction in lymph-node-negative breast cancer by image and flow cytometric analysis. *Mod Pathol* 1997;10(3):216–222.
159. Witzig TE, Ingle JN, Cha SS, et al. DNA ploidy and the percentage of cells in S-phase as prognostic factors for women with lymph node negative breast cancer. *Cancer* 1994;74(6):1752–1761.
160. Wingren S, Stal O, Sullivan S, et al. S-phase fraction after gating on epithelial cells predicts recurrence in node-negative breast cancer. *Int J Cancer* 1994;59(1): 7–10.
161. Stal O, Dufmats M, Hatschek T, et al. S-phase fraction is a prognostic factor in stage I breast carcinoma. *J Clin Oncol* 1993;11(9):1717–1722.
162. Merkel DE, Winchester DJ, Goldschmidt RA, et al. DNA flow cytometry and pathologic grading as prognostic guides in axillary lymph node-negative breast cancer. *Cancer* 1993;72(6):1926–1932.
163. Dressler LG, Eudey L, Gray R, et al. Prognostic potential of DNA flow cytometry measurements in node-negative breast cancer patients: preliminary analysis of an intergroup study (INT 0076). *J Natl Cancer Inst Monogr* 1992;11:167–172.
164. Clark GM, Mathieu MC, Owens MA, et al. Prognostic significance of S-phase fraction in good-risk, node-negative breast cancer patients. *J Clin Oncol* 1992; 10(3):428–432.
165. Clark GM, Dressler LG, Owens MA, et al. Prediction of relapse or survival in patients with node-negative breast cancer by DNA flow cytometry. *N Engl J Med* 1989;320(10):627–633.
166. Sigurdsson H, Baldetorp B, Borg A, et al. Flow cytometry in primary breast cancer: improving the prognostic value of the fraction of cells in the S-phase by optimal categorization of cut-off levels. *Br J Cancer* 1990;62(5):786–790.
167. Winchester DJ, Duda RB, August CZ, et al. The importance of DNA flow cytometry in node-negative breast cancer. *Arch Surg* 1990;125(7):886–889.
168. Remvikos Y, Beuzeboc P, Zajdela A, et al. Correlation of pretreatment proliferative activity of breast cancer with the response to cytotoxic chemotherapy. *J Natl Cancer Inst* 1989;81(18):1383–1387.
169. Bagwell CB, Clark GM, Spyratos F, et al. Optimizing flow cytometric DNA ploidy and S-phase fraction as independent prognostic markers for node-negative breast cancer specimens. *Cytometry* 2001;46(3):121–135.
170. Michels JJ, Duigou F, Marnay J. Flow cytometry in primary breast carcinomas. Prognostic impact of proliferative activity. *Breast Cancer Res Treat* 2000;62 (2):117–126.
171. Veronese SM, Maisano C, Scibilia J. Comparative prognostic value of Ki-67 and MIB-1 proliferation indices in breast cancer. *Anticancer Res* 1995;15(6B): 2717–2722.
172. Keshgegian AA, Cnaan A. Proliferation markers in breast carcinoma. Mitotic figure count, S-phase fraction, proliferating cell nuclear antigen, Ki-67 and MIB-1. *Am J Clin Pathol* 1995;104(1):42–49.
173. Seshadri R, Leong AS, McCaul K, et al. Relationship between p53 gene abnormalities and other tumour characteristics in breast-cancer prognosis. *Int J Cancer* 1996;69(2):135–141.
174. Haerslev T, Jacobsen GK, Zedeler K. Correlation of growth fraction by Ki-67 and proliferating cell nuclear antigen (PCNA) immunohistochemistry with histopathological parameters and prognosis in primary breast carcinomas. *Breast Cancer Res Treat* 1996; 37(2):101–113.
175. Veronese SM, Gambacorta M, Gottardi O, et al. Proliferation index as a prognostic marker in breast cancer. *Cancer* 1993;71(12):3926–3931.
176. Querzoli P, Albonico G, Ferretti S, et al. MIB-1 proliferative activity in invasive breast cancer measured by image analysis. *J Clin Pathol* 1996;49(11):926–930.
177. Railo M, Lundin J, Haglund C, et al. Ki-67, p53, Er-receptors, ploidy and S-phase as prognostic factors in T1 node negative breast cancer. *Acta Oncol* 1997; 36(4):369–374.
178. Jansen RL, Hupperets PS, Arends JW, et al. MIB-1 labelling index is an independent prognostic marker in primary breast cancer. *Br J Cancer* 1998;78(4):460–465.

179. Harbeck N, Dettmar P, Thomssen C, et al. Prognostic impact of tumor biological factors on survival in node-negative breast cancer. *Anticancer Res* 1998; 18(3C):2187–2197.
180. Domagala W, Markiewski M, Harezga B, et al. Prognostic significance of tumor cell proliferation rate as determined by the MIB-1 antibody in breast carcinoma: its relationship with vimentin and p53 protein. *Clin Cancer Res* 1996;2(1):147–154.
181. Tynninen O, von Boguslawski K, Aronen HJ, Paavonen T. Prognostic value of vascular density and cell proliferation in breast cancer patients. *Pathol Res Pract* 1999;195(1):31–37.
182. Midulla C, De Iorio P, Nagar C, et al. Immunohistochemical expression of p53, nm23-HI, Ki67 and DNA ploidy: correlation with lymph node status and other clinical pathologic parameters in breast cancer. *Anticancer Res* 1999;19(5B):4033–4037.
183. Nakagomi H, Miyake T, Hada M, et al. Prognostic and therapeutic implications of the MIB-1 labeling index in breast cancer. *Breast Cancer* 1998;5(3): 255–259.
184. Liu S, Edgerton SM, Moore DH 2nd, Thor AD. Measures of cell turnover (proliferation and apoptosis) and their association with survival in breast cancer. *Clin Cancer Res* 2001;7(6):1716–1723.
185. Pinder SE, Wencyk P, Sibbering DM, et al. Assessment of the new proliferation marker MIB1 in breast carcinoma using image analysis: associations with other prognostic factors and survival. *Br J Cancer* 1995;71(1):146–149.
186. Biesterfeld S, Kluppel D, Koch R, et al. Rapid and prognostically valid quantification of immunohistochemical reactions by immunohistometry of the most positive tumour focus. A prospective follow-up study on breast cancer using antibodies against MIB-1, PCNA, ER, and PR. *J Pathol* 1998;185(1):25–31.
187. Dettmar P, Harbeck N, Thomssen C, et al. Prognostic impact of proliferation-associated factors MIB1 (Ki-67) and S-phase in node-negative breast cancer. *Br J Cancer* 1997;75(10):1525–1533.
188. Gasparini G, Boracchi P, Verderio P, Bevilacqua P. Cell kinetics in human breast cancer: comparison between the prognostic value of the cytofluorimetric S-phase fraction and that of the antibodies to Ki-67 and PCNA antigens detected by immunocytochemistry. *Int J Cancer* 1994;57(6):822–829.
189. Pinto AE, Andre S, Pereira T, et al. Prognostic comparative study of S-phase fraction and Ki-67 index in breast carcinoma. *J Clin Pathol* 2001;54(7):543–549.
190. Wintzer HO, Zipfel I, Schulte-Monting J, et al. Ki-67 immunostaining in human breast tumors and its relationship to prognosis. *Cancer* 1991;67(2):421–428.
191. Hollstein M, Sidransky D, Vogelstein B, Harris CC. p53 mutations in human cancers. *Science* 1991;253 (5015):49–53.
192. Barnes DM, Dublin EA, Fisher CJ, et al. Immunohistochemical detection of p53 protein in mammary carcinoma: an important new independent indicator of prognosis? *Hum Pathol* 1993;24(5):469–476.
193. Saitoh S, Cunningham J, De Vries EM, et al. p53 gene mutations in breast cancers in midwestern US women: null as well as missense-type mutations are associated with poor prognosis. *Oncogene* 1994;9(10):2869–2875.
194. Thor AD, Moore DH II, Edgerton SM, et al. Accumulation of p53 tumor suppressor gene protein: an independent marker of prognosis in breast cancers. *J Natl Cancer Inst* 1992;84(11):845–855.
195. Eisinger F, Jacquemier J, Guinebretiere JM, et al. p53 involvement in BRCA1-associated breast cancer. *Lancet* 1997;350(9084):1101.
196. Allred DC, Clark GM, Elledge R, et al. Association of p53 protein expression with tumor cell proliferation rate and clinical outcome in node-negative breast cancer. *J Natl Cancer Inst* 1993;85(3):200–206.
197. Silvestrini R, Benini E, Daidone MG, et al. p53 as an independent prognostic marker in lymph node-negative breast cancer patients. *J Natl Cancer Inst* 1993; 85(12):965–970.
198. Gasparini G, Weidner N, Bevilacqua P, et al. Tumor microvessel density, p53 expression, tumor size, and peritumoral lymphatic vessel invasion are relevant prognostic markers in node-negative breast carcinoma. *J Clin Oncol* 1994;12(3):454–466.
199. Elledge RM, Allred DC. Prognostic and predictive value of p53 and p21 in breast cancer. *Breast Cancer Res Treat* 1998;52(1–3):79–98.
200. Elledge RM, Clark GM, Fuqua SA, Yu YY, Allred DC. p53 protein accumulation detected by five different antibodies: relationship to prognosis and heat shock protein 70 in breast cancer. *Cancer Res* 1994;54(14):3752–3757.
201. Jansson T, Inganas M, Sjogren S, et al. p53 Status predicts survival in breast cancer patients treated with or without postoperative radiotherapy: a novel hypothesis based on clinical findings. *J Clin Oncol* 1995; 13(11):2745–2751.
202. Silvestrini R, Veneroni S, Benini E, et al. Expression of p53, glutathione S-transferase-pi, and Bcl-2 proteins and benefit from adjuvant radiotherapy in breast cancer. *J Natl Cancer Inst* 1997;89(9):639–645.
203. Rozan S, Vincent-Salomon A, Zafrani B, et al. No significant predictive value of c-erbB-2 or p53 expression regarding sensitivity to primary chemotherapy or radiotherapy in breast cancer. *Int J Cancer* 1998; 79(1):27–33.
204. Stal O, Stenmark Askmalm M, Wingren S, et al. p53 expression and the result of adjuvant therapy of breast cancer. *Acta Oncol* 1995;34(6):767–770.
205. Elledge RM, Gray R, Mansour E, et al. Accumulation of p53 protein as a possible predictor of response to adjuvant combination chemotherapy with cyclophosphamide, methotrexate, fluorouracil, and prednisone for breast cancer. *J Natl Cancer Inst* 1995;87(16): 1254–1256.
206. Degeorges A, de Roquancourt A, Extra JM, et al. Is p53 a protein that predicts the response to chemotherapy in node negative breast cancer? *Breast Cancer Res Treat* 1998;47(1):47–55.
207. Goulding H, Abdul Rashid NF, Robertson JF, et al. Assessment of angiogenesis in breast carcinoma: an important factor in prognosis? *Hum Pathol* 1995; 26(11):1196–1200.
208. Ogawa Y, Chung YS, Nakata B, et al. Microvessel quantitation in invasive breast cancer by staining for factor VIII-related antigen. *Br J Cancer* 1995;71(6): 1297–1301.
209. Heimann R, Ferguson D, Powers C, et al. Angiogenesis as a predictor of long-term survival for patients

210. Vermeulen PB, Libura M, Libura J, et al. Influence of investigator experience and microscopic field size on microvessel density in node-negative breast carcinoma. *Breast Cancer Res Treat* 1997;42(2):165–172.
211. Horak ER, Leek R, Klenk N, et al. Angiogenesis, assessed by platelet/endothelial cell adhesion molecule antibodies, as indicator of node metastases and survival in breast cancer. *Lancet* 1992;340(8828): 1120–1124.
212. Toi M, Hoshina S, Yamamoto Y, et al. [Tumor angiogenesis in breast cancer: significance of vessel density as a prognostic indicator]. *Gan To Kagaku Ryoho* 1994;21 (suppl 2):178–182.
213. Weidner N, Semple JP, Welch WR, Folkman J. Tumor angiogenesis and metastasis—correlation in invasive breast carcinoma. *N Engl J Med* 1991;324(1):1–8.
214. Weidner N, Folkman J, Pozza F, et al. Tumor angiogenesis: a new significant and independent prognostic indicator in early-stage breast carcinoma. *J Natl Cancer Inst* 1992;84(24):1875–1887.
215. Weidner N, Folkman J. Tumoral vascularity as a prognostic factor in cancer. *Important Adv Oncol* 1996; 167–190.
216. Fox SB, Leek RD, Smith K, et al. Tumor angiogenesis in node-negative breast carcinomas—relationship with epidermal growth factor receptor, estrogen receptor, and survival. *Breast Cancer Res Treat* 1994;29(1): 109–116.
217. Fox SB, Gatter KC, Leek RD, et al. More about: Tumor angiogenesis as a prognostic assay for invasive ductal breast carcinoma. *J Natl Cancer Inst* 2000; 92(2):161–162.
218. Axelsson K, Ljung BM, Moore DH 2nd, et al. Tumor angiogenesis as a prognostic assay for invasive ductal breast carcinoma. *J Natl Cancer Inst* 1995;87(13): 997–1008.
219. Peters-Engl C, Frank W, Leodolter S, Medl M. Tumor flow in malignant breast tumors measured by Doppler ultrasound: an independent predictor of survival. *Breast Cancer Res Treat* 1999;54(1):65–71.
220. Hayes DF. Angiogenesis and breast cancer. *Hematol Oncol Clin North Am* 1994;8(1):51–71.
221. Normanno N, Ciardiello F, Brandt R, Salomon DS. Epidermal growth factor-related peptides in the pathogenesis of human breast cancer. *Breast Cancer Res Treat* 1994;29(1):11–27.
222. Fox SB, Smith K, Hollyer J, et al. The epidermal growth factor receptor as a prognostic marker: results of 370 patients and review of 3009 patients. *Breast Cancer Res Treat* 1994;29(1):41–49.
223. Klijn JG, Berns PM, Schmitz PI, Foekens JA. The clinical significance of epidermal growth factor receptor (EGF-R) in human breast cancer: a review on 5232 patients. *Endocr Rev* 1992;13(1):3–17.
224. Mansour OA, Zekri AR, Harvey J, el-Ahmady O. Epidermal growth factor receptors: status and effect on breast cancer patients. *Anticancer Res* 1997;17(4B): 3107–3110.
225. Sainsbury JR, Farndon JR, Harris AL, Sherbet GV. Epidermal growth factor receptors on human breast cancers. *Br J Surg* 1985;72(3):186–188.
226. Bolla M, Chedin M, Colonna M, et al. Prognostic value of epidermal growth factor receptor in a series of 303 breast cancers. *Eur J Cancer* 1992;28A(6–7): 1052–1054.
227. Walker RA, Dearing SJ. Expression of epidermal growth factor receptor mRNA and protein in primary breast carcinomas. *Breast Cancer Res Treat* 1999;53 (2):167–176.
228. Gerstein ES, Muaviia MA, Letiagin VP, Kushlinskii NE. [Prognostic significance of epidermal growth factor receptors in stage I-II breast cancer: results of a six-year follow-up]. *Vopr Onkol* 1998;44(4): 383–389.
229. Toi M, Tominaga T, Osaki A, Toge T. Role of epidermal growth factor receptor expression in primary breast cancer: results of a biochemical study and an immunocytochemical study. *Breast Cancer Res Treat* 1994;29(1):51–58.
230. Chrysogelos SA, Dickson RB. EGF receptor expression, regulation, and function in breast cancer. *Breast Cancer Res Treat* 1994;29(1):29–40.
231. Nicholson S, Richard J, Sainsbury C, et al. Epidermal growth factor receptor (EGFr);results of a 6 year follow-up study in operable breast cancer with emphasis on the node negative subgroup. *Br J Cancer* 1991;63(1):146–150.
232. Gasparini G, Boracchi P, Bevilacqua P, et al. A multiparametric study on the prognostic value of epidermal growth factor receptor in operable breast carcinoma. *Breast Cancer Res Treat* 1994;29(1):59–71.
233. Grimaux M, Romain S, Remvikos Y, et al. Prognostic value of epidermal growth factor receptor in node-positive breast cancer. *Breast Cancer Res Treat* 1989; 14(1):77–90.
234. Spyratos F, Delarue JC, Andrieu C, et al. Epidermal growth factor receptors and prognosis in primary breast cancer. *Breast Cancer Res Treat* 1990;17(2):83–89.
235. Spyratos F, Martin PM, Hacene K, et al. Prognostic value of a solubilized fraction of EGF receptors in primary breast cancer using an immunoenzymatic assay—a retrospective study. *Breast Cancer Res Treat* 1994;29(1):85–95.
236. Nicholson S, Wright C, Sainsbury JR, et al. Epidermal growth factor receptor (EGFr) as a marker for poor prognosis in node-negative breast cancer patients: neu and tamoxifen failure. *J Steroid Biochem Mol Biol* 1990;37(6):811–814.
237. Sainsbury JR, Farndon JR, Needham GK, et al. Epidermal-growth-factor receptor status as predictor of early recurrence of and death from breast cancer. *Lancet* 1987;1(8547):1398–1402.
238. Sainsbury JR, Farndon JR, Sherbet GV, Harris AL. Epidermal-growth-factor receptors and oestrogen receptors in human breast cancer. *Lancet* 1985;1(8425): 364–366.
239. Rios MA, Macias A, Perez R, et al. Receptors for epidermal growth factor and estrogen as predictors of relapse in patients with mammary carcinoma. *Anticancer Res* 1988;8(1):173–176.
240. Lewis S, Locker A, Todd JH, et al. Expression of epidermal growth factor receptor in breast carcinoma. *J Clin Pathol* 1990;43(5):385–389.
241. Eissa S, Khalifa A, el-Gharib A, et al. Multivariate analysis of DNA ploidy, p53, c-erbB-2 proteins, EGFR, and steroid hormone receptors for prediction of poor short term prognosis in breast cancer. *Anticancer Res* 1997;17(2B):1417–1423.

242. Nicholson RI, McClelland RA, Finlay P, et al. Relationship between EGF-R, c-erbB-2 protein expression and Ki67 immunostaining in breast cancer and hormone sensitivity. *Eur J Cancer* 1993;7(23):1018–1023.
243. Nicholson RI, McClelland RA, Gee JM, et al. Epidermal growth factor receptor expression in breast cancer: association with response to endocrine therapy. *Breast Cancer Res Treat* 1994;29(1):117–125.
244. Harris AL. What is the biological, prognostic, and therapeutic role of the EGF receptor in human breast cancer? *Breast Cancer Res Treat* 1994;29(1):1–2.
245. Ciardiello F. Epidermal growth factor receptor tyrosine kinase inhibitors as anticancer agents. *Drugs* 2000;60 Suppl 1:25–32;discussion 41–42.
246. Baselga J, Pfister D, Cooper MR, et al. Phase I studies of anti-epidermal growth factor receptor chimeric antibody C225 alone and in combination with cisplatin. *J Clin Oncol* 2000;18(4):904–914.
247. Mendelsohn J, Baselga J. The EGF receptor family as targets for cancer therapy. *Oncogene* 2000;19(56):6550–6565.

29

Prognostic Factors in Invasive Breast Cancer Using Histology

Sarah E. Pinder, Ian O. Ellis, Andrew H.S. Lee, and Christopher W. Elston

The fundamental role of the histopathologist, in the treatment of patients with breast cancer, has been in providing the correct diagnosis on excision biopsy material, with or without use of frozen section. Local regional lymph node examination, for the presence or absence of metastases, might or might not have been required. It was unusual for other prognostic information to be requested by clinicians and therefore it was not supplied. Over several decades, breast cancer treatment has changed dramatically. There are now a wide variety of therapeutic options, and choices have to be made by both patient and clinician regarding local and systemic treatments. However, all of the adjuvant treatments presently available have some kind of morbidity. It has become increasingly important, therefore, to assess individual patient prognosis and devise an appropriate therapeutic plan. The understanding of predictive factors, rather than prognostic factors, is becoming increasingly recognised as a role of the histopathologist. Predictive assays are used to identify individual tumors which are expected to respond to specific treatments.

Huge numbers of prognostic factors have been proposed in patients with invasive breast cancer. Many are reported to be of value in relatively small series using univariate analysis but do not withstand multivariate analysis. This chapter addresses those which appear to be of greatest importance.

TUMOR SIZE

Tumor size, which is in part a time-dependent factor, has been shown to influence prognosis in numerous series of patients with invasive breast carcinoma (1–5). Patients with small tumors are known to have better long-term survival than those with large primary lesions. In the long-term study from Memorial-Sloan Kettering Cancer Centre (MSK) (6), the projected relapse-free survival rates 20 years after initial treatment were, by tumor size: less than 10 mm, 88%; 11 mm to 13 mm, 73%; 14 mm to 16 mm, 65%; and 17 mm to 22 mm, 59%. More recent reports have similarly demonstrated that the survival of women with very small cancers is good. Analysis of the 8-year survival of women with node-negative breast cancers 1 cm or less in size from NSABP protocols B-6, B-13, B-14, B-19 and B20 indicates a 92% overall survival (7). The relapse-free survival in these series ranged from 79% for those women with estrogen receptor (ER) negative tumors receiving surgery ($\pm$ radiotherapy) to 94% for those with ER-positive tumors receiving surgery ($\pm$ radiotherapy) with tamoxifen and chemotherapy. In this same group of patients the overall survival did not improve significantly with the addition of adjuvant treatment.

The importance of tumor size as a prognostic factor is confirmed particularly in those series where local not central review pathologists have carried out the measurement of tumors, as even then strong correlations with prognosis are seen (2,3,5). Clinical tumor size is notoriously inaccurate compared with histological determination. Where estimate of tumor size is required for therapeutic reasons, it is best done using ultrasonography (8). To achieve an accurate assessment, the size of a breast cancer should be assessed on the excised pathological specimen. The size of any surgically excised tumor should be measured by the histopathology laboratory to the nearest millimeter, in three planes. This is done three times: first in the fresh state, second confirmed after fixation and finally re-checked on the histological section using the stage micrometer of the microscope. The greatest dimension of the invasive component is taken as the final tumor size, although the total dimension of invasive carcinoma plus ductal carcinoma in situ (DCIS) is also recorded. Confirmation of size from histological sections is particularly important for DCIS or tumors with a large in situ component and for small lesions measuring less than 1 cm in size. It is, however, clear that with decreasing size, the risk of errors in measurement increases and some studies have reported these inconsistencies (9,10).

It is imperative that tumor dimensions are measured as accurately as possible in order to provide accurate audit data. Tumor size is an important quality assurance measurement for breast screening programs (11–13) and is utilized to confirm radiologists' ability to detect mammographically impalpable invasive carcinomas. One target in the UK Breast Screening Programme prevalence cases is for 50% of invasive cancers to measure less than 15 mm in size (13).

LYMPH NODE STAGE

Local regional lymph node involvement in invasive breast cancer is well recognized as a powerful prognostic factor. Patients with metastatic deposits in local regional lymph nodes have a significantly poorer prognosis than those who are node negative (1,2,14–18). Ten-year survival is reduced from 75% for node-negative patients to as little as 25% to 30% for those with nodal disease. Clinical assessment of disease in axillary lymph nodes is inaccurate and certainly not sufficiently robust for therapeutic decision-making (19). Accurate evaluation of nodal involvement must be made on thorough histological examination of excised lymph nodes.

In addition to the presence of metastatic disease in the lymph nodes, it is also clear that patient outcome is also related to the number and the level of lymph nodes involved. The greater the number of nodes involved the poorer the patient survival (3,20). For therapeutic purposes, three groups of patients can be defined based on the number of nodes involved: node-negative, one to three positive nodes, and four or more metastatic nodes. Metastatic lymph nodes in higher levels of the axilla, specifically the apex, also carry a worse prognosis (18,21) as do metastatic deposits in the internal mammary nodes (21).

Axillary surgery in patients with breast cancer is still controversial. There are persuasive arguments in favor of both axillary sampling and axillary clearance (22–27). Sentinel lymph node biopsy (SLNB) for patients with invasive breast cancer has also been advocated and validated in the last few years (28–32).

The concept of SLNB relies on the premise that the first nodal deposit of metastatic disease will be dictated by the lymphatic system draining an individual tumor. When the sentinel lymph node contains metastatic tumor, further axillary surgery or radiotherapy should be undertaken. If negative (SLNB negative), the remaining lymph nodes in that area should be free from metastatic disease. Series have confirmed that if only one node contains metastatic carcinoma it is almost always the sentinel node. However, a weakness of many of the series published to date is that the sentinel node has often been examined more intensively than the other lymph nodes. Metastases in "non-sentinel" nodes could therefore be missed (33–35). The incidence of negative sentinel lymph nodes, when metastases have been found elsewhere in the axilla, have been reported to vary from 1% to 11% (31,33–37).

Debate remains regarding the most appropriate technique for examination of excised sentinel nodes to obtain the optimum prognostic information. The methodology is of clinical importance because historical prognostic data on axillary nodal status is based predominately on series which used routine stains on one slice from each lymph node. Clinical decisions continue to be made routinely based on this information.

Techniques exist to increase the sensitivity of detection of metastatic disease by examining a greater surface area of lymph nodes. This may be done either by embedding all of the node in multiple slices or examining serial sections (38–40). The use of immunohistochemistry also increases the chance of detection of small deposits of metastatic tumor (40–42), partly by increasing the surface area of the node examined and partly by making very small deposits easier to recognize. Immunohistochemistry and serial sections both increase the detection of metastases in sentinel lymph node biopsies (18,43). Using reverse transcriptase polymerase chain reaction (RT-PCR) has been proposed by some to increase sensitivity further.

The rationale for more sensitive methods to detect deposits remains unclear. Most prognostic data on node status in the literature is based on less extensive histological examination, and the prognostic implications of smaller deposits identified by new techniques remains uncertain. There is some evidence that the size of the lymph node deposit is of prognostic significance (40,42,44–46) but there is neither an agreed definition for these small deposits nor a universal methodology for their detection. The definition of "occult" or "micrometastases" includes a variety of lesions: (a) metastases less than a given size, often 2 mm, (b) metastases found on review that were initially missed, (c) deposits shown only in deeper histological sections or (d) metastases shown with immunohistochemistry for cytokeratins but not apparent on routine haematoxylin and eosin stains (H&E). Because of the varying definitions for these deposits of metastatic disease, comparison of published results is impossible and their significance remains unclear.

Some larger studies have shown poorer prognosis for patients with "micrometastases" compared with node-negative individuals, but only using univariate analysis (38,40–42,47). The effect is more apparent for disease-free survival than overall survival. This has not, however, been universally reported and other series have found no prognostic significance for tiny "occult" nodal metastases (48). Only one of seven larger series have found occult metastases to be an independent predictor of poor prognosis in multivariate analysis (42). There are also conflicting data on whether the position of the metastatic deposit, i.e., in the marginal sinus or parenchyma, is important (38,39,49,50). Series with strict adherence to well-described protocols and definitions are urgently required to clarify the optimum methodology for disease detection and to determine the impact on outcome of small SLN metastatic deposits.

Routine use of frozen sections for perioperative examination of lymph nodes has, in our view, an unacceptably high false negative rate from 10% to 30% (35,51–53). Frozen section may be appropriate when the node is thought clinically to contain tumor. If disease can be confirmed histologically, then immediate axillary surgery can be undertaken. Time-consuming, labor-intensive and expensive intraoperative assessment with serial sections and immunohistochemistry has been described but is not widely performed. Intraoperative imprint cytology has also been advocated by those who have found an acceptable low false negative rate of 2% to 3% (32,51) but many have not been able to achieve this remarkably high level of accuracy. Our own current routine practice is based on pragmatism (54); axillary lymph nodes are in general cut into slices about 3 mm thick perpendicular to the long axis (thus maximizing the assessment of the marginal sinuses). Each node is examined in a single cassette. The vast majority of nodes can be completely embedded, although larger nodes may have only alternate slices examined. Only one section is taken of very large obviously involved nodes.

Extranodal Spread

There remains uncertainty regarding the prognostic significance of extranodal spread of carcinoma into adipose tissue in the axilla surrounding the lymph nodes. Extranodal spread has been reported to carry a poor prognosis (55), particularly in patients with one to three nodes, but not those with four or more involved nodes (56). Other groups have found that extranodal disease confers no additional information to lymph node disease (57) and has no intrinsic prognostic significance (58,59).

LYMPHO-VASCULAR INVASION

Not surprisingly, lympho-vascular invasion is strongly related to local regional lymph node involvement (60–62). Some groups claim it can provide prognostic information which is as powerful as lymph node stage (63). The presence of vascular invasion predicts for both recurrence (22,63,64) and survival (60,65–67) in several studies. Conversely, earlier series found no correlation between lympho-vascular invasion and prognosis (68,69). Discrepancies may, in part, be explained by the wide variation in the reported frequency of vascular invasion in the literature (20% to 54%), which may reflect on the time and care spent looking at each section or the number of sections prepared.

Tumor emboli are examined histologically within the thin-walled vascular channels of a section. As it is impossible to reliably determine whether these spaces are capillaries, venules or lymphatic spaces, the broad term "vascular invasion" is used. Muscular blood vessels are rarely involved. The wide variation in reporting of vascular invasion might be, in part, explained by the difficulty in distinguishing true vessels from soft tissue spaces, which are artifacts most common in suboptimally fixed specimens. Both DCIS and shrinkage artefact have been misinterpreted as vascular invasion (60,61). However usage of strict criteria allows reproducible assessment (3,60,70).

In our hands, using multivariate analysis, vascular invasion relates to long-term survival independent of lymph node stage (60). In lymph node-negative patients, there is also correlation between presence of vascular invasion and early recurrence (63,64,71). The most important clinical application of vascular invasion lies, however, in its power to predict local recurrence after breast conservation surgery (22,60, 64,71,72) and of flap recurrence after mastectomy (73).

DIFFERENTIATION

Both lymph node stage and tumor size are, in part, time-dependent factors. Histological features can also be assessed to establish the individual aggressiveness of an invasive breast carcinoma. Histological classification of mammary cancer was historically restricted to *in situ* or invasive breast carcinoma. It is evident that invasive carcinomas can be further sub-divided according to their differentiation. This can be performed either by assessment of (a) histological grade or (b) histological type.

HISTOLOGICAL GRADE

The first recognized study of histological grading of invasive breast cancer was performed over 70 years ago by Greenhough (74). Eight morphological features were examined in, by today's standards, a somewhat subjective way and showed an association with "cure." Greenhough's method was re-assessed by Scarff and colleagues, who reported that only three factors, tubule formation, nuclear pleomorphism and hyperchromatism, were of importance (75). The majority of subsequent grading systems for invasive breast cancer have been based on this technique. Some use multiple histological features of the tumor (3,76–80); others include only assessment of nuclear appearances (81–83). Most studies have demonstrated significant association between grade and patient survival, despite the plethora and variety of methodology used. Histological grade has been convincingly proven to be associated with prognosis (84).

Histological grading needs to be carried out by trained histopathologists based on an agreed protocol. One of the fundamental problems with older systems was the lack of strictly defined written criteria. Although Bloom and Richardson (78) improved Patey and Scarff's method by adding numerical scoring (75), they did not define clear criteria for cut-off points. Additional modifications to their method were made to improve objectivity (80). The features routinely assessed are: tubule formation, nuclear pleomorphism, and mitotic count, as described in Patey and Scarff's original work, but each is scored from one to three based on strictly defined criteria. The amendments are both qualitative and quantitative.

Acceptance of the technique into routine practice has been slow, despite convincing evidence that histological grade is of prognostic value. This has largely been due to lack of clinical demand. In addition, there was the perception of poor reproducibility and consistency (85), although significant numbers of studies have reported acceptable levels of observer variability (86–90). The method has now been adopted for use in the pathological data sets of the U.K. NHSBSP (National Health Service Breast Screening Programme) (54), the rest of Europe (91), and the United States (92).

Histological grade is a predictive factor, in addition to a prognostic factor which can be used to indicate the likely response to chemotherapy. We reported that patients with lymph node-positive disease who had grade 3 tumors obtained a significant overall and disease-free survival benefit from prolonged compared to perioperative chemotherapy whilst those with grade 1 and grade 2 primary tumors did not (93).

HISTOLOGICAL TYPE

The widely varied histological appearances of invasive mammary carcinoma may also be subgrouped by means of large numbers of histological types (16,94,95). This provides additional prognostic information (94). Although criteria for diagnosis of different histological types of invasive breast carcinoma have been described in detail (54,94–97), the subjective element to histological typing should be recognized and there is not as yet any universal agreement. For example, in the U.K. NHSBSP pathology quality assurance scheme consistency of histological subtyping has been disappointingly low (9), suggesting that pathologists adhere poorly to the protocol criteria. However, as histological type is not used to determine clinical management, it may be that histopathologists concentrate their efforts on features perceived to have greater clinical implications.

This example of poor histological type reproducibility may, in part, explain the widely varying proportions of types reported in the literature. Few long-term comprehensive follow-up studies address survival of patients with different subtypes of invasive breast carcinoma, although it is well established that certain subgroups have good prognosis. Tubular (98–100) and invasive cribriform carcinoma (101,102), medullary carcinoma (103,104), mucinous carcinoma (105,106), infiltrating lobular carcinoma (108), and tubulo-lobular carcinoma (108) have all been reported to have a better prognosis than carcinomas of ductal/no special type (NST) or not otherwise specified (NOS) (68). It is also evident that there is a relative excess of some "special type" tumors in cancers detected in the prevalent round of mammographic breast screening (109,110).

Individuals presenting with invasive carcinoma of the breast can be stratified into broad prognostic groups according to their histological type (111). The excellent (more than 80% 10-year survival) prognosis group comprises mucinous, tubular, invasive cribriform and tubulolobular carcinomas. The 60% to 80% 10-year survival group is composed of mixed ductal/NST in association with a special type element, tubular mixed and also alveolar lobular carcinomas. The average prognosis group with 50% to 60% 10-year survival includes classical lobular, invasive papillary, medullary and atypical medullary carcinomas. The worst prognosis group with less than 50% 10-year survival is composed of ductal/NST, mixed ductal and lobular, solid lobular and lobular mixed carcinomas.

Subtyping adds to our understanding of the biology of breast carcinoma whilst adding relatively little prognostic information to histological grade. Some subtypes of carcinoma are likely to express certain markers or infiltrate in a particular fashion. For example, the pattern of metastatic spread is different in breast cancers of infiltrating lobular type (112,113) and these lesions are also more often ER-positive than tumors of ductal/NST (114). Similarly the identification of a relative excess of carcinomas of ductal/NST with medullary features in patients with BRCA1 compared to BRCA2 mutations adds to our knowledge of the link between tumor biology and genetics (115–117).

OTHER HISTOLOGICAL FACTORS

Various morphological features have been proposed, from time to time, as potential prognostic factors. In our experience these are of much less importance than those discussed above.

This includes factors such as extent of DCIS, stromal fibrosis, stromal elastosis, and tumor necrosis, amongst many others.

The percentage and extent of DCIS identified in association with an invasive tumor is extremely variable. Assessment of its degree remains subjective but it has been suggested that a prominent component of DCIS within an invasive carcinoma conveys a better prognosis for the patient and a decreased likelihood of nodal metastases (118,119). However, an extensive component of DCIS may be of greater clinical importance in the management of individuals undergoing breast-conserving therapy. Some years ago it was suggested that the principal risk factor for disease relapse after BCT was large residual tumor burden and that the main source of this burden might be extensive *in situ* component (EIC) (120). EIC has been defined as the presence of DCIS in an invasive breast cancer with the *in situ* component comprising 25% or more of the lesion and extending beyond the confines of the main invasive disease (121). Invasive breast carcinomas with EIC have been reported to have considerably higher local recurrence rate than those without extensive *in situ* disease. The Boston group have reported that the most powerful predictor of local recurrence was assessment of excision margins and that EIC was not of importance if complete excision was obtained (122). EIC did, however, predict the likelihood of margin involvement in this study.

Stromal fibrosis is common, in varying amounts, in invasive breast carcinoma. It has been variously reported to be associated with a poorer survival (123–124), a favorable prognosis (125) and to have no effect on outcome (68). This is almost certainly because an association with tumor type confounds the data.

There are similarly conflicting data on the prognostic significance of stromal elastosis which is also a feature of many breast lesions but can be seen diffusely through a tumor or in a periductal distribution (126). Studies have indicated that its presence is associated with an improved prognosis (127,128) but this has not been universally reported (129,130).

Tumor necrosis is a relatively common feature in invasive breast cancers, especially in grade 3 lesions, but its prognostic importance has been rarely addressed. Its presence has been reported to be related to poor outcome and early treatment failure (3,123,131). However, a precise definition is not included in many of the studies in which it is reported and terms such as "extensive" have been utilized, making reassessment impossible.

NOTTINGHAM PROGNOSTIC INDEX

Prognostic factor research, in invasive breast cancer, has grown exponentially over the last 10 years. Several histological features described above have been examined in numerous series. Prognostic factors can be used to select the most appropriate treatment for an individual invasive breast cancer patient. In particular, women with an excellent prognosis (comparable to those without breast cancer) can avoid the unnecessary side effects and morbidity of systemic adjuvant treatment and those with a poor prognosis can receive more aggressive therapies (132).

Lymph node stage is the most commonly proposed prognostic factor in mammary cancer but it is a relatively poor discriminator when used alone. Patients with near to 100% survival cannot be defined, neither can those with near to 100% mortality, based on nodal stage. Histological grade remains a complex morphological result of the losses and gains of a multitude of molecular markers but alone it is not sufficiently discriminatory to allow choices of definitive therapy.

The greatest prognostic relevance in multivariate analysis are histological grade, lymph node stage, and tumor size. These have been combined into the Nottingham prognostic index (NPI) (17), using appropriate weighting. This is calculated as:

$$\text{NPI} = \text{Tumor size} \times 0.2 \text{ (in cm)} \\ + \text{Lymph node stage } (1–3) \\ + \text{Histological grade } (1–3).$$

The NPI has been confirmed prospectively (14) in studies from Nottingham as providing robust information for women aged 70 or under with operable primary invasive breast carcinoma. Other groups have validated the findings in series using large numbers of patients (133–136). Cut-off points of 3.4 and 5.4 are used to group

(PG = Prognostic Group, Good PG < or = 3.4, Moderate PG 3.41-5.4, Poor PG >5.4)

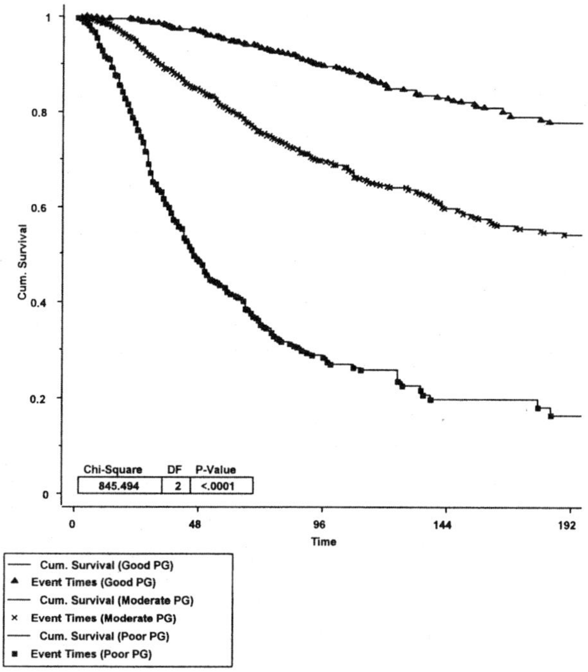

NUMBER AT RIST				
Time (months)	0	48	96	144
Good PG	1219	944	513	230
Moderate PG	1892	1234	581	278
Poor PG	590	194	57	17

Fig 29.1. Overall survival by Nottingham Prognostic Index Group.

the patients into three categories for management purposes (Fig. 29.1). Women with an NPI of 3.4 or less have a good survival and receive no adjuvant systemic treatment. Those patients with a score greater than this have systemic adjuvant treatment and receive hormone therapy when their tumor is estrogen receptor positive (see below).

PREDICTIVE FACTORS

Since the late 19th century, steroid hormones have been known to affect the growth of some tumors, particularly breast and prostatic cancer (137). Cytosol assays were used for determining hormone receptor levels in tumors but these required significant amounts of tissue and in premenopausal women were affected by endogenous hormones. Monoclonal antibodies raised to the nuclear estrogen receptor (ER) (138–140) allow *in situ* localization of receptor by immunocytochemistry. Immunohistochemical determination of ER status is now performed routinely on formalin-fixed paraffin-embedded material (141,142). A semi-quantitative scoring of the proportion and intensity of nuclear immunoreactivity is undertaken (139) or a simple categorical scoring system can be used (143,144). Either method of scoring can reliably predict response to hormone therapy (142,144).

We have not found that ER status assessment is an independent *prognostic* factor as it is associated closely with histological grade. ER status is, however, a *predictive* factor. Whilst approximately 30% of unselected patients with breast carcinoma will respond to hormone therapies, ER assays allow more accurate prediction with 50% to 60% of ER-positive tumors responding (145). However, no system for predicting response to hormone therapies is completely specific or sensitive; a small proportion of ER-negative tumors will respond to hormone manipulation (146,147) and approximately 30% of apparently ER-positive tumors will progress despite hormonal therapy (142).

New predictive factors are emerging in conjunction with new therapies such as the humanized anti-c-*erb*-B2 (HER-2) monoclonal antibody, trastuzumab (Herceptin). Suitable patients require preselection by determination of overexpression of the c-*erb*-B2 oncoprotein using immunohistochemistry or amplification of the gene by fluorescent *in situ* hybridization (FISH). There is now some data that the FISH technique appears better in predicting response to trastuzumab, although there is a close correlation between amplification of the gene and overexpression of the protein (148).

Molecular markers such as HER-2/c-erb-B2 protein expression (149), EGFR expression (150), and epithelial mucin immunohistochemistry (151) have not achieved significance as independent prognostic factors in multivariate analyses when included with histological grade, tumor size, and lymph node stage. The future is likely to prove, however, that some additional molecular markers will be predictive factors for particular therapies including chemotherapy, new novel targets, and possibly radiotherapy.

Histological grading is derived by combining the appearance of various morphological features and mitotic figure frequency (152). It provides, therefore, a summation of a variety of tumor-related variables and in essence gives an overview of various molecular events affecting morphological appearance. It is not surprising therefore that in multivariate analysis, no single molecular event can compete with histological grade for patient outcome. It would be surprising if any single molecular event could offer analogous information to careful histological evaluation of an invasive breast cancer. This is because traditional histopathological factors depend on a variety of complex variables including the time a tumor has been present (size and lymph node stage), differentiation (grade and type), proliferation (grade), and metastatic potential (lymph node stage and vascular invasion).

CONCLUSION

The most important prognostic factors in invasive breast cancer remain, thus far, traditional histological features of grade, lymph node stage, and tumor size. Routine decisions regarding the appropriateness of adjuvant therapy can be made once prognosis has been indicated by a combination of these features. Assessment of predictive factors including histological grade, estrogen receptor and HER-2 status enables prediction of the likely response to specific treatments and thus currently optimum therapy can be selected.

REFERENCES

1. Cutler SJ, Black MM, Mork T, et al. Further observations on prognostic factors in cancer of the female breast. *Cancer* 1969;24:653–657.
2. Elston CW, Gresham GA, Rao GS, et al. The Cancer Research Campaign (Kings/Cambridge) trial for early breast cancer—pathological aspects. *Br J Cancer* 1982;45:655–669.
3. Fisher ER, Sass R, Fisher B, et al. Pathologic findings from the National Surgical Adjuvant Project for breast cancer (protocol no 4). Discrimination for tenth year treatment failure. *Cancer* 1984;53:712–723.
4. Carter GL, Allen C, Henson DE. Relation of tumor size, lymph node status, and survival in 24,740 breast cancer cases. *Cancer* 1989;63:181–187.
5. Neville AM, Bettelheim R, Gelber RD, et al. Predicting treatment responsiveness and prognosis in node-negative breast cancer. *J Clin Oncol* 1992;10:696–705.
6. Rosen PP, Groshen S. Factors influencing survival and prognosis in early breast carcinoma (T1NOMO-T1N1MO). Assessment of 644 patients with median follow up of 19 years. *Surg Clin North Am* 1990;70:937–962.
7. Tan-Chiu E, Dignam J, Fisher B, et al. Prognosis of node-negative breast cancer patients with small (less than or equal to 1 cm) tumors: NSABP experience

from protocols B-06, B-13, B-14, B-19 and B-20. *Breast Cancer Res Treat* 1999;57:25 (Abstract).
8. Tresserra F, Feu J, Grases PJ, et al. Assessment of breast cancer size: sonographic and pathologic correlation. *Journal of Clinical Ultrasound* 1999;27:485–491.
9. Sloane JP, National Co-ordinating Group for Breast Screening Pathology. Consistency of histopathological reporting of breast lesions detected by screening: findings of the UK National External Quality Assessment (EQA) Scheme. *Eur J Cancer* 1994;30:1414–1419.
10. Beahrs OH, Shapiro S, Smart C, et al. Summary report of the Working Group to review the National Cancer Institute-American Cancer Society Breast Cancer Demonstration Detection Projects. *J Nat Cancer Inst* 1979;62:641–709.
11. Hartman WH. Minimal breast cancer: an update. *Cancer* 1984;53:681–684.
12. Tabar L, Duffy SW, Krusemo UB. Detection method, tumor size and node metastases in breast cancers diagnosed during a trial of breast cancer screening. *Eur J Cancer Clin Oncol* 1987;23:959–962.
13. Royal College of Radiologists. Quality Assurance Guidelines for Radiologists. January 1997. NHSBSP Publications no 15. 1997.
14. Galea MH, Blamey RW, Elston CW, et al. The Nottingham Prognostic Index in primary breast cancer. *Br Cancer Res Treat* 1992;22:207–219.
15. Ferguson DJ, Meier P, Karrison T, et al. Staging of breast cancer and survival rates: an assessment based on 50 years of experience with radical mastectomy. *JAMA* 1982;248:1337–1341.
16. Fisher ER, Gregorio RM, Fisher B. The pathology of invasive breast cancer. A syllabus derived from findings of the National Surgical Adjuvant Breast Cancer Project (protocol no 4). *Cancer* 1975;36:144–156.
17. Haybittle JL, Blamey RW, Elston CW, et al. A prognostic index in primary breast cancer. *Br J Cancer* 1982;45:361–366.
18. Veronesi U, Galimberti V, Zurrida S, et al. Prognostic significance of number and level of axillary node metastases in breast cancer. *Breast* 1993;2:224–228.
19. Barr LC, Baum M. Time to abandon TNM staging of breast cancer? *Lancet* 1992;339:915–917.
20. Nemoto T, Vana J, Bedwani RN. Management and survival of female breast cancer: results of a national survey by the American College of Surgeons. *Cancer* 1980;45:2917–2924.
21. Handley RF. Observations and thoughts on carcinoma of the breast. *Proc R Soc Med* 1972;65:437–444.
22. Locker AP, Ellis IO, Morgan DAL, et al. Factors influencing local recurrence after excision and radiotherapy for primary breast cancer. *Br J Surg* 1989;76:890–894.
23. Steele RJC, Forrest APM, Gibson T, et al. The efficacy of lower axillary sampling in obtaining lymph node status in breast cancer: a controlled randomised trial. *Br J Surg* 1985;72:368–369.
24. O'Dwyer PJ. Editorial. Axillary dissection in primary breast cancer;the benefits of node clearance warrant reappraisal. *Br Med J* 1992;302:360–361.
25. Cabanes PA, Salmon RJ, Vilcoq JR, et al. Value of axillary dissection in addition to lumpectomy and radiotherapy in early breast cancer. *Lancet* 1992;339:1245–1248.
26. Dixon JM, Dillon P, Anderson TJ, Chetty U. Axillary sampling in breast cancer: an assessment of its efficacy. *Breast* 1998;7:206–208.
27. Kutianawala MA, Sayed M, Stotter A, et al. Staging the axilla in breast cancer: an audit of lymph-node retrieval in one UK regional centre. *Eur J Surg Oncol* 1998;24:280–282.
28. Albertini JJ, Lyman GH, Cox C, et al. Lymphatic mapping and sentinel node biopsy in the patient with breast cancer. *JAMA* 1996;276:1818–1822.
29. Giuliano AE, Kirgan DM, Guenther JM, Morton DL. Lymphatic mapping and sentinel lymphadenectomy for breast cancer. *Ann Surg* 1994;220:391–401.
30. Giuliano AE. Sentinel lymphadenectomy in primary breast carcinoma: an alternative to routine dissection. *J Surg Oncol* 1996;62:75–77.
31. Nwariaku FE, Euhus DM, Beitsch PD, et al. Sentinel lymph node biopsy, an alternative to elective axillary dissection for breast cancer. *American Journal of Surgery* 1998;176:529–531.
32. Rubio IT, Korourian S, Cowan C, et al. Sentinel lymph node biopsy for staging breast cancer. *Am J Surg* 1998;176:532–535.
33. Borgstein P, Pijpers R, Comans EF, et al. Sentinel lymph node biopsy in breast cancer: Guidelines and pitfalls of lymphoscintigraphy and gamma probe detection. *J Am Coll Surg* 1998;186:275–283.
34. Giuliano A, Jones R, Brennan M, Statman R. Sentinel lymphadenectomy in breast cancer. *J Clin Oncol* 1997;15:2345–2350.
35. Veronesi U, Paganelli G, Viale G, et al. Sentinel lymph node biopsy and axillary dissection in breast cancer: Results in a large series. *J Natl Cancer Inst* 1999;91:368–373.
36. Krag D, Weaver D, Ashikaga T, et al. The sentinel node in breast cancer—A multicenter validation study. *N Engl J Med* 1998;339:941–946.
37. Miltenburg DM, Miller C, Brunicardi FC. Meta-analysis of sentinel lymph node biopsy in breast cancer. *Journal of Surgical Research* 1999;84:138–142.
38. International Breast Cancer Study Group. Prognostic importance of occult axillary lymph node micrometastases from breast cancers. *Lancet* 1990;335:1565–1568.
39. Wilkinson EJ, Hause LL, Hoffman RG, et al. Occult axillary lymph node metastases in invasive breast carcinoma: characteristics of the primary tumor and significance of the metastases. *Pathol Ann* 1982;17:67–91.
40. Nasser IA, Lee AKC, Bosari S, et al. Occult axillary lymph node metastates in 'node-negative' breast carcinoma. *Hum Pathol* 1993;24:950–957.
41. Hainsworth PJ, Tjandra JJ, Stillwell RG, et al. Detection and significance of occult metastases in node-negative breast cancer. *Br J Surg* 1993;80:459–463.
42. McGuckin MA, Cummings MC, Walsh MD, et al. Occult axillary node metastases in breast cancer: their detection and prognostic significance. *Br J Cancer* 1996;73:88–95.
43. Cserni G. Metastases in axillary sentinel lymph nodes in breast cancer as detected by intensive histopathological work-up. *J Clin Pathol* 1999;52:922–924.
44. Fisher ER, Palekar A, Rockette H, et al. Pathologic findings from the National Surgical Adjuvant Breast Project (protocol no 4). V. Significance of axillary nodal micro and macro metastases. *Cancer* 1978a;42:2032–2038.

45. Huvos AG, Hutter RVP, Berg JW. Significance of axillary macrometastases and micrometastases in mammary cancer. *Ann Surg* 1971;173:441–461.
46. Rosen PP, Saigo PE, Braun DW, et al. Axillary micro- and macrometastases in breast cancer. *Ann Surg* 1981; 194:585–591.
47. de Mascarel I, Bonichon F, Coindre JM, Trojani M. Prognostic significance of breast cancer axillary lymph node micrometastases assessed by two special techniques: re-evaluation with longer follow-up. *Br J Cancer* 1992;66:523–527.
48. Millis RR, Springall R, Lee AHS, et al. Occult axillary lymph node metastases are of no prognostic significance in breast cancer. *Br J Cancer* 2002; in press.
49. Friedman S, Bertin F, Mouriesse H, et al. Importance of tumor cells in axillary sinus margins ('clandestine' metastases) discovered by serial sectioning in operable breast cancer. *Acta Oncol* 1988;27:483–487.
50. Hartveit F, Lilleng PK. Breast cancer: two micrometastatic variants in the axilla that differ in prognosis. *Histopathology* 1996;28:241–246.
51. Fisher CJ, Boyle S, Burke M, Price AB. Intraoperative assessment of nodal status in the selection of patients with breast cancer for axillary clearance. *Br J Surg* 1993;80:457–458.
52. Galimberti V, Zurrida S, Zucali P, Luini A. Can sentinel node biopsy avoid axillary dissection in clinically node-negative breast cancer patients? *Breast* 1998;7: 8–10.
53. vanDiest PJ, Torrenga H, Borgstein PJ, et al. Reliability of intraoperative frozen section and imprint cytological investigation of sentinel lymph nodes in breast cancer. *Histopathol* 1999;35:14–18.
54. National Coordinating Group for Breast Screening Pathology. Pathology Reporting in Breast Screening Pathology. 2nd ed: NHSBSP Publications, no 3.; 1997.
55. Cascinelli N, Greco M, Bufalino R, et al. Prognosis of breast cancer with axillary node metastases after surgical treatment only. *Eur J Cancer Clin Oncol* 1987; 23:795–799.
56. Mambo NC, Gallager HS. Carcinoma of the breast. The prognostic significance of extranodal extension of axillary disease. *Cancer* 1977;39:2280–2285.
57. Fisher ER, Gregorio RM, Redmond C, et al. Pathologic findings from the National Surgical Adjuvant Breast Project (protocol no 4). III. The significance of extranodal extension of axillary metastases. *Am J Clin Pathol* 1976;65:439–444.
58. Hartveit F. Paranodal tumor in breast cancer: extranodal extension versus vascular spread. *J Pathol* 1984; 144:253–256.
59. Donegan WL, Stine SB, Samter TG. Implications of extracapsular nodal metastases for treatment and prognosis of breast cancer. *Cancer* 1993;72:778–782.
60. Pinder S, Ellis IO, O'Rourke S, et al. Pathological prognostic factors in breast cancer. III. Vascular invasion: relationship with recurrence and survival in a large series with long-term follow-up. *Histopathology* 1994;24:41–47.
61. Örbo A, Stalsberg H, Kunde D. Topographic criteria in the diagnosis of tumor emboli in intramammary lymphatics. *Cancer* 1990;66:972–977.
62. Davis BW, Gelber R, Goldhirsh A, et al. Prognostic significance of peritumoral vessel invasion in clinical trials of adjuvant therapy for breast cancer with axillary node metastases. *Hum Pathol* 1985;16: 1212–1218.
63. Bettelheim R, Penman HG, Thornton-Jones H, et al. Prognostic significance of peritumoral vascular invasion in breast cancer. *Br J Cancer* 1984a;50:771–777.
64. Roses DF, Bell DA, Fotte TJ, et al. Pathologic predictors of recurrence in stage 1 (T1NOMO and T2NOMO) breast cancer. *Am J Clin Pathol* 1982;78:817–820.
65. Nime FA, Rosen PP, Thaler HT, et al. Prognostic significance of tumor emboli in intramammary lymphatics in patients with mammary carcinoma. *Am J Surg Pathol* 1977;1:25–30.
66. Nealon TF, Nkongho A, Grossi CE, et al. Treatment of early cancer of the breast (T1NOMO and T2NOMO) on the basis of histologic characteristics. *Surgery* 1981;89:279–289.
67. Dawson PJ, Karrison T, Ferguson DJ. Histologic features associated with long-term survival in breast cancer. *Hum Pathol* 1986;17:1015–1021.
68. Dawson PJ, Ferguson DJ, Karrison T. The pathologic findings of breast cancer in patients surviving 25 years after radical mastectomy. *Cancer* 1982;50: 2131–2138.
69. Sears HF, Janus J, Levy W, et al. Breast cancer without axillary metastases. Are there subpopulations? *Cancer* 1982;50:1820–1827.
70. Gilchrist KW, Gould VE, Hirschl S, et al. Interobserver variation in the identification of breast carcinoma in intramammary lymphatics. *Hum Pathol* 1982;13:170–172.
71. Rosen PP, Saigo PE, Brown DW, et al. Predictors of recurrence in stage 1 (T1NOMO) breast carcinoma. *Ann Surg* 1981;193:15–25.
72. Sundquist M, Thorstenson S, Klintenberg C, et al. Indicators of local regional recurrence in breast cancer. The South East Swedish Breast Cancer Group. *Eur J Surg Oncol* 2000;26:357–362.
73. O'Rourke S, Galea MH, Euhus D, et al. An audit of local recurrence after simple mastectomy. *Br J Surg* 1994;81:386–389.
74. Greenhough RB. Varying degrees of malignancy in cancer of the breast. *J Cancer Res* 1925;9:452–463.
75. Patey DH, Scarff RW. The position of histology in the prognosis of carcinoma of the breast. *Lancet* 1928; 1:801–804.
76. Bloom HJG. Prognosis in carcinoma of the breast. *Br J Cancer* 1950a;4:259–288.
77. Bloom HJG. Further studies on prognosis of breast carcinoma. *Br J Cancer* 1950b;4:347–367.
78. Bloom HJG, Richardson WW. Histological grading and prognosis in breast cancer. A study of 1409 cases of which 359 have been followed for 15 years. *Br J Cancer* 1957;11:359–377.
79. Contesso G, Mouriesse H, Friedman S, et al. The importance of histologic grade in long-term prognosis of breast cancer: a study of 1010 patients, uniformly treated at the Institut Gustave-Roussy. *J Clin Oncol* 1987;5:1378–1386.
80. Elston CW, Ellis IO. Pathological prognostic factors in breast cancer. I. The value of histological grade in breast cancer: experience from a large study with long-term follow-up. *Histopathology* 1991;19:403–410.
81. Hartveit F. Prognostic typing in breast cancer. *Br Med J* 1971;4:253–257.
82. Black MM, Barclay THC, Hankey BR. Prognosis in breast cancer utilizing histologic characteristics of the primary tumor. *Cancer* 1975;36:2048–2055.

83. Le Doussal V, Tubiana-Hulin M, Friedman S, et al. Prognostic value of histologic grade nuclear components of Scarff Bloom Richardson (SBR). An improved score modification based on a multivariate analysis of 1262 invasive ductal breast carcinomas. *Cancer* 1989;64:1914–1921.
84. Fitzgibbons PL, Page DL, Weaver D, et al. Prognostic factors in breast cancer. College of American Pathologists Consensus Statement 1999. *Arch Pathol Lab Med* 2000;124:966–978.
85. Gilchrist KW, Kalish L, Gould VE, et al. Interobserver reproducibility of histopathological features in stage II breast cancer. An ECPG study. *Breast Cancer Res Treat* 1979;5:3–10.
86. Fisher ER, Redmond C, Fisher B. Histologic grading of breast cancer. *Pathol Annu* 1980;15:239–251.
87. Hopton DS, Thorogood J, Clayden AD, MacKinnon D. Observer variation in histological grading of breast cancer. *Eur J Surg Oncol* 1989;15:21–23.
88. Robbins P, Pinder S, de Klerk N, et al. Histological grading of breast carcinomas. A study of interobserver agreement. *Hum Pathol* 1995;26:873–879.
89. Frierson HF, Wolber RA, Berean KW, et al. Interobserver reproducibility of the Nottingham modification of the Bloom and Richardson histological grading scheme for infiltrating ductal carcinoma. *Am J Clin Pathol* 1995;105:195–198.
90. Dalton LW, Page DL, Dupont WD. Histologic grading of breast carcinoma: a reproducibility study. *Cancer* 1994;73:2765–2770.
91. European Commission. *European guidelines for quality assurance in mammography screening*, 2nd ed. Luxembourg: Office for Official Publications of the European Communities, 1996.
92. Connolly JL, Fechner RE, Kempson RL, et al. Recommendations for the reporting of breast carcinoma. *Hum Pathol* 1996;27:220–224.
93. Pinder SE, Murray S, Ellis IO, et al. The importance of histological grade in invasive breast carcinoma and response to chemotherapy. *Cancer* 1998;83:1529–1539.
94. Ellis IO, Galea M, Broughton N, et al. Pathological prognostic factors in breast cancer. II. Histological type. Relationship with survival in a large study with long-term follow-up. *Histopathology* 1992;20:479–489.
95. Page DL, Anderson TJ. *Diagnostic histopathology of the breast*. Edinburgh: Churchill Livingstone, 1987.
96. Pinder SE, Elston CW, Ellis IO. Invasive carcinoma—usual histological types. In: Elston CW, Ellis IO, eds. *Systemic pathology—the breast*, 3rd ed. London: Churchill Livingstone, 1998.
97. Eusebi V, Foschini MP. Rare carcinomas of the breast. In: Elston CW, Ellis IO, eds. *Systemic pathology. the breast*, 3rd ed. London: Churchill Livingstone, 1998: 339–364.
98. McDivitt RW, Boyce W, Gersell D. Tubular carcinoma of the breast. *Am J Surg Pathol* 1982;6:401–411.
99. Cooper HS, Patchefsky AS, Krall RA. Tubular carcinoma of the breast. *Cancer* 1978;42:2334–2342.
100. Carstens PHB, Greenberg RA, Francis D, Lyon H. Tubular carcinoma of the breast. A long-term follow-up. *Histopathology* 1985;9:271–280.
101. Page DL, Dixon JM, Anderson TJ, et al. Invasive cribriform carcinoma of the breast. *Histopathology* 1983;7:525–536.
102. Dixon JM, Page DL, Anderson TJ, et al. Long term survivors after breast cancer. *Br J Surg* 1985;72:445–448.
103. Bloom HJC, Richardson WW, Field JR. Host resistance and survival in carcinoma of the breast: a study of 104 cases of medullary carcinoma in a series of 1411 cases of beast cancer followed for 20 years. *Br Med J* 1970;3:181–188.
104. Ridolfi RL, Rosen PP, Port A, et al. Medullary carcinoma of the breast—a clinicopathologic study with a ten year follow-up. *Cancer* 1977;40:1365–1385.
105. Lee BJ, Hauser H, Pack GT. Gelatinous carcinoma of the breast. *Surg Gynecol Obstet* 1934;59:841–850.
106. Clayton F. Pure mucinous carcinomas of the breast: morphologic features and prognostic correlates. *Hum Pathol* 1986;17:34–38.
107. Haagensen CD, Lane N, Lattes R, Bodian C. Lobular neoplasia (so-called lobular carcinoma in situ) of the breast. *Cancer* 1978;42:737–767.
108. Fisher ER, Gregorio RM, Redmond C, et al. Tubulolobular invasive breast cancer: A variant of lobular invasive cancer. *Hum Pathol* 1977;8:679–683.
109. Anderson TJ, Lamb J, Donnan P, et al. Comparative pathology of breast cancer in a randomised trial of screening. *Br J Cancer* 1991;64:108–113.
110. Ellis IO, Galea MH, Locker A, et al. Early experience in breast cancer screening: Emphasis on development of protocols for triple assessment. *Breast* 1993;2:148–153.
111. Pereira H, Pinder SE, Sibbering DM, et al. Pathological prognostic factors in breast cancer. IV: Should you be a typer or a grader? A comparative study of two histological prognostic features in operable breast carcinoma. *Histopathology* 1995;27:219–226.
112. Lamovec J, Bracko M. Metastatic pattern of infiltrating lobular carcinoma of the breast: an autopsy study. *J Surg Oncol* 1991;48:28–33.
113. Harris M, Howell A, Chrissohou M. A comparison of the metastatic pattern of infiltrating lobular carcinoma and infiltrating duct carcinoma of the breast. *Br J Cancer* 1984;50:23–30.
114. Domagala W, Markiewski M, Kubiak R, et al. Immunohistochemical profile of invasive lobular carcinoma of the breast: predominantly vimentin and p53 protein negative, cathepsin D and oestrogen receptor positive. *Virchows Arch (A) Pathol Anat Histopathol* 1993;423:497–502.
115. Breast Cancer Linkage Consortium. Pathology of familial breast cancer: differences between breast cancer in carriers of BRCA1 or BRCA2 mutations and sporadic cases. *Lancet* 1997;349:1505–1510.
116. Marcus JN, Watson P, Page DL, et al. Hereditary breast cancer. Pathobiology, prognosis and BRCA1 and BRCA2 gene linkage. *Cancer* 1996;77:697–709.
117. Lakhani SR, Jacquemier J, Sloane JP, et al. Multifactorial analysis of differences between sporadic breast cancers and cancers involving BRCA1 and BRCA2 mutations. *J Natl Cancer Inst* 1998;90:1138–1145.
118. Matsukuma A, Enjoji M, Toyoshima S. Ductal carcinoma of the breast. An analysis of the proportion of intraductal and invasive components. *Pathol Res Prac* 1991;187:62–67.
119. Silverberg SG, Chitale AR. Assessment of the significance of the proportion of intraductal and infiltrating tumor growth in ductal carcinoma of the breast. *Cancer* 1973;32:830–837.

120. Van Dongen JA, Fentiman IS, Harris JR, et al. In situ breast cancer: the EORTC consensus meeting. *Lancet* 1989;2:25–27.
121. Schnitt SJ, Connelly JL, Harris JR, et al. Pathologic predictors of early local recurrence in stage I and stage II breast cancer treated by primary radiation therapy. *Cancer* 1984;53:1049–1057.
122. Gage I, Schnitt SJ, Nixon AJ, et al. Pathologic margin involvement and the risk of recurrence in patients treated with breast-conserving therapy. *Cancer* 1996;78:1921–1928.
123. Parham DM, Hagen N, Brown RA. Morphometric analysis of breast carcinoma: association with survival. *J Clin Pathol* 1988;41:173–177.
124. Black R, Prescott R, Bers K, et al. Tumor cellularity, oestrogen receptors and prognosis in breast cancer. *Clin Oncol* 1983;9:311–318.
125. Sistrunk WE, MacCarty WC. Life expectancy following radical amputation for carcinoma of the breast—a clinical and pathological study of 218 cases. *Ann Surg* 1922;75:61–69.
126. Parfrey NA, Doyle CT. Elastosis in benign and malignant breast disease. *Hum Pathol* 1985;16:674–676.
127. Shivas AA, Douglas JG. The prognostic significance of elastosis in breast carcinoma. *J Roy Coll Surg Edinb* 1972;17:315–320.
128. Masters JR, Millis RR, King RJB, Rubens RD. Elastosis and response to endocrine therapy in human breast cancer. *Br J Cancer* 1979;39:536–539.
129. Robertson AJ, Brown RA, Cree IA, et al. Prognostic value of measurement of elastosis in breast carcinoma. *J Clin Pathol* 1981;34:738–743.
130. Rasmussen BB, Pederson BV, Thorpe SM, Rose C. Elastosis in relation to prognosis in primary breast carcinoma. *Cancer Res* 1985;45:1428–1430.
131. Carter D, Elkins RC, Pipkin RD, et al. Relationship of necrosis and tumor border to lymph node metastases and 10 year survival in carcinoma of the breast. *Am J Surg Pathol* 1978;2:39–46.
132. Clark GM. Do we really need prognostic factors for breast cancer? *Breast Cancer Res Treat* 1994;30:117–126.
133. Brown JM, Benson EA, Jones M. Confirmation of a long-term prognostic index in breast cancer. *Breast* 1993;2:144–147.
134. Balslev I, Axelsson CK, Zedelev K, et al. The Nottingham Prognostic Index applied to 9,149 patients from the studies of the Danish Breast Cancer Cooperative Group (DBCG). *Breast Cancer Res Treat* 1994;32:281–290.
135. Sundquist M, Thorstenson S, Brudin L, Nordenskjold B. Applying the Nottingham Prognostic Index to a Swedish breast cancer population. South East Swedish Breast Cancer Study Group. *Breast Cancer Res Treat* 1999;53:1–8.
136. D'Eredita' G, Giardina C, Martellotta M, et al. Prognostic factors in breast cancer: the predictive value of the Nottingham Prognostic Index in patients with a long-term follow-up that were treated in a single institution. *Eur J Cancer* 2001;37:591–596.
137. Beatson JT. Treatment of inoperable cases of carcinoma of the mamma; suggestions for a new method of treatment with illustrative cases. *Lancet* 1896;2:104–107.
138. King WJ, Greene GL. Monoclonal antibodies localize oestrogen receptor in nuclei of target cells. *Nature* 1984;307:745–747.
139. McCarty KS Jr, Miller LS, Cox EB, et al. Estrogen receptor analyses: Correlation of biochemical and immunohistochemical methods using monoclonal antireceptor antibodies. *Arch Pathol Lab Med* 1985;109:716–721.
140. Greene GL, Nolan C, Engler JP, et al. Monoclonal antibodies to human estrogen receptor. *Proc Natl Acad Sci USA* 1980;77:5115–5119.
141. Snead DJR, Bell JA, Dixon AR, et al. Methodology of immunohistochemical detection of oestrogen receptor in human breast carcinoma in formalin fixed paraffin embedded tissue: a comparison with frozen section morphology. *Histopathology* 1993;23:233–238.
142. Goulding H, Pinder S, Cannon P, et al. A new immunohistochemical antibody for the assessment of estrogen receptor status on routine formalin-fixed tissue samples. *Hum Pathol* 1995;26:291–294.
143. Barnes DM, Millis RR. Oestrogen receptors: the history,the relevance and the methods of evaluation. In: Kirkham N, Lemoine NR, eds. *Progress in pathology*. Edinburgh: Churchill Livingstone, 1995:89–114.
144. Harvey JM, Clark GM, Osborne CK, Allred D. Estrogen receptor status by immunohistochemistry is superior to the ligand-binding assay for predicting response to adjuvant endocrine therapy in breast cancer. *J Clin Oncol* 1999;17:1474–1781.
145. NIH Consensus Development Conference. Steroid receptors in breast cancer. *Cancer* 1980;46:2759–2963.
146. Robertson JFR, Bates K, Pearson D, et al. Comparison of two oestrogen receptor assays in the prediction of the clinical course of patients with advanced breast cancer. *Br J Cancer* 1992;65:727–730.
147. McClelland RA, Berger U, Miller LS, et al. Immunocytochemical assay for oestrogen receptor in patients with breast cancer. Relationship to biochemical assay and to outcome of therapy. *J Clin Oncol* 1986;4:1171–1176.
148. Birner P, Oberhuber G, Stani J, et al. Evaluation of the United States Food and Drug Administration-approved scoring and test system of HER-2 protein expression in breast cancer. *Clin Cancer Res* 2001;7:1669–1675.
149. Lovekin C, Ellis IO, Locker A, et al. c-erbB-2 oncoprotein expression in primary and advanced breast cancer. *Br J Cancer* 1990;63:439–443.
150. Lewis S, Locker A, Todd JH, et al. Expression of epidermal growth factor receptor in breast carcinoma. *J Clin Pathol* 1990;43:385–389.
151. Ellis IO, Bell J, Todd J, et al. Evaluation of immunoreactivity with monoclonal antibody NCRC-II in breast carcinoma. *Br J Cancer* 1987;56:295–299.
152. Elston CW. Grading of invasive carcinoma of the breast. In: Page DL, Anderson TJ, eds. *Diagnostic histopathology of the breast*. Edinburgh: Churchill Livingstone, 1987:300–311.

PART IV

Issues for the Practicing Oncologist

…
SECTION 1

Supportive Care and Quality of Life

30

Science and Alternative Therapy: The Past, Present, and Future

Brent A. Bauer and Charles L. Loprinzi

The seemingly endless proliferation of alternative treatments for cancer sometimes seems to have developed in the past one or two decades. Much of this is due to the explosive growth of the World Wide Web in that same time period. Treatments that normally would have had to spread by word of mouth can now be disseminated to millions of potential users literally in seconds. Yet, in reality, alternative treatments have existed as long as there have been conventional treatments. As patient advocates, physicians must be able to sort through the hundreds of alternative treatments and thousands of claims that currently exist, and then, in turn, provide safe and honest counsel to our patients. To this end, it is instructive to first consider the past history of alternative treatments. Such knowledge helps place the current usage in context and can then be used to expand our understanding of the present. With such understanding, we can then look to a near future where physicians and patients work collaboratively to find the appropriate place for alternative therapy within an individual patient's treatment plan. Sifting the helpful from the harmful, based on sound scientific principles (but with recognition that improvements in quality of life are sometimes as important as changes in lab values), will be an ongoing task.

THE PAST

"It should be forbidden and severely punished to remove cancer by cutting, burning, cautery, and other fiendish tortures. It is from nature that the disease comes, and from nature comes the cure, not from physicians."
Paracelsus (1493–1541 AD)

This quote by Paracelsus is reflective of the state of conventional medicine at a time when diseases were often considered either an imbalance of essential humors or the result of occult forces. Attempts to cure ranged from the use of herbs to trepanning to exorcism. Any attempt at surgery—in a period lacking anesthesia or basic concepts of microbiology—was indeed apt to be a "fiendish torture." That conventional medicine had relatively little to offer the patient with cancer meant that any of a number of theories and practices coexisted. Thus, even at this early date, the concept of natural cures being superior was already evident.

By the 1700s, conventional medicine had evolved and was primarily "heroic medicine," a medical system founded on the theory that diseases resulted from an overabundance of fluids in the body. Treatments were therefore aimed at releasing these "excess" fluids, employing such means as purging, bleeding and blistering. Venisection, scarification, cupping, and blistering were all used to drain excess fluids. Calomel, a mercury compound, was commonly used as a purgative. Such treatments, however, were often far worse than the diseases they were intended to treat. Thus, the popularity of alternative therapies during that period of history is not surprising.

Arguing against the harsh (and generally ineffective) treatments of conventional physicians, alternative providers sprang up with innumerable theories and cures throughout the 1800s. Samuel Thomson (1769–1843) believed that disease was the result of a "clogged system" and was cured by purging and sweating. However, unlike the heroic doctors, he advocated vegetable and herbal tonics, vehemently opposing the use of harsh (and toxic) purgatives such as calomel. He also argued strongly against the value of blood letting. His system, known as Thomsonism, became very popular.

However it is the rise of patent medicines (and the traveling medicine shows frequently used to promote them) that seem to characterize this era best. One of the best-known traveling medicine shows was "The Kickapoo Indian Medicine Company." Its principal product, "Kickapoo Indian Sagwa," was advertised by stating:

> The germs of scrofula, salt rheum, and many other diseases, which sooner or later undermine the health, all arise from impure blood. To insure good health, this state of things must be changed; the blood must be cleansed from all impurities.... Indian Sagwa is the acknowledged Blood Renovator... In all cases of blood disease, Sagwa works like magic. (*Kickapoo Indian Medicine Company, Advertising Booklet, circa 1885.*)

The makers of Sagwa even used an equivalent to one of the commonest current themes, boosting the immune system:

> ... it stimulates and enlivens the vital functions, promotes energy and strength, restores and preserves health and infuses new life and vigor throughout the whole system..."

Like many of today's nostrums, Sagwa was "natural" and a "cure-all":

> It is compounded of the virtues of Roots, Herbs, Barks, Gums and Leaves... The sciences of Medicine and Chemistry have never produced so valuable a remedy, nor one so potent to cure all diseases.

By the 1840s, home medical guides were also flourishing, spurred by a growing mistrust of conventional physicians, populism and a degree of anti-intellectualism. "The Indian Vegetable Family Instructor" (1) addressed the issue of breast cancer as follows:

> To cure a real cancer... the whole system must be first cleared of canker. When this is done, there is nothing left to support what is called the cancer. My method of curing, is, first to clear the system with the emetic, &c., giving powders, bitters, &c., to help the digestion; and continue this course until the whole body is cleared of what makes and supports the cancer... apply the cancer plaster... the cancer eats the plaster instead of being drawn out by it... this is very simple, safe and generally effectual remedy.

Fear of conventional treatments also spawned a number of sanatoriums, devoted to gentle cures of cancer.

> Cancer Cured with Soothing Balmy Oils... Cancer of the nose, eye, lip, ear, neck, breast, stomach—in fact, all internal or external organs—cured without knife or burning plasters, but with soothing oils. (*Print advertisement, Dr. B.F. Bye Sanatorium, Indianapolis, Indiana circa 1900.*)

Thus, over a century ago, alternative providers were already playing on the fears that patients had regarding the "harshness" of conventional treatments (knife and plasters then, surgery and chemotherapy now).

The Nichol's Sanitarium (2) had an impressive record of treating cancer in the 1920s:

> To date, May 28th, 1928, we have treated 18,276 patients. Of this number, 75% have been cured.

Financial remuneration was secondary to the reward brought by helping patients:

> A cured patient means much more to us than the fee he pays us.

Fortunately, Nichols had knowledge of the true cure:

> Our method of treatment is the Escharotic... which has as many advantages over the plaster as an electric light has over a tallow candle, and has been successfully applied in a hundred situations where no one with either knife or plaster has ever dared to venture... When properly applied, it will kill any ordinary cancer upon the base in a few hours. Upon the breast, or in some very heavy growth, it will take from 2–5 days.

One popular program, Viavi Hygiene (3), promoted unusual ideas regarding causes and cures of cancer, along with a large list of proprietary Viavi products. For example, in regards to cancers of the breast:

> The cause of all such growth in the breast, is weakened vital action, such as should remove waste from the body instead of allowing it to accumulate (p. 356). The unnatural amount of blood sent to the breast did not pass from the body in the menstrual flow, and this occurs again and again until the breast takes on malignant degeneration.

Though such antique notions now appear quaint, it is well to consider that unusual ideas regarding causes and treatment of cancer have continued with us to the present day. In the 1970s, William Donald Kelley, a Dallas dentist, developed a mail-order system to cure cancer. After filling out a 3,200-question metabolic evaluation form, patients received a computer generated printout and tape-recorded message full of instructions on how to change their habits to produce a cure. Numerous nutritional supplements could be ordered from Dallas, including Kelley's brand of coffee (to be used for coffee enemas, which were prescribed for daily detoxification) (4). Also in the 1970s, Adele Davis wrote in *Let's Get Well:* "I have yet to know of a single adult who developed cancer who has habitually drunk a quart of milk daily." And John A. Richardson wrote in *Laetrile Case Histories:* "In our view, cancer . . . is a disease caused by a deficiency of vitamin B-17, pancreatic enzymes, or both."

Even more intriguing is the Nanoray device, produced by Nanoray, Inc., which became available in the mid-1970s. The manufacturer suggested that a "dangerous space frequency" had begun emanating from the sun on April 4, 1973, at 3 p.m. that was affecting health. Using the Nanoray, this frequency could be reversed and cure any disease, including "palladium poisoning, cancer, and tuberculosis" (pamphlet accompanying Nanoray device, dated 1976).

THE PRESENT

It appears well established that many of the attributes of today's alternative therapies ("natural," "safe," "gentle") were in fact claimed for the remedies of the 1800s and 1900s as well. Then, as now, these claims reflect the trepidation that conventional therapies did (and still do) engender in the general public. Cancer is feared greatly but, at times, only slightly more so than its treatment. Popular belief from the 1800s to the 2000s has imbued the conventional treatment of cancer with horrific side effects. Attributes claimed for the patent medicines and nostrums of the 1800s ("cleansing," "immune boosting") are again finding currency with today's health consumer.

Definition

As has been intimated already, the very concept of what is alternative therapy is debatable. The terminology has been anything but static, with many now favoring the broader term of "complementary and alternative medicine" (CAM). Others find the concept of alternative pejorative and argue for the use of "integrative medicine" (IM). This seems to imply broad endorsement to all therapies, making this terminology problematic as well.

Regardless of the rubric employed (alternative, CAM, or IM), the exact definition of what it is that is attempting to be named remains elusive. Many have struggled to provide definition to the concept of alternative medicine. David Eisenberg of Harvard suggested in 1990 that alternative medicine is defined by what it is not: "Interventions neither taught widely in medical schools nor generally available in hospitals" (5). Yet, since that time, much has changed and nearly two-thirds of medical schools offer some training in alternative medicine. Hospitals are slowly but increasingly also offering a number of alternative therapies in a bid to improve patient satisfaction. In 1995, a conference on complementary and alternative medicine convened by the then Office of Alternative Medicine (now the National Center for Complementary and Alternative Medicine-NIH) attempted to create a definition. That conference yielded the following: "A broad domain of healing resources that encompass all health systems, modalities and practices, and their accompanying theories and beliefs, other than those intrinsic to the politically dominant health system of a particular society or culture in a given historical period" (6). While comprehensive, this definition is somewhat unwieldy and difficult to apply in day-to-day practice. Another definition of CAM is "health-related behavior patterns and medications, which are used with the intention of curing and improving a respective illness, without the existence of valid proof of efficacy according to scientific criteria" (7). Cassileth (8) suggests that *complementary* treatments are used "*in addition to* mainstream care", while *alternative* therapies are "promoted for . . . use *instead of* mainstream therapy."

The plethora of definitions reflects the difficulties in reaching unanimous decisions regarding what alternative medicine actually is. Perhaps one of the simplest definitions recently advanced may also be the easiest to use as it is free of judgmental tone and encompasses most of what are generally thought to be alternative therapies. Stephen Strauss, MD, director of NCCAM, suggests that CAM is "health care practices that are not an integral part of conventional medicine" (9).

GENERAL USAGE

The lack of agreement on an exact definition of what constitutes an alternative treatment results in wide variations of the estimates of use. In 1990, according to the widely referenced work of Eisenberg and colleagues (5), 34% of the U.S. population (60 million people) was estimated to be using some form of alternative therapy. When the survey was reconducted in 1997, Eisenberg reported that usage had increased to 42% of the population (83 million people) (10). Expenditures for alternative therapies had increased from $22.6 billion in 1990 to $32.7 billion in 1997. Visits to practitioners of alternative therapies in 1997 were in excess of those to conventional practitioners by an estimated 243 million visits, further characterizing this explosion in interest in alternative therapies (10). Worldwide, the usage of CAM modalities by the general population has been estimated to be somewhere between 25% and 50% of most industrialized nations (11,12).

More recently, a national survey (13) found that of 1,148 U.S. adults surveyed, two-thirds had used alternative medicine at some point. Approximately 30% had tried each of the most popular alternative therapies (herbal medicine, chiropractic, and massage). The next most common therapy was meditation, which 14% of respondents had tried. Of the respondents, 23% had used herbs in the two-week period prior to the survey and 50% had used vitamin supplements. Women were more likely than men to have tried most of the alternative medicine treatments. Less than 10% had tried acupuncture, yoga, homeopathy, hypnosis, traditional Chinese medicine, or Tai chi.

Usage in Cancer Patients

An attempt to summarize current literature investigating the prevalence of CAM usage in patients with cancer was published in 1998 by Ernst and Cassileth (14). They reviewed 26 surveys that investigated the prevalence of CAM usage in patients with cancer. These surveys came from 13 different countries, including four studies that focused on pediatric patients. The use of CAM therapies in the adult populations ranged from 7% to 64% with an average prevalence across the adult studies of 31.4%.

Usage in Breast Cancer Patients

Specific information regarding the use of CAM therapies by patients with breast cancer is available from several studies (Table 30.1). Crocetti, in 1998 (15) used a mailed questionnaire to study 473 women who had undergone surgical intervention for breast cancer, with 242 responding. CAM had been used by 16.5% of the respondents after the diagnosis of cancer. The most commonly used modalities were homeopathy, manual healing, herbals, and acupuncture. Users were younger and more educated compared to nonusers. Of those patients who had used a CAM therapy, 73% said they were satisfied with these treatments.

A population-based study (16) of women who received the histological diagnosis of breast cancer, conducted in San Francisco found that 69% of the participants had used a CAM treat-

TABLE 30.1. Breast cancer patients' usage of complementary and alternative medicine

Author	Year	N	Usage	Therapies
Ernst/Cassileth (all cancers)	1998	26 (survey review)	31.4 % (range 7%–64%)	Multiple
Crocetti	1998	473	16.5%	Homeopathy, manual healing, herbs, acupuncture
Adler	1999	Population study	72% overall age 66–74, 58% age 35–49, 78%	Not listed
Gotay	1999	Unknown	36%	Religious/spiritual therapy, herbs
Wyatt (all cancers)	1999	699	33% age ≥ 64	Exercise, herbs, spiritual healing
Burstein	1999	480	28.1%	Megavitamins, herbs, massage, relaxation
Morris (all cancers)	2000	935 (breast) 1000 (other)	75% overall 84% breast 66% other	Nutrition, massage, herbs
Rees	2000	1,023	31.5%	Chiropractic, massage
Lee	2000	379	50%	Spiritual healing, herbs, dietary methods, massage and acupuncture
Boone	2000	555	66.7%	Vitamins/minerals, herbs, green tea, Essiac, acupuncture, chiropractic, traditional Chinese Medicine, naturopathy
Richardson (all cancers)	2000	453	83.3% overall 68.7% exc spiritual and psychotherapy	Spiritual practices, vitamins, herbs, movement/physical
Moschen	2001	117	47%	Special drinks, vitamins, whole foods, mistletoe, trace elements, homeopathy

Exc, excluding; N, number of patients analyzed.

ment before they were aware of their breast cancer diagnosis. They also found that after the diagnosis, usage increased to 72%. Patients were divided into two cohorts based on age (60 to 74 and 35 to 49). Usage in the older cohort was 58% while that in the younger cohort was 78%.

Gotay (17) found that 36% of Hawaiian breast cancer patients used some CAM modalities, most commonly religious/spiritual therapy and herbal treatments. Again, usage was associated with younger age and higher education levels. In interviews with several breast cancer patients, the authors found that satisfaction with medical care was generally rated quite high, suggesting that the use of CAM was not a reflection of dissatisfaction with conventional care.

Another survey (18) was used to ask 699 cancer patients, all age 64 or older, to assess their use of CAM modalities. Approximately 33% reported using CAM, with higher use in breast cancer patients and those with higher levels of education. The most frequently used therapies were exercise, herbal therapy, and spiritual healing.

Burstein (19) reported on the use of alternative therapies by women who had undergone standard therapy for early-stage breast cancer that was diagnosed between September 1993 and September 1995. Out of a cohort of 480 patients, they found that new use of alternative medicine after surgery for breast cancer was reported by 28.1% of the women. A total of 10.6% of the women had used alternative medicine prior to the diagnosis of breast cancer.

Morris (20) surveyed 1,935 random cancer patients from a tumor registry (935 breast cancer patients and 1,000 patients with other primary site diagnoses). A total of 617 responses (288 breast, 329 other) were received. Of those patients, 75% reported use of a complementary therapy (nutrition 63%, massage 53%, herbs 44%). Therapy was used consistently by 84% of the breast cancer patients versus 66% of patients with other cancers. Sixty-six percent felt that CAM improved their overall health and well-being. Interestingly, age and social economic levels were equally distributed among users and non-users.

Rees (21) sent a questionnaire to 1,023 women from the Thames Cancer Registry who had been diagnosed with breast cancer within the past seven years. Of the respondents, 22.4% had consulted a complementary practitioner in the prior 12 months and 31.5% had done so since their diagnosis of breast cancer. Women using complementary therapies were slightly younger, more educated, and more likely to have used complementary medicine before their initial diagnosis than those who did not use such therapies.

Lee (22) looked at the prevalence of CAM usage by women in four ethnic groups (Latino, white, black, and Chinese) who had been diagnosed with breast cancer between 1990 and 1992 in San Francisco, California. Three hundred seventy-nine participants completed a 30-minute telephone interview that showed that approximately 50% of the women used at least one type of CAM modality and approximately one-third used two types with duration of therapy use generally less than six months. Blacks most often used spiritual healing (36%), Chinese most often used herbal medicines (22%), and Latino women most often used dietary therapies (30%) and spiritual healing (26%). White patients used dietary methods (35%) and physical methods such as massage and acupuncture (21%). Women who had a higher educational level or income, or were of younger age, had private insurance, and exercised or attended support groups were more likely to be CAM users. More than 90% of the subjects found the therapies to be helpful and would recommend them to their friends.

Boone (23) used a mailed questionnaire to determine the prevalence of use of CAM by breast cancer survivors in Ontario, Canada and also to compare the characteristics between CAM users and CAM non-users. Five hundred fifty-five surveys were mailed with a response rate of 76.3%. This survey found that 66.7% of the respondents had used CAM, usually in an attempt to boost the immune system. CAM practitioners (chiropractors, herbalists, acupuncturists, traditional Chinese medicine practitioners, and/or naturopathic practitioners) had been visited by 39.4% of the respondents. Of the respondents, 62.0% reported use of CAM products (vitamins/minerals, herbal medicines, green tea, special foods, and Essiac). Interestingly, support group attendance was the only factor that was found to be significantly associated with the use of CAM in this survey.

Richardson (24) evaluated cancer patients at the University of Texas M.D. Anderson Cancer Center between December 1997 and June 1998. Participants completed a self-administered questionnaire. Four hundred fifty-three participants (response rate 51.4%) showed that 99.3% had heard of CAM, 83.3.% had used at least one CAM approach, with the greatest usage being for spiritual practices (80.5%, followed by vitamins and herbs 62.6%) and movement and physical therapies (59.2%). Usage was higher in women and in younger patients. When spiritual practices and psychotherapy were excluded, 95.8% of the participants were aware of CAM and 68.7% had used CAM.

Finally, Moschen (25) recently compared patients using CAM versus patients receiving only conventional treatment following the diagnosis of breast cancer. One hundred seventeen outpatients were surveyed. Fifty-five (47%) reported that they had used CAM in addition to conventional treatment. These included special drinks, vitamin preparations and whole foods (50%), mistletoe preparations (49%), trace elements (47%), and homeopathy (31%). Users of CAM tended to be younger and better educated.

Reasons for CAM Usage

Crocetti (15) noted that the main reason sited for using complementary and alternative medicine was physical distress. Gotay (17) found symptom control and psychological support to be the main benefits sought from CAM treatments. Many of the respondents suggested that they tried various therapies because they had "nothing to lose." Morris (20) found that the most common reason patients stated was to improve immune function (73%). The second most common reason for using CAM was to alleviate side effects (39%). Only 21% expressed hope that CAM would help cure their cancer. Boone (23) noted that the most common reason patients used CAM was to boost the immune system (63%). Other reasons included to:

- increase quality of life (53%)
- prevent recurrence of cancer (42.5%)
- provide a feeling of control (37.9%)
- aid conventional medical treatment (37.9%)
- treat breast cancer (27.9%)
- treat side effects of conventional treatments (21%)
- attempt to stabilize current condition (17.4%)
- compensate for failed conventional medical treatments (5%)

Disclosing CAM Usage

Adler (26) interviewed 86 San Francisco residents with recently diagnosed breast cancer. Approximately 72% of the participants were using at least one CAM therapy for breast cancer. Six months later, 65% of the participants were still using CAM. However, overall, only 33% disclosed their CAM use to their physicians. Reasons for not disclosing CAM use included:

- the impression of physician disinterest
- the anticipation of a negative response
- the conviction that the physician would be unwilling or unable to contribute useful information

In the study by Morris (20), breast cancer patients informed their conventional physician 63% of the time regarding their CAM use (while other cancer patients reported usage to their physicians 53% of the time). Lee (22) found that approximately 50% of users reported discussing their usage with their primary physician. Boone (23) also found that approximately 50% of patients had informed their physicians of their use of CAM. Metz (27) evaluated 106 consecutive patients presenting for consultation at the University of Pennsylvania with the general diagnosis of cancer. During the standard history and physical, five patients (4.7%) revealed that they had used CAM. Evaluation of the remaining 101 patients with directed questioning found an additional 39 patients (38.6%) who were actually using CAM as well. Thus, of the 44 patients using CAM, 89% were identified by direct questioning and only 11% by standard history and physical examination. Thus, the importance of a carefully worded and non-judgmental inquiry into patients' use of (or interest in) CAM cannot be overestimated. Failing to inquire of each and every cancer patient regarding this topic means opportunities to educate and inform will be missed. And as some therapies can be toxic in and of themselves, failure to learn of a patient's use of them can result in harm.

CAM Information Sources

In a large U.S. survey (13), respondents admitted that they tried alternative medicine because of the recommendations of a friend or family member (62%), recommendation from a doctor (22%), and information from a newspaper, magazine, or Internet source (20%). Crocetti (15) noted that major sources of information on the CAM modalities came from personal experience, relatives or friends, or from the patients' general practitioner. In the Boone study (23), 51% reported that they first learned about CAM from a friend or family member.

A potentially worrisome source of information for breast cancer patients appears to be health food stores, as indicated by the results of a unique study conducted by Gotay (28). A trained surveyor posed as the daughter of a breast cancer patient and visited 40 different health food stores that offered products for cancer patients. The surveyor asked for recommendations regarding her mother's case. Only five stores (13%) asked the surveyor questions about her mother before making recommendations. In 36 stores, one or more products were suggested. The most frequently recommended was shark cartilage oil. Other popular recommendations included maitake mushrooms, Essiac, co-enzyme Q10, and vitamin C. Eight stores (20%) suggested a change of diet (for example, macrobiotic diet, brown rice, minimizing animal proteins, etc.). Seven stores (18%)

directly or indirectly counseled against the use of orthodox cancer therapies.

Personnel frequently stated that CAM products worked by cleansing or bringing the body back into balance.

CAM and the Internet

One of the most wildly growing sources of information (and misinformation) has been the Internet. A growing number of Americans and individuals around the world are turning to the Internet to address questions regarding health. In March of 2001, 63% of American adults were online, and of those, 75% had used the Internet to find health information (29). According to another survey (30), on any given day, 6% of Internet users (or more than 5.5 million Americans) are seeking health information. Further, of all online health information seekers, 70% said that the information they found on the Internet influenced their decision about how to treat an illness. Fifty-two percent of users who have visited health sites online felt that "almost all" or "most" health information found on the Web is reliable.

Bonakdar (31) searched the World Wide Web using "herb" and "cancer," finding over 58,000 matches. Review of selected sites showed that 58.3% of the commercial sites discussed a cure for cancer and only 38.9% recommended consulting with a physician prior to use. Furthermore, the Dietary Supplement Health and Education Act of 1994 (DSHEA) warning disclaimer was found on only 36.1% of the sites. Dr. Bonakdar suggests that common tactics are employed on many of the sites promoting cancer cures. He has developed the acronym "TARGET YOU" to emphasize these recurring traits found on questionable sites:

T. *Testimonials*—many sites use testimonials, generally glowing and hopeful.
A. *Against the establishment*—sites are frequently critical of physicians, ACS, etc.
R. *Research is lacking*—rarely is solid research available to substantiate claims.
G. *Guarantee of success*—many sites offer guarantee (but difficult to collect).
E. *Everything can be cured*—the one drug "cures-all" claim is prevalent.
T. *Terminology used to impress*—scientific/scientific-sounding words used frequently.
Y. *You deserve better*—sites imply that conventional care is inadequate.
O. *Outrageous language*—e.g. "A miraculous breakthrough!!!"
U. *Urgency to treat*—sites imply that action is needed quickly.

Research on CAM and Breast Cancer

Since it is incumbent on physicians to be able to accurately counsel patients regarding CAM on a scientific basis, it is helpful to consider reviews which have attempted to do just that. In 2000, Jacobson (32) reviewed the biomedical literature from 1980 to 1997 that reported results of clinical research on CAM treatments, specifically focusing on therapies of interest to breast cancer patients. Despite retrieving more than 1,000 citations, the authors were only able to identify 51 articles that met their quality criteria. Only three were cancer-directed interventions. Two of these three involved the same treatment (melatonin). The authors noted that while several of the studies had encouraging results, none rose to the level of scientific proof of an improvement in disease progression. They did note that some modalities (e.g., acupuncture for nausea, pressure treatments for lymphedema) appeared to offer benefit in terms of quality of life. One helpful reference for current reviews of many of the CAM modalities most commonly employed by cancer patients is a web site maintained by the University of Texas (www.sph.uth.tmc.edu/utcam/default.htm). This site features reviews on ten common herbal cancer treatments (e.g., Essiac, green tea, mistletoe), ten biological therapies (e.g. shark cartilage, Coley toxins, and melatonin), and seven other miscellaneous therapies (714-X, antineoplastons, and hydrazine sulfate). Each review consists of a brief overview, a summary of the existing research (categorized into animal and human trials and by type of trial), an annotated bibliography and a comprehensive reference list. This is an excellent re-

Discussions with Patients Regarding CAM

So how does one approach a patient who is interested in (or perhaps already using) CAM therapies? Burstein (33) sets the stage by pointing out that, "In some, the interest in CAM is an understandable expression of the hopes, concerns, and symptoms experienced by cancer patients." He goes on to say that, "Such interest poses a challenge to oncologists: a challenge not to our scientific credentials or clinical intentions, but a challenge to be better doctors— to treat the disease and the patient. The use of complementary and health related practices is an opportunity to discuss the means that lie behind these practices, to share further in the experience of illness and well being and to focus clinicians on the genuine needs of cancer patients that neither surgery, radiation nor chemotherapy can satisfy."

Coss (34) attempted to delineate what issues were of greatest interest or most important to cancer patients regarding CAM. He surveyed 503 randomly selected patients who had been treated at the Sutter Cancer Center in Sacramento, California. Eighty-two (16%) had considered utilizing alternative therapy for cancer after a cancer diagnosis was made. Those most likely to consider such a treatment were young, female, college educated and more likely to have had a diagnosis of cancer for more than one year. Of those who were interested in alternative therapy, the greatest interest was expressed in:

- nutritional guidance
- support groups for families
- meditation
- patient support groups
- counseling
- spiritual care
- acupuncture
- herbal therapy

Eighty-five percent favored the idea of alternative care being offered as part of their oncology treatment. Seventy-five percent said that they would like to be able to ask their doctors for a referral to an alternative provider. Coss concluded, "Providing alternative therapy or referrals for alternative therapy within a cancer center ensures the availability of both the most advanced conventional treatment and care as well as accurate information and guidance with regard to alternative therapies" (34).

In regards to cancer patients seeking alternative therapies, Durant (35) states, "Physicians, especially oncologists, need to understand that many, maybe most, of their patients will be curious about, if not interested in, receiving such treatments. A willingness to talk openly about the specific approach being considered and to point out in a non-judgmental way the problems with it will likely not lead to a broken relationship and/or to the patient becoming non-compliant with standard therapy. Handling the complexities associated with unorthodox cancer therapies, no doubt, will continue to be most challenging in this era of excessive expectations and growing anti-science. Most communities require swimming pool owners to construct access barriers to their pools to protect the unsuspecting from the hazards of inadvertently drowning, so also we should protect the unsuspecting from the hazards of alternative medicine."

In summary, it seems advisable to view discussions of alternative therapies with patients as an opportunity to address needs that might not otherwise be expressed or discovered. It should be a time for scientific but compassionate evaluation of the treatments involved. It should be a time to fulfill the physician's role as patient advocate and it may be a time of learning for both physician and patient.

Reputable Sources of Information about Alternative Therapies

- American Cancer Society (www.cancer.org), ACS Guide to Complementary and Alternative Cancer Methods (888-227-5552)
- National Cancer Institute (www.nci.nih.gov)
- National Center for Complementary and Alternative Medicine (www.nccam.nih.gov)
- Memorial Sloan-Kettering Cancer Center (www.mskcc.org/mp.htm)

- University of Texas Center for Alternative Medicine Research in Cancer (www.chprd.sph.uth.tmc.edu/utcam/)
- National Counsel Against Health Fraud (www.ncahf.org)
- Quackwatch (www.quackwatch.com)
- Cancer Guide by Steve Dunn (www.cancerguide.org)
- Healthcare Reality Check (www.hcrc.org)

Resources on Herbs and Supplements

- Prescribers Letter Natural Medicine Database (www.naturaldatabase.com)
- FDA Division of Dietary Supplements (www.cfsan.fda.gov/~dms/supplement.html)
- IBIDS Dietary Supplement Database (http://ods.od.nih.gov/databases/ibids.html)

THE FUTURE

There are three possible avenues which alternative therapies for breast cancer may follow in the future: (a) wane in significance, (b) remain static, or (c) mature and evolve. The first scenario seems unlikely on many fronts. First, the past two decades have seen exponential growth in the interest in and use of CAM modalities, by healthy people and by those with serious illnesses. To postulate a mass repudiation of these therapies seems unlikely. The Internet constantly brings new ideas to the surface (and also repackages some old ones in modern lingo). Ideas can spread with mind-boggling speed and it seems improbable that any meaningful restriction of CAM information could be achieved, even if some regulatory agency were to try. In addition, CAM is a multibillion-dollar industry worldwide and growing. Thus, it seems unlikely that significant regulation will be forthcoming from the government sector. International travel is also increasing—which means all patients are going to be increasingly exposed to ideas, practices, and therapies that are currently not part of their culture. Many of these concepts will be considered alternative simply because they are new or different. With time, research, and education, some of these therapies will become part of our conventional armamentarium, some will be proven inert and some will be shown to be harmful. Taken in aggregate, these many factors argue strongly that CAM, at a minimum, is here to stay.

Is it possible that the second option could occur—that the realm of CAM will remain static. This suggests that the current state of affairs (thousands of therapies and practitioners, each claiming ownership of the truth, and each clamoring for the business of the sick and worried, all in a nearly free-for-all style of advertising on web sites and magazines and media of all types) will continue unchanged. This seems (fortunately) unlikely. Even now, glimmers of greater regulatory oversight of some of the more outlandish claimants is being seen. In the United States, the Federal Trade Commission has shown a willingness to enforce the provisions of the Dietary Supplement Health and Education Act of 1994 that preclude manufacturers from making medical claims for their products. The market is showing some evidence that it is serious about policing its own as various groups put forward Good Manufacturing Practice recommendations. In addition, the public is becoming savvier, no longer quite so willing to fall for every pitch for the next miracle cure.

In fact, forces seem very much aligned to ensure an evolutionary turn towards the realm of CAM which makes the third option the most likely scenario we will see unfold. Indeed, the realm of alternative therapies seems most likely poised to mature and evolve. Three major forces (the market, increasingly sophisticated consumers, and a growing research enterprise) will be the drivers behind this evolution.

The market is making itself felt already. In the Wired Age, so-called "fly-by-night" outfits can produce a slick web page overnight, make outrageous claims for their product, make substantial money, and disappear before legal action ensues. Such charlatanism is likely to always be a part of the CAM landscape. Yet there are rapidly evolving changes occurring. Perhaps the biggest is the entrance into the field of CAM products by large and respected manufacturers. For example, Warner Lambert has a line of herbal products (Quanterra) that are standardized. Glaxo Smith-

Kline recently launched Alluna—a standardized combination of valerian (*Valeriana officinalis*) and hops (*Humulus lupulus*) to aid with sleep problems. These and other pharmaceutical giants are responding to the public's demand for standardized and pure herbal products. As more and more large pharmaceutical companies move into the market, uncontrolled products will be squeezed increasingly into the periphery. Patients are already demonstrating increasing awareness of the issues surrounding herbal purity and standardization and the market may well continue to drive this move to quality in other CAM products as well.

This market change is, in turn, being driven by a growing percentage of consumers who are becoming more sophisticated in their approach to alternative therapies. CAM has been in the news and on the cover of almost every major news journal at some point in the past decade. Much of the early, uncritical acceptance has fallen by the wayside as wild claims have been shown to be just that. Weight loss agents, immune builders, and herbal breast size enhancers have been enjoying a heyday of sales and popular press. But the bloom is already off the rose and disappointment with products that did not live up to their promised miraculous performance has left a growing body of consumers more wary. These individuals are increasingly turning to the web, but now with a jaundiced eye and a goal of researching products before trying them.

Thus, the consumers are in turn driving the third engine of change, research. The U.S. Office of Alternative Medicine was formed by Congress in 1992, largely because of the persistent clamoring of constituents seeking reliable information about alternative therapies. It began with a budget of $2 million and rapidly grew in size and scope. In 1998, the Office became the National Center for Complementary and Alternative Medicine (NCCAM), a full NIH Center. In 2001, the budget for this enterprise was $92 million. The NCCAM's goal is "to build a new research enterprise dedicated to defining the effectiveness and safety of diverse complementary and alternative medical (CAM) practices" (37). Thus, studies are underway on topics as diverse as shark cartilage for the treatment of cancer to the role of massage to reduce cancer-related fatigue. Large academic centers (e.g., Mayo Clinic, Johns Hopkins and University of Pennsylvania) are meeting the need for quality information in this realm by conducting scientifically rigorous evaluations of some of the most popular (and often most promoted) therapies. Many more are being proposed. Within the next 5 years, it is highly probable that the physician who is approached by a patient with questions regarding an alternative therapy will be able to honestly respond with more than "I don't know" or "We don't have enough research to make an assessment." Tapping into a number of growing databases, such as "CAM on PubMed" (sponsored by the NCCAM and the National Library of Medicine), clinicians will increasingly be able to assess an ever-growing volume of scientific data regarding the most common alternative therapies. Sharing this information in a collaborative fashion with cancer patients can yield a partnership that provides the best opportunity for patients to make wise decisions regarding their use of CAM.

CONCLUSIONS

Any diagnosis of cancer can be overwhelming, striking at the very core of human existence. Breast cancer, perhaps more than most other cancers, may strike even deeper chords, as the afflicted woman may face additional struggles with issues of personal identity and societal views of femininity, etc. Perhaps this partly explains the tremendous interest in, and high usage of, CAM by patients with breast cancer. Confronted by a malady that threatens life and self, patients cannot be blamed for looking for any possible escape, or even a path of recovery that is less demanding or threatening. The siren songs of CAM (natural, safer, fewer side-effects, cleansing, immune building) exert a powerful influence on the mind of someone struggling with the enormity of the issue of breast cancer.

Rather than trying to shout down or eliminate the CAM voice, physicians need to supply a reasoned and evidence-based counterbalance, endorsing what is proven, condemning that which has been shown wanting or harmful, and holding judgment where evidence is not yet available.

REFERENCES

1. Bowker PF. *The Indian vegetable family instructor Utica,* published by Jared Doolittle, 1851.
2. Nichols H. *The value of escharotics: medicines which will destroy any living or fungus tissue in the treatment of cancer, lupus, sarcoma, or any other form of malignancy.* East Aurora, NY: The Roy Croft Shops, 1928.
3. *Viavi Hygiene: Explaining the natural principles upon which the Viavi system of treatment for men, women and children is based* (Revised edition). Published by the Viavi Co., San Francisco, CA, 1913:358.
4. Young JH. *American health: quackery selected essays.* Princeton, NJ: Princeton University Press, 1992:120.
5. Eisenberg DM, et al. Unconventional Medicine in the United States: prevalence, costs, and patterns of use. *N Engl J Med* 1993;328:246–252
6. Office of Alternative Medicine (OAM) expert panel at the Conference on CAM Research methodology, April 1995.
7. Schwarz R. Paramedizine in der arzt-patient-beziehung. *Zallgmed* 1989;65:871–875
8. Cassileth BR. Complementary therapies: The American experience. *Support Care Cancer* 2000;8:16–23.
9. Straus SE. Complementary and alternative medicine: challenges and opportunities for American medicine. *Acad Med* 2000;75:572–573.
10. Eisenberg DM, Davis RB, Ettner SL, et al. Trends in alternative medicine use in the United States, 1990–1997: results of a follow-up national survey. *JAMA* 1998;280(18):1569–1575.
11. Fisher P, Ward A. Complementary Medicine in Europe. *BMJ* 1994;309:107–111.
12. MacLennan AH, Wilson DH, Taylor AW. Prevalence and cost of alternative medicine in Australia. *Lancet* 1996;347:569–573.
13. InterSurvey, 2001 reviewed in Heme/Onc Today, Volume 2, Number 3. "Get more familiar with CAM; your patients already are." March 2001
14. Ernst E, Cassileth BR. The prevalence of complementary/alternative medicine in cancer. *Cancer* 1998;83(4):777–782.
15. Crocetti E, Crotti N, Feltrin A, et al. The use of complementary therapies by breast cancer patients attending conventional treatment. *Eur J Cancer* 1998;34(3):324–328.
16. Adler SR. Complementary and alternative medicine use among women with breast cancer. *Med Anthropol Q* 1999;13(2):214–222.
17. Gotay CC. Use of complementary and alternative medicine in Hawaii cancer patients. *Hawaii Med J* 1999;58(3):49–51, 54–55.
18. Wyatt GK, Friedman LL, Given CW, et al. Complementary therapy use among older cancer patients. *Cancer Pract* 1999;7(3):136–144.
19. Burstein HJ, Gelber S, Guadagnoli E, Weeks JC. Use of alternative medicine by women with early-stage breast cancer. *N Engl J Med* 1999;340(22):1733–1739.
20. Morris KT, Johnson N, Homer L, Walts D. A comparison of complementary therapy use between breast cancer patients and patients with other primary tumor sites. *Am J Surg* 2000;179(5):407–411.
21. Rees W, Feigel I, Vickers A, et al. Prevalence of complementary therapy use by women with breast cancer. A population-based survey. *Eur J Cancer* 2000;36(11):1359–1364.
22. Lee MM, Lin SS, Wrensch MR, et al. Alternative therapies used by women with breast cancer in four ethnic populations. *J Natl Can Inst* 2000;1992(1): 42–47.
23. Boon H, Stewart M, Kennard MA, et al. Use of complementary/alternative medicine by breast cancer survivors in Ontario: prevalence and perceptions. *J Clin Oncol* 2000;18(13):2515–2521.
24. Richardson M, Sanders T, Palmer J, et al. Complementary/alternative medicine use in a comprehensive cancer center and the implications for oncology. *J Clin Oncol* 2000;18(13):2505–2514.
25. Moschen R, Kemmler G, Schweigkofler H, et al. Use of alternative/complementary therapy in breast cancer patients—A psychological perspective support care. *Cancer* 2001;9:267–274.
26. Adler S, Fosket JR. Disclosing complementary and alternative medicine use in the medical encounter: a qualitative study in women with breast cancer. *J Fam Practice* 1999;48(6):453–458.
27. Metz JM, Jones H, Devine P, et al. Cancer patients use unconventional medical therapies far more frequently than standard history and physical examination suggests. *Proc ASCO* 2000;19:602a (Abstract 2368).
28. Gotay CC, Dumitriu D. Health food store recommendations for breast cancer patients. *Arch Fam Med* 2000; 9(8):692–698.
29. The Harris Poll, 2001
30. Fox S, Rainie L. The online health care revolution: How the Web helps Americans take better care of themselves. The Pew Internet and American Life Project, Washington, DC, 2000.
31. Bonakdar RA. Scripts Center for Integrative Medicine, International Conference on Complementary, Alternative and Integrative Medicine Research, May 18, 2001, San Francisco, CA, Abstract.
32. Jacobson JS, Workman SB, Kronenberg F. Research on complementary/alternative medicine for patients with breast cancer: A review of the biomedical literature. *J Clin Oncol* 2000;18(3):668–683.
33. Burstein HJ. Discussing complementary therapies with cancer patients: What should we be talking about? *J Clin Oncol* 2000;18(13):2501–2504.
34. Coss RA, McGrath P, Cagginano V. Alternative care: Patient choices for adjunct therapies within a cancer center. 1998;(6)3:176–181.
35. Durant JR. Alternative medicine: An attractive nuisance. *J Clin Oncol* 1998;16(1):1–2.
36. Strauss SE, Director NCCAM. Fiscal Year 2002 Budget Request; Statement to the House Subcommittee on Labor-HHS-Education Appropriations (May 16, 2001).

31

Ethics and Hereditary Cancer: Issues for Women and Families with Hereditary Breast/Ovarian Cancer

Lori d'Agincourt-Canning, Michael M. Burgess, and Barbara C. McGillivray

Scientific advances in molecular genetics have paved the way for genetic testing for hereditary breast/ovarian cancer. Already in clinical use, genetic testing provides the tested person with the knowledge that his or her risk for breast/ovarian cancer is higher or the same as that of the general population. While this advance has important implications for women and families living with hereditary cancer, it also raises serious social and ethical concerns. Genetic testing, for example, evokes questions about privacy, confidentiality and individual responsibility to family (1). Also germane to discussions of genetic testing is the potential for discrimination or social stigmatization based on genetic characteristics.

In this chapter, we provide a summary of ethical issues and challenges arising from genetic testing for hereditary breast/ovarian cancer. We also examine what empirical studies can add to the understanding and ethical analysis of new genetic technologies. We are among several research groups who have conducted empirical research designed to explore the various dimensions of people's concerns and experiences with this technology (2–7). We discuss some key findings here, including how this kind of research can inform conceptual analysis.

This chapter is organized into four sections. The first section provides a brief overview of genetic testing for hereditary breast/ovarian cancer: risk estimates, benefits and limitations of the technology and current standards of practice. The next section moves to an examination of ethical issues raised in the ethics and medical literature about genetic testing for hereditary breast/ovarian cancer. The third section describes additional ethical concerns raised by women and families in empirical work on experiences of inherited risk and genetic testing. We conclude by suggesting how practitioners can support patients' decisions about genetic testing in clinical practice.

SUSCEPTIBILITY TESTING FOR HEREDITARY BREAST/OVARIAN CANCER

The recent discovery of the genes responsible for hereditary breast/ovarian cancer offers the opportunity to identify those individuals within families who have inherited a strong predisposition to develop cancer. Most attention has been focused on two genes, BRCA1 and BRCA2. The work done thus far suggests that both BRCA genes, when present in mutated form, confer a risk of breast or ovarian cancer substantially higher than most women face. Available data suggest that women who inherit a mutated copy of either gene have an elevated risk of breast cancer, up to 87% by the age of 70 years (8–12). Similarly, the risk of developing ovarian cancer by age 70 is 16% to 63%, depending on the population studied (9,13). These inherited mutations are also associated with a 59% risk for second breast or ovarian primaries, respectively (14). In contrast, the corresponding population risk for North American women to develop breast and ovarian cancer is 10% and 1.4%, respectively (15,16).

Genetic testing for breast cancer susceptibility has been advanced in the hope that it will reduce cancer morbidity and mortality. Advocates of the technology promote genetic testing on the premise that women found to have the mutation can potentially reduce their cancer risks by using available detection and prevention strategies (17–19). This may take the form of increased surveillance such as breast self-examination, clinical breast examination, mammography and ultrasound of the ovaries. The rationale for screening high-risk women is that cancer may be detected at an early stage when the prognosis is better. Alternatively, it is proposed that women may decrease their risks by undergoing prophylactic surgery (bilateral mastectomy and/or oophorectomy) or chemoprevention (tamoxifen and potentially raloxifene treatment) (16). Two recent studies, as well as mathematical models, indicate that prophylactic bilateral mastectomy may reduce the incidence of breast cancer in women with known BRCA1/2 mutations (20–23). Although the numbers are small, more recent subgroup analysis of the National Breast Cancer Prevention Trial (NSABP P1 trial) suggests that tamoxifen reduces breast cancer incidence among healthy BRCA2 carriers, but not among healthy women with inherited BRCA1 mutations (24). This will be an important area to follow if these data are confirmed using larger sample sizes. Consequent action might also include an attempt at primary prevention through a change to a healthier lifestyle (25).

However, medical interventions offered to individuals with an inherited predisposition to breast cancer are imperfect and of uncertain efficacy (26). Mammographic screening is routinely recommended for high-risk women, but at younger ages, its sensitivity is much lower (27,28). Also of concern are the possible iatrogenic effects of radiation exposure in women with these or other genetic mutations (25,29). Further, genetic testing is limited by the probabilistic nature of the information. It can indicate whether someone is at increased risk for breast cancer, but in its statistical form, cannot predict when the cancer will develop, its clinical features or whether the person will get the disease at all.[1] It is also unclear what role modifying factors (hormonal, dietary, environmental, genetic) may play in determining whether a given mutation gives rise to cancer (26). Likewise, evidence to support the effectiveness or enduring nature of dietary changes or life style interventions is lacking.

The psychological impact of genetic testing has also raised concern. Initial reports do not provide evidence of long-term psychological effects, however, they suggest that BRCA1 carriers have higher levels of anxiety and distress after learning their risk status (30–33). In a more recent study, Kash et al. (34) reported that women who do not expect to be gene mutation carriers but have a positive test result exhibited the most emotional distress. In contrast, those who were at high risk and expected to test positive demonstrated less anxiety when learning they carried the mutation. Because genetic testing may impact an individual's psychological well-being, protocols for genetic testing include pretest and post-test counselling as well.

In Canada, genetic testing for breast cancer susceptibility is offered only at major teaching hospitals and research centres (35). Eligibility criteria vary amongst programs, but testing is usually restricted to those with significant family histories of the disease or particularly early presentation.[2] These programs have been designed to evaluate whether testing should be offered as part of routine care, as well as to determine the most appropriate methods of presenting risk information. At issue, however, is who will pay for the test and where testing will be done. Until recently, genetic testing was offered as a health service (usually in the context of global program funding) by most provincial health ministries at no direct cost to the patient. DNA analysis was conducted locally. As of July

---

[1] Penetrance is the extent to which a gene is expressed. Genetic mutations predisposing to breast and ovarian cancer are not fully penetrant, meaning that not everyone who has a mutation will actually be affected by the disease. Multiple factors—environmental, hormonal or interactions with other genetic factors—are necessary for the disease to become manifest (30).

[2] To provide an example, at this writing the BC Cancer Agency's eligibility criteria for genetic testing are as follows: women with breast cancer diagnosed at 35 years of age or younger, ovarian cancer diagnosed at age 50 or younger, or an Ashkenazi Jewish woman with breast or ovarian cancer at any age. Individuals are also eligible for genetic testing if their family history supports two of the following criteria: cancer in two or more closely related family members, cancer at an earlier age than expected in the general population (e.g., breast cancer before menopause), multiple primary cancers in one individual, and cancers associated with known hereditary syndromes.

2001, however, Myriad Genetics, Utah, sent out a legal notice asserting its patent rights for the BRCA1 and BRCA2 genes and stated that all genetic testing for these genes must be sent to Myriad (36). This translates into a three-fold increase in cost to perform the test ($2,600 US for the full sequencing of BRCA1 and 2 by Myriad, compared to approximately $760 to $960 U.S. for testing by Canadian provincial cancer laboratories). As a consequence of this legal action, the BC Ministry of Health Services has directed the BC Cancer Agency to suspend local testing (37). Patients who are eligible and are willing to pay for the test can obtain it through MDS Laboratories (the Canadian partner of Myriad Genetics). The Ontario government, on the other hand, has not suspended testing and is pursuing the matter legally (38). European countries, including France, Belgium, Denmark, Germany, the Netherlands, and the United Kingdom, are preparing legally to oppose the patent (39,40). It will take some time before this problem is resolved.

ETHICAL CONSIDERATIONS

Despite questions of cost (and who will pay), susceptibility testing for hereditary breast/ovarian cancer has generated considerable interest. The promise of earlier disease detection, more effective treatment or the potential for preventive action is alluring. Nonetheless, numerous organizations, health care professionals as well as lay critics have voiced concern that people may be harmed by information generated from DNA testing. Cited most often as key ethical issues are privacy, confidentiality, and the threat of genetic discrimination (41). Other concerns focus on the geneticization of disease, the implementation of tests of uncertain benefit, and the diversion of resources away from the other factors (i.e., the environment), which also contribute to cancer and other diseases (26,42–45).

H.J. McCloskey (46) identified ten opinions characterizing privacy. Of particular relevance to genetic testing is the definition of privacy "as the lack of disclosure, and the right to privacy as the right to selective disclosure." Here, privacy refers to the degree of control that we have or can maintain over what others know about us (47). It refers to an individual's authority to reveal or withhold information that is about her, in this case, to direct who may or who should not have access to presymptomatic information. Others stress that privacy is important, not just because of its legal implications, but because of its role in establishing moral personhood. Writing on ethical conduct for research involving humans, Michael McDonald et al. (48) state that privacy is a critical feature of personal relations.

> Privacy is valued not only because certain information is felt to be embarrassing, shameful or in other ways hurtful to the participant, but also because privacy is essential for intimate, personal and even spiritual relationships, that is, with what is thought to be "sacred" in a variety of ways.

Thus, privacy is a concept closely connected to constructions of self, identity and personal autonomy. It is also a central concept with respect to genetic testing.

As with any medical test, individuals are encouraged to exercise personal autonomy in deciding whether or not they wish to pursue genetic testing. From a clinical standpoint, autonomy is supported through standardized protocols that emphasize genetic counselling and informed consent (49). In pretest counselling, individuals discuss with genetic counsellors the possible benefits and potential harms of receiving genetic information. Patients must evaluate whether the risks are worth taking based on their own values and notions of welfare. Similarly, people's entitlement to privacy ensures that they are seen as knowing best with whom, when, and how to share this information.

At odds with traditional notions of autonomy, however, is the fact that predictive testing has serious implications for others. Genetic information is personal, but at the same time, familial. Because of shared DNA, one person's susceptibility to a genetic disease means that other biological relatives may also be at risk of developing the same disease. The discovery of inherited risk identifies other family members as well as the patient as potential beneficiaries of the information. Indeed, an individual's knowledge of being a carrier of a genetic mutation blurs the traditional boundaries of personal autonomy (50). Predictive testing for breast cancer reveals information about the tested individual, as well as the future health of her children, siblings and extended family. Individual privacy may conflict with benefiting other family members, and disclosure of inherited risk may affect the privacy of other family members.

Although genetic testing does not create substantively new dilemmas about patient confidentiality, problems may arise if an individual refuses to share information, which the clinician or other family members believe that she should share with them (51). Confidentiality is considered a hallmark of the clinician-patient relationship. Yet, ethical tensions may arise regarding who should or should not have access to genetic test results, especially if clinicians perceive this information as relevant to health care decisions faced by others. The problem becomes particularly salient if a genetic disorder or condition is thought to be preventable and a genetically at-risk individual chooses not to disclose information she possesses. In such situations, clinicians may find themselves torn between competing duties: the duty of confidentiality and the duty to protect others from potential harm (1,47,52). Currently in Canada, the speculative nature of the benefits is inadequate to justify a legal duty to warn relatives that they may have inherited an increased risk for breast/ovarian cancer (41,49,53). However, legal commentators caution this may change if more effective interventions are developed, and there is evidence that disclosure of genetic information could prevent harm (41,49,53).

Against the need to reconsider traditional notions of privacy, however, are equally problematic issues regarding discrimination. Critics warn that employers, insurance agencies, schools, government agencies and others, for various reasons, will want access to genetic information (1,45,52). Without appropriate safeguards in place, genetic information may be used as an exclusionary tool (54,55). Persons may be denied social opportunities and benefits based on genetic "difference" (50). Furthermore, the threat of discrimination may hinder people from seeking the benefits of some genetic tests (56).

Most risks associated with genetic testing have to do with the use and possible abuse of personal information by third parties. Although cases of exclusion are anecdotal, some studies indicate that genetic testing has been used to bar people diagnosed with genetic disorders from insurance coverage and employment (45, 50). Others warn that genetic knowledge may lead to reduced tolerance for diversity and, if unregulated, heighten inequities by labeling groups with particular genetic diseases or risks (44). Ethnic or racial issues may further augment the risk of stigmatization. Thus, a potential for genetic discrimination may be accompanied by a potential for "genetic elitism" (1) and some debate the possibility of a "genetic ghetto" (57).

Concerned about the potential misuse of genetic information, governments worldwide debate the nature of new legislation needed to ensure that DNA testing is used in appropriate ways (41,58). In the United States, an NIH-Department of Energy task force on genetic information and insurance clearly stated that genetic information should not be used to deny health care coverage or services to anyone (59). It also recommended that, until universal access to health coverage is made available, insurers should contemplate a moratorium on genetic testing in underwriting (41). In Canada, a study paper for the Law Reform Commission of Canada as well as the Science Council of Canada issued similar recommendations. They recommended that a guaranteed, basic form of life insurance be made universally available, with additional insurance optional and subject to genetic information supplied by the applicant (60).

Clearly, insurance companies, employers and multiple others hope to gain financially from knowledge of people's susceptibility to inherited cancer. While classical legal principles and human rights legislation afford broad protection to human rights, it is widely recognized that genetic testing will necessitate further legislation against social harms (41–50,61–63). In addition, ethical analysis needs to consider whether genetic technology may contribute to the oppression, either subtle or overt, of certain groups.[3] While such ethical issues are beyond the scope of clinical responsibility, they are relevant to informed consent and evaluation of the harms of genetic testing on patients, their families and their communities (64).

EMPIRICAL RESEARCH

This section extends ethical analysis by exploring what empirical research can bring to the understanding of moral issues around genetic testing.

Qualitative research has focused on the experiences of women who have undergone BRCA1/2 mutation testing (Burgess and d'Agincourt-Canning, personal communication; B. Koenig, Greely and Raffin, personal communication, January, 2002). Rather than examining clinical impact per se, much of this research seeks to identify the significance and impact of predictive testing on people's everyday lives. Understanding the perspectives of women seeking genetic testing will not only inform clinical care, but will help identify ethical concerns. Indeed, several studies suggest that women may be interested in BRCA testing initially, but interest often wanes when the uncertainties and limitations of the test are explained (2,3,7). While these study participants recognized that their family history put them at increased risk for breast cancer, they stated that genetic information would not alter their screening behavior or management of health care. They also perceived discrimination in insurance and employment as a considerable threat. The interest in genetic testing may increase, however, if studies continue to demonstrate that prophylactic surgery improves survival in women with an inherited predisposition to breast cancer or that tamoxifen reduces breast cancer incidence among healthy BRCA2 carriers (24). Nonetheless, the important message for clinicians is that family history should be taken seriously and women offered testing only with proper education, counselling and support.

Other studies have examined women's reasons for testing and with whom they disclose their results (Burgess & d'Agincourt-Canning, personal communication, January, 2002). Women often discuss genetic testing as having more than personal significance. For instance, even following diagnosis of breast cancer and therefore having risks not only of recurrence, but also possible new occurrence, women sometimes seek testing for the sake of their daughters or sisters. In some cases, women even described their primary motive for pre-symptomatic BRCA1 or BRCA2 testing as for the sake of their children—that they owe it to their children to know. Others worry about the risk to their children and about upsetting their family and elect not to be tested. Most testing programs first identify an index case, or a woman with a diagnosis and a mutation, before offering carrier testing to other family members without disease. Women at risk for hereditary breast cancer may become angry or frustrated with mothers or siblings who have been diagnosed with breast cancer, yet refuse the genetic testing.

Consider the following case:

Joanne was diagnosed at 42 with breast cancer and had her affected breast removed. Her mother and aunt both had premenopausal breast cancer. Joanne is now 47 and has been scheduled for prophylactic surgery to remove her other breast. She requests genetic testing to help reaffirm her decision to have the surgery. In counseling, Joanne explains that she is quite committed to the surgery but may change her mind if she is sure she is not at an increased risk due to a genetic predisposition. Joanne also wants to help her sister and two adult daughters, who will qualify for carrier testing if Joanne has a mutation. Joanne explains that one daughter says her physician does not take her seriously when she complains of lumps in one breast. Joanne is also concerned about the experience of one of the women in her cancer support group who says that her daughters were very upset that she went ahead and got tested. Joanne wants your advice about whether to be tested.

Joanne has two possible benefits that she seeks to achieve through genetic testing. One is to determine whether it would be good risk management to remove her remaining breast,

---

[3]For a summary of concerns regarding genetic testing of vulnerable groups, see references 41, 62, and 63.

and the other is to help her daughters to avoid breast cancer. Joanne's diagnosis and family history clearly qualifies for the BRCA1 and BRCA2 testing under most clinical criteria. Will the testing help achieve Joanne's goals? Are there negative effects of testing that might be greater in magnitude than the benefits of the testing for Joanne and her family?

Consider first how Joanne plans to use this information. A negative test result would be considered inconclusive, and an inherited risk could not be ruled out. Joanne has said that she would change her plan for prophylactic surgery only if she is certain that she does not have an inherited predisposition. So she needs to understand that a negative test result will not provide that kind of certainty, although it might encourage her to re-evaluate her risk and the surgery. If her test confirms a BRCA1 or BRCA2 mutation, then Joanne is reassured that prophylactic surgery is a reasonable choice based on both family history and genetic evidence. Further, a positive test result indicates an inherited predisposition to both breast and ovarian cancer. If she was found to be a BRCA1 or BRCA2 mutation carrier, she would be advised to undergo routine ovarian screening. Prophylactic oophorectomy would be discussed as a possible option as well.

Next, consider whether Joanne's test will help her daughters and sister lessen their risks of developing breast cancer. A positive test result may encourage her sister and/or daughters to be more vigilant about breast self-examinations. Yet, whether or not Joanne has a mutation, the family history alone raises serious concerns about her daughters' and sister's risk for breast cancer. Proper management for Joanne's daughters and perhaps her sister should include earlier mammography, five to ten years prior to Joanne's age of onset. That is appropriate management independent of the genetic test. As previously stated, a negative test result does not rule out the possibility of inherited mutation. However, a negative test result may lead to false reassurance and reduced breast cancer screening efforts. There are other risks associated with the genetic testing as well. Insurance discrimination and heightened anxiety related to breast cancer have been reported for both the tested individuals and their children. Confidentiality of test results is far from perfect. Moreover, genetic information is frequently misunderstood and/or confused with a diagnosis. Women who have undergone testing, as well as family members, may be confronted with the burden of changing misconceptions and explaining what the test means. Finally, since Joanne seeks to benefit her daughters and her sister, it is wise to assure that they will experience her seeking clarification of the inherited risk for breast cancer in the family as a positive and desirable action.

SUMMARY

This case study and the previous literature review highlight several important guidelines for the clinical management of women and families with a suspected inherited predisposition to breast cancer.

1. Testing for mutations on BRCA1 and BRCA2 is available, and can identify and/or confirm the presence of a mutation that may account for the predisposition to breast cancer in the family. The presence of a mutation is currently estimated to be associated with the following increased risks:
   - 50% to 87% accumulated lifetime risk of breast cancer,
   - 16% to 63% accumulated lifetime risk of ovarian cancer
   - 6% increased lifetime risk of breast cancer in males
   - 59% risk for second breast and ovarian primaries
2. Genetic counseling and informed consent are necessary to assure that the patient understands the nature, benefits, risks and limitations of genetic testing. It is standard practice that this is performed in the context of a counseling protocol. The health professional providing counseling must be able to provide current information about the following issues:
   - The established effectiveness of the strategies to manage risk that might be used following genetic testing.

- The significance of a result that does not identify a mutation.
- The significance of finding a mutation, or failing to find a mutation, for other family members.
- The confidentiality protections that will be used to protect the patient and family from inappropriate use of the information and discrimination.
- The risks of discrimination that might follow from disclosure of testing or the test result to the patient and family members.

3. Genetic counseling must support the patient in her assessment of whether the test will provide useful information. In particular:
   - Will the test change clinical care for the patient?
   - Will the test be useful in other ways that the patient expects, such as better access to testing and clinical management/surveillance for family members?
   - Is the test necessary to achieve these benefits? Counseling with screening recommendations based on family history is also of value.

4. Genetic counseling should also
   - Encourage the patient to reflect on family members' responses to the genetic test prior to testing.
   - Encourage consideration of with whom and how to discuss test results.
   - Inform the patient that the clinician has a duty to maintain confidentiality and will not disclose the test results to other family members. Advise the patient, however, that both information and banked DNA may be useful to family members. The patient and clinician should clearly record the patient's wishes about access to information by family members. If DNA is to be banked, the patient will need to consult the DNA bank's policy and consent to clarify access to the DNA by family members and researchers.

Acknowledgments: We would like to acknowledge the contributions and invaluable support of the Hereditary Cancer Program, BC Cancer Agency, and the Genetics and Ethics Research Group at UBC's Centre for Applied Ethics. Our research is supported by the Canadian Breast Cancer Foundation, the Huntington Society of Canada and the Earl and Jennie Lohn Foundation.

REFERENCES

1. Dickens B. Introduction—Genetics in life, disability and additional health insurance in Canada: A comparative legal and ethical analysis. In: Knoppers B, ed. *Socio-ethical issues in human genetics.* Quebec: Les Editions, Yvon Blais Inc., 1998, 109–114.
2. Bernhardt B, Geller G, Strauss M, et al. Toward a model of informed consent process for BRCA1 testing: A qualitative assessment of women's attitudes. *J Genet Counsel* 1997;6:207–222.
3. Geller G, Strauss M, Berhardt B, Holtzman N. "Decoding" informed consent: Insights from women regarding breast cancer susceptibility testing. *Hastings Center Report* 1997;27(2):28–33.
4. Green J, Richards M, Murton F, et al. Family communication and genetic counseling: the case of hereditary breast and ovarian cancer. *J Genet Counsel* 1997; 6:45–60.
5. Hallowell N. Reconstructing the body or reconstructing the woman? Perceptions of prophylactic mastectomy for hereditary breast cancer risk. In: Potts L, ed. *Ideologies of breast cancer: feminist perspectives.* London: Macmillan Press/St. Martin's Press, 2000a:153–180.
6. Hallowell N. A qualitative study of the information needs of high-risk women undergoing prophylactic oophorectomy. *Psycho-Oncology* 2000;9:486–495.
7. Tessaro I, Borstelmann N, Regan K, et al. Genetic testing for susceptibility to breast cancer: findings from women's focus groups. *J Women's Health* 1997;6:317–327.
8. Easton D, Narod S, Ford D, Steel M. The genetic epidemiology of BRCA1. *Lancet* 1994;344:761.
9. Easton D, Bishop D, Ford D, et al. Genetic linkage analysis in familial breast and ovarian cancer: Results from 214 families. *Am J Hum Genet* 1993;52:678–701.
10. Ford D, Easton D, Bishop D, et al. Risks of cancer in BRCA1-mutation carriers. *Lancet* 1994;343:692–695.
11. Shattuck-Eidens D, Oliphant A, McClure M, et al. BRCA1 sequence analysis in women at high risk for susceptibility mutations. *JAMA* 1997;278:1242–1250.
12. Wooster R, Bignell G, Lancaster J, et al. Identification of the breast cancer susceptibility gene, BRCA2. *Nature* 1995;378:789–792.
13. Struewing J, Hariga P, Wacholder S, et al. The risk of cancer associated with specific mutations of BRCA1 and BRCA2 among Ashkenazi Jews. *N Engl J Med* 1997;336:1401–1408.
14. Easton D, Ford D, Bishop T. Breast and ovarian cancer incidence in BRCA1-mutations. *Am J Hum Genet* 1995;56:265–271.
15. Greene MH. Genetics of breast cancer. *Mayo Clin Proc* 1997;72:54–65.
16. Foulkes W, Narod S. Cancers of the breast, ovary, and uterus. In: Foulkes W., Hodgson S, eds. *Inherited sus-*

ceptibility to cancer: clinical, predictive and ethical perspectives. Cambridge: Cambridge University Press, 1998:201–233.
17. Muto M. Genetic predisposition testing: Taking the lead. *Gynecol Oncol* 1997;67:121–122.
18. Olopade O. The human genome project and breast cancer. *Women's Health Issues* 1997;7:209–213.
19. Ponder B. Genetic testing for cancer risk. *Science* 1997; 278:1050–1054.
20. Hartmann L, Seller T, Schaid D, et al. Efficacy of bilateral prophylactic mastectomy in BRCA1 and BRCA2 gene mutation carriers. *J Natl Cancer Inst* 2001; 93:1633–1637.
21. Meijers-Heijboer H, van Geel B, van Putten W, et al. Breast cancer after prophylactic bilateral mastectomy in women with a BRCA1 or BRCA2 mutation. *N Engl J Med* 2001;345:159–164.
22. Shrag D, Kuntz K, Garber J, et al. Life expectancy gains from cancer prevention strategies for women with breast cancer and BRCA1 or BRCA2 mutations. *JAMA* 2000;283:617–624.
23. Shrag D, Kuntz K, Garber J, et al. Decision analysis-effects of prophylactic mastectomy and oophorectomy on life expectancy among women with BRCA1 or BRCA2 mutations. *N Engl J Med* 1997;336:1465–1471.
24. King M-C, Wieand S, Hale K, et al. Tamoxifen and breast cancer incidence among women with inherited mutations in BRCA1 and BRCA2. National Surgical Adjuvant Breast and Bowel Project (SNABP-P1) Breast Cancer Prevention Trial. *JAMA* 2001;286:2251–2256.
25. Cuckle H. Screening for cancer in those at high risk as a result of genetic susceptibility. In: Foulkes W, Hodgson S, eds. *Inherited susceptibility to cancer: clinical, predictive and ethical perspectives.* Cambridge: Cambridge University Press, 1998:20–29.
26. Koenig B, Greely H, McConnell L, et al. Genetic testing for BRCA1 and BRCA2: Recommendations of the Stanford Program in Genomics, Ethics and Society. *J Women's Health* 1998;7:531–545.
27. Fletcher S, Black W, Harris R, et al. Report of the international workshop on screening for breast cancer. *J Natl Cancer Inst* 1993;85:1644–1656.
28. Ferguson JH. National institutes of health consensus development conference statement: breast cancer screening for women ages 40–49, January 21–23, 1997. *J Natl Inst Health* 1997;89:1015–1025.
29. Burke W, Daly M, Garber J, et al. Recommendations for follow-up care of individuals with an inherited predisposition to cancer. *JAMA* 1997;277:997–1003.
30. Ponder B. Genetic testing for cancer risk. *Science* 1997;278:1050–1054.
31. Lerman C. Psychological aspects of genetic testing: Introduction to the special issue. *Health Psychol* 1997; 16:3–7.
32. Croyle RI, Smith KR, Botkin IR, et al. Psychological response to BRCA1 mutation testing: preliminary findings. *Health Psychol* 1997;16:63–72.
33. Lerman C, Narod S, Schulman K, et al. BRCA1 testing in families with hereditary breast-ovarian cancer. *JAMA* 1996;275:1885–1892.
34. Kash KM, Dabney MK, Holland JC, et al. Familial cancer and genetics: psychosocial and ethical aspects. In: Baider L, Cooper CL, Kaplan De-Nour A, eds. *Cancer and the family,* 2nd ed. 2000:389–403.
35. Sharpe N. *Making the most of genetic testing for breast cancer.* Scarborough, Ont.: Prentice Hall, 1997.
36. Hurst L. U.S. Firm calls halt to cancer test in Canada. *The Toronto Star,* 11 August 2001.
37. Kent H. Patenting move ends BC's gene-testing program. *CMAJ* 2001;165(6):812–814.
38. Mallan C. Gene tests for cancer won't stop. *The Toronto Star,* September 20, 2001.
39. Love J. Europeans fighting Myriad Genetics BRCA1 breast cancer gene. *PatNews,* October 26, 2001.
40. Wadman M. Europe's patent rebellion. *Fortune,* October 1, 2001.
41. Knoppers B, Godard B. Ethical and legal perspectives on inherited cancer susceptibility. In: Foulkes W, Hodgson S, eds. *Inherited susceptibility to cancer: clinical, predictive and ethical perspectives.* Cambridge: Cambridge University Press, 1998:30–45.
42. Asch A, Geller G. Feminism, bioethics, and genetics. In: Wolf S, ed. *Feminism & bioethics: Beyond reproduction.* Oxford: Oxford University Press, 1996: 318–350.
43. Sherwin S. Cancer and women: Some feminist concerns. In: Sargent C, Brettell C, eds. *Gender and health: international perspective.* Upper Saddle River, NJ: Prentice Hall, 1996:187–204.
44. Lippman A. The politics of health: geneticization versus health promotion. In: Sherwin S, ed. *The politics of women's health.* Philadelphia: Temple University Press, 1998:64–82.
45. Nelkin D, Lindee M. *The DNA mystique: the gene as a cultural icon.* New York: W.H. Freeman and Co., 1995.
46. McCloskey HJ. Privacy and the right to privacy. *Philosophy* 1980;55:22.
47. Stranc L, Evans J. Issues relating to the implementation of genetic screening programs. In: Knoppers B, ed. *Socio-ethical issues in human genetics.* Quebec: Les Editions, Yvon Blais Inc., 1998:43–105.
48. Report of the Tri-Council Working Group: Code of Conduct for Research Involving Humans (July 1997; 111–1). http:www.ethics.ubc.ca/code/July 97.
49. Burgess MM, Knoppers BM, Laberge CM. Ethics and genetics in medicine. In: Singer PA, ed. *Bioethics at the bedside: a clinician's guide.* Toronto: Canadian Medical Association, 1999:79–87.
50. Lemmens T, Bahamin P. Genetics in life, disability and additional health insurance in Canada: A comparative legal and ethical analysis. In: Knoppers B, ed. *Socio-ethical issues in human genetics.* Quebec: Les Editions, Yvon Blais Inc., 1998:107–275.
51. Sommerville A, English V. Genetic privacy: orthodoxy or oxymoron. *J Med Ethics* 1999;25:144–150.
52. Roy DJ, Williams JR, Dickens BM. *Bioethics in Canada.* Scarborough, Ont.: Prentice-Hall, 1994.
53. Dickens B, Pei N, Taylor K. Legal and ethical issues in genetic testing and counselling for susceptibility to breast, ovarian and colon cancer. *Can Med Assoc J* 1996;154:813–818.
54. Cox S. It's not a secret but . . ." Predictive testing and patterns of communication about genetic information in families at risk for Huntington disease. Unpublished Doctoral Dissertation. University of British Columbia, 1999.

55. Rowin L. Genetic testing in the workplace. *J Contemp Health Law Policy* 1998;4:375–413.
56. Ball B, Ondrusek N, Wiejer C. Report of a workshop for Canadian voluntary associations concerned with genetic diseases. In: Knoppers B, ed. *Socio-ethical issues in human genetics*. Quebec: Les Editions Yvon Blais Inc., 1998:425–434.
57. Buchanan A, Brock D, Daniels N, Winkler D. *From chance to choice: genetics and justice*. New York: Cambridge University Press, 2000:327–333.
58. McGleenan T, Wiesing U. Policy options for health and life insurance in the era of genetic testing. In: McGleenan T, et al., eds. *Genetics and insurance*. New York: Springer-Verlag, 1999:116–117.
59. NIH-DOE Working Group on Ethical, Legal, and Social Implications of Human Genome Research. Genetic information and health insurance, Washington, DC: Human Genome Project, NIH Pub. No. 93-3686, 1993.
60. Science Council of Canada. Genetics in Health Care: Report 42. Ottawa: Minister of Supply and Services Canada, 1992.
61. Knoppers B, *Socio-ethical issues in human genetics*. Quebec: Les Editions, Yvon Blais Inc., 1998.
62. Burgess MM, Brunger F. Collective effects of medical research. In: McDonald M, ed. *The governance of health research involving human subjects*. Law Commission of Canada 2000:141–175. http://www.lcc.gc.ca/en/papers/macdonald/macdonald.pdf.
63. Jonsen A. Genetic testing, individual rights and the common good. In: Campbell C, Lustig B, eds. *Duties to others*. Dordrecht, Netherlands. Kluwer Academic Publishers, 1994:279–291.
64. Burgess MM. Beyond consent: ethical and social issues in genetic testing. Nature Reviews. *Genetics* 2001;2:9–14.
65. d'Agincourt-Canning L. Experiences of genetic risk: disclosure and the gendering of responsibility. *Bioethics* 2000;15(3):231–247.
66. Hallowell N. Doing the right thing: genetic risk and responsibility. *Sociol Health Illness* 1999;21:597–621.
67. Hallowell N, Statham H, Murton F. Women's understanding of their risk of developing breast/ovarian cancer before and after genetic counselling. *J Genet Counsel* 1998;7:345–364.
68. Hallowell N. "You don't want to lose your ovaries because you think I might become a man." Women's perceptions of prophylactic surgery as a cancer risk management option. *Psychooncology* 1998;7(3):263–275.

32

Hematopoietic Growth Factor Support in Breast Cancer

Katia Tonkin, Douglas Stewart, and Stefan Gluck

One approach used in order to improve outcomes for women with breast cancer has been the use of higher doses of effective chemotherapeutic agents. These attempts have occurred both in the adjuvant and the metastatic setting. The rationale for this concept can be traced back to the original results from in vitro and animal tumor cell kill experiments supporting the thesis of increasing tumor cell death with increasing drug doses (1). Such models do, however, suggest a plateau, at which point higher doses do not lead to improved anti-tumor efficacy. It is not known, however, if this plateau is reached in patients at the known maximum tolerated dose (MTD) of a chemotherapeutic agent.

Since a large number of chemotherapy agents cause myelotoxicity as their dose-limiting toxicity, the development of hematopoietic growth factors has been a fundamental requirement in the exploration of increases in the dose intensity of chemotherapy for breast cancer.

ADJUVANT CHEMOTHERAPY AND ROLE OF ANTHRACYCLINES

The analysis of the Early Breast Cancer Trialists Collaborative Group (EBCTCG) has continued to demonstrate significant benefits in relapse-free and overall survival for the use of polychemotherapy versus no treatment and more recently for anthracycline regimens over CMF-based regimens (2). There is an overall 4.6% absolute survival advantage at 10 years for anthracyclines over standard oral CMF.

The analysis of anthracyclines regimens is complicated by inclusion of all types of regimens of varying doses. The AC regimen used in several large trials only contains doxorubicin (Adriamycin) 240 mg/m^2 and cyclophosphamide 2,400 mg/m^2 over four cycles given at 3-week intervals. This regimen has been shown by the NSABP B-15 trial (3) to be equivalent to CMF given for six cycles. More dose-intensive regimens use doxorubicin to a dose of 300 mg/m^2, such as FAC (5-fluorouracil, doxorubicin, cyclophosphamide) or epirubicin between 600 mg/m^2 to 720 mg/m^2 in the FEC100 and CEF regimens, respectively. Whether the overview analysis would prove more positive, with respect to the benefits of anthracyclines, if these regimens were divided into categories based on dose intensity is unknown.

THRESHOLD DOSE, DOSE INTENSITY AND DOSE-DENSITY ANTHRACYCLINES

The initial data on dose and response was produced by Skipper (4). More recent experimental studies have confirmed that there are several factors that can potentially influence this relationship. These include not only the chemotherapy agent and schedule but tumor factors such as tumor type and size. Using a sarcoma model (5), it was demonstrated that modest reductions in drug doses of cyclophosphamide and melphalan had no effect on the complete response (CR) rate but resulted in a significant decrease in long-term cures. This kind of data led to the concept of "threshold dose."

Initial clinical reports of the potential for dose intensity in adjuvant breast cancer were published in the early 1980s. A retrospective analysis of CMF (oral cyclophosphamide, methotrexate, and 5-fluorouracil) data in adjuvant therapy was published in 1981 (6). In this analysis, it was demonstrated that women who received less than 85% of the planned dose intensity had significantly worse relapse-free survival (RFS). At 5 years RFS was 48 versus 77% ($p < 0.0001$) for the less than 65% dose intensity group and more than 85% group, respectively. However, it was not possible to determine if the biological behavior of the tumor itself and thus its intrinsic prognosis was in any way responsible for the inability to treat to full dose and therefore the diminished outcome. As individuals who received less than 65% of intended dose did no better than the untreated control (48% versus 45%, respectively) this confirmed the concept of a threshold of effectiveness for the CMF regimen.

Hryniuk (7) defined the term "dose intensity" in oncology and developed a practical methodology for its application. His definition of dose intensity was the amount of drug divided by surface area divided by time, usually a week, to give units of mg/m^2/week. He used the term "average relative dose intensity" (RDI) and expressed the dose intensity of individual drugs in polychemotherapy regimens. The RDIs of the drugs in a regimen were then averaged to derive the average RDI of a regimen for purposes of comparison. It is now recognized to have major impact on breast cancer outcomes. More recent reevaluation of the methodology has led to the use of summation dose intensity (SDI) which requires calculation of unit dose intensity (UDI) for each drug. The UDI is defined as the dose required to produce a specified outcome when used as a single agent (8). The SDI is calculated by dividing the planned dose intensity by its UDI. For combination therapy the dose intensity is the fraction of the UDI of the drug with all values being added together to derive the SDI for that regimen.

The analysis of adjuvant chemotherapy trials in stage II breast cancer (9) revealed a measurable improvement in outcome for individuals who had received adequate dose CMF chemotherapy. This applied to various risk categories of age and nodal status. Although important, it was a retrospective analysis and hypothesis generating, rather than providing definitive answers concerning the importance of delivered dose-intensity. Similar data were generated from metastatic chemotherapy trials of CAF (oral cyclophosphamide, doxorubicin, and 5-fluorouracil) and CMF with respect to response (7). Review of treatment for metastatic disease using the SDI showed that an increase of one SDI unit resulted in an approximate 30% increase in response rate [CR plus partial response (PR)] 10% in CR and 3.75 months in median survival (8). However, the data are controversial as a result of methodological issues. A reanalysis of the adjuvant data (9) by Henderson et al. (10) using only CMF-based trials showed a negative correlation, in premenopausal women, between DFS and dose intensity.

With regard to outcome an analysis of dose intensity for node-positive adjuvant patients revealed that reduction in dose intensity to 50% resulted in inferior disease-free (DFS) and overall survival (OS) (11).

As a result of the retrospective hypothesis generating data of the early and mid-1980s, several prospective trials were designed to test the concept of dose and outcome. In metastatic disease a trial of CMF demonstrated that the lower dose arm had a poorer response rate (11% versus 26%) and shorter survival (12.8 versus 15.6 months), which was not, however, significantly different (12). In a similar trial the European Organization for Research and Treatment of Cancer (EORTC) demonstrated improved response and survival using an escalated oral dose of cyclophosphamide versus an intravenous schedule in the CMF regimen (13). These trials are notable more for the threshold effect demonstrated than the dose-intensity effect, as they did not use hematopoietic growth factor (G-CSF or filgrastim) support to enable escalated doses.

An EORTC study looked at a high-dose EC regimen (14) in locally advanced or metastatic disease. Patients received epirubicin (120 mg/m^2) and cyclophosphamide (9,830 mg/m^2) with filgrastim 4 μg/kg starting 24 hours after chemotherapy. The maximum schedule was chemotherapy given every 14 days with filgrastim given days 2 to 13. A total of 87% achieved response with a median duration of 18 months (range 4 to 52). The filgrastim allowed a 33% increase in dose intensity albeit with more chemotherapy-related toxicity such as mucositis and skin toxicity.

The CALGB (Cancer and Leukemia Group B) undertook an adjuvant trial using three dose levels of CAF (11). Over 1,500 node-positive women were treated using standard, moderate or low dose regimens. The 5-year OS was significantly improved in the moderate and standard groups. A further clinical practice database from the United States with review of 5,819 women treated with CMF, CAF or AC as adjuvant therapy reported that 21% of women received less than 85% of planned dose (15). The CMF dose reductions were higher than for AC (24 versus 11%) ($p < 0.0001$). Decreased dose intensity was also more likely in women over age 65.

The concept of dose density has been approached in several different ways. The idea was developed after it was demonstrated that tumor growth most closely fitted a Gompertzian model (16). The model revolves around the assumption that smaller tumors grow faster and thus tumor regrowth between cycles of chemotherapy is most rapid when cell kill is highest. Therefore, by decreasing time between cycles, the time available for tumors to regrow is diminished. Thus the model favors sequential administration of single agents at intensive doses rather than use of combinations. This more simply enables the incorporation of new agents than the use of combination regimens where dose of any single agent is usually compromised by the toxicity of the whole.

The Milan adjuvant trial (17) of doxorubicin 75 mg/m^2 for four cycles followed by classic oral CMF for eight cycles versus alternating doxorubicin and CMF was proof of principle. In this trial the outcome was improved for those receiving the four cycles of doxorubicin first. At a median follow up of 9 years the RFS was 42% versus 28% in favor of the sequential treatment and total survival was 58% versus 44% in the same direction. Both results were $p = 0.002$. The trial was by current standards quite small for an adjuvant study (N = 405), and there was an imbalance with 38% versus 29% of women with more than 10 positive nodes in the alternating versus sequential groups, respectively.

The alternative explanation, apart from the dose density principle, for the improvement in outcome might be that more cells were sensitive and thus killed by the sequential doxorubicin given for four cycles, thus leaving a smaller remaining cell population at the time the CMF was started. The dose of the doxorubicin was the same for both arms and the total doses for all drugs were the same in both groups.

In metastatic disease there are data to support improved response rates with use of filgrastim support. In a study of single-agent epirubicin a dose of 110 mg/m^2 was given either 2 weekly or 4 weekly (18) using filgrastim 5 µg/kg/day. There were 86 for high dose and 81 for lower dose. The CR rates were 17% versus 5% ($p = 0.011$) for dose intense versus 4 weekly treatment, respectively. Although direct outcome data are not available, it is also reported that achieving CR is a prognostic factor (19). In a review of 1,581 patients receiving first-line metastatic treatment with doxorubicin and an alkylating agent, 19% of the 263 patients achieving CR were disease free at more than 5 years and 10% at a follow-up of 191 months (20).

In a randomized study of 205 locally advanced or inflammatory patients, FEC or dose intense EC with filgrastim 5 µg/kg (21,22) was used, resulting in a trend to improved progression-free survival (PFS in the dose-intense arm, $p = 0.06$). The EC dose intensity was 119% and 75% more than the FEC-treated individuals. Toxicity was primarily hematological with neutropenia grade 3/4 at 85% and 77%, respectively; febrile neutropenia 14% and 18%, respectively; anemia grade 3/4 17% and 49%, respectively; and grade 3/4 thrombocytopenia 21% versus 32% for FEC and EC, respectively.

A small EORTC study treated 29 locally advanced or metastatic women with EC up to 120 mg/m^2 and 830 mg/m^2, respectively, using filgrastim 4 µg/kg. They report a response rate of 87% with an 18-month median duration (14). Another small study of 41 women showed that an increase of dose intensity of 59.5% was possible using filgrastim 5 µg/kg with EC chemotherapy with acceptable toxicity profile (23).

The development of growth factor support (G-CSF or filgrastim) has allowed dosing schedules to be given in such a way as to reflect the desire to maintain dose intensity, dose density, or ensure that treatment delays are minimized. There are several factors that may contribute to chemotherapy being delivered below the original planned dose intensity. Several are patient related such as tolerance to treatment and some are physician dependent such as guidelines for dose delays and/or reductions based upon neutrophil counts at treatment nadir or on the planned day of chemotherapy delivery.

A large pattern of practice study reviewed information on 20,000 women in more than 1,000 centers in the United States (24). In women more than 65 years old there were increased delays, reductions and suboptimal dose intensity. Dose intensity was not achieved in 18.4%, dose reductions occurred in 25.7% and dose delays were documented in 43.1%.

In a patterns-of-care study (25) a group of 1,111 women were reviewed from 13 U.S. practices including managed care, academic and community centers. Median age was 50 and CMF and AC accounted for 78% of the treatment given. Only 70% had delivered average relative dose intensity of more than or equal to 85%. Neutropenia complications resulted in modifications in 27.6% of patients and these recurred in 60.7%. AC was given most often close to target but when AC and CMF were both given to patients there were higher complication rates than for CMF given alone.

In a study reporting data from the Canadian Database Initiative (26) 444 women were reviewed. Average age was 47.7 and treatment was given from 1991 to 1996. Across all treatments, 42% experienced at least one neutropenic complication and 72% went on to have additional complications during additional cycles.

TAXANES

Early Breast Cancer

The studies of paclitaxel and filgrastim are not yet mature enough to determine if there is superiority for taxanes and dose intense anthracyclines. The CALGB have reported a pilot study of four cycles of paclitaxel given at 175 mg/m^2 as a 3-hour infusion after dose-intensive AC (75 mg/m^2 and 2,000 mg/m^2 respectively) with filgrastim. Just over half (54%) had more than four node-positive disease. The regimen led to 25% grade 4 leucopenia and at median follow-up of 2.4 years the RFS and OS are 87% and 89%, respectively (27).

In a further study of high-risk patients a dose-dense regimen of doxorubicin 90 mg/m^2 for three cycles, paclitaxel 250 mg/m^2, over 24 hours for three cycles and cyclophosphamide 3 g/m^2 for three cycles was given with filgrastim 5 μg/kg on days 3 through 10 (28). Each cycle was 2 weekly and the median dose intensity delivered was 92%. So far, in 42 patients followed for a median of 4 years, the DFS is 78%.

Neoadjuvant docetaxel with doxorubicin has also been reported to be active in several trials (29,30). Complete responses have been between 15% and 33% with overall responses of 85% to 93%. Doses of docetaxel were 50 to 75 mg/m^2 with doxorubicin 50 to 75 mg/m^2 using filgrastim for all cycles of therapy.

A further trial in 417 docetaxel-treated metastatic or localized patients has been completed (J.M. Nabholtz, personal communication). Patients were randomized in a double-blind phase 3 trial of G-CSF (filgrastim) compared to leridistim in the prevention of neutropenic complications of docetaxel, doxorubicin, and cyclophosphamide (TAC) (BCIRG 004 Trial). Leridistim (myelopoietin; MPO), which is a chimeric dual agonist that binds both G-CSF and interleukin-3 receptors, was given either daily or alternate days and compared to daily filgrastim. There was no difference in the cumulative incidence of patients with grade 4 neutropenia across the cohorts. Febrile neutropenia occurred in 7% of the filgrastim group compared to 19% ($p = 0.003$) in the daily and 22% ($p = < 0.001$) in the alternate day leridistim groups, respectively. There was no difference in the duration of febrile neutropenia or use of intravenous antibiotics in the three groups. The only other significant difference in toxicity was the occurrence of anemia (Hb less than 8.0 g/dL) which occurred in only 8% filgrastim patients versus 18% for the alternate day leridistim patients ($p = 0.02$). A total of 10% versus 20% of filgrastim versus alternate day leridistim patients ($p = 0.018$) discontinued due to adverse events. This trial suggests superiority for prophylactic use of filgrastim rather than its use secondarily, as the rate of febrile neutropenia reported was only 7%. This compares favorably to the historical untreated rate of 30% to 40% in doxorubicin-docetaxel combinations where filgrastim is not used as prophylaxis and may be due at least in part to prevention of severe neutropenia (absolute neutrophil count less than 100 cells/µL).

Metastatic Disease

In advanced disease using filgrastim support, paclitaxel has been used with a variety of drugs such as vinorelbine (31) and topotecan (32) or cisplatin (33,34) in anthracycline pretreated disease. Results have been encouraging, but no randomized trials are yet reported.

DOSE ESCALATION AND STEM-CELL TRANSPLANTATION

Chemotherapy resistance is multifactorial and may arise as a result of intrinsic tumor cell resistance, often resulting from the multidrug resistant phenotype, or as a result of extrinsic factors such as underexposure to appropriate drug levels. In experimental models it is possible to overcome cellular resistance by substantial increases in drug concentration (35,36). In experimental breast models there are data to suggest benefit of dose escalation, although there are numerous difficulties in the extrapolation of animal data to patients (37,38).

As there are drugs such as the alkylating agents that are known to have steep dose-response curves, the concept of dose escalation and stem cell transplantation has been extensively investigated in breast cancer patients both in the adjuvant and metastatic settings. The use of high-dose chemotherapy with stem cell rescue is the ultimate outcome of the dose-intensity paradigm and allows use of intensive treatments that were previously impossible to contemplate.

In reported large adjuvant studies of dose escalation with either doxorubicin or cyclophosphamide using filgrastim, there have not, however, to date been improvements in outcome, only increased toxicity (39–41).

The logical extension of increasing doses of chemotherapy was, as a result of the advent of hematopoietic growth factor support, use of high-dose therapy with stem cell transplant rescue. However, there have been numerous negative reports so far, and several trials have not used standard therapy as the control arm. This makes comparisons extremely complex. There are six published trials, with the Dutch trial, which is expected to report mature results in 2002, being the most promising (42). In these studies, the use of hematopoietic growth factors (G-CSF or filgrastim) is essential for stem cell mobilization and to improve post transplant granulocyte recovery.

Adjuvant studies include filgrastim-supported individually dose-escalated FEC versus FEC followed by stem cell supported high-dose cyclophosphamide, thiotepa, and carboplatin (43). Individual escalation for the FEC-only arm was done according to tolerance to the previous dose level. In the first 89 patients, 83 completed nine courses of treatment with median epirubicin 782 mg/m^2 and cyclophosphamide 10.33 g/m^2. In the two highest dose levels there was grade 0 to 1 non-hematological toxicity in 73% to 92% of courses. There was no difference in hematological toxicity between the highest and lowest dose intensities given, suggesting successful use of filgrastim for these individuals. An expanded study of 525 patients was presented in 1999 (44). No difference in outcome was reported.

In a further investigation (45), a multicenter study of dose-intensive and dose-dense therapy was reported. Individuals had either extracapsular lymph node spread or more than ten positive nodes and were treated with EC (90 mg and 600 mg/m^2 Q 3-weekly) followed by three cycles of oral CMF or dose-intensive and dose-dense EC (120 mg and 600 mg/m^2 Q 2-weekly) with prophylactic filgrastim. Patients also received locoregional radiation. A total of 144 patients, 95%, received their intended dose intensity and, as predicted, hematological toxicity was higher in the intensive arm. Only two patients did not complete planned therapy without any treatment-related mortality. No outcome is yet reported.

A third study in early breast cancer has compared CEF given 3-weekly or 2-weekly with filgrastim support (46). The 2-weekly arm represents a 50% increase in dose density but as yet no outcome data have been published.

NEUTROPENIA PREVENTION, NEUTROPENIC FEVER AND HEMATOPOIETIC GROWTH FACTOR SUPPORT

Several hematopoietic growth factors (HGFs) have been identified, sequenced, and cloned. Granulocyte colony-stimulating factor (G-CSF) is produced normally by monocytes, endothelial cells, and fibroblasts. Laboratory data suggest that G-CSF is crucial for maintaining the normal balance of neutrophil production during steady state granulopoiesis. It may also be involved in stimulating granulocyte production in infection. As a result of its action on the late progenitor cells committed to the neutrophil lineage, G-CSF stimulates the proliferation and maturation of neutrophils. It shortens bone marrow time-to-release of newly formed neutrophils from 5 days to 1 day (47). It also stimulates early pluripotent stem cells and committed progenitor cells to move from the bone marrow to the peripheral circulation. Other growth factors such as GM-CSF (granulocyte macrophage CSF), M-CSF (macrophage CSF), TPO (thrombopoietin), and SCF (stem cell factor) all play crucial and interdependent roles in hematopoiesis. Numerous interleukins (IL-3, IL-6, IL-7, and IL-11) are also involved (48).

The safety profile of filgrastim shows that it is well tolerated. Most common side effects are musculoskeletal pain, headache, and rash (49). Neutrophils produced after filgrastim stimulation appear to have normal *in vitro* function (49,50), and there is no evidence for stimulation of non-myeloid malignancies (51). Further data are required to determine if there are long-term sequelae.

G-CSF can be used to maintain planned-dose delivery and schedule of administration. In this manner the planned dose can be adhered to and thus minimize dose modifications. In a study of 123 premenopausal, node-positive women, filgrastim was used to maintain dose delivery after inadequate recovery from a prior cycle of therapy (52). This resulted in adequate white cell counts (WBC) in 83% of six cycles of oral CMF. In addition, 74% of patients received at least 85% dose intensity compared to 45% with low WBC who did not receive filgrastim ($p < 0.05$).

Secondary prophylaxis, which refers to administration of CSFs following neutropenia or febrile neutropenia to prevent recurrence, is commonly undertaken to prevent dose reductions and/or delays in administration. However, this secondary use of agents such as filgrastim involves the patient having already been exposed to a potentially fatal complication of therapy. It would be more rational to be able to identify the at-risk population and support full-dose therapy. However, thus far, these data are not available in a prospective and validated form.

A study has been performed in an attempt to validate pretreatment characteristics that would predict for neutropenia and its complications (53). Using a case series of 95 patients in a training set and a validation set of 80 patients, developmental models were constructed to predict neutropenia (absolute neutrophil count less than or equal to 0.250 µL), dose reduction less than or equal to 15% of scheduled dose, or delay less than or equal to 7 days. Pretreatment and post-cycle 1 data were used. The pretreatment data were unsuccessful. However, the depth of the first cycle nadir ($p = 0.0001$ to 0.004) or the use of chemotherapy with radiation ($p = 0.0011$ to 0.0901) were excellent predictors, and decline in hemoglobin also almost reached statistical significance.

There are reports of widespread variations according to practice patterns (25). One site reviewed had 8% hospitalization for febrile neutropenia and another reported only 2%. Significant dose modifications were reported 72% of the time with CAF, 68% with CMF, and only 27% with AC. More dose reductions were reported for one site than for another—4% versus 55% for CMF. It was noted that 55% of patients who experienced one neutropenia-related clinically significant dose modification were likely to have a second.

ECONOMIC IMPACT

A review of two national databases in the United States studied admissions for women with breast cancer. Length of stay and costs were estimated for 1994 to 1996 (54). Neutropenic and febrile neutropenic admissions were longer and incurred higher costs than non-neutropenic and afebrile admissions, respectively ($p < 0.05$). Thus, prophylaxis of neutropenia has the potential to reduce hospitalization costs. Of course, costs are likely to vary according to the different economic conditions of various countries and the method by which the economic impact is calculated.

A further analysis (55) studied hospitalization expenditure for patients admitted with febrile neutropenia (FN) over a 2-year period. Estimated total hospital costs were incorporated into a cost model for colony stimulation factors (CSFs). Incorporation of nonmedical indirect and intangible costs suggested that the cost of FN was greater than previously reported. This would result in reduction in the thresholds currently used for the use of CSFs.

FUTURE DIRECTIONS

The major downside for filgrastim is the need for daily injections and close monitoring of the white cell count. Some guidelines suggest use of filgrastim from the day after chemotherapy is given until the total white cell count is more than or equal to $10,000 \times 10^9$ per liter. However, there is some controversy, and changes have occurred over time since the introduction of filgrastim and publication of formal guidelines (56). As a result, a long-acting pegylated filgrastim preparation (SD/01, pegfilgrastim or Neulasta) has been developed. Several studies have shown that long-acting filgrastim can be given at a dose of 100 µg/kg as safely as filgrastim 5 µg/kg (57–59). In the recent Holmes study (57), a total of 310 patients were given docetaxel 75 mg/m^2 and doxorubicin 60 mg/m^2 for up to four cycles. Patients were randomized to day 2 treatment with pegfilgrastim or filgrastim given daily. Febrile neutropenic episodes were documented less often in the pegfilgrastim group and the neutrophil nadir was also less severe and lasted fewer days. The difference in median duration of severe neutropenia was less than 1 day, which is unlikely to be clinically relevant. Adverse event profiles for both compounds are similar.

SUMMARY

There have been experimental data to suggest the importance of dose intensity since the 1960s. From a clinical perspective, however, it has not been possible to exploit this route until the advent of hematopoietic growth factor support. There is level I evidence for the concept of threshold dosing in metastatic and adjuvant breast cancer. For dose intensity and stem cell transplantation, the data are much less clear, partly due to study design. The use of dose intensity and transplantation is certainly feasible but its value, from currently published prospective studies, remains less certain. More information from an important large Dutch study of stem cell transplantation should be available in 2002. In addition there are a number of other trials of dose intensity and dose density that are either continuing to accrue or mature results are not, as yet, published in peer-reviewed journals.

There is level II evidence (due to small numbers and unconfirmed data) for the dose-dense principle from the Milan study of sequential doxorubicin followed by CMF.

In locally advanced or metastatic disease there is similar level II evidence for dose-intense EC with filgrastim support with respect to PFS from an Intergroup study done by the EORTC National Cancer Institute of Canada Clinical Trials Group (NCIC-CTG) and the Scandinavian cooperative group (SAKK).

There is level I/II evidence for the ability to achieve dose-intensity, dose-dense and planned dose scheduling in both adjuvant and metastatic breast cancer.

The role of filgrastim (G-CSF) remains central to the further exploration of dose and scheduling in the treatment of breast cancer. Now that the long-acting version, pegfilgrastim, is available in the United States, more information on these long-acting growth factor molecules will undoubtedly become available in the near future.

REFERENCES

1. Schabel FM Jr, Griswold DP, Corbett TH, et al. Increasing the therapeutic response rate to anticancer drugs by applying the basic principles of pharmacology. *Cancer* 1984;50:1160–1167.
2. Early Breast Cancer Trialists Collaborative Group (EBCTCG). Polychemotherapy for early breast cancer: an overview of the randomized trials. *Lancet* 1998; 352:930–942.
3. Fisher B, Brown AM, Dimitrov NV, et al. Two months of doxorubicin-cyclophosphamide with and without interval reinduction therapy compared with 6 months of cyclophosphamide, methotrexate, and fluorouracil in positive-node breast cancer patients with tamoxifen-nonresponsive tumors. Results from the National Surgical Adjuvant Breast and Bowel Project B-15. *J Clin Oncol* 1990;8:1483–1496.
4. Skipper HE. Criteria associated with destruction of leukemia and solid tumor cells in animals. *Cancer Res* 1967;27:2636–2645.
5. McGowan AT, Fox BW. A proposed mechanism of resistance to cyclophosphamide and phosphoramide mustard in a Yoshida cell line in vitro. *Cancer Chemother Pharmacol* 1986;17:226.
6. Bonadonna G, Valagussa P. Dose-response effect of adjuvant chemotherapy in breast cancer. *N Engl J Med* 1981;304:10–15.
7. Hryniuk W, Bush H. The importance of dose intensity in chemotherapy of metastatic breast cancer. *J Clin Oncol* 1984;2:1281–1288.
8. Hryniuk W, Frei E III, Wright FA. A single scale for comparing dose-intensity of all chemotherapy regimens in breast cancer: summation dose-intensity. *J Clin Oncol* 1998;16:3137–3147.
9. Hryniuk W, Levine MN. Analysis of dose-intensity for adjuvant chemotherapy trials in stage II breast cancer. *J Clin Oncol* 1986;19:1162–1170.
10. Henderson IC, Hayes DF, Gelman R. Dose-response in the treatment of breast cancer: a critical review. *J Clin Oncol* 1988;6:1501–1515.
11. Wood WC, Budman DR, Korzun AH, et al. Dose and dose intensity of adjuvant chemotherapy for stage II, node-positive breast carcinoma. *N Engl J Med* 1994; 330(18):1253–1259.
12. Tannock IF, Boyd NF, DeBoer G, et al. A randomized trial of two dose levels of cyclophosphamide, methotrexate, and fluorouracil chemotherapy for patients with metastatic breast. *J Clin Oncol* 1988;6:1377–1387.
13. Engelman F, Klijn JCM, Rubens RD, et al. "Classical" CMF versus a 3-weekly intravenous CMF schedule in postmenopausal patients with advanced breast cancer. *Eur J Cancer* 1991;27:966–970.
14. Piccart MJ, Bruning P, Wildiers J, et al. An EORTC pilot study of filgrastim (recombinant human granulocyte colony stimulating factor) as support to a high-dose intensive epidoxorubicin-cyclophosphamide regimen in chemotherapy-naïve patients with locally advanced or metastatic breast cancer. *Ann Oncol* 1995; 6:673–677.
15. Smith GA, Fine MJ, Lenert LL, Newbold RC. Project ChemoInsight reveals physician practice patterns for adjuvant breast cancer chemotherapy and compares the dose intensity of CMF, AC and CAF. *Proc ASCO* 1999; 18:78a (Abstract 296).
16. Norton L. A gompertzian model of human breast cancer growth. *Cancer Research* 1988;48(24):7067–7071.
17. Bonadonna G, Zambetti M, Valagussa P. Sequential or alternating doxorubicin and CMF regimens in breast cancer with more than three positive nodes. Ten-year results. *JAMA* 1995;273:542–547.
18. Fountzilas G, Nicolaides C, Aravantinos G, et al. Dose-dense adjuvant chemotherapy with epirubicin monotherapy in patients with operable breast cancer and 10 positive axillary lymph nodes. A feasibility study. *Oncology* 1998;55:508–512.
19. Rahman ZU, Frye DK, Smith TL, et al. Results and long term follow-up for 1581 patients with metastatic breast carcinoma treated with standard dose doxorubicin-containing chemotherapy. *Cancer* 1999; 85:104–111.
20. Greenberg PAC, Hortobagyi GN, Smith TL, et al. Long-term follow-up of patients with complete remission following combination chemotherapy for metastatic breast cancer. *J Clin Oncol* 1996;14:2197–2205.
21. Therasse P, Tsitsa C, Sahmoud T, et al. Neoadjuvant chemotherapy in locally advanced breast cancer (LABC): FEC (5-FU, epirubicin, cyclophosphamide) versus high dose intensity EC + G-CSF (Filgrastim). An EORTC-NCIC-SAKK study. Preliminary results of dose intensity (DI). *Eur J Cancer* 1995;31A(suppl 5):S81 (Abstract 372).
22. Therasse P, Mauriac L, Welnicka M, et al. Neoadjuvant dose intensive chemotherapy in locally advanced breast cancer: and EORTC-NCIC-SAKK randomized phase III study comparing FEC (5-FU, epirubicin, cyclophosphamide) versus high dose intensity EC + G-CSF (filgrastim). *Proc ASCO* 1998;17:124a (Abstract 472).
23. Scinto AF, Ferraresi V, Campioni N, et al. Accelerated chemotherapy with high-dose epirubicin and cyclophosphamide plus r-met-HUG-CSF in locally advanced and metastatic breast cancer. *Ann Oncol* 1995; 6:665–671.
24. Hayes NA. Analyzing current practice patterns: lessons from Amgen's project chemoInsight. *Oncol Nurs Forum* 2001;28(suppl 2):11–16.
25. Link BK, Budd GT, Scott S, et al. Delivering adjuvant chemotherapy to women with early stage breast carcinoma. *Cancer* 2001;92(6):1354–1367.
26. Chang J. Chemotherapy dose reduction and delay in clinical practice: evaluating the risk to patient outcome in adjuvant chemotherapy for breast cancer. *Eur J Cancer* 2000;36:S11–S14.
27. Demetri GD, Berry D, Norton L, et al. Clinical outcomes of node-positive breast cancer patients treated with dose-intensified Doxorubicin/cyclophosphamide (AC) followed by taxol (T) as adjuvant systemic chemotherapy (CALGB 9141). *Proc ASCO* 1997;16:143a (Abstract 503).
28. Hudis C, Seidman A, Baselga J, et al. Sequential dose-dense doxorubicin, paclitaxel, and cyclophosphamide for resectable high-risk breast cancer: feasibility and efficacy. *J Clin Oncol* 1999;17:93–100.

29. Costa SD, von Minckwitz G, Raab G, et al. The role of docetaxel (Taxotere) in neoadjuvant chemotherapy of breast cancer. *Semin Oncol* 1999;26(3 suppl 9):24–31.
30. Biernat L, Flaherta L, Philip P, et al. A phase II study of the combination of taxotere, doxorubicin and 5-fluorouracil in the treatment of locally advanced breast cancer. Preliminary toxicity data. *Breast Cancer Res Treat* 1998;50:328 (Abstract 550).
31. Ellis G, Gralow JR, Pierce HI, et al. Infusional paclitaxel and weekly vinorelbine chemotherapy with concurrent filgrastim for metastatic breast cancer: high complete response rate in a phase I-II study of doxurubicin-treated patients. *J Clin Oncol* 1999;17(5):1407–1412.
32. Fleming GF, Kugler JW, Hoffmann PC, et al. Phase II trial of paclitaxel and topotecan with granulocyte colony-stimulating factor support in stage IV breast cancer. *J Clin Oncol* 1998;16:2032–2037.
33. Wasserheit C, Frazein A, Oratz R, et al. Phase II trial of paclitaxel and cisplatin in women with advanced breast cancer: An active regimen with limiting neurotoxicity. *J Clin Oncol* 1996;14:1993–1999.
34. Frasci G, Comella P, D'Aiuto G, et al. Weekly paclitaxel-cisplatin administration with G-CSF support in advanced breast cancer. A phase II study. *Breast Cancer Res Treat* 1998;49:13–26.
35. McGown AT, Fox BW. A proposed mechanism of resistance to cyclophosphamide and phosphoramide mustard in a Yoshida cell line in vitro. *Cancer Chemother Pharmacol* 1986;17:223–226.
36. McGown AT, Ward TH, Fox BW. Comparative studies of the uptake of daunorubicin in sensitive and resistant P388 cell lines of flow cytometry and biochemical extraction procedures. *Cancer Chemother Pharmacol* 1986;17:223–226.
37. Hortobagyi GN. The importance of dose reponse in cytotoxic therapy for breast cancer. In: Henderson IC, Borden EC, eds. *Advances in breast cancer treatment. Therapeutic changes in oncology.* London: Mediscript, 1990:47–69.
38. Skipper HE. In: Jacquillat C, Were M, Khayat D, eds. *Neo-adjuvant chemotherapy.* Colloque INSERM. 137th ed. London: John Libbey Eurotext, 1986:11–22.
39. Fisher B, Anderson S, Wickerman DL, et al. Increased intensification and total dose of cyclophosphamide in a doxorubicin-cyclophosphamide regimen for the treatment of primary breast cancer: Findings from the National Surgical Adjuvant Breast and Bowel Project B-22. *J Clin Oncol* 1997;15:1858–1869.
40. Fisher B, Anderson S, DeCillis A, et al. Further evaluation of intensified and increased total dose of cyclophosphamide for the treatment of primary breast cancer: findings from National Surgical Adjuvant Breast and Bowel Project B-25. *J Clin Oncol* 1999;17:3374–3388.
41. Henderson IC, Berry D, Demetri G, et al. Improved disease free (DFS) and overall survival (OS) from the addition of sequential paclitaxel (T) but not from escalation of doxorubicin (A) dose level in the adjuvant chemotherapy of patients (pts) with node-positive breast cancer (BC) (abstract). *Proc ASCO* 1998;17:101a.
42. Rodenhuis S, Bontenbal M, Beex L, et al. Randomized phase III study of high-dose chemotherapy with cyclophosphamide, thiotepa and carboplatin in operable breast cancer with 4 or more axillary lymph nodes (abstract). *Proc ASCO* 2000;19:74a.
43. Bergh J, Wiklund T, Erikstein B, et al. Dosage of adjuvant G-CSF (filgrastim)-supported FEC polychemotherapy based on equivalent haematological toxicity in high-risk breast cancer patients. *Ann Oncol* 1998;9:403–411.
44. The Scandinavian Breast Cancer Study Group 9401. Results from a randomized adjuvant breast cancer study with high dose chemotherapy with CTC_b supported by autologous bone marrow stem cells versus dose escalated and tailored FEC therapy. *Proc ASCO* 1999;18:2a (Abstract 3).
45. Untch M, Konecny G, Lebeau A, et al. Dose-intensification and c-erbB-2 overexpression in anthracycline-based adjuvant treatment of high-risk breast cancer. *Proc ASCO* 1998;17:103a (Abstract 395).
46. Venturini M, Del-Mastro L. More on dose-intensity of anthracyclines in breast cancer. *Ann Oncol* 1998;9:461.
47. Lord BI, Bronchud MH, Owens S, et al. The kinetics of human granulopoiesis following treatment with granulocyte colony-stimulating factor in vivo. *Proc Natl Acad Sci USA* 1989;86:9499–9503.
48. Lieschke GJ, Foote M, Morstyn G. Hematopoietic growth factors in cancer chemotherapy. In: Pindo HM, Longo DL, Chabner BA, eds. *Cancer chemotherapy and biological response modifiers annual 17.* New York: Elsevier Science, 1997:363–389.
49. Lindermann A, Hermann F, Oster W, et al. Hematologic effects of recombinant human granulocyte colony-stimulating factor in patients with malignancy. *Blood* 1989;74:2644–2651.
50. Bronchud MH, Potter MR, Morgenstern G, et al. In vitro and in vivo analysis of the effects of recombinant human granulocyte colony-stimulating factor in patients. *Br J Cancer* 1988;58:69–69.
51. Trillet-Lenoir V, Green JA, Manegold C, et al. Recombinant granulocyte colony stimulating factor in the treatment of small cell lung cancer, a long-term follow-up. *Eur J Cancer* 1995;31 A:2115–2116.
52. De Graaf H, Willemse PHB, Bong SB, et al. Dose intensity of standard adjuvant CMF with granulocyte colony-stimulating factor for premenopausal patients with node-positive breast cancer. *Oncology* 1996;53:289–294.
53. Silber JH, Fridman M, DiPaola RS, et al. First-cycle blood counts and subsequent neutropenia, dose reduction, or delay in early-stage breast cancer therapy. *J Clin Oncol* 1998;16:2392–2400.
54. Ghandi S, Arguelles L, Boyer G. Economic impact of neutropenia and febrile neutropenia in breast cancer: estimates from two national databases. *Pharmacotherapy* 2001;21(6):684–690.
55. Lyman GH, Kuderer N, Greene J, Balducci L. The economics of febrile neutropenia: implications for the use of colony-stimulating factors. *Eur J Cancer* 1998;34:1857–1864.
56. Bennett CL, Weeks JA, Somerfield MR, et al. Use of hematopoietic colony-stimulating factors: comparison of the 1994 and 1997 American Society of Clinical Oncology surveys regarding ASCO clinical practice guidelines. Health Services Research Committee of the American Society of Clinical Oncology. *J Clin Oncol* 1999;17:3676–3681.

57. Holmes F, O'Shaughnessy S, Vukelja S, et al. Blinded, randomized multicenter study to evaluate single administration pegfilgrastim once per cycle versus daily filgrastim as an adjunct to chemotherapy in patients with high-risk stage II or stage III/IV breast cancer. *J Clin Oncol* 2002;20:727–731.
58. Green M, Koelbl H, Baselga J, et al. A randomized, double-blind, phase 3 study evaluating fixed-dose, once-per-cycle pegylated filgrastim (SD/01) versus daily filgrastim to support chemotherapy for breast cancer. *Proc ASCO* 2001;20:23a (Abstract 90).
59. Holmes FA, Jones SE, O'Shaughnessy J, et al. Comparable efficacy and safety profiles of once-per-cycle pegfilgrastim and daily injection filgrastim in chemotherapy-induced neutropenia: a multicenter dose-finding study in women with breast cancer. *Ann Oncol* 2002;13:903–909.

33
Erythropoietin in the Management of Cancer Patients

Alexander H.G. Paterson and Mary-Ann Lindsay

ERYTHROPOIESIS

In adults, erythropoiesis occurs principally in the bone marrow. Pluripotent stem cells give rise to erythroid, granulocytic, and megakaryocytic precursors. Erythroid cells are derived from primitive cells known as burst-forming units (BFU-E) which differentiate into erythroid precursors, provided cofactors such as folate, B-12, and iron are available. Erythroblasts extrude their nuclei to become reticulocytes, which migrate from the bone marrow into the peripheral circulation and through maturation develop into normal red blood cells. The lower limits of normal for the level of red cell counts are 4.4×10^{12} and 3.9×10^{12} for men and women. Anemia is clinically defined as reported levels of hemoglobin, hematocrit, or red cell count below the generally accepted normal ranges.

ANEMIA OF CHRONIC DISEASE

Anemia arises from a variety of causes such as bleeding, hemolysis, and deficiency states. The anemia of chronic disease is associated with chronic infections and inflammatory or neoplastic diseases (1,2). It is distinguished from iron deficiency anemia by low-serum iron levels in the presence of normal iron stores. Plasma levels of the iron-transporting protein transferrin are low and the level of saturation of transferrin with iron is low; serum ferritin levels are normal or elevated, while in contrast, in iron deficiency anemia they are low (3).

The pathogenesis is not well understood. Red cell life span is shortened and there is defective production of new cells. Apoferritin in storage sites such as the bone marrow increases and this further diverts iron from serum to the storage pool. Inflammatory cytokines, such as interleukin-1 and tumor necrosis factor, are elevated and these may inhibit the production of transferrin (4).

THE ANEMIA OF CANCER

Anemia in cancer patients can be due to the same range of causality as in the patient without malignant disease, and it is important to make a proper hematological diagnosis, excluding causes such as bleeding, iron, B-12, folate deficiency, and hemolysis. In many patients, the anemia is due to the chronic malignant disease process.

Signs and symptoms of anemia include exertional dyspnea, palpitations, dizziness, depressive mood, impaired cognitive functions, anorexia, and, especially, fatigue (5). Fatigue affects patients physically, emotionally, and financially. In a recent survey of over 300 patients, a general feeling of debilitating weakness was regularly experienced by 76% of patients (6). The vast majority reported that this fatigue prevented them from leading a normal life and caused them to miss work, reduce their workload, or stop working altogether. It also caused those looking after these patients to reduce their own workload. Ashbury et al. (7) surveyed over 900 cancer patients and found fatigue was the most commonly reported symptom.

Fatigue is not necessarily due to the anemia of chronic disease and is often multifactorial. Cytotoxic drugs, pain-relieving medicines, antidepressants and anxiolytics, as well as paraneoplastic syndromes such as cancer-related myopathies, all contribute to the feeling of fatigue and lethargy. However, low hemoglobin levels are frequently found in cancer patients. Skillings et al. (8) found that 93% of lung cancer patients had a hemoglobin level less than

120 g/L and 50% were less than 100 g/L. Patients with other malignancies were frequently found to have low hemoglobin levels.

ENDOGENOUS HUMAN ERYTHROPOIETIN

Human erythropoietin was isolated from the urine of patients with aplastic anemia in the 1970s (9). It is a glycoprotein hormone with a 165 amino acid core and 4 oligosaccharide side-chains. It is produced chiefly in interstitial peri-tubular cells in the kidney with approximately 10% produced in the liver. Production is stimulated by hypoxia and, in a negative feedback mechanism, production is suppressed by successful erythropoiesis (10,11). Erythropoietin stimulates the growth of BFUs, colony-forming units (CFUs) and proerythroblasts, but not more mature erythroid cells. In iron-deficiency anemias, erythropoietin production increases proportionally to the degree of anemia; in chronic renal failure, the kidneys fail to produce sufficient quantities of erythropoietin; in chronic inflammatory and malignant diseases, erythropoietin levels increase somewhat, but not at levels sufficient to cause a rise in hemoglobin levels (12). The erythropoietin response appears to be blunted.

EPOIETIN ALPHA

Epoietin alpha was introduced into North America in 1990. It is now used extensively in patients with chronic renal failure. It has an amino acid sequence identical to endogenous human erythropoietin and is virtually indistinguishable from it. This recombinant product does not appear to be immunogenic (13).

Provided cofactor stores are intact, administration of epoietin alpha elevates reticulocyte counts within 10 days of initiating therapy. Red cell count, hemoglobin levels and the hematocrit starts to rise in 2 to 4 weeks (14). In a randomized, double-blind, placebo-controlled study, Abels et al. (15) showed that epoietin alpha (Eprex) increased the hematocrit significantly more than placebo whether patients were receiving no chemotherapy, cisplatinum-based chemotherapy, or non-platinum based therapy. The tumor type did not influence this response. That these changes in hematocrit had a beneficial effect on quality of life and functional capacity was suggested in a community-based study of epoietin alpha given to patients with a variety of cancers (16). Mean changes in FACT-An (functional assessment of cancer therapy—anemia) scores correlated very well with changes in hemoglobin levels (level III evidence). In double-blind, placebo-controlled trials, there appears to be no significant excess of adverse events in patients receiving epoietin alpha. Epoietin is contraindicated, however, in patients with uncontrolled hypertension or severe ischemic heart or cerebrovascular disease.

Prior to initiating therapy with epoietin alpha, patients' iron stores should be assessed since an erythropoietic response will lead to depletion of stores. Transferrin saturation should be at least 20% and serum ferritin levels at least 100 ng/mL. Serum B-12 and folate may require to be measured. If necessary, elemental iron may have to be supplemented; many physicians prescribe this routinely in patients commencing epoietin alpha therapy to avoid the potential of a mild deficiency state. Hypertension should also be controlled.

Epoietin alpha should be commenced at a dose of 150 IU/kg subcutaneously three times weekly. After 4 weeks, if the hemoglobin rise is equal to or greater than 10 g/L or the reticulocyte count is greater than 40,000 cells/µL, epoietin alpha can be continued until the hemoglobin returns to normal range. If these targets are not achieved after 4 weeks, the dose of epoietin alpha can be doubled to 300 IU/kg, but if no response is seen after 4 further weeks at the higher dosage, there is unlikely to be any benefit in persisting with therapy. Dose reduction of epoietin alpha is occasionally required as a result of hemoglobin levels rising greater than 20 g/L in a month.

BLOOD TRANSFUSIONS AND THE CANCER PATIENT

Blood transfusions are relatively easy to give in daycare units, but they can sometimes be associated with febrile reactions, urticarial reactions and fluid overload. In some jurisdictions, the availability of red cells for transfusions is decreasing, and patients' concerns regarding HIV, Creutzfeldt-Jacob, and cytomegalovirus are increasing. While these concerns are often of little relevance to the patient with advanced cancer, they are of concern in the adjuvant therapy setting.

There have been a number of clinical trials which have used blood transfusion requirements as a major outcome. All have shown that epoietin alpha reduces requirements for blood transfusions and most have shown significant elevations in mean hemoglobin levels. Abels et al. (11) showed that epoietin alpha given for 12 weeks compared to a placebo in patients receiving platinum-based chemotherapy with Hb less than 105 g/L led to significantly fewer blood transfusions.

Welch et al. (17), in a small, but well-performed study, showed that in patients with advanced ovarian cancer who were receiving platinum-based chemotherapy and who initially had normal hemoglobin levels, there was a significant difference in the mean Hb levels at cycles two through four ($p < 0.001$). Three of 15 patients in the epoietin arm required transfusions, compared to seven of 15 in the chemotherapy-only arm. Delmastro et al. (18) in breast cancer patients, Cascinu et al. (19) in platinum-based chemotherapy in patients with various malignancies, and Thatcher et al. (20) in lung cancer patients all showed that fewer blood transfusions were required in epoietin alpha treated patients (level II, grade A evidence).

TRIALS USING QUALITY OF LIFE AS AN OUTCOME

Reducing transfusion requirements may be useful in reducing the workload of busy daycare units and alleviating patients' concerns regarding the safety of the blood supply, but if these were the only outcomes of benefit, it would be unlikely that epoietin alpha would be widely used in cancer patients, principally because of cost. However, blood transfusion gives a rapid rise in Hb, followed by a decline, with recurrence of symptoms over a few weeks. If epoietin alpha can elevate and maintain Hb levels over time, one might expect quality of life to improve. This has been assessed in a number of studies.

Thatcher et al. (20), using a simple three-item questionnaire regarding energy level, daily activity, and quality of life, showed a significant improvement from baseline in overall quality of life in a group of lung cancer patients receiving epoietin alpha (level II evidence).

In the Abels et al. (15) study, there was an improvement in energy level, daily activities and overall quality of life, but the effects were small. The patients who experienced most improvement had an increase in Hb levels (level III evidence).

Gabrilove et al. (21), in an open-label single-arm study, showed that epoietin alpha given once weekly at 40,000 IU subcutaneously led to higher Hb levels ($p < 0.001$), a decrease in blood transfusions ($p < 0.001$) and an improvement in quality-of-life parameters (level III evidence).

Another study by Quirt et al. (22) was performed in patients with anemia of malignant disease who were not receiving concomitant chemotherapy: 183 patients received epoietin alpha 10,000 IU three times weekly. Response was defined as an increase of 20 g/L or more of Hb and was seen in 88 patients (48%). Quality of life improvement was seen only in those patients experiencing a hemoglobin response (level III evidence).

Two large non-randomized studies also confirm the relationship between a rise in Hb levels and improved quality of life (level III grade A evidence). Glaspy et al. (23) enrolled 2,342 patients with a variety of malignancies and therapies in a community-based study and showed that a rise in the Hb level correlated with an increase in mean energy levels, activity scores and quality-of-life scores. The magnitude of the increase in quality of life correlated with the magnitude of increase in the Hb levels, irrespective of tumor response.

Demetri et al. (16) enrolled 2,370 patients. Again, these patients had a variety of malignancies and therapies, but Hb rise correlated well with improved quality-of-life parameters.

Some intriguing data have been presented showing that erythropoietin crosses the blood-brain barrier and protects against experimental brain injury (24), suggesting other possible mechanisms for the mood and quality-of-life elevation than solely elevating Hb levels.

A RANDOMIZED, PLACEBO-CONTROLLED, MULTICENTER STUDY OF ANEMIC CANCER PATIENTS RECEIVING NON–PLATINUM-BASED CHEMOTHERAPY

A large phase 3 randomized, placebo-controlled trial of epoietin alpha has now been published (25). Study endpoints were the proportion of patients transfused (primary endpoint), changes in Hb levels, percent responders with Hb ≥ 2 g/L and changes in quality-of-life parameters (secondary endpoints). A supplemental endpoint of survival was added as a protocol amendment before unblinding of the study.

Patients receiving non–platinum-based chemotherapy for a variety of malignant diseases, including hematologic malignancies, were enrolled. Life expectancy was required to be at least 6 months with an Hb less than 10.5 g/dL or Hb more than 10.5 g/dL, but with a drop in Hb of 1.5 g/dL or more in a month. Randomization was on a 2:1 basis.

A total of 375 patients were enrolled: 251 in the epoietin arm and 124 in the placebo arm. The baseline patient characteristics were generally evenly distributed between treatment and placebo groups. The proportion of patients transfused (after day 28) was smaller in the epoietin alpha group than in the placebo group (24.7% versus 29.5%, $p = 0.0057$). This reduction in transfusion requirements occurred in both Hb strata (Hb less than 10.15 g/dL and Hb more than 10.5 g/dL). Mean Hb levels of the patients receiving epoietin alpha were higher throughout the first 28 weeks of the study ($p < 0.001$ for change from baseline to last value). This mean change in Hb levels occurred in both nonhematologic tumor patients and those with hematologic malignancies. The proportion of responders (Hb rise more than 2 g/dL) was 70.5% in the epoietin alpha arm compared to 19.1% in the placebo arm ($p < 0.001$). Linear analogue scores for energy ($p < 0.01$) were all improved significantly with epoietin alpha. FACT-An anemia scores ($p < 0.01$) and FACT-An fatigue scores ($p < 0.01$) were improved. Adverse events were comparable between the groups. A Kaplan-Meier estimate of survival shows an encouraging, but not statistically significant, improvement in survival in the epoietin alpha group with median survival of 17 months in the epoietin group compared to 11 months in the placebo group.

These results are very encouraging and warrant further studies of epoietin alpha in cancer patients, which should be sufficiently powered to demonstrate any survival advantage.

RADIOTHERAPY AND EPOIETIN ALPHA

Surprisingly, little work has been done with radiation therapy and epoietin alpha despite the well-known inverse relationship between hypoxia and cell kill from ionizing radiation. Grogan et al. (26) showed apparently improved outcomes in patients receiving blood transfusions when they became anemic during radiation for cervix carcinoma. Glaser et al. (27), in a small study of 37 patients with head and neck malignancies, showed that there appeared to be better local control at surgery in epoietin alpha-treated patients with 37% having residual cancer compared to 73% in the control group. At 17 months, local control was significantly better ($p < 0.03$; level II evidence). Other radiation trials are underway and this will undoubtedly provide a fertile ground for future clinical research.

PHARMACO-ECONOMICS

Costing of blood transfusion depends greatly on methods used. Costs have been reported to vary from $300 to $500 per unit of blood transfused. Eprex costs $0.08 to $0.09 per unit or $500 to $550 a month, and, therefore, if one-half to three-fourths of the patients who ordinarily would require blood transfusion avoid transfusions, incremental costs will be reduced somewhat. Nevertheless, there is a significant increase in costs to patients with an estimate of $16,000 to $18,000 per quality-of-life year gained. It is clear, however, that patients are willing to pay for this, and paying agencies across North America are being vigorously lobbied to provide this therapy which clearly improves life quality for cancer patients. Variations across Canada regarding access to Eprex programs, for example, are a cause for concern regarding fairness of application of the principle of equal access under the Canada Health Act.

RECOMMENDATIONS: CANADIAN CANCER AND ANEMIA GUIDELINE DEVELOPMENT GROUP

Broad recommendations for use of epoietin alpha therapy (28) are as follows:

1. Where the symptoms of anemia are sufficient to impair the patient's functional capacity or quality of life are present or anticipated.
2. Anemia sufficient to require red blood cell transfusion is present or anticipated.
3. Blood transfusion is not acceptable for medical, religious or patient choice reasons.

Specific guidelines for patient selection are as follows:

1. The anemia is directly or indirectly related to malignancy and is not caused by hemolysis, gastrointestinal bleeding, or Fe/B-12/folate deficiency.
2. There are low baseline Hb levels equal to or less than 100 g/L at start of chemotherapy.
3. Baseline Hb levels are less than or equal to 120 g/L, and symptoms are sufficient to impair functional capacity or quality of life are present or anticipated.
4. A drop in Hb of 10 g/L to 20 g/L per cycle of chemotherapy has occurred and where at least three remaining cycles remain to be administered.
5. Symptomatic anemia is present, affecting functional capacity or quality of life.

CONCLUSIONS

After its success in improving the quality of life of patients with chronic renal disease, erythropoietin has now been investigated in cancer patients with the anemia of chronic disease and the anemias associated with chemotherapy. There is now level I grade A evidence that epoietin alpha can reduce blood transfusion requirements, improve mean Hb levels of patients receiving chemotherapy (or not receiving chemotherapy) and improve quality-of-life parameters. There is level IV evidence of a survival gain which is being currently investigated in placebo-controlled trials.

Cost continues to be a concern of funding agencies, but given the obvious improvements in quality of life which occur, we believe it is just a matter of time before erythropoietin will become widely available for cancer patients throughout the Western Hemisphere.

REFERENCES

1. Means RT Jr, Krantz SB. Progress in understanding the pathogenesis of the anemia of chronic disease. *Blood* 1992;80(7):1639–1647.
2. Cash JM, Sears DA. The anemia of chronic disease: Spectrum of associated diseases in a series of unselected hospitalized patients. *Am J Med* 1989;87(6):636–644.
3. De Rienzo DP, Saleem A. Anemia of chronic disease: A review of pathogenesis. *J Tex Med* 1990;86(10):80–83.
4. Dinarello CA. Interleukin-1 and the pathogenesis of the acute-phase response. *N Engl J Med* 1984;311(24):1413–1418.
5. Ludwig H, Fritz E. Anemia in cancer patients. *Semin Oncol* 1998;25(3 suppl 7):2–6.
6. Curt GA, Breitbart W, Cella DF, et al. Impact of cancer-related fatigue on the lives of patients. *Proc ASCO* 1999;18:573a (A2214).
7. Ashbury FD, Findlay H, Reynolds B, et al. A Canadian survey of cancer patients' experiences: Are their needs being met? *J Pain Symptom Management* 1998;16(5):298–306.
8. Skillings JR, Rogers-Melamed I, Nabholtz JM, et al. An epidemiological review of anaemia in cancer chemotherapy in Canada. *The European Cancer Conference* 1995;31A(5):S183 (A879).
9. Ikegami S, Tamura S, Oide H. Simple purification procedure for human urinary erythropoietin. *Proc Soc Exp Biol Med* 1973;143(2):526–527.
10. McMahan FG, Vargas R, Ryan M, et al. Pharmacokinetics and effects of recombinant human erythropoietin after intravenous and subcutaneous injections in healthy volunteers. *Blood* 1990;76(9):1718–1722.
11. Abels RI, Rudnick SA. Erythropoietin: Evolving clinical applications. *Exp Hematol* 1991;19(8):842–850.

12. Miller CB, Jones RJ, Piantadosi S, et al. Decreased erythropoietin response in patients with the anemia of cancer. *N Engl J Med* 1990;322(24):1689–1692.
13. Egrie J. The cloning and production of recombinant human erythropoietin. *Pharmacotherapy* 1990;10(Pt 2):3S–8S.
14. Abels R. Review of hematologic effects of erythropoietin. *Semin Nephrol* 1990;10(2 suppl 1):1–10.
15. Abels RI, Larholt KM, Krantz DK, et al. Recombinant human erythropoietin (rHuEPO) for the treatment of the anemia of cancer. *Oncologist* 1996;1(3):140–150.
16. Demetri GD, Kris M, Wade J, et al. Quality-of-life benefit in chemotherapy patients treated with epoetin alfa is independent of disease response or tumor type: results from a prospective community oncology study. Procrit Study Group. *J Clin Oncol* 1998;16(10):3412–3425.
17. Welch RS, James RD, Wilkinson PM, et al. Recombinant human erythropoietin and platinum based chemotherapy in metastatic ovarian carcinoma. *Proc ASCO* 1993;12:254 (A804).
18. Del Mastro L, Venturini M, Garrone O, et al. Erythropoietin in the prevention of chemotherapy induced anemia: results from a randomized trial in early breast cancer patients. *Proc ASCO* 1995;14:256 (A697).
19. Cascinu S, Fedeli A, Del Ferro E, et al. Recombinant human erythropoietin treatment in cisplatin-associated anemia: A randomized, double-blind trial with placebo. *J Clin Oncol* 1994;12(5):1058–1062.
20. Thatcher N, DeCampos ES, Bell DR, et al. Epoetin alfa prevents anemia and reduces transfusion requirements in patients undergoing primarily platinum based chemotherapy for small cell lung cancer. *Br J Cancer* 1999;80(3–4):396–402.
21. Gabrilove JL, Einhorn LH, Livinstron RB, et al. Once-weekly dosing of epoietin alpha is similar to three-times-weekly dosing in increasing haemoglobin and quality of life. *Proc ASCO* 1999;18:574a (A2216).
22. Quirt I, Kovacs M, Burdette-Radoux S, et al. Epoietin alfa reduces transfusion requirements, increases hemoglobin (Hb) and improves quality of life in cancer patients with anemia who are not receiving concomitant chemotherapy. *Proc ASCO* 1999;18:594a (A2295).
23. Glaspy J, Bukowski R, Steinberg D, et al. Impact of therapy with epoetin alfa on clinical outcomes in patients with nonmyeloid malignancies during cancer chemotherapy in community oncology practice. Procrit Study Group. *J Clin Oncol* 1997;15(3):1218–1234.
24. Brines ML, Ghezzi P, Keenan S, et al. Erythropoietin crosses the blood-brain barrier to protect against experimental brain injury. *Proc Natl Acad Sci USA* 2000;12;97(19):10526–10531.
25. Littlewood TJ, Bajetta E, Nortier JW, et al. Effects of epoetin alfa on hematologic parameters and quality of life in cancer patients receiving nonplatinum chemotherapy: results of a randomized, double-blind, placebo-controlled trial. *J Clin Oncol* 2001;19(11):2865–2874.
26. Grogan M, Thomas GM, Melamed I, et al. The importance of hemoglobin levels during radiotherapy for carcinoma of the cervix. *Cancer* 1999;86(8):1528–1536.
27. Glaser C, Millesi W, Wanschitz B, et al. R-HuErythropoietin treatment increases efficacy of neoadjuvant radiochemotherapy and improves cancer free survival of patient with oral squamous cell carcinoma: A 17 month follow up. *Proc ASCO* 1999;18:399a (A1543).
28. Turner AR, Anglin P, Burkes R, et al. Epoetin alfa in cancer patients: Evidence-based guidelines. *J Pain Symptom Management* 2001;22(5):954–965.

34

The Place of Bisphosphonates in the Management of Breast Cancer

Alexander H.G. Paterson

Skeletal complications are major causes of morbidity in patients with metastatic breast cancer, despite recent advances in endocrine and cytotoxic therapy. These skeletal complications arise because of progressive focal or generalized osteolysis. Osteolysis occurs because of osteoclast activation, either directly by tumor products or as a result of products secreted by nearby host cells in response to tumor cell products (paracrine effect) (1). As the osteoclast plays a central role in focal or generalized osteolysis, inhibitors of osteoclast function can lead to clinically valuable palliation and, in some patients, to prevention of osteolytic destruction and its complications (2). It is also possible that the growth and development of bone metastases may be inhibited in some patients. The bone loss associated with adjuvant chemotherapy or hormones causing premature menopause and therefore an increased rate of new fractures (especially vertebral fractures) may be prevented.

THE CLINICAL PROBLEM

Skeletal pain, fracture and hypercalcemia are well recognized by oncologists as major causes of morbidity in patients with breast cancer. Vertebral fractures not only cause pain and disability, but are known to lead to spinal cord compression. In women, the problems of bone metastases are compounded by the propensity to osteoporosis. Women have a lower total bone mass than men and the threshold for developing fractures tends to be reached at an earlier age in women than in men. In addition, in premenopausal women with breast cancer, the increasing use of adjuvant cytotoxic chemotherapy leads to early menopause with subsequent earlier accelerated loss of bone. As evidence for the value of adjuvant LHRH analogues is accumulating and because these therapies (*a priori*) lead to bone loss, a new reason for bone complications is now evident.

NORMAL AND ABNORMAL BONE REMODELING

Bone remodeling is a dynamic process occurring in response to poorly understood physical and chemical forces along lines of stress (3). Remodeling may result from initial stimulation by osteoblastic cells which are derived from bone marrow stromal cells (4). Osteoclasts (derived from hematopoietic precursor cells) are recruited to an area of damaged or worn bone which is then broken down to form a bone resorption bay by the action of lytic substances secreted by the osteoclast. Osteoblasts then move into the bone resorption bay (Howship lacuna), and new bone precursor substances, largely consisting of type I collagen, are laid down in layers which, over time, become mineralized. The formation of new bone following orderly resorption in the resorption cavities is termed "coupling." Bone remodeling normally occurs, therefore, as the result of a balance between bone destruction and new bone formation.

When malignant cells infiltrate bone spaces, the balance of new bone formation and bone destruction is perturbed and bone remodeling and turnover become abnormal. Under these circumstances, three mechanisms contribute to abnormalities of bone remodeling (5). The first occurs when a wave of bone resorption is initiated, usually focally, but sometimes generally, leading to increased bone turnover; loss of bone occurs because the resorption phase precedes the formation phase. A second mechanism comes into play when the normal connection between bone resorption and formation is disrupted and new bone is formed at sites other than where resorption has recently taken place and erosion cavities are never subsequently repaired. A third mechanism, uncoupling, occurs when the amount of new bone formed in the resorption bays does not match quantitatively the amount of bone resorbed.

The pathophysiology of malignant osteopathy is extremely complex. Carcinoma cells can secrete a variety of substances, such as parathyroid hormone-related peptide (PTHrP), prostaglandin E, and transforming growth factors, which stimulate tumor growth by autocrine or paracrine mechanisms, but which also have stimulatory effects on osteoclast function. Most of these effects occur locally, but these substances can also be secreted into the circulation, and have a generalized effect on bone metabolism (6). In prostate cancer, where osteoblastic metastases predominate, the excessive, deranged and uncoupled new bone formation can lead to the "bone hunger syndrome," a situation in which Ca^{2+} entrapment in bone leads to lower than normal plasma Ca^{2+} levels, with subsequent elevation of parathyroid hormone. This secondary hyperparathyroidism can lead to further generalized bone loss (7). In breast cancer, PTHrP release also leads to increased proximal tubular reabsorption of Ca^{2+} within the kidney, and this is an important mechanism for the appearance of hypercalcemia in breast and other cancers (8).

SEED AND SOIL THEORIES

The concept of malignant cell-matrix interaction is an old one, and hypotheses have been developed to explain the appearance of metastases at specific sites. These have been termed "seed and soil" theories. Experiments designed to investigate the relationship between malignant cells and their surrounding tissues at sites of metastases suggest that chemical interactions form the basis of the association (9).

The association of breast cancer with the development of bone metastases was first expressed in print by Paget in 1889 when he wrote: "The evidence seems to be irresistible that in cancer of the breast, the bones suffer in a special way, which cannot be explained by any theory of embolism alone" (10). The notion that there might be a local reason for the development of metastases at specific sites beyond a chance colonization following embolism was further developed by Batson (11), who described the connection between the vertebral venous plexus and the bone marrow spaces, hypothesizing a retrograde spread that would allow metastases from a primary prostate cancer to lodge preferentially in the lower vertebrae. Once within the marrow space, metastases have a blood supply for further growth. Mundy has taken the "seed and soil" idea one step further by adding the concept of a "vicious cycle," with products from tumor-induced breakdown of bone leading to stimulation and further growth of malignant cells (12).

BONE METASTASES

Incidence and Morbidity

The association of osteolytic, osteosclerotic, and mixed lytic/sclerotic bone metastases with breast cancer is well known to clinicians. In the experience of a major clinical trials group, the National Surgical Adjuvant Breast and Bowel Project (NSABP) in the United States, bone metastases account for the highest proportion of first sites of distant relapse in breast cancer patients suffering recurrence of their disease after adjuvant therapy with hormones and/or chemotherapy. Approximately one-third of patients who develop distant metastases do so in bone either as the sole site of recurrence or simultaneously with other sites of disease. The rate of bone metastasis development is higher in node-positive patients (approximately 2% per annum) than in node-negative (approximately 1% per annum) and in ER-positive patients than in ER-negative (13). As the disease progresses, almost 70% of patients will develop bone metastases (14); the median survival from diagnosis of bone metastases is between 18 and 20 months (15). Recently, we have shown that patients presenting with breast cancer have a 4 to 5 times higher rate of vertebral fracture than an age-matched group of well women (16). This is most likely related to chemotherapy-induced premature menopause with accelerated bone loss.

Bone Pain

When malignant cells invade the intertrabecular spaces, the malignant cells may form a mass to a size where secreted substances have an impact on local physiology. It is too simplistic to explain bone pain on purely mechanistic grounds by suggesting that a bone metastasis causes pain because trabecular fractures occur and bone collapses, leading to compression and distortion of the periosteum, a site known to be innervated by pain fibers. It is difficult to understand how bone pain can occur in the absence of fracture, but this does happen commonly. Bone marrow spaces are innervated by nociceptive C-fibers sensitive to changes in pressure, and it is probable that the malignant cells secrete pain-provoking factors such as substance P, bradykinins, prostaglandins, and other cytokines, which lead to stimulation of C-type fibers within bone. Prostaglandins may also play a role by sensitizing free nerve endings to released vasoactive amines and kinins (17). The precise interaction between the tumor and bone microenvironment is unknown. The subject of bone pain due to metastases has been well reviewed (18).

GENERAL PRINCIPLES OF MANAGEMENT

Although this review focuses on the place of bisphosphonates in the treatment of bone metastases in breast cancer (mainly because this disease has provided some of the most exciting research in recent years), other modalities continue to provide the mainstay of therapy.

Bone pain management includes a thorough history and physical examination, full discussion with the patient about a plan of action, and attempts to modify the pathological process. These attempts include external beam radiotherapy (still the most effective remedy for alleviation of localized bone pain) and palliative systemic therapy. A good response to chemotherapy includes subjective relief of symptoms, including pain. Hormone therapy can provide a high-quality remission in breast cancer patients with bone metastases. Radionuclide therapy with strontium-89 can be effective in alleviating the bone pain of breast cancer. Patients may require sequential therapy with bisphosphonates and strontium-89. Trials of both modalities used together are overdue.

Elevation of the pain threshold with the use of nonpharmacological methods as well as analgesics, interruption of pain pathways by local or regional anaesthesia or neurolysis, and modification of lifestyle are all helpful, but invariably opiate and other adjuvant analgesic management will be required.

Prophylactic surgery and radiation therapy for patients with cortical erosion caused by metastasis in the femur and humerus may prevent the distress of a pathological fracture.

BISPHOSPHONATES

The geminal bisphosphonates are analogues of pyrophosphate characterized by a stable P-C-P bond. They bind with high affinity to hydroxyapatite crystals in bone, and are potent inhibitors of normal and pathological bone resorption (19). At the cellular level, several mechanisms of action seem to operate, the dominant mechanism differing in different compounds, but all appear to have a final common effect of inhibition of osteoclast function. The osteoblast might be the initial target cell for bisphosphonates, exerting an effect on the osteoclast by modulation of stimulating and inhibiting factors which control osteoclast function (20). TGF-β is known to induce osteoclast apoptosis, and its production by bone surface osteoblasts as a result of bisphosphonate stimulation may explain this phenomenon.

These agents appear to promote apoptosis in murine osteoclasts both *in vivo* and *in vitro*, the more potent bisphosphonates exhibiting the greatest apoptotic action (21). In the absence of apoptosis, inhibition of osteoclast function appears to be mediated by osteoblasts, which produce a factor that inhibits osteoclastic function (22). This action does not interfere with the ability of cells of the monocyte-macrophage lineage to produce colonies (23). Bisphosphonates can also inhibit the proliferation and promote the cell death of macrophages (24,25). Again, the process is one of apoptosis rather than necrosis and may, in part, explain the pain-relieving properties of bisphosphonates. More recently, Shipman et al. (26) have described the induction of apoptosis by bisphosphonates in human myeloma cell lines.

At the molecular level, bisphosphonates appear to fall into two broad classes: nitrogen-containing and nonnitrogen-containing bisphosphonates. These two groups have different molecular mechanisms of action. Nitrogen containing bisphosphonates, such as pamidronate, alendronate and ibandronate inhibit the mevalonate signally pathway in osteoclasts while nonnitrogen-containing bisphosphonates are incorporated into ATP forming nonhydrolyzable analogues (27). Differences in side-chain moieties account for the variation in potency between the various bisphosphonates, a feature much publicized by the marketing departments of pharmaceutical companies. As yet there is no level I evidence from clinical trials that these differences in potencies are anything more than quantitative (i.e., the amount of bisphosphonates required to achieve the same effect on bone turnover).

CLINICAL TRIALS OF BISPHOSPHONATES IN BREAST CANCER

Hypercalcemia

Many bisphosphonates have been assessed in the management of malignant hypercalcemia. These include etidronate, pamidronate, clodronate, residronate, mildronate, neridronate, alendronate, ibandronate, and zoledronate. Etidronate, pamidronate, and clodronate have been the most extensively tested bisphosphonates and are widely available for the treatment of hypercalcemia and Paget disease of bone. We have previously demonstrated the action and value of etidronate in the treatment of malignant hypercalcemia (28). Pamidronate, clodronate, and etidronate all lead to an effective lowering of serum calcium which is attributable to decreased bone resorption, but etidronate appears to impair the mineralization of bone and must be given intermittently to allow normal bone formation to occur (29). Pamidronate, an aminobisphosphonate, is not ideal for oral use because of dose-related gastrointestinal toxicity. There is some evidence that long-term pamidronate administered orally may also induce osteomalacia (30). Clodronate is effective when given intravenously for hypercalcemia and bone pain, and it can also be used orally. Its long-term administration appears not to be associated with a defect in the mineralization of bone (31).

As a result of secretion of factors from infiltrating malignant ductal cells acting focally and humorally, osteoclast activity is markedly increased, with a reduction in osteoblast activity, leading to uncoupling of bone resorption and formation (32). Parathyroid hormone related protein (PTHrP) appears to play a central role in the malignant hypercalcemia of breast cancer (33).

We have recently reviewed the evidence for the treatment of hypercalcemia and have offered some broad guidelines (34). Randomized trials in hypercalcemia patients are notoriously difficult to carry out due to the poor clinical status of most hypercalcemic patients, the questionable ethics of a non-treated control group, the difficulty in obtaining satisfactory consent, and the variable response rate which depends on the underlying primary malignancy. For example, the hypercalcemia of myeloma responds much more easily to treatment than the hypercalcemia associated with carcinoma of the lung. Saline rehydration will usually effect a median reduction of 0.25 mM but its effect is transient (35). Rehydration is useful for treating mild degrees of hypercalcemia but usually should be accompanied by bisphosphonate therapy. Symptomatic hypercalcemia, especially with levels of Ca^{++} greater than 3 mM, requires vigorous rehydration (N-saline 150 to 200 cc/hr with KCl 20 to 40 mEq/L added), and the administration of clodronate 1,500 mg in 500 cc physiological saline over 2 to 3 hours or pamidronate 60 to 90 mg in 500 cc physiological saline over 2 to 3 hours. Pamidronate may give a longer duration of maintenance of normocalcemia (36) than clodronate (28 days median versus 14 days) but in many countries is significantly more expensive. Newer bisphosphonates, such as ibandronate and zoledronate, are currently being studied. Ibandronate at doses of 4 mg to 6 mg i.v. (37) and zoledronate at 4 mg i.v. (38) appear to be at least as efficacious as pamidronate and it has been suggested that zoledronate may be superior to pamidronate in terms of duration of response with the added advantage of a shorter infusion time. These studies are difficult to assess, since results are heavily dependent on the clinical case mix, and are of low power (level II evidence).

Skeletal Complications

Early clinical investigations of bisphosphonates were carried out in uncontrolled trials of patients with advanced disease or small nonplacebo-controlled, open studies (39). Although these investigators were probably correct in their conclusions, it is difficult to determine the extent to which patient selection and the placebo effect influenced the positive results of the investigations.

One of the first randomized, controlled studies to be published was an open trial of the aminobisphosphonate, pamidronate, given orally for 2 years at 300 mg daily in patients with bone metastases from breast cancer (40). The investigators demonstrated a reduction in the skeletal complications of hypercalcemia and vertebral fractures. Radiation treatments for bone pain were also reduced, but there was difficulty in patient compliance due to a high rate of upper gastrointestinal side effects (level II evidence).

In a double-blind, randomized, placebo-controlled trial of oral clodronate, 1,600 mg given daily for two years, we confirmed this beneficial effect on skeletal morbidity in patients with bone metastases from breast cancer (41). The number of patients suffering from episodes of hypercalcemia and the total number of episodes were reduced; the number of major vertebral fractures and the vertebral deformity rate were also reduced; and the number of radiation therapy treatments was lower in the clodronate-treated patients. No survival benefit was evident (level I evidence). McCloskey et al. (42) reviewed the pre-entry and follow-up vertebral fracture prevalence in 163 of the 173 patients in this trial and found that 46% of the patients had evidence of vertebral fracture at trial entry. The patients deriving the greatest benefit from the oral clodronate were those who had already sustained vertebral fractures and were therefore at greatest risk for sustaining further fractures.

Pamidronate, which can occasionally induce sclerosis in osteolytic lesions when used as the only therapy (43), has been investigated in several trials. Measurement of response in bone is a difficult process and unless differences in the arms of a trial are large, small but significant differences can be missed. Tumor response in bone and duration of response were assessed in a double-blind, randomized trial, which showed similar response rates in bone but a significantly ($p = 0.02$) increased duration of response for patients receiving pamidronate 45 mg given intravenously every three weeks (249 days median time to progression compared to 168 days in controls) (44). Hortobagyi et al. (45) have reported a randomized trial of 380 patients with recurrent breast cancer in bone and demonstrated a convincing reduction in the skeletal complications of vertebral fracture, pain, and hypercalcemia with intravenous pamidronate 90 mg given monthly for 2 years. No survival benefit was apparent. A trial of intravenous pamidronate in 372 patients with bone metastases from carcinoma of the breast receiving hormone therapy has shown a similar reduction in skeletal complications (46).

As a result of these well-controlled trials giving level I, grade A evidence, we currently recommend the use of either oral clodronate 1,600 mg orally daily (preferably taken ½ to 1 hour before breakfast or at least 2 hours away from food) or intravenous pamidronate 90 mg every 4 weeks in patients with radiologically established bone metastases from breast cancer.

Bone Pain

The idea that bisphosphonates might decrease bone pain in some patients with bone metastases arose from clinical observations of patients receiving bisphosphonates for hypercalcemia. Patients experienced not only normalization of serum Ca^{2+} and relief of the symptoms of hypercalcemia, but also reported relief of pain.

Ernst et al. (47) demonstrated in a double-blind, cross-over trial of intravenous clodronate in patients with bone pain caused by a variety of malignancies that clodronate had useful analgesic properties (level II evidence). This was confirmed (level I evidence) in a larger randomized, double-blind, controlled trial of intravenous clodronate in patients with metastatic bone pain (48). No dose-response relationship was seen. Improvement in pain and mobility scores had been described in a previously reported trial of oral pamidronate, although these patients had not been selected specifically because of bone pain but because they had osteolytic metastases (49); however, the modest effect, coupled with its poor oral tolerability as demonstrated by Coleman et al. (50), make oral pamidronate unlikely to supercede its intravenous counterpart. Level I evidence of pain relief has also been described with intravenous pamidronate in the previously discussed placebo-controlled trial in patients with bone metastases from breast cancer (45). The mechanism of pain relief is unknown but may be related to osteoclast and macrophage apoptosis or an inhibition of pain-provoking cytokines.

TRIALS OF ADJUVANT BISPHOSPHONATES

Patients with Recurrent Disease but No Bone Metastases

Some intriguing pioneer data were generated in a small, randomized, placebo-controlled clinical trial of continuous oral clodronate in patients who had recurrent breast cancer but with no evidence of bone metastases on bone scanning and conventional radiology (51). Although overall survival in the two arms was similar, there was an expected significant reduction in skeletal complications. When the incidence of new bone metastases was assessed, a significant reduction in the number of new bone metastases in the clodronate treated group was found. However, the number of patients developing bone metastases, although lower in the clodronate-treated group, was not significantly different from the control group. This study is one of the first of its kind to suggest that the intervention of a bisphosphonate, which primarily acts on osteoclasts, can have an impact on the behavior of bone metastases.

One other trial has assessed oral pamidronate in a similar group of patients with advanced or recurrent disease but no bone metastases. The trial was randomized but not placebo-controlled, and was also relatively small, with an accrual of 124 patients. A large number of patients withdrew from the trial because of the gastrointestinal side effects of oral pamidronate and compliance was a problem. Results showed no effect on rate of development of skeletal metastases, quality-of-life, or survival (52). These two trials might be described as giving level II, grade C evidence.

Patients with Operable Breast Cancer: Pre-clinical Rationale

As Goldhirsch et al. (53) has pointed out in reviewing the trials of the International Breast Cancer Study Group, the main effect of the adjuvant therapy used in the group's trials has been to reduce local, regional, and distant soft-tissue recurrences. First recurrences in bone and viscera have been minimally affected.

At menopause, bone resorption accelerates in women and they reach the fracture threshold at an earlier mean age than men, largely because of their lower peak bone mass. Combination chemotherapy is now used in premenopausal women with all stages of breast cancer. Many women with multiple positive lymph nodes have received high-dose or dose-intense chemotherapy with stem cell rescue or cytokines (G-CSF or GM-CSF). One of the effects of these treatments, particularly when high-dose or dose-intensive chemotherapy is used, or when the protocol contains alkylating agents, is to cause ovarian ablation leading to premature menopause. The skeletal effects of oophorectomy in rats are predictable, and consist of an early acceleration of bone turnover with loss of bone substance, especially cancellous bone. This accelerated bone turnover can be reduced by estrogen or the bisphosphonate, residronate. The effect of estrogen is lost 90 days after cessation of estrogen therapy. In contrast, the bisphosphonate is still effective 180 days after withdrawal (54). The bone loss following premature menopause in patients can be substantial, reaching as much as 7% in the first year in some women, but can be prevented by clodronate (55) and residronate (56).

The results of adjuvant chemotherapy and hormone therapy show that there is room for improvement in dealing with bone metastasis as a site of recurrence of disease. Tamoxifen does appear to reduce the incidence of new bone metastases as well as metastases at other sites (57). This reduction of incidence of bone metastases as site of first recurrence is generally not seen with chemotherapy. Tamoxifen is also known to have a beneficial effect on reducing bone resorption in postmenopausal women (58). Early attempts to reduce the incidence of bone metastases in patients with operable breast cancer using prostaglandin inhibitors, such as aspirin and indomethacin, were unsuccessful. This was despite *in vitro* data from the Walker carcinoma cell lines and *in vivo* data in the osteolytic rabbit VX2 tumor, which suggested that osteolysis and bone metastases could be inhibited by early treatment with prostaglandin inhibitors (59). These agents, although useful for the relief of pain, have little effect on the skeletal complications of established bone metastases. Bisphosphonates, which have an established record in reducing the skeletal complications of bone metastases, are a more promising group of compounds for prevention trials.

If clodronate and pamidronate can reduce the skeletal complications of patients with breast cancer, myeloma, and possibly other malignancies, do they achieve this by means of a cytotoxic effect or by means of a protective "antiosteolytic" mechanism, as is implied by their known mechanisms of action; or is it possible that their final pathway mode of action, the inhibition of osteoclast function, has a feedback effect leading to inhibition of the growth of bone metastases? Can we, by affecting the "soil" of the microenvironment in which tumor cell deposits grow, influence the behavior of the "seeds," the tumor micrometastases themselves? Production of PTHrP by breast carcinoma cells in bone is enhanced by growth factors such as activated transforming growth factor β, produced as a result of both normal bone remodeling and accelerated osteolysis; this, as Mundy has suggested, sets up a vicious cycle (60). It is also known that breast cancer cells secrete low molecular-weight factors that specifically affect human osteoblast cell lines, inhibiting their proliferation and increasing their cAMP response to parathormone.

Is it possible that we are merely interfering with the mechanisms of diagnosis, for example, by inhibiting the uptake of radiolabeled technetium pertechnetate in the bone reaction surrounding a metastasis, thereby reducing the tumor background ratio of radionuclide uptake? This is unlikely, given the extensive experience of bone scanning in patients with bone metastases who have received oral or intravenous bisphosphonates. There have been no reports of inhibition of uptake of bone-seeking radionuclides by bisphosphonates. Pecherstorfer et al. (61) have demonstrated that there was no effect on bone scintigraphy in 11 patients with breast cancer scanned after receiving daily intravenous clodronate for 3 weeks. Similarly, there was no inhibition of uptake documented in post-bisphosphonate scans compared with baseline scans after intravenous pamidronate had been administered as little as 24 hours previously (62).

A body of animal experimental data suggests that bisphosphonates have an inhibitory effect on the development of bone metastases. Pretreatment with bisphosphonates protects against the development of bone metastases in rats. When the Walker 256B carcinosarcoma is implanted intraosseously into Wistar-Lewis rats, pretreatment with clodronate inhibits the development of bone metastases compared with controls (63). Shorter intervals between the bisphosphonate therapy and the inoculation of tumor cells gave the best results, suggesting that, in the human setting, early therapy might give better results. This protective effect diminished with time after inoculation. Low-dose, continuous therapy also provided protection against metastatic growth.

Cell adhesion molecules are likely to be involved in the growth and invasion of breast cancer cells in bone (64). Van der Pluijm et al. (65) have demonstrated that the more potent bisphosphonates can inhibit the adhesion of breast cancer cells to neonatal murine bone matrices (cortical bone slices and trabecular bone cryostat sections), although no effect was seen with etidronate or clodronate in this system. This anti-adhesion effect has been confirmed by Boissier et al. (66), who examined both prostate and breast cancer cells. No direct cytotoxicity on tumor cells was seen. Apoptosis of myeloma cells *in vitro* has been described (26) with several bisphosphonates, suggesting that this mechanism may emerge as an important cause of the clinical benefit in malignant disease.

These animal studies suggest that it is possible to use bisphosphonates not only as a treatment for skeletal complications of cancer in humans but also as a protector against the development of metastases in bone. However, the effects of bisphosphonates may last only as long as medication is continued or for a few months after stopping, unlike chemotherapy, which acts by cytotoxicity. Patients with operable breast cancer, although at risk for recurrence in bone, are essentially well women. It seems impractical to ask these patients to continue intravenous medications much past the period of their intravenous chemotherapy. Quite apart from the patient inconvenience, the utilization of resources is considerable. Either an i.v. medication with a long duration of action or a continuous oral medication would be preferred. Oral clodronate, which is reasonably well tolerated, has been the most studied. Another interesting possibility is oral ibandronate, a potent nitrogen containing bisphosphonate, which seems to be well tolerated at doses of 25 to 50 mg daily (67).

Trials have shown that bisphosphonates can prevent the accelerated bone loss following the menopause and that this might prevent the development of osteoporosis. Saarto et al. (68) demonstrated that 2 years of clodronate therapy reduced bone loss compared with controls in all groups of patients, including those receiving chemotherapy, although the effect was greatest in those women receiving Tamoxifen, some of whom gained bone density.

Patients with Operable Breast Cancer: Adjuvant Clinical Trials

The ideal setting for testing whether bisphosphonates can have a beneficial effect on the rate of development of bone metastases is in the adjuvant therapy of operable breast cancer. The diagnosis of new bone metastases and its differentiation from vertebral osteopenic fractures is possible in patients who are relatively fit, and the development of metastasis can be correlated with measurements of bone density and other parameters. Two small trials of adjuvant clodronate have been reported. In the first reported study (69), 142 patients with primary breast cancer and no evidence of distant metastases were randomized to receive 1,600 mg daily of oral clodronate, and a further 142 were randomized into a non-placebo control group. These patients all had bone marrow involvement, with tumor cells detectable using the technique described by this group (70). After a median follow-up of 3 years, 21 patients in the clodronate group had developed distant metastases, compared with 42 patients in the control group. There were ten patients relapsing in bone, with an average of 3.1 metastases per patient in the clodronate group, compared with 19 patients relapsing in bone, with an average of 6.3 metastases per patient in the control group. The relapse-free interval for bone was 23 months for the clodronate group, compared with 16 months for the control patients. Not only was there a reduction in new bone metastases but there was also a significant reduction in new visceral metastases and a survival advantage in the clodronate treated group.

In a recent update reanalysis, however, the advantage in nonosseous relapses is no longer significant in the clodronate arm (71). In a second, open-label trial in 299 patients with node-positive breast cancer, Saarto et al. (72) randomized 149 patients to adjuvant oral clodronate and 150 patients to a control group. At a median follow-up of 5 years, there was no difference in the rate of development of bone metastases between the arms. There was an increase in the rate of nonosseous metastases and a decreased disease-free and overall survival in the clodronate group.

The huge difference in outcome between these trials can be explained at least in part by differences in the patient population, trial design, and the small sample size of the studies (level II evidence, grade C). These two studies were also open label and it is not clear whether the threshold for launching diagnostic investigations for bone recurrence was the same in each arm. The German study (69) restricted recruitment to patients with evidence of bone marrow involvement; these patients may be at high risk for development of bone metastases and other recurrences and may constitute a group in which it is easier to detect a beneficial effect of bisphosphonate therapy. In the Finnish trial (72) it appears that there was a chance random allocation of poorer prognosis ER/PR negative and more than four node-positive patients to the clodronate arm despite the apparently similar distribution of clinical characteristics in the two arms. The final analysis of a larger, randomized, placebo-controlled trial in 1,079 operable breast cancer patients has just been presented (73). This suggests that the interpretation of outcomes may be more complex than previously considered. There appears to be a reduction in the incidence of new bone metastases for the 2 to $2\frac{1}{2}$ years that the patients are taking clodronate but by 5 years of follow-up the advantage is no longer significant. There is a trend to a reduction in nonosseous metastases and an improved survival at 5 years in the clodronate patients ($p = 0.047$). Of interest, there is a substantial reduction in the incidence of relapses in the bone marrow. This trial supplies level I evidence of an effect on outcomes of bone metastases and survival in breast cancer. But it requires confirmation. This is now being performed by the NSABP and other groups in patients with operable breast cancer.

At this point, therefore, we are unable to recommend the use of bisphosphonates specifically as antitumor agents for the prevention of bone metastases in patients with operable breast cancer.

CONCLUSIONS

The following suggestions are submitted for consideration by physicians treating patients with breast cancer:

- Malignant hypercalcemia: intravenous pamidronate or clodronate with rehydration as described in the text (level III, grade A evidence). Newer, more potent drugs, such as ibandronate or zoledronate may offer some advantages, but are more expensive.
- Presence of bone metastases (symptomatic or asymptomatic): oral clodronate 1,600 mg orally, daily (taken $\frac{1}{2}$ hour before breakfast) or pamidronate 90 mg every 4 weeks intravenously (level I, grade A evidence).
- Moderate to severe bone pain: pamidronate 90 mg intravenously every 4 weeks; clodronate 1,500 mg intravenously every 2 weeks (level I, grade A evidence).
- Postchemotherapy bone loss: oral clodronate 1,600 mg orally daily if, on bone densitometry, the T-score is more than 2.5 or the annual rate of bone loss more than 10%, or fragility fractures are documented (level II, grade A evidence from bone density studies).
- Operable breast cancer: further controlled trials are required, preferably with oral bisphosphonates (one trial has given level I evidence; two trials level II, grade C evidence).

REFERENCES

1. Mundy GR, Ibbotson KJ, DeSouza SM, et al. The hypercalcemia of cancer. Clinical Implication and pathogenic mechanisms. *N Engl J Med* 1984;310:1718–1727.
2. Taube T, Elomaa I, Blomqvist C, et al. Hisomorphometric evidence for osteoclast medicated bone resorption in metastatic breast cancer. *Bone* 1994;15(2):1616.
3. Kaplan FS. Osteoporosis: Pathophysiology and prevention. In: *Clinical Symposia No 4*. Published by Ciba-Geigy, 1987.

4. Mundy GR. Bone resorption and turnover in health and disease. *Bone* 1987;8(suppl 1):S9–16.
5. Kanis JA, McCloskey EV. Bone turnover and biochemical markers in malignancy. *Cancer* 1997;80(suppl 8): 1538–1545.
6. Mundy GR. Hypercalcemia of malignancy revisited. *J Clin Invest* 1988;82:1–6.
7. Berruti A, Sperone P, Fasolis G, et al. Pamidronate administration improves the secondary hyperparathyroidism due to 'bone hunger syndrome' in a patient with osteoblastic metastases from prostate cancer. *Prostate* 1997;1:252–255.
8. Kanis JA, Percival RC, Yates AJP, et al. Effects of diphosphonates in hypercalcemia due to neoplasia. *Lancet* 1986;I:615–616.
9. Kamenor B, Kieran MW, Barrington-Leigh J, et al. Homing receptors as functional markers for classification, prognosis, and therapy of leukemia and lymphomas. *Proceedings of the Society of Experimental Biology and Medicine* 1984;177:211–219.
10. Paget S. The distribution of secondary growths in cancer of the breast. *Lancet* 1889:I:571–573.
11. Batson OV. The function of the vertebral veins and their role in the spread of metastases. *Ann Surg* 1940; 112:138.
12. Mundy GR. Mechanisms of bone metastasis. *Cancer* 1997;80(suppl 8):1546–1556.
13. Smith R, Jiping W, Bryant J, et al. Primary breast cancer (PBC) as a risk factor for bone recurrence (BR): NSABP experience. *Proc ASCO* 1999;18:Abstract 457.
14. Coleman RE, Rubens RD. The clinical course of bone metastases from breast cancer. *Br J Cancer* 1987;55: 61–66.
15. Paterson AHG. Natural history of skeletal complications of breast cancer, prostate cancer and myeloma. *Bone* 1987;8(suppl 1):S17–S22.
16. Kanis JA, McCloskey EV, Powles T, et al. A high incidence of vertebral fractures in women with breast cancer. *Br J Cancer* 1999;79(7–8):1179–1181.
17. Ferreira SH. Prostaglandins: peripheral and central analgesia. *Adv Pain Res Ther* 1983;5:627–634.
18. Ernst DS. Role of bisphosphonates and other bone resorption inhibitors in metastatic bone pain. *Top Palliative Care* 1997;3:117–137.
19. Fleisch H. Bisphosphonates in bone disease—from the laboratory to the patient, 4th ed. San Diego: Academic Press, 2000.
20. Sahni M, Guenther HL, Fleisch H, et al. Bisphosphonates act on rat bone resorption through the mediation of osteoblasts. *J Clin Invest* 1993;91:2004–2011.
21. Hughes DE, Wright KR, Uy HL, et al. Bisphosphonates promote apoptosis in murine osteoclasts *in vitro* and *in vivo*. *J Bone Miner Res* 1995;10:1478–1487.
22. Siwec B, Lacroix M, DePllak C, et al. Secretory products of breast cancer cells specifically affect human osteoblastic cells: partial characterization of active factors. *J Bone Miner Res* 1997;12:552–560.
23. Nishikawa M, Akatsu T, Katayama Y. Bisphosphonates act on osteoblastic cells and inhibit osteoclast formation in mouse marrow cultures. *Bone* 1996;18: 9–14.
24. Selander KS, Monkkonen J, Karhukorpi EK, et al. Characteristics of clodronate-induced apoptosis in osteoclasts and macrophages. *Mol Pharmacol* 1996;50: 1127–1138.
25. Rogers MJ, Chilton KM, Coxon FP, et al. Bisphosphonates induce apoptosis in mouse macrophage-like cells in vitro by a nitric oxide independent mechanism. *J Bone Miner Res* 1996;11:1482–1491.
26. Shipman CM, Rogers MJ, Apperley JF, et al. Bisphosphonates induce apoptosis in human myeloma cell lines: a novel anti-tumor activity. *Br J Haematol* 1997;98: 665–672.
27. Rogers MJ, Gordon S, Benford HL, et al. Cellular and molecular mechanisms of action of bisphosphonates. *Cancer* 2000;88(S12):2961–2978.
28. Ryzon B, Martodam RR, Troxell M, et al. Intravenous etidronate in the management of malignant hypercalcemia. *Arch Intern Med* 1985;145:449–452.
29. Kanis JA, Urwin GH, Gray RES, et al. Effects of intravenous etidronate disodium on skeletal and calcium metabolism. *Am J Med* 1984;82(suppl 2A):55.
30. Adamson BB, Gallacher SJ, Byars J, et al. Mineralization defects with pamidronate therapy for Paget's disease. *Lancet* 1993;342:1459–1460.
31. Taube T, Elomaa I, Blomqvist C, et al. Comparative effects of clodronate and calcitonin in metastatic breast cancer. *Eur J Clin Oncol* 1993;29:1677–1681.
32. Body JJ, Delmas PD. Urinary pyridinium cross-links as markers of bone resorption in tumor-associate hypercalcemia. *J Clin Endocrinol Metab* 1992;74: 471–475.
33. Grill V, Ho P, Body JJ, et al. Parathyroid hormone-related protein: elevated levels in both humoral hypercalcemia of malignancy and hypercalcemia complicating metastatic breast cancer. *J Clin Endocrinol Metab* 1991;73: 1309–1315.
34. Body JJ, Bartl R, Burckhardt P, et al. Current use of bisphosphonates in oncology. International Bone and Cancer Study Group. *J Clin Oncol* 1998;16(12): 3890–3899.
35. Singer FR, Rich PS, Lad TE, et al. for the Hypercalcemia Study Group. Treatment of hypercalcemia of malignancy with intravenous etidronate. A controlled, multicenter study. *Arch Intern Med* 1991;151: 471–476.
36. Purohit OP, Radstone CR, Anthony C, et al. A randomised double-blind comparison of intravenous pamidronate and clodronate in the hypercalcemia of malignancy. *Br J Cancer* 1995;71:1289–1293.
37. Ralston SH, Thiebaud D, Hermann Z, et al. Dose response study of ibandronate in the treatment of cancer associated hypercalcemia. *Br J Cancer* 1997;75(2): 295–300.
38. Major P, Coleman RE. Zoledronic acid in the treatment of hypercalcemia of malignancy: results of the international clinical development program. *Semin Oncol* 2001;28(2 suppl 6):17–24.
39. Elomaa I, Blomqvist C, Porrka L, et al. Treatment of skeletal disease in breast cancer: a controlled clinical trial. *Bone* 1987;8(suppl 1):S53–S56.
40. van-Holten-Verzanvoort AT, Bijvoet OL, Cleton FJ, et al. Reduced morbidity from skeletal metastases in breast cancer patients during long-term bisphosphonates (APD) treatment. *Lancet* 1987;11:983–985.

41. Paterson AHG, Powles TJ, Kanis JA, et al. Double-blind controlled trial of oral clodronate in patients with bone metastases from breast cancer. *J Clin Oncol* 1993;11:59–65.
42. McCloskey EV, Spector TD, Eyres KS, et al. The assessment of vertebral deformity: a method for use in population studies and clinical trials. *Osteoporosis Int* 1993;3:138–147.
43. Coleman RE, Woll PJ, Miles M, et al. Treatment of bone metastases from breast cancer with (3-amino-1-hydroxypropylidene)-1, 1-bisphosphonate (APD). *Br J Cancer* 1988;58:621–625.
44. Conte PF, Latreille J, Mauriac L, et al. Delay in progression of bone metastases in breast cancer patients treated with intravenous pamidronate: results from a multinational randomised controlled trial. *J Clin Oncol* 1996;14:2552–2559.
45. Hortobagyi GN, Theriault RL, Porter L, et al. Efficacy of pamidronate in reducing skeletal complications in patients with breast cancer and lytic bone metastases. *N Engl J Med* 1996;335:1785–1791.
46. Theriault RL, Lipton A, Hortobagy GN, et al. Pamidronate reduces skeletal morbidity in women with advanced breast cancer and lytic bone lesions: a randomized placebo controlled trial. *J Clin Oncol* 1999;17(3):846–854.
47. Ernst DS, MacDonald N, Paterson AHG, et al. A double-blind cross-over trial of intravenous clodronate in metastatic bone pain. *J Pain Symptom Management* 1992;7:4–11.
48. Ernst DS, Brasher P, Hagen NA, et al. A randomised, controlled trial of intravenous clodronate in patients with metastatic bone disease and pain. *J Pain Symptom Management* 1997;13:319–326.
49. van-Holten-Verzanvoort AT, Zwinderman AH, Aaranson NK, et al. The effect of supportive pamidronate treatment on aspects of quality of life of patients with advanced breast cancer. *Eur J Cancer* 1991;27:544–549.
50. Coleman RE, Houston S, Purohit OP, et al. A randomized phase II evaluation of oral pamidronate for advanced bone metastases from breast cancer. *Eur J Cancer* 1998;34:820.4.
51. Kanis JA, Powles T, Paterson AHG, et al. Clodronate and skeletal metastases. *Bone* 1996;19:663–667.
52. van-Holten-Verzanvoort AT, Hermans J, Beex LF, et al. Does supportive pamidronate treatment prevent or delay the first manifestations of bone metastases in breast cancer patients? *Eur J Cancer* 1996;32a:450–454.
53. Goldhirsch A, Gelber RD, Price KN, et al. Effect of systemic adjuvant treatment on first sites of breast cancer relapse. *Lancet* 1994;343:377–381.
54. Wronski TJ, Dann LM, Qi H, et al. Skeletal effects of withdrawal of estrogen and diphosphonate treatment in ovariectomised rats. *Calcif Tissue Int* 1993;53:210–216.
55. Powles TJ, McCloskey E, Paterson AHG, et al. Oral clodronate will reduce the loss of bone mineral density in women with primary breast cancer. *Proc ASCO* 1997;16:460(abstr).
56. Delmas PD, Balena R, Confraveux E. The bisphosphonate residronate prevents bone loss in women with artificial menopause due to chemotherapy of breast cancer: a double-blind, placebo-controlled study. *J Clin Oncol* 1997;15:955–962.
57. Fisher B, Constantino J, Redmond C, et al. A randomised clinical trial evaluating tamoxifen in the treatment of patients with node-negative breast cancer who have oestrogen receptor-positive tumors. *N Engl J Med* 1989;320:479–484.
58. Turken S, Siris E, Seldin D, et al. Effects of tamoxifen on spinal bone density in women with breast cancer. *J Natl Cancer Inst* 1989;81:1086–1088.
59. Powles TJ, Muindi J, Coombes C. Mechanisms for development of bone metastases and effects of anti-inflammatory drugs. In: Powles TH, ed. *Prostaglandins and cancer: First International Conference*. New York: Alan R. Liss, 1982:541–543.
60. Mundy GR, Yoneda T. Bisphosphonates as anticancer drugs. *N Engl J Med* 1998;339(6):398–400.
61. Pecherstorfer M, Schilling T, Janisch S, et al. Effect of clodronate treatment on bone scintigraphy in metastatic breast cancer. *J Nucl Med* 1993;34:1039–1044.
62. Macro M, Bouvard G, LeGangneux E, et al. Intravenous aminohydroxy-propylidine bisphosphonate does not modify 99m Tc-hydroxy-methylene bisphosphonate bone scintigraphy. A prospective study. *Revue Du Rheumatisme English Edition* 1995;62:99–104.
63. Krempien B. Morphological findings in bone metastasis, tumorosteopathy and anti-osteolytic therapy. In: *Metastatic bone disease. Fundamental and clinical aspects* (Diel IJ, Kaufmann M, Bastert G, eds.), New York: Springer, 1994.
64. Yoneda T, Sasaki A, Mundy G. Osteolytic bone metastasis in breast cancer. *Breast Cancer Res Treatment* 1994;32:72–84.
65. van der Pluijm G, Vloedgraven H, van Beek E, et al. Bisphosphonates inhibit the adhesion of breast cancer cells to bone matrices in vitro. *J Clin Invest* 1996;98:698–705.
66. Boissier S, Magnetto S, Frappart L, et al. Bisphosphonates inhibit prostate and breast cancer cell adhesion to unmineralized and mineralized bone extracellular matrices. *Cancer Res* 2000;57:3890–3894.
67. Coleman RE, Purohit OP, Black C, et al. Double-blind, randomised, placebo-controlled, dose-finding study of oral ibandronate in patients with metastatic bone disease. *Ann Oncol* 1999;10(3):311–316.
68. Saarto T, Blomqvist C, Valimaki M, et al. Chemical castration induced by adjuvant cyclophosphamide, methotrexate and fluorouracil chemotherapy causes rapid bone loss that is reduced by clodronate: a randomised study in premenopausal breast cancer patients. *J Clin Oncol* 1997;15:1341–1347.
69. Diel IJ, Solomayer EF, Costa SD, et al. Reduction in new metastases in breast cancer with adjuvant clodronate treatment. *N Engl J Med* 1998;339(6):357–363.
70. Diel IJ, Kaufmann M, Costa SD, et al. Micrometastatic breast cancer cells in bone marrow at primary surgery: prognostic value in comparison with nodal status. *J Natl Cancer Inst* 1996;88:1652–1658.

71. Diel IJ. Bisphosphonates in the prevention of bone metastases: current evidence. *Semin Oncol* 2001;28(4 suppl 11):75–80.
72. Saarto T, Blomqvist C, Virkkunen P, Elomaa I. Adjuvant clodronate treatment does not reduce the frequency of skeletal metastases in node-positive breast cancer patients: 5 year results of a randomized controlled trial. *J Clin Oncol* 2001;18(1):10–17.
73. Powles T, Paterson A, Burstein H, et al. Randomized, placebo-controlled trial of clodronate in patients with primary operable breast cancer. *J Clin Oncol* 2002; 20:3219–3224.

35

Cutaneous Metastasis and Malignant Wounds

Valerie Nocent Schulz

Patients with malignant wounds have a constant reminder of the presence of their cancer increasing their risk for lowered quality of life. The life expectancy of this patient population has increased from 3 months (1) to 1 to 34 (average 21.7) months. Cutaneous metastasis was reported in 420 of 4,020 (10.5%) patients with metastatic disease (2). The incidence of patients with cutaneous metastasis is not rare and their life expectancy has increased significantly. This may be the result of improved treatment outcomes, data collection, or a combination of these. Therefore, patients with malignant wounds may require long-term assessment and management. Impeccable symptom management complements traditional oncology care to reduce physical, functional, emotional and social distress.

Patients with malignant wounds differ significantly from those with benign wounds in terms of wound cellular characteristics, growth patterns, treatment approaches, response to treatment, and the patient's response to the wound. In addition, patients often have a progressive underlying malignant disease process that requires specific local or systemic therapy.

DEFINITION OF TERMS DESCRIBING A MALIGNANT WOUND

Since the malignant wound is the central concern of this chapter, it is vital that the term be understood. The terms malignant wounds, malignant cutaneous wounds, fungating and ulcerating wounds, cutaneous metastases and tumor invasion to the skin, are often mingled, or interchangeably substituted in research and the literature. Clarification of these terms is necessary to avoid confusion of these overlapping concepts, with slightly different definitions, and patient populations.

Haisfield-Wolfe and Rund (3), cited Cooper (1993), who described a malignant wound as "a break in the epidermal integrity by infiltration of malignant cells." More recently, a staging system was reported for malignant cutaneous wounds (4), which were defined as "primary or metastatic skin lesions of cancerous infiltration that are different in location and progression from traditionally encountered wounds." Within the Haisfield-Wolfe et al. staging system, A—stage I—was a closed wound with intact skin. There remains a discrepancy within these two definitions as to whether a break in the epidermal integrity is required to diagnose a malignant wound. The term "malignant cutaneous wound" has redundancies within it, as cutaneous means "relating to the skin." Cutaneous metastases, in contrast to malignant wounds, have been defined as "lesions in the dermis or subcutaneous tissue that were noncontiguous with the primary neoplasm" and cutaneous involvement by direct extension has been defined as, "a skin lesion produced by the primary tumor mass" (5).

Malignant wounds are often reported as fungating wounds. Haller (6) stated, "fungating wounds were the result of cancerous infiltration of epithelium and the surrounding blood and lymphatic vessels." A concern with the use of the term "fungating" wound is that it is a description of one class of malignant wound rather than an all-inclusive term for the population of patients with cancer spread to the skin.

Since a clear definition for the term malignant wound does not exist, a broad, simple definition was used. For the purposes of this chapter and any research conducted by Schulz to date, the term malignant wound refers to "the invasion by cancer into the skin" (7). Future research may be required to clarify this medical term as it defines the patient population under study.

DEVELOPMENT OF MALIGNANT WOUNDS

Malignant wounds can arise from primary skin carcinomas, cutaneous metastases from internal malignancy, and direct tumor extension to the skin from internal malignancies. Internal malignancies with a tendency to cutaneous metastasis have been reported as: (a) breast, melanoma, ovarian, large intestine, lung, sarcoma, adenoma, and oral cavity in females, and (b) lung, large intestine, melanoma, kidney, stomach, esophagus, sarcoma, and pancreas in males (8). Breast cancer is the most common direct tumor extension to the skin reported for any internal malignancy, and head and neck cancers collectively are second only to breast in developing cutaneous metastases (2). Breast cancer patients represent 50% of all patients referred to a specialized malignant wound clinic (9).

The mechanism of dissemination of internal malignancies to the skin may dictate the location of the wound. Dissemination primarily occurs through the lymphatic system particularly in breast and oral cavity tumors and probably for lung and renal cell carcinomas (8). Tumors with distant skin metastasis such as melanoma may spread hematogenously. Anatomically, malignant wounds are most commonly located on the chest and abdomen, followed by head and neck regions, and occur rarely in the extremities, except in melanoma (10). This reflects the frequency of breast and head and neck malignancies as the primary lesions causing malignant wounds.

PREVENTION OF MALIGNANT WOUND DEVELOPMENT

Preventing the development of malignant wounds, if possible, facilitates long-term patient management. Adjuvant radiotherapy and systemic therapy in node-positive premenopausal (11) and postmenopausal (12) women with breast cancer administered after a modified radical mastectomy have demonstrated a significant reduction in locoregional relapse and improved survival (13).

Prevention of surgical malignant implantation, and therefore locoregional recurrence, is currently under discussion in the literature. Potential causes of locoregional recurrence are: (a) intraoperative wound contamination with tumor, and (b) residual microscopic tumor at the operative site. A xenograft model of tumor-cell wound contamination with human squamous cell carcinoma of the hypopharynx, using a total of 40 mice, was developed to demonstrate the effects of various surgical irrigation techniques. Wound recurrence rates were dependent on the intraoperative irrigant. On day 56, 80% of controls (no irrigation), 75% of water, 40% of saline ($p < 0.1$), and 35% ($p < 0.004$) of gemcitabine irrigated mice had recurrent disease. Wound healing was not effected by gemcitabine (14). Disaggregated human GW39 colon cancer cells were injected into hamster peritoneum to represent a model of tumor spillage that may occur during laparoscopic colectomy for resectable carcinoma of the colon. The hamsters were randomized for irrigation and at seven weeks the surgical sites were analyzed. No tumor was found in the group treated with 5mCi of (64) Cu-PTSM while 96% of the wound sites treated with saline had macroscopic tumor growth. There were no signs of toxicity in the surgically irrigated hamsters (15). These animal models demonstrate promise for studying methods to reduce local recurrence. Similar human trials may be beneficial particularly in breast and head and neck cancers as these disease sites are the most common internal malignancies to develop malignant wounds.

THE CLASSIFICATION OF MALIGNANT WOUNDS

The classification of malignant wounds remains vague in the available literature to date. The concept of classifying malignant wounds, however, is very important. It is unclear whether malignant wounds should be classified according to their appearance and behavior, or in terms of their primary tumor origins. A classification system based on appearance of the tumor is presented in Table 35.1 (7).

The nodules and induration classification includes subcutaneous nodules and subcutaneous spread to the skin (Fig. 35.1). Cutaneous metas-

TABLE 35.1. *Classification of malignant wounds based on wound appearance (7)*

Malignant wound classification	Wound types within the classification
Nodules and Induration	Subcutaneous nodules
Subcutaneous spread—flat, spreading wound, ± open areas	Carcinoma erysipeloides—(erythema, appearance of cellulitis)
	Carcinoma en cuirasse—(dry, flat indurated skin)
	Elephantiasic skin changes—(thick, raised, indurated skin)
	Schirrhous dermal reaction—(scleraderma-like tightness)
Fungating and ulcerating wounds	Fungating
	Ulcerating
Other	Zosteriform lesions (appearance similar to herpes zoster)
	Wounds that do not fall within the above descriptions
	Wounds with mixed appearances

tasis resulting in subcutaneous nodules may not develop into a problematic malignant wound unless the overlying skin develops direct invasion. Alopecia neoplastica, areas of scarring and hair loss on the scalp (16) may be associated with these nodules.

Subcutaneous spread is the contiguous spread of malignancy within the skin resulting from lymphatic spread of malignancy with invasion of the dermis. It has been described for breast cancer and may be a useful description for cutaneous metastasis from other tumor types. The phases of subcutaneous spread are: carcinoma erysipeloides, carcinoma en cuirasse, elephantiasic skin changes, and schirrhous dermal reactions (16).

Carcinoma erysipeloides is the initial phase of cutaneous spread (Fig. 35.2). It is the phase of inflammation. The tumor has the appearance of spreading sheets of erythema and inflammation and is light pink in color. This is frequently diagnosed as cellulitis. Patients describe being able to feel the progressive growth at the tumor margin (9). Biopsy reveals carcinoma in the dermis or lymphatics plus inflammation (16).

Carcinoma en cuirasse (Fig. 35.3) develops subsequent to carcinoma erysipeloides. It is a phase of induration as the skin and subcutaneous tissue harden. It appears as dry, flat, indurated skin. The tumor often grows in size and begins to involve large body surface areas. It may spread extensively; from unilateral to bilateral chest wall lesions, across the abdominal wall, shoulder, upper back, neck and to the upper extremities. Patients report tightness, pruritus, dryness, lymphedema typically distal to the wound (i.e., upper extremities), embarrassment as the wound becomes difficult to

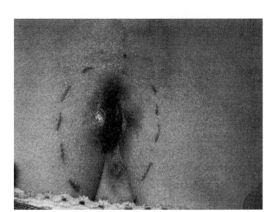

FIG. 35.1. Breast cancer with a suprasternal subcutaneous nodule. See color plate.

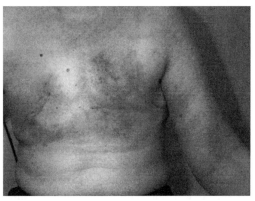

FIG. 35.2. Breast cancer with early subcutaneous metastasis presenting as inflammation known as carcinoma erysipeloides. See color plate.

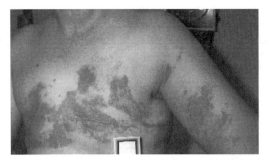

FIG. 35.3. Breast cancer with subcutaneous metastasis with induration of the skin called carcinoma en cuirasse. See color plate.

conceal under clothes, anxiety while watching the tumor progress, and changes in social interactions and intimacy (9). Patients may feel quite well and may have a significant life expectancy of 2 or more years even at this stage.

Some, but not all patients with carcinoma en cuirasse have progression of subcutaneous spread of malignancy resulting in elephantiasic skin changes (Fig. 35.4). This is associated with dermal stasis, hyperkeratosis, and papillomatosis (16). The tumor appears as thick, raised, indurated skin with shades of red and blue and sometimes purple discoloration. Patients frequently report tightness, pruritus, localized areas of skin breakdown, decreased mobility associated with lymphedema of the upper extremity or head and neck region, embarrassment, anxiety, and social withdrawal (9). This may progress to scirrhous dermal reaction, similar to morphea (16) appearing as localized scleroderma. All patient symptoms intensify at this stage.

Cutaneous metastasis may grow as fungating and/or ulcerating lesions (Table 35.1) (7). Fungating malignant wounds (Fig. 35.5) may show characteristics of both proliferation and ulceration. Inadequate blood supply to support the entire fungating mass results in infarcts, necrosis, and sloughing of the tumor allowing ulcerations to develop within the fungating mass (16). Therefore, fungating tumors are intimately associated with ulcerating features. Fungating tumors occur most commonly in breast cancer, but also in lung, stomach, head and neck, uterus, kidney, ovary, colon, bladder, melanoma, and

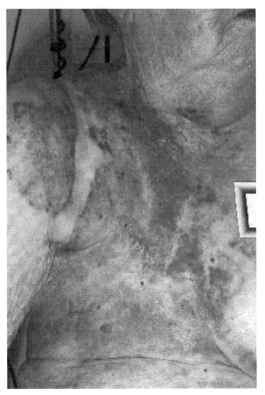

FIG. 35.4. Breast cancer with subcutaneous metastasis presenting as carcinoma en cuirasse with elephantiasic skin changes in the thickened tissue. This patient experienced lymphedema of the head and neck and upper extremity. See color plate.

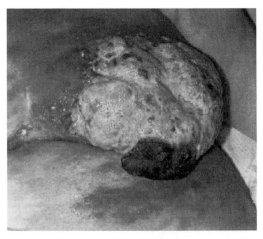

FIG. 35.5. Fungating malignant wound with surrounding carcinoma en cuirasse from breast carcinoma. See color plate.

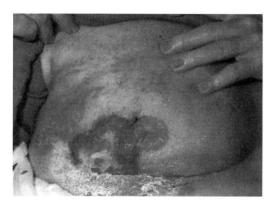

FIG. 35.6. Ulcerating malignant wound from carcinoma of the breast. See color plate.

lymphoma (16). Ulcerating malignant wounds are not always associated with fungating tumors (Fig. 35.6). Head and neck tumors, bowel, lymphoma (8,10), squamous cell, and basal cell carcinoma (10), amongst others, more commonly develop ulcers without fungating features. This process of ulceration can be so aggressive that fistulas may develop within the wound.

Zosteriform, zoster-like distribution of carcinoma (Fig. 35.7), results from perineural lymphatic spread of malignancy (17). Curiously, individual vesicular-like lesions may appear as miniature fungating tumors with a small central ulcer (9). The spread is not contiguous as there is normal-appearing skin between the lesions, although with disease progression the lesions can appear in broad clusters. Patients may experience exudate, pain, odor, emotional, and social concerns (9). Malignant wounds may have features of more than one category. Malignant wound classification would benefit from further research.

THE ASSESSMENT OF PATIENTS WITH MALIGNANT WOUNDS

A thorough patient assessment is the cornerstone to determining the best approach to investigation and management of patients with malignant wounds. Benign wound assessment cannot be applied to malignant wounds as these patient groups have unique features.

The clinical problems common to patients with malignant wounds as determined by caregivers report was recently identified (18). Data were collected from 136 health care providers, representing 136 patients. The symptom themes were analyzed using descriptive and exploratory analysis. The clinical problems for patients with malignant wounds identified in this study were: pain, odor, exudate, bleeding, edema, emotional stress, social concerns, functional compromise, and wound complications (e.g., fistulas and infection) (18). Individual patients generally experience some but not all of these symptoms. A patient assessment based on these common concerns is beneficial (18–21).

An organized, directed assessment guides patient management (18,20). The Schulz Malignant Wound Assessment Tool (S-MWAT) (7,22) was designed to be a comprehensive assessment for patients with malignant wounds (Table 35.2). A systematic method was used to gather evidence for construct and content validity within the S-MWAT (7,22) design. The assessment is based on understanding the individual patient concerns through addressing the population-based concerns common to these patients. It includes: (a) compiling general patient information such as gender, age, allergies, medications, medical problems, cancer history, oncology care in general and specific to the wound, wound dressing care, and

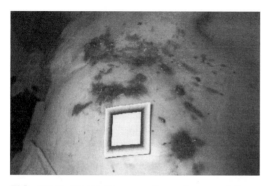

FIG. 35.7. Zosteriform malignant wound from carcinoma of the breast; this is the patient's left lateral chest wall. See color plate.

TABLE 35.2. *Schulz Malignant Wound Assessment Tool*

Patient Information: This information may be obtained from the chart or the patient

Name		Female ____ Male ____
Date	Date of birth	
Institution/location	Institution number	
Cancer diagnosis	Date of diagnosis	
Previous Radiation		
Chemotherapy		
Cancer surgery		
Current Radiation		
Chemotherapy		
Cancer surgery		
Other metastases		
Date patient first noticed the wound		
Rate wound changes / month / year		
Wound care is provided by: 1 = family 2 = health care, 3 = patient, 4 = other	Karnofsky performance status 0 – 100	
Method of cleaning wound: 1 = saline, 2 = water, 3 = cleaning products, 4 = other	Dressing changes #/day or #/week	
Name all dressings and wound treatments		
Is the appearance of the wound covering important? (dressing / clothing)		
Describe wound care effectiveness.		
State previous wound care attempted.		
Relevant medical problems		
Allergies		
Medications		

continued

family support systems; (b) understanding the individual patients' perspective of living with the wound based on assessing their physical, functional, emotional, and social concerns; and (c) completing a physical examination of the wound. The physical examination includes identifying the wound classification, location, size, and description of the wound and peri-wound skin. The examiner reports their observation of odor, exudate, bleeding, edema, and functional compromise such as limitations in mobility, swallowing, vision, and so on. Complications from the wound location, for example, fistulas, or incontinence, need to be identi-

TABLE 35.2. Continued

Schulz Malignant Wound Assessment Tool (SMWAT) Items relate to malignant wound concerns

Patient's Name		Date		Interviewer	
Answer 1 or more items per row		0 = not at all to 10 = overwhelming		Circle "na" if row not applicable	
1. Pain	During dressing changes 0 - 10	Between dressing changes 0 - 10	Burning 0 - 10	Sensitive to light touch 0 - 10	Itching 0 - 10
2. Patient describes	Smell 0 - 10	Drainage 0 - 10	Bleeding 0 - 10	Swelling 0 - 10	
3. Social issues	Family support 0 - 10	Friends support 0 - 10	Health care support 0 - 10	Social isolation 0 - 10	
4. Emotional concerns Does the patient feel:	Anxious 0 - 10	Depressed 0 - 10	Embarrassed 0 - 10	Fear 0 - 10	Frustration 0 - 10
5. What bothers the patient most?					
6. Wound classification	Fungating	Ulcerating	Subcutaneous a. Dry / b. Raised	Multiple nodules	
7. Wound bed	% Pink / red wound	% necrotic tissue covering	Describe		
8. Wound edges	Flat	Elevated wound	Elevated edge	Tunneling	
9. Odor - describe	na	Under dressing	Near patient	Moderate odor	Strong odor
10. Odor - cause	na	Necrotic tissue	Infection	Exudate	
11. Exudate amount	na	Dry	Moist	Wet	Copious
12. Exudate describe	na	Serous	Purulent	Fistula exudate	Brown
13. Bleeding amount	na	Minimal	Moderate	Severe	Intermittent
14. Bleeding cause	na	Dressing	Coagulation	Friable tumour	Blood vessels
15. Describe wound (include location)					
16. Measurement	Tracing	Photograph	Measurements (cms)		
17. Peri-wound skin	na	Treatment effects	Dry	Moist	Discoloured
18. Function altered R = right L=left	na	Circle all that apply: Shoulder – R / L Arm, hand – R / L	Eye – R / L Ear – R / L Leg, foot – R / L	Breathing Bowel	Mouth Opening Chewing Swallowing Bladder
19. Edema in or distal to wound	na	Circle edema location(s) : (a) arm R / L leg R / L	in wound Head	around wound Neck	distal to wound

fied. A tracing of the wound or a photograph supports the physical examination.

MANAGEMENT OF PATIENTS WITH MALIGNANT WOUNDS

A fundamental principle in managing patients with malignant wounds is to consciously focus on the entire individual (19,21,23) in keeping with a standard palliative care approach to patients. Management goals are based directly on the results of the patient assessment. Since these patients are so unique and standard treatments have not been identified, each patient must be considered individually. Providing treatment for the daily patient challenges is difficult with the paucity of evidence-based medicine (21). Case-based reports comprise most of the published information on patients with malignant wounds (24).

The malignant wound treatment goals of tumor reduction or cure requires radiation, systemic medical, and/or surgical oncology. Wound biopsy should be conducted only when necessary for diagnostic purposes until its benefit is studied. Promotion of tumor growth with open biopsies has been reported in the head and neck literature (25) and has been noted by this author after punch biopsy of malignant wounds. If a diagnostic test is necessary, perhaps fine-needle biopsy may be safer if it yields the required information.

Oncology treatment can provide palliative benefit for relief of symptoms with or without tumor reduction. Aggressive radiotherapy has been shown to provide locoregional control particularly in patients without prior treatment and with small, isolated chest wall recurrences (26). A note of caution: Anecdotal experience suggests that dressing and drug products with moisture, or heavy metals (zinc, iodine, charcoal, silver, etc.) may intensify radiation skin reaction. Always discuss the use of any products with the radiation oncologist if products are felt to be necessary during a course of radiation therapy, or remove the dressings during radiation treatment until their safety is established by clinical experience or trial data.

The option of surgical chest wall resection for 38 patients with locally recurrent breast cancer has recently been reviewed (27). Size of the largest tumor nodule (more than 4 cm, $p = 0.04$) and regional nodal disease ($p < 0.01$) were significant predictors of local postoperative recurrence. Lymph node metastasis was the only predictor of long-term survival ($p < 0.01$). Authors believed complete resection of all locally recurrent disease was unlikely to improve survival and the quality of palliation should be considered (27). Warzelhan et al. (28), however, also published results in 2000 and concluded that chest wall resection offered immediate relief of severe sequelae and contributed to long-term survival, especially in local recurrence after breast cancer. The fact that two recent papers offer apparently opposing advice may lie in patient selection defining patients suitable for resection. This underlies the difficulty of evaluating current malignant wound literature, as there is no widely accepted staging or descriptive terminology.

Photodynamic therapy appears to be a useful supplement to palliative oncology modalities in recurrent carcinoma of the breast, especially with skin metastases. It has a low side-effect profile (29). Photodynamic therapy may be used, where available, after failure of salvage surgery, radiation, and systemic therapy (30).

The use of intraarterial infusion chemotherapy into arteries supplying the fungating breast has been described. A case report (31) and a literature review (32) report some encouragement as a potential tumor reduction technique. As for photodynamic therapy, the use of intraarterial therapy is limited by its availability and the level of supporting evidence.

If cure, or control, of this metastatic manifestation of an underlying malignancy is not possible, the primary goal becomes optimizing quality of life (19,33). Impeccable symptom management with reduction in physical, functional, social, and emotional concerns is the central focus. Management is based on the assessment and the patient's primary concerns provide a starting point for treatment.

Judicious use of the general principles of benign wound care has been adapted to the malignant wound patients (19,21). Patients are des-

TABLE 35.3. *Concerns common to patients with malignant wounds and potential symptom management to complement appropriate oncology care (9)*

1. Pain
   - Pain *during* dressing—non-adherent dressings, barrier, cancer pain management, relief of incident pain
   - Pain *between* dressing changes—cancer pain management
   - Protect peri-wound skin
2. Odor from the wound—always treat odor if it concerns the patient
   - Necrotic tissue from tumor necrosis—clean wound regularly and change dressings more frequently, add charcoal dressings
   - Treat infections
3. Exudate from the wound
   - Quantify the amount of exudate—use effective dressings
   - Qualify the appearance of the exudate—rule out—infection and fistula
4. Bleeding in the wound
   - Identify the cause of the bleeding and treat the cause
     - Patient characteristics—abnormal tumor vasculature, congenital coagulation abnormality
     - Iatrogenic causes—infection, adherent dressings, anticoagulant therapy
5. Edema associated with the wound
   - Location of the edema is often distal to the wound. Elevation and gentle compression with massage therapy may be helpful, very limited evidence to support this treatment is available.
6. Functional compromise due to the location of the wound
   - Identify the patient's functional compromise, i.e., limited use of upper extremities with lymphedema. Design patient specific management based on the patient's concerns.
7. Emotional Issues
   - Identify the patient's emotional concerns from living with the wound. Fear, anxiety, frustration, embarrassment, and depression are common patient concerns.
8. Social concerns
   - Altered relationships with family, friends, and health care providers; social isolation, and time-consuming factors affect social integration.
   - Emotional and social issues can be decreased if recognized and addressed
     - Use cosmetically acceptable, effective dressings—an important link to society
     - Obtain oncology care
     - May require social work, psychology or psychiatry assistance

Note: The patient concerns listed in Table 35.3 are included in the S-MWAT.

perate regarding all aspects of immediate care for daily living. Future research is essential to advance wound care specific to individuals with malignant wounds and is more likely to occur with a consistent outcome measure such as the S-MWAT (7,22).

MANAGEMENT OF CLINICAL PROBLEMS

Pain

The management of pain is determined by identifying the cause of the pain. Caregivers and patients need to identify the timing of the pain, between or during dressing changes (Table 35.3). Pain between dressing changes is likely related to the wound itself, as a result of direct cancer pain or wound infection. Surprisingly, patients with large malignant wounds seldom have severe pain. The most painful wounds are typically shallow ulcers or those invading underlying structures (9).

Pain that occurs during dressing changes should be assessed for dressing adherence. The painful area may be in the wound or peri-wound skin. The use of premedication is appropriate where necessary. Adherent dressings may be soaked loose with sterile water, saline, a shower, or wound cleansing products. It is prudent that the dressings are not quickly, or forcibly, removed as it increases pain and the risk of damaging the wound causing bleeding from friable tumor tissue. Dry gauze should be avoided as a dressing in the wound bed. It embeds itself within the wound, has a minimum ability for absorption, and may promote infection. Change to a more suitable, non-adherent contact dressing can enable easier dressing changes (19–21). Non-adherent dressings include: skin protectants (spray, spread), gels (in dry wounds), foams, calcium alginates (may need to be soaked off), silicone-based dressings, and hydrofibers (in moist wounds). If pain occurs with exposure to air, have cleaning solutions at the temperature the patient prefers ready to cover the exposed wound as soon as the dressing is removed.

Pain may be located in the wound or in the peri-wound skin. If the pain is located in the peri-wound skin, the wound management changes. Peri-wound skin can be compromised by subcutaneous infiltration of tumor, cellulitis, maceration from wound exudate, repeated dressing applications, previous surgery, and radiation. Therefore, the peri-wound skin can be fragile and easily damaged. It is easier to avoid peri-wound skin problems than it is to treat them. Skin-barrier film spray and creams can be applied over the peri-wound skin for protection. Adhesives can be applied over the films once the film has dried. Barrier creams, some containing zinc, can be applied immediately around the wound to protect the peri-wound skin from maceration, but avoid this during a course of radiation therapy. Patients with dry, pruritic, peri-wound skin find moisturizers provide some symptomatic relief. Hydrocolloids have been used to protect the peri-wound skin by placing a thin strip of the hydrocolloid on the normal skin around the wound to secure the dressings. Elastic mesh is useful to hold dressings to avoid the use of adherent products. The elastic mesh can be held up with straps created from ribbon gauze or similar products.

Odor

The management of odor is based on its cause. The most common causes are necrotic tissue and infection. Cleaning is required on a regular basis, typically with each dressing change. Showering, normal saline, sterile water, and wound cleansing products are useful (8). Necrotic tissue can adhere to the wound. Gentle autolytic debridement with gels or chemical debridement that does not damage normal tissue may decrease excessive amounts of necrotic tissue. Some authors have recommended gentle surgical debridement of necrotic tissue (21). However, avoid aggressive debridement as abnormal blood vessels in malignant tissue may bleed significantly. There is concern that damaging the wound bed may enhance tumor growth. Future research will be necessary to determine the safety of debridement.

General measures to control odor, such as charcoal (19,21) within absorbent dressings or on top of the dressings, frequent dressing changes, bedding changes, and adequate ventilation, help reduce odor. Infection should be suspected with any malodorous wound and it is discussed below as a wound complication.

Exudate

Health care providers should view the undressed wound and report the quality and the quantity of the exudate in the wound. The quality can be described as: dry, moist, moderate, large, or copious amounts of exudate. The quality of the exudate can be described as: serous (clear or golden), serosanguinous (thin blood tinged), sanguinous (bloody), purulent (thick yellow or tan), or brown exudates (9). It is important to evaluate how well the dressings are controlling the exudates (34). The patients' evaluation of their exudate will reflect the ability of their dressings to control the exudate. Wounds with moderate amounts of exudate may be reported as 2/10 if the dressings control the exudates, or 8/10 if the dressings are inadequate. Infection may increase exudates and should be considered and treated if present. The absorbency of the dressing should match the quantity of exudate in the wound. Absorbent dressings include foams, composite dressings, alginates and hydrofibers, and so on. Dressings with salt have been shown to help dry a wound, however, must be evaluated for adherence to the wound (35).

Bleeding

Management of bleeding in a malignant wound is directed at resolving the cause of bleeding

(9,19,21). Patient-related and iatrogenic factors are the most important causes of bleeding. Patient-related factors include friable tumor with abnormal vasculature or coagulopathy. Friable tumor may be reduced with radiotherapy, surgery, or chemotherapy. Iatrogenic factors include adherent dressings and anticoagulants. Adherent dressings, in particular dry gauze, should be abandoned and non-adherent dressings should be substituted in its place. There are many non-adherent products available and the one chosen should correspond with the amount of exudate in the wound. Some calcium alginates have coagulant properties. Systemic anticoagulation therapy may cause exorbate or cause bleeding in a malignant wound. Arterial catherisation and embolisation to control severe, recurrent bleeding has been reported (36), but research is limited and it is only available in specific centers with expertise in this procedure.

Edema

Anecdotal observations reveal that edema associated with malignant wounds is nearly always located distal to the wound (9). This may be related to alterations in lymphatic drainage through the wound site. The management of edema is dependent on the extent and location of the edema. The edema may be lymphedema of the arm, legs or head and neck region. It can be a very complex clinical problem to manage. Compression may not be successful as it may shift the edema from the extremity into the wound. Elevation may be useful, particularly for head and neck edema. There is a paucity of information on the successful management of lymphedema in cancer patients, and even less in patients with a malignant wound and lymphedema.

Complications and Functional Compromise

Infection may occur with or without odor, although it should be suspected when the wound is malodorous. Antibiotics have been demonstrated to be useful. Topical antibiotics often complement oral or intravenous medications. A proper wound swab should be taken prior to instituting the antibiotic and if the patient is sufficiently unwell, antibiotic treatment may need to begin prior to the results in order to prevent sepsis from occurring. Antibiotics recommended for infections in ulcers, drainage, and fistulas should follow the benign wound infection literature (37).

Patients with open malignant wounds receiving chemotherapy have been noted to have an increased risk of infection (9). Consider a wound culture at the time of administration of chemotherapy in all malignant wound patients so that the potential pathogens have been identified prior to the development of infection. The wound culture should be repeated prior to the institution of antibiotics, along with all other required cultures such blood, urine, sputum, and so on, to be more certain of the actual infecting pathogen and its antibiotic sensitivities.

Fistula formation is caused by tumor spreading through the skin allowing an open communication of an internal organ. It occurs most commonly in relation to malignant wounds in the head and neck region or on the abdominal wall. An external fistula may cause incontinence of urine or stool when associated with internal fistulas. The fistulas tend to have an irregular shape that changes as the cancer grows and may have copious exudate. Fistulas alter normal function. Management is frequently very challenging. Treatment is aimed at restoring function and controlling the related symptoms. As an example, fistulas in the head and neck region might prohibit eating and drinking. Alternate approaches to feeding, such as a gastro-jejunostomy feeding tube may be appropriate. Occlusion of the fistula with dressings, or rarely with surgery, may restore function.

Functional compromise from the location of the wound has been reported to cause restriction of movement and compromised daily activities. Immobility or decreased mobility of the arms and legs may occur as a result of the tumor. This can be associated with limb weakness, lymphedema, and physical restrictions from the wound dressings. Management of these symptoms needs to be tailored to the individual patient. Improvement of mobility can significantly improve the patient's quality of life.

Emotional Stress

Emotional stress, the personal reaction to watching the tumor grow across their bodies, is a classic feature in this patient population. Emotional stress includes depression, discouragement, embarrassment, fear of "being replaced by cancer," fear of looking at the tumor, anxiety, frustration, altered self-image and body image, and managing the wound. It is important to acknowledge this stress (18,19,21). Referral for oncology treatment and dressings that are functional and cosmetically acceptable play a fundamental role in improving emotional well-being. It may be appropriate to involve other disciplines such as social work, psychology, or psychiatry.

Social Concerns

Social concerns result from changes in interaction with family, friends, colleagues, health care providers, and so on. It is important to recognise this potential problem and discuss it openly. Often, the situation improves once it has been acknowledged. This may occur more frequently when the signs of the wound are not controlled or concealed with effective, cosmetically acceptable dressings. Socially acceptable and functional dressings enhance the patient's degree of social interaction.

In one patient looked after by the author, a theatre make-up artist created a thin sheet of imitation skin to match a patient's skin colouring and it was applied to cover a large buccal mucosal fistula as a cosmetically acceptable covering for special occasions to enhance social interactions. Such innovative approaches are clearly related to the ingenuity, generosity, distinct abilities, and resources of a team approach to patients with malignant wounds.

Health care providers themselves often have some degree of difficulty dealing with patients with malignant wounds. This reaction to a wound can strain the interaction between the provider and patient. Simply regarding the wound as a symptom requiring management and reducing the number of effective dressing changes whenever possible may reduce this problem.

Effective, socially acceptable dressings may have a higher unit cost, while reducing the frequency of dressing changes, the labor costs, and stress associated with the dressing changes. Patients are often well enough to socialize and socialization if enhanced when the clinical concerns are controlled.

Malignant wound patients require complex care and assistance from a variety of providers may be of value. Oncology, palliative care, dermatology, community nursing, and enterostomal therapy nursing can all offer elements to assist in their care.

CONCLUSION

Patients with malignant wounds are a unique population as these wounds behave significantly different from benign wounds. It cannot be overemphasized the reason malignant wounds differ from benign wounds is because the wound bed is "cancer." The wound can result from primary skin tumors, the direct extension of an internal malignancy, and lymphatic spread of cancer. It may be shallow wound or be the surface of a large tumor mass.

Oncologists, surgeons, and researchers have attempted to prevent the development of locoregional recurrence with surgery, intraoperative irrigation agents, and postoperative systemic and radiation therapy. Physicians have strived for control of the recurrence of cancer with multimodal therapy including radiation and systemic therapy and, in addition, frequently unavailable treatments such as photodynamic therapy and intraarterial chemotherapy have been tried.

Oncology attempts for cure or control of tumor burden is complimented with excellence in symptom management as the cornerstone to patient care for patients with malignant wounds. Pain, odor, exudate, bleeding, edema, complications related to the location of the tumor, emotional distress, and social concerns are the most common clinical problems these patients develop. At the present time, there is a paucity of evidence-based information to support the management these patients require. A concerted effort to develop appropriate management must be conducted in order to avoid treatment related harm. The S-MWAT (7,22) is a specific assessment tool for patients with malignant wounds developed with construct and content validity. It is a potentially valuable outcome measure for clinical practice and research on this patient population.

It is essential that patients with malignant wounds have an opportunity for the highest quality of life as the average life expectancy is close to two years after developing cutaneous metastasis. As with any pioneering area of medicine, change is expected over time. While treatments are being developed, patients require the best available malignant wound assessment and management.

REFERENCES

1. Reingold IM. Cutaneous metastases from internal carcinoma. *Cancer* 1966;19:162–168.
2. Lookingbill D, Spangler N, Helm K. Cutaneous metastases in patients with metastatic carcinoma: A retrospective study of 4020 patients. *J Am Acad Dermatol* 1993;29:2, 228–236.
3. Haisfield-Wolfe ME, Rund C. Malignant cutaneous wounds: A management protocol. *Ostomy/Wound Management* 1997;43(1):56–66.
4. Haisfield-Wolfe ME, Baxendale-Cox L. Staging of malignant cutaneous wounds. A pilot study. *Oncology Nursing Forum* 1999;26(6):1055–1064.
5. Lookingbill D, Spangler N, Sexton FM. Skin involvement as the presenting sign of internal carcinoma. *J Am Acad Dermatol* 1990;22:19–26.
6. Hallett N. Fungating wounds. *Nursing Times* 1995; 91(39):81–83.
7. Schulz VN. The development of a malignant wound assessment tool. Unpublished thesis. University of Alberta, Edmonton, Alberta, Canada, 2001.
8. Holland J, Bast JR, Morton D, et al. *Cancer Medicine*, 4th ed. 1997:2459–2464.
9. Schulz VN. [Clinical experience and retrospective review of patients referred to a malignant wound clinic.] London Regional Cancer Centre, London, Canada, 2002. (unpublished raw data)
10. Abeloff M, Armitage J, Lichter A, Niederhuber J. In: *Clinical oncology.* New York: Churchill Livingstone, 1995: Management of Specific Malignancies/III p. 1026.
11. Ragaz J, Jackson SM, Le N, et al. Adjuvant radiotherapy and chemotherapy in node-positive premenopausal women with breast cancer. *N Engl J Med* 1997;337(14):956–962.
12. Overgaard M, Jensen M, Overgaard J, et al. Postoperative radiotherapy in high-risk postmenopausal breast-cancer patients given adjuvant tamoxifen: Danish Breast Cancer Cooperative Group DBCG 82c randomized trial. *Lancet* 1999;353:1641–1648.
13. Whelan TJ, Julian J, Wright J, et al. Does locoregional radiation therapy improve survival in breast cancer? A meta-analysis. *J Clin Oncol* 2000;18(6): 1220–1229.
14. Allegretto M, Selkaly M, Mackey JR. Intraoperative saline and gemcitabine irrigation improves tumour control in human squamous cell carcinoma-contaminated surgical wounds. *J Otolaryngol* 2001;30(2):121–125.
15. Lewis JS, Connett JM, Garbow JR, et al. Copper-64-pyruvaldehyde-bis(N(4)-methylthiosemicarbazone) for the prevention of tumor growth at wound sites following laparoscopic surgery: monitoring therapy response with micro PET and magnetic resonance imaging. *Cancer Res* 2002;15:62(2):445–449.
16. Mortimer PS. Management of skin problems: medical aspects. In: Doyle D, Hanks G, MacDonald N, eds. *Oxford testbook of palliative medicine,* 2nd ed. Oxford: Oxford University Press, Ch. 9.6:618–620.
17. Thiers B. Dermatologic manifestations of internal cancer. *CA Cancer J Clin* 1986;36(3):130–148.
18. Schulz VN, Triska O. Malignant wounds: caregiver determined clinical problems. *J Pain Symptom Manage* 2002; in press.
19. Haisfield-Wolfe ME. Malignant cutaneous wounds: A management protocol. *Ostomy/Wound Management* 1997;43(1):56–66.
20. Miller C. Management of skin problems: nursing aspects. In: Doyle D, Hanks G, MacDonald N, eds. *Oxford testbook of palliative medicine,* 2nd ed. Oxford: Oxford University Press, Ch. 9.6.3:642–657.
21. Fairbairn K. A challenge that requires further research: management of fungating breast lesions. *Professional Nurse* 1994;9:4;272–277.
22. Schulz VN, Triska OH, Tonkin K. The development of a malignant wound assessment tool. 2002; in press.
23. Grocott P. The palliative management of fungating malignant wounds. *Wound Care* 1995;4(6): 240–242.
24. Hastings D. Basing care on research. *Nursing Times* 1993;89(13):70–76.
25. Gleeson M, Herbert A, Richards A. Management of lateral neck masses in adults. *BMJ* 2000;320:1521–1524.
26. Halverson KJ, Perez CA, Kuske RR, et al. Isolated local-regional recurrence of breast cancer following mastectomy: radiotherapeutic management. *Int J Radiation Oncology Biol Phys* 1990;19:851–858.
27. Downe RJ, Rusch V, Hsu FI, et al. Chest wall resection for locally recurrent breast cancer: is it worthwhile? *J Thorac Cardiovasc Surg* 2000;119(3):420–428.
28. Warzelhan J, Stoelben E, Imdahl A, et al. Results in surgery for primary and metastatic chest wall tumors. *Eur J Cardiothorac Surg* 2000;19(5):584–588.
29. Koren H, Gerhart A, Gerlinde MS, Jindra RH. Photodynamic therapy—an alternative pathway in the treatment of recurrent breast cancer. *Int J Radiation Oncology Biol Physics* 1994;28(2):463–466.
30. Allison R, Mang T, Hewson G, et al. Photodynamic therapy for chest wall progression from breast carcinoma is an underutlilized treatment modality. *American Cancer Society* 2001;91(1):1–8.
31. Murakami M, Kuroda Y, Sano A, et al. Validity of local treatment including intraarterial infusion chemotherapy and radiotherapy for fungating adenocarcinoma of the

breast: case report of more than 8-year survival. *Am J Clin Oncol* 2001;24(4):388–391.
32. Bufill JA, Grace WR, Neff R. Intra-arterial chemotherapy for palliation of fungating breast cancer. A cast report and review of the literature. *Am J Clin Oncol* 1994;17(2):118–124.
33. van Leeuween BL, Houwerzijl M, Hoekstra HJ. Educational tips in the treatment of malignant ulcerating tumors of the skin. *Eur J Surg Oncol* 2000;26(5):506–508.
34. Grocott P. Exudate management in fungating wounds. *J Wound Care* 1998;7:9;445–448.
35. Upright C, Salton C, Roberts F, Murphey J. Evaluation of Mesalt dressings and continuous wet saline dressings in ulcerating metastatic skin lesions. *Cancer Nurs* 1994;17(2):149–155.
36. Rankin EM, Rubens RD, Reidy JF. Transcather embolization to control severe bleeding in fungating breast cancer. *Eur J Surg Oncol* 1998;15(2):199–200.
37. Finlay IG, Bowszyc J, Ramlou C, Gwiezdzinski Z. The effect of topical 0.75% metronidazole gel on malodorous cutaneous ulcers. *J Pain Symptom Management* 1996;11(3):158–162.

36
Chemotherapy-induced Nausea and Vomiting

Sheryl Koski and Peter Venner

The most common side effect from the cytotoxic chemotherapy used for the treatment of malignancy is nausea and vomiting. Approximately 70% to 80% of untreated patients will experience nausea and vomiting. Even in treated patients, it is estimated that 40% to 50% of patients will experience some degree of nausea or vomiting, which can have a significant impact on a patient's quality of life and compliance with treatment (1). Several factors, including the emetogenicity of the chemotherapeutic agent and patient risk factors, impact upon the incidence and severity of chemotherapy-induced emesis. Fortunately, the introduction of new antiemetic agents, in recent years, has resulted in significant improvements in the prevention and treatment of this almost universally feared side effect.

EMETOGENICITY OF CYTOTOXIC CHEMOTHERAPY

The definition of highly emetogenic chemotherapeutic agents are those that cause severe emesis in more than 90% of patients. Although cisplatin is considered the most highly emetogenic agent, there are other drugs in this category, including dacarbazine and high doses of cyclophosphamide (more than 1,500 mg/m^2). Moderately emetogenic agents are defined as those that lead to emesis in 30% to 90% of patients. Examples of frequently prescribed agents in this category are doxorubicin and cyclophosphamide at doses less than 1,500 mg/m^2. Mildly emetogenic agents induce emesis only in a minority of patients (10% to 30%) but may still warrant antiemetic prophylaxis. Examples include mitoxantrone and etoposide. Minimally emetogenic agents seldom require the use of prophylactic antiemetic therapy (e.g., the vinca alkaloids) (1,2). There is some controversy regarding the classification of combination chemotherapy regimens, with respect to emesis. The general consensus is that the emetogenicity of a combination should be the same as that of the most highly emetogenic drug within the regimen (3). Table 36.1 lists the emetogenic classification of some common chemotherapy regimens.

RISK FACTORS AND PATHOPHYSIOLOGY

Acute Emesis

Definition

Acute emesis is defined as nausea and vomiting occurring during the first 24 hours after chemotherapy. With most agents, it starts within 1 to 2 hours of receiving chemotherapy; however, with some agents there can be a late onset of acute emesis starting 9 to 18 hours after receiving chemotherapy (e.g., carboplatin, high-dose cyclophosphamide) (1).

Risk Factors

Risk factors for the development of acute emesis include: (a) the chemotherapeutic agent; (b) emesis experienced with prior chemotherapy cycles; (c) younger age; (d) female gender; and (e) low chronic ethanol intake (2,3).

Pathophysiology

The precise pathophysiology of chemotherapy-induced nausea and vomiting is not completely understood. The mechanisms for acute emesis have been studied more than those of delayed emesis. There are three pathways involved in the emetic response: the central nervous system (CNS), gastrointestinal tract and vestibular system. Traditionally it has been believed that there are two key areas within the CNS that are

TABLE 36.1. *Classification of emetogenicity* (1,3)

Highly emetogenic	Moderately emetogenic	Mildly emetogenic	Minimally emetogenic
Cisplatin > 50 mg/m^2	Cisplatin 20–50 mg/m^2	Mitoxantrone	5-fluorouracil
Cyclophosphamide > 1500 mg/m^2	Carboplatin	Etoposide	Bleomycin
Dacarbazine	Doxorubicin	Irinotecan	Vinca alkaloids
	Epirubicin	Docetaxel	Methotrexate
	Idarubicin	Paclitaxel	Hydroxyurea
	Cyclophosphamide	Gemcitabine	Chlorambucil
	Ifosfamide		Fludarabine
	Cytarabine		Cladribine
	CMF (IV or po)		
	FEC/FAC		

involved in the emetic response. The first area is the vomiting center, located in the lateral reticular formation of the medulla. The second, the chemoreceptor trigger zone (CTZ), is located in the area postrema (AP). The CTZ is outside the blood-brain barrier and senses humoral stimuli within the blood and cerebrospinal fluid. Signals are then transmitted to the vomiting center which coordinates the motor mechanisms of emesis. Other sources of stimulation to the vomiting center include the vestibular system, the pharynx, the GI tract, and higher cortical centers. However, while the vestibular system has a primary role in motion sickness, the higher cortical centers may play a role in anticipatory emesis (4). The CTZ, the GI tract, and higher cortical centers are known to be involved in the emetic response following cytotoxic chemotherapy (2). Recently, studies have suggested that the nucleus tractus solitarius (NTS) is also important in the emetic response. The NTS is located below the area postrema (AP) and coordinates the function of visceral and somatic afferents within the brainstem. The neurons of the NTS have been shown to terminate within the AP and it is possible that it may, in fact, be the NTS not the CTZ, which is important in the chemotherapy-induced emetic pathway (5).

A variety of neurotransmitters are involved in the emetic response. Those that are known to play a role in the pathophysiology of chemotherapy-induced emesis include dopamine, serotonin, and substance P. Receptors for these neurotransmitters are found in the CTZ, the vomiting center, and the GI tract. As early studies focused on the role of the dopamine receptor in chemotherapy-induced emesis, this resulted in the development of the dopamine receptor antagonists (e.g., metoclopramide, domperidone). The use of high-dose metoclopramide was the standard therapy for patients receiving cisplatin-based chemotherapy. However, in the 1970s it was discovered that the use of metoclopramide at high doses resulted in the inhibition of serotonin receptors, not dopamine receptors. This discovery led to the development of the serotonin receptor antagonists, which selectively inhibit the serotonin receptor (4,6).

Cytotoxic chemotherapy causes release of serotonin from the enterochromaffin cells of the GI tract which, in turn, stimulates serotonin receptors. The exact mechanism by which cytotoxic chemotherapy results in the release of serotonin from the enterochromaffin cells is not known, but it may occur via free radical generation (5). This stimulus is relayed up to the vomiting center in the CNS via abdominal vagal afferents. As serotonin receptors have also been identified within the AP, antagonists of the receptor may also act through these central receptors to mediate the development of chemotherapy-induced nausea and vomiting (2,6).

Research into emesis pathways in cancer patients receiving high-dose cisplatin has shown that there is an increase in the plasma level and urinary excretion of 5-hydroxyindolacetic acid (5-HIAA), a metabolite of serotonin, which parallels the onset of emesis. 5-HIAA levels return to baseline approximately 9 to 16 hours after the infusion of cisplatin. The increase in 5-HIAA is not affected by the use of serotonin receptor antagonists. Antiemetics acting on the serotonin pathway would seem not to prevent the release of serotonin but instead inhibit its action at the level of the serotonin receptor (2,7,8). Similar increases in plasma and urinary 5-HIAA are also seen following the administration of dacarbazine, cyclophosphamide, and low-dose cisplatin. The magnitude of the rise in 5-HIAA is similar for high-dose cisplatin and dacarbazine. In the cyclophosphamide and low dose cisplatin patients, the increase in 5-HIAA is smaller and more delayed in onset. Therefore, the emetogenicity of a chemotherapy regimen may be related to its ability to release serotonin (7).

Substance P (SP) is a neurokinin with widespread distribution both in the central and peripheral nervous systems and which selectively binds to the neurokinin-1 (NK-1) receptor. It was discovered that, when injected into ferrets, SP produced emesis. There have been a number of animal studies investigating the potential site of emetic activity for SP. In these various models, SP binding sites have been identified in the neurons of the solitary nucleus, vagal C-afferents, and medulla. The discovery of the role of SP in emesis led to the development of a series of selective NK-1 receptor antagonists as potential antiemetic agents. NK-1 receptor antagonists have been shown to prevent emesis caused by a wide variety of stimuli (copper sulfate, nicotine, cytotoxic chemotherapy, opioids, radiation, motion), suggesting a role for SP in the final common pathway of the emetic reflex (9,10).

Delayed Emesis

Definition

Delayed emesis is defined as nausea and vomiting occurring more than 24 hours after chemotherapy. This is most commonly seen in patients receiving cisplatin-based chemotherapy regimens.

Risk Factors

The single most important risk factor for the development of delayed emesis is poor control of acute emesis (3).

Pathophysiology

The pathophysiology of delayed emesis is not at all well understood. Studies, which followed the plasma and urinary levels of 5-HIAA following the infusion of cisplatin, found that the levels of 5-HIAA returned to baseline between 9 and 16 hours after cisplatin administration. Therefore, it is unlikely that serotonin plays a significant role in the etiology of delayed nausea and vomiting (8). This is supported by the finding that the serotonin receptor antagonists are less effective for the treatment of delayed emesis. One possibility is that alterations in gut motility may contribute to the development of delayed emesis (5). Recent studies have shown that the use of an NK-1 receptor antagonist can decrease the incidence of delayed emesis. Therefore, substance P, the ligand for the NK-1 receptor, may play a role in the pathophysiology of both delayed and acute emesis (11,12).

Anticipatory Emesis

Definition

Anticipatory nausea and vomiting (ANV) generally begins 24 hours prior to the onset of chemotherapy. Approximately 30% of patients report this phenomenon by the fourth cycle of chemotherapy (13). Two types of ANV have been described. The first is "clinic specific" which occurs only in response to sights or smells associated with drug injections. The second is "pervasive" and occurs during a specific time period prior to clinic visits and is not necessarily precipitated by specific sights or smells (14).

Risk Factors

Individuals experiencing ANV tend to be more psychologically distressed by chemotherapy than those who do not develop ANV. The occurrence of post-treatment nausea and vomiting is also a risk factor, since ANV is seldom seen in those who have not experienced post-treatment nausea and vomiting (1,13,14). Other characteristics of patients who tend to develop ANV is that they are younger and receive a greater number of chemotherapy drugs; in particular, agents with greater emetic potential (14).

Pathophysiology

ANV is believed to be a conditioned response, although its pathophysiology has not as yet been evaluated in detail. It is known only that its frequency increases with the number of chemotherapy cycles received and that ANV is related both to the frequency and severity of post-treatment nausea and vomiting.

CLASSES OF ANTIEMETIC AGENTS

Dopamine Receptor Antagonists

Prior to the development of the serotonin receptor antagonists in the 1980s, the dopamine receptor antagonists were the predominant class of agents used for the treatment of chemotherapy-induced emesis. This group of drugs can be classified into the substituted benzamides, phenothiazines, and butyrophenones.

1. *Substituted Benzamides.* Metoclopramide is the most well-known and thoroughly studied agent in this group of drugs. Early studies showed that high-dose metoclopramide was effective in the treatment of cisplatin-induced emesis, achieving complete control in 30% to 40% of patients where conventional doses are ineffective. For moderately emetogenic chemotherapy, high-dose metoclopramide is no more effective than use of conventional dosing schedules. Oral dosing of metoclopramide does not possess significant activity for acute chemotherapy-induced emesis (15).
2. *Phenothiazines.* This class of dopamine receptor antagonist includes chlorpromazine and prochlorperazine. This group of agents has a high affinity for the dopamine receptor, and antiemetic activity is mediated through this receptor, not the serotonin receptor. These agents are ineffective in the treatment of highly emetogenic chemotherapy. For moderately emetogenic chemotherapy, studies have demonstrated either equivalence or inferiority to a number of other of antiemetic agents including metoclopramide, cannabinoids, and corticosteroids. As single agents, phenothiazines are only effective for the treatment of emesis related to mildly emetogenic chemotherapy. Increasing doses can result in superior antiemetic efficacy, but at the cost of more frequent side effects (15).
3. *Butyrophenones.* This class of agents, including haloperidol, droperidol, and domperidone, possess antiemetic activity, but these drugs have been less well studied for the treatment of chemotherapy-induced emesis (15).

Serotonin Receptor Antagonists

As discussed previously, the discovery that high-dose metoclopramide achieved its antiemetic activity through the inhibition of the serotonin receptor led to the development of selective serotonin receptor antagonists. There are three commonly available agents in this class: ondansetron, granisetron, and dolasetron. The introduction of these agents in the 1980s revolutionized the treatment of acute emesis occurring as a result of either highly or moderately emetogenic chemotherapy regimens. Multiple studies and overviews have confirmed the superiority of the serotonin receptor antagonists for emetic control following highly and moderately emetogenic chemotherapy regimens (16,17). However, the lack of activity of the serotonin receptor antagonists for the prevention and treatment of delayed emesis has proven disappointing.

Neurokinin-1 (NK-1) Receptor Antagonists

The NK-1 receptor antagonists are the newest class of antiemetic agents. They are still under study, and their role in the treatment of chemotherapy-induced emesis is not yet clearly defined. These agents work by selectively binding to the NK-1 receptor, the receptor for the neurokinin transmitter, substance P. There have been two randomized phase 3 trials and one randomized phase 2 trial examining the efficacy of three different NK-1 receptor antagonists in the treatment of cisplatin-induced emesis (12,18, 19). In all three trials, the addition of the NK-1 receptor antagonists given prior to cisplatin and in combination with the standard therapy of a serotonin receptor antagonist and dexamethasone resulted in superior control of acute emesis over standard therapy alone. Only one study examined the role of the NK-1 receptor antagonist alone and found it to be inferior to standard therapy (18). All three studies also showed improved control of delayed emesis with the use of the NK-1 receptor antagonists in comparison to placebo. It is not clear whether a single dose of the NK-1 receptor inhibitor prior to chemotherapy is sufficient or whether continued dosing through the delayed phase (days 2 to 5) is necessary. Further study on the appropriate scheduling of the NK-1 receptor inhibitors is necessary. There also needs to be a comparison to the current accepted standard therapy for delayed emesis, a corticosteroid with or without metoclopramide or prochlorperazine.

Corticosteroids

The mechanism of action of corticosteroids in the emetic pathway is unknown. Hypotheses include alteration in permeability of the CTZ, stabilization of membrane/intracellular components, or decreasing inflammatory changes in the gut following chemotherapy. Activity through the release of endorphins has also been hypothesized (15). The role of corticosteroids in antiemetic therapy evolved when it was noted that chemotherapy protocols containing corticosteroids [e.g., MOPP (mechlorethamine, vincristine, procarbazine, and prednisone)] were better tolerated than similar protocols which did not contain corticosteroids. Multiple studies have confirmed the equivalence or superiority of corticosteroids to other classes of antiemetics. Additionally, when used in combination for the treatment of acute emesis, corticosteroids have been found to improve the antiemetic activity of both dopamine receptor antagonists and serotonin receptor antagonists. To date, no other class of agents has proven superiority to corticosteroids, for the treatment of delayed emesis.

Cannabinoids

The mechanism of antiemetic activity of the synthetic cannabinoids is not known, although receptors for cannabinoids have been identified in several areas throughout the CNS (cortex, hippocampus, and hypothalamus) (20). There are currently three agents of this class which are in common use: nabilone, dronabinol, and levonantradol. Recently, a meta-analysis of all randomized trials has been performed, evaluating the role of cannabinoids in the treatment of chemotherapy-induced nausea and vomiting. As these were older trials, the comparators were either placebo or a dopamine receptor antagonist. There have been no randomized comparisons of cannabinoids to either corticosteroids or the serotonin receptor antagonists. The results of this meta-analysis suggest that the cannabinoids are superior to placebo for the treatment of chemotherapy-induced emesis. Following moderately emetogenic chemotherapy the cannabinoids have been shown to be somewhat superior to standard therapy using a dopamine receptor antagonist. However, this improved control was at the cost of more side effects, including dysphoria, paranoia, hallucinations, and depression. In contrast, in both mildly emetogenic and highly emetogenic chemotherapy, the cannabinoids were no more effective than standard therapy. As a result of toxicity, there is currently no accepted role for the cannabinoids in the routine prophylaxis and treatment of chemotherapy-induced emesis.

Benzodiazepines

Benzodiazepines act by facilitating the inhibitory neurotransmitter GABA (gamma-aminobutyric acid) (20). Their primary role has been as an adjunct to other antiemetic agents. The addition of a benzodiazepine to a dopamine receptor antagonist and/or a corticosteroid-containing regimen has been shown to improve antiemetic efficacy in most studies (21–29). There are few studies using the combination of a benzodiazepine with a serotonin receptor antagonist but as yet there appears to be no clear advantage of this combination in the treatment of acute or delayed emesis (30–33). However, in a few studies, the addition of a benzodiazepine has resulted in less anticipatory nausea and vomiting (29,34).

TREATMENT OF ACUTE EMESIS

The serotonin receptor antagonists are the most effective antiemetic agents for the treatment of acute emesis secondary to both highly and moderately emetogenic chemotherapy. There has been very little study of the appropriate treatment of emesis associated with less emetogenic regimens. This section discusses the dosing guidelines and relative efficacy of available agents in addition to the use of adjunctive agents.

Highly Emetogenic Chemotherapy

The lowest effective doses for the serotonin receptor antagonists in the prophylaxis of acute emesis following highly emetogenic chemotherapy that have been reported are: (a) ondansetron 8 mg i.v.; (b) granisetron 10 µg/kg i.v. (approximately 1 mg i.v.); (c) dolasetron 1.8 mg/kg i.v.; (d) ondansetron 24 mg orally; and (e) granisetron 2 mg orally (45–49). The use of multiple-dose schedules or continuous infusion does not appear to confer any additional benefit (35–37,42,50,51). The three serotonin receptor antagonists have been shown to have equivalent efficacy (38,41,44,45,52–55). However, oral dosing of any one of the serotonin receptor antagonists has not been well studied in highly emetogenic chemotherapy regimens. The above recommendations for oral dosing are based, therefore, on current best evidence, but further study is warranted.

There has also been extensive study of the role of adjunctive corticosteroids. Multiple studies have confirmed that the addition of a corticosteroid to a serotonin receptor antagonist results in superior control of acute emesis (30,56–63). There have been no comparative studies of the different corticosteroids; however, dexamethasone is the agent most commonly used. Only one study has assessed the dose response of dexamethasone and found that dexamethasone 12 mg i.v. was superior to lower doses (4 mg i.v. or 8 mg i.v.) and equivalent to higher doses (20 mg i.v.) (64).

Moderately Emetogenic Chemotherapy

The lowest effective doses studied for the three serotonin receptor antagonists in the prophylaxis of acute emesis following moderately emetogenic chemotherapy are: (a) ondansetron 8 mg i.v.; (b) granisetron 10 µg/kg i.v. (approximately 1 mg i.v.); (c) ondansetron 8 mg orally twice a day; (d) granisetron 2 mg orally daily; (e) granisetron 1 mg orally twice a day; and (f) dolasetron 100 mg orally twice a day (65–73). The three serotonin receptor antagonists, predictably, appear to have equivalent efficacy (67,69,74–77).

As with the highly emetogenic chemotherapy regimens, the addition of a corticosteroid to a serotonin receptor antagonist results in improved control of acute emesis following moderately emetogenic chemotherapy (75,78–80). Dexamethasone is generally prescribed in doses of 8 mg to 12 mg i.v. but there have been no studies comparing the appropriate dosing of corticosteroids in this setting.

Mild and Minimally Emetogenic Chemotherapy

There have been few comparative trials of antiemetic agents for chemotherapy agents in this class. An expert panel convened by the American Society of Clinical Oncology (ASCO) has recommended that patients receiving mildly emetogenic chemotherapy should receive a single dose of corticosteroid, such as dexamethasone 4 mg to 8 mg orally, prior to chemotherapy. This should result in the control of acute emesis in approximately 90% of patients. No routine antiemetic prophylaxis is recommended for patients receiving minimally emetogenic chemotherapy (3).

Treatment of Delayed Emesis

The control of delayed emesis has long been a difficult treatment dilemma. Part of this difficulty is that the pathophysiology of delayed emesis is poorly understood. The only significant risk factor for the development of delayed emesis appears to be the development of acute emesis. Therefore, the best method to treat or prevent delayed emesis would seem to be to provide adequate prophylaxis for acute emesis.

Relevant studies on the treatment of delayed emesis should control for the type of antiemetic regimens administered during the acute phase. Since there are only a few studies which meet this criteria, these studies have been strongly influential in directing recommendations for the treatment of delayed emesis.

Highly Emetogenic Chemotherapy

Studies have demonstrated the superiority of dexamethasone, dopamine receptor antagonists, and serotonin receptor antagonists, in addition to various combinations of these agents in the control of delayed emesis, when tested against placebo (81–86).

At present only three well-designed trials address the optimal regimen for the treatment of delayed emesis following cisplatin-based chemotherapy. In all three trials, patients received a serotonin receptor antagonist and dexamethasone for the prophylaxis of acute emesis, and individuals were then randomized to one of two different antiemetic regimens during the delayed phase. In two of these studies, dexamethasone alone was compared to a combination of a serotonin receptor antagonist and dexamethasone (87,88), whereas in the third study a combination of dexamethasone and metoclopramide was compared to a combination of dexamethasone and a serotonin antagonist (89). In all three studies, addition of a serotonin receptor antagonist did not improve control of delayed emesis. The possible exception was in those patients who had less than complete control of acute emesis. Subgroup analysis performed in two of the studies suggested that this group of patients might respond better to a serotonin receptor antagonist-containing regimen (88,89).

Only one study has compared the use of single-agent dexamethasone to a combination of dexamethasone and metoclopramide, in the delayed phase (90). In this study, the combination of metoclopramide and dexamethasone resulted in better control of delayed symptoms. However, this was prior to the routine use of serotonin receptor antagonists for the prophylaxis of acute emesis, so patients in this study were treated with high-dose metoclopramide prophylaxis prior to chemotherapy administration. Whether the expectation of improved control of acute emesis with serotonin receptor antagonists would affect this result is unknown. There have not been any studies examining the dose or scheduling of corticosteroids or metoclopramide in the treatment of delayed emesis.

Moderately Emetogenic Chemotherapy

Dexamethasone, given singly or in combination with serotonin receptor antagonists, has been shown to be superior to placebo for the control of delayed emesis following moderately emetogenic chemotherapy (91,92).

There are only two well-designed trials comparing the use of serotonin receptor antagonists with standard antiemetic regimens in the treatment of delayed emesis following moderately emetogenic chemotherapy. In both studies, patients were given a combination of a serotonin receptor antagonist and dexamethasone for the prophylaxis of acute emesis. In the first study, patients were then randomized to receive dexamethasone either alone or in combination with a serotonin receptor antagonist. In this trial the complete control rate (no emesis, no worse than mild nausea and no use of rescue therapy) was equivalent in both arms of the trial. The combination of a serotonin receptor antagonist and dexamethasone resulted in a statistically superior control of delayed nausea. However, using a visual analogue score (VAS), the difference between the two arms was 6 of 100 mm versus 9 of 100 mm. Relative to other studies using VAS, this difference is unlikely to be clinically relevant (93).

In the second trial (94), after receiving prophylaxis for acute emesis, patients were categorized as low-risk if they achieve complete control of acute emesis, or high-risk if they achieved less than complete control. The low-risk group was randomized either to placebo, dexamethasone singly or in combination with a serotonin receptor antagonist, with no placebo arm in the high-risk subgroup. In the low-risk subgroup, both treatment arms were statistically superior to placebo, in the control of delayed nausea and vomiting. However, there was no significant difference between either treatment arms. In the high-risk subgroup there was no statistically significant difference between the two treatment arms. In the latter group the rate of complete control of acute emesis was higher than anticipated. As a result this study is not sufficiently powered to detect a difference between the two treatment arms used in the high-risk subgroup.

Mildly and Minimally Emetogenic Chemotherapy

There has been very little study on the incidence or prevention of delayed emesis following mildly and minimally emetogenic chemotherapy. The expert consensus panel convened by ASCO does not recommend routine use of antiemetics for the prevention of delayed emesis for patients receiving these chemotherapy regimens (3).

SUMMARY OF RECOMMENDATIONS

A summary of recommended antiemetic schedules and doses is listed in Table 36.2. For highly and moderately emetogenic chemotherapy, current best evidence supports the use of a serotonin receptor antagonist given in combination with dexamethasone for the prophylaxis of acute emesis. There is little evidence on which to base recommendations for mildly or minimally emetogenic chemotherapy. The guidelines are based on the expert consensus panel convened by ASCO.

During the delayed phase, evidence supports the use of dexamethasone, alone or in combination with metoclopramide, following highly and moderately emetogenic chemotherapy. If patients are refractory to this combination, or if there is poor control of acute emesis, then a combination of dexamethasone and a serotonin receptor antagonist can be considered. However, there is little trial evidence to support this

TABLE 36.2. *Dosing guidelines for antiemetic prophylaxis*

Chemotherapy regimen	Acute phase	Delayed phase
Highly emetogenic	One of: Ondansetron 8 mg i.v. Granisetron 1 mg i.v. Dolasetron 1.8 mg/kg i.v. Ondansetron 24 mg p.o. Granisetron 2 mg p.o. + Dexamethasone 12 mg i.v.	1st Line: Dexamethasone 8 mg p.o. b.i.d. days 2–4 +/- Metoclopramide 20 mg p.o. q.i.d. days 2–4 Refractory: Dexamethasone 8 mg p.o. b.i.d. days 2–4 + One of: Ondansetron 8 mg p.o. b.i.d. Granisetron 1 mg p.o. b.i.d. Dolasetron 100 mg p.o. q.d.
Moderately emetogenic	One of: Ondansetron 8 mg i.v. Granisetron 1 mg i.v. Ondansetron 8 mg p.o. b.i.d. Granisetron 2 mg p.o./1 mg p.o. b.i.d. Dolasetron 100 mg p.o. + Dexamethasone 8–12 mg i.v.	1st Line: Dexamethasone 4 mg p.o. b.i.d. days 2–4 Refractory: Dexamethasone 4 mg p.o. b.i.d. days 2–4 + One of: Ondansetron 8 mg p.o. b.i.d. Granisetron 1 mg p.o. b.i.d.
Mildly emetogenic	Dexamethasone 4–8 mg p.o.	No routine prophylaxis
Minimally emetogenic	No routine prophylaxis	No routine prophylaxis

latter recommendation. The dosing and scheduling of antiemetics during the delayed phase has not been well studied. The doses listed in Table 36.2 are the lowest effective doses used in current studies. There is no evidence to support the routine use of antiemetic agents for the prophylaxis of delayed emesis following mildly or minimally emetogenic chemotherapy.

The neurokinin-1 receptor antagonists show promise for the treatment of both acute and delayed emesis following highly and moderately emetogenic chemotherapy. Further study is necessary before these agents can be recommended for routine use.

TREATMENT OF ANTICIPATORY EMESIS

As discussed earlier, the etiology of anticipatory nausea and vomiting (ANV) appears to be a conditioned response. It generally occurs in individuals who have had poor control of acute or delayed emesis with previous cycles of chemotherapy and its incidence increases with increasing number of chemotherapy cycles received. The best approach for the treatment of ANV is prevention by administering optimal prophylaxis for acute and delayed emesis as described above. Once ANV develops it is generally unresponsive to antiemetic therapy. Low doses of benzodiazepines and behavioral therapy, such as hypnosis, biofeedback and systemic desensitization may be effective (3,13,14,34).

SUMMARY

A significant number of patients develop nausea and vomiting secondary to cytotoxic chemotherapy and it is one of the most feared side effects of anticancer therapy. Although the pathophysiology is poorly understood, significant headway in symptomatic control continues to be made. The advent of the serotonin receptor antagonists has resulted in a dramatic improvement in control of chemotherapy-induced acute emesis. However, delayed and anticipatory emesis still present treatment challenges. This chapter has presented guidelines for the optimal management of chemotherapy-induced emesis based on current evidence. Clearly, there remains room for improvement and research into this area, to identify newer more powerful anti-emetic regimens with fewer side effects and should continue.

REFERENCES

1. Osoba D, Warr D, Fitch M. Guidelines for the optimal management of chemotherapy-induced nausea and vomiting: a consensus. *Can J Oncol* 1995;5:381–399.
2. Gregory RE, Ettinger DS. 5-HT3 receptor antagonists for the prevention of chemotherapy-induced nausea and vomiting. A comparison of their pharmacology and clinical efficacy. *Drugs* 1998;55:173–189.
3. Gralla RJ, Osoba D, Kris MG, et al. Recommendations for the use of antiemetics: evidence-based, clinical practice guidelines. *J Clin Oncol* 1999;17:2971–2994.
4. Grunberg SM, Hesketh PJ. Control of chemotherapy-induced emesis. *N Engl J Med* 1993;329:1790–1796.
5. Andrews PLR, Naylor RJ, Joss RA. Neuropharmacology of emesis and its relevance to anti-emetic therapy. *Support Care Cancer* 1998;6:197–203.
6. Andrews PLR, Bhandari P. The 5-hydroxytryptamine receptor antagonists as antiemetics: preclinical evaluation and mechanism of action. *Eur J Cancer* 1993; 29A:S11–16.
7. Cubeddu LX. Mechanisms by which cancer chemotherapeutic drugs induce emesis. *Semin Oncol* 1992; 19:2–13.
8. Wilder-Smith OH, Borgeat A, Chappuis P, Fathi M, Forni M. Urinary serotonin metabolite excretion during cisplatin chemotherapy. *Cancer* 1993;72:2239–2241.
9. Bleiberg H. A new class of antiemetics: the NK-1 receptor antagonists. *Curr Opin Oncol* 2000;12:284–288.
10. Diemunsch P, Grelot L. Potential of substance P antagonists as antiemetics. *Drugs* 2000;60:533–546.
11. Kris MG, Roila F, De Mulder PHM, Marty M. Delayed emesis following anticancer chemotherapy. *Support Care Cancer* 1998;6:228–232.
12. Navari RM, Reinhardt RR, Gralla RJ, et al. Reduction of cisplatin-induces emesis by a selective neurokinin-1-receptor antagonist. *N Engl J Med* 1999;340:190–195.
13. Morrow GR, Roscoe JA, Kirshner JJ, et al. Anticipatory nausea and vomiting in the era of 5-HT3 antiemetics. *Support Care Cancer* 1998;6:244–247.
14. Redd WH, Andrykowski MA. Behavioral intervention in cancer treatment: controlling aversion reactions to chemotherapy. *J Consul Clin Psychol* 1982;50:1018–1029.
15. Herrstedt J, Aapro MS, Smyth JF, Del Favero A. Corticosteroids, dopamine antagonists and other drugs. *Support Care Cancer* 1998;6:204–214.
16. Jantunen IT, Kataja V, Muhonen TT. An overview of randomised studies comparing 5-HT3 receptor antagonists to conventional anti-emetics in the prophylaxis of acute chemotherapy-induced vomiting. *Eur J Cancer* 1997;33:66–74.
17. Fauser AA, Fellhauer M, Hoffmann M, et al. Guidelines for anti-emetic therapy: acute emesis. *Eur J Cancer* 1999;35:361–370.

18. Campos D, Pereira JR, Reinhardt RR, et al. Prevention of cisplatin-induced emesis by the oral neurokinin-1 antagonists, MK-869, in combination with granisetron and dexamethasone or with dexamethasone alone. *J Clin Oncol* 2001;19:1759–1767.
19. Hesketh PJ, Gralla RJ, Webb RT, et al. Randomized phase II study of the neurokinin receptor antagonist CJ-11, 794 in the control of cisplatin-induced emesis. *J Clin Oncol* 1999;17:338–343.
20. Mitchelson F. Pharmacological agents affecting emesis: a review (Part I). *Drugs* 1992;43:295–315.
21. Bishop JF, Olver IN, Wolf MM, et al. Lorazepam: a randomized, double-blind, crossover study of a new antiemetic in patients receiving cytotoxic chemotherapy and prochlorperazine. *J Clin Oncol* 1984;2:691–695.
22. Gordon CJ, Pazdur R, Ziccarelli A, et al. Metoclopramide versus metoclopramide and lorazepam. Superiority of combined therapy in the control of cisplatin-induced emesis. *Cancer* 1989;63:578–582.
23. Tsavaris N, Tsoutsos H, Bacoyannis C, et al. Antiemetic efficacy of alprazolam in carboplatin-induced emesis. *Chemotherapy* 1991;37:365–370.
24. Charak BS, Banavali SD, Iyer RS, et al. Low dose, oral lorazepam: a safe and effective adjuvant to antiemetic therapy. *Indian J Cancer* 1991;28:108–113.
25. Gonzalez Baron M, Chacon JI, Garcia Giron C, et al. Antiemetic regimens in outpatients receiving cisplatin and non-cisplatin chemotherapy. A randomized trial comparing high-dose metoclopramide plus methylprednisolone with and without lorazepam. *Acta Oncol* 1991;30:623–627.
26. Clerico M, Bertetto O, Morandini MP, et al. Antiemetic activity of oral lorazepam in addition to methylprednisolone and metoclopramide in the prophylactic treatment of vomiting induced by cisplatin. A double-blind, placebo-controlled study with crossover design. *Tumori* 1993;79:119–122.
27. Mori K, Saito Y, Tominaga K. Antiemetic efficacy of alprazolam in the combination of metoclopramide plus methylprednisolone. Double-blind randomized crossover study in patients with cisplatin-induced emesis. *Am J Clin Oncol* 1993;16:338–341.
28. Buzdar AU, Esparza L, Natale R, et al. Lorazepam-enhancement of the antiemetic efficacy of dexamethasone and promethazine. A placebo-controlled study. *Am J Clin Oncol* 1994;17:417–421.
29. Malik IA, Khan WA, Qazilbash M, et al. Clinical efficacy of lorazepam in prophylaxis of anticipatory, acute, and delayed nausea and vomiting induced by high doses of cisplatin. A prospective randomized trial. *Am J Clin Oncol* 1995;18:170–175.
30. Ahn MJ, Lee JS, Lee KH, et al. A randomized double-blind trial of ondansetron alone versus in combination with dexamethasone versus in combination with dexamethasone and lorazepam in the prevention of emesis due to cisplatin-based chemotherapy. *Am J Clin Oncol* 1994;17:150–156.
31. Tsavaris N, Charalambidis G, Pagou M, et al. Comparison of ondansentron (GR 38032F) versus ondansentron plus alprazolam as antiemetic prophylaxis during cisplatin-containing chemotherapy. *Am J Clin Oncol* 1994;17:516–521.
32. Meden H, Meissner O, Conrad A, Kuhn W. Improved control of nausea and emesis with a new bromazepam-containing ondansetron regimen in ovarian cancer patients receiving chemotherapy with carboplatin and cyclophosphamide. *Eur J Gynaecol Oncol* 1996;17:114–122.
33. Bauduer F, Coiffier B, Desablens B. Granisetron plus or minus alprazolam for emesis prevention in chemotherapy of lymphomas: a randomized multicenter trial. *Leuk Lymphoma* 1999;34:341–347.
34. Razavi D, Delavaux N, Farvacques C, et al. Prevention of adjustment disorders and anticipatory nausea secondary to adjuvant chemotherapy: a double-blind, placebo-controlled study assessing the usefulness of alprazolam. *J Clin Oncol* 1993;11:1384–1390.
35. Seynaeve C, Schuller J, Buser K, et al. Comparison of the anti-emetic efficacy of different doses of ondansetron, given as either a continuous infusion or a single intravenous dose, in acute cisplatin-induced emesis. A multicentre, double-blind, randomised, parallel group study. Ondansetron Study Group. *Br J Cancer* 1992;66:192–197.
36. Beck TM, Hesketh PJ, Madajewicz S, et al. Stratified, randomized, double-blind comparison of intravenous ondansetron administered as a multiple-dose regimen versus two single-dose regimens in the prevention of cisplatin-induced nausea and vomiting. *J Clin Oncol* 1992;10:1969–1975.
37. Hainsworth JD, Hesketh PJ. Single-dose ondansetron for the prevention of cisplatin-induced emesis: efficacy results. *Semin Oncol* 1992;19:14–19.
38. Ruff P, Paska W, Goedhals L, et al. Ondansetron compared with granisetron in the prophylaxis of cisplatin-induced acute emesis: a multicentre double-blind, randomised, parallel-group study. The Ondansetron and Granisetron Emesis Study Group [published erratum appears in Oncology 1994 May–Jun;51(3):243]. *Oncology* 1994;51:113–118.
39. Riviere A. Dose finding study of granisetron in patients receiving high-dose cisplatin chemotherapy. The Granisetron Study Group. *Br J Cancer* 1994;69:967–971.
40. Navari RM, Kaplan HG, Gralla RJ, et al. Efficacy and safety of granisetron, a selective 5-hydroxytryptamine-3 receptor antagonist, in the prevention of nausea and vomiting induced by high-dose cisplatin. *J Clin Oncol* 1994;12:2204–2210.
41. Navari R, Gandara D, Hesketh P, et al. Comparative clinical trial of granisetron and ondansetron in the prophylaxis of cisplatin-induced emesis. The Granisetron Study Group. *J Clin Oncol* 1995;13:1242–1248.
42. Harman GS, Omura GA, Ryan K, et al. A randomized, double-blind comparison of single-dose and divided multiple-dose dolasetron for cisplatin-induced emesis. *Cancer Chemother Pharmacol* 1996;38:323–328.
43. Yeilding A, Bertoli L, Eisenberg P, et al. Antiemetic efficacy of two different single intravenous doses of dolasetron in patients receiving high-dose cisplatin-containing chemotherapy. *Am J Clin Oncol* 1996;19:619–623.
44. Hesketh P, Navari R, Grote T, et al. Double-blind, randomized comparison of the antiemetic efficacy of intravenous dolasetron mesylate and intravenous ondansetron in the prevention of acute cisplatin-induced emesis in patients with cancer. Dolasetron Comparative Chemotherapy-induced Emesis Prevention Group. *J Clin Oncol* 1996;14:2242–2249.
45. Audhuy B, Cappelaere P, Martin M, et al. A double-blind, randomised comparison of the anti-emetic effi-

cacy of two intravenous doses of dolasetron mesilate and granisetron in patients receiving high dose cisplatin chemotherapy. *Eur J Cancer* 1996;32A:807–813.
46. Perez EA, Navari RM, Kaplan HG, et al. Efficacy and safety of different doses of granisetron for the prophylaxis of cisplatin-induced emesis. *Support Care Cancer* 1997;5:31–37.
47. Fumoleau P, Giovannini M, Rolland F, et al. Ondansetron suppository: an effective treatment for the prevention of emetic disorders induced by cisplatin-based chemotherapy. French Ondansetron Study Group. *Oral Oncol* 1997;33:354–358.
48. Krzakowski M, Graham E, Goedhals L, et al. A multicenter, double-blind comparison of i.v. and oral administration of ondansetron plus dexamethasone for acute cisplatin-induced emesis. Ondansetron Acute Emesis Study Group. *Anticancer Drugs* 1998;9:593–598.
49. Needles B, Miranda E, Rodriguez FM, et al. A multicenter, double-blind, randomized comparison or oral ondansetron 8 mg b.i.d., 24 mg q.d., and 32 mg q.d. in the prevention of nausea and vomiting associated with highly emetogenic chemotherapy. S3AA3012 Study Group. *Support Care Cancer* 1999;7:347–353.
50. Tsavaris N, Fountzilas G, Mylonakis N, et al. A randomized comparative study of antiemetic prophylaxis with ondansetron in a single 32 mg loading dose versus 8 mg every 6 h in patients undergoing cisplatin-based chemotherapy. *Oncology* 1998; 55:513–516.
51. Birch R, Weaver CH, Carson K, et al. A randomized trial of once vs twice daily administration of intravenous granisetron with dexamethosone in patients receiving high-dose cyclophosphamide, thiotepa and carboplatin. *Bone Marrow Transplant* 1998;22:685–688.
52. Noble A, Bremer K, Goedhals L, et al. A double-blind, randomised, crossover comparison of granisetron and ondansetron in 5-day fractionated chemotherapy: assessment of efficacy, safety and patient preference. The Granisetron Study Group. *Eur J Cancer* 1994;8:1083–1088.
53. Ondansetron versus granisetron, both combined with dexamethasone, in the prevention of cisplatin-induced emesis. Italian Group of Antiemetic Research. *Ann Oncol* 1995;6:805–810.
54. Gralla RJ, Navari RM, Hesketh PJ, et al. Single-dose oral granisetron has equivalent antiemetic efficacy to intravenous ondansetron for highly emetogenic cisplatin-based chemotherapy. *J Clin Oncol* 1998;16:1568–1573.
55. Spector JI, Lester EP, Chevlen EM, et al. A comparison of oral ondansetron and intravenous granisetron for the prevention of nausea and emesis associated with cisplatin-based chemotherapy. *Oncologist* 1998;3:432–438.
56. Roila F, Tonato M, Cognetti F, et al. Prevention of cisplatin-induced emesis: a double-blind multicenter randomized crossover study comparing ondansetron and ondansetron plus dexamethasone. *J Clin Oncol* 1991;9:675–678.
57. Smyth JF, Coleman RE, Nicolson M, et al. Does dexamethasone enhance control of acute cisplatin induced emesis by ondansetron? *BMJ* 1991;303:1423–1426.
58. Chevallier B, Marty M, Paillarse JM. Methylprednisolone enhances the efficacy of ondansetron in acute and delayed cisplatin-induced emesis over at least three cycles. Ondansetron Study Group. *Br J Cancer* 1994; 70:1171–1175.
59. Hesketh PJ, Harvey WH, Harker WG, et al. A randomized, double-blind comparison of intravenous ondansetron alone and in combination with intravenous dexamethasone in the prevention of high-dose cisplatin-induced emesis. *J Clin Oncol* 1994;12:596–600.
60. Joss RA, Bacchi M, Buser K, et al. Ondansetron plus dexamethasone is superior to ondansetron alone in the prevention of emesis in chemotherapy-naive and previously treated patients. Swiss Group for Clinical Cancer Research (SAKK). *Ann Oncol* 1994;5:253–258.
61. Latreille J, Stewart D, Laberge F, et al. Dexamethasone improves the efficacy of granisetron in the first 24 h following high-dose cisplatin chemotherapy. *Support Care Cancer* 1995;3:307–312.
62. Handberg J, Wessel V, Larsen L, et al. Randomized, double-blind comparison of granisetron versus granisetron plus prednisolone as antiemetic prophylaxis during multiple-day cisplatin-based chemotherapy. *Support Care Cancer* 1998;6:63–67.
63. Kleisbauer JP, Garcia-Giron C, Antimi M, et al. Granisetron plus methylprednisolone for the control of high-dose cisplatin-induced emesis. *Anticancer Drugs* 1998;9:387–392.
64. Double-blind, dose-finding study of four intravenous doses of dexamethasone in the prevention of cisplatin-induced acute emesis. Italian Group for Antiemetic Research. *J Clin Oncol* 1998;16:2937–2942.
65. Hacking A. Oral granisetron—simple and effective: a preliminary report. The Granisetron Study Group. *Eur J Cancer* 1992;28A:S28–32.
66. Bleiberg HH, Spielmann M, Falkson G, Romain D. Antiemetic treatment with oral granisetron in patients receiving moderately emetogenic chemotherapy: a dose-ranging study. *Clin Ther* 1995;17:38–51.
67. Stewart A, McQuade B, Cronje JD, et al. Ondansetron compared with granisetron in the prophylaxis of cyclophosphamide-induced emesis in out-patients: a multicentre, double-blind, double-dummy, randomised, parallel-group study. Emesis Study Group for Ondansetron and Granisetron in Breast Cancer Patients. *Oncology* 1995; 52:202–210.
68. Ettinger DS, Eisenberg PD, Fitts D, et al. A double-blind comparison of the efficacy of two dose regimens of oral granisetron in preventing acute emesis in patients receiving moderately emetogenic chemotherapy. *Cancer* 1996;78:144–151.
69. Massidda B, Ionta MT. Prevention of delayed emesis by a single intravenous bolus dose of 5-HT3-receptor-antagonist in moderately emetogenic chemotherapy. *J Chemother* 1996;8:237–242.
70. Davidson NG, Paska W, Van Belle S, et al. Ondansetron suppository: a randomised, double-blind, double-dummy, parallel-group comparison with oral ondansetron for the prevention of cyclophosphamide-induced emesis and nausea. The Ondansetron Suppository emesis study group. *Oncology* 1997;54:380–386.
71. Grote TH, Pineda LF, Figlin RA, et al. Oral dolasetron mesylate in patients receiving moderately emetogenic platinum-containing chemotherapy. Oral Dolasetron Dose Response Study Group. *Cancer J Sci Am* 1997; 3:45–51.
72. Rubenstein EB, Gralla RJ, Hainsworth JD, et al. Randomized, double blind, dose-response trial across four oral doses of dolasetron for the prevention of acute

emesis after moderately emetogenic chemotherapy. Oral Dolasetron Dose-Response Study Group. *Cancer* 1997;79:1216–1224.
73. Beck TM, York M, Chang A, et al. Oral ondansetron 8 mg twice daily is as effective as 8 mg three times daily in the prevention of nausea and vomiting associated with moderately emetogenic cancer chemotherapy. S3A-376 Study Group. *Cancer Invest* 1997;15: 297–303.
74. Fauser AA, Duclos B, Chemaissani A, et al. Therapeutic equivalence of single oral doses of dolasetron mesilate and multiple doses of ondansetron for the prevention of emesis after moderately emetogenic chemotherapy. European Dolasetron Comparative Study Group. *Eur J Cancer* 1996;32A:1523–1529.
75. Lofters WS, Pater JL, Zee B, et al. Phase III double-blind comparison of dolasetron mesylate and ondansetron and an evaluation of the additive role of dexamethasone in the prevention of acute and delayed nausea and vomiting due to moderately emetogenic chemotherapy. *J Clin Oncol* 1997;15:2966–2973.
76. Perez EA, Hesketh P, Sandbach J, et al. Comparison of single-dose oral granisetron versus intravenous ondansetron in the prevention of nausea and vomiting induced by moderately emetogenic chemotherapy: a multicenter, double-blind, randomized parallel study. *J Clin Oncol* 1998;16:754–760.
77. Perez EA, Lembersky B, Kaywin P, et al. Comparable safety and antiemetic efficacy of a brief (30-second bolus) intravenous granisetron infusion and a standard (15-minute) intravenous ondansetron infusion in breast cancer patients receiving moderately emetogenic chemotherapy. *Cancer J Sci Am* 1998;4:52–58.
78. Carmichael J, Bessell EM, Harris AL, et al. Comparison of granisetron alone and granisetron plus dexamethasone in the prophylaxis of cytotoxic-induced emesis [published erratum appears in Br J Cancer 1995 May;71(5):1123]. *Br J Cancer* 1994;70:1161–1164.
79. Dexamethasone, granisetron, or both for the prevention of nausea and vomiting during chemotherapy for cancer. The Italian Group for Antiemetic Research. *N Engl J Med* 1995;332:1–5.
80. Kirchner V, Aapro M, Terrey JP, Alberto P. A double-blind crossover study comparing prophylactic intravenous granisetron alone or in combination with dexamethasone as antiemetic treatment in controlling nausea and vomiting associated with chemotherapy. *Eur J Cancer* 1997;33:1605–1610.
81. Roila F, Baschetti E, Tonato M, et al. Predictive factors of delayed emesis in cisplatin-treated patients and antiemetic activity and tolerability of metoclopramideor dexamethasone. A randomized, single-blind study. *Am J Clin Oncol* 1991;14:238–242.
82. Gandara DR, Harvey WH, Monaghan GG, et al. Delayed emesis following high-dose cisplatin: a double-blind randomised comparative trial of ondansetron (GR 38032F) versus placebo. *Eur J Cancer* 1993;29A: S35–8.

83. Esseboom EU, Rojer RA, Borm JJ, Statius van Eps LW. Prophylaxis of delayed nausea and vomiting after cancer chemotherapy. *Neth J Med* 1995;47:12–17.
84. Navari RM, Madajewicz S, Anderson N, et al. Oral ondansetron for the control of cisplatin-induced delayed emesis: a large, multicenter, double-blind, randomized comparative trial of ondansetron versus placebo. *J Clin Oncol* 1995;13:2408–2416.
85. Matsui K, Fukuoka M, Takada M, et al. Randomised trial for the prevention of delayed emesis in patients receiving high-dose cisplatin. *Br J Cancer* 1996;73: 217–221.
86. Olver I, Paska W, Depierre A, et al. A multicentre, double-blind study comparing placebo, ondansetron and ondansetron plus dexamethasone for the control of cisplatin-induced delayed emesis. Ondansetron Delayed Emesis Study Group. *Ann Oncol* 1996;7:945–952.
87. Latreille J, Pater J, Johnston D, et al. Use of dexamethasone and granisetron in the control of delayed emesis for patients who receive highly emetogenic chemotherapy. National Cancer Institute of Canada Clinical Trials Group. *J Clin Oncol* 1998;16:1174–1178.
88. Goedhals L, Heron JF, Kleisbauer JP, et al. Control of delayed nausea and vomiting with granisetron plus dexamethasone or dexamethasone alone in patients receiving highly emetogenic chemotherapy: a double-blind, placebo-controlled, comparative study. *Ann Oncol* 1998; 9:661–666.
89. Ondansetron versus metoclopramide, both combined with dexamethasone, in the prevention of cisplatin-induced delayed emesis. The Italian Group for Antiemetic Research. *J Clin Oncol* 1997;15:124–130.
90. Kris MG, Gralla RJ, Tyson LB, et al. Controlling delayed vomiting: double-blind, randomized trial comparing placebo, dexamethasone alone, and metoclopramide plus dexamethasone in patients receiving cisplatin. *J Clin Oncol* 1989;7:108–114.
91. Kaizer L, Warr D, Hoskins P, et al. Effect of schedule and maintenance on the antiemetic efficacy of ondansetron combined with dexamethasone in acute and delayed nausea and emesis in patients receiving moderately emetogenic chemotherapy: a phase III trial by the National Cancer Institute of Canada Clinical Trials Group. *J Clin Oncol* 1994;12:1050–1057.
92. Koo WH, Ang PT. Role of maintenance oral dexamethasone in prophylaxis of delayed emesis caused by moderately emetogenic chemotherapy. *Ann Oncol* 1996;7:71–74.
93. Pater JL, Lofters WS, Zee B, et al. The role of the 5-HT3 antagonists ondansetron and dolasetron in the control of delayed onset nausea and vomiting in patients receiving moderately emetogenic chemotherapy. *Ann Oncol* 1997;8:181–185.
94. The Italian Group for Antiemetic Research. Dexamethasone alone or in combination with ondansetron for the prevention of delayed nausea and vomiting induced by chemotherapy. The Italian Group of Antiemetic Research. *N Engl J Med* 2000;342:1554–1559.

37

Quality-of-Life Data Interpretation: An Update on Key Issues in Advanced Breast Cancer

Andrew Bottomley

Health-related quality of life (HRQOL), a multidimensional construct, is generally regarded as encompassing clinical subjective perceptions of positive and negative aspects of cancer patient domains, including physical, emotional, social, and cognitive functions and perhaps most importantly, disease symptoms and treatment (1).

Only 20 years ago, not much literature reporting quality of life in cancer research existed. However, over recent years, there has been a significant increase in peer-reviewed publications of studies reporting the assessment of HRQOL. A recent review of the published literature indicates that the number of HRQOL studies supports this substantial increase. Furthermore, at present, some 10% of all randomized cancer clinical trials include HRQOL as a main endpoint (2).

Introducing HRQOL into the day-to-day clinical arena has not been without numerous difficulties. There are several conceptual, methodological, practical, and attitudinal explanations for the challenges that have faced HRQOL researchers (3–5). Today, many of these are slowly being overcome (6–8). While researchers are often faced with situations where patients may not gain benefits in terms of traditional endpoints, such as survival or disease-free survival, it is possible to see significant changes in HRQOL (9).

Despite the greater use of HRQOL in clinical trials, clinicians are still faced with challenges. In particular, these difficulties limit HRQOL study integration and can influence results. Realizing the subjective nature of HRQOL studies generates barriers to acceptance by clinicians (9). Furthermore, as Moinpour (62) points out, the high number of and unfamiliarity with HRQOL measures available presents a serious challenge to clinician's awareness of interpretation and subsequent understanding of the conclusions.

The purpose of this chapter is to assist clinicians interpreting HRQOL data from reported studies in advanced breast cancer. This is particularly important because the treatment of advanced breast cancer remains mainly palliative and although it is common to see high response rates and sometimes modest increases in survival, these are usually associated with treatment-related toxicity (10,11). Unlike early breast cancer where a significant number of HRQOL studies have been published (12–15), in advanced breast cancer, Carlson (16) and Overmoyer (17) suggest that only a limited number of studies are available. Fossati et al. (18) confirmed this when they reported the results of a systematic review of published literature on medical interventions used in the treatment of advanced breast cancer. Between 1975 and 1997, a total of 189 studies were identified, treating 31,510 patients. However, only 9% (2,995) of these patients were reported to have been involved in any quality-of-life assessment. Perhaps this low figure represents in part the complexities of a population where treatment is mainly palliative and thus studies can be fraught with difficulties in design and implementation.

DESIGN AND ANALYSIS INFLUENCES ON HRQOL DATA INTERPRETATION

Analysis of HRQOL data is difficult and represents a significant challenge to researchers (19). If researchers are to report on evidence-based studies, it is essential when producing (or reviewing) the results that attention be given to matters of appropriate design and analysis. It is fundamental to determine that certain precautions have been taken to ensure a well-designed trial.

One obviously key issue frequently raised concerns the appropriateness of the measures chosen. In many cases, if well-validated instruments have not been used in the correct manner, for example, appropriate populations, timing, and place of assessment, there are right from the beginning issues of concern regarding appropriate interpretation (19). If the HRQOL instrument is not well known, it needs to be examined in detail to ensure its psychometric properties of reliability and validity are suitable before useful interpretation of the results can be made. Kong and Gandhi (20) note that, of 265 articles reviewed reporting the assessment of HRQOL in clinical trials, only 23% provided reliability data, and only 21% provided validity data. Unfortunately, many of the studies in advanced breast cancer have not published such data, including Bernhard et al. (21) and Seidman et al. (22).

Given the multidimensional nature of HRQOL data, it is important that researchers provide information on all measures used, including the domain investigated, even if not significant. One early study conducted by Priestman and Baum (23) serves as an example of the problems that arise when robust measures are not used and data on the psychometric properties of the measures are not included. In this study, 29 women undergoing two different chemotherapy regimens were assessed using a linear analogue self-assessment (LASA) technique. This method simply required patients to mark, on a line, a point that most accurately described their symptoms or views, ranging from the best (e.g., no pain) to the worst (e.g., extremely severe pain). While this type of assessment can be valuable, Priestman and Baum apparently self-selected the questions for the LASA (e.g., feelings of well being, mood, anxiety, appetite and social activities) without any explicit rationale. This can have serious implications for interpreting the results: the researchers could have been assessing certain aspects of HRQOL that they believed to be important. It is also possible that other issues that patients believed were important (e.g., spirituality, social support, symptoms such as hair loss) might not have been assessed (24,25). If we are to ensure evidence-based practice in HRQOL studies, researchers should ensure that they provide as much detail as possible regarding the development of instruments used to avoid such criticisms.

Fayers et al. (26) suggest that HRQOL data analysis can be classified into two broad categories: confirmatory and descriptive/exploratory. If confirmatory data analysis is used, then specifically defined questions are asked to test the statistically significant differences as specified in the protocol. One key issue is the selection of the pretrial hypotheses. This proposes the key HRQOL domains to be investigated, to avoid the problem of significant results from multiple significance testing (27).

However, several studies of advanced breast cancer have not followed this approach. One example is the Seidman et al. phase 2 study where 30 metastatic breast cancer patients underwent quality-of-life evaluation with no rationale for selecting which quality-of-life domains were presented. Similarly, Tannock et al. (28) investigated the effects of two dose levels (high and low) of CMF in a sample of 133 metastatic breast cancer patients. Only a subset of 49 patients completed a LASA 34-item scale, since compliance was limited by the "availability of personnel to monitor completion of the quality-of-life measures." In addition, an unspecified number of patients completed the Profile of Mood States. While it is clearly very difficult to make any interpretation based on such methodological limitations, it is surprising to see no prior HRQOL hypothesis in such a study.

Bishop et al. (29) report the results of a study with metastatic breast cancer patients where 209 patients were randomized to receive either paclitaxel i.v. or a CMFP (cyclophosphamide, methotrexate, 5-fluorouracil, and prednisone) regimen. HRQOL results were presented after analyzing data from the QOL linear analogue scale and by clinicians using the Spitzer QOL index (30). While no overall significant differences were seen on any of the domains of physical well being, mood, pain, nausea, appetite, overall QOL, or physical-related QOL, the authors conclude that, "with the exception of pain, patients on the paclitaxel arm experienced slightly better QOL for each parameter during treatment than patients on the CMFP arm." Because the researchers proposed no prior hypothesis it is clearly problematic to undertake repeated analysis without a clear idea of the influence on which HRQOL domain one is looking for.

Failure to state a prior hypothesis is not always found to be a problem. Some researchers demonstrate clarity. Bernhard et al. (31) compared breast cancer patients who underwent two second-line endocrine treatments. Patients were randomized into formestane and megestrol acetate groups. Given that the aims were a comparison of global HRQOL between the two groups, the methodology clearly justified the use of a global HRQOL score as a prior hypothesis. Osoba and Burchmore (32) also reported a well-designed randomized phase 3 study with 469 metastatic breast cancer patients. In this study patients were allocated into two arms of either trastuzumab (Herceptin) combined with chemotherapy or chemotherapy alone. A clear priori was selected of four domains (global quality of life, physical role, social functioning, and fatigue) on the validated EORTC QLQ-C30 (33), and the results suggested that those patients on the combined treatment had a higher HRQOL than chemotherapy alone.

After this confirmatory analysis, in both the Bernhard et al. and Osoba and Burchmore studies, it was possible to undertake exploratory analysis on subscale and domains. This type of analysis is used to explore, clarify, describe, and, more importantly, help interpret HRQOL data. While such analysis can often reveal important information about the data and can help interpretation, one needs to be aware that results are often generated after multiple testing and analysis, and, as Douglas (34) points out, significant influences can often be seen under such circumstances. In essence, while exploratory/descriptive analysis can help in interpreting the data, ideally this should serve the later testing of hypotheses.

When interpreting HRQOL results, it is vital that attention be given to incomplete data. Although the assessment of HRQOL is critical in cases of advanced breast cancer, it is affected by the problems of rapidly diminishing patient numbers. Frequently, this is due to few patients completing a set of assessments in the weeks and days immediately preceding death. One example is the study reported by Kramer and colleagues (35), who investigated the effects of HRQOL on patients with advanced breast cancer. In this prospective randomized phase 2/3 crossover study, 166 patients were assigned to treatment with paclitaxel and 165 to treatment with doxorubicin. However, less than two-thirds of patients completed baseline assessment, and compliance rates deteriorated continually thereafter.

This is not the only study with such poor rates of compliance. For example, Coates et al. (36), in the investigation of HRQOL for advanced breast cancer patients, reports that only 44% of individuals (133 of 305) were available for analysis after three cycles of chemotherapy. Similarly, in the study by Richards et al. (37), patients with advanced breast cancer underwent two different schedules of doxorubicin; only 71% had data from baseline and at the end of the third cycle 3 months later. Therefore, failure to take missing data into consideration when interpreting HRQOL results can lead to incorrect conclusions. For example, treatment differences may be biased if large numbers of patients fail to complete the questionnaire, and several studies have failed to consider these issues (23,29).

In some studies, such as reported by Harper-Wynne et al. (38), the quality of the HRQOL information collected has been so limited by missing data that the planned analysis could not be performed. In other studies, such as that reported by Kristensen et al. (39), the results are so plagued with missing data that the analysis could only be undertaken on the initial two assessments, allowing limited follow-on. However, while it may be argued that it is impossible to get a good compliance rate with advanced breast cancer patients, there are some studies that have good compliance levels. One of the most impressive is the study conducted by Hakamies-Blomqvist et al. (40). In this multicentered trial, 283 metastatic breast cancer patients were randomized to receive either docetaxel or sequential methotrexate and 5-fluorouracil. While this study showed no quality-of-life benefits of one treatment over the other, the investigators were able to demonstrate compliance levels of 96% at baseline and an overall compliance of 82%. This suggests the feasibility of having high levels of compliance even with advanced cancer patients. Clearly, the problems outlined here limit the extent to which we can make any reasonable interpretations of data; thus it is imperative that robust methods be adopted to ensure that high-quality data are collected and appropriately analyzed (27).

CLINICAL SIGNIFICANCE

Experience in medicine has led to an understanding that certain clinical events are related to health outcomes. A classical example, often cited in the literature, concerns a blood pressure reading of 110/60 mm Hg being normal for a healthy, young adult but dangerously low for a trauma victim. A change in 2 or 3 mm Hg in blood pressure probably has little or no clinical significance, but a 10 to 20 mm Hg difference could indicate shock or hypertension, depending on the situation. However, while this is a well-established fact, this level of clarity has not been achieved in the interpretation of HRQOL scores (19). For clinicians, it must be stressed that what constitutes clinical significance on many standard, objective measures is based on years of experience, learning, and contact with large numbers of patients over time—something that researchers and clinicians have yet to gain to a substantial degree of accuracy in HRQOL assessment.

As clinicians continue to gain more experience, this leads to greater awareness of how to relate scores to meaning of and events in life. However, questions must be asked: What do scores of 20 or 40 or whatever mean clinically? What degree of change in a score is needed for a clinically meaningful change? While a 4-point difference on a HRQOL scale may be statistically significant, is this clinically relevant to patients or society? Can these scores actually reflect the need to use or to recommend noncontinuance of a treatment? Perhaps what is considered meaningful really depends on who is looking at the results of the studies. It is often relatively easy to conduct large-scale studies that could, with correct methodology, give statistically significant results even when there are only small differences in scores. When epidemiologists, policy makers, or statisticians view the results, they may appear valuable simply because they are statistically significant. Perhaps, from a clinician's point of view, the most important aspect of understanding the results is to make them meaningful in terms of the individual patient or population.

Often researchers refer to what is called "minimal clinical importance difference," noted as the smallest difference in a score in a domain of interest that a patient perceives as beneficial. This indicates, in the absence of adverse scale effects, a change in patient treatment and care (41).

However, even with such a useful definition, clinicians can face difficulty in interpreting data in accordance with this (42). For example, when simply comparing mean score differences between two groups, difficult interpretations could easily arise. That is, while it is intuitive to look for a mean difference, it is important to be aware that such a group mean could easily mask certain patients in the sample by ignoring the distribution about the mean. However, when examining most reported studies of advanced breast cancer, interpretation is generally focused on changes in mean scores as opposed to using other techniques of interpretation (22, 29,31).

This may be understandable, since clinicians have a long way to go in understanding the clinical significance of HRQOL scores. Fortunately, several methods have been proposed to assist in interpretation. Perhaps the most common approach is to anchor the changes seen in disease-specific questions to a global rating question—one that asks about overall HRQOL changes, such as, "In general, how would you rate your quality of life?" Then, researchers would look at changes in answers to such a global HRQOL question over time and compare these with changes seen on the disease-specific questionnaire (43). In effect, the changes in the disease specific measures are thus anchored to reported changes in overall health status.

Also, it is possible to use time as an anchor, or for that matter, changes in therapy. Changes in therapy or time can help in interpreting HRQOL scores. However, while these anchor-based interpretations can help clinicians to understand a little more about the meaning of HRQOL, it is important to recognize they only reflect changes in HRQOL; they do not reflect score distribution.

Osoba et al. (44) investigated this issue using a subjective significance questionnaire, asking patients about perceived changes in physical, emotional, social functioning, and global HRQOL using the EORTC QLQ-C30 (33). The patients were receiving chemotherapy for metastatic breast cancer or extensive-disease—small-cell lung cancer. Osoba et al. found it possible to rate, on the seven-point subjective significance question, the significance of the changes in QLQ-C30 scores, from "much worse" to "much better."

From the data, Osoba et al. were able to interpret changes on the QLQ-C30 as meaningful, to the point of proposing, on a scale of 1 to 100, with a difference of 5 to 10 considered little change; patients who fell in the 10 to 20 range experienced a moderate change; and those with a 20-plus change reported very much change. It is also important to bear in mind that, in using anchoring, the degree of change perceived to be clinically significant could well differ from population to population and from patient to patient.

Another common method used to interpret HRQOL data is the norm-based approach. Here, clinicians compare particular individual or group scores with the distribution of the instrument scores in different populations using known criteria, including a general population, gender, age, diagnosis, and clinical populations. For example, the EORTC QLQ-C30 is used extensively not only with different cancer populations (45) but also in the general population (26,46, 47). Thus, it becomes possible to explore, compare, and interpret these data with other groups (48,49). However, while some authors have used reference data to help in the interpretation of HRQOL scores, few studies of patients with advanced breast cancer have used this approach. It should also be noted that while reference data are often very useful, as in the case of the EORTC QLQ-C30 data, collection took place in the framework of a cancer clinical trial. In such cases there are clear subject-recruitment selection procedures (21); therefore, it is essential that such reference data be used carefully, ensuring that it is representative of the group(s) under study. When we examine the limited number of publications on advanced breast cancer, it is clear many authors do not consider this issue in their publications (29,31,40).

PREDICTIVE VALUE OF HRQOL

The growing body of evidence suggests that, in the near future, clinicians will be able to interpret the HRQOL scores as measures in context, predicting both survival rates and the effectiveness of HRQOL during treatment. While a number of studies in other cancer sites report that HRQOL predicts survival rates (50,51), few have been reported in advanced breast cancer. Coates et al. (36) found baseline scores in women who underwent chemotherapy for advanced cancer were interpreted to indicate a prognostic factor. Kramer et al. (35) also found, in patients undergoing chemotherapy, that scores on the EORTC QLQ-C30 were predictive of survival outcome. However, there is evidence that quality of life scores are only predictive in patients with advanced breast cancer (52). Patients' scores, when undergoing adjuvant chemotherapy, are likely to be obscured by chemotherapy itself as in other patient groups. It is possible that, if results continue to be generated in support of this prognostic value, then it will be possible to interpret HRQOL scores and use them as factors in important prognostic considerations, replacing the more conventional performance scales. Indeed such scores may eventually help to identify patients eligible for clinical trials thus, ensuring appropriate stratification.

WHETHER TO AGGREGATE SCORES OR USE DOMAINS IN INTERPRETATION

Some researchers argue for the aggregation of scores of various HRQOL domains as a way of expressing and interpreting overall HRQOL. The advantage of this is single-number representation. This can be easily understood and compared with other single-number representations, and can be useful in other situations, such as calculating quality-adjusted years of life (42). However, while it is intuitive to have a single number, there are ongoing questions, including whether it is realistic to expect that a single number can adequately reflect the various domains of HRQOL. Many assumptions are made. For example, when summed together, do these complex domains make an accurate, global interpretation? Clinicians might assume that the various domains added together have equal weight or importance. This is not necessarily true, and is not supported by any evidence. It is highly probable, given the subjective nature of HRQOL, that some patients place greater weight on the HRQOL physical rather than psychological domains. In addition to individual weighting of such concerns, it is also likely that there is not only this variation but also variation over time. Interpretation of a single score is difficult because it lacks any detailed information about how the various domains are influenced by the disease and treatment. As such, it is quite possible that certain effects of the disease and the treatment are hidden. These would not be hidden had the domain scores been examined.

One way to address this limitation is the method adopted by the EORTC Quality of Life Group, where researchers ensure that they are able to obtain both a single global score and a detailed knowledge of the various domains (33). Here, not only does the EORTC QLQ-C30 collect details on the domains, but also assessment of two global HRQOL items gives additional indication of global HRQOL, independent of the domain scores. This has the advantage of avoiding making assumptions about the weighting of domains and drawing conclusions.

Although global quality of life items have the advantage of being easy to interpret by clinicians, they can have disadvantages (53). Specifically, while the use of a global quality of life item is valuable for detecting change in general, it provides somewhat limited information; it is impossible for clinicians to identify the nature of the HRQOL change. Global items also represent an interpretative difficulty, because it is almost impossible to know how people are relating the change in global HRQOL to specific HRQOL issues. In advanced breast cancer patients, for example, it is quite possible that as their condition becomes more serious, patients focus on limited physical functioning and possibly spiritual or psychological issues (11).

LIMITATIONS AND CHALLENGES ON HRQOL INTERPRETATION

Given the potential difficulties faced by researchers in HRQOL studies, it is understandable that there are numerous potential limitations influencing the interpretation (54). There are the general and actual difficulties that must be considered by authors reporting HRQOL research results. As already mentioned, these include the following: making sure that the researchers have selected appropriate, valid and reliable instruments; ensuring that analysis of data is robust, taking into account the problem of missing data; and making sure that researchers are aware of potential bias from social desirability of cancer patients (the tendency to put oneself in a favorable light and endorse questionnaire statements), and that demographic factors are considered (27).

It is important that particular attention be paid, specifically in cancer clinical trials, to the potential problems of cultural bias; results of treatment in one group may not have the same weight or value in another culture (55). Indeed, even if cultural differences are reported in multinational trials, it is essential that researchers consider, for example, patient characteristics and institutional participation to avoid creating ecological fallacy whereby results are misinterpreted as cultural differences in HRQOL, when in reality they could simply be differences in patient selection in different cultural populations (56). In addition, clinicians are increasingly aware that patterns of response to HRQOL assessment do vary with marital status, education, income, race (57,58), geography (59), and a host of other extraneous psychological factors that need to be monitored carefully when reporting HRQOL results (43,60,61).

SUMMARY

Invaluable HRQOL data can be obtained when assessing a wide variety of interventions in patients suffering from advanced breast cancer. However, only a limited number of studies have been published to date, and many of these have suffered from a wide variety of methodological problems that limits the interpretation of the results. Adopting basic scientific principles of effective design and analysis of new studies should ensure that researchers collect reliable and robust data for accurate evidence based interpretation. This will result in improved HRQOL assessment in the field of advanced breast cancer and acquisition of a stronger scientific basis. HRQOL could then be used to a greater degree, in the future, for treatment decision making.

REFERENCES

1. Leplege A, Hunt S. The problem of quality of life in medicine. *JAMA* 1997;278(1):47–50.
2. Sanders C, Egger M, Donovan J, Tallon D, Frankel S. Reporting on quality of life in randomised controlled trials: bibliographic study. *BMJ* 1998;317(7167):1191–1194 Review.
3. Detmar SB, Aaronson NK. Quality of life assessment in daily clinical oncology practice: a feasibility study. *Eur J Cancer* 1998;34(8):1181–1186.
4. Feld R. Endpoints in cancer clinical trials: is there a need for measuring quality of life? *Support Care Cancer* 1995;3(1):23–27.
5. Muldoon MF, Barger SD, Flory JD, Manuck SB. What are quality of life measurements measuring? *BMJ* 1998;316(7130):542–545.
6. Osoba D. Lessons learned from measuring health-related quality of life in oncology. *J Clin Oncol* 1994;12(3):608–616.
7. Young T, Maher J. Collecting quality of life data in EORTC clinical trials—what happens in practice? *Psycho-oncology* 1999;8:260–263.
8. Bottomley A. Developing clinical trial protocols for quality of life assessment. *Applied Clinical Trials* 2001;10(1):40–44.
9. Velikova G, Stark D, Selby P. Quality of Life instruments in oncology. *Eur J Cancer* 1999;35(11):1571–1580.
10. Bull AA, Meyerowitz BE, Hart S, et al. Quality of life in women with recurrent breast cancer. *Breast Cancer Res Treat* 1999;54(1):47–57.
11. Groenvold M. Methodological issues in the assessment of health-related quality of life in palliative care trials. *Acta Anaesthesiol Scand* 1999;43(9):948–953.
12. Fisher B, Bauer M, Margolese R, et al. Five year results of a randomised clinical trial comparing total mastectomy and segmental mastectomy with or without radiation in the treatment of breast cancer. *N Engl J Med* 1985;312(11):665–673.
13. Levy SM, Herberman RB, Lee JK, et al. Breast conservation versus mastectomy: distress sequelae as a function of choice. *J Clin Oncol* 1989;7(3):367–375.
14. Shimozuma K, Ganz PA, Petersen L, Hirji K. Quality of life in the first year after breast cancer surgery: rehabilitation needs and patterns of recovery. *Breast Cancer Res Treat* 1999;56(1):45–57.
15. Pusic A, Thompson TA, Kerrigan CL, et al. Surgical options for the early-stage breast cancer: factors associated with patient choice and postoperative quality of life. *Plast Reconstr Surg* 1999;104(5):1325–1333.
16. Carlson RW. Quality of life issues in the treatment of metastatic breast cancer. *Oncology* (Huntingt) 1998;12(3 suppl 4):27–31.
17. Overmoyer BA. Chemotherapeutic palliative approaches in the treatment of breast cancer. *Semin Oncol* 1995;22(2 suppl 3):2–9.
18. Fossati R, Confalonieri C, Torri V, et al. Cytotoxic and hormonal treatment for metastatic breast cancer: a systematic review of published randomized trials involving 31,510 women. *J Clin Oncol* 1998;16(10):3439–3460.
19. Green SB. Does assessment of quality of life in comparative cancer trials make a difference? A discussion. *Control Clin Trials* 1997;18(4):306–310.
20. Kong SX, Gandhi SK. Methodologic assessments of quality of life measures in clinical trials. *Ann Pharmacother* 1997;31(7–8):830–836.
21. Bernhard J, Hurny CDT, Coates A, et al. Applying quality of life principles in international cancer clinical trials. In: Spilker B, ed. *Quality of life and pharmacoeconomics in clinical trials,* 2nd ed. Philadelphia: Lippincott-Raven, 1996.
22. Seidman AD, Hudis, CA, Norton L. Memorial Sloan-Kettering Cancer Center Experinece with paclitaxel in the treatment of breast cancer: from advanced disease to adjuvant therapy. *Semin Oncol* 1995;22(8):3–8.
23. Priestman TJ, Baum M. Evaluation of quality of life in patients receiving treatment for advanced breast cancer. *Lancet* 1976;24:899–900.
24. Calkins DR, Rubenstein LV, Cleary PD, et al. Failure of physicians to recognise functional disability in ambulatory patients. *Ann Intern Med* 1991;114(6):451–454.
25. Nelson E, Conger B, Douglass R, et al. Functional health status levels of primary care patients. *JAMA* 1983;249(24):3331–3338.
26. Fayers PM, Machin D. Summarizing quality of life data using graphical methods. In: Staquet MJ, Hays RD, Fayers PM, eds. *Quality of life assessment in clinical trials: methods and practice.* Oxford Medical Publications, 1998.
27. Staquet M, Berzon R, Osoba D, Machin D. Guidelines for reporting results of quality of life assessments in clinical trials. *Qual Life Res* 1996;5(5):496–502.
28. Tannock IF, Boyd NF, DeBoer G, et al. A randomized trial of two dose levels of cyclophosphamide, methotrexate, and fluorouracil chemotherapy for patients with metastatic breast cancer. *J Clin Oncol* 1988;6(9):1377–1387.

29. Bishop JF, Dewar J, Toner GC, et al. Initial Paclitaxel improves outcome compared with CMFP combination chemotherapy as front-line therapy in untreated metastatic breast cancer. *J Clin Oncol* 1999;17(8): 2355–2364.
30. Spitzer WO, Dobson AJ, Hall J, et al. Measuring the quality of life of cancer patients: a concise QL-index for use by physicians. *J Chronic Dis* 1981;34(12):585–597.
31. Bernhard J, Thurlimann B, Schmitz S, et al. Defining clinical benefit in postmenopausal patients with breast cancer under second-line endocrine treatment: does quality of life matter? *J Clin Oncol* 1999;17(6):1672–1679.
32. Osoba D, Slamon DJ, Burchmore M, et al. Effects on quality of life of combined trastuzumab and chemotherapy in women with metastatic breast cancer. *J Clin Oncol* 2002;20:3106–3113.
33. Aaronson NK, Ahmedzai S, Bergman B, et al. The European Organization for Research and Treatment of Cancer QLQ-C30: a quality-of-life instrument for use in international clinical trials in oncology. *J Natl Cancer Inst* 1993;85(5):365–376.
34. Douglas JA. Item response models for longitudinal quality of life data in clinical trials. *Stat Med* 1999; 18(21):2917–2931.
35. Kramer J, Curran D, Parridaens R. Quality of life assessment in patients with advanced breast cancer. 1999; in press.
36. Coates A, Gebski V, Stat M, et al. Improving the quality of life during chemotherapy for advanced breast cancer: a comparison of intermittent and continuous treatment strategies. *N Engl J Med* 1987;317(24):1490–1495.
37. Richards MA, Hopwood P, Ramirez AJ, et al. Doxorubicin in advanced breast cancer: influence of schedule on response, survival and quality of life. *Eur J Cancer* 1992;28A(6/7):1023–1028.
38. Harper-Wynne C, English J, Meyer L, et al. Randomized trial to compare the efficacy and toxicity of cyclophosphamide, methotrexate and 5-fluorouracil (CMF) with methotrexate mitoxantrone (MM) in advanced carcinoma of the breast. *Br J Cancer* 1999; 81(2):316–322.
39. Kristensen B, Ejlertsen B, Groenvold M, et al. Oral clodronate in breast cancer patients with bone metastases: a randomized study. *J Intern Med* 1999;246: 67–74.
40. Hakamies-Blomqvist L, Luoma M, Sjostrom J, et al. Quality of life in patients with metastatic breast cancer receiving either docetaxel or sequential methotrexate and 5-fluorouracil. A multicentre randomised phase III trial by the Scandinavian breast group. *Eur J Cancer* 2000;36(11):1411–1419.
41. Juniper EF, Guyatt GH, Willan A, Griffith LE. Determining a minimal important change in a disease-specific Quality of Life Questionnaire. *J Clin Epidemiol* 1994; 47(1):81–87.
42. Smith KW, Avis NE, Assmann SF. Distinguishing between quality of life and health status in quality of life research: a meta-analysis. *Qual Life Res* 1999;8(5): 447–459.
43. Koller M, Heitmann K, Kussmann J, Lorenz W. Symptom reporting in cancer patients II: relations to social desirability, negative affect, and self-reported health behaviors. *Cancer* 1999;86(8):1609–1620.
44. Osoba D, Rodrigues G, Myles J, Zee B, Pater J. Interpreting the significance of changes in health-related quality-of-life scores. *J Clin Oncol* 1998;16(1):139–144.
45. Hjermstad MJ, Fayers PM, Bjordal K, Kaasa S. Using reference data on quality of life-the importance of adjusting for age and gender, exemplified by the EORTC QLQ-C30 (+3). *Eur J Cancer* 1998;34(9): 1381–1389.
46. Hjermstad M, Holte H, Evensen S, et al. Do patients who are treated with stem cell transplantation have a health-related quality of life comparable to the general population after 1 year? *Bone Marrow Transplant* 1999;24(8):911–918.
47. King MT, Dobson AJ, Harnett PR. A comparison of two quality-of-life questionnaires for cancer clinical trials: the functional living index-cancer (FLIC) and the quality of life questionnaire core module (QLQ-C30). *J Clin Epidemiol* 1996;49(1):21–29.
48. Ringdal GI, Ringdal K. Testing the EORTC Quality of Life Questionnaire on cancer patients with heterogeneous diagnosis. *Qual Life Res* 1993;2(2):129–140.
49. Ringdal K, Ringdal GI, Kaasa S, et al. Assessing the consistency of psychometric properties of the HRQoL scales within the EORTC QLQ-C30 across populations by means of the Mokken Scaling Model. *Qual Life Res* 1999;8(1–2):25–43.
50. Ganz PA, Lee JJ, Siau J. Quality of life assessment. An independent prognostic variable for survival in lung cancer. *Cancer* 1991;67(12):3131–3135.
51. Kassa S, Mastekassa A, Lund E. Prognostic factors for patients with inoperable non-small cell lung cancer, limited disease. The importance of patients' subjective experience of disease and psychosocial well-being. *Radiother Oncology* 1989;15(3):235–242.
52. Coates AS, Hurny C, Peterson H, et al. Quality of life predict outcome in metastatic but not early breast cancer. *J Clin Oncol* 2000;15:3768–3774.
53. Mozes B, Maor Y, Shmueli A. Do we know what global ratings of health-related quality of life measure? *Qual Life Res* 1999;8(3):269–273.
54. Ware JF Jr, Keller SD. Interpreting general health measures. In: Spilker B, ed. *Quality of life and pharmacoeconomics in clinical trials*, 2nd ed. New York: Lippincott-Raven Publishers, 1996.
55. Browman GP. Science, language, intuition and the many meanings of quality of life. *J Clin Oncol* 1999; 17(6):1651–1653.
56. Padilla GV, et al. Quality of life—cancer. In: Spilker B, ed. *Quality of life and pharmacoeconomics in clinical trials*, 2nd ed. New York: Lippincott-Raven Publishers, 1996.
57. Juarez G, Ferrell B, Borneman T. Cultural considerations in education for cancer pain management. *J Cancer Educ* 1999;14(3):168–173.
58. Collins GS, Bottomley A, Fayers P, et al. Psychometric properties of the EORTC quality of life core questionnaire (QLQ-C30) in EORTC trials. Abstract accepted at ECCO 11, Lisbon, October 2001.
59. Wahl A, Moum T, Hanestad BR, Wiklund I. The relationship between demographic and clinical variables,

and quality of life aspects in patients with psoriasis. *Qual Life Res* 1999;8(4):319–326.
60. Bucquet C, Guillemin F, Briancon S. Nonspecific effects in longitudinal studies: impact on quality of life measures. *J Clin Epidemiol* 1996;49(1):15–20.
61. van Dam FS, Schagen SB, Muller MJ, et al. Impairment of cognitive function in women receiving adjuvant treatment for high risk breast cancer: high-dose versus standard dose chemotherapy. *J Natl Cancer Inst* 1998;90(3):210–218.
62. Moinpour CM. Do quality of life assessments make a difference in the evaluation of cancer treatments? *Control Clin Trials* 1997;18:311–317.

38

The Internet, the Evidence, and the Health Consumer

Lewis Rowett

MORE ROTTING FISH?

Back in the last century, writing for the first edition of this book, I felt obliged to begin by justifying a chapter about the Internet in a textbook on breast cancer. Now just 2 years on, and even with the intervening bursting of the dot.com bubble, it seems that we might more reasonably ask, "Why another textbook?" I will trust that if you have worked systematically through this book to here, my co-authors have already provided strong answers to that one. But you should know that some of what you have read is out of date. If, however, you are dipping into these conclusions in search of take-home messages before looking at the rest of the book, try this: *caveat lector:* Reader beware, the contents of this book have already started to rot. Which should, I believe, bring us back to . . .

THE INTERNET

The Internet, as a network of computer networks, has three fundamental components (1): (a) hardware, the cables, switches, satellites and computers that constitute the physical network; (b) software, the protocols, and programs that make the network work; and (c) the people who run the computers, write the programs, create the information, surf the Web, etc. There are elements of all three components that are important for our consideration. The widespread nature of the physical networks has made access practically universal. Anyone (and here we must acknowledge that we mean anyone with access to a computer, a modem, and a phone line, not a majority in world terms) can get on the Net. The Internet is a peer-to-peer network: unlike a television network, all points on the network can transmit and receive (2). The standard nature of the protocols and the broadly standard nature of much of the software and publishing languages mean that transmitted information can appear to the reader much as it did to the author. All this has not gone unnoticed: People have been making more and more information available on the Internet (3), databases, textbooks, practice guidelines, and systematic reviews (4), participating via e-mail, contributing to discussion groups and bulletin boards, and Web publishing. It is this last activity and the Web surfing that has accompanied it that has driven the recent rapid growth in Internet activities (from barely 200 Web servers in September 1993 to more than 31 million in July 2001) (5). And, as we shall see, this development of the Web has led to innovative approaches to conducting the business of research.

To Discover the Secrets of the Web, *Click Here*

But what's so special about the Web? The functioning of a hypertext, the ability to easily link, in context, between documents on the Web, underpins its success (6). Hypertext itself is not new; the term was coined in the 1960s and the concept is widely credited to VanneBush's 1948 article *As we may think.* Hypertext was already a feature of the Macintosh computer in the 1980s (7). But it is in combination with the Internet that hypertext truly shines: "[H]ypertext and the Internet permit unlimited linkages to related and supplementary material" (8). Moreover, the hypertext links can stretch across the entire Internet, between documents on the same computer or between documents on different continents (4), and can link to text, graphics, video, sound, even software, or can be used to call other Internet services such as e-mail and

FTP (6). That the development of the NCSA Mosaic browser allowed graphics to be displayed in line with text (6) and that the basics of hypertext markup language (HTML), the language that tells a Web browser how to display a document, can be learned in a few minutes (9) have probably also contributed to the success of the Web.

Key Issues

Key issues for any form of academic information on the Internet must be privacy, security, quality, access and archiving.

The issues of privacy and security are probably outside the scope of this chapter, though there are obvious implications for the use of medical information and particularly clinical data. [Those interested in privacy and security issues related to the Internet should consult the CPSR's *Electronic Privacy Principles* (www.cpsr.org/program/privacy/privacy8.htm), the *Privacy Resource Center* of the Massachusetts Health Data Consortium (www.mahealthdata.org), and Lincoln Stein's *WWW Security FAQ* (www.w3.org/Security/Faq/www-security-faq.html).]

The quality of Internet-based medical information has probably been more widely considered than any other issue (10–13). Here, we should remember the distinction between evidence, which cites original studies or reviews in support of statements, and information, which may not (8). When considering quality of Web sites, however, we might also draw a distinction between content and design; the latter is arguably a question relating to access and is considered below. As Coiera has noted, the creation of information content for Web sites may be the largest single associated cost; higher quality may incur higher costs (14). In the short term, this may place those who provide high-quality information at a disadvantage, and certainly poor-quality health information can be found (15,16). Nevertheless, in the long term those who can establish a level of trust with their audience should be able to establish a brand identity (10).

In medicine the development of portal sites, such as Health on the Net (www.hon.ch) and Omni (http://omni.ac.uk) and their associated Web site evaluation criteria, e.g., The HON Code of Conduct (www.hon.ch/HONcode), have done much to drive awareness of quality issues, particularly with respect to content. Emerging key criteria are as follows:

- Authorship, which should be clearly indicated with credentials and affiliations
- Attribution, i.e., clear referencing of source materials and indication of copyright
- Disclosure of ownership, sponsorship, advertising, and privacy policies, and potential conflicts of interest
- Currency, the freshness of the information and frequency of updates, with clear indications of posting and updating dates (10,17).

In a study of 29 published rating tools and evaluation criteria for health-related Web sites, design and aesthetics were the second and sixth most frequently cited points (17). A strength of the Web, if used wisely, is the stability of the user interface (9). Operation of the browser is standard, using browser default colors and fonts for text and links that can ease navigation through what may be large and unfamiliar structures. Careful organization of materials within a site, with adequate navigation, in-context links, and search facilities can do much to allow users to find the information they need. Such is the perceived importance of these issues in oncology that in 2000 the US National Cancer Institute, as part of its Extraordinary Opportunities in Cancer Communication program, established its own site, Usability.gov, specifically to promote careful Web site design.

Finding the sites on the Web in the first place is a still larger issue of access. Sizing the Web is, for the moment, a constant struggle; any published estimate of its size will be out of date by the time you read it. A 1999 estimate of the size of the publicly indexable Web placed it at 800 million pages, or about 6 terabytes of information, with no search engine indexing more than about 16% of it (3). By July 2000, Cyveillance.com, a Washington, D.C. Internet consultancy, was reporting 2.1 billion unique, publicly available pages and predicting that the figure would double by Spring 2001 (18). Meanwhile, Search Engine Watch, reporting in August 2001, estimated that the search engine Google had indexed over 1 billion pages, and through a function of its programming, could actually find listings for an additional 300,000 pages that it had not indexed (19).

However, there still seems little reason to disregard Lawrence and Giles's 1999 estimate that only 6% of indexed pages are scientific or educational materials. As the electronic journal advocate Stevan Harnad has put it, "In the huge growth of the Internet the relative proportion of research use has shrunk to the size of the flea on the tail of the dog" (20). Even so, 6% of 4 billion is still 240 million pages; clearly searching skills will be important to the health professional and reliable, trusted sites will be important to the health consumer. But technical developments, such as field-specific search engines using novel search technologies and the development of the Extensible Markup Language (XML) to allow Web designers to incorporate machine-readable descriptions of page content into their pages will be increasingly important too (21).

Archiving is a particularly important access issue: Will we be able to retrieve tomorrow what we have found today? And how about 10, 50, 200 years from now? Anyone who has spent time surfing the Web will be familiar with broken links and "Error 404 - file not found" messages. For research purposes the long-term availability of electronically published materials is vital. With the oldest exclusively electronic journals in medicine barely 10 years old, real long-term access has still to be proven. Surveying URLs contained in some 270,977 articles held in the Research Index database, Lawrence et al. (22) in 2000 found that 23% of URLs in articles from the previous year were invalid, while this figure rose to over half (53%) of the URLs for articles from 1994. Organizations considering electronic publication must be aware of this issue at the outset of a project and make a commitment to archiving, ideally without changing URLs, the major cause of those broken links.

Underpinning all these issues is the question of cost. If increased quality increases cost then the Web may still be the best place to publish since once a site has been established the additional costs related to the publishing of new materials are small relative to those of producing a paper supplement or a new CD. In considering evidence-based healthcare, we may find that this potential to reduce information costs has powerful implications for changing medical practice, since uptake may be hampered by perceived costs (23).

THE EVIDENCE

The Web, and the Internet generally, therefore, has many features that make it particularly attractive for practitioners and proponents of evidence-based healthcare. New materials can be published and distributed cheaply, and existing materials can be similarly updated. Related materials from diverse sources can be linked together, and Web-mounted databases, search engines, and directories can provide access to journals, abstracts, collaborative tools and still more databases, search engines, and directories. Evidence-based healthcare has indeed spawned a minor industry in associated products with the Web as a major repository; Andrew Booth's site, *Netting the Evidence* (www.nettingtheevidence.org.uk/), has links to over 200 sites spread over four continents in several languages. Consequently, strategies for interrogating the Web to provide appropriate evidence for specific clinical questions have themselves become a major publishing exercise (24,25).

It is, however, becoming increasingly apparent that the Internet is, and should be, more than just another publishing system. The combination of global access, peer-to-peer communication and low additional costs for additional materials open up possibilities that have been previously unthinkable.

The Prerequisites of Evidence

The processes of planning, coordinating, recruiting, treating, analyzing, and reporting of clinical trials represent significant areas where the Internet offers real opportunities (26). Organizations such as the NCI and EORTC already maintain online directories of clinical trials. A commercial metaregister of controlled trials established at www.controlled-trials.com has accrued over 6,400 trials (27), while the U.S. National Institutes of Health's (NIH) trial register, http://clinicaltrials.gov, has details of some 5,700 trials. Online patient registration and randomization is being done (e.g., http://random.eortc.be/). Trials groups may already operate their own password-protected Web sites, so promoting communication, and data submission via the Internet to a single centralized database is possible. With the possibility of presenting questionnaires online and conducting follow-up communications by e-mail, conducting quality-of-life studies via the Internet may seem particularly attractive, but care must be taken not to exclude patients without the required Internet access (28). The reduced cost and space constraints associated with Web publishing also present an opportunity for extended protocol publication and review. *The Lancet* has, since 1997, offered electronic publication of summaries of randomized trial and systematic review protocols associated with published studies (29). This had led, by summer 2001, to the submission of some 150 protocols, of which 46 had been accepted for publication on *The Lancet*'s Web site (27). Meinert (30) has taken this idea further by proposing that authors unwilling or unable to publish their protocol on a Web site should have their published articles annotated to indicate this. The possibility to pre-publish protocols under development for extended peer review also exists, and Chalmers and Altman in 1998 described this as an opportunity for primary prevention of poor research.

The Web may also be a resource where previously unpublished data may be found for systematic reviews. Testing this hypothesis, Eysenbach and Diepgen (31) in 1999 modified the search strategies of eight Cochrane Systematic Reviews to incorporate Web searching. These modified strategies identified information on unpublished and ongoing trials relevant to four of the reviews.

Completely new materials have also been generated by the accessibility of the Internet, most notably, perhaps, online groups, often with strong patient involvement, and patient narrative sites, normally developed and maintained by individual patients. Certain advantages of online groups are immediately clear: They can draw together geographically dispersed individuals, individuals with limited mobility are not excluded, and rare disease groups can be formed. Physicians visiting or even using such groups may gain new perspectives on an illness from those most directly affected by it (32). The proliferation of patient experience sites can also offer different perspectives to physicians, while offering advice and support to fellow patients. See, for example, *Dave's Happy Little Hodgkins Web Site* (www.davesite.com/hodgkins/), Dave Kristula's account of his teenage encounter with Hodgkin's disease:

"I got Hodgkins from a curse, most people just get it because. But heck, now we are both in the same boat, so who cares how I got it, let's get to getting rid of it! I was diagnosed with Stage 2b (to my best knowledge) on March somethingith 1997 when I was 15."

Attempts to bring such information together include the Association of Cancer Online Resources (www.acor.org) and the Database of Individual Patient Experiences (www.dipex.org).

A Web of Journals

But even as we acknowledge that as a publishing system the Web has reduced the cost of entry into the information marketplace, we still recognize that its potential for use in academic publishing is unparalleled. Many journals are now available free online (see www.freemedicaljournals.com), and many more are available online to subscribers. In 1998 the *British Medical Journal* announced that it wished its electronic version, which currently has open and free access, to be considered the primary version (33). Published articles on the site contain links within articles from citations to references and links to Medline abstracts or online articles, where available, from references; in addition, articles citing the article are noted and linked to, as is related correspondence. As online journals move to rolling publication of electronic articles as they become available, with the increasing use of electronic supplementary materials, such as *The Lancet*'s protocol summaries, increasing numbers of us will use electronic versions of articles without reference to a paper edition.

The Internet also provides ways to speed the editorial process, from fully automated online processing of manuscripts from submission to final decision (see, for example, www.espere.org), to simple communication by e-mail. Even the production of paper journals can be accelerated using the Internet to distribute proofs to authors using Adobe's portable document (PDF) file format, which can preserve the appearance of the printed page when displayed by the Adobe Acrobat software.

The Internet Versus the File-drawer Effect

More radical solutions to the editorial process also present themselves. Freed from constraints of paper budgets and print runs, why not simply publish everything? Electronic archives of articles not formally peer reviewed already exist and function well in fields such as physics and computer science. The development of an electronic archive for medicine, if it could achieve some respect in the broader medical community, might help to redress the oft-noted publication bias of existing journals towards positive studies. In 1999, then U.S. NIH Director Harold Varmus proposed E-biomed, a biomedical publishing site on the Web that would allow "instantaneous, cost-free access . . . to E-biomed's entire content" (34). The proposal further called on commercial publishers and learned societies to contribute their journals to that entire content. In addition the possibility of publication within the system without full, formal peer review was foreseen. After a 2-month consultation period, during which strong opinions, both pro and contra, were expressed in many areas, the NIH announced that the site, now renamed PubMed Central, would start operation in January 2000 (35). The peer-review-free element remained intact but it was made clear that the responsibility for the non-peer-reviewed materials would be devolved to screening organizations. By summer of 2001 PubMed Central (www.pubmedcentral.nih.gov) had accrued fewer than ten print journals, plus the online journals of the commercial-but-free service Biomedcentral.com, with a further ten journals listed as "forthcoming." Whether such a system really can promote publication of useful but otherwise neglected materials remains to be seen. What is much clearer is that the development of PubMed Central has promoted debate about freedom of access to the scientific literature; more recently this has led to the non-profit Public Library of Science (www.publiclibraryofscience.org) calling, in an open letter, for scientists to support only those journals that have agreed to grant unrestricted free distribution rights to all original research they publish (36). At the time of writing this chapter, the letter had acquired more than 28,000 signatories from over 170 countries.

THE HEALTH CONSUMER

With all this material available or potentially available on the Internet, what are the consequences for health consumers? What are the consequences for real medical practice? Anecdotal evidence abounds; here a patient self-diagnoses from poor quality information and presents too late to a physician, there a patient finds an important piece of information unknown to his physician. But both scenarios are not specific to the Internet. Despite the wealth and variety of information available on the Internet, conclusions about positive or negative impacts on public health outcomes are hard to draw (14). A systematic review of the literature, including Medline, Embase, Psyinfo, Cinahl, and Healthstar, performed in April 2001 searching for evidence of harm caused by inaccurate information on the Internet identified only two articles that met the criteria of harm associated with inaccurate information (37). One of these described poisoning in dogs related to misinformation obtained on the Internet, and the other described a lung cancer patient who self-medicated with an unproved drug and died as a result (38).

Implicit in all this is our assumption that health consumers are everywhere on the Internet. Patients are contributing to support groups and forums, producing their own sites, searching for information in online journals and highly publicized commercial sites such as Drkoop.com and Medscape.com. It seems that we may really be heading towards an age of evidence-based patient choice and consumer health informatics in which health consumers' information needs are studied and met with real evidence-based information (38,40). Certainly there are formidable obstacles to be overcome, problems of lack of access, varying public levels of scientific and health literacy, the volume of poor-quality information already available, and perhaps even some reluctance or fear on the part of medical professionals. Physicians certainly do report feeling poorly prepared to cope with patients armed with information from the Internet (41,42). Even so, the fear is surely misplaced and misconstrues the role of the physician in evidence-based practice. Healthcare practices based on finding, critically appraising and applying evidence appropriately must welcome collaboration from patients in finding information, and we must acknowledge that critical appraisal and application will largely remain the preserve of professionals. Professionals must nevertheless take real steps to involve patients by education (43), engagement, and partnership (44). Tools that educate and help patients to make assessments about information quality are already appearing on the Internet (39,45), notably Quick (the Quality Information Checklist at www.quick.org.uk/) and Discern (www.discern.org.uk/), and more seem certain to appear as expertise in delivery and design of such tools increases.

Wake Up and Smell the Bouillabaisse!

Beginning this chapter with a consideration of where I began in the previous edition, I find that my conclusion from that edition needs reconsideration too:

> 'The Internet is a veritable bouillabaisse for finding information, with a huge and outrageously expanding pot, and you never know when you stick your fork in what tasty morsel or bit of fish debris you will stab' (8). And so it will remain.

The American Medical Association reports that 70% of U.S. physicians used the Web in 2000, up from 20% in 1997 and 37% in 1999 (46). Could it be that the tasty morsels are starting to win through?

REFERENCES

1. [CPSR] Computer Professionals for Social Responsibility. (1998) One-planet, one-net fact sheet #1, CPSR, www.cpsr.org/onenet/whatis.html, accessed 11 October 2001.
2. Sterling B. (1993) Short history of the Internet, www.forthnet.gr/forthnet/isoc/short.history.of.internet accessed 4 October 2001.
3. Lawrence S, Giles L. Accessibility of information on the web. *Nature* 1999;400:107–109.
4. Hersh W. (1996) Evidence-based medicine and the Internet, ACP Journal Club, www.acponline.org/journals/acpjc/julaug96/jcjedit.htm accessed 4 October 2001.
5. Zakon RH. (2001) Hobbes' Internet Timeline v5.4, www.zakon.org/robert/internet/timeline/, accessed 16 October 2001.
6. Pallen M. Guide to the internet: the world wide web. *BMJ* 1995;311:1552–1556.
7. Rockwell G. (1998) Hypertext Places, http://cheiron.humanities.mcmaster.ca/≈htp/ accessed October 2001.
8. Sackett DL, Richardson WS, Rosenberg W, Haynes RB. *Evidence-based medicine—How to practice and teach EBM*. Edinburgh: Churchill Livingstone, 1997.
9. Greenspun P. (1999) Philip and Alex's guide to web publishing, Academic Press/Morgan Kaufmann, San Diego (www.photo.net/wtr/thebook/ accessed at 4 October 2001).
10. Silberg WM, Lundberg GD, Musacchio RA. Assessing, controlling, and assuring quality of medical information on the internet. *JAMA* 1997;277:1244–1245.
11. Eysenbach G, Diepgen TL. Use of the World-Wide-Web to identify unpublished evidence for systematic reviews. *J Med Internet Res* 1999;1(suppl 1):e25 (www.jmir.org/1999/1/suppl1/e25/index.htm accessed 16 October 2001).
12. Shepperd S, Charnock D, Gann B. Helping patients access high quality health information. *BMJ* 1999;319:764–766 (www.bmj.com/cgi/content/short/319/7212/764 accessed 4 October 2001).
13. Lissman TL, Boehnlein JK. A critical review of Internet information about depression. *Psychiatr Serv* 2001;54:1046–1050.
14. Coiera E. Information epidemics, economics and immunity on the internet. *BMJ* 1998;317:1469–1470 (www.bmj.com/cgi/content/full/317/7171/1469 accessed 4 October 2001).
15. Bower H. Internet sees growth of unverified health claims. *BMJ* 1996;313:497.
16. Impicciatore P, Pandolfini C, Casella N, Bonati M. Reliability of health information for the public on the world wide web: systematic survey of advice on managing fever in children at home. *BMJ* 1997;314:1875–1879.
17. Kim P, Eng TR, Deering MJ, Maxfield A. Published criteria for evaluating health related web sites: review.

BMJ 1999;318:647–649 (www.bmj.com/cgi/content/full/318/7184/647 accessed 4 October 2001).
18. Murray BH, Moore A. Sizing the Internet. Cyveillance, Inc. Washington DC, 2000.
19. Sullivan D. The Search Engine Report, August 15, 2001, www.searchenginewatch.com/reports/sizes.html accessed 17 September 2001.
20. Harnad S. (1997) How to fast-forward learned serials to the inevitable and the optimal for scholars and scientists, http://cogprints.soton.ac.uk/documents/disk0/00/00/16/95/cog00001695–00/harnad97.learned.serials.html accessed 16 October 2001.
21. Butler D. Souped-up search engines. *Nature* 2000; 405:112–115.
22. Lawrence S, Coetzee F, Glover E, et al. Persistence of web references in scientific research. *IEEE Computer* 2001;34;26–31.
23. Coiera E. Information epidemics, economics and immunity on the internet. *BMJ* 1998;317:1469–1470 (www.bmj.com/cgi/content/full/317/7171/1469 accessed 4 October 2001).
24. O'Rourke A. (1999) Finding suitable web sites, www.shef.ac.uk/uni/projects/wrp/ebpsem1.html accessed 13 October 2001.
25. Wyatt JC, Vincent S. Selecting computer-based evidence sources. *Ann Oncol* 1999;10:267–273.
26. Mross K, Marz W. Clinical trials: prerequisite of evidence-based oncology: reality, perspectives and a new tool recruited—the Internet. *Onkologie* 2001;24(suppl 1):24–34.
27. McNamee D. Review of clinical protocols at The Lancet. *Lancet* 2001;357:1819.
28. Treadwell JR, Soetkino RM, Lenart LA. Feasibility of quality-of-life research on the Internet: a follow-up study. *Qual Life Res* 1999;8:743–747.
29. Chalmers I, Altman DG. How can medical journals help prevent poor medical research? Some opportunities presented by electronic publishing. *Lancet* 1999; 353:490–493.
30. Meinert CL. Beyond CONSORT: need to improve reporting standards for controlled trials. *JAMA* 1998; 279:1487–1489.
31. Eysenbach G, Diepgen TL. Towards quality management of medical information on the internet: evaluation, labelling, and filtering of information. *BMJ* 1998; 317:1496–1502 (www.bmj.com/cgi/content/short/317/7171/1496 accessed 13 October 2001).
32. Lamberg L. Online support groups help patients live with, learn more about the rare skin cancer CTCL-MF. *JAMA* 1997;277:1422–1423.
33. Delamothe T, Smith R. The BMJ's website scales up. *BMJ* 1998;316:1109–1110 (www.bmj.com/cgi/content/full/316/7138/1109 accessed 16 October 2001).
34. Varmus H. (1999) Original proposal for E-biomed (draft and addendum) E-biomed: a proposal for electronic publications in the biomedical sciences, NIH, www.nih.gov/welcome/director/pubmedcentral/ebiomedarch.htm accessed 4 October 2001.
35. [NIH] National Institutes of Health. (1999) PubMed Central: An NIH-operated site for electronic distribution of life sciences research reports,www.nih.gov/welcome/director/pubmedcentral/pubmedcentral.htm accessed 13 October 2001.
36. Roberts RJ, Varmus HE, Ashburner M, et al. Information access. Building a "GenBank" of the published literature. *Science* 2001;291:2318–2319.
37. Crocco AG, Villasis-Keever M, Jadad A. Much ado about "nothing"? Looking for evidence on harm resulting from health information on the internet, Fourth International Congress on Peer Review in Biomedical Publication, abstract, 2001.
38. Black M, Hussain H. Hydrazine, cancer, the Internet, isoniazid, and the liver. *Ann Intern Med* 2000;133: 911–913.
39. Eysenbach G. Consumer health informatics. *BMJ* 2000; 320:1713–1716 (www.bmj.com/cgi/content/full/320/7251/1713 accessed 4 October 2001).
40. Eysenbach G, Jadad AR. Evidence-based patient choice and consumer health informatics in the Internet age. *J Med Internet Res* 2001;2:e19 (www.jmir.org/2001/2/e19/index.htm accessed 16 October 2001).
41. Coiera E. The Internet's challenge to healthcare provision. *BMJ* 1996;312:3–4.
42. Wilson SM. Impact of the Internet on primary care staff in Glasgow. *J Med Internet Res* 1999;1:e7 (www.jmir.org/1999/2/e7 accessed 16 October 2001).
43. Glass RM, Molter J, Hwang MY. Providing a tool for physicians to educate patients. *JAMA* 1998;279: 1309.
44. Jadad A. Promoting partnerships: challenges for the internet age. *BMJ* 1999;319:761–764 (www.bmj.com/cgi/content/full/319/7212/761 accessed 4 October 2001).
45. Charnock D, Sheppard S, Needham G, Gann R. DISCERN: an instrument for judging the quality of written consumer health information on treatment choices. *J Epidemiol Community Health* 1999;53:105–111.
46. [AMA] American Medical Association. Study on physicians use of the World Wide Web. *AMA* Chicago, Illinois, 2001.

SECTION 2

Prevention and Screening

39
Breast Screening

Anthony B. Miller

It has been believed for some time that mass screening for breast cancer can reduce mortality from the disease (1,2). Both single-view mammography alone and double-view mammography combined with physical examination have been regarded as effective screening modalities. Current data are insufficient to determine whether appreciable extra benefit in terms of mortality reduction derives from adding physical examination to mammography. Until recently it was not clear whether mammography adds appreciable extra benefit to screening by high-quality breast physical examination, a question raised by the working group to review the uncontrolled U.S. Breast Cancer Detection Demonstration Projects (3). This question now appears to be resolved by the Canadian National Breast Screening Study (CNBSS) in women age 50 to 59 on entry to the study (4–7).

The evidence that has accrued to justify the above statements, and the recommendations for national screening programs that have resulted from them, has, almost uniquely to date for screening, been derived from large randomized phase 3 screening trials (level I, category A evidence). Despite this, it is clear that there is no uniform view in the interpretation of the data from these trials, not only regarding screening for women age 40 to 49 (8), but also for older women (9). As a result, different organizations have accepted different levels of evidence in making recommendations for screening. For example, the American Cancer Society guidelines for breast cancer detection are that every woman should be urged to practice breast self-examination every month from the age of 20, that women should have a breast physical examination every three years from the age of 20 and every year from the age of 40, and that mammography should be given every one to two years from age 40 to 49 and every year from the age of 50 (10). No randomized trial data exist that relate to screening women under the age of 40, and with respect to women over age 70, only one trial actually included women over age 69. In contrast, although also from the United States, their Preventive Services Task Force (11) did not recommend mammography screening for women age 40 to 49. To add to the confusion, the U.S. National Cancer Institute, after accepting that the scientific evidence did not confirm efficacy of screening in women age 40 to 49 (12), later reversed that position despite recommendations by a consensus conference (8).

Canada and several countries in Europe (e.g., Finland, the Netherlands, Sweden, the United Kingdom) have organized breast screening programs, all involving mammography screening for women age 50 to 64 (or 69) but only some counties in Sweden actively invite women age 40 to 49 for screening. The majority invite women to return every 2 years, but in the United Kingdom, every 3 years. It is still too early to judge the effectiveness of these programs. Although it seemed likely that mortality reductions attributable to screening would be seen in those countries where the programs have achieved the planned (70% or more) level of compliance within a few years, this has become complicated because mortality reductions attributable to improved therapy have been seen in several countries since 1990 (13,14).

In the following sections, the evidence that has accrued on screening in the various age groups 40 to 49, 50 to 69 and 70 or more will be reviewed together with the recent controversies, and implications for the future discussed.

SCREENING AT AGES 40 TO 49

The hypothesis that the efficacy of screening for women under 50 was less than for women age 50 to 69 was initially raised by the 5-year report of the Health Insurance Plan (HIP) trial, because there was no evidence that breast screening was effective in women age 40 to 49, though the evidence was strong for women age 50 to 69 (15). Subsequently, long-term follow-up of the HIP study suggested efficacy in younger women, commencing about 9 years after initiation of screening (16,17). However, the numbers of breast cancers detected by mammography screening in women age 40 to 49 on entry were low, and the main reason for an apparent reduction of mortality in this age group appears to be a poorer survival of stage I cancers in the control group of the trial than both the screen-detected cancers and the non-screen detected cancers in the study group (18).

Because of the HIP finding, subsequent trials also examined analytically the efficacy of screening in women age 40 to 49, though with the exception of the CNBSS (19), none of them had been specifically designed to evaluate this issue. The majority of these trials recruited women over the whole of the 40 to 49 age span, though two, Edinburgh and Malmö, only recruited women from the age of 45. The initial reports of these trials largely repeated the HIP experience, with no early effect of screening noted, but as women aged, benefit began to be seen. Table 39.1 lists the trials, the degree of benefit at the time of the most recent report, and the year the benefit began to be seen. The table includes the U.K. trial, though this is strictly a quasi-experimental study, only the Edinburgh component being randomized. The Edinburgh trial reports therefore replicate the findings of the U.K. trial in terms of the Edinburgh screened group and the Edinburgh control group is only reported in the Edinburgh trial reports.

With the exception of the Gothenburg trial, all trials showed delayed efficacy, raising the suspicion that the effect is the result of continuing to screen women beyond 50 (20), especially the Edinburgh and Malmö trials. Even for the Gothenburg trial (21), there is room for concern over the anomaly of more cancers ascertained in the control than the screened groups (22).

A report on the 11- to 16-year follow-up of the CNBSS in women age 40 to 49 is now pending. There is still no evidence of efficacy of using annual mammography plus physical examination versus usual care following a single physical examination (Miller, personal communication, March, 2002). There is, however,

TABLE 39.1. *Screening trials of women age 40 (45)–49*

Trial	Age range	Year benefit first seen	Latest year of follow up	RR (95% CI)	Reference
HIP	40–49	7	18	0.77 (na)[a]	Shapiro et al. (16)
Two-county	40–49	8	16	0.87 (0.54–1.41)	Tabar et al. (61)
Malmö	45–49	7	17	0.64 (0.45–0.89)	Andersson & Janzon (46)
Stockholm	40–49	10	12	1.08 (0.54–2.17)	Frisell & Lidbrink (65)
Gothenburg	39–49	5	11	0.56 (0.31–0.99)	Bjurstam et al. (20)
Edinburgh	45–49	7	14	0.75 (0.48–1.18)[b]	Alexander et al. (42)
UK "Trial"	45–49	7	16	0.70 (0.57–0.86)	U.K. Trial of early . . . (38)
CNBSS-1	40–49	—	11–16	1.06 (0.80, 1.40)[c]	Miller et al. (22)

[a]Not available.
[b]Adjusted for socio-economic status.
[c]Adjusted for interval mammograms.

TABLE 39.2. Overview and meta-analyses of screening trials, women age 40–49

Author and year	Trials	Period	RR (95% CI)
Larsson et al. (24)	Swedish	12.8 years	0.77 (0.59–1.01)
Cox (25)	All 7[a]	10 years	0.93 (0.77–1.11)
Glasziou & Irwig (27)	All 7[a]	to 1996	0.85 (0.71–1.01)
Kerlikowske (30)	All 7[a]	7–9 years	1.02 (0.82–1.27)
		10–14 years	0.84 (0.71–0.99)
Hendrick et al. (28)	Swedish	to 1997	0.71 (0.57–0.89)
	All 7[a]	Average 12.7 years	0.82 (0.71–0.95)

[a]Not including the U.K. Trial. Hendrick et al. (28) counted the Swedish two county trial as two trials.

evidence of over-diagnosis of mammography-detected cancers when *in situ* cancers are included, amounting to more than 70% of those detected by mammography alone.

An overview analysis of the results of the Swedish trials has been reported (23) and updated (24), and meta-analyses of all trials have been performed and updated (25–31). These are summarized in Table 39.2. Only that of Kerlikowske et al. (29) and Kerlikowske (30) specifically addressed the issue of the time after initiation of screening that the effect was noted. In the analysis of Kerlikowske et al., the OR for 7 to 9 years follow-up was 1.02, and for 10 or more years, 0.84. The results of these meta-analyses are similar, but not identical, which is of interest given that they were all performed largely using the same data. Some of the differences relate to different time periods, e.g., that of Cox (25) was restricted to the first 10 years of follow-up. In addition, the methods used to combine the data varied. This is most strikingly seen for the analysis of Hendrick et al. (28), which produced the greatest estimate of reduction from all seven trials, and a larger estimate of effect for the Swedish trials than Larsson et al. (24), even though both authors presumably had the same or very similar data.

It is unlikely that further follow-up of any of the trials listed in Table 39.1 will solve the question of whether the delayed effect in women age 40 to 49 is due to screening after the age of 50. A trial has however been initiated in the United Kingdom, recruiting women age 40 to 41, and randomizing them to annual mammography screening for 7 years or unscreened control in a ratio of 1:2. When participants in both the screened and control groups reach age 50, they will be included in the U.K. National Programme. No results are expected from this trial until at least 2005. A similar trial planned for various other countries in Europe, the Eurotrial 40, has not been funded.

The studies that have evaluated the cost-effectiveness of screening women age 40 to 49 have invariably concluded that the cost-effectiveness is less than for screening women over the age of 50 (19,32,33). There are three reasons for this: the lower incidence and detection rates in younger women, a lesser degree of effect and the delay in the effect being seen. However, it seems likely that this differential would be less if screening was initiated at the age of 45.

Some observational data provide evidence for the efficacy of breast self-examination (BSE) in this age group. Two case-control studies have shown no overall benefit in the reduction of advanced disease (34,35), but one suggested benefit in BSE compliers (35). A cohort study of BSE compliers in Finland suggested a benefit in reducing breast cancer mortality (36), as did a case-control study nested within the CNBSS which showed benefit from good BSE practice in reducing breast cancer mortality and the cumulative prevalence of advanced (metastatic) breast cancer (37). The U.K. quasi-experimental study showed no reduction in breast cancer mortality in the BSE centres compared to the control though the proportion of women who attended the BSE classes was low in each area (38). There are two trials of BSE ongoing, one in Russia (39) and one in China (40). Neither have yet reached the stage of follow-up at which change in breast cancer mortality would be expected.

No randomized trial data relating to the efficacy of physical examinations of the breast exist, though there is some evidence that it may be helpful (41).

SCREENING AT AGES 50 TO 69

The HIP trial showed screening effectiveness with the combination of mammography plus physical examination annually in women age 50 to 64 on entry to the trial (14,15). This trial has been criticized by Gotzsche and Olsen (8) largely on the basis of an inequality in the numbers of breast cancers identified as being diagnosed and excluded prior to randomization with greater exclusions in the screened arm. This differential occurred because when those in the screened group attended for screening, previously diagnosed breast cancers were identified, but this was not possible for the controls. However, the process of follow-up over 18 years enabled all deaths from breast cancer to be identified comparably in both arms, and then it was possible to determine the date of diagnosis by collecting the relevant hospital records. Those diagnosed before randomization were then excluded. Although this process did not eliminate the inequality in the numbers of previously diagnosed breast cancer patients still living at 18 years, the small differential in person years of observation is very unlikely to have biased the results. Therefore I conclude that the results from this trial are valid, though they reflect an era when breast screening was applied with much larger numbers of large breast cancers being treated than now occurs, and an era when adjuvant chemotherapy and hormone therapy was not available. Therefore, their relevance to the present day is in doubt.

This effect of combined screening was later confirmed by the U.K. studies (38,42), and a case-control study in the Netherlands (43). The inference that mammography alone could replicate this benefit was confirmed by several Swedish trials, and case-control studies in Florence (44) and in the Netherlands (45), and further confirmed by the Swedish overview analysis (23). The trials of breast screening in this age group are summarized in Table 39.3. Updated data are not yet available for the Malmö and Stockholm trials, and have not yet been published for the Gothenburg trial, but are included in the Nyström et al. (23) overview analysis. Interestingly, there is some evidence of lesser effectiveness at age 50 to 54 than at older ages. This was first seen in one of the case-control studies in the Netherlands (43), is suggested by comparing the data for women age 39 to 49 for Gothenburg (20) with that published in the Swedish overview analysis for ages 40 to 59 (23) and is again suggested for Malmö by comparing the data published by Andersson et al. (46) for women age 45 to 54 with those later reported by Andersson and Janzon (47) for

TABLE 39.3. Screening trials of women age 50–69

Trial	Age range	Year benefit first seen	Latest year of follow-up	RR (95% CI)	Reference
HIP	50–64	3	18	0.68 (0.49–0.96)	Shapiro et al. (15)
Two-county	50–59	5	14	0.66 (0.46–0.93)	Tabar et al. (61)
	60–69	6	14	0.60 (0.42–0.82)	
Malmö	55–69	8	10	0.79 (0.51–1.24)	Andersson et al. (46)
Stockholm	50–64	2	7	0.57 (0.3–1.1)	Frisell et al. (66)
All Swedish trials	50–59	3	12	0.72 (0.58–0.90)	Nyström et al. (23)
	60–69	3	12	0.69 (0.54–0.88)	
Edinburgh	50–54	na[a]	14	0.99 (0.62–1.58)[b]	Alexander et al. (42)
	55–59	na	14	0.65 (0.43–0.99)[b]	
	60–64	na	14	0.80 (0.51–1.25)[b]	
U.K. "Trial"	50–54	10	16	0.79 (0.62–1.00)	UK Trial of Early . . . (38)
	55–59	6	16	0.71 (0.56–0.90)	
	60–64	8	16	0.72 (0.56–0.92)	
CNBSS-2	50–59	—	13	1.02 (0.78–1.33)	Miller et al. (6)

[a]Not available.
[b]Adjusted for socio-economic status.

women age 45 to 49. This was also seen in the Edinburgh trial (42), and to a lesser extent in the U.K. Trial as a whole (38). The published results of the Edinburgh and U.K. Trials do not provide RRs for the whole age group 50 to 64, but for the age group 45 to 64 the RRs were 0.79 (95% CI 0.60 to 1.02) (42) (adjusted for socio-economic status) and 0.73 (95% CI 0.63 to 0.84) (38), respectively.

Because there has been far less controversy as to the efficacy of screening women age 50 to 69, there have been far fewer meta-analyses than for screening women age 40 to 49. However, Kerlikowske et al. (29) reported an RR of 0.74 (95% CI 0.66 to 0.83) for all studies, with almost identical effects for 7 to 9 years (0.73, 95% CI 0.63 to 0.84) as for 10 to 12 years follow-up (0.76, 95% CI 0.67 to 0.87).

Controversy arose when Gotzsche and Olsen (8) published their review. Basically they concluded that all the trials that showed evidence of benefit were biased, except possibly for the Malmö trial, and that there was no reliable evidence for the effectiveness of breast screening at any age. Several have disputed this conclusion (48–53), with the main rebuttal being that the effect of the imbalances Gotzsche and Olsen observed is too small to abolish the beneficial effect of screening. Having already commented on the HIP trial, it is also worth noting that the acknowledged imbalance in the cluster-randomized Edinburgh trial, when corrected for, strengthened the evidence in favor of screening mammography. Perhaps most attention needs to be given to the Swedish two-county trial, which is relatively dominant in the Swedish overview analysis. Gotzsche and Olsen pointed out that there is evidence of imbalance in this cluster-randomized trial. Duffy and Tabar (48) maintained that this effect was likely to be small, and claimed that the analyses performed of all cause mortality by Gotzsche and Olsen were not valid. Further, when a separate analysis was performed taking careful note of the cluster randomization, the beneficial effect of screening was still seen (54). In other words, a cluster-randomized trial has to be analyzed according to its design. However, there is one possible imbalance that could be critical, of which there has been too little consideration. The controls in the two-county trial were only identified through the population register, they were not aware they were part of a trial. In contrast, the screened group was invited to attend special centres for screening, and 90% did so. The breast cancers that occurred in the screened group were largely managed at these special centres, and almost certainly, if stage II or more, would have received adjuvant therapy, only then being introduced in Sweden. The women who developed breast cancer in the control group would not have received specialized management, and it is likely that most did not receive adjuvant therapy. Therefore the differential in breast cancer mortality that eventually emerged could largely be due to the differential application of adjuvant therapy. This possibility must be evaluated before we can regain confidence in the results of the Swedish two-county trial.

An intriguing aspect of the results of the trials comparing screening with no screening (i.e., all except CNBSS-2 in Table 39.3), is the failure of the more recent studies using more modern mammography to demonstrate a larger breast cancer mortality reduction than in the HIP trial, in spite of greater compliance levels. There is some evidence, using surrogate indicators of efficacy, that double view mammography performs better than the single view mammography used in the majority of the early Swedish trials (55). However, that cannot be the whole explanation. The HIP trial used the combination of 1960s mammography with good physical examinations. Much of the benefit in that trial was attributable to the earlier detection of advanced cases, probably due as much to the physical examinations as to mammography (56). With the improvement in mammography, many, but not all, of the cancers detected by physical examination but missed by mammography in the HIP era are picked up by modern mammography, and the benefit of mammography alone is probably due to their detection. However, this does not tell us how much mammography adds to good physical examination (3).

CNBSS-2 was designed to provide an answer to this question. Thus, in women age 50 to 59, the primary objective of CNBSS-2 was to determine the additional contribution of routine annual mammography screening to screening by physical examination alone. Screening with yearly mammography in addition to physical examination detected considerably more node-negative and small breast cancers than screening with physical examination alone, but had no impact on mortality from breast cancer in the first 7 years from entry (5), even though mammography screening achieved its anticipated performance parameters (57,58). Nevertheless, the confidence intervals around this estimate of no effect were wide at seven years, and an effect of the order seen in the other trials could not be excluded. However, after a follow-up period that ranges from 11 to 16 years from entry, the numbers of events have more than doubled, and there is still no evidence of a breast cancer mortality reduction in the mammography-containing arm compared to those screened by physical examination and the teaching and reinforcement of BSE (13). This trial is not comparable to the trials evaluating screening compared to no screening. It does, however, reinforce the suggestion that the benefit derived from mammography alone is due to the earlier detection and treatment of palpable breast cancers, not the impalpable cancers as many have assumed.

As to the effect of BSE itself, all the evidence to date is observational, and is as reviewed above for those women age 40 to 49.

Most studies of the cost-effectiveness of screening for breast cancer have been made to compare screening among women age 40 to 49 and those age 50 to 69, although some have assessed different frequencies of rescreening (59,60). The studies that have assessed different frequencies of re-screening have tended to assume a similar degree of efficacy. This seems inherently unlikely, though the conclusion that the marginal benefit of annual screening versus two yearly, or two-yearly versus three-yearly may be small is probably correct. A UK trial is underway assessing different frequencies of screening (annual versus 3-yearly), though it uses surrogate indicators of benefit to estimate the effect, not mortality reduction.

SCREENING AT AGES 70 OR MORE

Only the Swedish two-county trial included women over the age of 70 (70 to 74), and only invited them to screening once, as the compliance was much lower than for younger women. After 14 years the RR in this age group was 0.79 (95% CI 0.51 to 1.22) (61).

There is no agreement as to whether women over the age of 70 should be screened. There is no evidence to suggest a lesser level of effectiveness in this age group than for those age 60 to 69 assuming a similar compliance with screening. However, there is clear evidence that compliance drops off with increasing age, and therefore it is quite likely that the population impact of screening at ages older than 70 will be small. Thus no program currently actively recruits women into screening over the age of 70, though, at least in North America, women who attend for screening over the age of 70 are not turned away. The same types of decisions are made in terms of cessation of screening for women age 69. There is evidence that the lead time gained from screening is longer for older women, thus even if screening stops at the age of 69, there will continue to be benefit well into their 70s. Therefore in most programs women are not re-invited from the age of 69 (some from the age of 65 in Europe).

A model-based evaluation of the relative effect of extending screening to an older age compared to changing the frequency of rescreening relative to the United Kingdom has been made (59). This suggests that it would be more cost-effective to increase the age range screened than to increase the frequency of re-screening from every 3 years to every 2 years.

DISCUSSION

Using the standard criteria, if the conclusions of Gotzsche and Olsen (8) are ignored, it may be concluded that there is level 1 evidence for the efficacy of mammography screening for the age group ages 50 to 69. The majority of studies have shown an early benefit of combined screening with mammography and physical examination or of mammography alone, though the evidence is strongest for those age 55 to 64 on initiation of screening.

For women age 40 to 49 the evidence is still at level 1, but the interpretation is less certain, largely because of the greater delay to evidence of effect, and the suspicion that at least some of the apparent benefit is due to continuing screening beyond 50. The NIH Consensus Panel (7) discussed the various issues other than economic, in some depth, that led to their recommendation that in this age group currently available data does not warrant universal recommendation of mammography for all women in their forties. Berry (62) later provided some of the statistical underpinning for such a conclusion.

It has often been assumed that the improvement in mammography quality in the last decade or so must inevitably result in a greater degree of benefit. However, Kerlikowske et al. (63) have demonstrated the variability that exists in mammography interpretation, suggesting that the improvement in mammography quality is not being reflected in greater diagnostic efficiency. Further, the cancer-detection rates reported for breast screening programs in the 1990s seem to be no better than from the randomized trials of the 1980s. For example, Wald et al. (55) reported a cancer detection rate at the first screen for women age 50 to 64 with two-view mammography of 6.84 per 1,000. This compares with the CNBSS-2 rate at first screen for women age 50 to 59 of 7.20 per 1,000. Major improvements in results, therefore may have to await improved technology.

The evidence in support of other modalities of screening is far less than for mammography. So far, breast self-examination has only level 3 evidence in support of its efficacy. Evidence in support of breast physical examination is even more indirect. However, the CNBSS-2 findings suggest another viable option for screening women over the age of 50. This option may prove to be of substantial interest in countries where breast cancer is an increasing problem, but where mammography services are almost nonexistent. Nevertheless, it has to be emphasized that the physical examinations performed in the CNBSS involve far more skilled attention to relatively minor signs than those often rather casually performed by health care workers who have not been trained to recognize the signs of minimal breast cancer. The protocol for physical examinations and the teaching of breast self-examination has been fully described by Bassett (64). Currently, the only breast screening program which uses this method is the Ontario Breast Screening Program, which, significantly, has similar cancer detection rates for women age 50 to 59 on initial examination as for CNBSS-2.

The recent declines in breast cancer mortality in the United Kingdom, Canada, and the United States, with lesser declines in other countries including Sweden, suggest that the widespread application of adjuvant chemotherapy and hormone therapy, which occurred before breast screening programs were introduced, has had a very important population impact. It is unclear at present whether there will be additional reductions from the breast screening programs. On present evidence, it is also unclear whether a differential effect of therapy in the two-county trial in Sweden accounts for the benefit seen in that trial. If so, it is likely that the anticipated population impact of screening will turn out to be much less than has been anticipated in the planning for these programs.

REFERENCES

1. Day NE, Baines CJ, Chamberlain J, et al. UICC project on screening for cancer: Report of the workshop on screening for breast cancer. *Int J Cancer* 1986;38:303–308.
2. Miller AB, Chamberlain J, Day NE, et al. Report on a workshop of the UICC project on evaluation of screening for cancer. *Int J Cancer* 1990;46:761–769.
3. Beahrs O, Shapiro S, Smart C. Report of the working group to review the National Cancer Institute American Cancer Society Breast Cancer Detection Demonstration Projects. *J Natl Cancer Inst* 1979;62:640–709.
4. Miller AB, Howe GR, Wall C. The National Study of Breast Cancer Screening: protocol for a Canadian randomized controlled trial of screening for breast cancer in women. *Clin Invest Med* 1981;4:227–258.
5. Miller AB, Baines CJ, To T, et al. Canadian National Breast Screening Study 2. Breast cancer detection and death rates among women aged 50 to 59 years. *Can Med Assoc J* 1992;147:1477–1488.

6. Miller AB, To T, Baines CJ, Wall C. Canadian National Breast Screening Study-2: 13-year results of a randomized trial in women age 50–59 years. *J Natl Cancer Inst* 2000;92:1490–1499.
7. Miller AB, To T, Baines CJ, Wall C. The Canadian National Breast Screening Study: Update on breast cancer mortality. *Monogr Natl Cancer Inst* 1997;22:37–41.
8. National Institutes of Health Consensus Development Panel. Consensus statement. *Monogr Natl Cancer Inst* 1997;22:vii–xviii.
9. Gotzsche PC, Olsen O. Is screening for breast cancer with mammography justifiable? *Lancet* 2000;355:129–134.
10. Mettlin C, Smart CR. Breast cancer detection guidelines for women aged 40–49 years: rationale for the American Cancer Society reaffirmation of recommendations. *Ca* 1994;44:248–255.
11. Preventive Services Task Force. Guide to clinical preventive services. (Washington, DC, Department of Health and Human Services) 1989:26–31.
12. Kaluzny AD, Rimer B, Harris R. The National Cancer Institute and guideline development: lessons from the breast cancer screening controversy. *J Natl Cancer Inst* 1994;86:901–903.
13. Blanks RG, Moss SM, McGahan CE, et al. Effect of NHS breast screening programme on mortality from breast cancer in England and Wales, 1990–8: comparison of observed with predicted mortality. *BMJ* 2000; 321:665–669.
14. Miller AB. Effect of screening programme on mortality from Breast cancer. Benefit of 30% may be substantial overestimate. *Br Med J* 2000;321:1527.
15. Shapiro S, Strax P, Venet L. Periodic breast cancer screening in reducing mortality from breast cancer. *JAMA* 1971;215:1777–1785.
16. Shapiro S, Venet W, Strax P, Venet L. *Periodic screening for breast cancer. The Health Insurance Plan Project and its sequelae, 1963–1986.* Baltimore: The Johns Hopkins University Press, 1988.
17. Shapiro S. Periodic screening for breast cancer: the HIP randomized controlled trial. Health Insurance Plan. *J Natl Cancer Inst Monogr* 1997;22:27–30.
18. Miller AB. Is routine mammography screening appropriate for women 40–49 years of age? *Am J Prev Med* 1991;7:55–62.
19. Miller AB, Baines CJ, To T, et al. Canadian National Breast Screening Study 1. Breast cancer detection and death rates among women aged 40 to 49 years. *Can Med Assoc J* 1992a;147:1459–1476. [Published erratum appears in *Can Med Ass J* 1993;148:718]
20. de Koning HJ, van Ineveld BM, van Oortmarssen GJ, et al. Breast cancer screening and cost-effectiveness; policy alternatives, quality of life considerations and the possible impact of uncertain factors. *Int J Cancer* 1991;49:531–537.
21. Bjurstam N, Björneld L, Duffy SW, et al. The Gothenburg breast screening trial. First results on mortality, incidence and mode of detection for women ages 39–49 years at randomization. *Cancer* 1997;80:2091–2099.
22. Miller AB, Baines CJ, To T. The Gothenburg Breast Screening Trial. First results on mortality, incidence and mode of detection for women ages 39–49 years at randomization. *Cancer* 1998;83:186–188.
23. Nyström L, Rutqvist LE, Wall S, et al. Breast cancer screening with mammography: overview of Swedish randomized trials. *Lancet* 1993;341:973–978.
24. Larsson L-G, Andersson I, Bjurstam N, et al. Updated overview of the Swedish randomized trials on breast cancer screening with mammography: Age group 40–49 at randomization. *Monogr Natl Cancer Inst* 1997; 22:57–61.
25. Cox B. Variation in the effectiveness of breast screening by year of follow-up. *Monogr Natl Cancer Inst* 1997; 22:69–72.
26. Glasziou PP, Woodward AJ, Mahon CM. Mammographic screening trials for women aged under age 50. A quality assessment and meta-analysis. *Med J Aust* 1995;162:625–629.
27. Glasziou P, Irwig L. The quality and interpretation of mammographic screening trials for women ages 40–49. *Monogr Natl Cancer Inst* 1997;22:73–77.
28. Hendrick RE, Smith RA, Rutledge JH, Smart CR. Benefit of screening mammography in women aged 40–49: A new meta-analysis of randomized controlled trials. *Monogr Natl Cancer Inst* 1997;22:87–92.
29. Kerlikowske K, Grady D, Rubin SM, et al. Eficacy of screening mammography. *JAMA* 1995;273:149–154.
30. Kerlikowske K. Efficacy of screening mammography among women aged 40 to 49 years and 50 to 69 years: Comparison of relative and absolute benefit. *Monogr Natl Cancer Inst* 1997;22:79–86.
31. Smart CR, Hendrick RE, Rutledge JH III, Smith RA. Benefit of mammography screening in women ages 40 to 49 years. Current evidence from randomized controlled trials. *Cancer* 1995;75:1619–1626. (Published erratum appears in *Cancer* 1995;75:2788.)
32. Eddy DM, Hasselblad V, McGivney W, et al. The value of mammography screening in women under age 50 years. *JAMA* 1988;259:1512–1519.
33. Salzmann P, Kerlikowske K, Phillips K. Cost-effectiveness of extending screening mammography guidelines to include women age 40 to 49 years of age. *Ann Intern Med* 1997;127:955–965.
34. Muscat JE, Huncharek MS. Breast self-examination and extent of disease: A population-based study. *Cancer Detect Prev* 1991;15:155–159.
35. Newcomb PA, Weiss NS, Storer BE, et al. Breast self-examination in relation to the occurrence of advanced breast cancer. *J Natl Cancer Inst* 1991;83:260–265.
36. Gastrin G, Miller AB, To T, et al. Incidence and mortality from breast cancer in the Mama Program for breast screening in Finland, 1973–1986. *Cancer* 1994; 73:2168–2174.
37. Harvey BJ, Miller AB, Baines CJ, Corey PN. Effect of breast self-examination techniques on the risk of death from breast cancer. *Can Med Assoc J* 1997;157:1205–1212.
38. UK Trial of early detection of breast cancer group. 16-year mortality from breast cancer in the UK trial of early detection of breast cancer. *Lancet* 1999;353: 1909–1914.
39. Semiglazov VF, Sagaidak VN, Moiseyenko VM, Mikhailov EA. Study of the role of breast self-examination in the reduction of mortality from breast cancer: The Russian Federation/World Health Organization Study. *Eur J Cancer* 1993;29A:2039–2046.
40. Thomas DB, Gao DL, Self SG, et al. Randomized trial of breast self-examination in Shanghai: Methodology and preliminary results. *J Natl Cancer Inst* 1997;89: 355–365.

41. Baines CJ, Miller AB. Mammography versus clinical examination of the breasts. *Monogr Natl Cancer Inst* 1997;22:125–129.
42. Alexander FE, Anderson TJ, Brown HK, et al. 14 years of follow-up from the Edinburgh randomised trial of breast-cancer screening. *Lancet* 1999;353:1903–1908.
43. Collette HJA, Day NE, Rombach JJ, de Waard F. Evaluation of screening for breast cancer in a non-randomized study (the Dom project) by means of a case-control study. *Lancet* 1984;i:1224–1226.
44. Palli D, del Turco R, Buiatti E, et al. A case-control study of the efficacy of a non-randomized breast cancer screening program in Florence (Italy). *Int J Cancer* 1986;38:501–504.
45. Verbeek ALM, Hendriks JHCL, Holland R, et al. Mammographic screening and breast cancer mortality: Age-specific effects in Nijmegen project, 1975–82. *Lancet* 1985;i:865–866.
46. Andersson I, Aspergren K, Janzon L, et al. Mammographic screening and mortality from breast cancer: The Malmö mammographic screening trial. *Br Med J* 1988;297:943–948.
47. Andersson I, Janzon L. Reduced breast cancer mortality in women under age 50: Updated results from the Malmö mammographic screening program. *Monogr Natl Cancer Inst* 1997;22:63–67.
48. Duffy SW, Tabar L. Screening mammography re-evaluated. *Lancet* 2000;355:747–748.
49. Moss S, Blanks R, Quinn MJ. Screening mammography re-evaluated. *Lancet* 2000;355:748.
50. Nyström L. Screening mammography re-evaluated. *Lancet* 2000;355:748–749.
51. Hayes C, Fitzpatrick P, Daly L, Buttimer J. Screening mammography re-evaluated. *Lancet* 2000;355:749.
52. Law M, Hacksaw A, Wald N. Screening mammography re-evaluated. *Lancet* 2000;355:749–750.
53. Cates C, Senn S. Screening mammography re-evaluated. *Lancet* 2000;355:750.
54. Nixon RM, Prevost TC, Duffy SW, et al. Some random-effects models for the analysis of matched-cluster randomised trials: application to the Swedish two-county trial of breast cancer screening. *J Epidemiol Biostat* 2000;5:349–358.
55. Wald NJ, Murphy P, Major P, et al. UKCCCR multicentre randomized trial of one- and two-view mammography in breast cancer screening. *Br Med J* 1995;311:1189–1193.
56. Miller AB. Mammography: A critical evaluation of its role in breast cancer screening, especially in developing countries. *J Publ Health Policy* 1989;10:486–498.
57. Fletcher SW, Black W, Harris R, et al. Report of the International Workshop on Screening for Breast Cancer. *J Natl Cancer Inst* 1993;85:1644–1656.
58. Narod SA. Re: Canadian National Breast Screening Study-2: 13-year results of a randomized trial in women aged 50–59 years. *J Natl Cancer Inst* 2001;93:396.
59. Boer R, de Koning H, Threlfall A, et al. Cost effectiveness of shortening the screening interval or extending age range of NHS breast screening programme: computer simulation study. *Br Med J* 1998;317:376–379.
60. Woodman CBJ, Threlfall AG, Boggis CRM, Prior P. Is the three year breast screening interval to long? Occurrence of interval cancers in NHS breast screening programme's north western region. *Br Med J* 1995;310:224–226.
61. Tabar L, Fagerberg G, Chen H-H, et al. Efficacy of breast screening by age. New results from the Swedish two-county trial. *Cancer* 1995;75:2501–2517.
62. Berry DA. Benefits and risks of screening mammography for women in their forties: a statistical appraisal. *J Natl Cancer Inst* 1998;90:1431–1439.
63. Kerlikowske K, Grady D, Barclay J, et al. Variability and accuracy in mammographic interpretation using the American College of radiology breast imaging reporting and data system. *J Natl Cancer Inst* 1998;90:1801–1809.
64. Bassett AA. Physical examination of the breast and breast self-examination. In: Miller AB, ed. *Screening for Cancer.* Orlando, FL: Academic Press, 1995:271–291.
65. Frisell J, Lidbrink E. The Stockholm mammographic screening trial: Risks and benefit in age group 40–49 years. *Monogr Natl Cancer Inst* 1997;22:49–51.
66. Frisell J, Eklund G, Hellstrom L, et al. Randomized study of mammography screening—preliminary report on mortality in the Stockholm trial. *Breast Cancer Res Treat* 1991;18:49–56.

40

Chemoprevention Studies in Italy and the United Kingdom

Andrea Decensi, Jack Cuzik, and Umberto Veronesi

TAMOXIFEN STUDIES

As follow-up continues, and more events are observed, the initial differences between the NSABP P1 trial (1) and two European trials have become less evident (2,3). More importantly, the initial results of the International Breast Cancer Intervention Study (IBIS) I trial as they were presented in a preliminary report (4) indicate the efficacy of tamoxifen in reducing the incidence of breast cancer in at-risk women based on family history.

The Italian Study

The Italian study was a multicenter, double-blind, placebo-controlled chemoprevention trial, initiated in October 1992, to evaluate the effect of a daily dose of 20 mg oral tamoxifen for 5 years, on the prevention of breast cancer in healthy women (2). Eligible subjects were healthy women aged 35 to 70 years old who had prior hysterectomy for nonmalignant conditions and the primary endpoint of this study is the incidence of breast cancer. Recruitment was stopped on December 31, 1997 with 5,408 women randomized. The updated results of the Italian study after a median of 81 months have recently been published (2). At a mean observation time of 81 months, a 25% reduction of breast cancer was noted in the tamoxifen arm compared with placebo (45 versus 34 events, HR = 0.75, 95% CI 0.48–1.18). While there is no difference in the subset of women who never took HRT before or during the trial (HR = 1.01, 95% CI 0.60–1.70), women who had ever taken HRT at some point before or during the study (n = 1,584) had fewer breast cancers in the tamoxifen arm (six on tamoxifen versus 17 on placebo, HR = 0.35, 95% CI 0.14–0.89). Among the women continuously on HRT during the trial (n = 754), breast cancer events were three on tamoxifen versus 11 on placebo, respectively (HR = 0.30, 95% CI 0.08–1.06). Importantly, 76.9% of HRT users received transdermal unopposed ERT and further 6.5% took transdermal ERT combined with progestins.

The Royal Marsden Trial

An updated analysis of the Royal Marsden pilot prevention trial has also been published within a meta-analysis of all prevention trials with SERMs (5). In the Marsden study, 2,494 healthy women, aged between 30 and 70 at increased risk of breast cancer because of family history were accrued between 1986 and 1996. Each participant had at least one first-degree relative aged under 50 with breast cancer, or one first-degree relative with bilateral breast cancer, or one affected first-degree relative of any age plus another first-degree or second-degree relative. Women with a history of benign breast biopsy who had a first-degree relative with breast cancer were also eligible. They were randomized in a double blind fashion to receive tamoxifen 20 mg a day or placebo for up to 8 years. The primary endpoint was the occurrence of breast cancer.

In the initial report after a median follow-up of 70 months, when the study had adequate power to detect a 50% reduction of breast cancer in the tamoxifen arm, the results demonstrated the same overall frequency of breast cancer in both arms (tamoxifen 34, placebo 36, RR 1.06 [95% CI 0.7–1.7], $p = 0.8$) (3). Interestingly, women who were already on HRT (mostly using the oral route) when they entered the trial showed an increased risk of breast cancer compared with non-users, while the subjects who started HRT while on trial had a significantly reduced risk. However, no interaction was noted between ever use of HRT and any tamoxifen effect on breast cancer occurrence. There were 12 cancers in the 523 ever users of HRT (mostly started HRT during the study) on tamoxifen compared with 13 of 507 HRT ever users on placebo. The occurrence of severe adverse events was low. There were four cases of endometrial cancer in the tamoxifen arm versus one in the placebo arm and seven cases versus four of DVT and pulmonary embolism. Importantly, there were 18 cases of menstrual abnormalities in the tamoxifen arm and six in the placebo arm, indicating that tamoxifen can safely be administered to HRT users with a low rate of bleeding complications.

The updated analysis refers to a median of months. There is now a 10% reduction in the incidence of breast cancer in the tamoxifen arm compared with placebo (5).

The International Breast Intervention Study (IBIS) Trial

In the IBIS trial (4), 7,134 women age 35 to 70 at an increased risk for breast cancer were recruited, ranging from a two-fold relative risk for ages 45 to 70 to a 10-fold relative risk for ages 35 to 39, for a double-blind–placebo-controlled tamoxifen study between 1992 to 2001. The mean age was 58.8 years, and 54.7 % were between 45 to 54. Sixty percent were from the United Kingdom, 37% from Australia and New Zealand, and 3% from the rest of Europe. Notably, 49% were postmenopausal and 41% had previously been treated with HRT. Nearly all the women (97%) had some breast cancer family history. The single largest risk group (62%) had two or more first- or second-degree relatives with breast cancer. The median follow up was 50 months, and a total of 29,967 women-years of follow-up were accrued. Full compliance to 5 years was estimated to be 65% and 75%, respectively, in the tamoxifen and placebo arm.

A total of 169 cases of breast cancer were observed in the two groups. A 33% reduction of breast cancer was seen in the tamoxifen group, when compared to the placebo group (68 versus 101, $p = 0.01$). The combined data from other trials predicts a 38% reduction, which is comparable to the 33% found in this trial (4). A reduction in breast cancer was evident in both noninvasive and invasive cancers (69%, 5 versus 16 and 26%, 63 versus 85, respectively). There was a significantly greater reduction in DCIS ($p = 0.02$). There was no evidence that HRT use, age, or level of risk affected the tamoxifen benefit.

A non-significant two-fold relative increase (11 versus 5) of endometrial cancer was observed ($p = 0.20$). The rate of endometrial-cancer in the controls ($34/10^5$ women years [WY]) was similar to the rates in the general population in the United Kingdom. Most of the cancers were observed in women over 50 years at randomization. All cancers were adenocarcinomas except one case of low-grade sarcoma in the placebo group. Overall tumors were of low or intermediate grade. Moreover, there was no evidence that endometrial cancer was linked to HRT or of an interaction between HRT and tamoxifen. Ten (63%) of the patients had never used HRT, and only four (25%) of the patients had only used it during the trial. The incidence of all other cancers were equal between the two arms. Thromboembolic events increased significantly (43 versus 17, OR = 2.5, 95% CI 1.4–4.8, $p = 0.001$). Twenty-four (40%) of these events occurred within 3 months of major surgery or following immobility, and 19 of these were in the tamoxifen arm. Even in these cases, there was no indication of synergy between tamoxifen and HRT and actually in some instances there was evidence for negative interaction. Vasomotor events and gynecological reports increased by about 21% in patients taking tamoxifen, while breast complaints were 22% lower, and benign breast disease was reduced by 21% ($p = 0.001$). In osteoporotic or nonosteoporotic fractures, no differences were observed in tamoxifen users; similarly, no difference was found in the incidence of cataracts.

The death rate in the tamoxifen arm was significantly higher (25 versus 10, $p = 0.016$). This was due to other cancers (10 versus 4), thromboembolic events (3 versus 1), and other vascular (3 versus 1) and cardiac deaths (5 versus 0). However, cancer cases were detected at a wide range of different sites and there was no increase in cancer incidence, suggesting that they are not linked to tamoxifen. On the contrary, the excess of thromboembolic events could be attributed to tamoxifen.

The results of this study confirm that tamoxifen reduces the risk of breast cancer in healthy women in the active treatment phase. This is consistent with the combined results of all the prevention trials (4,5). Similarly, the doubling of endometrial cancer and 2.5-fold relative risk for vascular events was previously observed (7). Only for thromboembolic disease was there clear evidence of an increase in mortality, as supported by the excess in the thromboembolic event rate and the small but significant excess mortality from pulmonary embolism. This is at variance with respect to other studies, and should be viewed in the totality of information now available. The relatively low breast cancer death rate highlights the importance of a full evaluation of side effects, which this study addressed. The most important complication emerging from the IBIS and P1 trial is an excess of thromboembolic events. Since most of the risk occurred after surgery, a wise precaution to follow would be to cease the use of tamoxifen before and at least and four weeks after a surgical procedure to ensure that appropriate antithrombotic measures are provided. A similar treatment regimen should be given to women that become immobilized.

RESEARCH IMPLICATIONS FROM CURRENT DATA ON HRT AND TAMOXIFEN

From the biological point of view, the increased risk of breast cancer associated with HRT use is linked to an increased expression of estrogen receptors in the breast tissue (8), thus leading to an enhanced sensitivity to the mitogenic effect of estrogen. The addition of a SERM capable of reducing this growth-promoting effect could therefore blunt ER positive breast cancer risk. Consistent with these findings, tamoxifen appears to be beneficial also in women at increased risk for ER positive breast cancer due to hormonal and reproductive factors such as early menarche, delayed first pregnancy, preserved ovarian function and height (9,10). Notably, previous studies have also shown that the combination of HRT and tamoxifen does not adversely affect their biological effects, including bone density and clotting factors (11,12).

Similarly, no evidence for a positive interaction between tamoxifen and ERT was noted on venous thromboembolic events (VTE) (14). A summary of the effect of tamoxifen in HRT users among the three different trials is illustrated in Table 40.1. It is evident that for all three major endpoints (breast cancer, endometrial cancer, and VTE), the combination of HRT and tamoxifen seems to reduce risks while re-

TABLE 40.1. *Effect of tamoxifen on breast cancer, endometrial cancer, and venous thromboembolic events by HRT use in primary prevention trials*

		Breast cancer		Endometrial cancer		VTE	
		Tam	Plac	Tam	Plac	Tam	Plac
IBIS-I	HRT	37	59	4	2	12	9
	No HRT	31	42	7	3	31	8
Italian trial	HRT	6	17	n.a.	n.a.	0	3
	No HRT	29	28	n.a.	n.a.	11	8
Marsden trial	HRT	12	13	4	1	7	4
	No HRT	22	23				

HRT, hormone replacement therapy; IBIS, International Breast Intervention Study; VTE, vascular thromboembolic events.

taining benefits of either agent alone. Altogether, these findings provide strong justification for studying the effect of the combination of HRT and tamoxifen in order to reduce the risks while retaining the benefit of either agent. The HOT study (HRT Opposed by Tamoxifen), a phase 3 trial addressing this issue is taking place (15).

TAMOXIFEN AT A LOWER DOSE

The use of tamoxifen as a chemoprevention agent may be problematic because of the risk of endometrial cancer. This risk appears to be dose- and time-dependent. A relationship between the length of tamoxifen treatment and endometrial cancer incidence is evident in the meta-analysis of all adjuvant trials of tamoxifen (16).

The effect of 2 months of tamoxifen at lower doses (10 mg per day and 10 mg on alternate days) on the change in serum biomarkers regulated by the estrogen receptor was compared with 20 mg per day (17,18). No evidence for a concentration-response relationship was observed on most of the biomarkers. The concept of a dose reduction is further supported by the observation that tamoxifen has a very high tissue distribution, ranging from 5 to 60 times its blood concentrations, and a prolonged half-life (9 and 13 days for tamoxifen and metabolite X, respectively (19). Also, the breast tissue level attainable with 10 mg per alternate days still exceeds the growth inhibitory concentration of tamoxifen in breast cancer cell lines. Interestingly, a recent cross-sectional study conducted in older, nursing home residents in the New York State long-term facilities has shown a significant reduction of bone fracture rate among breast cancer women taking 10 mg day of tamoxifen (7). Altogether, these findings provide a strong rationale to assess a lower dose of tamoxifen in a preventive context.

AROMATASE INHIBITORS

The new third-generation aromatase inhibitors have shown good efficacy in advanced breast cancer and have a low toxicity profile. They offer another approach to local control, prevention of recurrence and the prevention of primary breast cancers, which may be superior and/or complementary to the use of SERMs.

A very large trial (ATAC) is currently evaluating the role of anastrozole both alone and in combination with tamoxifen compared to tamoxifen in the adjuvant setting for early breast cancer. This trial has recruited 9,366 patients and more than 1,000 recurrences or deaths have now been recorded. After a median follow-up of 33 months, the initial result has been publicly announced (San Antonio meeting, 10 December 2001). Significantly fewer recurrences have been reported on the anastrozole arm compared to tamoxifen (HR = 0.83, $p = 0.013$). New contralateral tumors were also reduced by 58% ($p = 0.007$). There are no significant differences in distant recurrence or survival. The side effect profile was generally favorable, with fewer endometrial cancers, thromboembolic events, strokes, and hot flushes than tamoxifen. However, there were significant increases in musculoskeletal complaints (primarily arthralgia) and fractures.

A multicenter, randomized placebo-controlled clinical trial of anastrozole in 6,000 postmenopausal women aged 40 to 70 years who are at increased risk for breast cancer will be conducted (IBIS-II). Increased risk is determined from family history, previous benign disease with evidence of proliferation, mammographic dysplasia, and nulliparity.

A parallel trial of 4,000 women with DCIS receiving local treatment will also be conducted as described above, except that randomization will only be between tamoxifen and anastrozole.

CONTROL OF ER-NEGATIVE BREAST CANCER

Tamoxifen and other SERMs can reduce breast cancer incidence in at-risk women. However, the incidence of estrogen receptor (ER)-negative cancers is not affected. Furthermore, some ER-positive precancerous lesions might be resistant to tamoxifen intervention. Since approximately one-third of all invasive cancers are ER-negative and women with a family history of breast and ovarian cancer have a higher risk of developing ER-negative breast cancer compared with the general population, strategies to prevent ER-negative tumors are actively being searched.

A favorable trend to a reduction of contralateral breast cancer in BRCA-1 mutation carriers undergoing adjuvant tamoxifen compared with carriers not receiving tamoxifen has been demonstrated (20). Conversely, recent data from the P1 trial indicate that tamoxifen does not reduce the risk of a primary breast cancer in BRCA 1 carriers (1). This is consistent with the notion that BRCA-1 carriers have approximately 90% ER-negative tumors which display a peculiar gene expression profile. Interestingly, certain pathological features can help to distinguish breast tumors with BRCA1 mutations (high-grade cancers, high mitotic index, lymphocytic infiltrate, negative HER-2, and estrogen/progesterone negative receptors). Women with BRCA1 mutation, ER-negative DCIS, or prior ER negative breast cancer have a high risk of developing an ER-negative tumor. Thus, they are potential candidates for phase 1 and phase 2 chemoprevention trials with novel agents.

A number of new potential chemopreventive agents are currently evaluated or planned in clinical prevention trials in women at increased risk for ER-negative breast cancer. These include inhibitors of tyrosine kinase, cyclin dependent kinase inhibitors, PPARγ ligands (glitazones), RXR selective ligands (rexinoids), COX-2 selective inhibitors, demethylating agents, histone deacetylase inhibitors, Vit D3 derivatives, etc. Morphological and molecular biomarkers can be used to select candidates at higher short-term risk, to predict the response to a particular class of agents, and assess the response in phase 2 prevention trials.

REFERENCES

1. Fisher B, Costantino JP, Wickerham DL, et al. Tamoxifen for prevention of breast cancer: report of the National Surgical Adjuvant Breast and Bowel Project P-1 Study. *J Natl Cancer Inst* 1998;90:1371–1388.
2. Veronesi U, Maisonneuve P, Costa A, et al. Prevention of breast cancer with tamoxifen: preliminary findings from the Italian randomised trial among hysterectomised women. Italian Tamoxifen Prevention Study. *Lancet* 1998;352:93–97.
3. Powles T, Eeles R, Ashley S, et al. Interim analysis of the incidence of breast cancer in the Royal Marsden Hospital tamoxifen randomised chemoprevention trial. *Lancet* 1998;352:98–101.
4. Cuzick J. International Breast Cancer Intervention Study. A brief review of the International Breast Cancer Intervention Study (IBIS), the other current breast cancer prevention trials, and proposals for future trials. *Ann N Y Acad Sci* 2001;949:123–133.
5. Cuzick J, et al. *Lancet* 2002; in press.
6. Breuer B, Wallenstein S, Anderson R. Effect of Tamoxifen on bone fractures in older nursing home residents. *J Am Geriatr Soc* 1998;46:968–972.
7. Fisher B, Costantino JP, Redmond CK, et al. Endometrial cancer in tamoxifen-treated breast cancer patients: findings from the National Surgical Adjuvant Breast and Bowel Project (NSABP) B-14. *J Natl Cancer Inst* 1994;86:527–537.
8. Lawson JS, Field AS, Tran DD, et al. Hormone replacement therapy use dramatically increases breast oestrogen receptor expression in obese postmenopausal women. *Breast Cancer Res* 2001;3:342–345.
9. Fabian CJ. Breast cancer chemoprevention: beyond tamoxifen. *Breast Cancer Res* 2001;3:99–103.
10. Fabian CJ, Kimler BF. Chemoprevention for high-risk women: tamoxifen and beyond. *Breast J* 2001;7:311–320.
11. Wu F, Ames R, Clearwater J, et al. Prospective 10-year study of the determinants of bone density and bone loss in normal postmenopausal women, including the effect of hormone replacement therapy. *Clin Endocrinol (Oxf)* 2002;56:703–711.
12. Winkler UH, Altkemper R, Kwee B, et al. Effects of tibolone and continuous combined hormone replacement therapy on parameters in the clotting cascade: a multicenter, double-blind, randomized study. *Fertil Steril* 2000;74:10–19.
13. Effects of hemostasis of hormone replacement therapy with transdermal estradiol and oral sequential medroxyprogesterone acetate: a 1-year, double-blind, placebo-controlled study. The Writing Group for the Estradiol Clotting Factors Study. *Thromb Haemost* 1996;75:476–480.
14. Boschetti C, Cortellaro M, Nencioni T, et al. Short- and long-term effects of hormone replacement therapy (transdermal estradiol vs oral conjugated equine estrogens, combine with medroxyprogesterone actetate) on blood coagulation factors in post menopausal women. *Thromb Res* 1991;62:1–8.
15. Cushman M. Effects of estrogen and selective estrogen receptor modulators on hemostasis and inflammation: potential differences among drugs. *Ann N Y Acad Sci* 2001;949:175–180.
16. Early Breast Cancer Trialists' Collaborative Group. Tamoxifen for early breast cancer: an overview of the randomized trials. *Lancet* 1998;351:1451–1467.

17. Guerrieri-Bonzaga A, Bagliecto L, Johanson H, et al. Correlation between tamoxifen elimination and biomarker recovery in a primary prevention trial. *Cancer Epidemiol Biomarkers Prev* 2001;10:967–970.
18. Decensi A, Bonanni B, Guerrieri-Gonzaga A, et al. Biologic activity of tamoxifen at low doses in healthy women. *J Natl Cancer Inst* 1998;90:1461–1467.
19. Decensi A, Gandini S, Guerrieri-Gonzaga A, et al. Effect of blood tamoxifen concentrations on surrogate biomarkers in a trial of dose reduction. *J Clin Oncol* 1999; 17:2633–2638.
20. Fuchs WS, Leary WP, van der Meer MJ, et al. Pharmacokinetics and bioavailability of tamoxifen in postmenopausal healthy women. *Arzneimittelforschung* 1996;46: 418–422.
21. Narod SA, Brunet JS, Ghadirian P, et al. Tamoxifen and risk of contralateral breast cancer in BRCA1 and BRCA2 mutation carriers: a case-controlled study. Hereditary Breast Cancer Clinical Study Group. *Lancet* 2000;356:1876–1881.

41
Breast Cancer Prevention: The U.S. Viewpoint

D. Lawrence Wickerham and Joseph Costantino

This chapter will review the current status of breast cancer prevention strategies in the United States, where it is estimated that there will be more than 200,000 new invasive breast cancers in the year 2002 and more than 20,000 additional cases of non-invasive intraductal carcinoma (1). Due in large part to screening and improvements in treatment, the number of deaths from breast cancer in the United States decreased during the 1990s, but despite these improvements more than 39,000 women in the United States will die from the disease in 2002. The concept of breast cancer prevention is an attractive addition to screening and treatment in the fight against breast cancer.

PROPHYLACTIC MASTECTOMY

The use of prophylactic mastectomy as an option for the prevention of breast cancer is a drastic and irreversible step. There are no randomized controlled studies of this procedure and only limited information about its long-term effectiveness. However, even when a prophylactic mastectomy is performed by highly experienced surgeons, residual breast tissue will remain, and such remnants are thought to be the source of subsequent cancers. Case reports have appeared in the literature of women developing primary breast cancer after total or subcutaneous mastectomies, cancer that presumably resulted from residual tissue (2).

In 1999 Hartmann et al. (2) published a retrospective review of bilateral prophylactic mastectomy cases from the Mayo Clinic; 639 women with a family history of breast cancer who had undergone bilateral prophylactic mastectomy were identified and divided into two categories, 214 at high risk and 425 at moderate risk. These cases were compared to a control group of sisters of those in the high-risk group and Gail Model scores of the predicted number of breast cancers for the moderate-risk group. The authors performed a thoughtful analysis using a variety of methods designed to minimize bias and identified a statistically significant decrease in the incidence of breast cancer and death from breast cancer after prophylactic mastectomy in the high-risk group. Compared to the expected incidence of breast cancer for women with a family history who did not have the procedure, the reduction in incidence of breast cancer was 90%, and the reduction in the risk of death ranged from 81% to 94%. In the moderate-risk group, similar reductions were noted.

In a related paper, 176 of the 214 high-risk women from Hartmann's 1999 study (3) underwent BRCA1 and BRCA2 testing (3). Mutations were identified in 26 of the women, none of whom had developed a breast cancer after a median follow-up of 13.4 years. These two studies demonstrate that prophylactic mastectomy does result in a substantial reduction in breast cancer incidence in both women at high risk (based on family history of breast cancer) and in those with known BRCA1 and BRCA2 alterations. Although these evaluations are retrospective, randomized trials of prophylactic mastectomy would be difficult if not impossible to conduct given ethical considerations of treatment versus no treatment in these high- or moderate-risk individuals.

CHEMOPREVENTION

Chemoprevention has been defined as pharmacologic intervention with specific nutrients or chemicals to suppress or reverse carcinogenesis and to prevent the development of invasive cancer (4,5). Among the various agents that have been evaluated as chemoprevention therapies for breast cancer, the most highly studied is the selective estrogen receptor modulator (SERM) tamoxifen, with more than 14 million patient years of experience with this drug in the treatment of breast cancer. Tamoxifen has been clearly demonstrated to reduce the risk of recurrence and the risk of dying from breast cancer (6). In the clinical trials that have evaluated tamoxifen as a treatment for the disease, a substantial reduction in new primary cancers of the opposite breast has also been shown. It was this clinical observation and substantial preclinical data that led to the initial large randomized breast cancer prevention studies.

Design of the NSABP Breast Cancer Prevention Trial

The National Surgical Adjuvant Breast and Bowel Project is a North American multi-center cooperative trials group that is funded by the National Cancer Institute of the United States. For more than 40 years the group has conducted phase 3 randomized trials evaluating therapies for primary breast and bowel cancer. In 1992 the group expanded its research agenda to include chemoprevention trials, the first of which was the Breast Cancer Prevention Trial (BCPT), also referred to as P-1.

The BCPT was a clinical trial in which women were randomized in a double-blinded fashion to receive either 20 mg of tamoxifen or placebo for a duration of five years (7). The primary objective of the trial was to determine the efficacy of tamoxifen in the reduction of the incidence of invasive breast cancer. To be eligible for participation in the trial, women had to have no prior history of invasive breast cancer or ductal carcinoma *in situ* and had to be at high risk for the occurrence of breast cancer. "High risk" was defined as: (a) being at least 60 years of age; and (b) having a five-year projected breast cancer risk of at least 1.66% as determined by the modified Gail model (8) for breast cancer risk prediction; or (c) having a history of lobular carcinoma *in situ*. Eligibility also required no history of deep-vein thrombosis or pulmonary embolism, and no history of having taken hormone replacement therapy, oral contraceptives, or androgens for at least three months prior to randomization. In addition, the protocol required that trial participants not use these hormones during the course of the study.

The primary endpoint of the trial from which the sample size and statistical power were determined was the incidence of invasive breast cancer. Several other endpoints were included *a priori* as a means to obtain a full identification of the potential benefits and risks associated with the use of tamoxifen among relatively healthy women. As therapy was randomized, double-blinded, and placebo-controlled, the trial design was maximized in terms of obtaining unbiased information about the efficacy of tamoxifen and potential detrimental outcomes required to determine the therapeutic benefit/risk ratio. The specific secondary endpoints included the incidence of: (a) all other invasive cancers; (b) non-invasive breast and endometrial cancers; (c) myocardial infarction, angioplasty, coronary artery bypass graph, new Q-wave on electrocardiogram, elevated serum enzymes indicative of infarction, and angina requiring hospitalization without surgery, as measures of heart disease; (d) hip, spine, and Colles fractures, as measures of fractures, associated with osteoporosis; and (e) any death. In addition to these secondary endpoints, the trial required the reporting and documentation of the discharge diagnosis of all inpatient and outpatient visits. The study also included the systematic collection at baseline, at 3 months, and at every 3 months thereafter of quality-of-life information using a series of questionnaires composed of 104 items (9–11). Among others, instruments that were used included the CES-D (Center for Epidemiological Studies—Depression) and the MOS SF-36 (Medical Outcomes Study Short Form).

The trial was monitored by an independent data monitoring committee (DMC) that employed formal interim monitoring for early stopping based on the incidence of invasive breast cancer. The stopping rule of Fleming et al. (12) was employed. In addition, as an informal tool to facilitate the monitoring of the composite of all of the multiple beneficial and detrimental endpoints included in the trial, the DMC employed a global index modeled after that of Freedman (13). In March 1998, because it was deemed that the efficacy of tamoxifen to reduce the incidence of invasive breast cancer had been proven beyond any reasonable doubt ($p < 0.0001$), the DMC directed the study leadership to stop the trial, announce the findings, and unblind all participants. Subsequently, the analyses of the study findings were published in September 1998 (7). All analyses by treatment group were based on the treatment assigned at the time of randomization employing the intention-to-treat principle. Average annual event rates for the study endpoints were determined for each treatment group, and the groups were compared using relative risk with 95% confidence intervals (14). Cumulative incidence rates across time of follow-up were determined using the method of Korn and Dorey (15).

Description of the Study Population

A total 13,388 randomized participants entered the trial. At the time of the publication of results, follow-up information was available for 13,175 of these women, 6,599 in the placebo group and 6,576 in the tamoxifen group, providing more than 52,400 person years of follow-up. The median follow-up time was 54.6 months, with 67% followed for more than 4 years and 37% followed for more than 5 years. The characteristics of the study participants are summarized in Table 41.1. The population was comprised primarily of white women (96.5%). The average five-year projected risk of breast cancer among the women was 3.6%. Women younger than 50 made up 39.3% of the population; 31.7% were between the ages of 50 and 59; and 30.0% were 60 or older. The average body mass index of the women was 27.5. Three-fourths of the women had at least one first-degree relative with breast cancer, 6.3% had a history of lobular carcinoma *in situ,* and 9.1% had a history of atypical hyperplasia of the breast. Thirty-seven percent had undergone hysterectomy, and 12.5% were current smokers.

Summary of Findings: Disease Outcomes

Table 41.2 displays the results from the BCPT for 13 disease outcomes that were shown to be affected by treatment with tamoxifen. The risk of breast cancer among those treated with tamoxifen was one-half the risk among those treated with placebo. There were 175 cases of invasive breast cancer in the placebo group compared to 89 in the tamoxifen group (relative risk [RR] comparing tamoxifen to placebo, 0.50, with 95% confidence intervals [95% CI] of 0.39 to 0.66), and 69 cases of noninvasive breast cancer in the placebo group and 35 in the tamoxifen group (RR of 0.50 [95% CI = 0.33–0.77]). The cumulative incidence plots for the breast cancer events are shown in Figure 41.1. The most notable feature of the breast cancer effect of tamoxifen was that the drug reduced only the risk of estrogen-receptor (ER)-positive disease; there was no difference between treatment groups in terms of the inci-

TABLE 41.1. *Characteristics of the study population included in the report of the NSABP Breast Cancer Prevention (P-1) Trial*

Population characteristic	Placebo	Tamoxifen	Total
Number of women	6,599	6,567	13,175
Age (years)			
< 50	39.3	39.2	39.2
50–59	30.6	30.9	30.7
60 +	30.1	29.9	30.0
% Caucasian	96.4	96.5	96.4
Mean 5-year projected breast cancer risk (%)	3.59	3.61	3.60
% with at least one first-degree relative with breast cancer	75.8	76.6	76.2
% with Hx of lobular carcinoma	6.2	6.3	6.3
% with Hx of atypical hyperplasia of the breast	9.3	8.8	9.1
% with prior hysterectomy	36.4	37.7	37.1
Mean body mass index	27.5	27.6	27.5
% currently smoking	12.4	12.6	12.5

TABLE 41.2. *Summary of disease outcome findings from the NSABP Breast Cancer Prevention (P-1) Trial*

Endpoint	Number of events		Rate per 100 women		Relative risk	95% confidence interval
	Placebo	Tamoxifen	Placebo	Tamoxifen		
Cancer						
Invasive breast cancer	175	89	6.76	3.43	0.51	0.39–0.66
Noninvasive breast cancer	69	35	2.68	1.35	0.50	0.33–0.77
Invasive endometrial cancer	15	36	0.91	2.30	2.53	1.35–4.97
Heart disease						
Myocardial infarction[a]	28	31	1.07	1.19	1.11	0.65–1.92
Severe angina[b]	14	13	0.53	0.50	0.93	0.40–2.14
Acute ischemic syndrome[c]	20	27	0.77	1.03	1.36	0.73–2.55
Fractures						
Hip	22	12	0.84	0.46	0.55	0.25–1.15
Spine	31	23	1.18	0.88	0.74	0.41–1.32
Colles	26	14	0.88	0.54	0.61	0.29–1.23
Vascular						
Deep vein thrombosis	22	35	0.84	1.34	1.60	0.91–2.86
Pulmonary embolism	6	18	0.23	0.69	3.01	1.15–9.27
Stroke	24	38	0.92	1.45	1.59	0.93–2.77
Cataracts	507	574	21.72	24.82	1.14	1.01–1.29

[a]International classification of disease codes 410 to 411.
[b]Requiring angioplasty or coronary artery bypass graft.
[c]New Q-wave on electrocardiogram without angina or elevation of serum enzymes or angina requiring hospitalization without surgery.

dence of ER-negative disease, but a 69% reduction of the incidence of ER-positive disease (RR = 0.31; 95% CI = 0.22–0.45). Tamoxifen treatment also reduced the risk of fractures associated with osteoporosis; there were 79 fractures in the placebo group compared to 49 in the tamoxifen group. The RR was 0.55 (95% CI = 0.25–1.15) for hip fracture, 0.74 (95% CI = 0.41–1.32) for spine fracture, and 0.61 (95% CI-0.29–1.23) for Colles fracture. As a result of a low total number of events, none of these risk reductions is statistically significant.

Because tamoxifen treatment is known to reduce blood lipid levels, it was theorized that the risk of heart disease would be reduced in the tamoxifen group. However, no effect of therapy was evident for the incidence of myocardial infarction. There were 28 cases of myocardial infarction in the placebo group and 31 in the tamoxifen arm (RR = 1.11, 95% CI = 0.65–1.92). No statistically significant effect was evident for the other two heart disease endpoints included in the study. There were 14 cases of severe angina in the placebo group compared to 13 in the tamoxifen group (RR = 0.93; 95% CI = 0.40–2.14), and 20 cases of acute ischemic syndrome in the placebo group compared to 27 in the tamoxifen group (RR = 1.36, 95% CI = 0.73–2.55). To determine if there was a relationship between tamoxifen treatment and heart disease among those with a history of heart disease, subset analysis was performed based on a stratification of the BCPT population into those who did and did not report a history of heart disease at the time of randomization (16). No significant differences between the treatment groups were seen for any of the three heart disease endpoints:

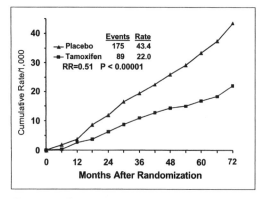

Fig 41.1. Commutative Incidence of Invasive Breast Cancer among Women in the NSABP Breast Cancer Prevention (P-1) Trial

combining all these endpoints, the RR was 0.96 (95% CI = 0.63–1.46) for those without a history of heart disease and 1.39 (95% CI = 0.73–2.67) for those with a history.

Tamoxifen was also shown to affect some outcomes in a detrimental manner. At the initiation of the BCPT, an association between therapy and an increase in the risk of endometrial cancer had already been documented from the results of several treatment trials. The elevation in risk seen in the BCPT for this endpoint was similar to that noted in the treatment trials. The RR for endometrial cancer was 2.53 (95% CI = 1.35–4.97), with 15 cases occurring in the placebo group compared to 36 in the tamoxifen group. This increased risk occurred predominantly among those who were age 50 or older at the time of randomization (Fig. 41.2). There was no evidence to suggest that the endometrial cancer cases that occurred among women who received tamoxifen were any different in terms of pathology or pathogenicity from those that occurred among women who received placebo. As with endometrial cancer, before the BCPT, tamoxifen therapy had been associated with increased risk of pulmonary embolism and deep vein thrombosis. Again, the elevations in risk seen in the BCPT for these endpoints were similar to what had been noted previously. There was a 60% increase in the risk of deep vein thrombosis (RR = 1.60, 95% CI = 0.91–2.86), with 22 cases occurring in the placebo group and 35 in the tamoxifen group. The risk of pulmonary embolism was increased threefold (RR = 3.01; 95% CI = 1.15–9.27), with six and 18 cases occurring in the placebo and tamoxifen groups, respectively. Although not statically significant, there also appeared to be an increased risk of stroke of about 59% (RR = 1.59; 95% CI = 0.93–2.77). There were 24 strokes among women in the placebo group and 38 in the tamoxifen group. As was noted for endometrial cancer, the increased risk of all of these vascular events occurred predominantly among women 50 years of age or older at the time of randomization (Fig. 41.2). Lastly, the risk of cataracts was increased 14% (RR = 1.14, CI = 1.01–1.29) in the tamoxifen group.

Recently the results of the International Breast Cancer Intervention Study (IBIS) I trial, a study that involved more than 7,000 women, and was similar in design to the BCPT, confirmed the findings of the BCPT about the chemopreventive effects of tamoxifen. The IBIS I trial reported findings that were strikingly similar to those seen in the BCPT. A significant breast cancer risk reduction was noted, with the incidence rate in the tamoxifen-treated group being about one-third less than in the placebo-treated group. This study also reported increased risks of thromboembolic effects associated with tamoxifen use that were similar to those seen in the BCPT (17).

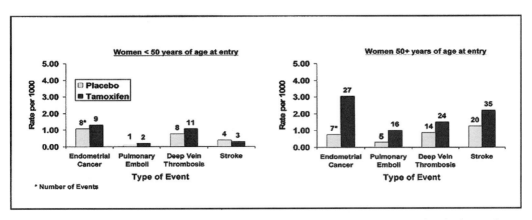

FIG 41.2. Comparison by age group of the incidence rates per 1,000 women for detrimental outcomes experienced in the Breast Cancer Prevention (P-1) Trial.

Quality-of-Life Endpoints

In addition to information on the effects on disease outcome described above, data from the BCPT were analyzed to determine the effects of tamoxifen on several quality-of-life endpoints (9–11). There was no difference between the tamoxifen and placebo groups in terms of scoring on the CES-D, in MOS SF-36 summary physical and mental scores, or on numerous subscales including physical functioning, bodily pain, vitality, mental health, general health perception, social functioning, role-physical, or role-emotional. The relationship of tamoxifen and depression was assessed extensively (10,11), and despite several reports in the literature of a possible relationship between tamoxifen use and depression (18–22), data from the BCPT did not support this. Even when the groups were stratified by depression risk (based on conditions reported at baseline) and the effects evaluated by time of follow-up, there was no evidence to suggest that tamoxifen increases the rate of depression. For all periods of follow-up studied, the RR of depression, as measured by a score of 16 or higher on the CES-D, was found to be very close to 1 or less than 1 (Table 41.3). This contrast in findings from earlier reports in the literature and those of the BCPT illustrate the importance of randomized clinical trials as an unbiased method to ascertain the true existence and magnitude of any treatment effect. Weight gain is another effect that has been anecdotally associated with tamoxifen. Again, the evidence from the BCPT does not support the existence of such an association; it was found that the proportion of women reporting weight loss during the first three years of treatment was slightly higher among women in the tamoxifen group (44.9%) than among those in the placebo group (42.0%).

Several symptoms were shown to be associated with tamoxifen use. The most frequent of these were vasomotor effects (hot flashes, night sweats, cold sweats) and gynecologic symptoms (vaginal dryness, vaginal discharge, vaginal itching). There also was a slight increase in reported problems of sexual functioning among women in the tamoxifen group, which ranged from 1% to 2% higher for women in the tamoxifen group, depending on the time of follow-up and the nature of the specific complaint.

BRCA1 and BRCA2

Information about the breast cancer risk reduction effect of tamoxifen among women who are carriers of BRCA1 or BRCA2 mutations is limited (23). Among all the breast cancer cases reported in the BCPT, there were only 19 women who were known carriers of these mutations. Of these 19, 11 were placebo patients and eight were tamoxifen patients. The distribution of these cases by mutation type, treatment group, and ER status is presented in Table 41.4. Overall, there was a greater risk reduction effect among BRCA2 carriers (RR = 0.38, 95% CI = 0.06–1.56) than among BRCA1 carriers (RR = 1.66, 95% CI = 0.32–10.70), although neither was statistically significant. We postulated that the lack of effect among BRCA1 mutation carriers was due to the propensity for the development of ER-negative tumors in these women.

TABLE 41.3. *Relative risk of depression observed in the NSABP Breast Cancer Prevention (P-1) Trial by follow-up time and categories of depression risk established at baseline*[a]

Period of follow-up	Depression risk category					
	Low		Medium		High	
	RR	95 % CI	RR	95 % CI	RR	95 % CI
12 months	1.02	0.86–1.22	0.99	0.81–1.22	0.62	0.41–0.92
24 months	0.96	0.80–1.13	1.04	0.82–1.30	0.83	0.54–1.28
36 months	0.86	0.71–1.03	1.01	0.64–1.54	1.00	0.64–1.57

[a]Relative risk, comparing tamoxifen to placebo of scoring 16 or higher on the CES-D depression scale.

TABLE 41.4. *Distribution of BRCA1 and BRCA2 mutation carriers among breast cancer patients in the NSABP Breast Cancer Prevention (P-1) Trial by mutation type, estrogen receptor status, and treatment group*

Estrogen receptor status	BRCA1		BRCA2	
	Placebo	Tamoxifen	Placebo	Tamoxifen
Total	3	4	8	3
ER positive	0	1	4	2
ER negative	3	3	2	1
ER unknown	0	1	2	0
RR (95% CI)[a]	1.66	(0.23–10.70)	0.38	(0.06–1.56)

[a]Relative risk and 95% confidence intervals of the relative risk for total.

INCORPORATION OF TAMOXIFEN PREVENTION INTO ROUTINE PRACTICE

Risks and Benefits of Tamoxifen Therapy to Reduce the Risk of Breast Cancer

When there are numerous beneficial and detrimental effects of a drug, as with tamoxifen, the determination of who is or is not likely to benefit from risk reduction therapy is complex. The risks and benefits of tamoxifen have been studied in depth, and the results of detailed risk/benefit analysis have been described (24–26). Risk/benefit assessment can be carried out for any individual; a summary sheet is used as a tool for reviewing the results of such assessments, and tables are provided to identify values of potential risk and potential benefit for women of specific age categories, racial groups, and levels of projected breast cancer risk, from which information can be abstracted onto the summary sheet.

The net effect of tamoxifen is primarily a function of the individual's age, race, and level of projected breast cancer risk. Age is a factor because the baseline risk of potential detrimental outcomes (stroke, pulmonary embolism, deep vein thrombosis, and endometrial cancer) increases with age. Thus, the older one is, the higher the risk of these outcomes. Race is a factor because the baseline risk of the potential detrimental outcomes varies substantially by race. For example, the risk of these detrimental outcomes is generally higher among African-American women than among white women. The level of projected risk is important because the potential gain from risk reduction therapy increases directly with increasing level of breast cancer risk.

Generally speaking, women who are highly likely to benefit from tamoxifen therapy include those who: (a) are under age 50 with a five-year projected risk of breast cancer of at least 1.66% as determined by the Gail model (8); (b) have a history of non-invasive breast cancer (ductal carcinoma *in situ,* lobular carcinoma *in situ*); or (c) have a five-year projected risk of breast cancer of at least 6.5%. Women who are highly likely to suffer detriment from tamoxifen therapy are those who: (a) have a five-year projected risk of breast can less than 1.66%; (b) have a history of stroke or clotting disorders; or (c) have a pattern of risk factors that puts them at high risk for stroke or clotting disorders (hypertension, smoking, obesity, etc), particularly if they are over 50 years of age. Women who do not fall into these categories have a potential net-effect that ranges between that of likely to benefit and likely to experience detriment. As it is not possible to easily identify a simple pattern of factors that defines the net effect for this latter portion of women, a full risk/benefit assessment using risk/benefit methodology should be performed for these individuals.

History of Tamoxifen Use and Risk Assessment in Breast Cancer

In December 1998, the U.S. Food and Drug Administration (FDA) approved tamoxifen for the reduction of breast cancer incidence in high-risk women. "High risk" women were defined as those at least 35 years of age who had a five-year predicted risk of breast cancer more than or equal to 1.66% as calculated by the Gail model. Physicians were instructed, "After an assessment of the risk of developing breast cancer, the decision regarding therapy with tamoxifen for the reduction in breast cancer incidence should be based upon an individual assessment of the benefits and risks of tamoxifen therapy." The NCI estimated at that time that there were as many as 29,000,000 women in the United States who were potential candidates for tamoxifen.

Precise data on the use of tamoxifen for prevention/risk reduction are not available. AstraZeneca, the manufacturer of tamoxifen in the United States, has seen an increase of 20% in the sales of the drug, but this is unlikely to be due only to its use in prevention. During the same time period, tamoxifen was approved for the adjuvant therapy of ductal carcinoma *in situ* (DCIS), and the 10-year Oxford Overview results were published, which demonstrated the appropriateness of using tamoxifen for a 5-year period for the treatment of invasive breast cancer (6). However, even if all the increased use of this drug were attributed to prevention, this would still indicate that substantially fewer women than the estimated 29 million potential candidates are receiving the drug.

Why would this be true? It is likely that there are many reasons, none of them dominant. Although tamoxifen provided substantial benefit in reducing the number of both invasive and noninvasive breast cancers as well as fractures, it was also associated with increased risk for several serious conditions including endometrial cancer, thromboembolic events, and cataracts. The decision to use this therapy is complex and requires a thorough evaluation of both benefit and risk.

In an effort to make the Gail model available to health care professionals and the general public, the U.S. National Cancer Institute began to distribute its Breast Cancer Risk Assessment Tool in both IBM and Mac formats. A web-based version of the program was also posted at http://bcra.nci.nih.gov/brc/, and AstraZeneca distributed a version of the model on a handheld calculator.

At the same time, physicians and potential tamoxifen users were receiving mixed messages about tamoxifen's usefulness in prevention. Not long after the announcement of the NSABP P-1 results, two European trials were published in *The Lancet* that also compared tamoxifen to placebo in a high-risk population (27,28). Neither demonstrated benefit from tamoxifen in reducing invasive breast cancers, and many individuals, including breast cancer advocates, expressed concern about the drug's potential toxicities and what they described as "mixed trial results." Although none of the studies was designed to evaluate survival as a primary endpoint, the lack of a documented survival benefit was widely discussed as a reason not to use tamoxifen. There has also been uncertainty about what type of physician should be advising women about breast cancer prevention and prescribing chemoprevention therapies. Oncologists are familiar with both breast cancer and tamoxifen, but do not traditionally see healthy women. Primary care physicians, including gynecologists, routinely follow healthy women who may be candidates for chemoprevention and are familiar with preventive medicine but are not as familiar with breast cancer and tamoxifen.

Anecdotal reports suggest that clinicians have prescribed tamoxifen with increasing frequency for two general groups of individuals: (a) women with biopsy-proven risk factors (LCIS or atypical hyperplasia of the breast), which are known to increase substantially the risk for future breast cancer; and (b) premenopausal women with substantial risk of future breast cancer but who, based on the P-1 data, have little or no risk of endometrial cancer or thromboembolic disease that could result from taking tamoxifen. Women who have had a hysterectomy and thus have no risk of endometrial cancer are also more likely to be prescribed tamoxifen than those who have not had a hysterectomy.

OTHER CHEMOPREVENTION AGENTS UNDER EVALUATION

Although the NSABP's P-1 study has demonstrated that tamoxifen is effective in reducing the incidence of breast cancer, the drug's toxicities are a barrier to its routine use for this purpose. Identifying more effective agents with less toxicity is an appropriate goal, and several possible drugs are or will soon be under evaluation as possible breast cancer chemoprevention therapies.

Raloxifene

Of all the newer SERMs, raloxifene has received the most attention with regard to its potential use for breast cancer chemoprevention. Raloxifene is a benzothiophene SERM that has been shown to increase bone density in postmenopausal women and is approved in the United States for both the treatment and the prevention of osteoporosis.

MORE Trial

The Multiple Outcomes of Raloxifene Evaluation (MORE) Trial was a randomized, placebo-controlled, double-blinded study designed to determine whether raloxifene would reduce the risk of fracture in postmenopausal women with osteoporosis (29,30). Each of the 7,704 women enrolled (mean age = 66.5 years) was assigned to receive either 60 mg raloxifene, 120 mg raloxifene, or a placebo. The development of breast cancer was a secondary endpoint of the trial, and women were not selected because of their breast cancer risk. The four-year results of the trial demonstrated a 62% overall breast cancer risk reduction with raloxifene (RR 0.28, 95% CI 0.17–0.46). This drug also reduced the risk of estrogen-receptor-positive invasive breast cancer by 84% (RR 0.16, 95% CI 0.09–0.30). Thromboembolic disease occurred more frequently in the raloxifene-treated group than in the placebo-treated group ($p = 0.003$), but there was no excess risk of endometrial cancer among raloxifene-treated women.

Treatment with raloxifene, like treatment with tamoxifen, results in a reduction of total cholesterol. Overall, the MORE trial found no reduction in cardiovascular disease; however, in a highly selected subgroup at increased risk for cardiovascular problems, a benefit has been identified (31).

ASCO TECHNOLOGY ASSESSMENT ON BREAST CANCER RISK REDUCTION STRATEGIES: TAMOXIFEN AND RALOXIFENE

The results of the NSABP Breast Cancer Prevention Trial and the MORE study results prompted the American Society of Clinical Oncology to conduct a technology assessment of both tamoxifen and raloxifene as a breast cancer risk reduction strategy (32). The technology assessment process determines whether a procedure is appropriate for broad-based use in clinical practice. A working group comprised of representatives of the Health Services Research Committee and selected ad hoc members including breast cancer patient advocates reviewed the data available on both tamoxifen and raloxifene. It was their conclusion that for women with a defined 5-year projected risk of breast cancer equal to or more than 1.66% (the risk eligibility utilized by the NSABP BCPT), tamoxifen 20 mg per day for up to 5 years may be offered to reduce the risk of breast cancer. The committee thought it was premature to recommend raloxifene's use to lower the risk of developing breast cancer outside a clinical trial setting.

STAR Trial

In July 1999, the NSABP began accrual to its second breast cancer prevention trial, the Study of Tamoxifen and Raloxifene (STAR). This is a randomized, double-blinded trial to compare the proven benefits of tamoxifen to the promising results of raloxifene (Fig. 41.3). Eligible participants are postmenopausal women at increased risk for the future development of breast cancer based on a five-year breast cancer risk estimate from the Gail model of more than or equal to 1.66%. Participants will be assigned to receive 20 mg tamoxifen plus a placebo or 60 mg raloxifene plus a placebo daily for 5 years. They will undergo breast examinations every six months as well as yearly mammograms, gynecologic examinations, and screening blood work. The goal is to determine whether raloxifene is as good as or better than tamoxifen in

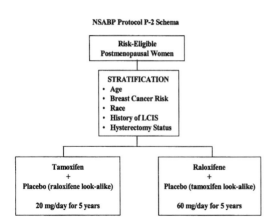

FIG 41.3. NSABP Protocol P-2 (the STAR Trial) schema.

preventing breast cancer with fewer side effects. The sample size required to complete the study is 22,000 women.

There are currently 500 sites participating in the STAR Trial in the United States, Canada, and Puerto Rico. As of January 31, 2002, 12,387 participants had been randomized into the trial, which represents 56.2% of the sample size. Accrual at present is limited to postmenopausal women; raloxifene has not been evaluated extensively in premenopausal women, and there are no safety or efficacy data available for the drug in such women. The age distribution of current participants reflects this postmenopausal group: 10% of the population is under the age of 50, 50% is age 50 to 59, and 40% is age 60 or older. Eleven percent of the women have a 5-year breast cancer risk as estimated by the Gail model of less than 2%; 62% have an estimated risk between 2% and 4.9%; and 27% have an estimated risk of 5%. Of the participants randomized, 8.3% (1,033) have a history of lobular carcinoma *in situ,* and 19.2% (2,377) have a history of breast biopsy demonstrating atypical hyperplasia. Seventy-five percent of the participants have one or more first-degree relatives (mother, sister, or daughter) have or who have had breast cancer. More than half (52.5%) have histories of hysterectomy with or without oophorectomy; this is more than the 37% of women in the P-1 trial who had had a hysterectomy prior to entry.

More than 105,000 women have filled out NSABP Risk Assessment Forms (RAFs) to determine their Gail model scores and to establish their risk eligibility for the STAR trial. Of the women who completed RAFs, 59,472 (56.2%) are risk-eligible. All these women take part in one-to-one discussions about breast cancer and breast cancer risk. Many are pleasantly surprised that their breast cancer risk is not as high as they had imagined. In addition to the Gail model score, each woman receives a summary of benefits and risks associated with SERM use based on data from the P-1 trial. Each potential participant also receives a table that shows certain medical events that would be expected during the next 5 years among 10,000 women not receiving SERM therapy, matched by age, race, and breast cancer risk. These numbers are then compared to the number of expected events that would be prevented or caused by 5 years of SERM use. Life-threatening events listed include invasive breast cancer, hip fracture, endometrial cancer, stroke, and pulmonary embolus; severe events that are projected include *in situ* breast cancer and deep vein thrombosis; other events include wrist fractures and spine fractures, and the increased occurrence of cataracts. When the breast cancer risk scores are examined alongside the risk/benefit tables, a skewed distribution of participants randomized from the various Gail score categories is evident: only 2.3% of the women with 5-year Gail scores under 2% have been randomized into the trial, but 35% of the women with scores over 5% have been randomized. The higher the Gail score, the more likely a woman will be to have a more favorable risk/benefit ratio. Women who are interested in obtaining their breast cancer risk assessment and the risk/benefit projection will find a list of participating STAR sites at www.nsabp.pitt.edu/STAR/index.html.

Anastrozole

There are several third-generation aromatase inhibitors that are currently in development for the treatment of breast cancer. The selective aromatase inhibitors are frequently divided into steroidal and nonsteroidal categories and differ in potency as well as in their type of inhibition. The selective nonsteroidal aromatase inhibitors have already become established as second-line endocrine therapy in advanced postmenopausal breast cancer. Anastrozole, which has been available in the United States since 1996 for the treatment of advanced breast cancer, is one of these. Results of the Arimidex and Tamoxifen, Alone or in Combination (ATAC) trial were recently announced (33). This multicenter, randomized, double-blinded study involved 9,366 postmenopausal women from 380 centers in 21 countries, more than 2,200 of whom were from the United States. Women completed primary surgery and chemotherapy (when applicable) prior to study entry and were required to be a candidates for adjuvant hormonal therapy. Patients were randomly assigned to anastrozole (Arimidex), tamoxifen, or a combination of anastrozole and tamoxifen. The trial was designed to determine if anastrozole was equal to, or more effective than, tamoxifen, and whether anastrozole offered additional safety and tolerability benefits. The study also included a combination treatment arm (tamoxifen and anastrozole) to determine if both medications together were more effective than tamoxifen alone. Participating patients were randomized to receive anastrozole (1 mg daily), tamoxifen (20 mg daily), or a combination of the two treatments for 5 years or until recurrence of the disease. Primary trial endpoints were disease-free survival and safety. Secondary endpoints were time to distant recurrence, survival, and contralateral breast cancers. Results were based on a median of 33.3 months of follow-up and a median duration of treatment of 30.7 months. Of the 3,125 women in the anastrozole group, 317 had a relapse of breast cancer and died, compared with 379 of the 3,116 women in the tamoxifen group ($p = 0.0129$). This represents a 17% reduction in relative risk of disease recurrence in all women who developed recurrence when the anastrozole treatment was compared to tamoxifen, and an absolute risk reduction of 2.2%. In women with confirmed estrogen-receptor-positive tumors, when anastrozole treatment was compared to tamoxifen, the reduction in the relative risk of recurrence was 22% ($p = 0.0054$). The absolute risk reduction in this group of women was 2.7%. There was no additional benefit seen in the combination group, in which 383 of 3,125 women had a relapse of breast cancer and died, compared to 379 of the 3,116 women in the tamoxifen group. Survival results were not reported and are not yet significant.

In the prevention setting, there is currently little information available about anastrozole and its effect on breast cancer in the long term. In the ATAC trial, the incidence of invasive and non-invasive contralateral breast cancer was decreased by 58% in the anastrozole group compared to the tamoxifen group (14 versus 33 cases). According to Dr. Michael Baum, professor emeritus of surgery at the University College London, England, anastrozole does appear to be a good candidate to study in the chemoprevention arena.

Based in large part on the ATAC results, the Imperial Cancer Research Fund has announced that an international multicenter randomized double-blinded controlled trial known as the International Breast Cancer Intervention Study (IBIS) II, will evaluate anastrozole as a chemopreventative agent in women at increased risk for breast cancer and in those with DCIS. The trial will include 10,000 women who have a moderate-to-high risk of breast cancer and an additional 6,000 women with DCIS. Accrual is planned to begin in late 2002.

SUMMARY

Prophylactic Mastectomy

Level of evidence III, category B: Results on incidence and death reported in the two papers by Hartmann et al. (2,3) are consistent with the results from reported series of individuals undergoing prophylactic mastectomy and are in keeping with the biological understanding of the development of breast cancer. It is unlikely that results from randomized clinical trials will ever be available in the foreseeable future, so the level of evidence for this procedure is unlikely to change. With the increasing availability of genetic testing for inherited mutations and better knowledge of the clinical outcomes of specific mutations, the use of prophylactic mastectomy can be reserved for individuals with clearly identified high levels of risk, and can be utilized with a reasonable assurance that it is effective in dramatically reducing but not totally eliminating the risk of breast cancer.

Chemoprevention

Level of evidence I, category A: The results of NSABP P-1 have now been confirmed by the data from the IBIS I Trial and both clearly demonstrate that tamoxifen is an effective chemopreventative agent. These clinical data are in keeping with the extensive experience with tamoxifen in the treatment of breast cancer that demonstrates reduction in opposite breast cancers that persist through 15 years and are in keeping with laboratory evidence that demonstrates that tamoxifen prevents both the initiation and the promotion of breast cancer. The two smaller European studies with negative findings noted in this paper that have less power are the exception, but as a group the tamoxifen trials combined are compatible with a positive outcome for tamoxifen.

The MORE Trial, in which breast cancer was a secondary endpoint, further supports the concept of selective estrogen receptor modulators as effective chemopreventative agents. At present, the use of raloxifene outside clinical trials for the prevention of breast cancer does not seem justified. However, the STAR Trial is well under way and should allow for future demonstration of the effectiveness of this agent.

Information on aromatase inhibitors as chemopreventative agents is limited but sufficient to justify randomized trials to evaluate its use as a chemopreventative agent. Such trials are planned to begin in the near future.

As a concept, chemoprevention of breast cancer has been demonstrated. The goal now is to identify more effective agents that possess less toxicity, allowing a broader population of women access to such agents.

This chapter has not discussed diet or exercise as a method to reduce breast cancer risk. Although there are extensive laboratory and epidemiologic data evaluating various regimens, controlled clinical trials with outcome data in this area are extremely limited, and meaningful recommendations cannot be made at this time.

Acknowledgment: The authors thank Barbara C. Good, PhD, for editorial assistance with this manuscript.

REFERENCES

1. Jemal A, Thomas A, Murray T, Thun M. Cancer statistics, 2002. *CA Cancer J Clin* 2002;52(1):23–47.
2. Hartmann LC, Schaid DJ, Woods JE, et al. Efficacy of bilateral prophylactic mastectomy in women with a family history of breast cancer. *New Eng J Med* 1999; 340:77–84.
3. Hartmann LC, Sellers TA, Schaid DJ, et al. Efficacy of bilateral prophylactic mastectomy in BRCA1 and BRCA2 gene mutation carriers. *J Natl Cancer Inst* 2001;93(21):1633–1637.
4. Lotan R. Retinoids in cancer chemoprevention. *FASEB J* 1996;10(9):1031–1039.
5. Mavne ST, Lippman SM. Retinoids and and carotenoids. In: DeVita VT, Hellman S, Rosenberg SA, eds. *Cancer principles & practice of oncology,* 5th ed. Philadelphia: Lippincott-Raven, 1997:585–599.
6. Tamoxifen for early breast cancer: An overview of the randomised trials. Early Breast Cancer Trialists' Collaborative Group. *Lancet* 1998;351(9114):1451–1467.
7. Fisher B, Costantino JP, Wickerham DL, et al. Tamoxifen for prevention of breast cancer: Report of the National Surgical Adjuvant Breast and Bowel Project P-1 Study. *J Natl Cancer Inst* 1998;90(18):1371–1388.
8. Costantino JP, Gail MH, Pee D, et al. Validation studies for models projecting the risk of invasive and total breast cancer incidence. *J Natl Cancer Inst* 1999;91 (18):1541–1548.
9. Ganz PA, Day R, Ware JE Jr, et al. Base-line quality-of-life assessment in the National Surgical Adjuvant Breast and Bowel Project Breast Cancer Prevention Trial. *J Natl Cancer Inst* 1995;87:1372–1382.
10. Day R, Ganz PA, Costantino JP, et al. Health-related quality of life and tamoxifen in breast cancer prevention: A report from the National Surgical Adjuvant Breast and Bowel Project P-1 Study. *J Clin Oncol* 1999;17(9):2659–2669.
11. Day R, Ganz PA, Costantino JP. Tamoxifen and depression: More evidence from the National Surgical Adjuvant Breast and Bowel Project's Breast Cancer Prevention (P-1) Randomized Study. *J Natl Cancer Inst* 2001; 93(21):1615–1623.
12. Fleming TR, Harrington DP, O'Brien PC. Designs for group sequential tests. *Control Clin Trials* 1984;5(4): 348–361.
13. Freedman L, Anderson G, Kipnis V, et al. Approaches to monitoring the results of long-term disease prevention trials: Examples from the Women's Health Initiative. *Controll Clin Trials* 1996;17(6):509–525.
14. Rosner B. *Fundamentals of biostatistics.* 4th ed. Boston: Duxbury Press, 1995:590–594.

15. Korn EL, Dorey FJ. Applications of crude incidence curves. *Stat Med* 1992;11(6):813–829.
16. Reis SE, Costantino JP, Wickerham DL, et al. Cardiovascular effects of tamoxifen in women with and without heart disease: Breast Cancer Prevention Trial. *J Natl Cancer Inst* 2001;93(1):16–21.
17. Pritchard KI. Prevention of breast cancer: Results from the IBIS I Study. 3rd European Breast Cancer Conference, 2002, Barcelona, Spain, Abstr.
18. Anelli TF, Anelli A, Tran KN, et al. Tamoxifen administration is associated with a high rate of treatment-limiting symptoms in male breast cancer patients. *Cancer* 1994;74–77.
19. Cathcart CK, Jones SE, Pumroy CS, et al. Clinical recognition and management of depression in node negative breast cancer patients treated with tamoxifen. *Breast Cancer Res Treat* 1993;27(3):277–281.
20. Love RR, Cameron L, Connell BL, Leventhal H. Symptoms associated with tamoxifen treatment in postmenopausal women. *Arch Intern Med* 1991;151(9):1842–1847.
21. Pluss JL, DiBella NJ. Reversible central nervous system dysfunction due to tamoxifen in a patient with breast cancer. *Ann Intern Med* 1984;101:652.
22. Shariff S, Cumming CE, Lees A, et al. Mood disorder in women with early breast cancer taking tamoxifen, an estradiol receptor antagonist. An expected or unexpected effect? *Ann N Y Acad Sci* 1995;761:365–368.
23. King MC, Wieand S, Hale K, et al. Tamoxifen and breast cancer incidence among women with inherited mutations in BRCA1 and BRCA2: National Surgical Adjuvant Breast and Bowel Project (NSABP P-1) Breast Cancer Prevention Trial. *JAMA* 2001;286(18):2251–2256.
24. Gail MH, Brinton LA, Byar DP, et al. Projecting individualized probabilities of developing breast cancer for white females who are being examined annually. *J Natl Cancer Inst* 1989;81(24):1879–1886.
25. Gail MH, Costantino JP, Bryant J, et al. Weighing the risks and benefits of tamoxifen treatment for preventing breast cancer. *J Natl Cancer Inst* 1999;91(21):1829–1846.
26. Costantino JP, Vogel VG, Wickerham DL. Prescribing therapy to reduce the risk of breast cancer: balancing the risk-benefit analogies. *Prevent Care Cancer* 2001;21(9):13–21.
27. Powles T, Eeles R, Ashley S, et al. Interim analysis of the incidence of breast cancer in the Royal Marsden Hospital tamoxifen randomised chemoprevention trial. *Lancet* 1998;352(9122):98–101.
28. Veronesi U, Maisonneuve P, Costa A, et al. Prevention of breast cancer with tamoxifen: Preliminary findings from the Italian randomised trial among hysterectomised women. Italian Tamoxifen Prevention Study. *Lancet* 1998;352(9122):93–97.
29. Cummings SR, Eckert S, Krueger KA, et al. The effect of raloxifene on risk of breast cancer in postmenopausal women: Results from the MORE randomized trial. Multiple Outcomes of Raloxifene Evaluation. *JAMA* 1999;281(23):2189–2197.
30. Cauley JA, Norton L, Lippman ME, et al. Continued breast cancer risk reduction in postmenopausal women treated with raloxifene: 4-year results from the MORE trial, Multiple Outcomes of Raloxifene Evaluation. *Breast Cancer Res Treat* 2001;65(2):125–134.
31. Cummings SR, Duong T, Kenyon E, et al. Serum estradiol level and risk of breast cancer during treatment with raloxifene. *JAMA* 2002;287:216–220.
32. Chlebowski RT, Collyar DE, Somerfield MR, et al. American Society of Clinical Oncology technology assessment on breast cancer risk reduction strategies: tamoxifen and raloxifene. *J Clin Oncol* 1999;17(6):1939–1955.
33. Baum M, on behalf of the ATAC Trialists' Group. The ATAC (Arimidex, Tamoxifen, Alone or in Combination) adjuvant breast cancer trial in post-menopausal women. San Antonio Breast Cancer Symposium, 2001, Abstract #8.

PART V

Clinical Data Analysis: Current and Future Standards

42

Evidence Analysis: Historical and Contemporary Perspectives

Jean-Marc Nabholtz, Linda Harris, David M. Reese, and Katia Tonkin

We have to ask ourselves, then, by what standard we can measure the chance of success.
Theodor Billroth

The whole art of medicine is in observation.
William Osler

THE ORIGINS OF BREAST CANCER MEDICINE

By historical standards, the oncologist of today possesses an enviable armamentarium of treatments for breast cancer. Relying primarily on the four pillars of surgery—radiation therapy, endocrine therapy and chemotherapy—contemporary doctors are able to cure more than half of all women with the disease, a result obtainable only in the last two decades. Yet, despite advances in the local and systemic treatment of breast cancer, substantial progress remains to be made. Metastatic breast cancer is still largely incurable, and a substantial number of patients with early breast cancer will ultimately relapse and succumb to the disease. It is undeniable that much has been done, but that many problems must be solved.

There is now considerable optimism among clinical investigators as we embark on a new millennium of breast cancer care. This stems from the fact that, after 30 years of intense effort, the breast cancer cell is finally yielding up its secrets to the methods of molecular biology. Indeed, there is a great deal we already know about the molecular pathogenesis and progression of breast cancer. Nearly every breast tumor cell contains various alterations in oncogenes, tumor suppressor genes, components of the cell cycle, apoptotic molecules, and angiogenesis. Translating what we have discovered about these pathway alterations into effective new therapies is our greatest current challenge.

Evaluating new breast cancer treatments and using them effectively in the clinic is a complex business, one that requires both science and art. The researcher must identify a precise clinical problem, develop a treatment strategy in response to that problem, and then test the treatment in a fashion that will provide definitive answers as to its effectiveness. Ultimately, these research observations must be applied to a specific patient. As modern physicians, we accept this paradigm, and rarely think to question the merits of a scientific approach.

But the use of controlled evidence in cancer medicine—in all of medicine—is a relatively recent phenomenon. To be sure, the birth of Western medicine itself nearly 2,500 years ago contained the seeds of our burgeoning ability to eradicate breast cancer. Many long centuries would pass, however, before bedside observations would be formalized into what we know as the clinical trial. To appreciate where we are and where we need to go, it is worthwhile to see how far we've come.

Oncology can trace its origins to Hippocrates, author of the famous oath and widely regarded as the founder of bedside medicine. Most of what we believe about the legendary healer is myth, shrouded in the embellishments of later generations. We do know that Hippocrates was the son and grandson of physicians and was born in 460 B.C.E. on Cos, a small Mediterranean island situated off the coast of Asia Minor. He was supposedly the nineteenth lineal descendant of Asclepius, the Greek god of medicine and healing. After an illustrious career during which he treated patients throughout Greece, Hippocrates died at the age of one hundred; the inscription on his tomb declared that he "gained many victories over disease, and won great glory not by chance but by science" (1).

Outside the oath, Hippocrates's legacy endures because of 60-odd texts, known as the Hippocratic Corpus, for which we give him credit. Ranging from ethics to epidemics to abstract philosophy, these fascinating books are crammed with case reports, general medical advice, and specific treatment recommendations (2). It is in the Corpus that we find the first clinical description of cancer as a distinct disease with a characteristic natural history.

Greek physicians were forbidden by religious tradition to dissect the human body. As a result, the Hippocratics were most familiar with growths located on the skin or in areas that could be easily palpated. In one brief passage, Hippocrates set down a vivid picture of cancer that scarcely has been surpassed:

> Cancer is a roundish, unequal, hard, and livid tumor, generally seated in the glandular parts of the body, supposed to be so called because it appears at length with turgid veins shooting out from it, so as to resemble the crab; or, as others say, because like a crab, where it has once got, it is hardly possible to drive it away (3).

This succinct characterization, rendered in poetic prose, also, as every clinical oncologist recognizes, reflects certain biologic fact. Indeed, Hippocrates could have been—and probably was—describing locally advanced breast cancer. Because they were the first to identify cancer, the Hippocratics had to invent a vocabulary for what they saw. Accordingly, Hippocrates coined the term *karkinoma* (from *karkinos,* the crab) to denote malignant growths; the word was later Latinized to carcinoma. The Greek word *onkos* (tumor) gave our field its name (4).

In addition to his other appellations, Hippocrates has justly been called the father of oncology (5). Unfortunately, he was also the father of a gross inaccuracy that hindered the development of cancer medicine for over two millennia. According to ancient Greek physiology, four essential humors—blood, yellow bile, black bile, and phlegm—were the primary constituents of the body. In health, these humors were in harmony, combining in just the right proportions; illness resulted from a humoral imbalance. Cancer itself was thought to represent an overproduction of black bile (6). While this notion seems fanciful to us, once the humoral theory was codified by Galen, a Greek physician practicing in Rome during the apogee of the Roman Empire, it was accepted as immutable fact for over a thousand years. As William Osler noted, Galen spoke, and "fifteen centuries stopped thinking and slept" (7).

Medicine's slumber meant that there was no scientific approach to evaluating cancer treatments. The Hippocratics, and Galen after them, advocated a combination of bloodletting (to drain black bile) along with dietary manipulations, warm baths, and other "supportive care" interventions. Cancer surgery was occasionally performed, but, until the introduction of anesthesia and antisepsis in the mid-nineteenth century, the procedure was unbearable and almost uniformly fatal. No one thought to test the utility of these cancer treatments.

Late in the nineteenth century, the notion of formally evaluating the effectiveness of a therapy finally made its way into cancer medicine. Of course, clinical trials of sorts had been performed earlier. Around 1200 C.E., Frederick II, Emperor of Rome, decided to study the effects of digestion on food. He gave two knights an identical meal; one was told to sleep and the other went hunting. After a number of hours the emperor had both killed, and discovered that the sleeping knight had digested more food than the one who had exercised (8). Five hundred years later, Jean Baptiste van Helmont, a celebrated Belgian physician and chemist, outlined a study in which 200 to 500 people with fever would be divided into two groups (bloodletting or no bloodletting) by casting lots. Outcome was then to be ascertained (9). The randomized design was superb, but, unfortunately, van Helmont's trial never took place.

One of the first efforts to track outcome in cancer medicine was recorded by Theodore Billroth, the leading surgeon in Europe in the late nineteenth century. Billroth performed simple mastectomies on several hundred women (n = 548) with breast cancer, and then paid an assistant to conduct long-term follow-up on these patients. After three years, fewer than 5% remained alive, a dismal testament to the fact that most of these patients presented with far advanced local disease and, almost certainly, undiagnosed systemic metastases (10). It was not until 1954 that the first randomized trial in oncology occurred. Emil Frei and his associates studied the effects of 6-mercaptopurine and methotrexate on childhood acute lymphoblastic leukemia (11). The resounding success of this study led to the development of cooperative groups for the investigation of new cancer therapies and the widespread adoption of randomized, controlled clinical trials in oncology research. Ten years later, Sir Austin Bradford-Hill and Sir Richard Doll published "Mortality in Relation to Smoking: Ten Years' Observation on British Doctors" (12). Implicit in this trial was an emphasis on rigorous statistical analysis, which further paved the way for the modern generation of oncology clinical trials beginning in the early 1970s.

The triumph of the clinical trial, raised on the foundation of sophisticated statistical methodologies, raised a crucial issue. Just how do we evaluate medical evidence? What constitutes good evidence, and what should be thrown out? The answers to these questions are fundamental to the approach to presenting material we have taken in this book.

EVALUATING MEDICAL EVIDENCE

Evidence-based medicine (EBM) was developed to answer clinical questions facing treating physicians. This approach is especially useful when a clinician must choose between two treatments for a condition that arise from opposing viewpoints on therapy. Conceptually, EBM is the integration of research evidence with clinical expertise and patient values. From a practical standpoint, EBM requires the following:

1. The conversion of information needs into answerable questions.
2. The ability to search for the best available evidence with which to answer the question.
3. Critical appraisal of the literature, understanding its validity, applicability, and importance.
4. Integration of the evidence with clinical knowledge and individual patient needs.
5. Continuing evaluation of the first four steps to improve them for future needs.

In recent years EBM has become more prevalent, especially in light of the rise of clinical trials in the last three decades. There are now at least six journals devoted to EBM, and the literature is growing almost exponentially. However, the adoption of practices advocated by EBM remains imperfect. Part of the reason surely lies in the fact that it is not often easy to use EBM at the bedside, when confronted with the particularities of an individual patient's situation (13). In addition, we are (and always will be) influenced by expert opinion, which is driven not only by scientific considerations but also the personal philosophies and experience of the experts in question.

This second edition of *Breast Cancer Management*, as was the first volume, is intended to help the practicing clinician determine which therapies should be selected for an individual patient. In compiling the chapters in this book, we have focused on addressing questions a busy clinician needs to answer when evaluating the breast cancer literature. What information is relevant to a particular patient or group of patients? What related information must also be considered? Are new data consistent with, or contrary to, previously published observations? In assessing new findings, is confirmatory evidence necessary—and, practically, will it be available—from other ongoing or planned clinical trials? It is our hope that the approach used in this book will provide an easily accessible, pertinent, up-to-date source of information for the breast cancer physician confronted with the realities of clinical practice and the enormity of a complex literature.

This book grew out of the work of the Breast Cancer International Research Group (BCIRG), the first academic global translational cooperative group. We believe that the model of the academic global translational group is a potent tool to help us rapidly test new ideas in the clinical arena. The goal is to bring new therapies from the laboratory to the clinic as quickly as possible. Key factors in the success of academic virtual translational groups include:

1. Scientific and academic control of the clinical development of new treatments. Rather than relying on industry or the government to dictate the research agenda, BCIRG wishes to define, in collaboration with research partners and sponsors, multi-step global strategies of development, in order to streamline the process necessary to obtain definitive scientific answers and focus on the ultimate therapeutic role of new compounds.
2. Globalization of research operations and processes. This allows worldwide access to patients and subgroups of patients, to conduct specific scientific studies within the context of a global development strategy. A consequence of this approach is speed, which is its great strength. The potential weakness is the quality of data. Therefore, to ensure the highest level of quality, BCIRG has implemented extraordinarily strict processes for systematic source documentation and data validation.
3. Cultivation of close working relationships with all the parties needed to most rapidly translate biologic discoveries into new therapies that benefit patients. These groups include patients, clinical researchers (academic and community-based), academic basic scientists, a variety of experts from the pharmaceutical and biotechnology industries, and government representatives. The most important task is to create the conditions by which these groups can be integrated, to most effectively translate scientific information to the bedside.
4. Use of modern techniques of communication and cutting-edge scientific tools and informatics. This permits the creation of a worldwide virtual group capable of conducting high-quality clinical research and effectively evaluating new translational therapies.

We stand at a historic juncture, a time when numerous new cancer drugs are entering clinical trials. The explosion of drug discovery, however, creates new problems for those engaged in clinical research. There are a limited number of patients, for instance, and a limited number of physicians trained in clinical research methodologies. Thus, to most effectively evaluate the various new agents making their way into the clinic, there is a need for global organizations such as BCIRG, which are dedicated to a focused, science-driven research agenda. Academic virtual translational groups will become especially important as we attempt to identify subpopulations of patients who, based on the bi-

TABLE 42.1. Levels of evidence in evaluating clinical trials (13)

Level	Type of evidence for recommendation
I	Evidence obtained from meta-analysis of multiple, well-designed, controlled studies; randomized trials with low false-positive and low false-negative errors (high power)
II	Evidence obtained from at least one well-designed experimental study; randomized trials with high false-positive and/or negative errors (low power)
III	Evidence obtained from well-designed quasi-experimental studies, such as non-randomized controlled, single-group pre-post, cohort, time or matched case-control series
IV	Evidence from well-designed, non-experimental studies, such as comparative and correlation, descriptive and case studies
V	Evidence from case reports and clinical examples
Category	Grade of evidence
A	There is evidence of type I or consistent findings from multiple studies of types II, III, or IV
B	There is evidence of types II, III, or IV, and findings are generally consistent
C	There is evidence of types II, III, or IV, but findings are inconsistent
D	There is little or no systemic evidence
NG	No grade given

ology of their tumors, will most benefit from specific targeted therapies. Indeed, the identification of key signaling pathways and the development of reliable predictive factors will be essential to optimize the use of most of the new biologics.

To provide a framework for the evaluation of evidence in this book, we have used a system endorsed by the American Society of Clinical Oncology (14). This system, which relies on pragmatic criteria, categorizes evidence into different levels based on the nature of the clinical studies that provided data (Table 42.1). Of course, the five-level system is not the only method available to evaluate evidence, but we believe it provides a practical way to weight information being used to make clinical decisions. In addition, we have included in this second edition a new section on the evolving basic science of breast cancer, to provide relevant translational research findings in a format clinicians can understand. This is intended to introduce the next generation of therapeutics, stimulate collaborations among clinical and basic scientists, and, not least, demonstrate how far along the path to truly individualized therapy we have come. Ultimately, the success of *Breast Cancer Management* will depend on its effectiveness in improving the care of breast cancer patients around the world.

REFERENCES

1. Jounna J. *Hippocrates*. Translated by M. B. Debevoise. Baltimore: Johns Hopkins University Press, 1999.
2. Hippocrates. *The collected works of Hippocrates*. Translated by J. Chadwick. Springfield, IL: Charles C. Thomas, 1950.
3. Kardinal CG, Yarbro JW. A conceptual history of cancer. *Semin Oncol* 1979;6:396–408.
4. Keil H. The historical relationship between the concept of tumor and the ending -oma. *Bull Hist Med* 1950; 24:352–357.
5. Shimkin M. *Contrary to nature*. Washington: U.S Department of Health, Education, and Welfare, 1977.
6. Porter R. *The greatest benefit to mankind: a medical history of humanity*. New York: W. W. Norton, 1998.
7. Osler W. The master-word in medicine. In: Osler W, ed. *Aequanimitas, with other addresses to medical students, nurses, and practitioners of medicine*, 3rd ed. New York: McGraw-Hill, 1906.
8. Greenhalgh T. *How to read a paper: the basics of evidence based medicine*. London: BMJ Books, 1997.
9. van Helmont JB. *Oriatrike, or physick refined: the common errors therein refuted, and the whole art reformed and rectified*. London: Lodowick-Lloyd, 1662.
10. Cooper WA. The history of the radical mastectomy. *Ann Med Hist* 1941;3:36–54.
11. Frei E, Holland JF, Schneiderman MA, et al. A comparative study of two regimens of combination chemotherapy in acute leukemia. *Blood* 1958;13:1126–1148.
12. Doll R, Bradford-Hill A. Mortality in relation to smoking: ten years' observation of British doctors. *BMJ* 1964; 1:1399–1410.
13. Straus SE, McAlister FA. Evidence based medicine: past, present, and future. *Ann R Coll Physicians* 1999; 32:260–264.
14. American Society of Clinical Oncology. Recommended breast cancer surveillance guidelines. *J Clin Oncol* 1997; 15:2149–2156.

43
Clinical Practice Guidelines

George P. Browman

DEFINITIONS

"Clinical practice guidelines" have been defined as systematically developed statements to assist practitioner and patient decisions about appropriate health care for specific clinical circumstances (1).

The definition implies many important principles. It prescribes a systematic and, therefore transparent, process for developing guidelines. It acknowledges guidelines as tools, not rules, for practice that are intended to assist clinical judgments, not replace them. The definition respects the input of patients in clinical decision making. Finally, in addressing "specific" clinical circumstances, the definition suggests that guidelines be designed to avoid vague generalizations that focus on the generic patient at the expense of the specific circumstances in question.

"Evidence-based medicine" has been defined as the explicit, systematic, and judicious application of the best available evidence from health research in the management of individual patients (2).

This definition likewise implies principles that are often forgotten in the formulaic approach used by many guideline developers and decision-makers. As with guidelines, the definition demands a systematic process that implies transparency in how recommendations from evidence are built. The definition calls for the "judicious" use of the evidence, thus respecting the role of clinical judgment; it is implied that clinicians will value other inputs into their decisions that place a context around the evidence. The term "best available" evidence should be distinguished from "truth." In making our decisions, we can only do the best with the evidence that is before us. We cannot predict how the evidence might change; thus, decisions based on high-quality evidence cannot be fairly judged in retrospect. However, the phrase "best available evidence" also holds decision-makers accountable for considering all the evidence rather than selecting the evidence based on personal beliefs or based solely on their informal awareness of some of the evidence. Finally, the definition of "evidence-based medicine" clearly places emphasis on evidence from the research domain, which is not intended to exclude information of other types.

Thus, decision-makers ought to be accountable only for *considering* the evidence within a context, because it cannot always be applied in the specific clinical situation of concern. Thus, a better definition of evidence-based medicine might be: the explicit *consideration* of the best available research evidence and its judicious application in the management of individual patients.

EVIDENCE-BASED CLINICAL PRACTICE GUIDELINES

Several methods have been used to develop clinical practice guidelines (CPGs). These can be generally classified as "opinion based," "consensus-based," and "evidence-based" (3). Although even evidence-based guidelines require expert opinion for the proper interpretation and application of the evidence, the problem with purely opinion-based CPGs is that they generally are not transparent in stating how the evidence was considered along the path to making recommendations. The lack of transparency makes it difficult to know whether all the evidence was considered, whether the right evidence was considered, and whether there was bias in how the evidence was acquired, evaluated, considered and applied. While expert opinion alone is legitimate as a clinical decision process for one's own patients with whom implicit contractual arrangements exist, it is insufficient for making broader recommendations that may affect the treatment of others outside of one's own practice. Here, the level of accountability ought to be greater. The role of the clinical expert is to provide input into the interpretation of evidence that has been synthesized using explicit and rigorous methods. As the evidence-based movement evolves, however, more and more clinical experts are becoming sophisticated consumers of research information with methodological expertise.

Consensus-based CPGs rely mainly on group consensus methods that may or may not include the explicit consideration of best available evidence for making clinical recommendations. One of the criticisms of purely consensus-based methods is that when consensus is the main goal of the process, it may often be achieved at the expense of what the evidence suggests (4). The strength of consensus methods is that they harness the views of a variety of legitimate stakeholders. Consensus processes should be considered useful for improving evidence-based CPGs because evidence does not necessarily speak for itself. Consensus approaches can assist with the interpretation of the evidence from different perspectives, and for defining the clinical circumstances to which the evidence can be generalized. Consensus approaches also allow for the input of patients as stakeholders, who have much to say about clinical recommendations. Breast cancer survivors can contribute to group processes in sorting out which outcomes matter most to patients and their families, the magnitude of benefits from trials that have clinical meaning to them, and how recommendations can be framed in order to promote shared decision-making. Therefore, the combination of consensus and evidence-based methods is ideal for CPG development.

The process of evidence-based CPG development simply means that there was an explicit and systematic consideration of the best available evidence using rigorous methods such as the systematic review of the literature, which is designed to minimize bias in the location, selection and synthesis of the evidence; it also means that these processes are reported to ensure transparency (5).

A simplistic evaluation of the evidence-based approach would question whether all the effort is worth it if, in the end, the recommendations produced are the same as those generated by other, less costly approaches. It is fair to assume that evidence-based and expert-based (or opinion-based) CPG development strategies are likely to produce the same or similar recommendations for a very high proportion of topics. After all, experts do not practice in willful neglect of the evidence. However, accountability demands that we be more explicit in how we consider evidence when making recommendations.

In the longer term, evidence-based approaches may be more efficient than those that are opinion-based if we recognize that CPGs are living documents that require continuous refreshing (i.e., updating) as the evidence evolves. Explicit and transparent documents that were developed systematically are more amenable to modification over time using the same methods that were originally applied. In the absence of documented systematic methods for arriving at recommendations, new evidence that is based on expert opinion alone would not be able to benefit from a baseline inventory of processes and knowledge. This would require starting from scratch, especially if different experts are consulted when updating is needed.

One of the criticisms of the evidence-based approach is the labor-intensiveness, expense and time required to produce valid guidelines. This issue has recently been raised, with a challenge for guideline developers to find a more reasonable balance between scientific rigor and pragmatism, so that we can be more efficient in producing valid guidelines (6).

THE HALLMARK OF THE EVIDENCE-BASED GUIDELINE AND LEVELS OF EVIDENCE

How would one judge whether a CPG is evidence-based? The hallmark of an evidence-based CPG is the use of the systematic review, with an explicit method for synthesizing the entire body of evidence (using either qualitative or quantitative methods) in informing the clinical recommendations. A systematic review is not a CPG. It is only that part of the CPG that brings the clinical research evidence into the mix of other inputs. Furthermore, systematic reviews, like randomized trials themselves, can be of variable quality (7).

Any CPG that does not provide a list of citations to support its clinical recommendations based on evidence cannot be considered to be evidence-based because it asks the reader to trust the author(s). Evidence-based CPGs ought to allow readers to delve into the evidence as deeply as they are able to, in the same way the guideline developers did.

The use of levels of evidence (8) is not the hallmark of an evidence-based approach, and the absence of the use of levels of evidence is not sufficient to reject a guideline because it is not evidence-based. (Actually, the term evidence-informed is probably better than evidence-based in conveying the role of research evidence in clinical decisions or recommendations).

The phrase "levels of evidence" was conceived as descriptive shorthand. It was intended to convey or categorize the quality of evidence, based on the rigor of the design used to generate it. This speaks to the validity of the conclusions based on the research. Levels of evidence can be thought of as an ordinal classification of the quality of the research information available.

The use of levels of evidence is furthermore intended to convey the nature of the best available evidence that addresses a particular problem. For example, if there are results from large randomized controlled trials of drug X versus control for a given condition, then the level of evidence is level I by most classifications used. This evidence trumps lower quality evidence so that it is unnecessary, in fact redundant, to classify such a recommendation as having, for example, level I plus levels II, III and IV evidence. Yet, many existing guidelines use this approach.

The use of levels of evidence as a shorthand descriptive tool was never intended to provide only positive support for interventions. For example, level V evidence (case reports or case series, depending on the classification used) is usually a flag that the evidence ought to be seriously challenged as a support for a positive recommendation. Yet, many guideline developers in their enthusiasm use level V evidence as justification to recommend an intervention, as opposed to justifying its rejection. Some guideline development groups actually categorize expert opinion as level V evidence. This serves only to suggest a veneer of rigor that does not actually exist, and reduces the usefulness of the levels of evidence approach. Level V evidence has also been used to attach to a recommendation a level of evidence for the apparent sake of completeness. Often, such a recommendation (such as a chest x-ray for staging breast cancer) will never be tested in a trial, and does not require slavish adherence to a formula. On the other hand, a recommendation such as an annual chest x-ray in otherwise healthy low-risk people ought to be supported by rigorous evidence before it is implemented.

Because of these concerns, the use of levels of evidence has been curtailed by at least one guideline development group in favor of meaningful narrative that provides more than an ordinal scale descriptor regarding the strength of the available evidence (9). Shorthand monikers are useful communications tools when properly used, but can deteriorate to a level of absurdity when abused.

THE BENEFITS AND LIMITATIONS OF THE CLINICAL PRACTICE GUIDELINE AS A DECISION AID

Benefits

Clinical practice guidelines serve as useful reference tools for helping clinicians and patients make clinical decisions. Evidence-based CPGs provide a valid and reliable summary of the available evidence. Given that the peer-reviewed literature is poorly organized for clinical decision making, the CPG can be the vehicle for consolidating evidence related to a particular clinical problem, highlighting the gaps in knowledge and indicating where further research is needed.

CPGs may be useful to those responsible for organizing and paying for healthcare services. An inventory of properly developed, credible clinical guidelines serves to highlight where investments in health services are needed and justified.

CPGs also serve as a baseline inventory of knowledge that can foster dialogue among clinicians, patients, the public, healthcare managers and payers so that appropriate healthcare can be debated on the substantive issues. The experience has also been that evidence-based cancer guideline initiatives when applied on a programmatic basis (9) can elevate the level of discussion among several stakeholder groups. This has resulted in increases rather than reductions in funding for cancer care services in Ontario, especially in the approval for new and emerging chemotherapy and supportive care agents (10–12).

Evidence-based guideline processes can use consensus methods as an educational tool to influence the culture of an organization by promoting critical examination of evidence by groups of practitioners and other stakeholders. This may improve communication among oncologists, and increase the expertise of clinicians in searching for, evaluating and interpreting the evidence from healthcare research. Guideline development panels can be a rich educational environment and an opportunity for research productivity by trainees in cancer care disciplines. Some oncology residency and fellowship training programs have used Ontario cancer guidelines as part of their educational materials. In sum, it could be argued that the process of a rigorous and inclusive guideline development program adds at least, if not more, value to the system than the final product, the guideline itself.

Limitations

The main limitations of evidence-based guidelines relate to: (a) the effort and cost of their development; (b) duplication of effort; (c) inadequate investments in implementation strategies; (d) difficulties in evaluation; (e) slow adoption of innovations as a side effect; and (f) guideline abuse, as discussed below.

a. Properly constructed evidence-based CPGs take a lot of time to develop. This means relatively high costs. Those who commission CPGs and expect high-quality products need to be patient. There are few available short cuts that will not in some way erode either the validity or the credibility of a guideline and therefore its effectiveness. Thus, cheap CPGs will not add value to the health system. However, we need to find ways to produce evidence-based guidelines more efficiently while maintaining their validity (6).

b. Given the cost of their development, one of the most frustrating aspects of the guideline development industry is the current lack of cooperation among interested groups. This has led to unnecessary duplication of efforts in aspects of CPG development where cooperation is possible and preferable. Lack of cooperation has led to wastage of funding for a very expensive resource. Given that CPGs need to be continuously updated, continued independent programs will waste even more resources on their updating processes. Strategies can be developed to pool resources and cooperate in the development and updating of CPGs, and in their implementation and evaluation. A national workshop planned for September 2002 addressed collaboration for guideline development and aftercare across Canada, and similar approaches are being pursued actively in Europe (Dr. Beatrice Fervers, personal communication).

c. While tremendous efforts and resources have been expended by a variety of groups to develop CPGs, these commitments have not been matched by support for implementation or evaluation. Like any other healthcare innovation, CPGs will not be adopted if they are not made available to clinicians at the point of care to assist them with their decision making. Passive dissemination and peer-reviewed publications are insufficient strategies to ensure that CPGs get used. The importance of implementation has been highlighted in a recent review about why physicians don't follow guidelines (14).

d. Efforts to evaluate the influence of CPGs on either practice patterns, or patient outcomes, or both are currently in their early stages, and such evaluations are difficult to design and expensive to carry out. Strategies such as clinician surveys are very prone to bias, as it has been shown that how clinicians think they practice is quite different from how they do practice (13,14). Audits of clinical records (15–17) and population data examining patterns of practice in relation to the timing of the release of a CPG may provide valuable information on the consistency of practice with a CPG but will not provide direct evidence of whether a CPG is being consulted in the clinic. Only rigorous trials and, eventually, clinical information systems in the form of electronic medical records will yield direct information on whether clinicians consult CPGs, whether they abide by their recommendations, and the reasons why recommendations are not followed. Such information could in the longer term be related to patient outcomes. It is reasonable to ask at this time whether large investments in complex trials to evaluate CPGs can be justified when we are facing imminent dramatic changes in health records systems that will do the same job at less expense.

e. The evidence-based approach can legitimately be criticized for its conservatism in recommending the adoption of new and promising, but not proven, interventions. The evidence-based proponents would argue that for these interventions, research is what is required. This is a reaction to legitimate concerns in healthcare of the premature adoption of many innovative ideas that subsequently were found to be less beneficial than advertised and often harmful to patients. Notwithstanding the validity of the latter claim, the evidence-based approach may be casting a pall over the spirit of innovation in oncology. Cancer is as much an investigative discipline as it is an evidence-based discipline. While evidence-based principles embrace the investigative spirit in theory, there is concern that its application in practice may be having a dampening effect on innovation and its adoption, especially in publicly funded systems. This issue should not be minimized, and may contribute to the unwillingness of payers to support research-based practice in oncology, which is the lifeblood of the discipline.

f. The definitions of CPGs and evidence-based medicine are consistent in relating these concepts to the management of individual patient care. However, CPGs are being promoted more by managers and payers as vehicles to control practice and reduce costs. Nonetheless, in Ontario, CPGs have actually resulted in increased funding to the cancer care system. While CPGs are intended as clinical tools, they are being used as policy tools. It is still not clear whether the decisional context of the clinical encounter can be scaled up to the boardroom in terms of the utility of the evidence-based approach. In a recent article, it was pointed out how identical interpretation of the same research evidence by a clinician in a clinical context and a manager in a policy context could produce opposite courses of action, but of which are defensible (18). We are still in the early learning phase in knowing how best to apply CPGs in clinical practice and policy.

Simplistic notions of evaluation of clinical practice also threaten CPGs. It seems perfectly clear, at this time, that the same research evidence can produce conflicting clinical recommendations, and that conflicts between clinical and policy recommendations can be defensible and legitimate (discussed below). Nonetheless, some managers and payers are intent on developing intrusive strategies that can interfere with good judgment about how to manage an individual patient. Data about variations between practice and guidelines ought to be interpreted as flags to the practitioner, not judgments of the practitioner. A well-implemented CPG that is not influencing practice is as likely to signal a badly designed CPG as it is inappropriate practice.

In an instructive example, recommendations for the surgical management of stage I breast cancer according to the Canadian Steering Committee identifies lumpectomy (breast-conserving surgery) followed by local radiation as the preferred option (19). At the same time, Ontario's CPG recommends that either mastectomy or lumpectomy followed by radiation is acceptable; but the patient should be offered a choice (20). These CPGs are consistent with one another, but clearly have different implications in terms of how they would be evaluated. Of interest, when a decision tool was developed in Ontario to help patients decide with their surgeons about which approach to take, the rate of breast conserving surgery (BCS) actually fell for those surgeons who were more often offering BCS prior to the development of the decision aid.

CONTRASTING CANADIAN AND AUSTRALIAN GUIDELINES ON BREAST CANCER

To highlight some of the principles discussed above, it is instructive to examine differences between guidelines on the same topic produced by different organizations, both of which used a rigorous evidence-based approach. Here, I have selected national guidelines from Canada and Australia for the management of early-stage breast cancer. For additional insights, I have also included some guideline statements from the Cancer Care Ontario guideline initiative.

TABLE 43.1. *Contrasting Canadian and Australian breast cancer guidelines*

Canadian breast cancer guidelines tend to be more prescriptive
Australian guidelines present the evidence
Canadian breast CPGs follow a more traditional medical orientation
Australian guidelines stress communication, psychosocial issues
Canadian breast CPGs are formatted for quick reference to be used at the point of care
Australian CPGs serve more as background reference material, although selected issues are highlighted
Australian guidelines are more comprehensive in the material they cover
Recommendations from both countries are generally consistent with the evidence
Differences seem to reflect local organizational and cultural (medical and societal) issues and perspectives

TABLE 43.2. *Contrasting guideline statements (mastectomy or lumpectomy)*

Mastectomy or lumpectomy

Canada:
For patients with stage I or II breast cancer, BCS followed by radiotherapy is generally recommended

Ontario:
Women with stage I or II breast cancer who are candidates for BCS should be offered the choice of either BCS or modified

Australia:
There is no difference in the rate of survival or distant metastasis between women having mastectomy and those having BCS where appropriate

The following examples are for illustrative purposes only. Updates of these documents since the preparation of this chapter may render certain specific information obsolete.

Table 43.1 highlights some of the fundamental differences between the Australian and Canadian national guidelines, both of which are evidence-based. The most obvious feature distinguishing the sets of guidelines in this example is that those from Australia did not make any prescriptive statements at all, but simply described the nature of the evidence. Thus, they shy away from recommendations. In contrast,

TABLE 43.3. *Contrasting guideline statements (radiotherapy following lumpectomy) (BCS)*

Radiotherapy following lumpectomy (BCS)

Canada:
Women who undergo BCS should be advised to have postoperative breast RT. Omission of RT increases risk of local recurrence. Local breast RT should begin no later than 12 weeks, but optimal interval not defined.

Ontario:
Women who have undergone BCS should be offered postoperative breast irradiation. Optimal schedule not established. RT should begin within 12 weeks, but window of safety is unknown.

Australia:
Radiotherapy after lumpectomy significantly reduces the risk of local recurrence. Omission of RT leads to increased risk of local recurrence. "While it is not uncommon clinical practice to omit RT in…selected cases…the decision requires the woman to weigh . . ."

TABLE 43.4. *Contrasting Canadian and Australian guideline topics for early stage breast cancer*

Canadian consensus document	Australian NHMRC guidelines
Early-stage disease	
1. The palpable breast lump	1. Counseling issues
2. Investigation of mammography detected lesions	2. Volume/outcome considerations
3. Mastectomy or lumpectomy?	3. Navigating the health system
4. Axillary dissection	4. Role of surgery in mammography
5. Management of DCIS	5. Simple vs. radical mastectomy
6. Breast radiotherapy after BCS	6. Mastectomy vs. BCS
7. Adjuvant systemic therapy for node-negative disease	7. Local radiotherapy after BCS
8. Adjuvant systemic node-positive	8. Adjuvant therapy for node-positive and node-negative disease
9. Follow-up after treatment for . . .	9. Management of DCIS & LCIS
10. Management of chronic pain	10. Follow-up after treatment

both the Canadian and Ontario guidelines did make recommendations for practice. The guideline statements in Tables 43.2 and 43.3 illustrate these differences. Note also in Figure 43.2 how the difference in the recommendations for the surgical management of early stage breast cancer reveals different values for patient choice between Canada and Ontario.

Table 43.4 demonstrates interesting differences in perspective between Australian and Canadian guidelines at that time in terms of the topics included for the management of early-stage breast cancer. The medical orientation of the Canadian guideline contrasts with the broader perspective of those produced in Australia. However, despite these noticeable differences in approach and style, there is overall consistency in the substance of the guidelines from the two countries. Furthermore, it is likely that the examples from each country will influence future guideline approaches by others.

TOOLS FOR GUIDELINES

Well conceived, cancer-related, evidence-based CPGs are produced by a variety of sources, many of which have developed their own Web sites for reference. Useful Web sites for consulting guidelines on breast cancer include the Cancer Care Ontario Guideline Initiative at http://hiru.mcmaster.ca/ccopgi/, the American Society of Clinical Oncology at www.asco.org/, and the Australian NHMRC National Breast Cancer Centre www.nbcc.org.au/. The National Comprehensive Cancer Network (NCCN) in the United States produces useful guidelines in the form of clinical algorithms. These guidelines are developed through expert consensus, and their publication does not include a comprehensive list of citations so that to date they cannot be formally classified as evidence-based.

A Web site sponsored by the U.S. Agency for Health Research & Quality (AHRQ) uses specific eligibility criteria for evidence-based guidelines before it will include them in its Web site. The Web site promises to help clinicians and policy makers be aware of guidelines and determine the strengths and weaknesses among several different CPGs on the same topic so that the most appropriate can be used in the circumstances. The Web site address for the U.S. Guideline Clearinghouse is www.guideline.gov/index.asp. The Canadian Medical Association also provides an inventory of guidelines in Canada, with links to original Web sites. The CMA Web site address is www.cma.ca/cpgs/index.htm. Some guideline programs produce CD-ROM versions of their products. One such program is the *Standards, Options and Recommendations* of the excellent evidence-based French oncology guideline initiative, which also provides a Web site, www.fnclcc.fr/. A commercial CD-ROM product with an extensive inventory of guidelines is available from Faulkner & Gray, and guidelines are regularly updated at www. guidelines.faulknergray.com.

CONCLUSION

Clinical practice guidelines share the characteristics of other healthcare innovations. Their introduction will be associated with some benefits, and their limitations will be recognized. But, like other innovations, they need to be allowed to evolve as we learn more about how to use them in the most appropriate way. Progress in the application of clinical practice guidelines will require research if they are to evolve and improve like other healthcare technologies (21).

REFERENCES

1. Field MJ, Lohr KM, eds. Institute of Medicine. Guidelines for medical practice: from development to use. Washington, DC: National Academy Press, 1992.
2. Sackett DL, Rosenberg WMC, Gray MJA, et al. Evidence-based medicine: what it is and what it isnt. *BMJ* 1996;312:71–72.
3. Browman GP. Evidence-based paradigms and opinions in clinical management and cancer research. *Semin Oncol* 1999;26(suppl 8):9–13.
4. Wortman PM, Vinokur A, Sechrest L. Do consensus conferences work? A process evaluation of the NIH consensus development program. *J Health Politics Policy Law* 1988;13:469–498.
5. Mulrow CD. Rationale for systematic reviews. *BMJ* 1994;309:597–599.
6. Browman G. Development and aftercare of clinical guidelines. The balance between rigor and pragmatism. *JAMA* 2001;286:1509–1511.
7. Jadad AR, Cook DJ, Jones A, et al. Methodology and reports of systematic reviews and meta-analyses: a comparison of Cochrane reviews with articles published in paper-based journals. *JAMA* 1998;280:278–280.
8. Cook DJ, Guyatt GH, Laupacis A, et al. Clinical recommendations using levels of evidence for antithrombotic agents. *Chest* 1995;108(4 suppl):227S–230S
9. Browman GP. Background to clinical guidelines in cancer: SOR, A programmatic approach to guideline development and aftercare. *Br J Cancer* 2001;84:1–3.
10. Browman GP, Levine MN, Mohide EA, et al. The practice guidelines development cycle: A conceptual tool for practice guidelines development and implementation. *J Clin Oncol* 1995;13:502–512.
11. Evans WK, Newman TE, Graham I, et al. Lung cancer practice guidelines: Lessons learned and issues addressed by the Ontario Lung Cancer Disease Site Group. *J Clin Oncol* 1997;15:3049–3059.
12. Browman GP, Newman TE, Mohide EA, et al. Progress of clinical oncology guidelines development using the practice guidelines development cycle: The role of practitioner feedback. *J Clin Oncol* 1998;16:1226–1231.
13. Cabana MD, Rand CS, Powe NR, et al. Why don't physicians follow clinical practice guidelines? *JAMA* 1999;282:1458–1465.
14. Lomas J, Anderson GM, Domnick-Pierre K, et al. Do practice guidelines guide practice? The effect of a consensus statement on the practice of physicians. *N Engl J Med* 1989;321:1306–1311.
15. Rosser WW. Dissemination of guidelines on cholesterol. Effect on patterns of practice of general practitioners and family physicians in Ontario. *Can Fam Physician* 1993;39:280–284.
16. Ray-Coquard I, Philip T, Lehmann M, et al. Impact of a clinical guidelines program for breast and colon cancer in a French cancer center. *JAMA* 1997;278:1591–1595.
17. Ray-Coquard I, Philip T, de Laroche G, et al. A controlled before-after study: Impact of a clinical guidelines programme and regional cancer network organization on medical practice. *Br J Cancer* 2002;86:313–320.
18. Browman GP. Essence of evidence-based medicine: A case report. *J Clin Oncol* 1999;17:1969–1973.
19. Steering Committee on Clinical Practice Guidelines for the Care and Treatment of Breast Cancer. Mastectomy or lumpectomy? The choice of operation for clinical stage I and II breast cancer. *Can Med Assoc J* 1998;158(3 suppl):S15–21.
20. Mirsky D, OBrien SE, McCready DR, et al. Surgical management of early stage invasive breast cancer (stage I and II). *Cancer Preven Control* 1997;1:10–16.
21. Browman GP, Levine MN, Graham I, et al. The clinical practice guideline: an evolving health care technology. *Cancer Prevent Control* 1997;1:7–8.

44

RECIST: Response Evaluation Criteria in Solid Tumors

Janet Dancey, Patrick Therasse, Susan G. Arbuck, and Elizabeth A. Eisenhauer

All clinical trials should be prospectively planned and conducted under controlled conditions to provide definitive answers to well-defined questions. Yet, despite careful planning and execution, the results of non-randomized trials evaluating the same agent or combination of therapies in the same tumor type often vary widely. Some of this variability is due to differences in patient characteristics, and reflects a true spectrum of benefit that can be expected from the treatment of patients with a given disease. It is due to this variability that treatment benefit can only be determined definitively through randomized controlled trials. Because of the cost, complexity and duration of randomized studies, preliminary evidence of antitumor activity is often determined in smaller, single-arm phase 2 studies. These trials usually use the surrogate endpoint of tumor response. Phase 2 studies are important in setting the direction of cancer research as they determine whether an agent or regimen is worthy of further evaluation. With an expanding number of agents and combinations for evaluation and a limited number of patients available for clinical trials, the efficient use of these resources is increasingly important. An accurate estimate of drug activity is essential to efficiently use drug development resources; however, the reliability of the estimate not only depends on patient, disease and treatment related factors, but also on the methods of assessing, analyzing and reporting the endpoint of interest.

Phase 2 trials are not designed to be formally compared to the results of other studies; rather, they are designed to identify an absolute level of biologic activity of interest based on historical data so that decisions regarding further development can be made. As a result, it is imperative that the methods of evaluating the endpoint of interest are consistent across studies. The purpose of this chapter is to describe the limitations of older response criteria and to present the recently revised Response Criteria in Solid Tumors (RECIST), which were developed to address these limitations and provide new standards for assessing and reporting response rates.

TUMOR RESPONSE AS AN ENDPOINT OF CLINICAL TRIALS:

The primary goal of phase 2 trials in oncology is to estimate the antitumor activity of either a novel cytotoxic agent or combined therapeutic regimen against a specific cancer. The most commonly used endpoint of these trials is the objective response rate.

There are at least three reasons for using tumor response as an endpoint in a phase 2 study. First, tumor regression implies some degree of antitumor activity of the agent being evaluated. Second, it is an outcome measure available early in the trial; thus, studies require smaller numbers of patients followed for shorter durations than studies assessing survival. Third, improvements in tumor response rates correlate, to some extent, with improvements in more definitive measures of patient benefit such symptom palliation or prolongation of survival (1). Although there are many examples of agents with promising response rates in phase 2 studies that were not found to be beneficial in phase 3 studies, all standard cytotoxic and hormonal treatments currently available were selected for phase 3 evaluation based on promising phase 2 results. Until better methods of assessing antitumor activity are available, some measure of change in tumor size will continue to be used as an endpoint for phase 2 studies assessing anticancer agents that are expected to induce tumor regression.

To identify the most promising agents for phase 3 evaluation, it is essential to obtain an accurate estimate of drug activity in phase 2 studies. However, the reported tumor response rate may be influenced by a number of factors. These factors include not only the choice of patients, disease stage, and the details of treatment, but also the criteria for assessment of therapeutic effect and the analysis of results. The definition of tumor response, the techniques for assessing tumor size and their associated errors of measurement, the sample size of the trial, and the frequency with which treated patients are excluded from analysis all influence the reported response rates obtained from phase 2 studies (2–5). In fact, the definition and criteria for determining objective response affect the response rate, response duration, progression-free survival and time to treatment failure. While unknown patient and tumor-related factors may vary from study to study despite careful planning, using common definitions and criteria can reduce variability in assessing and reporting clinical outcomes.

Response criteria which have been published for breast cancer trials are those of the National Cancer Institute (NCI) (6), Union Internationale Contre le Cancer (UICC) (7), and British Breast Cancer Group (8). For solid tumors, response criteria have been developed by the World Health Organization (WHO), Eastern Co-operative Oncology Group (ECOG), Southwest Oncology Group (SWOG), and European Organization for Research and Treatment of Cancer (EORTC) (9–12). These criteria were developed by consensus among experts. Unsurprisingly, as different individuals were involved in the development of these criteria, specific definitions and recommendations vary. Which tumor deposits are considered assessable, the number of lesions that should be assessed and the changes in measurable and nonmeasurable disease that define significant tumor regression or growth are some of the areas of discrepancy.

The WHO criteria have been the most commonly used in phase 2 trials of solid tumors worldwide. These classify disease as bidimensionally and unidimensionally measurable, nonmeasurable evaluable, and unevaluable. The WHO criteria also stipulate the method for determining tumor burden and define four categories of tumor response: complete response (CR), partial response (PR), stable disease (SD), and progressive disease (PD). Although the WHO criteria include both unidimensional and bidimensional disease as measurable, over time, various research groups redefined measurable disease to mean measurable in two dimensions because of difficulties integrating uni- and bidimensional lesions into response definitions. Thus, in most trials, tumor burden is calculated by summing for each measured lesion the products obtained by multiplying the largest diameter by its largest perpendicular diameter. The definition of complete response is the disappearance of all evidence of disease for a minimum of four weeks. Partial response is defined as a 50% or more decrease in total tumor load of the lesions that have been measured for a minimum of 4 weeks without evidence of progression in other sites. The advantages of specifying a minimum duration for CR or PR are twofold: a response of short duration is unlikely to be of clinical benefit and requiring a confirmatory assessment before declaring response may reduce the likelihood of misclassification of response due to measurement error. Progressive disease is defined as an increase of 25% in the size of one or more measurable lesions or the appearance of new lesion(s). Changes in tumor load that do not fit the definitions for CR, PR, or PD are classified as stable disease.

Since the effect of therapy on tumor burden reflects a continuum from the complete disappearance of all tumor to utterly unimpeded tumor growth, the cut-offs used to create the four response categories are arbitrary. The definitions are based on assumptions regarding the magnitude of tumor reduction that would be measurable, unlikely to occur spontaneously and likely to provide patient benefit. Similarly, the definition of progression was thought to be the minimum change in tumor growth that should prompt the discontinuation of a usually toxic and clearly ineffective therapy.

The assumptions underlying these definitions, that objective tumor response results in patient benefit and the changes in tumor burden can be accurately and reliably determined, are questionable. A 50% reduction in tumor area represents a cut-off in the spectrum of changes in tumor size that can occur while patients are receiving treatment. There is no reason to believe that clinical outcome will be substantially different for patients with somewhat lesser or greater changes in tumor burden. It is not surprising, therefore, that phase 3 studies have shown that higher response rates may or may not be associated with improved survival, or that the survival of patients with partial responses or stable disease has been found to differ modestly or not at all (13). While many studies have shown that responders live longer than nonresponders, such comparisons do not prove that the survival of responders was prolonged as a result of treatment, because such an analysis is confounded and biased. Patients with disease sensitive to cytotoxic or hormonal therapy may have been destined to do well anyway because of favorable prognostic factors or disease biology. Patients who die early, even those who die of treatment-related complications, are included among the nonresponders (1,14).

The classification of response requires repeated measurements of tumor nodules; thus, the accuracy of the results will depend on the method of assessment. The definition of CR, the disappearance of all evidence of disease for a minimum of four weeks, is straightforward although it will be influenced by the sensitivity of the tests used to identify and follow sites of disease. However, PR, PD, and SD are defined by "cut-offs" and may therefore be influenced by errors in measurement. Various studies of simulated tumor nodules (3,5,15), neck nodes (5), and lung metastases on x-ray (5,16) have indicated there is up to an 8% chance of falsely declaring a PR and a 30% chance of falsely declaring progression. The chance of error is higher when lesions are small, physical examination is the method of assessment and different observers make the measurements. These errors are so serious and common that independent review panels are often employed by pharmaceutical companies to standardize the reporting of tumor response in clinical trials. Independent review panel reports can disagree with "home radiologists" in 50% of cases, with major disagreements in up to 40% of cases (17). As lesions are assessed at multiple intervals during treatment, the chance of a false progression being recorded is probably higher during a clinical trial (15). Measuring more than one lesion and requiring sequential measurements at least 4 weeks apart can reduce the number of false PRs; however, these safeguards are not uniformly applied to the determination of progression. The use of such small changes in tumor area based on a single observation can lead to premature discontinuation of a potentially effective therapy due to measurement error (5).

To provide more reproducible and objective assessments of change in tumor size, response assessment has become more rigorous and technology-based. Most studies now use chest x-ray, computed tomography (CT) and magnetic resonance imaging (MRI) in preference to physical examination, ultrasound (US), and nuclear medicine studies. Cross-sectional imaging techniques such as CT and MRI allow accurate lesion assessment and independent review at a later date (18). However, even sophisticated technologies such as CT and MRI vary in quality and interpretation. Factors such as the level of technology, expertise, quantity, timing and method of injecting intravenous contrast material and the choice of slice thickness and pulse sequences (for MRI) may result in differences between the quality of the generated image and its subsequent interpretation (19).

As CT and MRI imaging procedures have improved and sophisticated software for calculating tumor volume is becoming more generally available, there is increasing interest in using volumetric tumor measurement. This has led to some confusion about how to integrate tridimensional measures into response assessment. A 50% reduction in tumor volume is not as strict a criterion for response as a 50% reduction in tumor cross-sectional area (20). In fact, a 65% reduction in volume would be required to be equivalent of a 50% reduction in cross-sectional area. While these technologies may more accurately assess change in tumor burden, whether this improvement in precision of measurement will translate into more reliable estimates of antitumor effect and correlate better with patient-related outcomes is uncertain.

Since their development, the WHO criteria have been adapted by different research organizations to integrate measurable and evaluable disease into response evaluation, define the minimum size and number of lesions to be measured, and modify the definition of progression. The lack of standardization in these areas among research organizations, as well as the development of new imaging technologies and other modalities of assessing tumor burden, eventually led to the realization that a revision of existing standards for evaluating tumor response was required.

THE RECIST CRITERIA

Over a period of 5 years, representatives of research organizations, industry and regulatory authorities from North America, Europe and Japan revised the WHO criteria. The result of this international collaboration is the RECIST. RECIST includes new definitions of measurable disease and tumor response, as well as recommendations for assessing tumor burden and for reporting results. These guidelines are more specific than the WHO criteria on a number of points that aid those evaluating solid tumors. RECIST gives specific size requirements for measurable lesions at baseline, distinguishes target from nontarget lesions, and gives the maximum number of target lesions to be followed up to a total of ten. Also, RECIST specifies a baseline tumor burden (smallest sum of long diameters from the start of treatment) for determining progressive disease and states that all target lesions should be measured to determine progressive disease instead of "one or more measurable lesions" as described in the WHO criteria. While standardization and simplification were priorities, the new criteria were also devised to allow results of future studies to be compared to historical data. The following discussion highlights some of the significant elements of RECIST. For a complete description of RECIST, readers are referred to the full publication (21). Answers to questions can be found at the RECIST Questions & Answers Web site at www.eortc.be/recist or sent by e-mail to recist@eortc.be.

MEASURABLE AND NONMEASURABLE DISEASE

Since objective response is determined by comparing overall tumor burden assessed at baseline to subsequent measurements, only patients with at least one measurable lesion should be eligible for studies in which objective tumor response is the primary endpoint. If the measurable disease is restricted to a solitary lesion, its neoplastic nature should be confirmed by tissue diagnosis (cytology or histology). The definitions of measurable and nonmeasurable disease are the first significant change to be found in RECIST and the rationale for this change will be discussed in detail.

According to RECIST, tumor lesions are categorized as either measurable or nonmeasurable. Measurable lesions must have a longest diameter more than or equal to 20 mm with conventional techniques or more than or equal to 10 mm with spiral CT scan. Measurements should be recorded in metric notation, using a ruler or callipers. Nonmeasurable lesions include small lesions as well as bone lesions, leptomeningeal disease, ascites, pleural/pericardial effusion, inflammatory breast disease, lymphangitis cutis/pulmonis, abdominal masses that are not confirmed and followed by imaging techniques, and cystic lesions. Nonmeasurable disease is recorded as present or absent. All baseline evaluations should be performed as close as possible to the treatment start and never more than 4 weeks before the beginning of treatment.

All measurable lesions, to a maximum of five lesions within an organ and ten lesions representative of all involved organs, should be measured and recorded at baseline. These "target" lesions should be selected on the basis of their size and suitability for accurate repetitive measurements. A sum of the longest diameter (LD) for all target lesions should be calculated and reported as the baseline sum LD. The baseline sum LD will be used to determine objective tumor response of the measurable dimension of the disease. All other lesions or sites of disease should be identified as nontarget lesions; these are recorded at baseline and followed to determine whether they are "present" or "absent."

Clearly, the use of a single measurement, the longest diameter, rather than the product of two measurements, the longest diameter and its largest perpendicular diameter, from each tumor nodule is a significant change from the other response criteria. However, both theoretical and practical considerations as well as data from clinical trials support the use of the sum of the longest diameter rather than the sum of the products to estimate change in tumor burden. Assuming that a tumor nodule approximates a sphere, there is a fixed mathematical relationship between its diameter, surface area and volume. A 50% decrease in area is equivalent to a 30% decrease in diameter or a 65% decrease in volume. Alternatively, a 25% increase in area corresponds to a 12% increase in diameter and 40% increase in volume. As most tumor deposits are spherical, the maximum diameter correlates well with the longest perpendicular diameter, the surface area and tumor perimeter (16). The maximum diameter becomes very inaccurate as an estimate of tumor size only when the length is more than twice its width (22). For spherical tumors 1 cm to 10 cm in diameter, the relationship between tumor diameter and the logarithm of cell number is more proportional than is the product of the longest perpendicular diameters (23). Thus, changes in diameter are approximately independent of initial tumor size, whereas changes in the sum of the products of larger tumors are the result of smaller log cell reduction compared to changes in smaller lesions. Theoretically, the sum of the diameters may be a better approximation of change in tumor burden because of its more linear relationship to the logarithm of cell number (24), although the clinical significance of this is uncertain.

Retrospective analyses of clinical trial data to determine response rates using either unidimensional or bidimensional measurements yielded remarkably similar results. James et al. (24) analyzed tumor response rates by the WHO criteria and unidimensional RECIST from data obtained on 569 patients enrolled in eight clinical trials. With few exceptions, the same patients were considered responders by either method and, without exception, the same conclusions about the efficacy of the regimen under study were reached. These results were confirmed in a much larger data set of 4,614 patients obtained from industry and American and Canadian cooperative group studies (21). In this analysis, best response for each patient was calculated using WHO criteria and RECIST. Because falsely declaring progression due to errors in measurement was a concern, a 20% increase in diameter, equivalent to a 44% increase in area and 73% increase in volume, was chosen to define progression by RECIST. Whether the calculations were based on WHO criteria or RECIST, the response rates and progressive disease rates were essentially identical: 25.6% versus 25.4% and 30.3% versus 29%, respectively. These results suggest that the use of unidimensional measurements should not result in active drugs being discarded because of perceived inactivity.

Since the RECIST guidelines require a greater change in tumor size for the classification of PD, the date progressive disease is declared should be later by RECIST compared to WHO criteria. To determine the magnitude of the difference, time-to-progression as defined by WHO criteria and RECIST was compared using a subset of trials obtained from SWOG. SWOG criteria define progression as a 50% increase in the sum of the products of bidimensional measurements, an absolute increase of 10 cm^2 or the appearance of new lesions. Based on results obtained from 234 patients with breast, colorectal, melanoma, or lung cancers, the same date of progression was found for 91.2% of cases. Unsurprisingly, an earlier date of progression with WHO criteria was obtained for 7.3% of patients. For the majority of these cases, the difference between the dates of progression was unknown, as RECIST was not reached at the time the data was censored. These results suggest there is no meaningful difference in response and progression categorization by WHO criteria or RECIST.

One concern may be that the initial evaluation of the concordance between unidimensional and bidimensional measurements was largely based on a retrospective statistical evaluation of measurements rather than original imaging data. However, two small studies have evaluated the concordance between unidimensional and bidimensional measurement criteria on serial CT imaging (25,26). In the assessment of treatment response, there was 90% and 100% agreement between one-dimensional and two-dimensional measurements. Thus, CT assessment of tumor response using uni- or bidimensional measures had limited influence on the classification of treatment response.

The similarity of results obtained, whether WHO criteria or RECIST are used, supports using the sum of the longest diameters instead of the sum of the products to simplify response evaluation. There are a number of advantages to requiring only a single measurement of each tumor nodule. Time and effort are saved by not calculating products of individual tumor nodules. More importantly, simplifying tumor assessment encourages measuring more lesions in an individual patient, reducing the risk of errors (27). The rate of accrual and completion time of phase 2 studies may be improved as patients with only unidimensionally measurable disease, who would have been excluded from phase 2 studies using older criteria, are eligible for studies using RECIST. There is little risk that including patients with only unidimensional disease or measuring change in the sum of the longest diameters will result in promising therapies being rejected (24,28).

MEASUREMENT OF LESIONS

The RECIST document includes a number of recommendations for evaluating disease to minimize measurement error. Because of the unreliability of repeated physical examination, clinically assessable lesions should only be considered measurable when they are superficial (e.g., skin nodules, palpable lymph nodes). In the case of skin lesions, documentation by color photography, including a ruler to estimate the size of the lesion, is recommended.

Measurements obtained from imaging studies are preferred to evaluation by clinical examination when both methods have been used to assess the antitumor effect of a treatment. Care must be taken as radiographic measurement may also be subject to errors introduced by differing techniques in sequential radiographic studies. The same method of assessment and the same technique should be used to characterize each identified and reported lesion at baseline and during follow-up. Chest x-ray may be used to assess lesions that are clearly defined and surrounded by aerated lung. However, CT and MRI are the most accurate and reproducible methods to measure target lesions selected for response assessment (18,19,29).

Ensuring consistent quality of enhancement and precise matching of lesions and measurements are important. To evaluate lesions within the chest, abdomen and pelvis, conventional CT and MRI should be performed with contiguous cuts of 10 mm or less in slice thickness, and spiral CT should be performed using a 5-mm contiguous reconstruction algorithm. Evaluation of lesions in the head and neck and extremities usually requires specific protocols. While it is not necessary for centers participating in studies to standardize their CT and MRI imaging protocols, it is important that, within each center, standards are used to ensure comparability of sequential studies.

Some modalities, such as US, nuclear medicine scans, endoscopy and tumor markers, should not be used to estimate changes in tumor burden in clinical trials using objective response as the primary endpoint, because they are unreliable or lack validity. Since US examination is subjective and highly operator dependent, accurate lesion assessment on subsequent examinations and independent review at a later date is difficult (18). Ultrasound can be an alternative to clinical measurements for superficial lymph nodes, subcutaneous lesions, and thyroid nodules, and may be used to confirm the complete disappearance of superficial lesions assessed by clinical examination. Laparoscopy and endoscopy may be useful to confirm complete pathological response when biopsies are obtained. However, their use for assessing changes in tumor size has not yet been fully validated, and requires sophisticated equipment and a high level of expertise that may only be available in some centers. Therefore, the utilization of such techniques for objective tumor response should be restricted to validation purposes in reference centers. Specific additional criteria for standardized evaluation of changes in prostate-specific antigen (30,31) and CA-125 (32,33) have been developed and can be incorporated into objective response evaluations once fully validated.

DETERMINING BEST OVERALL RESPONSE

The best overall response is defined as the best response recorded from the start of treatment until disease progression or recurrence. The increase in size is based on the smallest measurements recorded since treatment started. In general, the patient's best response assignment will depend on the achievement of both measurement and confirmation criteria.

Complete response is defined as disappearance of all target and non-target lesions and normalization of tumor markers. In some circumstances it may be difficult to distinguish residual disease from normal tissue (e.g., fibrosis) or tumor necrosis. When the evaluation of complete response depends upon this determination, it is recommended that the residual lesion be investigated by fine-needle aspirate or excisional biopsy to confirm complete response status.

Partial response is at least a 30% decrease in the sum of baseline LD of target lesions, without evidence of progression in non-target lesions. Thus, the persistence of one or more non-target lesions and/or maintenance of tumor marker levels above normal limits, even in the presence of a complete response of measurable lesions, results in the designation of overall tumor response of PR. Progression is at least a 20% increase over the smallest sum LD recorded or the appearance of one or more new lesions. Changes in sum LD that do not meet criteria for PR or PD are classified as SD.

Occasionally, a patient's physical status worsens without objective documentation of progressive disease. Patients with a global deterioration of health status requiring discontinuation of treatment without objective evidence of disease progression at that time should be reported as "symptomatic deterioration." Every effort should be made to document objective progression, even after discontinuation of treatment, to confirm that clinical deterioration is due to worsening disease rather than treatment toxicity or other illness.

The main goal of confirmation of objective response is to minimize the risk of overestimating the response rate. Designations of PR or CR require confirmation by repeat studies performed no less than 4 weeks after the criteria for response are first met. Longer intervals as determined by the study protocol may also be appropriate. Repeat studies to confirm changes in tumor size may not always be feasible or may not be necessary for protocols in which progression-free survival and overall survival are the key endpoints. These patients should be reported as having "unconfirmed responses." For SD, measurements must have met the SD criteria at least once after study entry at a minimum interval that is defined in the study protocol. This time interval should take into account the expected clinical benefit that such a status may bring to the population under study.

All patients included in the study must be assessed for response to treatment, even if there are major protocol treatment deviations or if they are ineligible. Each patient should be assigned one of the following categories: CR, PR, SD, PD, early death (whether due to malignant disease, toxicity or other causes), or unknown due to insufficient data. All patients who met the eligibility criteria should be included in the main analysis of the response rate. Those patients removed from treatment early should be considered as treatment failures. Incorrect treatment schedule or drug administration is not a cause of exclusion from the analysis of the response rate. Thus, to determine objective response rate, the numerator should be composed of the number of patients with confirmed CRs and PRs, and the denominator should include all eligible patients. It is preferable that the response rate be reported with 95% confidence limits. Subanalyses may then be performed on a subset of patients, excluding those for whom major protocol deviations have been identified. Reasons for excluding patients from the analysis should be clearly reported. However, these subanalyses should not serve as the basis for drawing conclusions concerning treatment efficacy; all conclusions should be based on analyses of the outcome of all eligible patients.

For trials in which the response rate is the primary endpoint, it is strongly recommended that all responses be reviewed by an expert(s) independent of the study. Consistent application of response criteria by an independent panel may significantly reduce response rates but should produce greater consistency and reproducibility of results (15,18).

Since the type and schedule of treatment can dictate the frequency of tumor re-evaluation, the RECIST guidelines stipulate that the frequency of reassessment be specified in the protocol. Follow-up every other cycle (i.e., 6 to 8 weeks) seems a reasonable norm; however, smaller or greater time intervals may be justified for specific regimens or circumstances. After treatment is completed, the need for repetitive tumor evaluations depends on whether the primary endpoint of the phase 2 trial is the response rate or "time to an event" (progression/death). If "time to event" is the main endpoint of the study, then routine re-evaluation of patients is warranted at frequencies to be determined by the protocol.

DURATION OF RESPONSE

The duration of overall response is measured from the time measurement criteria are met until the first date that recurrent or progressive disease is objectively documented. The duration of overall CR is measured from the time measurement criteria are first met for CR until the first date that recurrent disease is documented. Stable disease is measured from the start of the treatment until the criteria for progression are met. It is worth emphasizing that the baseline pretreatment examination may not always serve as the reference study to determine the date of progression. Instead, progressive disease is defined as a 20% increase in sum of LD over the smallest measurements recorded since the treatment started. The durations of response, SD and progression-free survival are influenced by the frequency of follow-up after baseline evaluation. Any comparisons among trials must take into account the lack of precision of the measured endpoint.

APPLICATION OF RECIST TO CLINICAL TRIALS

When response rate is the primary outcome measure of a trial, rigorous evaluation of tumor response as outlined in RECIST is justified. However, applying these criteria to evaluate tumor response in phase 3 trials, in which objective response is not the primary endpoint, is not required. For example, in such trials it might not be necessary to measure as many as ten target lesions, or to confirm response with a follow-up assessment after 4 weeks or more. Methods to evaluate response should be specified in the protocol and these deviations from RECIST should appear in reports of the trial. However, if response rate is the primary endpoint of a phase 3 trial because there is a direct relationship between objective tumor response and a real therapeutic benefit for the population to be studied, the same criteria as those used in phase 2 trials should be employed.

CONCLUSIONS AND FUTURE DIRECTIONS

It is undeniable that the expeditious clinical development and approval of new anticancer therapies beneficial to patients are matters of high priority. The decision to proceed with definitive phase 3 trials, with their added complexity and intensive use of resources, depends on informal comparisons of phase 2 trial results. Variability in the reporting of response rates for a given set of data due to differences in measurement and reporting criteria is detrimental as it makes judgements about the relative merits of experimental treatments difficult. To evaluate the results of clinical trials depends upon consistent definitions of tumor response and the use of reliable and reproducible methods of tumor measurement. The use of standard assessment criteria is not only desirable but also imperative.

Since the development of the WHO criteria, our understanding of issues related to study design and patient assessment has evolved, and this evolution will undoubtedly continue in the years to come. The RECIST guidelines are meant to resolve discrepancies which have arisen as research organizations have sought to overcome various limitations of the WHO criteria. In addition to the English language publication, RECIST has been translated into French and Japanese and has been adapted for pediatric oncology. These guidelines are not meant to discourage development and validation of new techniques that may provide more reliable surrogate endpoints than objective tumor response to predict therapeutic benefit for cancer patients. New techniques to better establish objective tumor response will be integrated into these criteria when they are fully validated. In the interim, these guidelines advocate a more rigorous and technology-based assessment of tumor response to improve the reliability of phase 2 trial results. They are the standard to which newer techniques should be compared.

REFERENCES

1. Buyse M, Piedbois P. On the relationship between response to treatment and survival time. *Stat Med* 1996; 15:2797–812.
2. Davis HL Jr, Multhauf P, Klotz J. Comparisons of cooperative group evaluation criteria for multiple-drug therapy for breast cancer. *Cancer Treat Rep* 1980;64: 507–517.
3. Moertel CG, Hanley JA. The effect of measuring error on the results of therapeutic trials in advanced cancer. *Cancer* 1976;38:388–394.
4. Tonkin K, Tritchler D, Tannock I. Criteria of tumor response used in clinical trials of chemotherapy. *J Clin Oncol* 1985;3:870–875.
5. Warr D, McKinney S, Tannock I. Influence of measurement error on assessment of response to anticancer chemotherapy: proposal for new criteria of tumor response. *J Clin Oncol* 1984;2:1040–1046.
6. Breast Cancer Force Treatment Committee. National Cancer Institute: Report from the Combination Chemotherapy Trials working Group. US Department of Health, Education and Welfare. DHEW Publication No. (NIH) 1977:77–1192.
7. Hayward JL, Carbone PP, Heuson JC, et al. Assessment of response to therapy in advanced breast cancer: a project of the Programme on Clinical Oncology of the International Union Against Cancer, Geneva, Switzerland. *Cancer* 1977;39:1289–1294.
8. Anonymous. Assessment of response to treatment in advanced breast cancer. British Breast Group. *Lancet* 1974;2:38–39.
9. Miller AB, Hoogstraten B, Staquet M, Winkler A. Reporting results of cancer treatment. *Cancer* 1981;47: 207–214.
10. Oken MM, Creech RH, Tormey DC, et al. Toxicity and response criteria of the Eastern Cooperative Oncology Group. *Am J Clin Oncol* 1982;5:649–655.
11. Green S, Weiss GR. Southwest Oncology Group standard response criteria, endpoint definitions and toxicity criteria. *Invest New Drugs* 1992;10:239–253.
12. van Oosterom AT. Tumor eligibility and response criteria for phase II and phase III studies and (sub)acute toxicity grading (with suggested amendments to the WHO criteria) EORTC Data Center Manual, Brussels, 1992: 84–86.
13. Torri V, Simon R, Russek-Cohen E, et al. Statistical model to determine the relationship of response and survival in patients with advanced ovarian cancer treated with chemotherapy. *J Natl Cancer Inst* 1992; 84:407–414.
14. Anderson JR, Cain KC, Gelber RD. Analysis of survival by tumor response. *J Clin Oncol* 1983;1:710–719.
15. Lavin PT, Flowerdew G. Studies in variation associated with the measurement of solid tumors. *Cancer* 1980; 46:1286–1290.
16. Gurland J, Johnson RO. How reliable are tumor measurements? *JAMA* 1965;194:973–978.
17. Thiesse P, Ollivier L, Di Stefano-Louineau D, et al. Response rate accuracy in oncology trials: reasons for interobserver variability. Groupe Francais d'Immunotherapie of the Federation Nationale des Centres de Lutte Contre le Cancer. *J Clin Oncol* 1997;15:3507–3514.
18. Gwyther S, Bolis G, Gore M, et al. Experience with independent radiological review during a topotecan trial in ovarian cancer. *Ann Oncol* 1997;8:463–468.
19. Gwyther SJ. Response assessment using radiological methods. *Crit Rev Oncol Hematol* 1999;30:45–62.
20. Clamon G, Clamon L. Relationship between tumor area, tumor volume, and criteria of response in clinical trials. *J Clin Oncol* 1993;11:1839.
21. Therasse P, Arbuck SG, Eisenhauer EA, et al. New guidelines to evaluate the response to treatment in solid tumors. *J Natl Cancer Inst* 2000;92:205–216.
22. Spears CP. Volume doubling measurement of spherical and ellipsoidal tumors. *Med Pediatr Oncol* 1984;12: 212–217.
23. Collins VP, Loeffler RK, Tivey H. Observations on growth rates of human tumors. *Am J Roentgenol* 1956; 78:988–1000.

24. James K, Eisenhauer E, Christian M, et al. Measuring response in solid tumors: unidimensional versus bidimensional measurement. *J Natl Cancer Inst* 1999;91:523–528.
25. Sohaib SA, Turner B, Hanson JA, et al. CT assessment of tumor response to treatment: comparison of linear, cross-sectional and volumetric measures of tumor size. *Br J Radiol* 2000;73:1178–1184.
26. Werner-Wasik M, Xiao Y, Pequignot E, et al. Assessment of lung cancer response after nonoperative therapy: tumor diameter, bidimensional product, and volume. A serial CT scan-based study. *Int J Radiat Oncol Biol Phys* 2001;51:56–61.
27. James K, Eisenhauer E, Therasse P. Re: Measure Once or Twice Does It Really Matter? *J Natl Cancer Inst* 1999;91:1780.
28. Jett JR, Su JQ, Krook JE, et al. Measurable or assessable disease in lung cancer trials: does it matter? *J Clin Oncol* 1994;12:2677–2681.
29. Gwyther SJ, Aapro MS, Hatty SR, et al. Results of an independent oncology review board of pivotal clinical trials of gemcitabine in non-small cell lung cancer. *Anticancer Drugs* 1999;10:693–698.
30. Bubley GJ, Carducci M, Dahut W, et al. Eligibility and response guidelines for phase II clinical trials in androgen-independent prostate cancer: recommendations from the Prostate-Specific Antigen Working Group. *J Clin Oncol* 1999;17:3461–3467.
31. Dawson NA. Response criteria in prostatic carcinoma. *Semin Oncol* 1999;26:174–184.
32. Cruickshank DJ, Terry PB, Fullerton WT. CA125-response assessment in epithelial ovarian cancer. *Int J Cancer* 1992;51:58–61.
33. Rustin GJ, Nelstrop AE, Bentzen SM, et al. Use of tumor markers in monitoring the course of ovarian cancer. *Ann Oncol* 1999;10(suppl 1):21–27.

45

Need for Large-Scale Randomized Evidence to Assess Moderate Benefits Reliably

Richard Peto and Colin Baigent

THE NEED TO ASSESS MODERATE DIFFERENCES IN OUTCOME

Many interventions produce only moderate effects (with proportional reductions of about 10% to 20%) on major outcomes such as death, or distant recurrence of early breast cancer. But even a moderate effect of treatment, if demonstrated clearly enough for that treatment to be adopted widely, could prevent substantial numbers of premature deaths. Moreover, if more than one moderately effective treatment can eventually be identified for a particular type of patient, then the combination of two or three individually moderate improvements in outcome may collectively result in substantial gains. For reliable identification of moderate effects on major outcomes, there is often no reliable alternative to large-scale randomized evidence from meta-analyses of many trials.

TWO FUNDAMENTAL REQUIREMENTS FOR THE RELIABLE ASSESSMENT OF MODERATE TREATMENT EFFECTS: NEGLIGIBLE BIASES AND SMALL RANDOM ERRORS

If any clinical study is to assess moderate treatment effects reliably, then it must ensure that any biases and any random errors that are inherent in its design are both substantially smaller than the effect that is to be measured. This limits the range of study designs that can be informative (Table 45.1) (1).

Negligible Biases

If moderate differences are being assessed, then the study design must guarantee the exclusion of moderate biases, and this generally requires appropriate analysis of properly randomized evidence. This is essential because if the allocation of treatment is not properly randomized, then characteristics of the disease (or the patient) that affect the prognosis may also affect the choice of treatment. Such pre-existing differences could well bias a nonrandomized study. It may well be difficult or impossible to avoid such biases altogether, or to adjust fully for their effects. Even if nonrandomized comparisons happen to get the right answer, nobody will really know that they have done so. This is true unless the difference in outcome is extraordinarily large or the outcome is one that could not plausibly be associated with those aspects of the disease that might influence the choice of treatment. Thus, as nonrandomized study designs cannot generally be guaranteed to exclude moderate biases, they are of little practical value if the primary aim is to assess moderate treatment effects (whether beneficial or adverse) particularly if long-term outcome is of interest.

In the current medical literature (and from presentations at many clinical conferences) a particularly important source of bias is unduly data-dependent emphasis on particular trials or on particular subgroups of the randomized patients. Such emphasis is often entirely inadvertent, arising from a perfectly reasonable desire to understand the randomized trial results in terms of exactly who to treat, or exactly which treatments are preferable. But, whatever its origins, unduly selective emphasis on particular parts of the evidence can often lead to seriously misleading conclusions, as reliable identification of categories of patients for whom treatment is particularly effective (or ineffective) requires surprisingly large quantities of data. Even if the real sizes

TABLE 45.1. *Requirements for reliable assessment of moderate treatment effects*

1. *Negligible biases* (i.e., guaranteed avoidance of moderate biases)
   —Proper randomization (nonrandomized methods cannot guarantee the avoidance of moderate biases)
   —Analysis by allocated treatment (i.e., an "intention-to-treat" analysis)
   —Chief emphasis on overall results (with no unduly data-derived subgroup analyses)
   —Systematic meta-analysis of all the relevant randomized trials (with no unduly data-dependent emphasis on the results from particular studies)
2. *Small random errors* (i.e., guaranteed avoidance of moderate random errors)
   —Large numbers (with minimal data collection, because detailed statistical analyses of large amounts of data on prognostic features generally add little to the effective size of a trial)
   —Systematic meta-analysis of all the relevant randomized trials

of the effects of treatment do vary substantially among different subgroups of patients, subgroup analyses are so statistically insensitive that they may well fail to demonstrate these differences. On the other hand, if the real proportional risk reductions are about the same for everybody, the results from subgroup analyses can vary so widely just by the play of chance that the apparent findings in selected subgroups may be grossly distorted. Even when highly significant interactions are found, they may be a poor guide to the sizes (or even the directions) of any genuine differences in the proportional improvements, in particular outcomes among specific categories of patients. More extreme, such results may still owe more to the play of chance than to reality. This is particularly the case when such interactions have emerged after an examination of multiple subgroups.

Despite these difficulties, such subgroup analyses still get widely reported, and widely believed, in such a manner that may lead to the inappropriate management of hundreds of thousands of patients. For further discussion of this key issue, see reference 1, or see the analyses of the 1988 ISIS-2 report (2) that, if interpreted incautiously, would have indicated that aspirin works only for patients with acute MI who were not born under the astrological star signs of Libra or Gemini!

Appropriate meta-analyses help to avoid unduly data-dependent emphasis on especially striking results within particular trials, and hence to provide a better guide to the true effects of treatments. Occasionally, when detailed information on individual patients is available within a really large meta-analysis that includes several thousand major outcomes, such as death or cancer recurrence (3), it may be feasible to identify particular groups of individuals in whom the benefits or hazards of treatment really are especially great. Sometimes, however, even a meta-analysis of all the trials in the world is too small for reliable subgroup analyses—indeed, in many meta-analyses the total number of randomized patients is too small for even the main analyses to be statistically reliable, let alone the analyses of subgroups.

Small Random Errors

While avoidance of moderate biases chiefly requires careful attention both to the randomization process and to the analysis and interpretation of the available trial evidence, the avoidance of moderate random errors chiefly requires large numbers of events, and hence even larger numbers of patients. For many therapeutic questions, the scale of randomized evidence that is necessary for the assessment of major outcomes may well not yet be available even through a meta-analysis of all of the completed randomized trials in the world. In that case, the key need is to find some practicable way of generating new trials that do provide really large-scale evidence.

RANDOMIZED TRIALS CAN BE LARGE IF THEY ARE KEPT SIMPLE

If trials of the effects of treatments on major outcomes are to become substantially larger, then as many as possible of the main barriers to rapid recruitment need to be removed. One of the most effective ways to ensure failure to recruit large numbers is to burden busy clinicians with obtaining large amounts of information. The information that really needs to be recorded at entry can often be surprisingly brief (including at most only a few major prognostic factors and only a few variables that are thought likely to influence substantially the benefits or hazards of treatment). Similarly, the information recorded at follow-up can sometimes be limited largely to a few major outcomes and approximate measures of compliance. (Other outcomes that are of interest but do not need to be studied on such a large scale may best be assessed in separate smaller studies, or in subsets of these large studies when this is practicable.) Often, less information per patient may mean much larger trials, and hence better science.

THE UNCERTAINTY PRINCIPLE: ETHICALITY, HETEROGENEITY, AND MAXIMAL SAMPLE SIZE

For ethical reasons, randomization is appropriate only if both the doctor and, to the extent that they are part of the process of determining which treatments to use, the patient feel substantially uncertain as to which trial treatment is best. The "uncertainty principle" (Table 45.2) maximizes the potential for recruitment within this ethical constraint (1,4).

If many hospitals are collaborating in a trial, then wholehearted use of the uncertainty principle as the fundamental eligibility criterion en-

TABLE 45.2. *The Uncertainty Principle*

The "uncertainty principle": A patient can be entered if, and only if, the responsible physician is substantially uncertain as to which of the trial treatments would be most appropriate for that particular patient. A patient should not be entered if the responsible physician or the patient are for any medical or non-medical reasons reasonably certain that one of the treatments that might be allocated would be inappropriate for this particular individual (either in comparison with no treatment or in comparison with some other treatment that could be offered to the patient in or outside the trial).

courages clinically appropriate heterogeneity in the resulting trial population and this, in large trials, may add substantially to the practical value of the results. Homogeneity of those randomized may be a serious defect in clinical trial design, while heterogeneity may be a scientific strength: After all, trials need to be relevant to a very heterogeneous collection of future patients.

The uncertainty principle not only ensures ethicality and clinically useful heterogeneity but also is easily understood and remembered by the busy collaborating clinician. This, in turn, helps the randomization of large numbers of patients. There is scope, therefore, for many more trials to adopt this as their eligibility criterion.

CAN ALTERNATIVE STUDY DESIGNS SUBSTITUTE FOR LARGE-SCALE RANDOMIZED EVIDENCE?

Might it be possible to circumvent the need for large trials? First one might use routinely collected observational data sometimes referred to as "outcomes research." Second, one could analyze previously published randomized trials that are, even in aggregate, of only limited size with small-scale meta-analyses.

Outcomes Research

Outcomes research means various things to various people; but, as commonly used, the term refers to the use of routinely collected nonrandomized data to compare the effects of various treatments. Even within a carefully designed observational study, where specific arrangements to minimize sources of bias and confounding are planned and monitored, the guaranteed avoidance of biases that would correspond to a moderate increase or decrease in risk may well not be feasible. In nonrandomized studies, the effects of uncontrolled, and often uncontrollable, biases or confounding may therefore be at least as big as the sort of moderate effect that is to be assessed. This is the case for the so-called "indication bias" that occurs when there is a tendency to use particular treatments for particular types of patients who are considered to have specific indications. It follows, therefore, that routinely collected data from outcomes research projects are unlikely to be able to assess reliably any moderate effects on outcome, and should generally not be considered as providing credible evidence if attempts are made to use them for this purpose. This is particularly important when nonrandomized (phase 2) studies suggest that certain treatments have surprisingly large effects, since such findings are often refuted when those treatments are assessed in large randomized (phase 3) trials.

BIASES AND RANDOM ERRORS IN SMALL-SCALE META-ANALYSES

Since meta-analyses are appearing in medical journals with increasing frequency, it is important to be able to judge the reliability of such reviews—and, in particular, the extent to which confounding, biases or random errors could lead to mistaken conclusions. In a randomized trial, "confounding" exists when a comparison of some particular treatment in one group versus a control group involves the routine co-administration in one group, but not the other, of some co-intervention that might affect the outcome. To avoid any possibility of confounding, and to avoid any flexibility in the question of which trials to include, those who perform or interpret meta-analyses should generally adopt the rule that they will include only unconfounded properly randomized trials. The main problems that then remain are those of biases and random errors.

Two types of bias could affect the reliability of a meta-analysis: those that occur within individual trials, and those that relate to the selection of trials. Such defects have unpredictable consequences for particular trials, however, and no reliable generalizations about the likely size, or even direction, of the resultant biases are possible.

Selection bias can arise when some relevant trials are not identified (or are excluded once they have been identified). Unfortunately, the subset of trials that are eventually published (and, hence, are conveniently available) is often a biased sample of the trials that have been done. Trials may well be more likely to be submitted or accepted for publication if their results are strikingly positive than if they are negative or null. Such publication bias can, along with other sources of bias, produce surprisingly impressive-looking evidence of effectiveness for treatments that are actually useless. The particular circumstances in which publication bias has contributed to producing misleading estimates of treatment are difficult to identify, and it is even more difficult to generalize about the size of any such bias.

The problem of incomplete ascertainment is likely to be particularly acute within small meta-analyses that contain no more than a few major outcomes, and consist chiefly of small published trials. This is because results from trials with only a limited number of endpoints are subject to large random errors and such trials are therefore particularly likely to generate implausibly large effect estimates. If publication bias then results in unduly selective emphasis on the more promising of these small trial results, the resulting meta-analysis will be unreliable. Hence, unless the particular circumstances of a small-scale meta-analysis suggest that publication bias is unlikely, it may be best to treat such results as no more than "hypothesis-generating." On the other hand, a thoroughly conducted meta-analysis that in aggregate contains sufficient numbers of major outcomes to constitute large-scale, randomized evidence (3) is unlikely to be materially affected by publication bias. Provided there are no serious uncontrolled biases (see above) within the individual component trials, it is likely to be fairly trustworthy, at least in its overall conclusions—although, even then, inappropriate subgroup analyses may generate wrong answers.

CONCLUSION: THE PAST 50 YEARS AND THE NEXT 50 YEARS OF RANDOMIZED EVIDENCE

At present we are still not getting the correct answers to many therapeutic questions, chiefly from nonrandomized evidence, from inappropriately small randomized trials, or from small meta-analyses. During the past 50 years, the principle of doing randomized trials and, more recently, meta-analyses to avoid moderate bias has been widely accepted. In recent years the need for such studies to be large enough to avoid moderate random errors has also begun to be accepted, though there is still far to go. If the trend towards really large-scale randomized evidence can be maintained, then over the next 50 years the true potential of randomization will at last begin to be realized, with substantial patient benefits. An example of such a trial with early results is the ATAC study (Adjuvant Tamoxifen versus Arimidex or Combination) with more that 9,000 women randomized.

To argue the need for some large, simple, randomized trials is not to argue that all other trials are useless; indeed, small (or complicated) trials will continue to be needed for certain purposes, as will many other types of clinical research. But, for many important questions about moderate therapeutic improvements in the common causes of death or serious disability, there is no reliable alternative to large-scale randomized evidence.

REFERENCES

1. Collins R, Peto R, Gray R, Parish S. Large-scale randomized evidence: trials and overviews. In: Weatherall D, Ledingham JGG, Warrell DA, eds. *Oxford textbook of medicine*. Vol. 1. Oxford University Press, 1996: 21–32.
2. ISIS-2 (Second International Study of Infarct Survival) Collaborative Group. Randomized trial of intravenous streptokinase, oral aspirin, both, or neither among 17,187 cases of suspected acute myocardial infarction: ISIS-2. *Lancet* 1988;ii:349–360.
3. Early Breast Cancer Trialists' Collaborative Group. Systemic treatment of early breast cancer by hormonal, cytotoxic, or immune therapy: 133 randomized trials involving 31,000 recurrences and 24,000 deaths among 75,000 women. *Lancet* 1992;339:1–15 (Part I) & 71–85 (Part II).
4. Collins R, Doll R, Peto R. Ethics of clinical trials. In: Williams CJ, ed. *Introducing new treatments for cancer: practical, ethical and legal problems*. New York: John Wiley & Sons, 1992:49–65.

46

Economic Evaluation Analysis in Breast Cancer Therapy: From Evidence to Practice

Philip Jacobs, Katia Tonkin, and Barbara Conner-Spady

Economic evaluation analysis deals with the study of interventions, the focus of which is on the quantity of resources used in the management of patients in relation to outcomes. As a result of the rapidly changing technologies that are used in breast, as well as in other, cancer therapies, costs of treatment have risen substantially in recent years. In response to these cost increases, governments and insurers around the world have been seeking various means of containing costs. Drug formularies and clinical practice guideline programs are examples of initiatives that have been undertaken to control the use of new technologies. Economic analysis is an information tool that can be used by those who undertake these initiatives.

When we deal with resource issues, there are several different types of questions that we can address. First, we can compare alternative interventions that are focused on the same indications (e.g., metastatic breast cancer), addressing the question, "What are the cost and outcome implications of using different interventions?" Alternatively, we can compare different interventions that focus on different indications of disease (e.g., breast cancer and colorectal cancer). The research question would be the same as above, but the context would differ. Finally, we can address the issue of whether we should treat breast cancer at all. The research question in this instance might be phrased as, "Are the benefits that are gained from treating the patient (with a given technology) greater than the costs?"

In this chapter we focus on the first of these questions, which deals with the comparison of alternative interventions in breast cancer therapy. We discuss the comparison of costs and outcomes for these interventions. However, when addressing this question, we face some daunting problems. We first provide an overall framework for dealing with the general research question that we have just identified. Next, we summarize the results from the literature on cost-effectiveness in breast cancer therapy for specific interventions (taxanes). In particular, we demonstrate how these results can be interpreted by users of data.

ELEMENTS OF COST-EFFECTIVENESS ANALYSIS IN BREAST CANCER THERAPY

Overview

The general elements for a cost-effectiveness analysis are set out in several textbooks (1–3) and in guidelines that have been issued to standardize methodologies (4,5). The authors of the guidelines recommend that the following analytical elements be specified in a cost-effectiveness analysis:

- Treatment indications should be identified.
- Alternative interventions should be clearly specified, including a do-nothing alternative, if appropriate.
- A perspective or viewpoint should be chosen; this can be the patient's own perspective, the viewpoint of the payer (whether the third party insurers or the government health program), that of a single provider, or the societal perspective, which include all who incur costs, including the patient and caregivers.
- A time horizon that incorporates beginning and ending time lines of the study should be

selected. It is recommended that the time frame of the study be long enough to capture all downstream events (i.e., events subsequent to the intervention) that are associated with the study interventions.
- Appropriate outcome measures should be selected (see below).
- Sources of clinical data, which have been used to derive efficacy or effectiveness measures, should be specified.
- Resources and their related costs should be specified.

Following the application of these guidelines, a cost-effectiveness ratio, which summarizes the differences in costs and outcomes, can be derived. This ratio is made up of the net difference in costs between interventions divided by the net difference in outcomes between interventions.

Quality of Information

Cost effectiveness analyses can be conducted with data from both randomized clinical trials and administrative databases, or they can be constructed in the form of a "decision analysis," which is a modeling exercise using data from diverse sources (including clinical trials). However conducted, these analyses are subject to validity criteria, which are similar to the standards used to gauge other clinical and economic data. These criteria can be used to gauge the level of evidence and fall into three groups: the criterion used to assess the method of establishing effectiveness, the measure of outcome used, and the method of measuring cost (6).

Methods of Establishing Effectiveness

Most investigators accept the view that large, well-designed, randomized clinical trials are the gold standard in terms of establishing efficacy (7). Recently, however, investigators in the area of critical care medicine have put forward the view that studies that use observational databases can, if appropriately conducted, approach the level of evidence of randomized clinical trials (8). Indeed, in recent years, observational databases have improved dramatically in terms of control for self-selection bias and have been adopted in ground breaking studies (9). Data based on clinical opinion, rather than observation, are on the bottom rung in terms of quality of evidence. Further, clinical trials measure "efficacy" rather than "effectiveness." Effectiveness refers to net differences in outcomes under actual, rather than experimental, conditions. Observational data are considered to be a better source with which to measure effectiveness.

Outcome Measures

Although the definitions of health-related quality of life (HRQL) vary, most HRQL measures assess three broad areas of health: physical, psychological, and social functioning (10–13). Authors of health economics guidelines recommend that three different types of outcome measures be used in economic evaluations: generic health quality-of-life measures, disease-specific measures, and preference-based measures.

Generic measures or non-condition-specific measures are designed to apply to a wide variety of populations and conditions and contain a broad spectrum of items. They are generally not as responsive as disease-specific instruments, but can be used to compare relative impacts of health programs across various populations. Preference-based measures are types of generic measures that are based on subjects own evaluations of their own health states; they produce a single index score for use in economic evaluation. Preference-based measures (sometimes called utility measures) require a weighting system to be applied to a health state. This process involves a number of steps, which are used to derive the single index score: the measurement of HRQL of the target population, the measurement of preferences, and the assignment of preferences to the health states of individuals (10).

A special kind of index is the quality adjusted life year (QALY) index, which assigns the number zero to a health state of death and the number one to the state of perfect health. A QALY can be derived from generic or preference measures, using processes that require the investigator to make additional assumptions. Although these assumptions are often artificial, QALY indexes have an advantage of allowing the investigator to incorporate the health status of the patient while he or she is alive (usually valued at more than 0) with that after death (valued at 0) up to the final point of observation. Thus, the QALY is a very useful tool to use when comparing outcomes of individuals with varying survival times.

Instruments of HRQL should be chosen so that the inferences drawn from the scores are valid and not open to misinterpretation (11–14).

There has been considerable discussion about the source of the HRQL data. There is a general consensus that HRQL indices should represent the views of the patients, not those of the providers. However, the argument has been put forward that the general public, who pay for health care, should have their preferences for different health states expressed. One problem with this viewpoint is that the general public may not be able to imagine what certain illness experiences are really like; thus, their preferences for imaginary health states might differ considerably from those that were actually experienced.

Examples of Outcome Measures in Breast Cancer

The Functional Living Index–Cancer (FLIC) and the QLQ-C30 (15,16) are two examples of cancer-specific HRQL tools. The FLIC is a 22-item, cancer-specific tool which was designed to produce an overall global measure of the effect of cancer on patient function. It has acceptable reliability, and the evidence supports responsiveness, and convergent and discriminant validity in the breast cancer population. The QLQ-C30, a 30-item instrument, was designed for evaluating the quality of life of patients participating in international clinical trials. It includes six functional subscales, three symptom scales and six single items. Although the initial psychometric studies for the QLQ-C30 were conducted in lung cancer patients, several studies have supported aspects of validity in the breast cancer population. The QLQ-B23 (17), a supplementary module to the QLQ-C30 for use in breast cancer patients, measures body image, sexuality, and symptoms specific to breast cancer.

The EQ-5D, a generic, preference-based HRQL tool, was designed to be used alongside condition-specific measures as an outcome measure in evaluative studies (18). It has five questions and an accompanying visual analogue scale. Although reliability estimates of the EQ-5D are acceptable, validity evidence is inconsistent and its usefulness as an HRQL measure in clinical trials of breast cancer patients has not been established. Several measurement issues affect the validity of EQ-5D index scores, including: broadness of levels (19), ceiling effects in patient and population groups (20,21), less responsiveness than other measures (22–24), and unresolved issues in the measurement of preferences.

In spite of the weak validity evidence, an increasing number of studies are being published using the EQ-5D in economic analyses in cancer patients (25–28) and other patient groups. Few of these studies have examined the validity of EQ-5D scores in the cancer population. The only study that has employed the EQ-5D in breast cancer patients (29) used just the visual analogue scale. There is an eagerness to employ these tools in economic analyses despite the fact that there are still unresolved measurement issues. Just as the measurement of HRQL arose out of an important gap in the traditional outcome measures of mortality and morbidity, so the development of preference-based measures has arisen out of gaps in traditional HRQL measures.

Costs

The cost of a service is the product of the resources (labor, medicines, equipment, services) that are used to produce it and the monetary price paid for these resources (or the value that the resources would have in their best alternative use, if they are unpaid). Laupacis et al. (6) identify several criteria that can be used for the assessment of costs, including the direct measurement of resource use (rather than measures based on professional opinion) and the measurement of costs (resources and their prices) in the setting in which the services are provided. These criteria address internal validity issues. In addition, there are external validity criteria

Grades of Recommendation

The topic of "grades of recommendation" is related to the interpretation of the results. Assuming that a high-quality study was done, one is then faced with the task of interpreting the results. Cost-effectiveness analysis provides only the numbers. Investigators or policymakers must develop their own standards in order to evaluate these numbers. For example, assume that we have two drug therapies, A and B: the cost of A is $40,000 per patient and the cost of B is $50,000 per patient. Therapy A has a 40% chance of a positive response, whereas B has a 70% chance. Referring to our definition of the cost-effectiveness ratio as the ratio of differences in costs to the differences in outcomes, the differences in cost between the two interventions is $10,000 and the difference in the probability of a response is 0.3. The cost-effectiveness ratio is $10,000 for a 0.3 increase in response. For each positive response, the cost would be $10,000 per 0.3 or $33,333 per positive response.

Is it worth it? There are some instances in which this answer would be easy. If B cost less and had better outcomes, then B would be the dominant intervention and would be the more acceptable alternative. However, in this case, B costs more and is better, and so the policymaker is faced with a dilemma. The cost-effectiveness ratio in this case tells us how much more we have to spend and what we get for this additional expenditure. Policy-makers must develop standards to help them interpret these results. Cost-effectiveness analysis, by itself, cannot tell someone whether or not it is worth spending the additional $33,000 to achieve the additional benefits.

Some investigators have devised their own standards for cost-utility analysis (6). These standards stated that, if an intervention achieved an additional QALY for under $20,000, then there was strong evidence for its adoption. Moderate evidence was provided if the cost effectiveness ratio fell in the range $20,000 to $100,000 per QALY. These standards are useful in setting up some kind of benchmark. However, they are the results of the authors' own valuations, and should be recognized as such.

Further, it has been suggested that a high grade of recommendation might result from a very favorable cost effectiveness ratio but a lower quality study. A low-quality study will generate a lower level of confidence in the results, whether these are favorable or not.

THE LITERATURE

Method

We conducted a review of the cost-effectiveness analysis literature on breast cancer therapy, focusing on the use of alternative taxanes in breast cancer chemotherapy. We searched the Pub Med database from 1993 to 2001. The searches were restricted to English and human studies only. The subject word used was "breast neoplasms"; it was searched together with "cost-effectiveness" in the title. There were 129 citations using this search strategy. We also searched manually for additional articles using the bibliographies of any articles that we identified.

We selected three studies as examples of economic analyses comparing alternative chemotherapies for breast cancer (30–32). Two of the studies (30,31) were similar in structure. Both models were focused on the use of chemotherapy as a second-line therapy for metastatic breast cancer, following an unsuccessful treatment with anthracyclines. The models track hypothetical patients through successive time blocks, beginning with the use of second line treatments. The treatments which are compared in these studies are docetaxel, paclitaxel, and vinorelbine.

The models contain four components: the first, a basic structure which involves the identification of health states. The models in the two studies differ somewhat in their depiction of the disease process, but both contain time blocks of mild and severe infection, different specific toxicities, and stages of disease (response, stable, disease progression and death).

In the model, the patient progresses through the disease process, from time block to time block, according to transitional probabilities between the cycles. These probabilities form the second component of the model. Eventually, all persons in the model die. The transitional probabilities are derived from clinical studies and professional judgment. In the two studies under consideration, these probabilities come from clinical studies.

The third component of the model is the health status or utilities for each cycle or time block. In both studies the utilities were obtained from doctors and nurses; the same utilities were used in both studies.

The fourth component is the cost of care in each cycle. These costs include costs for chemotherapy, treatment for infections and toxicities, and prophylactics. The costs in Launois et al. (31) were based on observational data, while those in Brown et al. (30) were based on professional opinion.

The results of the two studies were similar. Launois et al. showed that docetaxel is dominant in relation to paclitaxel; that is, the cost of treatment is lower, and the outcome is better. Brown et al. showed that treatment with docetaxel is less costly and the outcome is better. The cost-effectiveness ratio is $8,615 per quality-adjusted life-year saved. This is a very favorable ratio, and would be recommended in most policy areas.

The third study (32) is also a Markov model, based on much the same efficacy information as the other two models, but using actual cost information from patients in a Canadian cancer center. The results are very different from the other two studies, and show vinorelbine to be the more cost-effective alternative. However, the assumptions used in this model are very different. The response rate for docetaxel is 21%, as compared with 41.7% in the Brown study and 57.1% in the Launois study. The post-treatment cost of care is much lower for vinorelbine in the Leung study (32) than in the Launois study; it is not reported on in the Brown study. These differences have led to different results for the studies.

However, a high level of evidence cannot be attributed to any of the three studies. The selection of the studies on which efficacy was based was not formally presented in any of the studies. In Brown et al., costs were obtained using professional opinion, not directly observed data. Leung used directly observed data, though from a somewhat different patient population; their measures may be of a higher quality.

The differences between these studies suggest further analysis will be necessary before a level of evidence recommendation can be made. A recent review of the literature from the United Kingdom (33) indicated that, especially when comparing docetaxel with vinorelbine, results were not robust. Whatever the results showed, the main issue remains inadequate quality of evidence. A more careful analysis, even with existing data, might yield some agreement on efficacy. There would still be considerable disagreement on costs, as no sound evidence currently exists in this regard.

REFERENCES

1. Drummond M, O'Brien B, Stoddart GI, et al. *Methods for the economic evaluation of health care programmes.* Toronto: Oxford University Press, 1997.
2. Jefferson T, Demicheli V, Mugford M. *Elementary economic evaluation in health care.* London: BMJ Publishing Group, 1996.
3. Gold MR, Siegel JE, Russel LB, Weinstein MC. *Cost-effectiveness in health and medicine.* New York: Oxford University Press, 1996.
4. Canadian Coordinating Office for Health Technology Assessment. *The use of G-CSF in the prevention of febrile neutropenia.* Ottawa: Canadian Coordinating Office for Health Technology (CCOHTA), 1997. [Technology overview: pharmaceuticals, issue 9.0, available from: http://www.ccohta.ca]
5. Brown M, Glick HA, Harnell F, et al. Integrating economic analysis into cancer trials: the National Cancer Institute—American Society of Clinical Oncology Economics Workbook. *J Natl Cancer Inst Monogr* 1998; 24:1–28.
6. Laupacis A, Feeny D, Detsky AS, Tugwell PX. How attractive does a new technology have to be to warrant adoption and utilization? Tentative guidelines for using clinical and economic evaluations. *Can Med Assoc J* 1992;146:473–481.
7. Jovell AJ, Navarro-Rubio MD. Evaluacion de la evidencia cientifica. *Med Clin* 1995;105:740–743.
8. Rubenfeld GD, Angus DC, Pinsky MR, et al. Outcomes research in critical care. Results of the American Thoracic Society Critical Care Assembly Workshop on Outcomes Research. *Am J Respir Crit Care Med* 1999; 160:358–367.
9. Connors AF Jr, Speroff T, Dawson NV, et al. The effectiveness of right heart catheterization in the initial care of critically ill patients. *JAMA* 1996;276:889–897.

10. Patrick DL, Eickson P. *Health status and health policy.* New York: Oxford University Press, 1993.
11. Schipper H, Clinch JJ, Olweny CLM. Quality of life studies: Definitions and conceptual issues. In: Spiler B, ed. *Quality of life and pharmacoeconomics in clinical trials,* 2nd ed. Philadelphia: Lippincott-Raven, 1996: 11–23.
12. Osoba D. *Effect of cancer on quality of life.* Boca Raton, FL: CRC Press, 1991.
13. Ware JE. Standards for validating health measures: Definition and content. *J Chronic Dis* 1987;40:473–480.
14. Messick S. Validity. In: Linn R, ed. *Educational measurement,* 3rd ed. New York: Macmillan Publishing Co, 1989:13–103.
15. Schipper H, Clinch JJ, McMurray A, Levitt M. Measuring the quality of life of cancer patients: the functional living index—cancer: development and validation. *J Clin Oncol* 1984;2:472–473.
16. Aaronson NK, Ahmedzai S, Bergman B, et al. The European Organization for Research and Treatment of Cancer QLQ-C30: A quality-of-life instrument for use in international clinical trials in oncology. *J Natl Cancer Instit* 1993;85:365–376.
17. Sprangers MAG, Groenvold M, Arraras JI, et al. The European Organization for Research and Treatment of Cancer breast-cancer specific quality-of-life questionnaire module: First results from a three-country field study. *J Clin Oncol* 1996;14:2756–2768.
18. Anonymous. EuroQol—a new facility fir the measurement of health-related quality of life. The EuroQol Group. *Health Policy* 1990;16:199–208.
19. Wolfe F, Hawley DJ. Measurement of the quality of life in rheumatic disorders using the EuroQol. *Br J Rheumatol* 1997;36:786–793.
20. Brazier J, Jones N, Kind P. Testing the validity of the EuroQol and comparing it with the SF-36 Health survey questionnaire. *Quality of Life Research* 1993;2: 169–180.
21. Essink-Bot ML, Krabbe PF, Bonsel GJ, Aaronson NK. An empirical comparison of four generic health status measures. The Nottingham Health Profile, the Medical Outcomes Study 36-item Short-Form Health Survey, the COOP/WONCA charts, and the EuroQol instrument. *Medical Care* 1997;35:522–537.
22. Hollingworth W, Mackenzie R, Todd CJ, Dixon AK. Measuring changes in quality of life following magnetic resonance imaging of the knee: SF-36, EuroQol or Rosser index? *Quality of Life Research* 1995;4:325–334.
23. Jenkinson C, Stradling J, Petersen S. How should we evaluate health status? A comparison of three methods in patients presenting with obstructive sleep apnoea. *Quality of Life Research* 1998;7:95–100.
24. Jenkinson C, Gray A, Doll H, et al. Evaluation of index and profile measures of health status in a randomized controlled trial. Comparison of the Medical Outcomes Study 36-Item Short Form Health Survey, EuroQol, and disease specific measures. *Medical Care* 1997; 35:1109–1118.
25. Norum J, Vonen B, Olsen JA, et al. Adjuvant chemotherapy (5-flourouracil and levamisole) in Dukes' B and C colorectal carcinoma. A cost-effectiveness analysis. *Ann Oncol* 1997;8:65–70.
26. Norum J, Angelsen V, Wist E, Olsen JA. Treatment costs in Hodgkin's disease: a cost-utility analysis. *Eur J Cancer* 1996;32A:1510–1517.
27. Uyl-de Groot CA, Vellenga E, de Vries EGE, et al. Treatment costs and quality of life with granulocyte-macrophage colony-stimulating factor in patients with antineoplastic therapy-related febrile neutropenia: Results of a randomized placebo-controlled trial. *Pharmacoeconomics* 1997;12:351–360.
28. Vellenga E, Uyl-de Groot CA, de Wit R, et al. Randomized placebo-controlled trial of granulocyte-macrophage colony-stimulating factor in patients with chemotherapy-related febrile neutropenia. *J Clin Oncol* 1996;14:619–627.
29. Glick HA, Shpall EJ, LeMaistre CF, et al. Empirical criteria for the selection of quality-of-life instruments for the evalutation of peripheral blood progenitor cell transplantation. *Int J Technol Assessment Health Care* 1998;14:419–430.
30. Brown RE, Hutton J, Burrell A. Cost effectiveness of treatment options in advanced breast cancer in the UK. *PharmacoEconomics* 2001;19(1):1091–1102.
31. Launois R, Reboul-Marty J, Henry B, Bonneterre J. A cost-utility analysis of second-line chemotherapy in metastatic breast cancer. Docetaxel versus paclitaxel versus vinorelbine. *Pharmacoeconomics* 1996;10(5): 504–521.
32. Leung PP, Tannock IF, Oza AM, et al. Cost–utility analysis of chemotherapy using paclitaxel, docetaxel, or vinorelbine for patients with anthracycline-resistant breast cancer. *J Clin Oncol* 1999;17(10):3082–3090.
33. Lister-Sharp D, McDonagh MS, Khan KS, Kleijnen J. A rapid and systematic review of the effectiveness and cost effectiveness of the taxanes used in the treatment of advanced breast and ovarian cancer. *Health Technology Assessment* 2000;4(17):1–108.

PART VI

High-Dose Chemotherapy

47

High-Dose Chemotherapy in the Adjuvant Therapy of Breast Cancer: The Argument for Further Investigation

John Crown

It is not possible, on the basis of existing data, to make, in the year 2002, any case for high-dose chemotherapy as a standard treatment for any patient with breast cancer at any stage. The apparent benefits that the results of single-arm studies suggested that this form of treatment might offer to patients with high-risk, early stage disease, or in metastatic cancer, have not been confirmed, despite a data-set which now includes fourteen random assignment trials. Furthermore, the fact that two of the early, and reportedly positive, randomized trials were subsequently shown to be marred by fraud delivered what many considered to be a coup de grace to an already tottering, and fatally wounded therapeutic strategy.

However it must be acknowledged that many of these trials were methodologically flawed, and moreover, until recently, all of them tested a single model of high-dose therapy (i.e., late intensification) out of the several that had been advanced. The results of at least one study also suggest the possibility that a putative benefit for high-dose therapy might only emerge with longer follow-up than has been reported for many of these trials. Thus, a case for continued investigation of high-dose chemotherapy can still be made. However, the hard question for investigators is whether any priority should be given to investigation of this modality in an era when new molecularly specific therapeutics are entering our clinical investigative armamentarium.

CHEMOTHERAPY OF BREAST CANCER: THEORY AND PRACTICE

Breast cancer is in many ways the prototype of a partially chemotherapy-sensitive neoplasm. Patients with metastases will usually achieve a degree of tumor shrinkage, with amelioration of the distressing symptoms of cancer, and some degree of survival prolongation. Most responses are partial, however, and in all but exceptional cases, are temporary. Durable complete remissions and cures are rare (1,2).

Chemotherapy is also given as an adjuvant to definitive locoregional therapy in patients with earlier-stage disease. This strategy was prompted by the classic experiments of Skipper and Schabel (3), which suggested that tumors grew exponentially with a constant growth rate, and that chemotherapy killed a constant proportion of cells. These investigators also found that there was an invariably inverse relationship between the size of a tumor and its curability by chemotherapy. Their model had profound implications for the concept of adjuvant systemic therapy, and appeared to be particularly relevant to breast cancer therapeutics. The same chemotherapy that produces responses in patients with metastases should produce a much greater survival impact when given as an adjuvant to patients with earlier stage disease (4). While several generations of studies have confirmed that adjuvant chemotherapy has a beneficial impact in patients with both node-positive and node-negative breast cancer, the impact has been less than might have been expected on the basis of the Skipper-Schabel model (5).

In attempting to explain why the impact of chemotherapy had not been more substantial, Norton and Simon (6) hypothesized that tumors grew, and regressed according to Gompertzian kinetics. The essential feature of Gompertzian growth is that the rate of growth is not constant, as had been predicted in the exponential model, but, rather, varied inversely with the size of the tumor. Thus, large tumors had lower growth fractions than did smaller ones, and hence were less sensitive to cytotoxics. They also proposed that the cell-kill induced by a chemotherapy drug was directly related to the size of the dose, and to the growth rate of the unperturbed tumor at that point in its growth curve. According to this model, patients with overt cancer should first be treated with chemotherapy to reduce their tumor burden, which would place them in the more sensitive phase of their growth curve. At this point tumor eradication might be attempted. Paradoxically, the same rapid regrowth that enhances the chemo-sensitivity of smaller populations, could, in the case of very small amounts of residual cancer cells, also make tumor eradication more difficult, in that any minimal residual populations of cells which survive a given cycle of treatment would undergo rapid, but wholly clinically in-apparent regrowth prior to the next cycle. Thus, the late phase of the treatment should be intensified. Several randomized trials have tested this hypothesis. The CALGB randomized patients with node-positive breast cancer to receive either intensification (i.e., anthracycline-containing chemotherapy) or further CMF (cyclophosphamide, methotrexate, and 5-fluourouracil) as crossover therapy following a phase of CMF induction (7). The Italian GOIRC group performed a similar study in patients with metastases (8). Both studies showed advantages for crossover late-intensification therapy.

Further support for the Norton-Simon model came from the work of Buzzoni et al. (9), who tested alternating putatively non-cross resistant chemotherapy (an approach based on the Goldie-Coldman hypothesis [10]) versus sequential administration of the same regimens, in node-positive breast cancer. Sequential chemotherapy was highly statistically significantly superior.

CHEMOTHERAPY DOSE-RESPONSE EFFECT

The frustrating partial chemotherapy sensitivity of breast cancer prompted a critical evaluation of dose escalation or intensification in the therapy of both early-stage and late-stage disease. There is ample experimental evidence that a relationship exists between the concentration of a drug to which a cancer cell is exposed, and the likelihood that the cell will be killed. Skipper and Schabel, and Teicher et al. (11) demonstrated that there was a relationship between dose and cell-kill. In these studies, the degree of dose escalation which was required to fully eradicate cancers was in general substantial, typically of a log order of magnitude. It would obviously be very difficult to replicate this degree of escalation in routine clinical practice due to toxicity. It is, thus, scarcely surprising that in the clinic (as will be discussed), minor degrees of dose escalation within the conventional range (i.e., to levels which do not require hematopoietic autograft support) have had a modest and inconsistent effect on antitumor endpoints. The concept of dose intensity relates to dose-per-unit time. Some, but not all, retrospective studies have suggested that there is a relationship between dose intensity and survival in breast cancer (12). The colony-stimulating factors (CSFs) facilitate somewhat more substantial increases in dose and intensity, although for most drugs and combinations, it does not approximate the level which the preclinical models predicted to be sufficient (13). For the purposes of this section, we will define moderate dose escalation or intensification as increases in dose and/or dose intensity which do not require autograft support, and will include both agents and combinations which are given with, and those which are given without, CSFs.

Retrospective studies have indicated that there may be a relationship between dose and anticancer effect, but do not prove causality. Similarly, single-arm studies of moderately intensified therapy in both early and late-stage breast cancer raised the possibility that this strategy might produce superior outcomes compared to standard dose therapy (14).

A number of prospective random assignment trials have now addressed the issue of moderate dose escalation or intensification in the clinical treatment of either metastatic or early stage breast cancer. These studies have produced inconsistent results, with generally higher response rates reported for higher-dose therapy in metastatic disease, but limited survival impact in either this setting or in patients with early stage disease (15–22). One conclusion which can be reached on the basis of these studies, however, is that arbitrary reductions below standard dose should be avoided.

Advances in supportive care, in particular in the area of hematopoietic support have allowed the investigation of very high doses of chemotherapy in the clinic (23), doses of an order of magnitude which appear to mimic those which were necessary for cure in experimental systems. Very high-dose chemotherapy with hematopoietic autograft support has been reported to produce exceptionally high rates of complete remission in patients with metastatic breast cancer, although the real clinical benefit of this treatment in this setting remains controversial (24).

HEMATOPOIETIC SUPPORT OF HIGH-DOSE CHEMOTHERAPY

It has long been known that it is possible to harvest bone marrow, and to cryo-preserve it for subsequent reinfusion following intensive chemotherapy or radiotherapy. In some early studies of HDC with autologous bone marrow support, treatment-related mortality was as high as 20%. The introduction of the hematopoietic CSFs had a powerful impact on the field of autograft-supported, high-dose chemotherapy. The administration of these CSFs following marrow reinfusion resulted in a dramatic abbreviation of the period of neutropenia, and a consequent fall in mortality (25). It was also discovered that the administration of CSFs to patients, either at steady state or following myelosuppressive chemotherapy resulted in the mobilization of large numbers of hematopoietic progenitors into the peripheral blood (26). These progenitors (PBPs) could in turn be harvested by leukapheresis, and used as a substitute for autologous bone marrow (ABM). These PBPs were demonstrated to be superior to growth factors alone, or to marrow in prospective random assignment trials (27,28). The dramatic improvement in the toxicity profile of HDC now allowed systematic investigation of this modality in a number of clinical settings, including breast cancer. It was observed in single-arm trials that high-dose chemotherapy with autograft support produced complete remission more than four times more frequently than did conventionally dosed therapy. There is fairly general agreement that high-dose therapy is indeed more active than is low-dose therapy, i.e., it produces more frequent and more complete responses. The controversies surrounding this modality relate to claims that it improves survival, or indeed that it cures. Investigators have attempted to harness this activity using one or other of a number of different high-dose strategies. Before studying the history of high-dose chemotherapy in this disease, we will first discuss these strategies.

HIGH-DOSE CHEMOTHERAPY STRATEGIES

Primary High-dose Chemotherapy

In this strategy, HDC is administered as one (or uncommonly, two or more) definitive cycles of stand-alone treatment to patients with cancer. This approach predominated in early studies. Toxicity in these early programs was substantial. High rates of usually short-lived response were reported in several studies, in metastatic breast cancer. It was noted that patients who underwent this treatment for cancer which had been resistant to prior conventionally dosed therapy had very poor outcomes (24). Primary high-dose chemotherapy has had rather little investigation, and late intensification rapidly became the dominant strategy for high-dose chemotherapy (29).

Late Intensification

This model is an adaptation of the work of Norton and Simon. As has been outlined above, these researchers suggested that curative chemotherapy should consist of a phase-of-induction treatment, which would induce response, and thus "shift," the tumor to the left along its Gompertzian growth curve. The smaller tumor would have a higher growth fraction and would hence be more sensitive to chemotherapy. It would, however, have a propensity for rapid regrowth according to the principles of Gompertzian mechanics. In order to ensure eradication of the left-shifted tumor, it should now be treated with a "clinically tolerable dose-intensification." As has been mentioned, the types of intensification which were available in the 1970s, when the Norton-Simon model was first formulated, were not, in fact, very intensive. Obviously, marrow or peripheral blood progenitor autografting allowed a much more substantial degree of dose escalation, and during the 1980s, late intensification became the most widespread application of high-dose chemotherapy.

In addition to the kinetic rationale, several other clinical arguments were advanced in support of using high-dose chemotherapy as a form of late-intensification. It was proposed that the cytoreduction which was achieved by conventional chemotherapy might increase the ability of the subsequent high-dose cycle to eradicate the cancer by presenting it with a smaller tumor burden. In addition, as early studies of high-dose chemotherapy in a variety of disease types had indicated, that HDC seldom produced cures in patients with disease that was resistant to conventional chemotherapy; the early, conventionally dosed induction phase of the program would allow the identification of those patients whose cancer was resistant, and who should be spared the rigors of therapy which was toxic and expensive and which would be ultimately futile. Thus, according to this interpretation, conventional chemotherapy acted as an *in vivo* chemo-sensitivity assay, which determined which patients would proceed to HDC. Conventional chemotherapy might also improve the performance status of patients with advanced cancer prior to their being subjected to high-dose treatment.

The only precise validation for the use of high-dose chemotherapy as a form of late intensification would come from a random assignment trial in which primary high-dose chemotherapy was compared to the use of the same regimen as intensification following conventional therapy. None have as yet been carried out, but a historical comparison using identical HDC regimens did not suggest a major benefit for the induction component of a late-intensification regimen (29,30).

High-dose Sequential

The innovative high-dose sequential approach devised by Gianni and colleagues in Milan enables very high doses of drugs to be delivered in a fashion which does not predispose to overlapping toxicity, and which also attempts to deal with the clonal heterogeneity predicted by Goldie and Coldman (10). In this approach, patients are treated with a number of different drugs and regimens given at, or close to, maximum dose. High-dose sequential therapy has produced highly promising results in the treatment of aggressive lymphoma (31) and high-risk stage 2 breast cancer (32). It is the subject of a number of randomized trials in these diseases. High-dose sequential therapy has also been studied in metastatic breast cancer. A principal theoretical argument against the high-dose sequential approach is that single cycles of any therapy have not been shown to be an efficient means of eradicating cells which are sensitive to those agents.

Multi-cycle High-dose Chemotherapy

The multi-cycle high-dose chemotherapy (MCHDC) model represents another attempt to improve on the promising but somewhat marginal clinical results which were reported in early trials of high-dose chemotherapy. It has its origins both in a critical analysis of the general development of clinical chemotherapy theory and practice, and in an alternative interpretation of the Norton-Simon model.

It will be apparent that, viewed in the context of the curative therapy programs that have evolved for the treatment of lymphoma, Hodgkin disease, early stage breast cancer and testicular germ cell cancer, induction/consolidation and high-dose sequential programs look very odd. Curative chemotherapy has generally involved the identification of a highly active regimen, and then, the application of a sufficient number of cycles of the regimen to achieve tumor eradication. Thus, in the early MOPP program of chemotherapy for Hodgkin disease from the U.S. National Cancer Institute, patients achieved remission after, on average, three cycles of therapy. Similarly in the chemotherapy of germ cell tumors, it has been demonstrated that three cycles of cisplatin-etoposide therapy was inferior to four.

Another observation that emerged in early chemotherapy studies in Hodgkin disease was the finding that pretreatment with largely ineffective single-agent therapy compromised the ability of subsequent active combination regimens to effect cure. It can thus be argued then that primary single-cycle high-dose chemotherapy, late-intensification high-dose chemotherapy, and high-dose sequential therapy all represent substantial departures from classic chemotherapy theory and practice. Multi-cycle high-dose chemotherapy, on the other hand, appears to be more consistent with successful precedents.

The original Norton-Simon interpretations of the kinetics of tumor growth and chemotherapy-induced regression were that tumor regression was directly related both to the dose of drug administered and to the growth rate of the unperturbed tumor at the time of treatment. It was nowhere stated that the dose-response relationship only existed for the late, intensified part of therapy. Rather, the greatest curative impact of intensified therapy might be at a time of minimal residual disease. As has been discussed, at the time of their formulation of these recommendations, the supportive care of the patient undergoing intensive chemotherapy was relatively primitive compared to that which is currently available. The degree of intensification which was possible was modest. In addition, it would not have been feasible to administer multiple cycles of highly intensive therapy.

The basic assumption underlying MCHDC is that single applications of an active drug or regimen have not been generally effective in eradicating even sensitive cancers. In those cancers which are successfully treated with chemotherapy, multiple cycles of effective regimens have been administered. For Hodgkin disease, the median number of cycles of MOPP chemotherapy which produced complete remission in the original NCI study was between two and three. It is thus reasonable to assume that the cure rate in this series would have been low if only a single cycle of MOPP had been administered. Similarly, is it not possible that single applications of high-dose chemotherapy would not represent the optimal use for this technology in patients with breast cancer? Should we not instead try to administer multiple high-dose cycles? Another consideration is that the Norton-Simon model emphasizes the potential for accelerated regrowth of surviving cells in between cycles of effective therapy. This acceleration would, according to the model, have its greatest impact in patients who harbored very small, subclinical populations of cells. Thus, according to this interpretation of tumor kinetics, the intercycle interval between such high-dose treatments might be of crucial importance. The essential difference between MCHDC and HDS chemotherapy is that the latter attempts to overcome drug resistance by introducing a number of different drugs and regimens, whereas MCHDC is designed to ensure that the therapeutic effects of effective therapy are maximized by administering an optimum number of cycles (33). Investigators in New York demonstrated the feasibility of accelerated, progenitor-supported, multi-cycle, high-dose chemotherapy in breast and ovarian cancer (34). Conventional dose-induction therapy might in theory allow the proliferation of those cells which are resistant to conventional doses, and sensitive only to high doses. Thus, the later application of high-dose chemotherapy might result in the high-dose therapy "confronting" a higher burden of cancer than it would have done had it been applied at the outset.

Single-Arm Trials of High-dose Chemotherapy with Autograft Support in Metastatic Breast Cancer

Only a small number of trials explored primary high-dose therapy as initial treatment for metastatic disease. The group at Duke University treated newly diagnosed patients with metastatic disease with a single cycle of high-dose cyclophosphamide, BCNU and cisplatin. The rate of complete remission was 54%, and one-fourth of these remissions were durable at 5 years. It was in an attempt to improve on these promising results that most investigators turned to the late-intensification model, and the overwhelming majority of trials which were conducted over the next 10 years used this model.

Typically, patients in such studies were treated with four to six cycles of an anthracycline-containing induction therapy, and those patients who had achieved either a partial or complete response were then consolidated with single, or in a few cases, tandem, cycles of high-dose therapy. Patients with highly resistant disease were thus spared the rigors of high-dose therapy, and the cytoreduction achieved with conventional therapy might contribute to ultimate cure by presenting the high-dose therapy with a smaller tumor burden to eradicate. Typically, approximately 50% to 70% of patients responded to induction therapy, and proceeded to "transplant." Some patients in partial response following induction were converted to complete remission, and of course patients were consolidated while already in CR from induction. In most of these studies, approximately 50% to 70% of patients achieved CR overall following both phases of therapy. The great majority of these remissions ended in relapse, but a proportion, generally 10% to 15% of patients subjected to the induction-consolidation approach, remained in CR for 5 years.

While there were no direct randomized comparisons of late intensification versus primary high-dose therapy, it is not immediately obvious that the results of the former were superior.

The "high-dose sequential" model has also had little study in metastatic breast cancer. Patrone et al. (35) treated patients with stage 4 disease with a regimen which was similar to that employed by Gianni. Again, a small proportion of patients achieved durable remissions.

The approach of accelerated MCHDC was studied by investigators at Memorial Sloan-Kettering Cancer Center in New York. Patients in a state of ongoing response following conventional chemotherapy were treated with a sequence of high-dose single-alkylating agents. In the first trial, 42 patients received tandem cycles of cyclophosphamide followed by tandem cycles of autograft-supported thiotepa. There were no treatment-related deaths, and overall, 20% of patients achieved prolonged remission (36). In a second trial, the therapy was further intensified by substituting autograft-supported high-dose melphalan for one of the cyclophosphamide cycles. The regimen was active but toxic, and three of 17 patients died from an unanticipated syndrome of fulminant interstitial pneumonitis. A fourth patient developed late leukemia. Five patients, however, remained alive and in continued remission at up to 5 years from treatment (37).

While historical comparisons seem to suggest a substantial survival advantage compared to conventional chemotherapy (38), the possibility that case selection bias might be an important contributory factor to the apparent success of HDC in this setting mandated prospective random assignment trials (39).

Single-arm Trials of High-dose Chemotherapy with Autograft Support as an Adjuvant Treatment for High-risk Early-stage Breast Cancer

Peters and colleagues (40) treated patients with breast cancer involving at least ten axillary lymph nodes with an aggressive doxorubicin-based regimen followed by a single cycle of high-dose, late-intensification chemotherapy supported by an autograft of bone marrow or peripheral blood. These authors reported that 70% of patients remained free of relapse at 5 years. Interestingly, many of the relapses that did occur in this study were locoregional recurrences before the routine introduction of radiotherapy consolidation. Gianni and colleagues (32) studied high-dose sequential chemotherapy (see below) in patients with stage 2 breast cancer involving ten or more axillary lymph nodes. In their study, 65% of patients remained free of relapse.

Randomized Trials of High-dose Chemotherapy with Autograft Support in Metastatic Breast Cancer

The results of seven random assignment trials in which HDC was compared to CDC in the treatments of patients with overtly metastatic disease have been reported. In summary, none of these studies have shown a survival advantage for high-dose therapy, but six revealed statistically significant advantages for HDC in terms of prolonged progression-free survival (41–45). One was entirely negative (46). Six utilized the late intensification approach. The only study which addressed primary multi-cycle HDC was positive for PFS. The data from the Bezwoda study (47) primary multi-cycle HDC were found to be unverifiable by an international audit team.

Randomized Trials of High-dose Chemotherapy with Autograft Support in Early-stage Breast Cancer

At this point in time, the results of eight randomized trials in which the role of high-dose chemotherapy in the treatment of high-risk early-stage breast cancer were studied have been reported. The results of one of these, by Bezwoda et al. (47), have been found to be unsafe following audit.

In the Scandinavian study of Berg et al., patients with high-risk disease were randomly assigned to receive either FEC chemotherapy followed by a single high-dose cycle or, in the "low-dose" arm, "individually tailored" doses of FEC chemotherapy. Patients on the low-dose arm in fact received substantially higher doses of anthracycline, cyclophosphamide and 5-fluorouracil than did patients on the high-dose arm. This study was negative, but it was in fact a comparison between two high-dose strategies, and as such contributes little to the debate concerning the merits of high-dose therapy. It is also noteworthy that there was an excess of treatment-related leukemia on the low-dose arm (49).

The CALGB attempted to validate the earlier cited Peters' adjuvant single-arm study in a large random assignment trial. Patients received aggressive doxorubicin-based induction, followed by either high-dose cisplatin, BCNU, cyclophosphamide with an autograft, or lower, but still aggressive, doses of the same triplet with filgrastim support. At a median follow-up of 5.1 years, the event-free and overall survival rates for the two arms were virtually identical. Interestingly, there was a significantly lower rate of disease relapse on the high-dose arm, but the unusually high (8%) rate of treatment-related mortality undermined any benefit. It is tempting to speculate that this study might in fact have been positive, if a more typical rate of toxic death (generally 1%–2% in other trials) had occurred (50).

Two other very small studies in which late-intensification HDC was compared to conventionally dosed therapy were also negative (51,52).

The recently reported Anglo-Celtic trial was a large (607 patients) study in which patients with four or more involved axillary lymph nodes were randomly assigned to receive either CMF chemotherapy or high-dose treatment following a phase of doxorubicin induction. With a median follow-up of 4 years, there is no difference between these arms in either disease-free or overall survival, despite a low rate of treatment-related death (53).

In the Dutch National Study, patients with four or more involved axillary lymph nodes were randomly assigned to receive either five cycles of FEC chemotherapy or four cycles followed by a single cycle of high-dose therapy. While differences in survival for the entire cohort did not reach statistical significance, a prospectively mandated sub-group analysis of the earliest patients with longest follow-up compellingly suggested a late emerging difference (54).

In the only random assignment trial addressing the use of high-dose sequential chemotherapy in breast cancer, Gianni et al. (55) compared this approach to the A-CMF regimen, and reported no survival differences.

RESEARCH PRIORITIES AND FUTURE DIRECTIONS

Even to the most misty-eyed transplanter, high-dose therapy could never have been anything other than "best chemotherapy." The truth is, oncologists have always dreamed of the end of the chemotherapy era anyway. We have long anticipated the availability of rationally designed molecularly targeted treatments for breast and other cancers. The first such agents have now become available, and it is likely that more will soon join trastuzumab, STI-571 and rituxamab.

However, several possible scenarios mandate keeping at least an open mind on the subject of high-dose treatment. It is possible that some of the currently negative studies may yet prove positive with longer follow-up. In addition, better understanding of biological predictive factors might allow for the identification of populations in whom high-dose therapy might be most advantageously studied.

In the event that ongoing studies ultimately demonstrate meaningful clinical benefits for the high-dose approach, two broad strategies will need to be addressed in successor trials. Attempts will have to be made attempting to improve on this treatment. The impact of new high-dose regimens versus existing programs, engineered versus unmanipulated autograft products (56,57), adjuvant immunotherapy (58), gene therapy (59), multiple versus single high-dose cycles, and of late-intensification versus high-dose sequential and primary high-dose chemotherapy strategies could all be studied. Antiangiogenesis factors might usefully be employed to maintain HDC-induced remissions (60). Allogeneic transplantation is also under investigation (61,62).

REFERENCES

1. Cold S, Jensen NV, Brincker H, Rose C. The influence of chemotherapy on survival after recurrence in breast cancer—a population-based study of patients treated in the 1950s, 1960s and the 1970s. *Eur J Cancer* 1993; 29A:1146–1152.
2. Greenberg PAC, Hortobagyi GN, Smith TL, et al. Long-term follow-up of patients with complete remission of patients with complete remission following combination chemotherapy for metastatic breast cancer. *J Clin Oncol* 1996;14:2197–2205.
3. Skipper HE, Schabel FM. Quantitative and cytokinetic studies in experimental tumor systems. In: Holland J, Frei FE, eds. Cancer medicine. Philadelphia: Lea and Febiger, 1988:663–684.
4. Early Breast Cancer Trialist's Collaborative Group. Systemic treatment of early breast cancer by hormonal, cytotoxic or immune therapy: 133 randomized trials involving 31,000 recurrences and 24,000 deaths among 75,000 women. *Lancet* 1992;339:1–15.
5. Norton L, Simon R. The Norton-Simon hypothesis revisited. *Cancer Treat Rep* 1986;70:163–169.
6. Norton L, Simon R, Brereton HD, et al. Predicting the course of Gompertzian growth. *Nature* (Lond.) 1976; 264:542–545.
7. Perloff M, Norton L, Korzun AH, et al. Post surgical adjuvant chemotherapy of stage II breast carcinoma with or without crossover to a non-cross-resistant regimen: a Cancer and Leukemia Group B Study. *J Clin Oncol* 1996;14:1589–1598.
8. Cocconi G, Bisagni G, Bacchi M, et al. A comparison of continuation versus late intensification followed by discontinuation of chemotherapy in advanced breast cancer. A prospective randomized trial of the Italian Oncology Group for Clinical Research (G.O.I.R.C.). *Ann Oncol* 1990;1(1):36–44.
9. Buzzoni R, Bonnadonna G, Vallagussa P, et al. Adjuvant chemotherapy with doxorubicin plus cyclophosphamide, methotrexate, and flurouracil in the treatment of resectable breast cancer with more than 3 positive axillary nodes. *J Clin Oncol* 1994;9:2134–2140.
10. Goldie J, Coldman AJ. A mathematical model for relating the drug sensitivity of tumors to their spontaneous mutation rate. *Cancer Treat Rep* 1979;63:1727–1773.
11. Teicher BA, Holden SA, Cucchi CA, et al. Combination thiotepa and cyclophosphamide in vivo and in vitro. *Cancer Res* 1988;48:94–100.
12. Hryniuk W, Bush H. The importance of dose intensity in chemotherapy of metastatic breast cancer. *J Clin Oncol* 1984;2:81–88.
13. O'Dwyer PJ, LaCreta FP, Schilder R, et al. Phase I trial of thiotepa in combination with recombinant human granulocyte-macrophage colony-stimulating factor. *J Clin Oncol* 1992;10:1352–1358.
14. Bronchud MH, Howell A, Crowther D, et al. The use of granulocyte colony-stimulating factor to increase the intensity of treatment with doxorubicin in patients with advanced breast and ovarian cancer. *Br J Cancer* 1989; 60:121–125.
15. Bastholt L, Dalmark M, Gjedde S. Dose-response relationship of epirubicin in the treatment of postmenopausal patients with metastatic breast cancer: a randomized study of epirubicin at four different dose levels performed by the Danish Breast Cancer Cooperative Group. *J Clin Oncol* 1996;14:1146–1155.
16. Hortobagyi GN, Buzdar AU, Bodey GP, et al. High-dose induction chemotherapy of metastatic breast cancer in protected environment units: a prospective randomized study. *J Clin Oncol* 1987;5:178–184.
17. Ardizzoni A, Venturini M, Sertoli MR, et al. Granulocyte-macrophage colony-stimulating factor (GM-CSF) allows acceleration and dose-intensity increase of CEF chemotherapy: a randomized study in patients with advanced breast cancer. *Br J Cancer* 1994;69:385–391.

18. Henderson IC, Berry D, Demetri G, et al. Improve disease-free survival and overall survival from the addition of sequential Paclitaxel but not from the escalation of doxorubicin dose in the adjuvant chemotherapy of patients with Node-positive primary breast cancer. Proc ASCO 1998;17:101a.
19. Fisher B, Anderson S, Wickerham DL, et al. Increased intensification and total dose of cyclophosphamide in a doxorubicin-cyclophosphamide regimen for the treatment of primary breast cancer: Findings from National Surgical Adjuvanrt Breast and Bowel Project B-22. J Clin Oncol 1997;15:1858–1869.
20. Levine MN, Gent M, Hryniuk WM, et al. A randomized trial comparing 12 weeks versus 36 weeks of adjuvant chemotherapy in stage II breast cancer. J Clin Oncol 1990;8(7):1217–1225.
21. Bonneterre J, Roché J, Bremond A, et al. Results of a randomized trial of adjuvant chemotherapy with FEC 50 vs FEC 100 in high-risk node positive breast cancer patients. Proc ASCO 1998;17:124a.
22. Tannock IF, Boyd NF, Deborer G, et al. A randomized trial of two dose levels of CMF chemotherapy for patients with metastatic breast cancer. J Clin Oncol 1988; 6:1377–1387.
23. Lazarus H, Reed MD, Spitzer TR, et al. High-dose iv thiotepa and cryopreserved autologous bone marrow transplantation for therapy of refractory cancer. Cancer Treat Rep 1987;71:689–695.
24. Eder JP, Antman K, Peters WP, et al High-dose combination alkylating agent chemotherapy with autologous marrow support for metastatic breast cancer. J Clin Oncol 1986;4:1592–1597.
25. Peters WP, Rosner G, Ross M, et al. Comparative effects of granulocyte-macrophage colony-stimulating factor (GM-CSF) and granulocyte colony-stimulating factor (G-CSF) on priming peripheral blood progenitor cells for use with autologous bone marrow after high-dose chemotherapy. Blood 1993;81:1709–1719.
26. Socinski MA, Elias A, Schnipper L, et al. Granulocyte-macrophage colony-stimulating factor expands the circulating haemopoietic progenitor cell compartment in man. Lancet 1988;i:1194–1198.
27. Beyer J, Schwella N, Zingsem J, et al. Bone marrow versus peripheral blood stem cells as rescue after high-dose chemotherapy. Blood 1993;82(suppl 1):454a.
28. Kritz A, Crown J, Motzer R. Beneficial impact of peripheral blood progenitor cells in patients with metastatic breast cancer treated with high-dose chemotherapy plus GM-CSF: A randomized trial. Cancer 1993;71: 2515–2521.
29. Peters WP, Shpall EJ, Jones RB, et al. High-dose combination alkylating agents with bone marrow support as initial treatment for metastatic breast cancer. J Clin Oncol 1988;6:1368–1376.
30. Jones RB, Shpall EJ, Ross M, et al. AFM induction chemotherapy followed by intensive alkylating agent consolidation with autologous bone marrow support for advanced breast cancer. Current results. Proc ASCO 1990;9:9.
31. Gianni AM, Bregni M, Siena S, et al. High-dose chemotherapy and autologous bone marrow transplantation compared with MACOP-B in aggressive B-cell lymphoma. N Engl J Med 1997;336(18):1290–1297.
32. Gianni AM, Siena S, Bregni M, et al. Growth factor supported high-dose sequential adjuvant chemotherapy in breast cancer with >10 positive nodes. Proc ASCO 1992;11:60.
33. Crown J, Norton L. Potential strategies for improving the results of high-dose chemotherapy in patients with metastatic breast cancer. Ann Oncol 1995;6(suppl 4): s21–s26.
34. Crown J, Wasserheit C, Hakes T, et al. Rapid delivery of multiple high-dose chemotherapy courses with G-CSF and peripheral blood-derived haemopoietic progenitor cells. J Natl Cancer Inst 1992;84:1935–1936.
35. Patrone F, Ballestrero A, Ferrando F. Four-step high-dose sequential chemotherapy with double hematopoietic progenitor-cell rescue for metastatic breast cancer, J Clin Oncol 1995;13:840–846.
36. Vahdat L, Raptis G, Fennelly D, et al. Rapidly cycled courses of high-dose alkylating agents supported by filgrastim and peripheral blood progenitor cells in patients with metastatic breast cancer. Clin Cancer Res 1995;1:1267–1273.
37. Crown J, Raptis G, Vahdat L, et al. Rapidly administration of sequentail high-dose cyclophosphamide, melphalan, thiotepa supported by filgrastim and peripheral blood progenitors in patients with metastatic breast cancer: a novel and very active treatment strategy. Proc ASCO 1994;13:110 (abst).
38. Antman K, Ayash L, Elias A, et al. A phase II study of high-dose cyclophosphamide, thiotepa, and carboplatin with autologous marrow support in women with measurable advanced breast cancer responding to standard-dose therapy. J Clin Oncol 1992;10:102–110.
39. Rahman ZU, Frye DK, Buzdar AU. Impact of selection process on response rate and long-term survival of potential high-dose chemotherapy candidates treated with standard-dose doxorubicin-containing chemotherapy in patients with metastatic breast cancer. J Clin Oncol 1997;15:3171–3177.
40. Peters WP, Ross M, Vredenburgh JJ, et al. High-dose chemotherapy and autologous bone marrow support as consolidation after standard-dose adjuvant therapy for high risk primary breast cancer. J Clin Oncol 1993; 11:1132–1144.
41. Peters WP, Jones RB, Vredenburgh J, et al. A large, prospective, randomized trial of high-dose combination alkylating agents (CBP) with autologous cellular support as consolidation for patients with metastatic breast cancer achieving complete remission after intensive doxorubicin-based induction therapy (AFM). Proc ASCO 1996;15:121.
42. Lotz J-P, Cure H, Janvier M, et al. High-dose chemotherapy (HD-CT) with hematopoietic stem cells transplantation (HSCT) for metastatic breast cancer: results of the French Protocol Pegase 04. Proc ASCO 1999;18:43a.
43. Biron P, Durand M, Roche H, et al. High dose thiotepa, cyclophosphamide, and stem cell transplantation after 4 FEC 1000 compared with 4 FEC alone allowed a better disease free survival but the same overall survival in first line chemotherapy for metastatic breast cancer. Results of the PEGASE 03 French protocol. Proc ASCO 2002;21:42a.
44. Crump M, Gluck S, Stewart D, et al. A randomized trial of high-dose chemotherapy with autologous peripheral blood stem cell support compared to standard therapy in women with metastatic breast cancer: A National

Cancer Institute of Canada Clinical Trials Group Study. *Proc ASCO* 2001;20:21a.
45. Schmid P, Samonigg H, Nitsch T, et al. Randomized trial of up front tandem high-dose chemotherapy cokmpared to standard chemotherapy with doxorubicin and paclitaxel in metastatic breast cancer. *Proc ASCO* 2002;21:43a.
46. Stadtmauer EA, O'Neill A, Goldstein LJ, et al. Phase III randomized trial of high-dose chemotherapy (HDC) and stem sell support (SCT) shows no difference in overall survival or severe toxicity compared to maintenance chemotherapy with cyclophosphomide, methotrexate and 5-fluorouracil (CMF) for women with metastatic breast cancer who are responding to conventional induction chemotherapy: The Philadelphia Intergroup Study (PBT-01). *Proc ASCO* 1999;18:1a.
47. Bezwoda WR, Seymour L, Dansey RD. High-dose chemotherapy with hematopoietic rescue as primary treatment for metastatic breast cancer: a randomised trial. *J Clin Oncol* 1995;13:2483–89.
48. Peters W, Rosner G, Vredenburgh J, et al. A prospective, randomized comparison of two doses of combination alkylating agents as consolidation after CAF in high-risk primary breast cancer involving ten or more axillary lymph nodes: Preliminary results of CALGB 9082/SWOG 9114/NCIC MA-13. *Proc ASCO* 1999; 18:1a.
49. The Scandinavian Breast Cancer Study Group 9401. Results from a randomized adjuvant breast cancer study with high-dose chemotherapy with CTC_b supported by autologous bone marrow stem cells versus dose escalated and tailored FEC therapy. *Proc ASCO* 1999;2a.
50. Peters WP, Rosner G, Vredenburgh J, et al. Updated results of a prospective, randomized comparison of two doses of combination alkylating agents as consolidation after CAF in high-risk primary breast cancer iinvolving ten or more axillary lymph nodes: CALGB 9082/SWOG 9114/NCIC Ma-13. *Proc ASCO* 2001;20:21a.
51. Hortobagyi GN, Buzdar AU, Champlin R. Lack of efficacy of adjuvant high-dose tandem combination chemotherapy for high-risk primary breast cancer a randomised trial. *Proc ASCO* 1998;17:123a.
52. Bezwoda WR. Randomised, controlled trial of high dose chemotherapy (HD-CNVp) vs. standard dose (CAF) chemotherapy for high risk, surgically treated, primary breast cancer. *Proc ASCO* 1999;18:2a.
53. Crown JP, Lind M, Gould A, et al. High-dose chemotherapy with autograft support is not superior to cyclophosphamide, methotrexate and 5-FU following doxorubicin inductrion in patients with breast cancer and 4 or more involved axillary lymph nodes: the Anglo-Celtic I study. *Proc ASCO* 2002;21:42a.
54. Rodenhuis S, Bontenbal M, Beex L, et al. Randomized phase III study of high-dose chemotherapy with cyclophosphamide, thiotepa, and carboplatin in operable breast cancer with 4 or more axillary lymph nodes. *Proc ASCO* 2000;286a.
55. Gianni A, Bonadonna G. Five year results of the randomized clinical trial comparing standard versus high-dose myeloablative chemotherapy in the adjuvant treatment of breast cancer with >3 positive nodes. *Proc ASCO* 2001;20:21a.
56. Brugger W, Heimfeld S, Berenson RJ, et al. Reconstitution of haematopoiesis after high-dose chemotherapy by autologous progenitor cells generated ex vivo. *N Engl J Med* 1995;333:283–287.
57. Shpall EJ, Jones RB, Bearman SI, et al. Transplantation of enriched CD34-positive autologous marrow into breast cancer patients following high-dose chemotherapy: influence of CD34-positive peripheral-blood progenitors and growth factors on engraftment. *J Clin Oncol* 1994;12:28–36.
58. Kennedy MJ, Vogelzang G, Beveridge R, et al. Phase I trial of intravenous cyclosporine to induce graft versus host disease in women undergoing autologous bone marrow transplantation for breast cancer. *J Clin Oncol* 1993;11:478–484.
59. Hesdorffer C, Ayello J, Ward M, et al. Phase I trial of retroviral-mediated transfer of the human MDR1 gene as marrow chemoprotection in patients undergoing high-dose chemotherapy and autologous stem-cell transplantation. *J Clin Oncol* 16.
60. O'Reilly MS, Holmgren L, Chen C, Folkman J. Angiostatin induces and sustains dormancy of human primary tumors in mice. *Nat Med* 1996;2(6):689–692.
61. Ueno N, Rondón G, Mirza NQ. Allogeneic peripheral-blood progenitor-cell transplantation for poor-risk patients with metastatic breast cancer. *J Clin Oncol* 16:986–993.
62. Chan S, Friedrichs K, Noel D, et al. Prospective randomized trial of docetaxel versus doxorubicin in patients with metastatic breast cancer. *J Clin Oncol* (in press).

PART VII

Summary Statement

48

The Future of Breast Cancer Medicine

Jean-Marc Nabholtz, Katia Tonkin, Matti S. Aapro,
Aman U. Buzdar, and David M. Reese

Experience is the name everyone gives to their mistakes.

Oscar Wilde

In a hundred years' time they'll laugh and call us savages.

Alexander Solzenitsyn, *Cancer Ward*

In 1856, shortly after joining the faculty at the University of Berlin, the German pathologist Rudolf Virchow delivered a series of lectures designed to enlighten his colleagues and students about the latest developments in medical science. These lectures, which brilliantly elucidated the cellular theory of disease—in the process casting aside misguided notions such as the existence of evil humors, prevalent since the days of Hippocrates and Galen—were edited and published as a book. Like Newton's *Principia* two hundred years earlier, Virchow's *Cellular Pathology* caused an immediate sensation in Europe. For 20 centuries physicians had been struggling to understand the root causes of illness; now, they had a new paradigm, one that taught them to focus on the cell and rely for progress on what Virchow called "the stronghold of scientific medicine." Nowhere was the cellular doctrine more important than in attacking the scourge of cancer.

As can be seen from the pages of this book, the international enterprise of scientific medicine has made substantial headway in the fight against breast cancer since Virchow's revolutionary opus was published. Surgery has evolved from the days of radical mastectomy to a time when the majority of patients undergo breast-conserving procedures, often with sentinel node dissection. We have learned that breast cancer is more often than not a systemic disease at the outset, and, as a result, most patients now receive some form of adjuvant therapy. While we still are unable to cure all but a few patients with metastatic disease, recently there has been measurable progress with the introduction of new cytotoxics such as the taxanes and trastuzumab, the first targeted therapy apart from hormonal treatment.

But it is clear that much remains to be learned and done. Simply evaluating the mass of information currently available is complicated and time-consuming. Moreover, in spite of the explosive growth in the number of randomized trials, often there are insufficient data to answer a specific clinical question. Thus, clinicians must look critically at imperfect evidence and decide what is best for individual patients. In this book we have outlined the available tools, applying the concept of "application of evidence to patient care" to the treatment of breast cancer. These data summarize where we stand and where we need to go.

One inescapable conclusion is that our traditional method of empirically testing new therapies is no longer a viable development strategy. Much of the evidence described in this book relating to systemic treatment, for example, was generated by adding new drugs to existing standards in traditional phase 1, 2, and 3 clinical trials. The scientific knowledge necessary to proceed differently did not exist. In the near future, however, we will have available numerous novel biologic therapies directed at multiple molecular alterations in the cancer cell. The trick will be to combine them rationally, for which we require reliable preclinical models to direct our efforts in the research clinic. There are a finite number of patients who are willing to participate in clinical research, and, with a huge number of potential combinations, we will need to focus on those regimens that have their foundations in science. Random combinations of new agents will no longer be feasible.

Another crucial area in which we must make progress is in our ability to predict which patients will benefit from a specific therapy, as well as to determine who requires therapy at all. Among women with high-risk node-negative breast cancer, for instance, approximately 30% will relapse without systemic therapy. While standard prognostic factors such as tumor size, grade, and hormone receptor status help to categorize the risk of disease recurrence, these are not completely reliable. Thus, to increase the cure rate from 70% to the currently achievable 76% to 78%, we currently must treat 100% of patients. It is imperative that we identify prognostic factors that tell us who will relapse without systemic therapy; we must also know which therapies are likely to succeed in a given patient, based on the biologic characteristics of the tumor. The ultimate goal is to be able to precisely characterize each tumor at the molecular level, and then use this information to individualize therapy.

We also need to adjust our approach to the evaluation of new therapeutics. Many of the angiogenesis inhibitors may be expected to produce stable disease, for example, at least in the short term. Failure to observe objective tumor responses according to traditional phase 2 criteria, then, may not indicate a lack of efficacy of these agents. In addition, based on the biology of tumor progression, anti-angiogenics will probably have their greatest utility in the treatment of early stage disease. Locally advanced or metastatic tumors often elaborate multiple pro-angiogenic growth factors, and use of a single agent such as an anti-VEGF inhibitor may not be sufficient to thwart tumor growth. It may make more sense to develop these drugs in the adjuvant setting.

In short, we must be creative in deciding which endpoints should be used to assess new molecular therapies, and we must test these new drugs in the appropriate stage of disease. This will entail abandoning the current paradigm, in which novel therapies are first used as second-line therapy in patients with metastatic disease, and then tested as first-line therapy and in the adjuvant setting if there is evidence of activity. Indeed, some drugs may most appropriately be evaluated first as preventive agents, bypassing altogether their use for the treatment of established disease.

Finally, we need to develop truly new systems for the management and dissemination of information. The Internet has opened up new ways of communication, making us a genuinely global research community. The Breast Cancer International Research Group (BCIRG) relies extensively on the information superhighway in its daily operations. As we move forward, it will be essential to capture and record in an easily retrievable fashion detailed information about each patient entered on a clinical trial. Ranging from standard demographics to gene expression profiles derived from microarray technologies, these data, linked to known clinical outcome, will be a fertile ground in which to generate new hypotheses. Just as the field of informatics is becoming indispensable to analyze the data generated by genomics and proteomics, so must the informatics expert be integrated into the clinical research operations of cooperative groups such as BCIRG.

The English poet William Cowper famously wrote that "knowledge and wisdom, far from being one, have oft-times no connection." Molecular biology is generating knowledge about the fundamental alterations that drive the proliferation and spread of cancer cells. Combinatorial chemistry and rational drug design are daily adding to the number of candidate compounds. The present challenge is to translate that knowledge of targets and potential new agents into the wisdom of effective therapies, quickly and efficiently. If we are sufficiently flexible in our approach, and lucky, they will indeed laugh and call our current therapies savage a hundred years from now—or even earlier.

Index

A
A-CMF regimen, 595
Absolute risk reduction
  anastrozole vs. tamoxifen and, 545
Absolute tumor-associated blood volume
  calculation of, 294
ABX-EGF
  esophageal cancer and, 277
  overview of, 277
Acromioclavicular joint
  irradiation and, 16
Acupuncture
  Complementary and Alternative
    Medicine (CAM) and, 428
Acute emesis
  overview of, 489
  pathophysiology of, 489–490
  prophylaxis for, 494
  risk factors of, 489
  serotonin receptor antagonists and, 494
Adenovirus
  E1A and, 314
Adenovirus vector
  gene therapy delivery and, 312
Adhesion signaling
  cancer cells and, 386
Adjuvant bisphophonates
  trials of
    recurrent disease with no metastases
      and, 468
Adjuvant breast cancer therapy
  dose-intensity potential in, 447–448
Adjuvant chemo/hormonal therapy
  final conclusions on, 104–105
Adjuvant chemotherapy (CT). *See also*
    Dose dense/intense adjuvant
    chemotherapy
  bone loss and, 463
  endocrine non-responsive disease and, 367
  final conclusions, 104–105
  hormonal therapy with, 103
  node-negative breast cancer (NNBC)
    and, 101
  predictive markers for, 370
  relapses and, 122
  role of anthracyclines and, 447
Adjuvant cytotoxic chemotherapy
  loss of bone and, 463
Adjuvant doxorubicin
  HER-2/*neu* and, 397
Adjuvant exemestane
  studies of, 208
Adjuvant hormone therapy (hormono-
    therapy)
  anastrozole (Arimidex) and, 545
  blockade of ER-signaling pathway and, 347
  CHOP and, 92
  EGFR tyrosine kinase inhibitors and, 278t
  final conclusions, 104–105

node-negative breast cancer (NNBC)
    and, 100
  predictive factors for, 395–396
  predictive markers for, 368–370
  pulmonary embolism, 530
  research implication from current data
    on, 531–532
Adjuvant immunotherapy
  future directions and, 596
Adjuvant RCTs of dose dense CT, 126t
Adjuvant tamoxifen, 532
  HER-2/*neu* and, 369t
Adjuvant therapy
  blood transfusions and, 459
  morbidity and, 411
  node positive breast cancer and
    summary of evidence for, 140–141
  tamoxifen and, 212–213
  taxanes and, 159–161
  taxanes and trastuzumab in, 163
  tumor size and, 393
Adjuvant trastuzumab
  early stage breast cancer and, 256
ADR-529, 190
Adrenalectomy
  non-selective aromatase inhibitors and, 205
Adriamycin/CMF
  mastectomy and, 87
Advanced breast cancer
  combination regimens for, 158
  docetaxel monotherapy and, 152
AF-1
  overview of, 233
AIDS
  myocardial biopsies and, 191
Alkylating agents, 451
  CALGB 9082 trial and, 137
Allen and Chonn study
  liposomes and, 190
Allogenic transplantation
  future directions and, 596
Alluna
  alternative therapies and, 434–435
ALND. *See* Axillary lymph node
    dissection
Alopecia
  paclitaxel vinorelbine regimen and, 158
  toxicities of paclitaxel and, 148
Alopecia neoplastica
  nodules and, 477
Alpha subunit, 288
Alpha tocopherol, 190
Alternative therapies
  breast cancer patients usage of, 428–429
  cancer patients usage of, 428
  cancer treatments and, 425
  definition of, 427–428
  future avenues for, 434–435
  general usage of, 428
  reputable sources for, 433
American Intergroup trial
  fenretinide and, 114

American Society of Clinical Oncology
    (ASCO)
  adjuvant tamoxifen and, 370
  breast cancer reduction strategy and
    raloxifene and, 543
  docetaxel and, 161
  HER-2 and, 370
  raloxifene and, 229
Amifostine, 190
Aminobisphosphonate
  studies of, 467
Aminoglutethimide, 209, 215
  non-selective aromatase inhibitors and, 204
  overview of, 205
  tamoxifen and, 111–112
Aminoglutethimide therapy
  vorzole *vs.*, 209
Analysis
  appropriate for evidence, 575
Anastrozole (Arimidex), 204
  adjuvant hormonal therapy and, 545
  adjuvant setting and, 213
  aromatase inhibitors and, 112
  conclusions from trials with, 215
  contralateral breast cancer and, 113
  first-line therapy with, 210–211
  fulvestrant and, 237
  megestrol acetate (MA) *vs.*, 211t
  overview of, 210, 544
  second-line therapy with, 210
  vs. tamoxifen and, 545
Anemia
  leridistim and, 450
  signs and symptoms of, 457
Anemia of chronic disease
  fatigue and, 457
  overview of, 457
Aneuploidy
  prognosis and, 99
Angiogenesis
  EGFR tyrosine kinase inhibitors and, 278t
  in breast cancer, 294t
  overview of, 287, 400
  positive and negative regulators of, 288t
  potentials for therapy target of, 290
  soluble measures of, 291–292
  surrogate endpoints of, 291
  tumor cell and, 551
  tumor growth and, 287
  tumor-associated, 287
Angiogenesis Foundation, 296
Angiogenesis inhibitors, 602
  clinic and
    preliminary data in, 296
Angiogenic signaling
  tumor growth and, 291
Angiogenic switch
  tumors and, 288
Angiogenic tumors
  micrometastases and, 388

603

Angiostatin
  mechanism of, 299–300
Angiozyme, 298–299
Anthracenedione, 190
Anthracycline-based chemotherapy (CT), 181
  CMF and, 370
  markers predicting activity of, 374
  overview of, 115
  risk and, 115
Anthracycline-containing induction therapy, 594
Anthracycline-containing regimens
  breast cancer therapy and, 189
  CMF vs., 118t
  toxicity and, 189
Anthracycline-cyclophosphamide plus trastuzumab
  heart failure and, 162
Anthracyclines, 10, 450
  adjuvant chemotherapy and, 27, 447
  Billingham scale and, 191, 191t
  cardiomyopathy and, 121
  drug-efflux pumps resistance to, 375
  high dose intensity, 124
  metastatic disease and, 124–125
  node-negative breast cancer (NNBC) and, 102
  non-randomized studies and, 89
  postmenopausal women and, 118
  suboptimal dose intensity and, 122–124, 123t
  trastuzumab and, 252
  vs. CMF, 116t, 125
  vs. non-anthracycline-based chemotherapy and, 102
Anti VEGF inhibitor
  tumor growth and, 602
Anti-EGF receptor therapies
  challenges in compound development in, 281–282
Anti-EGFR antibodies
  cisplatin and, 276
  overview of, 274–277
Anti-HER-2
  cisplatin and, 252
Anti-HER-2/neu
  cancer cell resistance to, 314
Anti-vascular endothelial growth factor (VEGF) receptor 2 antibodies, 263
Antiangiogenic activity
  chemotherapeutic agents and, 295
Antiangiogenic agents
  current trials with, 297t–298t
  two categories of, 290
Antiangiogenic chemotherapy, 261, 262
  conclusions on, 300–301
  overview of, 291
  tumor dormancy and, 389
Antiangiogenic drugs
  drug resistance and, 261
Antiangiogenic schedule
  cyclophosphamide and, 295
Antibody humanization, 249
Antibody-dependent, well-mediated cytotoxicity (ADCC)
  trastuzumab and, 250
Anticipatory emesis. See Anticipatory nausea and vomiting (ANV)
Anticipatory nausea and vomiting (ANV)
  chemotherapy and, 491
  definition of, 491
  pathophysiology of, 492

risk factors of, 491–492
  treatment of, 497
Antiemetic agents
  classes of, 492–494
Antiemetic prophylaxis
  dosing guidelines for, 496t
Antiepidermal growth factor receptor (EGFR/HER-1) antibodies, 252
Antiestrogens
  breast cancer therapy with, 223
  mechanism of action of, 237f
  mechanisms of action in, 225
  past or potential clinical value of, 226t
  preclinical and clinical assessment of, 225t
  three classes of, 226, 237
  effects of, 238t
Antigen retrieval
  Her-2 and, 247
  method for, 247
Antimetabolites
  trastuzumab with, 252
Antioxidants, 190
Antireceptor therapy, 274
Antitumor agents
  bisphosphonates and, 471
Apoferritin, 457
Apoptosis
  cancer cells and, 387
  E1A and, 318
  taxanes and, 147
  tumor cells and, 318
  tumor formation and, 323
  UCN-01 (7-hydroxystaurosporine) and, 360
Apoptotic index (AI)
  chemotherapy and, 93
Apoptotic molecules
  tumor cell and, 551
Aromatase inhibitors
  vs. megestrol acetate, 211t
Archiving
  Internet and, 513
Area postrema (AP), 490
Area under the curve (AUC)
  anthracycline and, 154
  Caelyx and, 191
  paclitaxel and, 147
Arimidex
  vs. EM-800, 230
Arimidex Tamoxifen Alone or Combination (ATAC), 213
  disease free survival in, 214t
  patient characteristics in, 213t
  postmenopausal women and, 112–113
  results from, 545
Arimidex-Nolvadex (ARNO) trial
  adjuvant trials and, 214
Aromatase enzyme, 203
  inhibitors and, 205
Aromatase inhibitors, 204–205, 204t
  breast cancer and, 532
  chemopreventive agent and, 546
  conclusions on, 219
  low toxicity profile of, 532
  new generation of, 112–113
  node-positive (NP) disease and, 107
  summary of evidence for, 140
  tamoxifen vs., 212t
Arthralgia
  toxicities of paclitaxel and, 148

Arzoxifene
  overview of, 229–230
  phase 1 and 2 studies with, 229t
Assessment
  criteria for cost, 583–584
  moderate treatment effects and requirements for, 576t
  requirements for, 575–576
ATAC. See Arimidex Tamoxifen Alone or Combination
ATP-dependent proteolysis
  cell cycle and, 356
AUC. See Area under the curve
Australian NHMRC National Breast Cancer Centre
  web sites for reference and, 563
Autologous bone marrow (ABM), 591
Autologous stem cell transplantation, 197
  high dose chemotherapy combined with, 195
Axilla
  recurrence of cancer in, 4
Axillary lymph node dissection (ALND)
  chemotherapy and, 78
  morbidity and, 79
  SLNB and, 61
Axillary lymph node staging
  chemotherapy and, 77–78
Axillary lymph nodes, 5
  disease in, 412
  irradiation and, 16, 17
  mammary nodes and, 4
  status of
    prognostic factor in determining, 392–393
Axillary node metastases
  sentinel lymph nodes and, 394

B

B-mode ultrasound
  breast tumors and, 293
BAD
  cell death regulation and, 273
Basic fibroblast growth factor (bFGF)
  breast carcinoma and, 312
Basset
  breast physical examination and, 525
Bcl-2 protein expression
  apoptosis inhibitor ER and, 395
  chemotherapy and, 93
BCIRG 006
  TCH and, 163
BCL-2
  cell death regulation and, 273
BCPT, 539
BCT. See Breast conserving treatment
Benzamides
  chemotherapy-induced emesis and, 492
Benzodiazepines
  chemotherapy-induced emesis an, 493
Benzopyrane
  diagram of, 228f
  overview of, 230
Benzothiophenes
  overview of, 228, 228f
Best available evidence, 557
Best overall response
  definition of, 571
  determining, 571
Beta subunit, 288
Billingham scale
  cardiomyopathy and, 191, 191t

Billroth, Theodore
  outcome in cancer and, 552
Biologic therapies
  taxane integration with, 161–163
Biological response modifiers
  therapies with, 97
Biomolecular Interaction Data-base (BIND)
  microarray data and, 328
Biopsy
  lobular carcinoma in situ (LCIS) and, 30
  relevance of, 78
  RNA degradation and, 324
  sentinel lymph node (SLN) and, 394
  tumor growth with open, 482
Bispecific antibodies
  overview of three, 277
Bisphosphonates
  bone metastases in breast cancer and, 465
  decrease in bone pain with, 467–468
  macrophages and, 466
  molecular level of, 466
  placebo effect and, 467
Bladder cancer
  EGFR expression and correlation with, 273
  VEGF concentrations (urinary) and, 292
Bleeding
  hormone replacement therapy and, 530
  management of, 484–485
Blood brain barrier
  erythropoietin and, 460
Blood flow
  color doppler ultrasonography (CDUS) and, 293
  lymph node metastases and, 293
Blood supply
  cancer and, 400
Blood transfusions
  epoetin alpha therapy and, 459
  pharmaco-economics, 460–461
BMS-275291
  overview of, 296
Bonadonna regimen, 128
  chemotherapy drugs and, 114
  six cycles of, 115
Bone fracture
  morbidity in breast cancer and, 463
Bone hunger syndrome
  parathyroid hormone and, 464
Bone marrow
  tumor staging and, 394
Bone marrow harvesting
  marrow reinfusion and, 591
Bone Marrow Transplant Registry (ABMTR)
  stem cell transplantation results with, 195–196
Bone metastases, 34
  conclusions on treatment of, 471
  hormonal therapy and, 469
  incidence and morbidity of, 464–465
  prostaglandin inhibitors and, 469
Bone mineral density (BMD)
  exemestane and, 208
Bone pain
  conclusions on treatment of, 471
  management of, 465
  overview of, 465
Bone remodeling
  abnormal and normal, 463–464
  mechanisms of, 463–464

Bone scintigraphy
  clodronate and, 469
Bone turnover
  estrogen and, 469
Brachial plexopathy, 12
Brachytherapy
  tumor bed and, 29
Brain metastases, 34
BRCA-1
  diagnosis of, 325, 326
  distribution of mutation carriers of, 541t
  hereditary breast and ovarian cancer and, 437
BRCA-2
  diagnosis of, 325, 326
  distribution of mutation carriers of, 541t
  hereditary breast and ovarian cancer and, 437
BRCA1 carriers
  risk status and, 438
BRCA1 mutation, 533
BRCA1/2
  qualitative research in genetic testing and, 441
BRCA1/2 mutations
  risk status and, 438
Breast
  lymphatic drainage of, 5
  radiotherapy and, 5–6
Breast cancer (BC)
  aromatase inhibitors and, 532
  bone loss and, 468
  bone metastasis and, 464
  carcinoma en cuirasse and, 478f
  cell cycle inhibitors and, 362
  Complementary and Alternative Medicine (CAM) and, 428, 429, 429t, 432–433
  conclusions on treating patients with, 471
  deregulation of cell cycle in, 357–358
  diagnosis and classification, 324
  direct tumor extension to skin and, 476
  doxorubicin and, 189
  early subcutaneous metastasis and carcinoma erysipeloids and, 477f
  EGFR expression and correlation with, 273
  EIA gene and, 311
  epidermal growth factor receptor (EGFR) and, 400–401
  fibrocystic lesions and, 288
  five classes of, 325
  genetic changes and, 323
  genetic testing and, 437
  history of tamoxifen use, 541–542
  hypercalcemia and mechanism for, 464
  inherited predisposition to summary of, 442–443
  predictive testing for, 440
  proteomics in identification of molecular markers in, 331–332
  role of angiogenesis in
    clinical evidence of, 288–290
    preclinical evidence of, 287–288
  S-phase fraction (SPF) and, 398
  suprasternal subcutaneous nodule and, 477f
  tamoxifen and
    effect of, 531t
  tamoxifen risk assessment in, 541–542

  taxanes and, 119
  tumor size and, 393
  ulcerating malignant wound from, 479f
Breast cancer cells
  growth factors stimulating proliferation of, 337
  mitogens for, 347
Breast cancer gene expression profiling
  DNA microarray-based, 323–324
Breast Cancer International Research Group (BCIRG)
  factors in success of, 554–555
  trastuzumab with docetaxel and platinums and, 256
Breast Cancer International Study Group (BCISG)
  clinical trials and, 602
Breast Cancer Intervention Study (IBIS)
  chemopreventive effects of tamoxifen and, 539
Breast Cancer Management
  physician aide in therapies and, 553
Breast cancer medicine
  origins of, 551–553
Breast cancer microarray
  future of, 327–328
Breast cancer prevention strategies
  overview of, 535
Breast cancer, early stage
  Canadian *vs.* Australian guidelines for, 563t
  summary of therapies, 401–402
Breast conserving treatment (BCT), 68
  primary tumors and, 67
Breast examinations
  Basset and, 525
  efficacy of, 525
  genetic testing and, 438
Breast International Group
  Herceptin and, 120
Breast neoplasia
  proteomic analysis and, 332
Breast radiotherapy
  lumpectomy and, 49–50
Breast screening
  ages 40-49 and, 520–522
    meta-analysis of trials, 521t
    trials of, 520t
  ages 50-69 and
    trials of, 521, 521t
  ages 70 or more and, 524
  discussion on, 524–525
  overview of, 519
  studies on cost-effectiveness and, 521
Breast self-examination, 519
  efficacy of, 525
Breast tumor
  analysis of, 324
Breast-conserving surgery (BCS)
  clinical guidelines for, 562
  invasive breast cancer and, 49
  randomized trials of, 25, 26, 26t
  vascular invasion and, 414
Breast-conserving therapy
  DCiS and, 416
British Breast Cancer Group
  response criteria published for breast cancer trials and, 566
British Columbia trial, 45
  radiation in association with chemotherapy, 42
British Medical Journal
  Internet and, 514

Burst-forming units–erythroid (BFU-E), 457
Butyrophenones
 chemotherapy-induced emesis and, 492

C

c-erb-B2
 predictive factors and, 418
 prognosis and, 99
C-erb-B2 gene
 breast cancers and, 245
C-erb-B2 overexpression
 NNBC patients and, 104
C-type fibers
 bone and, 465
Caelyx (Doxil)
 Kaposi's sarcoma and, 190
 liposomes and, 190
CAF (oral cyclophosphamide, Doxorubicin and 5-fluorouracil), 448
Calcine-AM
 cancer cell markers and, 384
CALGB (Cancer and Leukemia Group B)
 9082 trial
  alkylating agents and, 137
 9344 trial
  overview of, 159
  CMF induction and, 590
  dose levels of CAF, 449
  Duke high-dose chemotherapy requiring bone marrow transplant trial
   overview of, 44, 47
  node-negative breast cancer (NNBC) and, 101
  phase 3 studies and, 175–176
  study results from, 198
  taxane and, 118–119
Camptosar
 low-dose chemotherapy and, 269
Camptothecin
 UCN-01 (7-hydroxystaurosporine) and, 361
Canada Health Act
 fairness of application under, 461
Canadian cancer and anemia guideline development group
 recommendations of, 461
Canadian Medical Association
 web sites for reference and, 563
Cancer and Leukemia Group B. See CALGB
Cancer Care Ontario Guideline
 web sites for reference and, 563
Cancer cell labeling
 nanospheres and, 385
Cancer cells
 abnormalities presented by, 357
 cytokine interleukin 1α and, 386
 fluorescent labeling of
  for detection of non-dividing cells, 385
 genetic instabilities of, 261
 IVVM detection of, 383–384
 labeling of, 384
 metastasis and, 383
 preangiogenic micrometastases and, 387–388
 quantification of fate of solitary metastatic process and, 385

secondary sites and, 387
vascular adhesive molecules and, 386
vascular circulation and, 386
Cancer gene therapy
 classification of, 312
 future directions and, 596
 gene delivery systems in, 312, 313t
 immunologic, 311
 MD Anderson Center and, 311
 nonimmunologic, 311
 nonviral delivery of, 315
 overview of, 311
 viral delivery of, 315
Cancer patient
 blood transfusions and, 458–459
Cancer Research Campaign
 tamoxifen and, 108
Cancer treatments.
 overview of past, 425–427
Cancer(s)
 anemia of, 457–458
 epoetin alpha and, 458
 genetic disease overview of, 323
 locoregional recurrence of, 31–32
Cannabinoids
 chemotherapy-induced emesis and, 493
Capecitabine
 clinical mouse study of oral, 266
 enzymatic activation of, 170
 MD Anderson study on dosing patterns of, 171
 metastatic breast cancer and, 176
 overview of, 169
 pharmacokinetic studies of, 169
 phase 2 studies, 170–171, 171t
 randomized phase 2 studies and, 172–173
 renal involvement of, 170
 standard chemotherapy vs., 172–173
 summary of single-agent, 175
 taxanes and, 159
 toxicity with, 173
Capecitabine-Taxane combination therapy, 174, 174t
 conclusions for, 175
 metastatic disease and, 174
 overall survival (OS) and, 175
Carbonic anhydrase IX, 288
Carboxylic acid moiety, 227
Carcinoma en cuirasse
 breast cancer with, 478f
 subcutaneous spread and, 477
Carcinoma erysipeloids
 cutaneous spread and, 477
 subcutaneous spread and, 477
Carcinoma in situ
 lesions and, 26
Cardiac disease
 ovarian oblation and, 137
Cardiomyopathy
 anthracyclines and, 121
 Billingham scale and, 191, 191t
 taxane and, 118
Cardiotoxicity
 anthracycline regimen and, 189
 computer tomography (CT) and, 9
 cytotoxic drugs and, 121
 irradiation and, 6, 7t, 9, 10
 liposomes and, 191
 monitoring of, 191
 risk factors for, 115
 trastuzumab and, 255

Cathepsin-D levels
 prognosis and, 99
Cationic liposome
 gene therapy delivery and, 315
CBP (cyclophosphamide, carmustine and cisplatinum)
 trials with, 195
CBT. See Contralateral breast
CCI-779
 proteins and, 362
 trials with, 362
CD-Roms
 web sites for reference and, 563
CD31
 microvessel density (MVD) and, 400
CD34
 microvessel density (MVD) and, 400
CD64
 trials with, 277
CDK enzymes
 cell cycle and, 358
CDK inhibitors, 361
 cell cycle and, 358
Cell adhesion molecules
 breast cancer cells in bone and, 470
 tumorigenesis and, 292
Cell cycle, 356f
 based strategies for treatment of cancer, 358
 chemotherapeutic agents and, 358
 DNA damage and, 356
 examples of agents targeting, 359t
 molecular pathogenesis of cancer and, 357
 overview of, 355
Cell proliferation
 cancer cells and, 387
Cell, solitary
 metastasis and, 389
Cell-kill
 dose and, 590
Cellular protein kinases, 236
Cellular senescence
 cell cycle and, 356
Central venous catheter
 complications of, 169
CES-D (Center for Epidemiological Studies-Depression)
 cancer prevention trial and, 536
Checkpoint failure
 cancer cells and, 357, 358
Chemo-endocrine therapy, 86
 endocrine therapy vs., 129
 node positive breast cancer and, 126
 NP breast cancer and, 131
 summary of evidence for, 140–141
Chemoprevention
 evaluation of agents for, 542–543
 overview of, 535–536
 selective estrogen receptor modulator (SERM) and, 535–536
Chemoprophylaxis
 lobular carcinoma in situ (LCIS) and, 30
Chemoreceptor trigger zone (CTZ)
 emetic response and, 490
Chemoresistant breast cancer
 trastuzumab and, 253
Chemotherapeutic agents
 DNA and, 358
 higher doses of, 447
Chemotherapy (CT)
 below planned dose-intensity of, 450
 bone marrow suppression and, 312

INDEX

breast cancer and, 589
combination
   premenopausal women and, 468
   ZD1839 with, 280
cosmesis and, 76
dormant cells and, 390
dose-response effect in, 590
Doxorubicin-based, 28
EGFR tyrosine kinase inhibitors and, 278t
failure rates of, 4t
first line
   Herceptin and, 254
HER-2 protein and, 161
high-dose
   markers predicting activity of, 377
highly emetogenic, 494, 495
IMC-C225 and, 276
low-dose metronomic, 263
lower-dose regimen in, 263
mild emetogenic, 494
minimally emetogenic, 496
moderately emetogenic, 495
   dexamethasone for, 495
MTD-based, 263–264
non-randomized studies and, 89
ovarian ablation and, 134–135
overview of, 46, 261
overview of high dose, 195
preoperative
   rationale for, 68t
resistance to
   intrinsic tumor cell resistance and, 451
   tamoxifen and, 370
UCN-01 (7-hydroxystaurosporine) and, 361
Chemotherapy drugs (oral)
   clinical studies for metronomic chemotherapy and, 266
Chemotherapy-induced emesis
   overview of, 489, 490
Chest wall
   cancer recurrences and, 32
   irradiation of, 15–16
   postmastectomy recurrences in, 32
   recurrence of cancer in, 4
   regional lymph nodes and, 33
Chlorambucil (oral)
   node-negative breast cancer (NNBC) and, 101
Chlorpromazine
   chemotherapy-induced emesis and, 492
Choroidal metastasis
   treatment for, 34–35
Chromosome 17q21
   HER-2/*neu* and, 245
CI-1033
   EGF receptor family and, 281
Circulation. *See* Vascular circulation
Cisplatin (ECisF), 253, 594
   anti-EGFR antibodies and, 276
   anti-HER-2 and, 252
   anti-tumor effects of, 265
   emesis and, 489
   Marsden study and, 88
   mastectomy and, 87
   neurokinin-1 (NK-1) receptor antagonists and, 492–493
   paclitaxel and, 451
   UCN-01 (7-hydroxystaurosporine) and, 361
   urinary 5-HIAA and, 491

Cisplatin based therapy
   IMC-C225 and, 277
Cisplatin-etoposide therapy
   three *vs.* four cycles of, 593
Classical CMF
   survival and, 267
Clinical decisions
   evaluation and validation methodologies for, 391–392
   recommendations using principle of evidence based medicine and, 392t
Clinical practice guidelines (CPGs)
   Australian *vs.* Canadian breast cancer, 562–563, 562t
   benefits of, 559–560
   consensus-based, 558
   conclusions for, 563
   consensus methods and, 559–560
   defined, 557
   evidence-based, 557–558
   limitations of, 560–562
   tools for, 563
Clinical trials and studies
   anti-EGFR monoclonal antibodies and, 274
   bisphosphonates in
      breast cancer and, 466–467
   blood transfusions in
      quality of life as outcome and, 459–460
   British Columbia trial, 42
   Caelyx and, 191–192
   Complementary and Alternative Medicine (CAM) and, 432–433
   conclusions from, 161
   conservative breast cancer management and, 29
   conservative treatment *vs.* mastectomy and, 25
   Danish premenopausal study, 42
   directories for clinical trials on Web and, 513–514
   docetaxel-anthracycline combinations, 157
   epoetin alpha in phase 3, 460
   epoetin alpha therapy and sited, 459–460
   gemcitabine, epirubicin, and paclitaxel (GET) therapy, 159
   genetic testing and, 441
   health-related quality of Life (HRQOL) and, 501
   IMC-C225 and, 276
   irradiation and, 20
   large tumors and, 393
   levels of evidence in evaluating, 554t
   mammary carcinoma metastasis model, 388
   melanoma cells in mouse liver and, 388
   Memorial-Sloan Kettering Cancer Centre (MSK) and, 411
   models for cost-effectiveness and, 584
   nucleic acids
      protein chip technologies and, 341
   ongoing or unreported trials in, 90
   operable breast cancer, 470
   OSI-774 (Tarceva) and, 280
   outline of individual, 46–47
   phase 2 VNB and, 179–180
   prerequisites of evidence on Web and, 513–514

   single institution reports of SLNB in, 62
   Swedish trial, 42
   trastuzumab and phase 2, 253
   tumor xenografts using metronomic chemotherapy combined with antibody and, 265f
   University of Pennsylvania and, 32
   vorozole and, 209
   ZD 1839 and, 279
Clodronate, 470
   analgesic properties of, 467
   bone metastasis, 471
   postchemotherapy bone loss and, 471
   studies of, 467
Clomel
   disease treatment and, 425
Cluster analysis
   doxorubicin therapy and, 325
   overview of, 324
   tumors and, 325
CMF (cyclophosphamide, methotrexate, 5-fluorouracil)
   amenorrheic outcome and, 133
   based therapy, 31
   dose intensity and, 447, 448
   epirubicin and, 117
   node positive disease and, 115
   premenopausal women and, 132
   vs. anthracycline-containing regimens, 118t
   vs. anthracyclines, 115, 116t, 125
CMFP
   health-related quality of Life (HRQOL) and, 501
CNBSS-2
   ages 50–59 and
      breast screening and, 523, 524
Collagenase
   E1A and, 314
   impaired survival and, 289–290
Colleoni
   clinical study of low dose chemotherapy and, 267
Colloid carcinomas, 98
Colon cancer
   capecitabine and, 169–170
Colony-stimulating factors, 590
Color doppler ultrasonography (CDUS)
   tumor blood flow and, 293
Colorectal carcinoma
   CPT-11 and, 276
   EGFR and, 282
   IMC-C225 and, 276
Comedo necrosis
   breast tumor and, 52
Complementarity determining region (CDR)
   murine monoclonal antibodies and, 249
Complete pathological response (pCR)
   primary tumor and, 91, 92
Complete response (CR) rate, 447
   definition of, 571
Complementary and Alternative Medicine (CAM)
   cancer patients usage of, 428, 429t
   conclusions on, 435–436
   disclosing usage of, 431
   general usage of, 428
   information sources for, 431–432
   overview of, 427
   patients and discussions regarding, 432–433

Complementary and Alternative Medicine (CAM) (contd.)
  reasons for usage, 430–431
  shark cartilage oil and, 431
Computed tomography (CT)
  heart and, 9
  tumor size and, 567
Confirmation of objective response
  goal of, 571
Congestive heart failure (CHF)
  combined treatment and, 121
  toxicity and, 161
  trastuzumab and, 255
Consensus methods, 558
  clinical practice guidelines (CPGs) and, 560
Contralateral breast (CBT)
  events in, 55f
Contralateral breast cancer (CLBC)
  anastrozole and, 113
  CT and, 121
  tamoxifen (TAM) and, 110
Controls (CONTR), 40
Conventional dose therapy
  clinical study with, 199
Core biopsy
  systemic therapy and, 100
Cortical erosion
  radiation therapy and, 465
  surgery and, 465
Corticosteroids
  chemotherapy-induced emesis and, 492
Cost-effectiveness analysis
  elements of, 581–582
  literature on breast cancer therapy and, 584
  methods of establishing effectiveness and, 582
  policy makers and, 584
  quality of information and, 582
Cost-effectiveness ratio
  guidelines and, 582
Coumadin
  capecitabine and, 171
Coupling
  new bone and, 463
Cox regression analysis
  nodal status and, 92
COX-2 selective inhibitors, 533
  ER-Negative breast cancer and, 533
CPT-11
  IMC-C225 and, 276
CT (cyclophosphamide and thiotepa), 195
  premenopausal women and, 136–137
CTCb (cyclophosphamide, thiotepa and carboplatinum), 199
  clinical trials and, 195
Curative chemotherapy, 592–593
Cutaneous metastases
  clarification of, 475
  fungating lesions and, 478
  internal malignancy and, 476
  metastatic disease and, 475
Cyclic AMP response element-binding protein (CREB)
  cell death regulation and, 273
Cyclin D
  cell cycle and, 357
Cyclin dependent kinase inhibitors
  ER-Negative breast cancer and, 532–533
Cyclin E, 355
  cell cycle and, 357

Cyclin-dependent kinases (cdk)
  cell cycle progression and, 355
Cyclophosphamide, 254, 447, 594
  anti-tumor effects of, 265
  chemotherapy trial and, 74
  CHOP and, 92
  clinical mouse study of oral, 266
  dose-escalation with toxicity and, 451
  higher dose intensity of, 124
  highly emetogenic agents and, 489
  low-dose chemotherapy drugs and, 267
  metastatic disease and, 124–125
  node-negative breast cancer (NNBC) and, 101
  ongoing or unreported trials using, 90
  ovarian ablation (OA) and, 113
  patient survival and, 76–77
  PNU-145156E and, 299
  preoperative vs. postoperative chemotherapy and, 86
  proliferating fraction (PF) and, 93
  randomized studies with, 89, 90
  response of human MDA-MB-231 breast tumor to contrasting, 267f
  Spanish Group for Breast Cancer and, 102
  study of, 262
  suboptimal doses of, 124
  taxane studies and, 156
  urinary 5-HIAA and, 491
Cytochrome P-450 enzymes, 203, 205
Cytochrome P-450 nicotinamide adenine dinucleotide phosphate (NADPH), 203
Cytokines
  gene therapy and, 311
Cytosine deaminase
  suicide genes and, 311–312
Cytoskeletal elements
  breast cancer cells and, 335
Cytosol assays
  predictive factors and, 417
Cytotoxic agents
  liposomes and, 194
  side effects of, 121
  taxanes and, 163
  therapies with, 97
  tumors and, 590
Cytotoxic chemotherapy, 174
  emetogenicity of, 489
  metastatic disease and, 34
  ovarian ablation and, 134–135
  serotonin and, 490
  side effects of, 489
  trastuzumab (Herceptin) combined with, 252–253
Cyveillance.com, 512

D

Dacarbazine
  highly emetogenic agents and, 489
  urinary 5-HIAA and, 491
Dana-Farber Cancer Institute
  study results from
Danish Breast Cancer Cooperative Group
  radiation trials and, 46–47
Danish premenopausal study
  analysis of recurrence in, 43t
  chemotherapy and, 42
  tamoxifen and, 43

Danish-Swedish Breast Cancer Cooperative Group trial
  CMF and, 115–116
Databases
  bioinformatics in, 328
  linked, 328
Daunorubicin hydrochloride
  liposomal preparation and, 193
DaunoXome (daunorubicin citrate liposome)
  toxicity and, 193
DC-Chol cationic liposome
  cytokines and, 319
  gene therapy delivery and, 315
DC101 antibody
  mouse study with, 266
DCIS. See Ductal carcinoma in situ
Death rate
  tamoxifen and, 530
Deaths
  adjuvant chemotherapy and, 121
Delayed emesis
  definition of, 491
  pathophysiology of, 491
  risk factors of, 491
  treatment of, 494–495
Demethylating agents
  ER-Negative breast cancer and, 533
Deoxyhemoglobin
  intrinsic imaging methods and, 294
Depression risk
  NSABP Breast Cancer Prevention (P-1) trial and, 540t
Dermal stasis
  subcutaneous spread and, 478
Detrimental Outcomes Experienced in Breast Cancer Prevention (P-1) trial
  comparison by age group on incidence rates for women in, 539f
Dexamethasone, 496
  acute emesis and, 494
DFS
  anthracycline-based trials and, 117
  goserelin acetate and, 133
Diarrhea
  capecitabine and, 171
Diet
  Complementary and Alternative Medicine (CAM) and, 431
Dietary Supplement Health and Education Act of 1994 (DSHEA)
  Complementary and Alternative Medicine (CAM) and, 432
Diethylstilbestrol (DES), 235
Differentiation
  invasive carcinomas and, 414
Dihydropyrimidine dehydrogenase (DPD)
  human cancers and, 169
Direct tumor extension to skin
  breast cancer and, 476
Discern
  patient education on Web and, 516
Disease-free survival (DFS), 34
  adjuvant therapies in NNBC trials and, 104t
  microvessel density (MVD), 400
  node-negative breast cancer (NNBC) and, 98
  postoperative adjuvant chemotherapy and, 85
  tumor grading and, 395
  tumor staging and, 394

Disease-specific measures
  outcomes measures and, 582
DNA
  chemotherapeutic agents and, 358
  end-replication problem, 357f
  ER phosphorylation and, 348
  gene therapy delivery and, 315
  Ligand binding domain (LBD) and, 236
  transcription activation and, 236
DNA binding domain (DBD), 233
DNA flow cytometry
  S-phase fraction (SPF) and, 398
DNA microarray analysis
  conclusions about, 328
  genetic testing and, 438–439
  transcriptosome and, 323
DNA probe
  HER-2 gene and, 248
DNA repair enzymes
  tumor formation and, 323
DNA-fluorescence in situ hybridization (FISH)
  detection of HER-2 gene and, 247, 248
DNA/Cationic liposome complex
  gene therapy delivery and, 315
Docetaxel, 280, 376
  adjuvant setting and, 93
  chemotherapy trial and, 74
  comparison of alternative chemotherapies and, 584
  health-related quality of Life (HRQOL) and, 503
  metastatic trials and, 119
  NSABP B-27 study and, 160, 161
  overview of, 147
  randomized studies with, 90
  regimens in combination with, 158–159
  studies with, 174, 174t
  vinorelbine and, 158
Docetaxel Adjuvant Rhone-Poulenc-GEICAM Trial
  breast cancer patients and, 102
Docetaxel monotherapy
  conclusions of studies with, 153–154
  phase 1 trials and, 151–152
  phase 2 trials and, 152, 152t
  phase 3 trials and, 152–153, 153t
Docetaxel, platinum, and trastuzumab (TCH)
  triple therapy and, 162
Docetaxel-anthracycline combinations
  advanced breast cancer and, 156–158, 156t, 157t
  clinical conclusions regarding, 158
Docetaxel-gemcitabine combination
  overview of, 159
Dolasetron
  acute emesis and, 494
Domperidone
  chemotherapy-induced emesis and, 492
Dopamine
  emetic response and, 490
Dopamine receptor antagonists
  chemotherapy-induced emesis and, 490, 492
Dormancy, cell
  390
Dose and response
  factors affecting, 447
Dose dense/intense adjuvant chemotherapy
  summary of evidence for, 141

Dose density
  overview of, 449
  summary of, 453–454
Dose escalation
  benefit of, 451
Dose intense chemotherapy, 590
  anthracyclines and, 122–124
  methodology for application of, 448
  stem cell rescue (G-CSF) and, 468
Dose intensive chemotherapy
  multicenter study of, 451
Dose of radiation
  metastatic disease and, 34
Dose-dense therapy
  multicenter study of, 451
Dose-intensity
  paradigm for, 451
  survival in breast cancer and, 590
Dosing patterns
  efficacy of, 172
  irradiation and, 18–19
Doxorubicin (Adriamycin), 199, 254, 376, 447
  anti-EGFR antibodies and, 276
  anti-tumor effects of, 265
  breast cancer therapy and, 189
  cardiotoxicity and, 10
  chemotherapy and, 28, 74
  CHOP and, 92
  cluster analysis and, 325
  conclusions of evidence for, 151
  congestive heart failure and, 157
  dose dense regimen of, 450
  dose intensity and, 122
  dose-escalation with, 451
  mechanisms of antitumor effects of, 189
  microarray-determined gene expression and, 327
  ongoing or unreported trials using, 90
  patient survival and, 76
  preoperative vs. postoperative chemotherapy and, 86
  randomized studies with, 89, 90
  Spanish Group for Breast Cancer and, 102
  stage 3 breast cancer and, 92
  toxicity and, 151
  trastuzumab and, 255
Doxorubicin monotherapy
  breast cancer and, 325
DrdU index
  proliferative activity and, 397
Droloxifene
  osteoporosis and, 227
  overview of, 227
Droperidol
  chemotherapy-induced emesis and, 492
Drug release
  increasing rate of, 190
Drug resistance
  dosing and frequency of drug application and, 263
  strategies to circumvent, 261
Drug target enzymes
  tumor formation and, 323
Drug-efflux pumps
  resistance to anthracyclines and, 375
Drugs
  expression profiling and, 326
Ductal carcinoma in situ (DCIS)
  breast conserving surgery and, 49
  comparative studies and, 30t
  diversity of gene expression and, 325

EORTC 10853 trial and, 52
  management of, 29–30, 49
  protein profile of, 334, 335f
  relapse and, 32
  tamoxifen and, 49
  tumor measurement with, 412
  vascular patterns and, 288
Duration of overall response
  measurement criteria for, 572
Dutch National Study
  lymph nodes and, 595

E
E1A
  biology of, 314
  inhibition of HER-2/neu with, 314
  tumor necrosis factor (TNF) and, 314
  tumor suppressor factor of, 315
E1A gene therapy
  final thoughts on, 319–320
  human breast cancer and
    preclinical findings of, 315–316
  metastatic breast or ovarian cancer and, 316, 316f
  radiation therapy and, 319
E1A plasmid
  toxicity and, 317
E1A/DC-Chol complex
  gene therapy delivery and, 315
  HER-2/neu overexpressing ovarian cancer cells and, 315
  M.D. Anderson study and, 317
  final thoughts on, 319
E7070
  toxicities of, 362
Early Breast Cancer Trialists' Collaborative Group. See EBCTCG
Eastern Cooperative Oncology Group (ECOG), 56
  node-negative breast cancer (NNBC) and, 101
  tamoxifen and, 109
EBCTCG (Early Breast Cancer Trialists' Collaborative Group), 10
  anthracycline regimens and, 447
  meta-analysis of, 100
  tamoxifen and, 107, 108
EBCTCG meta-analysis
  ovarian ablation vs. no hormonal maneuver and, 132
EBCTCG radiation (RT) meta-analysis 200
  reanalysis of data from, 41, 41t
EC regimen
  Belgian trial and, 117
ECOG-2196, 296
Economic analysis
  comparison of alternative chemotherapies and, 584
  overview of, 581
Edema
  compression and elevation with, 485
  malignant wounds and, 485
Edinburg and Malmo trials
  breast screening and, 520, 523
Editorial process
  Internet and, 515
Effectiveness, 582
EGF receptor blockade, 274
EGF receptors, 345
  overview of, 273, 279–281
  tumor cells and, 347

EGFR receptor (HER-1)
  activation of, 273
EGFR signaling pathway, 275f
EGFR tyrosine kinase inhibitors
  ER and, 348
  mechanisms of antitumor activity with, 278
  overview of, 277–278, 281
EIA gene
  breast cancer and, 311
  ovarian cancer and, 311
EKB-569
  EGFR and, 281
Elderly
  trastuzumab and, 255
Electronic journals in medicine, 513
Elephantiasic skin changes
  subcutaneous spread and, 477, 477f
ELISA (Enzyme-linked immunosorbent assay), 254
  early stage breast cancer and, 247
  HER-2 protein and, 246
EM-652, 230
EM-800
  overview of, 230
EMD-7200
  phase 1 studies of, 277
Emesis
  summary of, 497
Emesis pathways
  cisplatin and, 490
Emetic response
  three pathways in, 489
Emetogenic chemotherapy
  summary of recommendations for, 496–497
Emetogenicity
  classification of, 490t
Emotional stress
  overview of, 486
Empirical testing
  development strategy and, 601
Endocrine therapy
  goals of, 203
  HER-2 receptor and, 345, 350t
  neoadjuvant therapy and, 208
  node-positive (NP) disease and, 107–108
  predictive markers and, 370
  summary of evidence for, 140
Endoglin (CD105)
  breast tumors and, 293
  growth factor and, 292
Endoglin (CD105) signaling
  vascular development and, 292–293
Endometrial cancer
  raloxifene and, 543
  tamoxifen and, 111, 530
    effect of, 531t, 532
  toremifene and, 227
Endomyocardial biopsy
  cardiomyopathy and, 191
Endoscopy, 571
Endostatin
  overview of, 300
  phase 1 studies of, 300
Endothelial cells
  Trastuzumab (Herceptin) and, 251
  tumor angiogenesis and, 262
  VEGF and, 263
Endothelial toxins
  TNP-470 and, 299
Enzyme-linked immunosorbent assay.
  See ELISA

EORTC 10853 trial
  DCIS and, 51, 52
Epidermal growth factor (EGF), 337
  receptors and, 246f
Epidermal growth factor receptor (EGFR), 274
  biology and overview of, 273–274
  overview of, 400–401
Epirubicin, 190, 447
  CMF and, 117
  dose intensity and, 122
  Marsden study and, 88
  mycete vs., 193
  proliferating fraction (PF) and, 93
  study with dose intensity of, 449
Epirubicin and cyclophosphamide (EC)
  United Kingdom study with, 156
Epirubicin and Taxol (ET)
  United Kingdom study with, 156
Epirubicin hydrochloride
  mastectomy and, 87
  paclitaxel and, 154
Epithelial cells
  carcinomas and, 394
  HER-2/neu and, 245
  proteomic analysis and, 332, 333
Epithelial tumors
  epidermal growth factor receptor (EGFR) and, 273
Epoetin alpha
  blood transfusions and, 459
  conclusions on quality of life with, 461
  overview of, 458
  quality of life and, 459–560
  radiotherapy and, 460
  reticulocyte counts and, 458
Eprex
  cost of, 460–461
EQ-5D
  health-related quality of life (HRQL) and, 583
ER-Negative breast cancer
  control of, 532–533
ER-positive tumors
  endocrine therapy and, 211
ERa
  distribution in tissues of, 234, 235
  ERβ interaction with, 234
Era-923
  overview of, 230
erb-B
  subversion of growth factor receptor function and, 345
Erb-B family
  Ras-Raf-MAP-kinase pathway and, 273
  signaling route of, 273
ErbB receptors, 273
ERβ
  ERa interaction with, 234, 235
ERβ positive tumors
  tamoxifen and, 236
Erythroblasts
  biogenesis of, 457
Erythroid cells
  biogenesis of, 457
Erythropoiesis
  overview of, 457
Erythropoietin, 119, 461
  blood brain barrier and, 460
  overview of, 458
Esophageal cancer
  ABX-EGF and, 277

Estradiol, 300
  differential effects of antiestrogens and, 235, 235f
Estrogen
  alternative pathways of, 349–350
  biological effects with, 236
  breast tumor cells and, 223
  cancer microsatellites and, 113
  effects on target tissues of, 224t
  endocrine therapy and, 203
  estrogen receptor effects on, 232
  human breast tissue growth and, 345
  node-positive (NP) disease and, 107
  overview of, 232–235
  transcription of genes and, 236
Estrogen biosynthesis pathways, 204f
Estrogen positive disease, 107
Estrogen receptor (ER)-positive
  breast cancers presenting, 345
Estrogen receptor-negative cells, 335
Estrogen receptors (ERs), 223
  adjuvant tamoxifen and, 368
  antiestrogen interaction with, 235–236
  biological effects of, 236–237
  cross-communication between growth factor receptor and, 346t
  cross-talk between growth factor receptor pathways and clinical significance to, 350
  estrogen and, 232
  functional domains of, 346f
  ligand-independent activation of, 347
  molecular mechanisms of growth factor receptor signaling and, 347f
  node-negative breast cancer (NNBC) and, 100
  overview of, 345
  predictive factors and, 417–418
  relevance of knowledge of, 237–238
  structure of, 232–233, 233f, 346
  tumors and, 395
Estrogen responsive genes
  control mechanisms for, 237
Estrogen-receptor (ER) positive disease, 203
Estrogen-response pathway
  tumor and, 395
Estrogen-responsive elements (ERE), 233
  DNA and, 346
Ethical constraints
  uncertainty principle and, 577, 577t
Ethidium bromide
  cancer cells and, 386
Etidronate
  bone formation and, 466
Etoposide
  clinical mouse study of oral, 266
  mildly emetogenic agents and, 489
  non-small cell lung cancer, 262
Eukaryotic cells
  cell cycle and, 356
  essentials for growth of, 336
European Organization for Research and Treatment of Cancer (EORTC), 27
  high-dose regimen and, 448
  oral cyclophosphamide and, 295–296
  response criteria published for breast cancer trials and, 566
Evidence-based medicine (EBM)
  criteria for recommendations using principle of, 392t
  evaluating, 553–555, 557

guidelines for, 392
Internet and, 513
Ewing sarcoma
E1A and, 314
Exemestane, 204
aromatase inhibitors and, 112
conclusions of study on, 208
first-line therapy with, 208
overview of, 207
second-line therapy with, 207
Expression profiling
drugs and, 326
Expression proteomics, 336
Extensible Markup Language (XML)
Internet and, 513
Extensive intraductal component (EIC), 26
Extranodal spread
prognosis and, 413
Extraordinary Opportunities in Cancer
Communication program, 512
Extravasation
secondary sites and, 386–387
Exudate
quantity and quality of wound, 484

F

FACT-L
quality of life and, 279
Factor VIII-related antigen
microvessel density (MVD) and, 400
Fadrozole, 204
overview of, 208–209
second-line therapy and, 209
False negative (FN) rate, 61, 62
Faslodex. *See* Fulvestrant
Fatigue
anemia and, 457
docetaxel monotherapy and, 151
toxicities of paclitaxel and, 148
FDA (Food and Drug Administration)
capecitabine and, 170–171, 171*t*
Febrile neutropenia, 452
cost and duration of stay studies and, 453
filgrastim and, 450, 451
low-dose chemotherapy and, 267
taxane and, 118
toxic deaths and, 121
VNB and, 181
Femara-Tamoxifen Breast International
Group (FEMTABIG) trial, 218
Fenretinide
tamoxifen and, 114
Fever
docetaxal and, 174–175
FGF-2 (fibroblast growth factor-2), 337
overexpression of, 337, 338
protein tyrosine phosphorylation
induced by, 338*f*
proteomic analysis of, 337–338
signaling pathways for, 339*f*
transcriptionally controlled tumor
protein (TCTP) and, 339
Fibroblast growth factors
overview of, 337
tumor cells and, 287–288
Filgrastim (G-CSF), 449, 451
dose-escalated FEC and, 451
dose intensity and, 181
downside for, 453
febrile neutropenia and, 450
functions of, 452
guidelines for use of, 453

overview of, 452
side effects of, 452
summary and conclusions on,
453–454
Fine needle aspiration biopsy, 71, 93
malignant wounds and, 482
First-line therapy
formestane and, 207
FISH, 374
overall survival (OS) with Herceptin in,
255*f*
FISH-positive patients
combination therapy and, 256
Fistula
formation of, 485
management of, 485
5-flourouracil (CMF)
ongoing or unreported trials using, 90
5-fluorouracil
health-related quality of Life (HRQOL)
and, 503
mastectomy and, 87
randomized studies with, 89
5-fluorouracil (5-FU)
metastatic breast cancer and, 169
5-fluorouracil (LMF)
node-negative breast cancer (NNBC)
and, 101
5-fluorouracil (TMF)
breast cancers and, 86
5-fluorouridine-5-triphosphate (FUTP)
RNA and, 169
5-FU (EcisF)
Marsden study and, 88
Fixed-ring compounds, 238
overview of, 228–232
Flavopiridol
breast cancer and, 360
cdk inhibitors and, 361
cdks and, 358–359
cell cycle, 358
human MCF-7 breast cancer model
and, 359
overview of, 358–359
phase 1 clinical trials of, 359–360
Flk-1
tumor angiogenesis and, 298
Fluid retention
docetaxel monotherapy and, 151
Fluorescence labeling
cancer cell detection and, 385
Fluoropyrimidine carbonate
tumor site and, 169
Fluoro-2-Deoxyglucose (FDG)
Positron Emission Tomography (PET)
and, 293
Fluorouracil-based regimens
markers predicting activity of, 376
Folinic acid (MFL)
node-negative breast cancer (NNBC)
and, 101
Folkman
angiogenesis and, 287
Forkhead transcription factors
cell death regulation and, 273
Formestane, 204, 206–207
aromatase inhibitors and, 112
conclusions of studies for, 207
injectable formulation of, 206
side effects of, 206
4D5
antibody humanization and, 249
HER-2 and, 248

14-3-3 proteins
potential clinical marker, 335
14-3-3 sigma
2D-patterns and, 336, 336*f*
as biomarker, 340
Free radical damage
doxorubicin and, 189
Frei, Emil
6-mercaptopurine and methotrexate
trial and, 553
French Adjuvant Study Group (FASG)
anthracycline and, 134
French Institut Bergonie trial
cancer recurrence and, 87
Friable tumor
bleeding and, 485
Frozen section
tumor and, 413
Fulvestrant
agonist activity of, 231
anastrozole and, 232, 237
metastatic hormone responsive disease
and, 113
phase 1 study and, 231
Functional compromise
management of, 486
Functional Living Index-Cancer (FLIC)
cancer specific tool for, 583
Functional proteomics, 336
Fungating tumors
ulcerating features and, 478
Fungating wounds
clarification of, 475
malignant
breast carcinoma and, 478*f*
characteristics of, 478

G

G-CSF (granulocyte colony stimulating
factor). *See* Filgrastim
Gail model
tamoxifen and, 542
Gail Model scores
Study of Tamoxifen and Raloxifene
(STAR) trial and, 544
Galen
blood-letting and, 552
Gamma detection probe (GDP)
SLNB and, 59, 60*t*, 62
Gastric cancer
ZD1839 with, 280
Gastrointestinal tract
emesis and, 489
Gelatinases
breast cancer and, 293
tumor angiogenesis and, 293
Geldanamycin
HSP90 and, 340
Gemcitabine
IMC-C225 and, 277
Gemcitabine, epirubicin, and paclitaxel
(GET) therapy
phase 3 trial of, 159
Gemicitabine, 158–159
trials of taxane and, 158–159
Geminal bisphosphonates
pathophysiology of, 465
Gene amplification, 245
detection of, 246
HER-2/*neu* and, 396
Gene expression
issues involved in, 313*t*

Gene expression profiling
  tumors and, 324
Gene therapy. *See* Cancer gene therapy.
Gene transcripts
  DNA samples and, 323
Generic health quality of life measures
  outcomes measures and, 582
Genetic counseling
  genetic testing and, 443
Genetic discrimination
  genetic testing and, 440
Genetic disease
  cancer as, 323
Genetic testing
  costs of, 441
  detection mechanisms and, 438
  ethical considerations with, 439–441
  overview of, 437
  psychological impact of, 438
Genomics
  proteomics and, 331
GFP (green fluorescent protein)
  cancer cell markers and, 384
Glioblastomas
  EGF receptors and, 273
Glitazones
  ER-Negative breast cancer and, 532–533, 533
Glucocorticoid receptor interacting protein (GRIP), 233
Glycolipids (GMI), 190
  liposomes and, 190
Glycoproteins, 273
Glycosylation
  protein function and, 341
Goldie-Coldman hypothesis, 590
Gompertzian kinetics
  overview of, 589–590
Goserelin acetate
  CMF and, 132–133
Goss clinical study
  vorozole and, 209
Gothenburg trial
  breast screening and, 520
Gotzsche and Olsen
  breast screening and, 521
Grades of recommendation
  results and, 584
Granisetron
  acute emesis and, 494
Granulocyte colony stimulating factor. *See* G-CSF
Granulocyte-macrophage colony-stimulating factor (GM-CSF)
  gene therapy and, 311
  trials with, 197
Granulopoiesis, 452
Green fluorescent protein. *See* GFP
Growth factor receptor
  estrogen receptor signaling pathways cross-communicating with, 346*t*
Growth factor support (G-CSF or filgrastim)
  dosing schedules and, 449–450
Growth factors
  cancer microsatellites and, 113
Grupo Español de investigación en Cáncer de Mama, 117
Guideline statements
  mastectomy or lumpectomy and, 562*t*
  radiotherapy following lumpectomy (BCS) and, 562*t*

GW 5638
  overview of, 227–228

H

H22-EGF
  tumor cell growth and, 277
Hakamies-Blomqvist study
  health-related quality of Life (HRQOL) and, 503
Haloperidol
  chemotherapy-induced emesis and, 492
Hand and foot syndrome
  capecitabine and, 171, 172
Hardman study, 11
Hartmann's 1999 study
  bilateral prophylactic mastectomy cases and, 535
HDC-induced remissions
  future directions and, 596
Head and neck tumors
  CPT-11 and, 276
  EGFR and, 282
  OSI-774 (Tarceva) and, 280
Health consumer
  Internet and, 515–516
Health Insurance Plan (HIP) trial
  age related breast screening and, 520
Health on the Net, 512
Health-related quality of life (HRQOL), 583
  data analysis of, 501–502
  categories of, 502
  interpreting results of data for, 503
  limitations and challenges of interpretation of, 506
  overview of, 501
  summary of, 507
  three areas of health and, 582
Health-related quality of Life (HRQOL) assessment
  clinical significance of, 504–505
  domains in interpretation *vs.* aggregate scores and, 505–506
  predictive value of, 505
Heat shock proteins (HSPs), 232
Helix 12, 235
Hellenic Cooperative Oncology Group
  epirubicin and paclitaxel and, 156
Hematocrit
  epoietin alpha and, 458
Hematologic malignancies
  epoietin alpha and, 460
Hematologic toxicity
  G-CSF and, 162
  phase 2 VNB and, 179–180
Hematopoetic stem cells, 254
Hematopoietic autograft support
  metastatic breast cancer and, 591
  remission and, 591
Hematopoietic growth factors (HGFs), 452
  dose-intensity of chemotherapy and, 447
Hematopoietic stem cell harvest and rescue reinfusion (SCT)
  positive nodes and, 137
Hematopoietic support
  high dose chemotherapy and, 591
Hemoglobin levels
  cancer and, 457
  epoietin alpha therapy and, 458
Hepatocyte growth factor (HGF), 337

HER family
  transmembrane proteins and, 246
HER-1
  activation of, 273
HER-2, 254, 279, 281
  CMF and, 371, 372*t*
  overexpression of, 350–351
  trastuzumab and, 282
HER-2 epitope
  trastuzumab binding to, 250*f*
HER-2 MAb combination
  model with chemotherapy for, 252*f*
HER-2 overexpression, 325
  adjuvant trastuzumab and, 257
  clinicopathologic variables and, 248*t*
  prognostic factor of, 245–246
  tamoxifen and, 370
  Trastuzumab (Herceptin) and, 246, 251
HER-2 positive tumors
  taxanes and, 375
HER-2 protein
  primary breast tumors and, 161
HER-2 tyrosine kinase receptor, 347, 349
  breast cancers and, 345
  endocrine therapy and, 345
  mechanisms linking ER and, 347, 348*t*
  overview of function of, 345–346
HER-2/c-erb-B2
  prognostic factors and, 418
HER-2/*neu*, 402
  activation of, 273
  adjuvant
    anthracycline-based chemotherapy and, 373*t*
    doxorubicin and, 397
    tamoxifen and, 369*t*
  breast carcinoma and, 312
  detection techniques for, 246
  E1A inhibition of, 314
  gene amplification and, 396
  IHC and, 396–397
  MCF7 breast carcinoma cells and, 246*f*
  MD Anderson Cancer Center study with, 316
  phase 1 trail outcome in, 317
  overview of, 245–246
  pathophysiology of malignancies and, 246
  receptor epitopes and, 247
  tumor specimens and, 246
HER-2/*neu* downregulation
  breast cancer and, 318*f*
HER-4
  activation of, 273
Herbal healing
  Complementary and Alternative Medicine (CAM) and, 428, 429, 429*t*
Herbs
  resources on, 434
HercepTest
  HER-2 overexpression and, 247
Herceptin. *See* Trastuzumab (Herceptin)
Herpes simplex virus thymidine kinase (HSV-tk)
  suicide genes and, 311–312
Heterodimerization
  receptors and, 273
HIF-1α
  progression of, 288
High dose therapy with SCS
  summary of evidence for, 141

INDEX

High-dose chemotherapy
  autograft support and, 591
    remission and, 591
  comparative trials of, 200t
  conclusions and future directions for, 201
  overview of, 589
High-dose chemotherapy and stemcell transplant
  early pilot trials of, 196t
High-dose chemotherapy with autograft support
  randomized trials of
    early-stage breast cancer and, 595
    metastatic breast cancer and, 595
High-dose sequential chemotherapy, 592
Highly emetogenic chemotherapy
  serotonin receptor antagonist and, 494
Hippocrates
  oncology and, 551–552
Histological examination
  excised lymph nodes and, 412
Histological grading, 416
  ER and, 395
  invasive breast cancer and, 414
  overview of, 395
  PgR and, 395
  prognosis and, 414
  prognostic factors and, 418
Histologic type
  criteria for diagnoses of, 415
  mammary carcinoma and, 415
Histone deacetylase inhibitors
  ER-Negative breast cancer and, 533
Histopathologist
  histological grading and, 414
  role of, 411
Histopathology laboratory
  tumor measurement protocol in, 411–412
Hodgkin's disease
  curative therapy programs and, 592
Højris study, 9
Homeopathy
  Complementary and Alternative Medicine (CAM) and, 428
Homodimerization
  receptors and, 273
HON Code of Conduct
  key criteria in, 512
Hormone receptors
  prognosis of NNBC and, 98
Hormone replacement therapy (HRT)
  ER and, 396
  ER-positive tumors and, 418
  metastatic disease and, 34
  PgR and, 396
  relapses and, 122
  resistance of breast tumors to, 349
Hormone therapy, 34
  tamoxifen and, 33
Hormonotherapy. See Adjuvant hormone therapy
HRT. See Hormone replacement therapy
HSP-inhibitory complex, 233
HSP90, 339
  geldanamycin and, 340
Human anti-humanized antibodies (HAHA)
  trastuzumab and, 250
Human anti-murine antibodies (HAMA)
  tumor targets and, 248
Human antibodies against chimeric antibodies (HACAs)
  IMC-C225 and, 276

Human genome
  sequencing of, 323, 331
Human genome sequence data, 328
Hydrocortisone
  tamoxifen and, 111–112
Hydrogen peroxide
  doxorubicin and, 189
Hydroxyl radicals
  doxorubicin and, 189
Hyperbilirubinemia
  capecitabine and, 171
Hypercalcemia, 466, 467
  morbidity in breast cancer and, 463
Hyperchromatism
  histologic grading and, 414
Hyperkeratosis
  subcutaneous spread and, 478
Hyperplastic Murine breast papillomas
  angiogenesis and, 287
Hypertest
  Internet and, 511
Hypnosis
  Complementary and Alternative Medicine (CAM) and, 428
Hypophysectomy
  non-selective aromatase inhibitors and, 205
Hypoxia
  angiogenesis and, 288
Hypoxia-inducible factors (HIF-1 and HIF-2)
  overview of, 288

I

Ibandronate, 470
  studies of, 467
IBT. See Ipsilateral breast
IBTR. See Ipsilateral breast tumor recurrence
ICI 182,780
  characteristics of, 231
IDEAL 1 study
  ZD 1839 and, 279
Idoxifene
  overview of, 227
IGF-1 (insulin growth factor) receptor, 335
IHC
  measurement of proliferation by, 399
  overexpression of p53 and, 399
  proliferative activity and, 397
  steroid receptor levels and, 396
IMC-C225 (Cetuximab), 281
  antitumor effects of, 275–276
  chemotherapy augmentation and, 276
  overview of, 274
  phase 2 studies and, 276
  side effects of, 276
IMC. See Internal mammary chain
Immune effector cells
  trastuzumab and, 250
Immunohistochemistry
  node examination and, 412–413
In situ cancer
  summary data regarding radiation therapy (RT) for, 30
In situ estrogen synthesis
  letrozole and, 219
In vitro anticancer effects, 326
In vivo studies
  detection of cancer cells and, 385

In vivo treatment
  IMC-C225 and, 276
In vivo videomicroscopy. See IVVM
Induction chemotherapy, 199
  comparison trials of, 196
Infection
  docetaxel-anthracycline combinations, 158
  granulocyte production in, 452
  malodorous wounds and, 484
  overview of wounds and, 485
  taxane and, 118
Inferior disease free (DFS), 448
Infiltrating lobular carcinoma
  prognosis and, 415
Inflammatory breast cancer
  prognosis for, 70–71
  systemic chemotherapy and, 70–71
Informed consent
  genetic testing and, 442
Inhibitors
  types of, 205
Inhibitors of tyrpsine kinase
  ER-Negative breast cancer and, 532–533
Inhibitory neurotransmitter GABA
  benzodiazepines and, 493
Institute of Canada Clinical Trials Group (NCIC CTG)
  tamoxifen and, 218
Insulin-like growth factor receptor 1, 282
Integrative medicine (IM)
  overview of, 427
Intensity modulated radiation therapy (IMRT)
  tissue overdose and, 19–20
Interferon
  gene therapy and, 311
Interferon alpha treatment
  hemangiomas and, 261
Intergroup Trial 0100
  treatment related events in, 128t
Interleukin-1
  anemia and, 457
Interleukin 1α
  cancer cells and, 386
Interleukin-12
  gene therapy and, 311
Interleukin-2
  gene therapy and, 311
Interleukin-6, 293
Internal malignancies
  mechanism of dissemination of, 476
Internal mammary chain (IMC), 31
Internal mammary lymphoscintigraphy, 18, 18f
Internal mammary nodes
  breast radiotherapy and, 17
  recurrence of cancer in, 4
International Breast Cancer Intervention Study (IBIS) 1 trial
  tamoxifen
    breast cancer based on family history and, 529, 530–531
International Breast Cancer Study Group (IBCSG)
  toremifene and, 113
International Collaborative Cancer Group (ICCG)
  exemestane and, 208
  low-dose epirubicin and TAM study and, 129
  tamoxifen and, 208

International Commission of Radiation
    Units and Measurements
    (ICRU), 15
Internet
    archiving and, 513
    British Medical Journal on, 514
    Complementary and Alternative
        Medicine (CAM) and, 432
    evidence-based healthcare and, 513
    fundamental components of, 511
    graphics and, 512
    health consumer and, 515–516
    key issues with academic information
        on, 512
Internet-based medical information
    medicine of, 512
    quality of, 512
Intraarterial infusion chemotherapy
    fungating breast and, 482
Intracellular signaling
    proteomics and, 336
Intrinsic protein tyrosine kinase
    receptors and, 273
Invasive breast carcinoma
    histological features and, 414
    histological subtype, 394–395
    lymph node stage and, 412
    treatment of, 28, 28t
    tumor size and, 411
Invasive cribriform carcinoma
    prognosis and, 415
Invasive ductal carcinomas, 98
Ipsilateral breast (IBT)
    events in, 55f
Ipsilateral breast tumor recurrence
    (IBTR), 26, 27, 28
    invasive vs. non-invasive, 50f
    mastectomy and, 73
    prognostic markers for, 51–52
    radiation therapy and, 27, 28
    relapse and, 32
Ir (Iridium) implant, 15
Irradiation
    cardiac morbidity and, 6
    chest wall and, 15–16
    cosmetic results of, 12–15
    dosing schedules for, 18
    indications for, 19f
    intact breast and, 13–14, 13f
    late toxicity and, 6
    postmastectomy, 3, 31
    pulmonary function and, 8t
    supraclavicular field and, 16
    surgery adjuvant to, 3
    whole-breast and
        alternatives to, 29
Irradiation fields
    treatment techniques for, 19t
Isosulfan blue dye
    use of, 59
Istituto Nazionale Tumori
    node-negative breast cancer (NNBC)
        and, 101
Italian Breast Cancer Adjuvant Study
    Group
    oral CMF and, 134
IVVM *(In vivo* videomicroscopy)
    fate of cancer cells and, 389
    metastases and, 383, 384

J
Joint Center for Radiation Therapy
    (JCRT), 28

Journals
    Internet and, 514
Juxtamembrane epitope
    trastuzumab and, 250

K
Kaposi's sarcoma (KS)
    Caelyx (Doxil) and, 190, 191
Karkinoma
    Hippocrates and, 552
Karnofsky performance score, 196
Keoxifene. *See* Raloxifene
Ki-67 expression, 318
Ki-67 proliferation index
    IHC and, 399
Ki-S2
    proliferative activity and, 397
Kimsey study, 11, 16

L
LABC (locally advanced breast cancers)
    treatment modalities and, 67
LABC, non-inflammatory
    strategy for management of, 70f
Laminin
    microvessel density (MVD) and, 400
Lancet
    protocol summaries on Internet, 514
Laparoscopic colectomy
    tumor spillage and, 476
Laparoscopy, 571
Lasofoxifene, 230
Late-intensification HDC
    vs. conventional dose therapy, 595
LBD. *See* Ligand binding domain
LCIS. *See* Lobular carcinoma in situ
Left ventricular ejection fraction
    (LVEF)
    cardiac monitoring and, 191
    doxorubicin and, 156, 255
    trastuzmab and, 256
Leridistim, 450
    anemia and, 450
Lesions
    measurement of, 570–571
Letrozole, 204
    adjuvant setting and, 218
    aminoglutethimide *vs.*, 216t
    aromatase inhibitors and, 112
    conclusions as second-line therapy for,
        219
    efficacy rates of, 217–218, 217t
    first-line therapy with, 217t
    overview of, 215
    second-line therapy and, 215–216
Leukemia
    cytotoxic drugs and, 121
Leukopenia
    dose intensity and, 122
Leuprolide acetate, 133
Lewis lung carcinoma model, 295
LHRH (luteinizing hormone-releasing
    hormone)
    CMF and, 132–133
Ligand binding, 347–348
Ligand binding domain (LBD), 233
    DNA and, 236
Ligand TGF-α
    EGFR expression and correlation with,
        273–274
Ligand-binding essay
    tumor specimens and, 396

Ligands, 236
    HER-2/*neu* and, 245
Lind study, 11
Lingos study
    radiation pneumonitis and, 10
Lipids
    tamoxifen (TAM) and, 110
Liposomal daunorubicin
    liposomes and, 190
Liposomes
    water soluble drugs and, 190
Liver metastases, 196
    breast cancer and, 180
    phase 2 VNB and, 179–180
Lobular carcinoma in situ (LCIS)
    prognosis of, 395
    radiation therapy (RT) in, 30
Locally advanced breast cancers. *See*
    LABC
Locoregional radiation (RT)
    frequency of death in, 44t
    impact of, 43t
    studies of, 40
    survival impact of, 39
Locoregional recurrence
    irradiation and, 5
    metastasis and, 5
    potential causes of, 476
    risk factors for, 5
Locoregional relapse, 33
    summary of data regarding
        management of, 33–34
Locoregional therapy
    node-negative disease (NNBC) and, 97
Longest diameter (LD)
    tumor measurement and, 569
Low dose metronomic anti-angiogenic
    chemotherapy
    concluding remarks regarding, 268
    phase 2 summary of, 268t
Low-dose metronomic chemotherapy
    antiangiogenic drug combined with,
        264–266
Ludwig Breast Cancer Study Group
    node-negative breast cancer (NNBC)
        and, 101
Lumpectomy
    breast conservation after primary
        chemotherapy and, 75
    ductal carcinoma in situ (DCIS) and,
        29–30
    lobular carcinoma in situ (LCIS) and,
        30
    NSABP B-trial and, 49–51, 50f
    Ontarios CPG and, 562
    post chemotherapy, 77
    radiation therapy (RT) and, 25, 49–50
    relapse following, 32
    vs. lumpectomy and radiation, 28t
Lung cancer
    EGFR expression and correlation with,
        273
    hemoglobin levels and, 457–458
Lung cancer subscale (LCS)
    disease related symptoms and, 279
Lung fibrosis
    dosimetry of breast irradiation and, 14f
Lung irradiation
    intact breast and, 13–14, 13f
Lung radiation dosimetry
    pulmonary function tests and, 10
Luteinizing hormone (LH), 203
Luteinizing hormone-releasing hormone
    (LHRH), 203

INDEX

Lymph node staging
　invasive breast cancer and, 412
　mammary cancer and, 416
Lymph nodes
　supraclavicular, 5
　treatment of, 5
　tumor size and, 393
Lymphadenectomy
　melanoma and, 59
Lymphatic drainage and
　irradiation and, 16–18
Lymphatic system
　internal malignancies and, 476
Lymphedema
　surgery and, 12
Lympho-vascular invasion
　regional lymph node involvement and, 413–414
Lymphoma
　curative therapy programs and, 592
Lymphoscintigraphy (LS), 61

M

M.D. Anderson clinical studies
　ALND and, 78
　anthracycline study and, 119
　clinical trials and, 76
　dosing patterns, 172
　inflammatory breast cancer and, 71
　survival figures following chemotherapy from, 92
Macromolecular contrast agents
　tumors and, 294
Magnetic resonance imaging (MRI)
　tumor associated vasculature, 294
　tumor size and, 567
Malignant cells
　bone
　　breakdown of, 464
　　formation and, 463
　　remodeling and, 463
　　proteomic analysis and, 332
Malignant disease
　anemia and, 457
　angiogenesis and, 287
　erythropoietin and, 458
　p53 alterations and, 399
Malignant ductal cells
　osteoclast and, 466
Malignant hypercalcemia
　conclusions on treating patients with, 471
Malignant melanoma cells
　extravasation kinetics and, 387
Malignant osteopathy
　pathophysiology of, 464
Malignant wound care
　principle of benign wound care and, 482
Malignant wounds
　appearance of
　　classification of, 477t
　assessment of patients with, 479–480
　bleeding and, 485
　classification of, 476–477
　concerns common to patients with
　　symptom management for, 483t
　conclusions on, 486–487
　definition clarification of, 475
　development of, 476
　overview of, 475
　prevention of development of, 476
　quality of life and, 486–487
　staging system for, 475

Mammary carcinoma
　histological type of, 415
Mammary carcinoma cells
　tumor dormancy and, 388–389
Mammary hyperplasia
　angiogenesis and, 287
Mammary nodes
　axillary lymph nodes, 4
Mammography. See also Breast Screening
　ductal carcinoma in situ (DSIS) and, 49
　genetic testing and, 438
　node-negative disease and, 97
　physical examination combined with, 519
Manual healing
　Complementary and Alternative Medicine (CAM), 428
MAP-Kinase signaling pathway, 275f
MAPK activation, 279
Marimastat
　overview of, 296
Markers
　IVVM for cancer cells using, 384
　proliferative activity and, 397
MARKs
　phosphorylation cascade and, 273
Marsden study
　non-randomized studies and, 88–89
Mass spectrometry analysis, 337
　protein identification and, 331
Mastectomy. See also Modified radical mastectomy (MRM); Radical mastectomy
　alternatives to, 25
　inflammatory breast cancer and, 71
　non-responders to chemotherapy and, 73
　Ontarios CPG and, 562
　primary chemotherapy and, 69
　radiotherapy and, 6
　relapse and, 32
　treatments with, 3
Mastectomy rate
　preoperative chemotherapy and, 88
Mastectomy, modified radical
　recurrence and, 3, 4, 4t
Mastectomy, prophylactic
　overview of, 535
Mastectomy, radical
　failure rates of, 4t
　recurrence and, 3
Mastectomy, total
　criteria for benefit from, 51
Matrix metaloproteinase (MMP), 293
　angiogenesis and, 287
Maximum tolerated dose (MTD), 262, 263
　chemotherapeutic agents and, 447
MCF-7 tumors
　tamoxifen and, 295
McGuire and Clark
　criteria for adjuvant therapy in node-negative breast cancer, 393–394
MD Anderson Cancer Center
　gene therapy study and, 311
　metastatic breast or ovarian cancer and, 316
　phase 1 trial outcome in, 317
MDA-MB-231
　cyclophosphamide (CTX) and, 267f
MDS Laboratories
　genetic testing and, 439
Mean microvessel density (MVD)
　metastases and, 288

Median overall survival
　anastrozole and, 212
Medical practice
　Internet access relating to, 515
Medicine
　evidence based, 292
　Internet-based medical information and, 512
Medline abstracts
　Internet and, 514
Medscape.com, 516
Medullary carcinomas, 98
　prognosis of, 395, 415
Megestrol acetate, 215, 216
　aromatase inhibitors vs., 211t
MEK kinases
　proteins and, 335
Melanoma cells
　early metastases and, 388
　tumor dormancy and, 388–389
Melphalan, 447
　vs. VNB
Memorial Visual Analog Scale
　pain intensity and, 171
Menopause
　adjuvant tamoxifen and, 111
　bone resorption and, 468
　cytotoxic drugs, 121
Meta-analysis
　effects of treatments and, 576
　Oxford, 40
　tested interventions and, 39
Meta-analysis, small scale
　biases and random errors in, 578
Metastases
　angiogenesis and, 287
　bone, 34
　chemotherapy and, 589
　clinical implications of experimental studies on, 389–390
　extravasation and, 387
　growth in secondary sites and, 387
　In vivo studies
　　detection of cancer cells and, 385
　lymph nodes and, 5, 6
　tumors and, 393
　overview of, 383
　prognostic factors of, 391
　tumors and, 85
Metastases, systemic
　chest wall and, 33
Metastatic breast cancer (MBC)
　5-fluorouracil (5-FU) and, 169
　aminoglutethimide and, 206
　Caelyx trial and, 191
　capecitabine and, 171
　docetaxel-anthracycline combinations, 158t
　doxorubicin and, 189
　hematopoietic autograft support and, 591
　HER-2 overexpression and, 247
　prognostic factors for, 402
　single-arm trials of high-dose chemotherapy
　　autograft support and, 593
　skeletal complications
　　morbidity secondary to, 463
　taxanes and, 124–125
　toremifene and, 227
　trastuzumab (Herceptin) and, 119–122
　VNB and, 185–186
Metastatic disease
　capecitabine and taxane studies and, 174
　dose intense regimen and, 453

Metastatic disease (*contd.*)
　filgrastim and, 451
　radiation therapy and, 34
　response rates and, 449
　sites of, 34
　symptomatic, 34
Metastatic lymph nodes
　prognosis and, 412
Metastatic process
　tools for studying, 383, 384*f*
Methotrexate (MTX), 257
　clinical mouse study of oral, 266
　mouse study with oral, 266
　node-negative breast cancer (NNBC) and, 101
　ongoing or unreported trials using, 90
　Spanish Group for Breast Cancer and, 102
Methotrexate plus 5 fluorouracil
　trials with, 153
Methotrexate sodium
　breast cancers and, 86
　node-negative breast cancer (NNBC) and, 101
Methoxypolyethylene glycol (MPEG), 190
　liposomes and, 190
Metoclopramide
　chemotherapy-induced emesis and, 492
Metronomic antiangiogenic chemotherapy
　origins of concept of, 262–264
Metronomic chemotherapy, 261
Metronomic chemotherapy combined with antibody
　clinical studies of, 265*f*
Metronomic dosing
　neuroblastoma xenografts and, 264
Metronomic low-dose vinblastine
　anti-tumor efficacy and toxicity in, 264*f*
Metronomic therapy, 295
Michelangelo Cooperative Group
　stem cell transplant and, 139
Microarray, 323
　breast cancer, 327
　classification of breast cancers with, 324–325
　DNA, 327
　overview of, 323
Microarray analysis
　disease prognosis and, 325–326
　drug development and, 325
　therapeutic benefit from, 325
　tumor clonality and, 325
Microarray data
　biomolecular Interaction Data-base (BIND) and, 328
　Cancer Genome Anatomy Project (CGAP) and, 328
Microarray experiments
　tumor handling and sampling in, 324
Microcalcifications, 77
Micrometastases
　angiogenic tumors and, 388
　cancer cells and, 388
　definition of, 413
　primary tumor and, 85
Microspheres
　cancer cell detection and, 385
Microtubule function
　taxanes and, 147
Microtubule-associated parameters (MTAP)
　taxane treatment and, 376

Microvessel density (MVD), 288, 289
　angiogenesis and, 400
　color doppler ultrasonography (CDUS) and, 293
　prognostic information and, 400
Milan adjuvant trial
　doxorubicin and, 449
Milan group studies, 88, 91
Mitogen activated protein-kinases (MAPK), 348
　gene expression and, 336–337
　receptors and, 275
Mitogenic signaling
　receptors and, 273
　trastuzumab (Herceptin) and, 250
Mitomycin-C
　trials using, 153
Mitosin
　proliferative activity and, 397
Mitotic count
　histological grading and, 414
Mitotic index (MI)
　overview of, 398
　proliferative activity and, 397
Mitoxantrone
　cardiotoxicity and, 190
　mildly emetogenic agents and, 489
Mixed lytic and sclerotic bone metastases
　breast cancer and, 464
MMP inhibitor
　tumor regrowth and, 296
Moderate dose escalation, 590
　random assignment trials and, 590
Modified radical mastectomy (MRM), 11
　chemotherapy and, 73
　recurrence and, 3, 4, 4*t*
Molecular genetics
　genetic testing for cancer and, 437
Molecular markers
　prognostic factors and, 418
Molecular pathogenesis
　breast cancer and, 551
Molecular therapies
　appropriate stage of disease and, 602
Molecule Bcl-2
　response to tamoxifen and, 370
Monoclonal antibodies
　EGFR and, 274
　p53 and, 399
　predictive factors and, 417
Morbidity
　osteolysis and, 463
MORE trial
　estrogen receptor modulators and, 546
MR parameters
　vs. angiogenesis in breast cancer, 294*t*
mRNA
　gene therapy and, 312
MTD-based therapy, 262
Mucinous carcinomas
　prognosis and, 395, 415
Mucositis
　Caelyx and, 192
　docetaxel monotherapy and, 151
　low-dose chemotherapy and, 267
Multi-cycle high-dose chemotherapy (MCHDC), 592–593
　Memorial Sloan-Ketting Cancer Center and, 594
Multiagent regimens
　vinorelbine and, 181–185, 182*t*–184*t*

Multiple Outcome of Raloxifene Evaluation (MORE)
　breast cancer incidence and, 113
Multiple *vs.* single high-dose chemotherapy
　future directions and, 596
Multivariate analysis
　prognostic factors and, 411
　prognostic relevance in, 416
　vascular invasion and, 414
Murine monoclonal antibodies
　tumor targets and, 248
Musculoskeletal disorders
　tamoxifen and, 214
Myalgias
　docetaxel and, 174–175
Myeloablative chemotherapy, 254
Myeloma cells
　apoptosis and, 470
Myelosuppression (neutropenia)
　cancer patients and, 261
　docetaxel monotherapy and, 151
　docetaxel-Anthracycline combinations, 157
　toxicities of paclitaxel and, 148
Myelotoxicity
　chemotherapy agents and, 447
Myocardial cells
　doxorubicin and, 189
Myocardium
　HER-2/*neu* and, 245

N
Nafoxidene, 230
Nanospheres
　cancer cell labeling, 385
Napthalenes
　overview of, 230
National Breast Cancer Prevention Trial
　BRCA2 carriers
　prophylactic tamoxifen and, 438
National Cancer Institute (NCI)
　flavopiridol and, 359–360
　response criteria published for breast cancer trials and, 566
National Cancer Institute of Canada (NCIC), 27
　clinical trials and, 20
National Cancer Institute of Canada Clinical Trials Group
　study results from, 198
National Cancer Institute of Milan
　chemotherapy regimens and, 72
National Center for Complementary and Alternative Medicine (NCCAM), 435
National Surgical Adjuvant Breast and Bowel Project. *See* NSABP
Nausea
　cytotoxic chemotherapy and, 489
NCIC-CTG trial
　CEF regimen and, 117
Necrotizing inflammation of colon
　low-dose chemotherapy and, 267
Negligible biases
　moderate differences and, 575
Neoadjuvant docetaxel with doxorubicin, 450
Neoadjuvant therapy
　anastrozole and, 214
　letrozole and, 218–219
　VNB-containing regimens and, 185

INDEX

Nerve growth factor (NGF), 337
Neulasta, 453
Neuregulins/heregulins
  HER-2/*neu* and, 245
Neuroblastoma xenografts
  metronomic chemotherapy and antiangiogenic drug with, 264
Neurokinin-1 (NK-1) receptor
  emesis and, 491
Neurokinin-1 (NK-1) receptor antagonists
  chemotherapy-induced emesis an, 492–493
Neuropathy
  toxicities of paclitaxel and, 148
Neurotransmitters
  emetic response and, 490
Neutropenia (myelosuppression), 452
  cost and duration of stay studies and, 453
  CSFs following marrow reinfusion and, 591
  docetaxel-Anthracycline combinations, 157
  prevention of, 452
  taxane and, 118
  toxicities of paclitaxel and, 148
Neutropenic fever, 452
Neutrophils
  G-CSF (granulocyte colony stimulating factor), 452
NGF (nerve growth factor), 337
Nichol's sanatorium
  disease treatment and, 426
NIH 3T3 cells, 337
NIH Consensus Conference on Adjuvant Therapy of Breast Cancer
  adjuvant therapy and, 97
NNBC. *See* Node-negative breast cancer
No special type (NST)
  prognosis and, 415
Nodal status
  breast cancer and, 401
  risk of recurrence and, 107
Node-negative breast cancer (NNBC)
  adjuvant hormone therapy (hormonotherapy) and, 100
  chemotherapy *vs.* no treatment and, 101–102
  crucial points in deciding treatment for, 97–98
  definition of risk categories for, 99t
  disease-free survival and, 98
  high mitotic count and, 398
  incidence of, 97
  prognostic factors in determination of recurrence risk in, 98–100
  summary of, 103–104
  systemic adjuvant therapy in, 100
Node-positive (NP) breast cancer
  adjuvant RCTs in postmenopausal women with, 127t
  adjuvant treatments for, 107–108
  SCT and, 138t–139t
Node-positive tumors
  postmenopausal women and, 127
Non-adherent dressings, 484
Non-Hodgkin's lymphoma
  flavopiridol and, 360
Non-invasive breast cancer
  management changes in, 49
Non-platinum based chemotherapy
  anemic cancer patients and, 460
Non-randomized study
  bias and, 575

Non-selective aromatase inhibitors
  ablative procedures and, 205
Non-small cell lung cancer
  PS-341 and, 361–362
Non-steroidal aromatase inhibitors, 208–209
Noninflammatory LABC, 68–72
Nonosseous metastases
  rate of, 471
Nonviral vectors
  gene therapy delivery through, 313
Normocalcemea, 467
Northern analysis, RT-PCR
  HER-2 protein and, 246
Northern blotting
  gene expression and, 337
Not otherwise specified (NOS)
  prognosis and, 415
Nottingham combined histological grade (NCHG)
  tumors and, 395
Nottingham prognostic index (NPI)
  overall survival by, 417f
  overview of, 416
Novel anti-estrogens
  endometrium and, 113
NSABP (National Surgical Adjuvant Breast and Bowel Project)
  characteristics of study population, 537t
  chemotherapy *vs.* post-operative therapy and, 73, 74
  data monitoring committee (DMC) and, 536
  design of cancer prevention trial and, 536–537
  doxorubicin and cyclophosphamide (AC) and, 175
  sentinel node resection and, 61
  study population description, 537
  study schema for protocol of, 74f
  summary of finding and disease outcomes from, 537–538, 538t
  tamoxifen and, 109
NSABP B-13
  node-negative breast cancer (NNBC) and, 101
NSABP B-17 trial, 49–50
NSABP B-18 study, 91
  lumpectomy and, 88
  preoperative *vs.* postoperative chemotherapy and, 86
  tumor response and, 89
NSABP B-20 protocol
  combination chemotherapy with tamoxifen and, 103
NSABP B-24 trial
  tamoxifen and, 53–56, 54f
NSABP B-27 study
  docetaxel and, 160
NSABP B-28 trial
  overview of, 159
NSABP B-32 protocol, 63
NSABP B-trial
  lumpectomy and, 49–51
  radiotherapy of breast and, 49–51
NSABP Breast Cancer Prevention (P-1) trial
  Commutative Incidence of Invasive Breast Cancer among Women in, 538f
  depression risk and, 540t
  quality of life endpoints and, 540

NU 6102
  cdk and, 361
Nuclear pleomorphism
  histological grading and, 414
Nucleus tractus solitarius (NTS)
  emetic response and, 490

O

O water
  tracers and, 293
  uptake in tumors and, 294
OBCSG trial II
  CMFp *vs.* surgical oophorectomy and, 135
Observational data
  effectiveness and, 582
  randomized clinical trials and, 582
Observed (O), 40
Occult
  definition of, 413
Octreotide
  growth factor and, 113
Odor
  management of, 484
Omni, 512
Oncogenes
  tumor cell and, 551
  tumor formation and, 323
Oncologists, 4
Oncology
  malignant wounds and, 482
  reference web sites for, 563
Ondansetron
  acute emesis and, 494
185kD surface membrane, 245
Oophorectomy
  skeletal effects of, 458
Operable breast cancer
  conclusions on treatment of, 471
Oral squamous cancer
  PKI-166 and, 280–281
Orthodox cancer therapies
  complementary and Alternative Medicine (CAM) and, 432
OS (overall survival)
  SCT and, 139
OSI-774 (Tarceva), 279
  overview of, 280
Oslo trial of postoperative irradiation, 9
Osteoblasts, 463, 465
Osteoclast apoptosis
  TGF-β, 465
Osteoclast function
  mechanisms of, 465
Osteoclasts, 463
Osteolysis
  morbidity and, 463
  prostaglandin inhibitors and, 469
Osteolytic bone metastases
  breast cancer and, 464
Osteoporosis (OP)
  droloxifene and, 227
  estrogen levels and, 223
  Multiple Outcome of Raloxifene Evaluation (MORE) and, 113
  premature menopause and, 137
  raloxifene and, 228
  supplemental calcium with biphosphonates and, 137
  tamoxifen (TAM) and, 110
Osteosclerotic bone metastases
  breast cancer and, 464

Outcome
  assessment of moderate differences in, 575
Outcome measures
  different types of, 582
Outcome research
  data analyses and, 577–578
Ovarian ablation (OA), 126
  adjuvant CMF and, 134
  chemotherapy and, 134–135
  comparative study with, 136t
  cyclophosphamide and, 113
  no adjuvant therapy vs., 131–132
  node-positive (NP) disease and, 107
  risks associated with, 137
  summary of evidence for, 140
  TAM versus chemotherapy and, 132–134
  tamoxifen and, 100–101
  techniques for achieving, 137
Ovarian carcinoma, 268
  Caelyx (Doxil) and, 190
  EGFR and, 282
  EIA gene and, 311
  epoietin and, 459
  genetic testing and, 437
  OSI-774 (Tarceva) and, 280
Overall survival (OS), 34, 448
  anthracycline vs. CMF regimens and, 447
  anthracycline-based trials and, 117
  capecitabine-Taxane combination therapy and, 175
  HER-2/neu and, 245
  letrozole and, 216, 218
  NNBC and, 98
  Nottingham prognostic index (NPI) and, 417f
  polychemotherapy vs. no treatment and, 447
  progesterone receptor (PgR) and, 396
  tamoxifen and, 218
  trastuzumab-vinorelbine combination and, 185
  vascular density and, 400
Oxford meta-analysis
  breast cancer treatment and, 367
Oxford study
  OA and, 134
  overview of, 40

P

P-13 kinase
  proteins and, 335
P13K/AKT signaling pathway, 275f
p185HER-2 tyrosine kinase
  trastuzumab (Herceptin) and, 250
p53 status
  prognosis and, 99
p53 tumor suppressor gene
  overview of, 399–400
Paclitaxel, 119, 199, 295, 450
  anti-EGFR antibodies and, 276
  anti-tumor effects of, 265
  breast cancer and, 360
  comparison of alternative chemotherapies and, 584
  metastatic disease and, 124–125
  non-randomized studies and, 89
  overview of, 147
  pharmacokinetics of, 147–148
  phase 2 trials, 172, 173
    in advanced breast cancer with, 148t
    with prolonged infusion times, 149t
  phase 3 trials, 150t
    with chemotherapy vs., 150–151
  premedication with, 148
  randomized trials, 149t
  regimens in combination with, 158–159
Paclitaxel IV
  health-related quality of life (HRQOL) and, 501
Paclitaxel monotherapy
  phase 1 trials and, 148
  phase 2 trials and, 148–150
Paclitaxel vinorelbine regimen
  toxicities of, 158
Paclitaxel-Anthracycline combinations
  efficacy of, 154, 155t
  randomized trials as first-line therapy of, 156t
Pain
  adherent dressings and, 483
  management of, 483–484
Palliative radiation
  goals of, 34
Palmar plantar erythrodysthesia
  Caelyx and, 192
Pamidronate
  malignant hypercalcemia and, 471
  serum calcium and, 466
  skeletal complications and, 469
  studies of, 467
PAN-HER (irreversible) tyrosine kinase inhibitors
  overview of, 281
PAN-HER (reversible) tyrosine kinase inhibitors
  overview of, 281
Pancreatic carcinoma
  gemcitabine and, 277
Papillary carcinomas, 98
Papillomatosis
  subcutaneous spread and, 478
Parathormone related peptide (PTHrP)
  carcinoma cells and, 464
Partial response (PR)
  defined as, 571
  dose rate and, 448
Pathologic complete response (pCR), 214
Pathologic partial response (pPR), 214
Pathological node-negative (pN-)
  breast cancer risk and, 59
Patient confidentiality
  genetic testing and, 440
Patient management
  assessment of malignant wounds and, 479, 482
PBT-1
  overall survival and toxicity studies and, 196
PC3 prostate tumors
  cyclophosphamide in mice and, 265
PCR-based techniques
  HER-2 protein and, 246
PEGASE 3
  study results from, 198
Pegfilgrastim, 453
  summary and conclusions on, 453–454
Pegylated liposomal doxorubicin
  cardiotoxicity and, 191
Peptide growth factors
  human breast tissue growth and, 345
Peri-wound skin, 484
Peripheral aromatase inhibitors (AIs)
  adjuvant tamoxifen and, 111
Peripheral blood progenitor autografting, 592
Peripheral blood progenitor cell (PBPC) transplantation
  stage 2 and 3 patients and, 137–139
Peripheral nervous system
  substance P and, 491
Peripheral neuropathy
  paclitaxel vinorelbine regimen and, 158
PgR. See Progesterone receptor
Pharynx
  vomiting center and, 490
Phase 2 trials
  goal of, 565
Phenothiazines
  chemotherapy-induced emesis and, 492
Phenytoin
  capecitabine and, 171
Pheochromocytoma PC12 cells
  2DE and, 337
Philadelphia Bone Marrow Transplant Group (PBT)
  chemotherapy-untreated breast cancer and, 196
Phosphatidylinositol 3-kinase (PI3K)
  EGF receptors and, 273
Phosphoinositide 3-kinase signaling
  resistance in human glioblastoma cells and, 282
Phosphorylation
  protein function and, 341
Phosphorylation cascade
  MAPKs and, 273
Phosphorylation of tyrosine 537, 233
Phosphorylation sites, 233f
Photodynamic therapy
  skin metastases and, 482
Physical
  health-related quality of life (HRQL) and, 582
PKI-166
  overview of, 280–281
Placebo effect
  bisphosphonates and, 467
Plasminogen activator
  E1A and, 314
Plasminogen activator inhibitor-1
  impaired survival and, 289–290
Plasminogen activator/inhibitor type 1 (PAI-1)
  node-negative breast cancer (NNBC) and, 101, 102
Platelet-derived growth factor (PDGF), 337
Pneumonitis
  radiation and, 10, 11
PNU-145156E
  antitumor activity and, 299
Polyacrylamide gel electrophoresis, 335
Polychemotherapy
  deaths and, 120–121
  summary of evidence for, 140
  systematic overview of, 114
Positron Emission Tomography (PET)
  Fluoro-2-Deoxyglucose (FDG) and, 293
Post-mastectomy
  radiation and, 30–31
Postchemotherapy bone loss
  conclusions on treatment of, 471
Postmastectomy irradiation
  role of, 5
  target for, 5

Postmenopausal women
  anastrozole and, 210
  anthracyclines and, 118
  aromatase inhibitors and, 205
  ATAC (Arimidex, Tamoxifen, Alone, or in Combination) Trialists' Group trial and, 112–113
  ER positive tumors and, 127
  low risk tumors and, 127
  tamoxifen and, 44
  vorozole and, 209
Postoperative adjuvant chemotherapy
  early breast cancer management and, 85
Postoperative adjuvant systemic therapy
  systemic disease and, 59
Preangiogenic micrometastases
  cancer cells and, 387–388
Predictive factors
  identification of, 367–368
  metastases and, 391
  overview of, 367, 417–418
  summary of recommendations for breast cancer, 401t
Predictive markers
  adjuvant hormonal therapy and, 368–370
  conclusions on, 377–378
Predictive value
  epidermal growth factor receptor (EGFR) and, 400–401
Prednisolone (CVAP)
  randomized studies with, 90
Prednisone, 129
  node-negative breast cancer (NNBC) and, 101
Preference-based measures
  outcomes measures and, 582
Premenopausal NP breast cancer, 136t
Premenopausal women
  chemotherapy and, 130–131
  estrogen production mechanism in, 203
  RCTs of, 133t
  relapse risk and, 121–122
  tamoxifen and, 108, 130–131
Preoperative chemotherapy
  aims of, 85
  biological predictive factors, 92
  clinical predictive factors in, 91
  effect of, 87, 87t
  pathological predictive factors, 91
  predictive factors for, 90–93
  primary operable breast cancer and summary of benefits for, 93–94
  rationale for, 68t
  survival effect of, 85–86, 86t
  tumor response and, 88–90
Primary breast cancer
  HER-2 and, 161
  prognostic factors of, 391
Primary chemotherapy
  breast conservation and, 72–75
  primary tumor response and, 67
  role of mastectomy after, 68
  schematic for alternative hypotheses during, 74f, 76
  summary of surgical issues after, 80t
  surgical issues related to, 67–68
Primary high-dose chemotherapy
  late-intensification of, 591–592
  overview of, 591
Primary physician
  Complementary and Alternative Medicine (CAM) and, 431

Primary skin carcinomas
  malignant wounds and, 476
Primary tumor
  micrometastases and, 85
  preoperative chemotherapy and, 9
Primary tumor vascularization
  surgery and, 289
Primary tumors
  relapse and, 32
Princess Margaret Hospital data, 10
Pro-angiogenic growth factor receptor antagonists
  overview of, 298–299
Prochlorperazine
  chemotherapy-induced emesis an, 492
Progelatinase-B
  tumor growth and, 288
Progenitors
  leukapheresis and, 591
Progesterone (PgR)
  growth factors and, 349
  node-positive (NP) disease and, 107
Progesterone receptor (PgR), 369, 370
  tumors and, 395
Progesterone-receptor (PgR) positive tumors, 203
  endocrine therapy and, 211
Prognosis
  histological grade and, 414
Prognostic factors
  axillary lymph nodes and, 392–393
  breast cancer and, 411
  conclusions on, 418
  metastasis and, 391
  morphological features and, 415
  overview of, 367
  summary of recommendations for breast cancer, 401t
  tumor size and, 411
  vs. predictive factor, 368f
Prognostic groups
  histological type and, 415
Prognostic value
  epidermal growth factor receptor (EGFR) and, 400–401
Progression-free survival
  paclitaxel and, 151
Proliferating cell nuclear antigen (PCNA)
  proliferative activity and, 397
Proliferating fraction (PF)
  tumor cells and, 93
Proliferation (Ki67 nuclear antigen)
  chemotherapy and, 93
Proliferation index
  overview of, 397–398, 399
Prophylactic antiemetic therapy
  chemotherapy and, 489
Prophylactic mastectomy
  overview of, 535
  summary of, 545
Prostaglandin E
  carcinoma cells and, 464
Prostaglandin inhibitors
  osteolysis and, 469
Prostate cancer
  osteoblastic metastases and, 464
  ZD1839 with, 280
Protease cathepsin D
  breast cancer and, 332
Protease inhibitors
  overview of, 296
Protein analysis
  gene expression and, 327

Protein chip technologies
  nucleic acids and, 341
Protein phosphorylation, 339
Protein tyrosine phosphorylation
  FGF-2 and, 338f
Proteins
  strategies for identification of, 334, 334f
Proteolysis
  prognosis and, 99
Proteomic analysis
  goals for, 331
  illustration of, 332f
  methodologies for, 331
  molecular markers identified by, 333f
  perspectives for, 340–342
Proteomic data
  molecular markers and, 340–341
  therapeutic targets and, 340–341
Proteomics
  growth-signaling pathways and, 336–337
  overview of, 331
Proteosome inhibitors
  cell cycle and, 358
PS-341
  overview of, 361–362
  proteosome inhibitor of, 361
Psychological
  health-related quality of life (HRQL) and, 582
PTEN function, 362
PTHrP
  production of, 469
Pulmonary embolism
  hormone replacement therapy and, 530
Pulmonary function
  irradiation and, 8t
  trastuzumab and, 253
Pulmonary function tests
  toxicity and, 10, 11
Pulmonary toxicity, 10

Q
Q10
  Complementary and Alternative Medicine (CAM) and, 431
QLQ-B23
  QLQ-C30 and supplement of, 583
QLQ-C30
  breast cancer specificity of, 583
  overview of, 583
  QLQ-B23 as supplement to, 583
Qualitative methods, 558
Quality adjusted life year (QALY) index
  overview of, 582–583
Quality of life
  conclusions regarding epoetin alpha and, 461
  criteria for, 197
  management of functional compromise and, 485
Quanterra
  alternative therapies and, 434–435
Quantitative methods, 558

R
Radiation, 45
  breast cancer and, 25–35
  breast cancer mortality and, 45
  breast-conservation surgery and, 27

Radiation (contd.)
　clodronate (oral) and, 467
　dose dense therapy and, 451
　E1A gene therapy and, 319
　EGFR tyrosine kinase inhibitors and, 278t
　IBTR and, 75
　IMC-C225 and, 276, 277
　　carcinoma of oropharynx and, 277
　impact of, 43t
　Ontarios CPG and, 562
　p53 and
　palliation of metastatic disease and, 34
　pneumonitis and, 10, 11
　post-mastectomy and, 30–31
　surgery and, 25–27
　systemic recurrences and, 45
　toxicity and, 6
　trials and, 45, 46
Radiation pneumonitis, 10
　Lind study and, 11–12
Radiation target volumes, 5
Radiation therapy (RT)
　lumpectomy and, 25
　patient groups and contraindications for, 27–28
Radiation Therapy Oncology Group (RTOG), 56
　clinical trial of, 29
Radiation toxicity
　avoidance of, 12–13
Radiation, adjuvant
　breast-conserving surgery and, 5–6
Radical mastectomy
　recurrence and, 3
Radiocolloid administration
　alternative routes of, 62–63
Radiocolloid diffusion zone
　intersurgeon variation and, 61
Radiosurgery
　brain irradiation and, 34
Radiotherapy, 39–40, 49
　breast cancer, 3
　comedo necrosis and, 52
　mastectomy, 6
　NSABP B-trial, 49–51, 50f
Raloxifene
　endometrium and, 113
　Multiple Outcomes of Raloxifene Evaluation (MORE) trial and, 543
　overview of, 228, 543
　total cholesterol and, 543
Random errors
　data analysis and, 576, 578
Randomized evidence
　data analysis and, 577
　past and next 50 years and, 578–579
Randomized trials, 575
　data analysis and, 576–577
Rapamycin
　mechanism of action with, 362
　signal transduction pathway of, 362f
Ras-Raf-MAP-kinase pathway
　Erb-B family and, 273
Razoxane
　renal cell carcinoma and, 292
Reagents
　angiogenesis and, 400
Receptor activation
　mechanisms of, 274f
Receptor enhanced chemosensitivity (REC)
　antibody with drug interaction studies and, 252

Receptor tyrosinase inhibitors, 274
Receptor-enhanced chemosensitivity
　trastuzumab (Herceptin) combined with, 252–253
Recurrence
　lympho-vascular invasion and, 414
Regional lymph nodes
　breast cancer prognosis and, 59
　chest wall and, 33
　treatment for recurrence in, 33
Regional nodal irradiation
　role of, 27
Rehydration
　hypercalcemia and, 466
Relapse-free survival rates, 411
Relative dose intensity (RDI)
　polychemotherapy regimens and, 448
Remission
　single cycle high-dose chemotherapy and, 594
Renal cell carcinoma
　EGFR and, 282
　razoxane and, 292
Renal dysfunction
　capecitabine and, 170
RERG
　breast tumorigenesis and, 327
Response Criteria in Solid Tumors (RECIST)
　assessing and reporting response rates and, 565
　classification of tumors and, 568
　criteria of, 568
Response rate
　analysis of, 571
Reticuloenclothelial system (RES)
　liposome breakdown and, 190
Retinoic acid
　cell proliferation and, 114
Retrospective analyses
　clinical trial data on measurements and, 569
Retroviral vectors
　gene therapy delivery and, 312
Reverse transcriptase polymerase chain reaction (RT-PCR)
　node examination and, 413
Ribozymes, 298
Risk Assessment Forms (RAF)
　Study of Tamoxifen and Raloxifene (STAR) trial and, 544
Risk reduction therapy
　tamoxifen and, 541
Rituximab, 596
RNA
　5′fluorouridine-5′-triphosphate (FUTP) and, 169
　microarray experiments and, 324
Rothwill study, 10
ROW trial, 232
Royal Marsden study
　survival and Milan study, 9192
RU 58668
　agonist activity of, 231
Rutqvist study, 9

S
S-phase fraction (SPF)
　DNA flow cytometry and, 398
　proliferative activity and, 397
San Antonio Breast Cancer Symposium
　anastrozole study and, 214

Sanatoriums
　disease treatment and, 426
Sarcoplasmic reticulum
　doxorubicin and, 189
Scandinavian Breast Cancer Study Group (SBG)
　Node Positive breast cancer and, 139
Scandinavian study
　single high dose vs. individually tailored doses of FEC, 595
Scarff-Bloom-Richardson (SBR) grading system, 395
Schulz Malignant Wound Assessment Tool, 480t
　items relating to malignant wound concerns and, 481t
Scirrhous dermal reactions
　subcutaneous spread and, 477
SCT (stem cell transplant)
　chemotherapy and, 261
　conclusions and future directions for, 201
　dose escalation and, 451–452
　high dose chemotherapy combined with, 195
　high-dose cyclophosphamide and, 451
　mortality and, 137
　Scandinavian Breast Cancer Study Group (SBG) and, 139
　trials with, 137, 138t–139t
SDS-PAGE (sodium dodecyl sulfate-polyacrylamide gel electrophoresis)
　tyrosine phosphorylation and, 337
Second-line therapy
　formestane and, 207
Secondary prophylaxis, 452
Seed and soil theories, 464
Selective estrogen receptor down-regulators, 223
Selective estrogen receptor modifiers (SERMs)
　adjuvant tamoxifen and, 111
　chemoprevention therapies and, 535–536
Selective inhibitor of cyclooxygenase-2 (COX-2), 267
Sentinel lymph node (SLN) hypothesis
　melanoma patients and, 59
Sentinel lymph node biopsy (SLNB)
　accuracy of, 60
　multicenter registry studies of, 60t
　single institution experience with, 60t
　surgeons and, 59
　tumor staging and, 394
Sentinel lymph node mapping
　relevance of, 78–79
Sentinel lymph nodes (SLN)
　biopsy of, 394
　metastatic tumor and, 412
　nodal pathology for status of, 79
　procedures for mapping, 78–79
　tumor staging and, 394
Sentinel node evaluation
　learning curve of surgeon and, 100
Sepsis
　toxic deaths and, 121
Sequential chemotherapy, 590
Serine phosphorylation
　estrogen binding and, 233
Serine threonine kinase Akt
　EGF pathways and, 273
Serine-104, 348

SERM 1, 223
SERM 3, 229
SERM 3 (arzoxifene), 223
SERM therapy
  Study of Tamoxifen and Raloxifene (STAR) trial and, 544
SERMs
  raloxifene and, 543
Serotonin
  emetic response and, 490
Serotonin pathway, 490–491
Serotonin receptor antagonists
  acute emesis and, 494
  chemotherapy-induced emesis an, 492
Serum erbB-2 antibodies
  clinical studies and, 93
Serum erbB-2 extracellular domain
  clinical studies and, 93
Sex hormone-binding globulin (SHBG), 206
Shark cartilage, 435
Shark cartilage oil
  complementary and Alternative Medicine (CAM) and, 431
Shorthand monikers, 559
Shrinkage artifact
  vascular invasion and, 414
Siddon study, 16
Signaling molecules, 274f
Signature-gene profile
  unnecessary treatments and, 326
Single-agent VNB. *See* Vinorelbine tartrate
Single-strand conformation polymorphism assays (SSCP)
  p53 and, 399
Skeletal complications, 467
  morbidity in patients with metastatic cancer and, 463
Skeletal pain
  morbidity in breast cancer and, 463
Skin barrier film spray
  peri-wound skin and, 484
Skin fibrosis
  breast cancer complications and, 12, 13f
Skin rash
  docetaxel monotherapy and, 151
Skin toxicity
  Caelyx and, 191–192
SLN marking agent
  SLNB and, 59
SLNB
  conclusions on, 64
  methodological development in, 62–63
  University of Vermont multicenter validation study and, 61
Social concerns
  malignant wounds and, 486
Social functioning
  health-related quality of life (HRQL) and, 582
Southwest Oncology Group (SWOG)
  node-negative breast cancer (NNBC) and, 101
  response criteria published for breast cancer trials and, 566
Spanish Group for Breast Cancer and cyclophosphamide and, 102
SR 16234
  agonist activity of, 231
SRC-1
  tamoxifen and, 236

St. Gallen Consensus Conference of 2001
  recurrence of cancer and, 99, 99t
Staging
  tumor-node-metastasis (TNM) and, 394
Steady state serum concentration (Css)
  receptor inhibition and, 280
Stem cell transplant. *See* SCT
Steroid biosynthesis pathways, 204f
Steroid hormone receptor status
  breast cancer and, 401
Steroid hormone receptors
  cross-communication with growth factor receptors and, 349
Steroid hormones
  human breast tissue growth and, 345
  predictive factors and, 417
Steroid prophylaxis
  docetaxel monotherapy and, 151
Steroid receptor coactivator (SRC), 233
Steroid receptor levels, 396
Steroidal antiestrogens
  chemical chain of, 227f
  lists of newer, 225t, 226
  overview of, 230–231
Steroidal aromatase inhibitors, 206–207
Steroidal compounds, 238
STI-571, 596
  cancer cell resistance to, 314
Stilboestrol
  estrogen and, 223
Stockholm breast radiotherapy trial, 9
Stomatitis
  capecitabine and, 171
Stress proteins
  tumor biopsies and, 335
Stromelysin
  E1A and, 314
Study of Tamoxifen against Raloxifene (STAR)
  postmenopausal women and, 229
Study of Tamoxifen and Raloxifene (STAR) trial and, 544f
  Gail Model scores and, 544
  overview of, 543–544
SU-5416
  inhibition of human tumor growth and, 298
  toxicity and, 298
Sub-typing
  histological type and, 415
Subcutaneous nodules, 476
Subcutaneous spread
  phases of, 477
  skin and, 476
Substance P
  emetic response and, 490
Subtyping
  invasive breast cancer and, 395
Suicide genes
  enzymes and, 311–312
  HER-2/*neu* and, 311–312
Summation dose intensity (SDI)
  unit dose intensity (UDI) and, 448
Superoxide anions
  doxorubicin and, 189
Supervised learning, 324
Supplements, 434
Supportive care, 591
Supraclavicular field
  irradiation of, 16, 16f, 17, 17f
Supraclavicular lymph nodes, 5
  recurrence of cancer in, 4

Suprasternal subcutaneous nodule
  breast cancer and, 477f
Surgery
  radiation and role of, 25–27
Surgery, axillary, 412
Surgery, breast-conserving
  relapse following, 32
Surgery, prophylactic
  genetic testing and, 438
Surgical chest wall resection
  recurrent breast cancer and, 482
Surgical learning curve
  vital blue dye and, 61–62
Surgical staging, 80
Surveillance, Epidemiology, and End Results (SEER)
  tumor grading and, 395
  tumor size and, 393
Survival
  clinical and pathological response to, 91t
Susceptibility testing
  hereditary breast and ovarian cancer and, 437–439
Sutter Cancer Center in Sacramento
  Complementary and Alternative Medicine (CAM) and, 432–433
Swedish trial
  breast screening and, 521
  outline of, 46
  radiation in absence of chemotherapy, 42
SWOG
  adjuvant CMFVp and, 135
Systematic review
  evidence-based guideline and, 558–559
Systemic adjuvant therapy
  node-negative breast cancer (NNBC) and, 100
Systemic chemotherapy, 39
  inflammatory breast cancer and, 70–71
  RT in trials with, 44
Systemic disease
  postoperative adjuvant systemic therapy and, 59

T
TAC (docetaxel, Adriamycin, and Cyclophosphamide)
  vs. FAC, 119
Tai Chi
  Complementary and Alternative Medicine (CAM) and, 428
Tamoxifen (TAM), 114, 126, 209, 211, 223, 237, 470, 530
  adjuvant RCTs and, 112t
  advantages *vs.* disadvantages, 224–225
  anastrozole and, 532
  aromatase inhibitors *vs.*, 212t
  benefits and risks of, 541
  bone resorption
    in postmenopausal women and, 469
  breast cancer and
    effect of, 531t
  breast cancer risk reduction effect and
    BRCA1 and, 540–541
    BRCA2 and, 540–541
  breast cancer trials and, 107–110
  clinical studies with, 128
  contralateral breast cancer (CLBC) and, 110
  Danish premenopausal study and, 43, 43t
  delayed, 110

Tamoxifen (TAM) (contd.)
    ductal carcinoma in situ and, 49
    duration of therapy with, 108–110
    elderly patients and, 108
    endometrial cancer and, 530
        effect of, 531t
    ER-negative tumors and, 130, 396
    ERβ positive tumors and, 236
    estrogen-independent mechanisms of
        action, 295
    HER-2 overexpression and, 370
    hormonal therapy and, 33
    imaging and, 294–295
    lipids and cardiovascular mortality
        with, 110
    lower dose of, 532
    lumpectomy and, 88
    National Surgical Adjuvant Breast and
        Bowel Project (NSABP) and, 536
    negative impact of, 110–111
    NNBC and, 99
    node-negative breast cancer (NNBC)
        and, 100
    NSABP B-24 trial and, 53–56, 54f
    opposite breast cancers and, 546
    overall survival (OS) and, 100, 102
    overexpressing HER-2 resistance to, 350
    postmenopausal women and, 44, 130
    premenopausal women and, 130–131
    reduction in risk of recurrence and
        dying with, 536
    response to antiestrogens as treatments
        vs., 229t
    stem cell transplant and, 196
    studies with, 135, 136
    total cholesterol and, 543
    venous thromboembolic events and
        effect of, 531t
Tamoxifen studies
    breast cancer based on family history
        and, 529
    Italian
        HRT and, 529
        overview of, 529
    overview of, 529
    Royal Marsden trial and
        analysis of, 529
        HRT and, 529
Tamoxifen therapy, 10, 214
    final conclusions with level of evidence
        recommendations and, 104–105
    ICI 182,780 and, 231
    research implication from current data
        on, 531–532
Tandem transplantation
    comparison trials of, 199
Tangenial irradiation fields, 13–14, 13f, 14f
    patterns of dose specification and, 15f
Target volumes, 6
TAT-59
    overview of, 227
Taxane monotherapy
    significance of, 154
Taxane(s), 159
    adjuvant
        RCTs with, 120t
        setting and, 159–161
        trials incorporating, 160t
    advanced breast cancer and, 148–153
    biologic therapies and, 161–163
    combination regimens for advanced
        disease and, 154
    conclusions of efficacy in studies, 163

early breast cancer and, 450–451
HER-2 positive tumors and, 375
lower doses of, 263
overview of, 147
patient survival and, 76
pharmacokinetics of, 147–148
risks of, 118
trastuzumab and, 252
trials with results, 118t
VNB and, 185
vs. non-taxane-containing
    chemotherapy and, 102–103
Taxane-based regimens
    markers predicting activity of, 375–376
Taxus baccata
    docetaxel and, 147
Taxus brevifolia
    paclitaxel and, 147
TCH. See Docetaxel, platinum, and
    trastuzumab
Technetium sestamibi
    tracers and, 293
    uptake in tumors and, 294
Telangectasia
    breast cancer complications and, 12, 13f
Testicular germ cell cancer
    curative therapy programs and, 592
Testolactone
    limited efficacy of, 205
TGF-β
    osteoclast apoptosis and, 465
TGFα
    EGFR and, 282
Thalidomide
    urine VEGF and, 292
Thallium (TL)
    tracers and, 293
Therapeutic interventions
    levels of scientific evidence about, 40
Therapy
    salvage mastectomy and, 32
Thiamidine labeling index
    node-negative breast cancer (NNBC)
        and, 101, 102
Thiotepa
    breast cancers and, 86
Thomson, Samuel
    disease treatment and, 426
Threshold dose, 447
Thromboembolic events
    aromatase inhibitors and, 112
    fulvestrant and, 232
    tamoxifen (TAM) and, 111, 213, 530
Thrombospondin-1
    tumor growth and, 288
Thymidine phosphorylase (TP)
    CMF and, 376
    pharmacokinetics of, 169
    predictive marker and, 376
Thymidine-labeling index
    proliferative activity and, 397
Thymidylate synthase (TS)
    fluorouracil and, 376
    pharmacokinetics of, 169
Time to treatment failure (TTF), 207
Tissue inhibitor of metaloproteinase-4
    (TIMP-4)
    tumor growth and, 288
Tissue remodeling
    breast cancer metastases and, 290
TLC D-99 (Myocet)
    5-flourouracil and, 192
    Adriamycin vs., 193

liposomes and, 190
phase two trials of, 192
toxicity and, 192
TNP-470
    endothelial toxins and, 299
Tolerance doses, 12
TOPIC 1 study
    chemotherapy regimen in, 89–90
Topoisomerase II alpha, 374
    proliferative activity and, 397
Topoisomerase II inhibitors
    trastuzumab with, 252
Topotecan
    anti-EGFR antibodies and, 276
    paclitaxel and, 451
    UCN-01 (7-hydroxystaurosporine) and,
        361
Toremifene citrate, 237
    endometrium and, 113
    overview of, 226–227
Total cholesterol
    raloxifene and, 543
Toxicity. See also Radiation toxicity
    angiogenesis and, 287
    anthracenedione and, 190
    anthracycline regimen and, 189
    antitumor drug and, 267
    cyclophosphamide and
        dose-escalation with, 451
    cytotoxic drugs and, 121
    docetaxel-Anthracycline combinations,
        157
    docetaxel-gemcitabine combination
        and, 159
    E7070 and, 362
    epirubicin and, 190
    flavopiridol and, 359
    HER-2 protein and, 161
    high-dose sequential chemotherapy
        and, 592
    IMC-C225 and, 276
    irradiation and, 6
    mitoxantrone and, 190
    multicenter RCT outcomes with, 129
    PS-341 and, 361–362
    studies of, 40
    SU-5416 and, 298, 299
    trastuzumab and, 253
    UCN-01 (7-hydroxystaurosporine) and,
        360
Transcriptional activation
Transcriptionally controlled tumor protein
    (TCTP)
    FGF-2 and, 339
Transcriptosome, 323
Transforming growth factors
    carcinoma cells and, 464
Transverse rectus abdominis
    myocutaneous (TRAM) flap
    irradiation and, 32
Trastuzumab (Herceptin), 596
    anthracyclines with, 252
    antiangiogenic effect in vivo of, 251f
    antimetabolites with, 252
    cardiotoxicity of, 255
    chemotherapy plus, 119–122
    cytotoxic chemotherapy combined
        with, 252–253
    development of, 248–250
    dose-dependent preclinical antitumor
        activity of, 249f
    future clinical development of,
        256–257

health-related quality of Life (HRQOL) and, 503
HER-2 and, 282
HER-2 overexpression and, 246
HER-2 protein and, 161, 162
  adjuvant trials with, 163t
HER-2-overexpressing xenografts and, 251
human anti-humanized antibodies (HAHA) and, 250
markers predicting activity of, 377
mechanism of action of, 250–252
metastatic breast cancer and, 397
pharmacokinetics and serum levels of HER-2 protein and, 253
phase 1 clinical trials of, 249t
phase 2 clinical trials with, 253
synergistic cytotoxicity with, 252t
taxanes with, 252
therapies with, 97
topoisomerase II inhibitors with, 252
transduction of, 250f
vinca alkaloids with, 252
Trastuzumab-vinorelbine combination, 185
Trilostane, 206
  non-selective aromatase inhibitors and, 204
Triphenylbromoethylene
  estrogen and, 223
Triphenylchloroethylene
  estrogen and, 223
Triphenylethylene antiestrogens, 224f, 226
  lists of new, 226
Triphenylethylenes, 226
  overview of, 226
Tru-Cut biopsy, 93
Tubular carcinomas, 98
  prognosis of, 395, 415
Tubule formation
  histological grading and, 414
Tubulin
  VNB binding to, 179
Tubulo-lobular carcinoma
  prognosis and, 415
Tumor(s)
  angiogenesis and, 287
  aromatase inhibitors and, 112
  axillary lymph node involvement and, 392–393
  BCT and, 74
  bone microenvironment and, 465
  Caelyx and, 191
  classification of, 325
  epidermal growth factor receptor (EGFR) and, 400–401
  endocrine therapy and, 401
  ER-negative, 33
  ER-positive, 33
  grading and, 395
  growth fractions and, 590
  HER-2 positive and, 374
  lumpectomy post chemotherapy and, 77
  measurable or nonmeasurable
    characterization of, 568
  metastases and, 383
  microarray experiments and, 324
  overexpressing HER-2 and, 371
  postmenopausal women and, 127
  prognosis in breast and axillary nodes and, 78
  prognosis with size of, 98

recurrence of, 4
response to letrozole, 218
Tumor angiogenesis
  markers of, 99
Tumor biomarkers
  response and outcome response and, 93
Tumor blood flow
  color doppler ultrasonography (CDUS) and, 293
Tumor burden, 570
  effect of therapy on, 566
Tumor cell apoptosis
  increase drug dose and, 447
Tumor cells, 274–275
  apoptosis and, 318
  vascular dependence and, 262
Tumor dormancy
  cancer cells and, 388–389
Tumor emboli
  examination of, 414
Tumor eradication, 593
Tumor formation
  genes and, 323
Tumor growth
  angiogenesis and, 287
  antiangiogenic therapies and, 291
  proteomics and, 336
Tumor histology
  cancer diagnosis and
Tumor invasion to skin
  clarification of, 475
Tumor kinetics
  high dose treatments and, 593
Tumor Marker Utility Grading System (TMUGS)
  tumor markers and, 391–392
Tumor markers
  clinical decisions on, 391
  Tumor Marker Utility Grading System (TMUGS) and, 391–392
Tumor microvessel density, 289
  color doppler ultrasonography (CDUS) and, 293
Tumor, muted, 53
  neoadjuvant chemotherapy and, 376
Tumor, primary
  overview of, 383
  patterns of blood flow from, 386
  vascularization of
    cancer cells and, 385
Tumor necrosis
  prognostic factors and, 416
Tumor necrosis factor (TNF)
  anemia and, 457
  E1A and, 314
Tumor necrosis factor alpha (TNFα), 293
Tumor nodules
  classification of response and, 567
Tumor-node-metastasis (TNM)
  staging and, 394
Tumor response
  clinical predictive factors for, 91
  effect of preoperative chemotherapy on, 89t
  endpoint in phase 2
    reasons for using, 565
  evaluation criteria, 565
  factors affecting, 566
  RECIST guidelines and, 572
  traditional phase 2 criteria and, 602
Tumor samples
  formalin fixation of, 247
Tumor, second primary, 12

Tumor shedding
  micrometastases and, 289
  surgery and, 289
Tumor size
  assessment of change in, 567
  prognostic factor and, 411
  survival rate projected by, 411
  tumor behavior and, 393–394
Tumor specimens
  HER2/neu and, 246
Tumor spillage
  laparoscopic colectomy and, 476
Tumor staging
  new aspects of, 394
Tumor suppresser genes, 399
  tumor cell and, 551
Tumor suppression
  tumor formation and, 323
Tumor vasculature
  imaging of, 293
Tumorigenesis
  cell adhesion molecules and, 292
  RERG and, 327
TUNEL assay
  apoptotic tumor cells in, 318f
Two-dimensional electrophoresis (2DE)
  proteomic analysis and, 331
2D-patterns
  down-regulation of 14-3-3 sigma, 336f
2DE
  action of growth factors in cancer cells and, 337
2DE analysis
  cancer cell growth and, 334
2DE. See Two-dimensional electrophoresis
2ME1
  overview of, 330
2ME2 treatment
  mechanisms of action with, 300
Type I inhibitors
  overview of, 205
Type IV collagen
  microvessel density (MVD) and, 400
Tyrosine kinase inhibitors
  anti-EGF receptor family and, 278t
  mechanisms of action with, 277–278
Tyrosine kinase receptors
  inhibition of, 340
Tyrosine kinase-membrane receptors
  eukaryotic cell growth and, 336
Tyrosine phosphorylation
  SDS-PAGE (sodium dodecyl sulfate-polyacrylamide gel electrophoresis) and, 337
Tyrosine-kinase inhibitor STI-571
  gene therapy and, 313

U

U.S. Agency for Health Research and Quality (AHRQ)
  web sites for reference and, 563
U.S. Breast Cancer Detection Demonstration Projects
  mammography and, 519
U.S. Guideline Clearinghouse
  web sites for reference and, 563
U.S. National Cancer Institute
  web sites for, 512
U.S. National Institutes for Health (NIH)
  directories for clinical trials on Web and, 513–514

U.S.A. Office of Alternative Medicine, 435
Ubiquinated proteins, 355–356
Ubiquitin-proteasome pathway, 355
Ubiquitination
 trastuzumab (Herceptin) and, 250
UCLA Community Oncology Research Network
 trastuzumab with docetaxel and platinums and, 256
UCN-01 (7-hydroxystaurosporine)
 apoptosis and, 360
Ulcerating malignant wound
 breast cancer and, 479f
Ulcerating wounds
 clarification of, 475
Ultrasound, 570
 genetic testing and, 438
 tumor size and, 567
Uncertainty principle
 data analyses and, 577, 577t
Union Internationale Contre le Cancer (UICC)
 response criteria published for breast cancer trials and, 566
Unit dose intensity (UDI)
 summation dose intensity (SDI) and, 448
Univariate analysis
 prognostic factors and, 411, 413
University of Vermont multicenter validation study
 SLNB and, 61
Up-front transplantation
 comparison trials of, 199
Urinary 5-HIAA, 491
Urokinase
 E1A and, 314
Urokinase-type plasminogen activator (uPA)
 impaired survival and, 289–290
 node-negative breast cancer (NNBC) and, 101, 102

V

Vaginal bleeding
 fulvestrant and, 232
Vallis study, 9–10
Van Nuys Prognostic Index (VNPI)
 DCIS and, 52, 53
Vascular cell adhesion molecule-1 (VCAM-1)
 metastases and, 292
Vascular circulation
 cancer cell survival in, 386
Vascular endothelial growth factor (VEGF)
 Trastuzumab (Herceptin) and, 251
 tumor growth and, 288
Vascular patterns
 ductal carcinoma in situ and, 288
Vasculostatins
 microvasculature and, 290–291

Vasculostatins agents
 microvasculature and, 290
Vasculotoxins, 290
VCAM-1 (soluble)
 cancer with increased concentrations of, 292
VEGF, 298, 300
 Flt-1, 292
 KDR (kinase domain region), 292
 negative prognostic value of, 290t
 overview of, 291–292
VEGF concentrations (urinary)
 bladder cancer and, 292
VEGF expression
 impaired response to tamoxifen and, 289
VEGF mRNA
 Trastuzumab (Herceptin) and, 252
VEGF receptor inhibitors, 269
VEGF type 2 receptors, 263
VEGFR-2 antibody
 multidrug-resistant breast cancer and, 265
Venous thromboembolic events
 tamoxifen and
  effect of, 531t
Vertebral fractures
 bone metastases and, 463
Vertebral osteopenic fractures
 metastasis and, 470
Vessels
 cancer cells in, 386
Vestibular system
 emesis and, 489
 vomiting center and, 490
Vimentin
 normal cells and, 335
Vinblastine sulfate, 268
 anti-tumor effects of, 265, 266
 trials with, 153
Vinblastine sulfate, low-dose
 anti-tumor efficacy and toxicity in, 264f
Vinca alkaloids
 laboratory data and, 179
 trastuzumab with, 252
Vincristine, 179
 CHOP and, 92
 randomized studies with, 90
Vindesine, 179
Vinorelbine tartrate (VNB)
 clinical trials with, 180t
 comparison of alternative chemotherapies and, 584
 conclusions on studies of, 185–186
 dosing of, 180
 malignancies and, 179
 multiagent regimens and, 181–185, 182t–184t
 paclitaxel and, 451
 pharmacokinetic profile of, 179
 trials using, 153
Virchow, Rudolf
 cellular theory of disease, 601

Vit D3 derivatives
 ER-Negative breast cancer and, 533
Vitamin C
 Complementary and Alternative Medicine (CAM) and, 431
VNB-containing regimens, 181–185, 182t–184t
 conclusions of studies on, 185–186
 neo-adjuvant treatment and, 185
VNB. See Vinorelbine tartrate
Vomiting
 cytotoxic chemotherapy and, 489
Vomiting center
 emetic response and, 490
Vorozole
 overview of, 209

W

West Midlands Oncology Association
 node-negative breast cancer (NNBC) and, 101
Western blot
 HER-2 protein and, 246
White cell counts (WBC)
 oral CMF and, 452
Whole-tumor analysis
 breast cancer and, 324
Women (older)
 endocrine-responsive disease and, 121
World Health Organization (WHO)
 criteria for phase 2 trials and, 566
 response criteria published for breast cancer trials and, 566, 569
 study design and patient assessment and, 573
Wound biopsy
 diagnostic purposes for, 482
Wound healing
 gemcitabine and, 476
Wounds
 pain and, 483

X

X-ray
 tumor size and, 567

Y

Yoga
 Complementary and Alternative Medicine (CAM), 428

Z

ZD 1839, 279
 phase 1 trials with, 280
 phase 2 study of, 276f, 279
Zoledronate
 studies of, 467
Zosteriform malignant wound
 carcinoma of breast and, 479f